Clinical Cardiology

Clinical Cardiology

Current Practice Guidelines

Demosthenes G. Katritsis, MD, PhD, FRCP, FACC
Athens Euroclinic, Athens, Greece
Bernard J. Gersh, MB, ChB, DPhil, FRCP, FACC
Mayo Medical School, Rochester, MN, USA
A. John Camm, MD, FRCP, FACC
St George's University of London, UK

OXFORD
UNIVERSITY PRESS

OXFORD
UNIVERSITY PRESS

Great Clarendon Street, Oxford, OX2 6DP,
United Kingdom

Oxford University Press is a department of the University of Oxford.
It furthers the University's objective of excellence in research, scholarship, and education by publishing worldwide. Oxford is a registered trade mark of Oxford University Press in the UK and in certain other countries

First Edition published in 2013

Impression: 2

Published in the United States of America by Oxford University Press
198 Madison Avenue, New York, NY 10016, United States of America

British Library Cataloguing in Publication Data

Data available

Library of Congress Control Number: 2013944647

ISBN 978-0-19-968528-8

Printed in Great Britain by
Ashford Colour Press Ltd

Foreword

Over the years I have had the pleasure of writing forewords for a number of books that I considered to be timely and to fulfill important objectives. Without hesitation, I would say that *Clinical Cardiology: Current Practice Guidelines*, by D.G. Katritsis, B.J. Gersh, and A.J. Camm, is the most outstanding book for which I have had the pleasure to write a foreword. Further, this is probably the book that better serves the cardiovascular specialist in day-to-day practice than any other written in the last two decades. This is not just a textbook; it is an extraordinary "toolkit" in the context of an evidence-based cardiovascular practice in the midst of rapidly evolving scientific knowledge and guidelines.

Because of the need to integrate current knowledge on evidence-based cardiology, about three years ago, under the auspices of the American Heart Association, we published a book that included the most recent guidelines by both the ACCF/AHA and the ESC. I believe that such integration was a step forward for the practicing cardiologist; indeed, in a "synopsis" fashion, this aspect is well served in *Clinical Cardiology: Current Practice Guidelines.* However, in the excellent compendium of my colleagues, three new components are incorporated, which we can describe as the "jewel" of the book: a very succinct definition, classification, pathophysiology, diagnosis, management, and need of specific clinical investigation (including genetics and molecular biology) of the various disease entities; a regularly updated online version on the most recent developments; and, most importantly a "user friendly, at a glance" presentation. These additional three components, that make *Clinical Cardiology: Current Practice Guidelines* so unique, deserve a brief description.

1) In regard to the various disease entities, general textbooks tend to employ, from definition to management, a rather long and descriptive format. In contrast, *Clinical Cardiology: Current Practice Guidelines* consolidates many of the topics, regardless of their complexity, from definition to management, in a clear, concise and instructive way, intermixed with the most recent guidelines. Thus, over 600 easily accessible tables dissect and summarize the key points of all the latest ACCF/AHA and ESC guidelines.
2) Rapidly evolving scientific knowledge, including the value of new diagnostic and management approaches and their incorporation in practicing guidelines, makes it difficult for the cardiovascular specialist to be aware of the latest clinical evidence-base. Written by three leading authorities in the field, its biannually updated online version provides the solution.
3) A novelty of this book is the "user-friendly, at glance" way of presentation that it makes it very useful to the practicing cardiovascular specialist. Useful because of its combination of succinctness and clarity, the book is up to date in every aspect of the cardiovascular science, and particularly on the most recent recommendations from both sides of the Atlantic. Thus, these recommendations are summarized in tables derived from the guideline documents and incorporated in the appropriate diagnostic or management sections of the 85 comprehensive chapters. For example, when confronted with complicated clinical issues that appear in everyday clinical practice (such as modern antiplatelet therapy of ACS, differential diagnosis of wide complex tachycardia, or management of stable CAD in view of COURAGE, FREEDOM or STICH) physicians consult general textbooks or, often several journal articles, in order to obtain this information in a rather loose form. In contrast, *Clinical Cardiology: Current Practice Guidelines* consolidates such topics in a summarized, succinct, and clear way.

This book is a tribute to the skill of the three editors who also served as the only authors. This limited, but unified and hardworking internationally known authorship is, without doubt, a great part of the success. It is with great pleasure that I pen these words to relate my enthusiasm for their work as a remarkable addition to the cardiovascular field.

Valentin Fuster
Physician-in-Chief, Mount Sinai Medical Center
Director, Mount Sinai Heart

ΠΑΝΤΕΣ ΑΝΘΡΩΠΟΙ ΤΟΥ ΕΙΔΕΝΑΙ ΟΡΕΓΟΝΤΑΙ ΦΥΣΕΙ
All humans by nature desire to know

Aristotle
The Metaphysics

Prologue

The entire field of cardiovascular medicine has witnessed an era of rapid scientific progress, accompanied by continuous technological and applied innovation. This occurs against a backdrop of increasing emphasis on the importance of evidence-based practice, and rapid development of guidelines by major professional societies. The resultant expansion of our body of knowledge by evidence-based recommendations interjects a new set of challenges for the practicing clinician with ever-extensive clinical responsibilities.

In order to practice evidence-based medicine, information must be easily accessible and, more importantly, easily retrievable when the need arises; this may not always be easy with the current pace of dissemination of knowledge. The rationale for writing this book reflects exactly this need, both ours and that of our potential readers: to organize our continually evolving knowledge on often diverse cardiology issues, in our environment of networked and facilitated communication. In other words, to provide a clinical tool that can be used in everyday clinical practice as a concise guide to what we know and, more importantly, what we do not know, and what we think we know. To quote Mark Twain, "what gets us into trouble is not what we don't know, it is what we know for sure that just ain't so."

The prerequisites of informed clinical practice are: a satisfactory background of basic knowledge of disease entities, remaining up-to-date on important clinical trials and emerging scientific evidence that shape current diagnosis and therapy, and acquaintance with current practice guidelines from established professional societies such as the American College of Cardiology Foundation/American Heart Association (ACCF/AHA) and the European Society of Cardiology (ESC), among many others.

Each chapter of this book has therefore been structured around the following parts:

1. **A clear definition and modern classification of disease entities, followed by updated, focused information on recent developments on the epidemiology and pathophysiology of each condition.** Recent original articles and reviews from leading journals were consulted and a summary of the most relevant information is included. Special care was taken not to omit the most recent information on medical genetics, an expanding and promising aspect.
2. **A description of the clinical presentation of the disease, with instructions on necessary clinical investigations.** Clinical investigations are presented in the context of recent evidence that dictates their current value or obsolescence. An effort has been made to include the very latest published knowledge on the clinical value of existing and evolving tests, based on recent randomized clinical trials and guidelines by both ACCF/AHA and ESC.
3. **Recommendations on management as derived from the most recent evidence available to the authors.** Because of the comprehensive nature of guidelines offered by learned societies, it was decided to provide the most recent recommendations in a summarized, tabulated format. These are not readily accessible since overlapping guidelines may appear on the same condition from different working groups, and updated documents are continually appearing. Thus, all guideline documents and their updates published in the US and Europe were scrutinized and classified according to year of publication. The most recent recommendations were defined, extracted and tabulated. The resulting tables provided in the book offer the most recent recommendations on each disease entity by both ACCF/AHA and ESC. Where appropriate, new evidence that questions the validity of specific recommendations, as well as the opinions of established experts, and other data, such as FDA alerts are included.
4. **Practical advice on "what and why to do".** Therapies, drug doses and selection of procedures are presented in a clear and user-friendly way.
5. **Carefully chosen references.** Major randomized clinical trials and seminal scientific studies that define evidence-based practice are included for further reference. In addition, recent, scholarly reviews are provided, which together with the contents of the book should allow in-depth study of specific entities that may interest the individual reader.
6. **Presentation of all recent guidelines.** Guidelines are referenced and presented separately in order to guide the reader to the most recent publications by ACCF/AHA and ESC.

An inherent disadvantage of a medical textbook is inability to keep up-to-date with recent developments. To overcome the problem, the online version of this book will be updated, initially on a 6-monthly basis.

This book would have never been possible without the wholehearted support and commitment of Helen Liepman, our Senior Editor at Oxford University Press. We are grateful for her acceptance of our view of a "next generation textbook". We also thank Imogen Lowe, Mark Knowles, and Richard Martin of Oxford University Press. Their professionalism and assistance throughout the production process is much appreciated.

Demosthenes G. Katritsis
Bernard J. Gersh
A. John Camm

Contents

Part 12 Syncope and sudden cardiac death

Part 13 Implantable devices

Part 14 Diseases of the aorta

List of abbreviations

<	less than
>	more than
≥	equal to or greater than
≤	equal to or less than
~	approximately
≈	approximately equal to
=	equal to
α	alpha
β	beta
δ	delta
γ	gamma
$	Dollar
€	Euro
ACC	American College of Cardiology
ACCP	American College of Chest Physicians
ACE	angiotensin-converting enzyme
ACEI	angiotensin-converting enzyme inhibitor
ACHD	adult congenital heart disease
ACS	acute coronary syndrome
ACT	activated clotting time
ADP	adenosine diphosphate
AF	atrial fibrillation
AH	atrial-His
AHA	American Heart Association
AHF	acute heart failure
AIDS	acquired immunodeficiency syndrome
AMI	acute myocardial infarction
AMP	adenosine monophosphate
ANP	atrial natriuretic peptide
Ao	aorta
AoD	aortic dissection
AP	action potential
APB	atrial premature beat
aPTT	activated partial thromboplastin time
AR	aortic regurgitation
ARB	angiotensin receptor blocker
ARF	acute rheumatic fever
ARVC/D	arrhythmogenic right ventricular cardiomyopathy or dysplasia
AS	aortic stenosis
ASD	atrial septal defects
ASO	arterial switch operation
AT	atrial tachycardia
AT1	angiotensin II type 1
AV	atrioventricular; aortic valve
AVNRT	atrioventricular nodal reentrant tachycardia
AVR	aortic valve replacement
AVRT	atrioventricular reentrant tachycardia
BAV	bicuspid aortic valve
bd	twice daily
BLS	basic life support
bpm	beat per minute
BMS	bare metal stent
BMV	balloon mitral valvotomy
BNP	brain natriuretic peptide
BP	blood pressure
bpm	beats per minute
BrS	Brugada syndrome
BSA	body surface area
BUN	blood urea nitrogen
Ca^{++}	calcium
CABG	coronary artery bypass grafting
CAD	coronary artery disease
cAMP	cyclic adenosine monophosphate
CAVF	coronary arteriovenous fistula
CCB	calcium channel blocker
CCD	cardiac conduction disease
CCF	congestive heart failure
CCS	Canadian Cardiovascular Society
CCT	coronary artery computed tomography
CCTGA	congenitally corrected transposition of the great arteries
CCU	Coronary Care Unit
CDT	catheter-directed thrombolysis
cGMP	cyclic guanine monophosphate
CHB	congenital heart block
CHD	congenital heart disease
CHF	chronic heart failure
CIED	cardiovascular implantable electronic device
CKD	chronic kidney disease
CL	cycle length
cm	centimetre
CMR	cardiac magnetic resonance
CMV	cytomegalovirus
CO_2	carbon dioxide
CoA	coarctation of the aorta
COPD	chronic obstructive pulmonary disease
CPAP	continuous positive airway pressure

CPET	cardiopulmonary exercise testing
CPVT	catecholaminergic polymorphic ventricular tachycardia
CrCl	creatinine clearance
CRP	C-reactive protein
CRT	cardiac resynchronization therapy
CSNRT	corrected sinus nodal recovery time
CSM	carotid sinus massage
CSS	carotid sinus syndrome
CT	computed tomography
CTEPH	chronic thromboembolic pulmonary hypertension
CTI	cavotricuspid isthmus
CUS	compression ultrasonography
CVA	cerebrovascular accident
Cx	circumflex
d	day
2D	two-dimensional
3D	three-dimensional
4D	four-dimensional
Da	Dalton
DAD	delayed after-depolarization
DAPT	dual oral antiplatelet therapy
DC	direct current
DCC	direct current cardioversion
DCM	dilated cardiomyopathy
DES	drug-eluting stent
DFT	defibrillator threshold
dL	decilitre
DNA	deoxyribonucleic acid
DSE	dobutamine stress echocardiography
DTI	direct thrombin inhibitor
DVT	deep vein thrombosis
dyn	dyne
EAD	early after-depolarization
EBV	Epstein–Barr virus
ECG	electrocardiogram
ECS	elastic compression stocking
EHRA	European Heart Rhythm Association
ELISA	enzyme-linked immunosorbent assay
ELT	endless loop tachycardia
EMA	European Medicines Agency
EP	electrophysiology
EPS	electrophysiological study
ERA	endothelin receptor antagonist
ERO	effective regurgitant orifice (area)
ERS	early repolarization syndrome
ESC	European Society of Cardiology
ESR	erythrocyte sedimentation rate
FA	Friedreich's ataxia
FDA	Food and Drug Administration
FDC	familial dilated cardiomyopathy
FFR	fractional flow reserve
FMC	first medical contact
FIRM	focal impulse and rotor modulation
g	gram
GAS	group A Streptococcus
GDF	growth differentiation factor
GFR	glomerular filtration rate
GI	gastrointestinal
GP	glycoprotein
GRACE	Global Registry of Acute Coronary Event
GUCH	grown-up congenital heart (disease)
h	hour
HA	His-atrial
HBV	hepatitis B virus
HCM	hypertrophic cardiomyopathy
Hct	haematocrit
HCV	hepatitis C virus
HDL	high density lipoprotein
HELLP	haemolysis, elevated liver enzymes, low platelet (count)
HF	heart failure
HIV	human immunodeficiency virus
HIT	heparin-induced thrombocytopenia
HLA	human leucocyte antigen
H_2O	water
HOCM	hypertrophic obstructive cardiomyopathy
HRS	Heart Rhythm Society
HRV	heart rate variability
Hz	hertz
IABP	intra-aortic balloon pump
IART	intra-atrial reentrant tachycardia
ICD	implantable cardioverter-defibrillator
IDC	idiopathic dilated cardiomyopathy
IE	infective endocarditis
IFDVT	iliofemoral deep vein thrombosis
IHD	ischaemic heart disease
ILR	implantable loop recorder
IM	intramuscular
IMH	intramural haematoma
IMT	intima-media thickness
INR	international normalized ratio
IOCM	iso-osmolar contrast media
IPAH	idiopathic pulmonary arterial hypertension
ISDN	isosorbide dinitrate
IU	international unit
IV	intravenous

IVC	inferior vena cava
J	Joule
JVP	jugular venous pressure
K	potassium
KCl	potassium chloride
kDa	kilodalton
kg	kilogram
km	kilometre
kPa	kilopascal
L	litre
LA	left atrium
LAA	left atrial appendage
LAH	left anterior hemiblock
lb	pound
LBBB	left bundle branch block
LDL	low density lipoprotein
LDL-C	low density cholesterol
LGE	late gadolinium enhancement
LIMA	left internal mammary artery
LMWH	low molecular weight heparin
LOCM	low osmolar contrast media
Lp(a)	lipoprotein (a)
LPH	left posterior hemiblock
LQTS	long QT syndrome
LVAD	left ventricular assist device
LVEDD	left ventricular end-diastolic diameter
LVEDP	left ventricular end-diastolic pressure
LVEF	left ventricular ejection fraction
LVESD	left ventricular end-systolic diameter
LVH	left ventricular hypertrophy
LVNC	left ventricular non-compaction
LVOT	left ventricular outflow tract
LVOTO	left ventricular outflow tract obstruction
m	metre
MAT	multifocal atrial tachycardia
MBC	mitral balloon commissurotomy
MBG	myocardial blush grade
MCT	multidetector computed tomography
MDCT	multidetector computed tomography
MDRD	modification of diet in renal disease
MEN	multiple endocrine neoplasia
mEq	milliequivalent
METS	metabolic equivalents
mg	milligram
mGy	milligray
MI	myocardial infarction
MIC	minimum inhibitory concentration
min	minute
μL	microlitre
mL	millilitre
μm	micron
mm	millimetre
mmHg	millimetre mercury
mmol	millimole
μmol	micromole
mo	month
mPAP	mean pulmonary artery pressure
MPI	myocardial perfusion imaging
MPS	myocardial perfusion stress
MRA	magnetic resonance angiography; mineraloco-rticoid receptor antagonist
MRI	magnetic resonance imaging
MRSA	methicillin-resistant *Staphylococcus aureus*
ms	millisecond
MS	mitral stenosis
mSv	milliSievert
mV	millivolt
MVA	mitral valve area
MVP	mitral valve prolapse
MVR	mitral valve replacement
Na	sodium
NaCl	sodium chloride
ng	nanogram
NIPPV	non-invasive positive pressure ventilation
NIV	non-invasive ventilation
NO	nitric oxide
NSAID	non-steroidal anti-inflammatory drug
NSTEMI	non-ST elevation myocardial infarction
NSVT	non-sustained ventricular tachycardia
NSTEACS	non-ST elevation acute coronary syndrome
NTG	nitroglycerin
NYHA	New York Heart Association
O_2	oxygen
OAC	oral anticoagulant
od	once daily
OH	orthostatic hypotension
OPAT	outpatient parenteral antibiotic therapy
OPCAB	off-pump beating heart bypass surgery
oz	ounce
p	probability
PA	pulmonary artery
PAH	pulmonary artery hypertension
PaO_2	partial pressure of oxygen
PAPVC	partial anomalous pulmonary venous connection
PAU	penetrating atherosclerotic ulcer
PAWP	pulmonary artery wedge pressure

PBV	percutaneous balloon valvuloplasty
PCC	prothrombin complex concentrate
PCDT	pharmacomechanical catheter-directed thrombolysis
PCWP	pulmonary capillary wedge pressure
PCI	percutaneous coronary intervention
PCR	polymerase chain reaction
PDA	patent ductus arteriosus
PDE	phosphodiesterase
PDE-5I	phosphodiesterase-5 inhibitor
PE	pulmonary embolism
PEEP	positive end-expiratory pressure
PES	programmed electrical stimulation
PFO	patent foramen ovale
pg	pictogram
PH	pulmonary hypertension
PHV	prosthetic heart valve
PISA	proximal isovelocity surface area
PJRT	permanent junctional reciprocating tachycardia
PMBV	percutaneous mitral balloon valvotomy
PMC	percutaneous mitral commissurotomy
po	oral route
PO_2	partial pressure of oxygen
POTS	postural orthostatic tachycardia syndrome
PPCM	post-partum cardiomyopathy
PPM	permanent pacemaker
PMT	pacemaker-mediated tachycardia
PR	pulmonary regurgitation
PV	pulmonary vein
PVARP	post-ventricular pacing atrial refractory period
PVC	premature ventricular contraction
PVOD	pulmonary veno-occlusive disease
PVR	pulmonary vascular resistance; pulmonary valve replacement
Qp	pulmonary flow
Qs	systemic flow
RA	right atrium; rheumatoid arthritis
RADT	rapid antigen detection test
RAO	right anterior oblique
RAAS	renin-angiotensin-aldosterone system
RBBB	right bundle branch block
RBC	red blood cell
RCA	right coronary artery
RCM	restrictive cardiomyopathy
RCT	randomized controlled trial
RF	radiofrequency; rheumatic fever
RNA	ribonucleic acid
rPA	rateplase
RVSP	right ventricular systolic pressure
RV	right ventricle
RVEF	right ventricular ejection fraction
RVOT	right ventricular outflow tract
RVOTO	right ventricular outflow tract obstruction
RWPT	R wave peak time
s	second
SAECG	signal-averaged electrocardiogram
SAM	systolic anterior motion
SaO_2	oxygen saturation
SBP	systolic blood pressure
SC	subcutaneous route
SCD	sudden cardiac death
SCL	sinus cycle length
SDCT	standard definition computed tomography
SIHD	stable ischaemic heart disease
SLE	systemic lupus erythematosus
SND	sinus node dysfunction
SNP	single-nucleotide polymorphism
SNRT	sinus nodal recovery time
SOBOE	shortness of breath on exertion
SPECT	single photon emission computed tomography
SPERRI	shortest pre-excited RR interval
sPESI	simplified pulmonary embolism severity index
SpO_2	saturation of peripheral oxygen
spp.	species
SQTS	short QT syndrome
SR	sinus rhythm
SSS	sick sinus syndrome
SSRI	selective serotonin reuptake inhibitor
STEMI	ST elevation myocardial elevation
SVC	superior vena cava
SVR	systemic vascular resistance
SVT	supraventricular tachycardia
TAPSE	tricuspid annular plane systolic excursion
TAPVC	total anomalous pulmonary venous connection
TAVI	transcatheter aortic valve implantation
TdP	torsade de pointe
tds	three times daily
TEVAR	thoracic endovascular aortic repair
TGA	transposition of great arteries
TIA	transient ischaemic attack
TIC	tachycardia-induced cardiomyopathy
TIMI	thrombolysis in myocardial infarction
TLR	target lesion revascularization
TnI	troponin I
TNK-tPA	tenecteplase

TnT	troponin T
TOE	transoesophageal echocardiogram
TOF	tetralogy of Fallot
tPA	tissue plasminogen activator
TR	tricuspid regurgitation
TS	tricuspid stenosis
TTE	transthoracic echocardiography
TV	tricuspid valve
TWA	T wave alternans
U	unit
UA	unstable angina
UFH	unfractionated heparin
ULN	upper limit of normal
URL	upper reference limit
USA	United States of America
V	volt
VA	ventricular arrhythmia
VD	valve disease
VEGF	vascular endothelial growth factor
VF	ventricular fibrillation
VHL	von Hippel–Lindau
VKA	vitamin K antagonist
VPB	ventricular premature beat
V/Q	ventilation perfusion
VSD	ventral septal defect
VT	ventricular tachycardia
VTE	venous thromboembolism
WBC	white blood cell
WPW	Wolff–Parkinson–White
WU	Woods unit
y	year

Part I

Grown-up congenital heart disease

Relevant guidelines

ACC/AHA 2008 guidelines on GUCH

ACC/AHA 2008 guidelines for the management of adults with congenital heart disease. *J Am Coll Cardiol.* 2008;**52**:e1–e121.

ESC 2010 guidelines on GUCH

ESC Guidelines for the management of grown-up congenital heart disease (new version 2010). *Eur Heart J.* 2010;**31**:2915–57.

ACCF/AHA 2010 guidelines on aortic disease

2010 ACCF/AHA/AATS/ACR/ASA/SCA/SCAI/SIR/STS/SVM Guidelines for the diagnosis and management of patients with thoracic aortic disease. *J Am Coll Cardiol.* 2010;**55**:e27–e129.

ACC/AHA 2008 guidelines on valve disease

Focused update incorporated into the ACC/AHA 2006 guidelines for the management of patients with valvular heart disease. *J Am Coll Cardiol.* 2008;**52**:e1–142.

ESC 2011 guidelines on pregnancy

ESC Guidelines on the management of cardiovascular diseases during pregnancy. *Eur Heart J.* 2011;**32**:3147–97.

AHA/ASA 2011 guidelines on Stroke and TIA

Guidelines for the Prevention of Stroke in Patients With Stroke or Transient Ischemic Attack: a guideline for healthcare professionals from the American Heart Association/American Stroke Association. *Stroke.* 2011;**42**:227–276.

Chapter 1

Grown-up congenital heart disease: general principles

Definition

Congenital heart disease refers to a defect in the structure of the heart and great vessels, which is present at birth.

Epidemiology

Approximately 0.8% of the population is born with congenital heart disease. Up to 40% of them are cured spontaneously (mainly small VSDs) and, with current surgical and interventional techniques, 85% survive into adulthood (grown-up congenital heart disease—GUCH) (Table 1.1).[1–4] According to data of the European Surveillance of Congenital Abnormalities, the live birth prevalence of congenital heart disease is 7/1000 births.[1]

Survival after operation is better in patients without heterotaxy, i.e. randomized variation in the left-right asymmetry of visceral organs that differs from complete situs solitus and situs inversus. This is probably due to ciliary dysfunction that is associated with heterotaxy.[5] Adult congenital heart disease comprises a population that is currently estimated at one million in the USA and 1.2 million in Europe, and admission rates in hospital are twice higher than in the general population.[6–8] In adults, VSD and ASD are the most common defects (each of them approximately 20% of all defects), followed by PDA and pulmonary valve stenosis.[2]

Aetiology

Environmental factors are rare: congenital rubella, maternal diabetes, paternal exposure to phthalates, maternal smoking, alcohol and drug abuse, air pollutants, and pesticides.[2]

Genetic factors Disruption at any point during cardiac primary morphogenesis (i.e. ornation of the heart tube, looping, septation, and resultant systemic and pulmonary circulations) results in the large spectrum of congenital heart defects. Genetic disorders responsible for these alterations can be classified into three types: chromosomal disorders, single-gene disorders, and polygenic disorders.

Chromosomal disorders (5–8% of congenital heart disease patients), caused by absent or duplicated chromosomes, include trisomy 21 (Down's syndrome), 22q11 deletion (di George syndrome), and 45X deletion (Turner's syndrome). Recurrence risk in an offspring is that of the chromosomal disorder.

Single-gene disorders (3% of congenital heart disease patients) are caused by gene deletions, duplications, or mutations. These disorders follow autosomal dominant, autosomal recessive, or X-linked inheritance patterns. Some examples are Holt–Oram syndrome, atrial septal defect with conduction abnormalities, and supravalvular aortic stenosis. Recurrence risk is high in first-degree relatives of patients with these disorders.

Polygenic disorders result from environmental and genetic factors.

Clinical problems in GUCH

Patients with complex lesions and/or complications should be managed in experienced GUCH centres.[9, 10]

Peripheral cyanosis may due to peripheral vasoconstriction, polycythaemia, or poor cardiac output.

Central cyanosis (arterial saturation <85% or >5g reduced haemoglobin) may be due to right to left shunting or reduced pulmonary flow. Differential cyanosis may be seen with PDA and pulmonary hypertension or interrupted aortic arch. In cyanosis from pulmonary causes, there is an increase of PO_2 to, at least, >21 kPa (160 mmHg) after breathing 100% O_2 for 5 min.

In patients with GUCH, cyanosis and chronic hypoxaemia leads to marked erythrocytosis and, frequently, to low platelet counts (<100 000), which may predispose to bleeding. The absence of erythrocytosis (e.g. haemoglobin >17.0 g/dL) in such patients suggests a 'relative anaemia'. Phlebotomy should be undertaken with haemoglobin >20 g/dL and Hct >65%, associated with headache, increasing fatigue, or other symptoms of hyperviscosity in the absence of dehydration or anaemia (ACC/AHA guidelines on GUCH 2008, Class I-C), under careful volume replacement with normal saline. Multiple phlebotomies result in iron deficiency that is associated with impaired small-vessel blood flow and an increase in the risk of reversible ischaemic neurological deficits and stroke. The use of anticoagulation and antiplatelet agents is controversial and should be confined to well-defined indications.

Digital clubbing Apart from GUCH, it may be seen in pulmonary malignancy, chronic infection, and primary hypertrophic osteoarthropathy.

Renal function Sclerotic renal glomeruli leading to increased creatinine levels, proteinuria, and hyperuricaemia.

Gallstones Increased breakdown of red cells results in increased risk of calcium bilirubinate gallstones.

Hypertrophic osteoarthropathy with thickened periosteum and **scoliosis** that may compromise pulmonary function.

Table 1.1 Adult patients with congenital heart disease

Complex conditions
Eisenmenger syndrome Double-outlet ventricle
Fontan procedure Mitral atresia
Pulmonary atresia
Pulmonary vascular obstructive diseases
Single ventricle (double inlet or outlet, common or primitive) Transposition of the great arteries
Tricuspid atresia
Truncus arteriosus/hemitruncus Other rare complex conditions include abnormalities of atrioventricular or ventriculoarterial connection, such as criss-cross heart, isomerism, heterotaxy syndromes, and ventricular inversion.
Moderate conditions
Anomalous pulmonary venous drainage (partial or total) Aortic valve disease (valvar, supravalvar, subvalvar) Atrioventricular septal defects Coarctation of the aorta Coronary fistulae Ebstein's anomaly Mitral valve disease Patent ductus arteriosus Pulmonary valve disease (valvar, supravalvar, subvalvar) Pulmonary arteriovenous malformations Sinus of Valsalva fistula/aneurysm Tetralogy of Fallot Ventricular septal defects
Simple conditions
Isolated aortic valve disease Isolated mitral valve disease (not parachute valve or cleft leaflet) Small patent ductus arteriosus Mild pulmonary stenosis Small ASD Small VSD

1. Conditions may start acyanotic and become cyanotic with time: Fallot's tetralogy, Ebstein's anomaly, and left-to-right shunts, resulting in Eisenmenger syndrome.
2. Cardiac dextroversion with situs solitus (i.e. normal position of viscera—gastric bubble on the left) is associated with congenital defects (TGA mainly, VSD, PS, tricuspid atresia) in 90% of cases. Dextrocardia with situs inversus (gastric bubble on the right) carries a low incidence of congenital heart disease, whereas situs inversus with levocardia is invariably associated with complex congenital abnormalities.
Warnes CA, Liberthson R, Danielson GK, *et al.* Task force 1: the changing profile of congenital heart disease in adult life. *J Am Coll Cardiol* 2001;**37**:1170–5.

Cerebrovascular events (embolic or haemorrhagic), **brain abscess, cognitive and psychological problems** are also common.

Atrial fibrillation is usually a late finding, and restoration of sinus rhythm may be difficult.

Atrial tachycardia (usually macroreentrant) is often seen in tetralogy of Fallot and following Fontan, Mustard, and Senning procedures. These arrhythmias can be treated with catheter ablation, usually assisted by electroanatomic mapping.

Atrioventricular reentrant tachycardia (accessory pathways) in Ebstein's anomaly and corrected transposition.

Sick sinus syndrome in ASD, post-operatively Fontan, Mustard, Senning.

AV block in ASD, corrected transposition, VSD closure, AVR.

Ventricular tachycardia Conditions with the greatest known risk of late sudden cardiac death are tetralogy of Fallot, d- or l-transposition, aortic stenosis, and univentricular hearts.[9]

ICD is recommended to any patient who has had a cardiac arrest or experienced an episode of haemodynamically significant or sustained ventricular tachycardia. Indications for ICD are discussed in detail in the chapter on ventricular arrhythmias.

Imaging techniques and investigations

Two- or three-dimensional echocardiography with Doppler imaging and **cardiac magnetic resonance** have now replaced cardiac catheterization as a diagnostic tool in most patients with GUCH.[11]

MRI is considered superior to echocardiography for:

- Quantification of RV volume and function, and PR
- Evaluation of the RVOT, RV-PA conduits, and great vessels
- Tissue characterization (fibrosis, fat, iron, etc.).

CT is superior to MRI for:

- Collaterals, arteriovenous malformations, and coronary anomalies
- Evaluation of intra- and extracardiac masses.

Haemodynamic assessment

Haemodynamic measurements of cardiac output and systemic and pulmonary flow are derived by Doppler echocardiography that has replaced calculations by the Fick method. However, verification of pressures by direct measurement at **cardiac catheterization** is necessary for therapeutic decision-making in the presence of pulmonary hypertension (>½ of systemic pressure) and for angiographic delineation of defects and selection of appropriate closure devices.

Pulmonary vascular (arterial) resistance (PVR) = (PA pressure–wedge pressure)/cardiac output (Normal range: 0.25–1.5 Wood units (mmHg/L/min) or 20–120 dyn/s/cm^5)

Systemic vascular (arterial) resistance (SVR) = (Ao pressure–RA pressure)/cardiac output (Normal range: 9–20 Wood units (mmHg/L/min) or 700–1600 dyn/s/cm^5)

If PVR is greater than two-thirds of SVR, vasodilating challenge, either acute in the catheter laboratory or chronic, with oxygen, nitric oxide, adenosine, epoprostenol, calcium channel blockers, endothelin antagonists, and phosphodiesterase inhibitors, is indicated to investigate the responsiveness of the pulmonary vascular bed. With fixed values, irreversible damage and Eisenmenger syndrome have developed.

Pulmonary flow/systemic flow (Qp/Qs)—usually derived by echocardiography.

According to the Fick method, Qp/Qs is calculated by oximetry as:

$$Qp/Qs = (\text{Ao saturation} - \text{mixed venous saturation}) / (\text{PV} - \text{PA saturation}), \text{ where}$$

$$\text{Mixed venous saturation} = (3 \times \text{SVC saturation} + \text{IVC saturation})/4$$

If PV saturation is not available, the value of 98 is used instead.

Routine **saturation run** during catheterization for exclusion of shunt involves blood sampling from: high SVC, RA/SVC junction, high RA, mid-RA, low RA, IVC, RV inflow, RV body, RV outflow, main PA, PV and LA if possible, LV, and Ao.

A step-up of saturation >10% indicates shunt.

Coronary angiography

Is indicated preoperatively in patients >40 years, postmenopausal women, adults with multiple risk factors for coronary artery disease, and children with suspicion of congenital coronary anomalies.

Spirometry

There is a high prevalence of markedly abnormal forced vital capacity (FVC) in patients with GUCH, and reduced FVC is associated with increased mortality.[12]

Cardiopulmonary exercise testing

It provides strong prognostic information in adult patients with congenital heart disease. Peak oxygen consumption (VO_2) is one of the best predictors of morbidity and mortality.[13, 14]

Principles of management

General measures are presented in Table 1.2. Specific management is discussed in relevant chapters.

Table 1.2 ESC 2010 GL on GUCH. Risk reduction strategies in patients with cyanotic congenital heart disease

Prophylactic measures are the mainstay of care to avoid complications. The following exposures/activities should be avoided:
• Pregnancy
• Iron deficiency and anaemia (no routine, inappropriate phlebotomies to maintain predetermined haemoglobin)
• Dehydration
• Infectious disease: annual influenza vaccination, pneumovax (every 5 years)
• Cigarette smoking, recreational drug abuse including alcohol
• Transvenous PM/ICD leads
• Strenuous exercise
• Acute exposure to heat (sauna, hot tub/shower)
Other risk reduction strategies include:
• Use of an air filter in an intravenous line to prevent air embolism
• Consultation of a GUCH cardiologist before administration of any agent and performance of any surgical/interventional procedure
• Prompt therapy of upper respiratory tract infections
• Cautious use or avoidance of agents that impair renal function
• Contraceptive advice

ESC Guidelines for the management of grown-up congenital heart disease (new version 2010). *Eur Heart J*. 2010;**31**:2915–57.

Permanent pacing and ICD

The most common indications for permanent pacemaker implantation in children, adolescents, and patients with congenital heart disease are symptomatic sinus bradycardia, the bradycardia–tachycardia syndromes, and advanced second- or third-degree AV block, either congenital or postsurgical.[15] Recommendations for ICD are not, in general, different than that to other patients with cardiac disease. Recommendations by ACCF/AHA/HRS and ESC are presented in the chapters on bradyarrhythmias (Chapters 63–65), SVT (Chapter 50), and ventricular arrhythmias (Chapter 55).

Endocarditis prophylaxis

Prophylaxis is now indicated only in high-risk patients and only before dental procedures that involve manipulation of gingival tissue or the periapical region of teeth or perforation of the oral mucosa, or before vaginal delivery.[9, 10] Congenital conditions for which endocarditis prophylaxis is recommended before the aforementioned procedures are presented in Table 1.3. A detailed discussion and specific recommendations is provided in the chapter on infective endocarditis.

Non-cardiac surgery

Preoperative evaluation and surgery for patients with congenital heart disease should be performed in specializing centres with experienced surgeons and cardiac anaesthesiologists. The ACC/AHA recommendations are provided in Table 1.4.

Table 1.3 ACC/AHA 2008 GL on GUCH

Recommendations for infective endocarditis (IE) prophylaxis in patients with adult congenital heart disease	
Patients must be informed of their potential risk for IE and should be provided with the AHA information card with instructions for prophylaxis.	I-B
When patients present with an unexplained febrile illness and potential IE, blood cultures should be drawn before antibiotic treatment is initiated to avoid delay in diagnosis due to 'culture-negative' IE.	I-B
Transthoracic echocardiography (TTE) when the diagnosis of native-valve IE is suspected.	I-B
Transoesophageal echocardiography if TTE windows are inadequate or equivocal, in the presence of a prosthetic valve or material or surgically constructed shunt, in the presence of complex congenital cardiovascular anatomy, or to define possible complications of endocarditis.	I-B
Patients with evidence of IE should have early consultation with a surgeon with experience in adult congenital heart disease (ACHD) because of the potential for rapid deterioration and concern about possible infection of prosthetic material.	I-C
Antibiotic prophylaxis before dental procedures that involve manipulation of gingival tissue or the periapical region of teeth or perforation of the oral mucosa, in patients with CHD with the highest risk for adverse outcome from IE:	IIa-B
a. Prosthetic cardiac valve or prosthetic material used for cardiac valve repair.	
b. Previous IE.	
c. Unrepaired and palliated cyanotic CHD, including surgically constructed palliative shunts and conduits.	
d. Completely repaired CHD with prosthetic materials, whether placed by surgery or by catheter intervention, during the first 6 months after the procedure.	
e. Repaired CHD with residual defects at the site or adjacent to the site of a prosthetic patch or prosthetic device that inhibits endothelialization.	
Antibiotic prophylaxis against IE before vaginal delivery at the time of membrane rupture in select patients with the highest risk of adverse outcomes:	IIa-C
a. Prosthetic cardiac valve or prosthetic material used for cardiac valve repair.	
b. Unrepaired and palliated cyanotic CHD, including surgically constructed palliative shunts and conduits.	
Prophylaxis against IE is not recommended for non-dental procedures (such as oesophagogastroduodenoscopy or colonoscopy) in the absence of active infection.	III-C

ACC/AHA 2008 guidelines for the management of adults with congenital heart disease. *J Am Coll Cardiol* 2008; **52**:e1–e121.

Risk factors of non-cardiac perioperative risk are:

- Cyanosis and/or pulmonary hypertension
- LVEF <35% and/or NYHA III or IV
- Prior Fontan procedure
- Complex congenital heart disease with heart failure, severe left-sided obstructive lesions, malignant arrhythmias, or the need for anticoagulation.

Exercise

Adults with congenital heart disease have subnormal exercise tolerance. However, participation in regular exercise is beneficial for fitness and psychological well-being.[13] In a recent statement, AHA recognized the importance of physically active lifestyles to the health and well-being of children and adults with congenital heart defects.[16] There is no evidence regarding whether or not there is a need to restrict recreational physical activity among patients with congenital heart defects, apart from those with rhythm disorders. Counseling to encourage daily participation in appropriate physical activity should be a core component of every patient encounter. As a general recommendation, dynamic exercise is more suitable than static exercise. Conditions that are not compatible with competitive sports are:

Table 1.4 ACC/AHA 2008 GL on GUCH

Recommendations for non-cardiac surgery in patients with adult congenital heart disease (ACHD)	
Preoperative assessment with systemic arterial oximetry, ECG, chest X-ray, TTE, and blood tests for full blood count and coagulation screen.	I-C
When possible, the preoperative evaluation and surgery for ACHD patients should be performed in a regional centre specializing in congenital cardiology, with experienced surgeons and cardiac anaesthesiologists.	I-C
High-risk patient should be managed at centres for the care of ACHD under all circumstances, unless the operative intervention is an absolute emergency. High-risk categories:	
a. Prior Fontan procedure.	I-C
b. Severe pulmonary arterial hypertension.	I-C
c. Cyanotic CHD.	I-C
d. Complex CHD with residua, such as heart failure, valve disease, or the need for anticoagulation.	I-C
e. Patients with CHD and malignant arrhythmias.	I-C
Consultation with ACHD experts regarding the assessment of risk for patients with CHD who will undergo non-cardiac surgery.	I-C
Consultation with a cardiac anaesthesiologist for moderate- and high-risk patients.	I-C

ACC/AHA 2008 guidelines for the management of adults with congenital heart disease. *J Am Coll Cardiol* 2008; **52**:e1–e121.

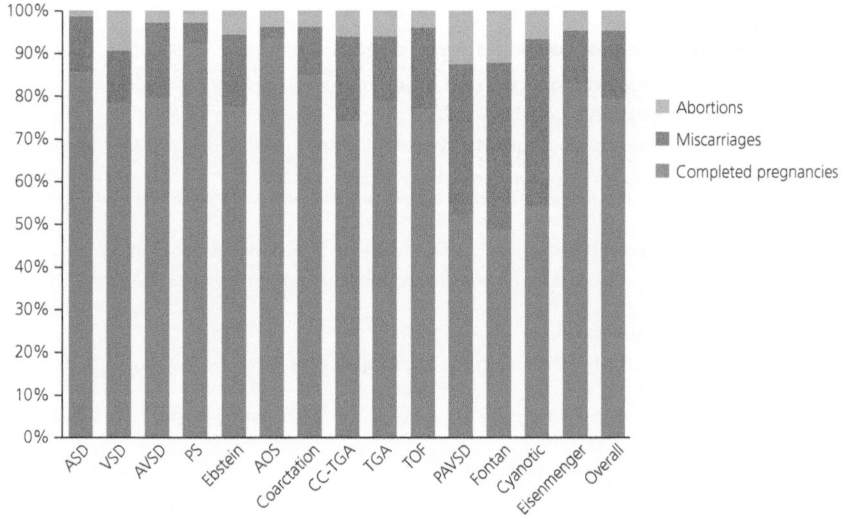

Figure 1.1 Distribution of miscarriages, completed pregnancies (>20 weeks pregnancy duration), and elective abortions for each congenital heart disease separately and the overall rates (from ESC 2011 guidelines on pregnancy).

ASD: atrial septal defect; AVSD: atrioventricular septal defect; AOS: aortic stenosis; CC-TGA: congenital corrected transposition of the great arteries; coarctation: aortic coarctation; Ebstein: Ebstein's anomaly; Eisenmenger: Eisenmenger syndrome; Fontan: patients after Fontan repair; PAVSD: pulmonary atresia with ventricular septal defects; PS: pulmonary valve stenosis; TGA: complete transposition of the great arteries; TOF: tetralogy of Fallot; VSD: ventricular septal defect.

ESC Guidelines on the management of cardiovascular diseases during pregnancy. *Eur Heart J*. 2011;**32**:3147–97

- Eisenmenger syndrome
- Pulmonary hypertension
- Univentricular heart physiology
- Ebstein's anomaly
- Transposition of great arteries
- Coronary artery anomalies.

Maximal exercise testing is contraindicated in all patients with pulmonary hypertension.

Long-distance flights

Cyanotic patients should use only pressurized commercial airplanes and should drink non-alcoholic and non-caffeinated fluids frequently on long-distance flights to avoid dehydration. Oxygen therapy, although often unnecessary, may be suggested for prolonged travel in cyanotic patients. Similarly, residence at high altitude is detrimental for patients with cyanosis.

Pregnancy

Generally, pregnancy is not recommended in Eisenmenger syndrome. In women with congenital defects not complicated by Eisenmenger syndrome, significant pulmonary hypertension or Marfan's syndrome (and Ehlers–Danlos or Loeys–Dietz syndromes) with aortic root >40 mm, pregnancy can be tolerated (Figure 1.1). The most prevalent cardiac complications during pregnancy are arrhythmias, heart failure, and hypertensive complications. Risk factors are discussed in the chapter on pregnancy (miscellaneous topics).

The **recurrence rate** of congenital heart disease in offspring ranges from 2% to 50% and is higher when the mother, rather than the father, has congenital heart disease. Diseases with a single-gene disorder and/or chromosomal

Table 1.5 ACC/AHA 2008 GL on GUCH

Recommendations for pregnancy and contraception	
Consultation with an expert in adult congenital heart disease (ACHD) before patients plan to become pregnant.	I-C
Patients with intracardiac right-to-left shunting should have fastidious care taken of intravenous lines to avoid paradoxical air embolus.	I-C
Pre-pregnancy counselling is recommended for women receiving chronic anticoagulation with warfarin.	I-B
Meticulous prophylaxis for deep venous thrombosis, including early ambulation and compression stockings, for all patients with an intracardiac right-to-left shunt. Subcutaneous heparin or LMWH for prolonged bed rest. Full anticoagulation for high-risk patients.	IIa-C
The oestrogen-containing oral contraceptive pill is not recommended in ACHD patients at risk of thromboembolism, such as those with cyanosis related to an intracardiac shunt, severe pulmonary arterial hypertension (PAH), or Fontan repair.	III-C

ACC/AHA 2008 guidelines for the management of adults with congenital heart disease. *J Am Coll Cardiol* 2008;**52**:e1–e121.

Table 1.6 ESC 2011 GL on pregnancy

Recommendations for the management of congenital heart disease	
Pre-pregnancy relief of stenosis (usually by balloon valvulotomy) in severe PV stenosis (peak Doppler gradient >64 mmHg).	I-B
Follow-up should range from twice during pregnancy to monthly.	I-C
Symptomatic patients with Ebstein's anomaly with cyanosis and/or heart failure should be treated before pregnancy or advised against pregnancy.	I-C
Pre-pregnancy pulmonary valve replacement (bioprosthesis) in symptomatic women with marked dilatation of the RV due to severe pulmonary regurgitation (PR).	I-C
Pre-pregnancy pulmonary valve replacement (bioprosthesis) in asymptomatic women with marked dilatation of the RV due to severe PR.	IIa-C
All women with a bicuspid aortic valve should undergo imaging of the ascending aorta before pregnancy, and surgery should be considered when the aortic diameter is >50 mm.	IIa-C
Anticoagulation during pregnancy in Fontan patients.	IIa-C
Anticoagulation in pulmonary arterial hypertension (PAH) with suspicion of pulmonary embolism as the cause (or partly the cause) of the pulmonary hypertension.	IIa-C
In patients who are already taking drug therapy for pulmonary arterial hypertension before becoming pregnant, continuation should be considered after information about the teratogenic effects.	IIa-C
Women with pulmonary hypertension should be advised against pregnancy.	III-C
Women with an oxygen saturation <85% at rest should be advised against pregnancy.	III-C
Patients with TGA and a systemic RV with more than moderate impairment of RV function and/or severe TR should be advised against pregnancy.	III-C
Fontan patients with depressed ventricular function and/or moderate to severe atrioventricular valvular regurgitation or with cyanosis or with protein-losing enteropathy should be advised against pregnancy.	III-C

ESC Guidelines on the management of cardiovascular diseases during pregnancy. *Eur Heart J*. 2011;**32**:3147–97.

abnormalities are associated with a high recurrence rate. In Marfan's, Noonan's, and Holt–Oram syndromes, there is a 50% risk of recurrence. In VSD and ASD, the estimated risk is 6–10%, in AS 8%, and in Fallot's tetralogy 3%.

Oestrogen-only contraceptives potentially increase the thrombotic risk and should be avoided.

The ACC/AH recommendations, as well as the ESC guidelines on pregnancy,[17] are presented in Tables 1.5 and 1.6.

References

1. Dolk H, *et al.* Congenital heart defects in Europe: prevalence and perinatal mortality, 2000 to 2005. *Circulation.* 2011;**123**, 841–9.
2. Go AS, *et al.* Heart disease and stroke statistics—2013 update: a report from the american heart association. *Circulation.* 2013;**127**:e6–245.
3. Hoffman JI, *et al.* The incidence of congenital heart disease. *J Am Coll Cardiol.* 2002;**39**:1890–900.
4. Warnes CA, *et al.* Task Force 1: the changing profile of congenital heart disease in adult life. *J Am Coll Cardiol.* 2001;**37**:1170–5
5. Nakhleh N, *et al.* High prevalence of respiratory ciliary dysfunction in congenital heart disease patients with heterotaxy. *Circulation.* 2012;**125**:2232–42.
6. Hoffman JI, *et al.* Prevalence of congenital heart disease. *Am Heart J.* 2004;**147**:425–39.
7. Moons P, *et al.* Delivery of care for adult patients with congenital heart disease in Europe: results from the euro heart survey. *Eur Heart J.* 2006;**27**:1324–30.
8. Verheugt CL, *et al.* The emerging burden of hospital admissions of adults with congenital heart disease. *Heart.* 2010;**96**:872–8.
9. Baumgartner H, *et al.* ESC guidelines for the management of grown-up congenital heart disease (new version 2010). *Eur Heart J.* 2010;**31**:2915–57.
10. Warnes CA, *et al.* ACC/AHA 2008 guidelines for the management of adults with congenital heart disease: a report of the American College of Cardiology/American Heart Association Task Force on practice guidelines (writing committee to develop guidelines on the management of adults with congenital heart disease). Developed in collaboration with the American Society of Echocardiography, Heart Rhythm Society, International Society for Adult Congenital Heart Disease, Society for Cardiovascular Angiography and Interventions, and Society of Thoracic Surgeons. *J Am Coll Cardiol.* 2008;**52**:e143–263.
11. Hundley WG, *et al.* ACCF/ACR/AHA/NASCI/SCMR 2010 expert consensus document on cardiovascular magnetic resonance: a report of the American College of Cardiology Foundation Task Force on expert consensus documents. *J Am Coll Cardiol.* 2010;**55**:2614–62.
12. Alonso-Gonzalez R BF, *et al.* Abnormal lung function in adults with congenital heart disease: Prevalence, relation to cardiac anatomy, and association with survival. *Circulation.* 2013;**127**:882–90.
13. Inuzuka R, *et al.* Comprehensive use of cardiopulmonary exercise testing identifies adults with congenital heart disease at increased mortality risk in the medium term. *Circulation.* 2012;**125**:250–9.
14. Rhodes J, *et al.* Exercise testing and training in children with congenital heart disease. *Circulation.* 2010; **122**:1957–67.
15. 2012 ACCF/AHA/HRS focused update incorporated into the ACCF/AHA/HRS 2008 guidelines for device-based therapy of cardiac rhythm abnormalities. *J Am Coll Cardiol.* 2013;**61**:e6–75.
16. Longmuir PE *et al.* on behalf of the American Heart Association Atherosclerosis, Hypertension and Obesity in Youth

Committee of the Council on Cardiovascular Disease in the Young. Promotion of physical activity for children and adults with congenital heart disease: A scientific statement from the American Heart Association. *Circulation*. 2013; **127**:2147–59.

17. Regitz-Zagrosek V, *et al.* ESC guidelines on the management of cardiovascular diseases during pregnancy: the Task Force on the management of cardiovascular diseases during pregnancy of the European Society of Cardiology (ESC). *Eur Heart J*. 2011; **32**: 3147–97.

Chapter 2

Ventricular septal defects

Definition and classification

The ventricular septum can be divided into two morphological components, the membranous septum and the muscular septum. The ***membranous septum*** is small and located at the base of the heart between the inlet and outlet components of the muscular septum, behind the septal leaflet of the tricuspid valve and below the right and non-coronary cusps of the aortic valve. Defects that involve the membranous septum are the most common VSD (70–80%) and are called **perimembranous, paramembranous, or infracristal**. Perimembranous defects may extend into the adjacent muscular septum and, in this case, are called **perimembranous inlet, perimembranous muscular,** and **perimembranous outlet** (Figure 2.1).[1,2]

The ***muscular septum*** can be divided into inlet, trabecular, and infundibular components. Defects in the inlet muscular septum, i.e. inferoposterior to the membranous septum, are called **inlet VSD** (usually part of a complete AV canal defect) (5%). A defect in the trabecular septum is called **muscular VSD** if the defect is completely rimmed by muscle (15–20%). Muscular VSDs may be multiple and can be acquired after a septal myocardial infarction. Defects in the infundibulum (5%) are called **infundibular, outlet, supracristal, conal, conoventricular, subpulmonary**, or **doubly committed subarterial** defects. Perimembranous or infundibular VSDs are often associated with progressive AR due to prolapse of an aortic cusp.

Epidemiology

VSD is the most common congenital heart defect after the bicuspid aortic valve, occurring in 40% of all children with congenital heart disease and with an estimated prevalence of 5% in newborn babies.[2] With paternal VSD, the recurrence risk in an offspring is 2%. Maternal VSD has a recurrence risk of 6–10%.

Aetiology

The origins of VSD are not known, and as in most cases of GUCH, they are most probably multifactorial (see Chapter 1). Recently a locus on chromosome 10p15 was associated with familial ventricular aneurysms and VSDs,[3] and mutations in the transcription factors TBX5 and GATA4 have been identified in familial cases of VSD.[2] No direct genetic testing at this time for VSD exists. **Associated disorders** are tetralogy of Fallot, AV canal, and aortic coarctation.

Pathophysiology

The shunt volume in a VSD depends on the size of the defect and the pulmonary vascular resistance. Without pulmonary hypertension or obstruction to the right ventricle, the direction of shunt is left to right, with decreased LV output and compensatory intravascular volume overload. Thus, pulmonary artery, left atrial, and left ventricular volume overload develop. Moderate or large VSDs result in the transmission of LV pressure to pulmonary vascular bed with increased shear forces. This combination of high volume and pressure contributes to the development of irreversible pulmonary vascular disease.[5] VSD is the most common cause of pulmonary hypertension. Eventually, the elevated pulmonary vascular resistance becomes irreversible and leads to reversal of shunt and cyanosis, and Eisenmenger syndrome develops. In the setting of elevated pulmonary vascular resistance or right ventricular obstruction resulting from muscle bundles or pulmonary stenosis, the shunt volume is limited and may be right to left, depending on the difference in pressure.

Spontaneous closure Muscular or membranous VSDs can undergo spontaneous closure, usually in the first years of

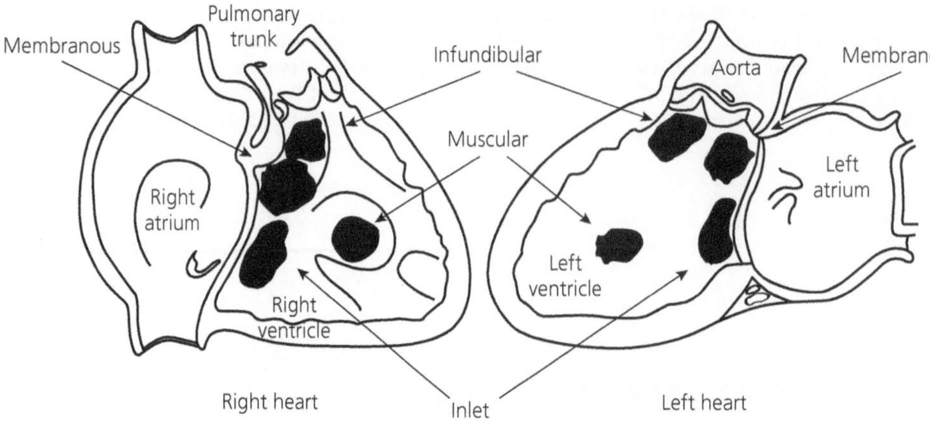

Figure 2.1 Location of VSDs.

Minette MS, *et al*. Ventricular septal defects. *Circulation*. 2006;**114**:2190–7

life. Up to 90% of such defects close spontaneously by one year of age.[5]

Presentation

Adults with small defects and normal pulmonary artery pressure are generally asymptomatic. Patients with large defects who survive to adulthood usually have left ventricular failure or pulmonary hypertension with associated RV failure.[6]

Physical examination

- Physical signs depend on the size of VSD.
- **Holosystolic (pansystolic) murmur**, with or without a **thrill**, with moderate or large defects. The grade of murmur depends on the velocity of flow. **Very small or large defects** with no shunt and defects with Eisenmenger physiology and right-to-left shunt may not have a VSD murmur. **Muscular** defects can be heard along the lower left sternal border and may vary in intensity, as the defect size changes with muscular contraction throughout systole. **Infundibular** defects close to the pulmonary valve can be heard best at the left upper sternal border.
- Short, **mid-diastolic apical rumble** (increased mitral flow) may be heard.
- **Decrescendo murmur** in the presence of AR.
- **Cyanosis** with **clubbing** and **peripheral oedema** due to right-sided heart failure gradually appear.

Investigations

- **ECG** is normal in small VSD. With large defects, there is LA and LV hypertrophy. When pulmonary hypertension develops, there is right axis deviation and RV hypertrophy.
- **Chest radiography** is normal with small VSDs. With large defects, there is 'shunt vascularity', i.e. well-visualized small pulmonary arteries in the periphery of both lungs. When pulmonary hypertension develops, there is marked enlargement of the proximal PAs, rapid tapering of the peripheral arteries (pruning), and oligaemic lung fields.
- **Transthoracic** or **transoesophageal echocardiography** with colour flow mapping are used for quantification of the shunt, assessment of pulmonary artery pressure, distortion of the aortic valve, and obstruction of the right ventricular outflow tract (double-chamber RV). **Three-dimensional echocardiography** is useful for defects that are difficult to evaluate by two-dimensional imaging.
- **Cardiac magnetic resonance** is very useful with complex associated lesions.
- **Cardiac catheterization** is no longer necessary. However, it can be used to determine Qp/Qs by oximetry, and pulmonary artery pressure and resistance in case of anticipated closure (Table 2.1). It can also assess response to pulmonary vasodilators that can guide therapy and evaluate coexistent AR, dual-chamber RV, or multiple VSDs.

Therapy

Medical

Adult patients with small VSD without evidence of left ventricular volume overload or AR do not require intervention.[7] These patients, as well as patients who had VSD repair, need surveillance for AR (perimembranous and infundibular VSDs) and endocarditis. Endocarditis a lifelong risk in unoperated patients, being six times higher than in the normal population, but is primarily associated with

Table 2.1 ACC/AHA 2008 GL on GUCH

Recommendations for cardiac catheterization	
Cardiac catheterization to assess the operability of adults with VSD and PAH should be performed in an ACHD regional centre in collaboration with experts.	I-C
In adults with VSD in whom non-invasive data are inconclusive and further information is needed for management. Data to be obtained include the following:	
a. Quantification of shunting.	IIa-B
b. Assessment of pulmonary pressure and resistance in patients with suspected PAH. Reversibility of PAH should be tested with various vasodilators.	IIa-B
c. Evaluation of other lesions, such as AR and double-chambered right ventricle.	IIa-C
d. Determination of whether multiple VSDs are present before surgery.	IIa-C
e. Performance of coronary arteriography is indicated in patients at risk for coronary artery disease.	IIa-C
f. VSD anatomy, especially if device closure is contemplated.	IIa-C

ACC/AHA 2008 guidelines for the management of adults with congenital heart disease. *J Am Coll Cardiol* 2008;**52**:e1–e121.

the associated valve disease rather than the VSD itself.[7] Routine **endocarditis prophylaxis**, however, is not recommended any more for unrepaired VSDs. For closed VSDs, prophylaxis is recommended for 6 months after the procedure.[8, 9] Instead, patients are advised on dental hygiene, and the physician should be alert of suspicious symptoms (see Chapter 1 and Chapter 79 on endocarditis). In adults with inoperable VSDs with progressive/severe pulmonary vascular disease, pulmonary vasodilator therapy may be considered (ACC/AHA guidelines on GUCH 2008, Class IIb-B).

Indications for closure

Indications are presented in Tables 2.2 and 2.3.[8, 9] Main indications are:

- Qp/Qs >1.5
- History of endocarditis
- Progressive AR
- LV volume overload.

Contraindications for closure

Irreversible pulmonary arterial hypertension, i.e. PA pressure >2/3 systemic pressure or PVR >2/3 SVR at baseline or after oxygen or vasodilation.

Catheter closure

Currently, defect-specific devices are in the investigational stage and have been used both for congenital and post-MI VSD. They may interfere with AV or TV and carry a higher risk for AV block than surgical closure. Recent experience with closure of perimembranous VSDs indicates a <1% risk of complete AV block, which is comparable to that after surgical closure.[10, 11]

Table 2.2 ACC/AHA 2008 GL on GUCH

Recommendations for Ventricular Septal Defect Closure	
Surgeons with training and expertise in CHD should perform VSD closure operations.	I-C
Closure of VSD when there is a Qp/Qs ≥2.0 and clinical evidence of LV volume overload.	I-B
Closure of VSD with a history of endocarditis.	I-C
Closure of VSD with net left-to-right shunting and PA pressure <2/3 systemic pressure and PVR <2/3 SVR.	IIa-B
Closure of VSD with net left-to-right shunting and Qp/Qs >1.5 and LV systolic or diastolic failure.	IIa-B
Device closure of a muscular VSD may be considered, especially if the VSD is remote from the tricuspid valve and the aorta, if the VSD is associated with severe left-sided heart chamber enlargement, or if there is PAH.	IIb-C
VSD closure in severe irreversible PAH.	III-B

ACC/AHA 2008 guidelines for the management of adults with congenital heart disease. *J Am Coll Cardiol* 2008;**52**:e1–e121.

Table 2.3 ESC 2010 GL on GUCH

Indications for intervention in VSD	
Surgical VSD closure in patients with symptoms that can be attributed to L–R shunting through the (residual) VSD and who have no severe pulmonary vascular disease.	I-C
Surgical VSD closure in asymptomatic patients with evidence of LV volume overload attributable to the VSD.	I-C
Surgical VSD closure in patients with a history of IE.	IIa-C
Surgery for patients with VSD-associated prolapse of an aortic valve cusp, causing progressive AR.	IIa-C
Surgery for patients with VSD and PAH when there is still net L–R shunt (Qp/Qs >1.5) present and PAP or PVR are <2/3 of systemic values (baseline or when challenged with vasodilators, preferably nitric oxide, or after targeted PAH therapy).	IIa-C
Surgery in Eisenmenger VSD and when exercise-induced.	III-C
Surgery if the VSD is small, not subarterial, does not lead to LV volume overload or pulmonary hypertension, and if there is no history of IE.	III-C

ESC Guidelines for the management of grown-up congenital heart disease (new version 2010). *Eur Heart J*. 2010;**31**:2915–57.

Pregnancy

Contraindicated in Eisenmerger syndrome.[8,9] Women with large shunts and pulmonary arterial hypertension may have arrhythmias, LV dysfunction, and progression of pulmonary hypertension. Combinations of epoprostenol and sildenafil may improve outcome in pregnant women with severe pulmonary hypertension who choose to continue pregnancy (see also General principles).[2] The estimated recurrence rate in the offspring is 6–10%.[8]

References

1. Minette MS, *et al.* Ventricular septal defects. *Circulation.* 2006;**114**:2190–7.
2. Penny DJ, *et al.* Ventricular septal defect. *Lancet.* 2011;**377**:1103–12.
3. Tremblay N, *et al.* Familial ventricular aneurysms and septal defects map to chromosome 10p15. *Eur Heart J.* 2011;**32**:568–73.
4. Sommer RJ, *et al.* Pathophysiology of congenital heart disease in the adult: part I: shunt lesions. *Circulation.* 2008;**117**:1090–9.
5. Hoffman JI, *et al.* The incidence of congenital heart disease. *J Am Coll Cardiol.* 2002;**39**:1890–1900.
6. Brickner ME, *et al.* Congenital heart disease in adults. Second of two parts. *N Engl J Med.* 2000;**342**:334–42.
7. Gabriel HM, *et al.* Long-term outcome of patients with ventricular septal defect considered not to require surgical closure during childhood. *J Am Coll Cardiol.* 2002;**39**:1066–71.
8. Baumgartner H, *et al.* ESC guidelines for the management of grown-up congenital heart disease (new version 2010). *Eur Heart J.* 2010;**31**:2915–57.
9. Warnes CA, *et al.* ACC/AHA 2008 guidelines for the management of adults with congenital heart disease: a report of the American College of Cardiology/American Heart Association Task Force on practice guidelines (writing committee to develop guidelines on the management of adults with congenital heart disease). Developed in collaboration with the American Society of Echocardiography, Heart Rhythm Society, International Society for Adult Congenital Heart Disease, Society for Cardiovascular Angiography and Interventions, and Society of Thoracic Surgeons. *J Am Coll Cardiol.* 2008;**52**:e143–263.
10. Yang J, *et al.* Transcatheter device closure of perimembranous ventricular septal defects: mid-term outcomes. *Eur Heart J.* 2010;**31**:2238–45.
11. Zhang GC, *et al.* Transthoracic echocardiographic guidance of minimally invasive perventricular device closure of perimembranous ventricular septal defect without cardiopulmonary bypass: initial experience. *Eur Heart J Cardiovasc Imaging.* 2012;**13**:739–44.

Chapter 3

Atrioventricular septal defects

Definitions and classification of AVSDs

The primordial single atrium divides into right and left sides by formation and fusion of the septum primum and septum secundum. The septum primum grows from the primordial atrial roof toward the endocardial cushions, and the septum secundum grows from the ventrocranial atrial wall on the right side of the septum primum.

- **Atrioventricular septal defects (AV canal or endocardial cushion defects)** are **complete** (large VSD, common AV junction, and common AV valve with five leaflets) or **partial** (ostium primum ASD with a common AV junction but two separate AV valves) (Figure 3.1).[1,2]
- **Ostium primum defect** at the lower part of the atrial septum is a partial atrioventricular septal defect and may, or may not, have a VSD component (15% of ASDs).
- **Ostium secundum defect** involves the region of the fossa ovalis (80%).
- **Sinus venosus defect** at the junction of the right atrium and superior vena cava (5%).
- **Coronary sinus septal defect** ('unroofed' coronary sinus) and **inferior sinus venosus defect** (at the junction of right atrium and inferior vena cava): very rare (<1%).
- **Patent foramen ovale** is the incomplete septal partition (usually an oval-shaped window) at the point where the septum secundum overlaps perforations of the septum primum (i.e. the foramen secundum).

Complete AV canals rarely reach adulthood without Eisenmenger syndrome. Partial AV canal defects (including ostium primum ASD) are not uncommon in adults.

Ostium primum ASD

Epidemiology

All kinds of ASD, in general, represent one-third of the cases of congenital heart disease detected in adults.[3]

Aetiology

Approximately 40% of patients with Down's syndrome have an AV septal defect, usually complete. Primum ASD

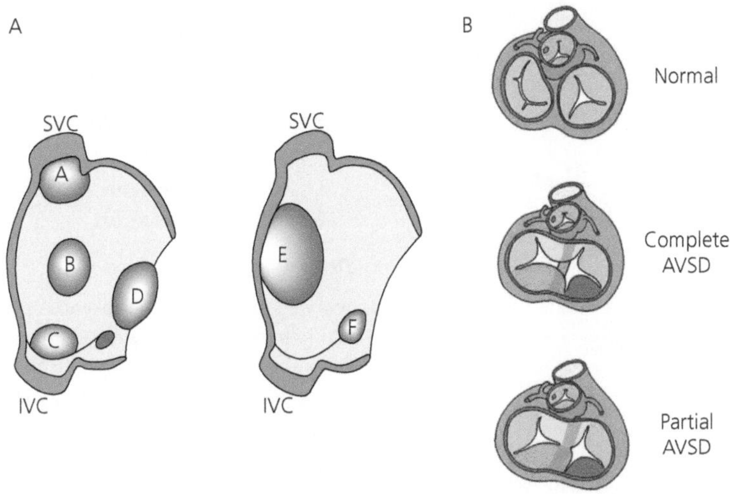

Figure 3.1 Anatomy of ASDs. A: superior sinus venosus ASD; B: secundum ASD; C: inferior sinus venosus ASD; D: ostium primum ASD or partial AV septal defect; E, secundum ASD without posterior septal rim; F: coronary sinus ASD.
Webb G, *et al*. Atrial septal defects in the adult: recent progress and overview. *Circulation*. 2006;**114**:1645–53

may also be associated with di George, Ellis-van Creveld, and Noonan's syndromes. Gender distribution is equal for ostium primum ASD. Adults with AV septal defects have an approximate 3–10% risk of recurrence in their offspring (excluding familial ASD and heart-hand syndromes with autosomal dominant inheritance).[4, 5]

Pathophysiology

In ostium primum ASD, there is a cleft (trileaflet) mitral valve and results in variable degrees of regurgitation.[1, 5] The shorter distance from the left AV valve annulus to the left ventricular apex compared to that from the apex to the aortic annulus, combined with the cleft mitral valve, creates the characteristic 'gooseneck' deformity that used to be a major diagnostic feature on left ventriculography. The elongation of the left ventricular outflow tract as well as the chordal attachments of the left AV valve to the ventricular septum is the reason for the development of LV outflow tract obstruction which may occur even late after successful repair of the defect and require reoperation. The abnormal AV junction affects the AV conduction tissue, which, in turn, produces the characteristic left axis deviation and predisposes these patients to heart block. Most primum ASDs are relatively large and lead to right heart dilation. Right atrial dilation and stretching predisposes to the development of atrial flutter and fibrillation. The pathophysiology of isolated primum ASD is similar to that of a large secundum ASD (see Chapter 4).

Presentation

Depending on the severity of dysfunction of the left AV valve, adult patients with ostium primum ASD may become symptomatic at a much younger age than patients with other types of ASD.

Physical examination

Physical signs as in secundum ASD (see Chapter 4), but there is usually an additional **pansystolic murmur** due to MR (or TR). If there is also a ventricular defect, signs resemble those found in large VSD with MR or TR. **Cyanosis** suggests pulmonary hypertension or pulmonary stenosis.

Investigations

- **Chest radiography** in ostium primum ASD may be normal; otherwise resembles that of secundum ASD. Coexistent VSD usually is associated with cardiomegaly and pulmonary plethora.
- **ECG** Long PR (unless if AF or flutter), left axis deviation, RBBB with RV hypertrophy. Development of right axis deviation in primum ASD suggests pulmonary hypertension.
- **Echocardiography** and **cardiac magnetic resonance** have replaced angiography as the main diagnostic tool for documentation of the type and size of the ASD, direction of the shunt and pulmonary venous return.
- Maximal **exercise testing** can be useful to document exercise capacity in patients with symptoms that are discrepant with clinical findings or to document changes in oxygen saturation in patients with pulmonary hypertension (Class IIa-C, ACC/AHA guidelines on GUCH 2008).
- **Cardiac catheterization** is used only to assess pulmonary hypertension and test vasoreactivity in patients with repaired or unrepaired ASD.[6]

Therapy

Primary surgical repair is recommended for partial AV canals, provided there is no irreversible pulmonary hypertension (Tables 3.1 and 3.2). In cases of residual interatrial or interventricular communications, endocardial pacing causes an elevated risk of paradoxical emboli, and epicardial pacing may be required.[7]

Table 3.1 ACC/AHA 2008 GL on GUCH. Management of atrioventricular septal defect (AVSD)

Recommendations for surgical therapy	
Surgeons with training and expertise in CHD should perform operations for AVSD.	I-C
Surgical reoperation is recommended in adults with previously repaired AVSD, with the following indications:	I-B
1. Left AV valve repair or replacement for regurgitation or stenosis that causes symptoms, atrial or ventricular arrhythmias, a progressive increase in LV dimensions, or deterioration of LV function.	
2. LVOT obstruction with a mean gradient >50 mmHg or peak instantaneous gradient >70 mmHg or a gradient <50 mmHg in association with significant mitral regurgitation or AR.	
3. Residual/recurrent ASD or VSD with significant left-to-right shunting.	

ACC/AHA 2008 guidelines for the management of adults with congenital heart disease. *J Am Coll Cardiol* 2008;**52**:e1–e121.

Table 3.2 ESC 2010 GL on GUCH. Indications for intervention in AVSD

Complete AVSD	
Cardiac surgery in patients with Eisenmenger physiology. In case of doubt, PVR testing is recommended.	III-C
Partial AVSD	
Surgical closure in case of significant volume overload of the RV.	I-C
AV valve regurgitation	
Symptomatic patients with moderate to severe AV valve regurgitation should undergo valve surgery, preferably AV valve repair.	I-C
Valve surgery for asymptomatic patients with moderate or severe left-sided valve regurgitation and LVESD >45 mm and/or impaired LV function (LVEF <60%) when other causes of LV dysfunction are excluded.	I-B
Surgical repair in asymptomatic patients with moderate or severe left-sided AV valve regurgitation who have signs of volume overload of the LV and a substrate of regurgitation that is very likely to be amenable for surgical repair.	IIa-C

ESC Guidelines for the management of grown-up congenital heart disease (new version 2010). *Eur Heart J.* 2010;**31**:2915–57.

Endocarditis prophylaxis

It is recommended only in high-risk patients with repaired ASDs. Revised indications are discussed in Chapter 1 and Chapter 79 on endocarditis.

Pregnancy

It is well tolerated in the absence of severe pulmonary arterial hypertension but with an increased risk of paradoxical embolus and stroke, arrhythmia, and heart failure (see Introduction). All women with a history of AVSD should be evaluated before conception to ensure that there are no significant residual haemodynamic lesions that might complicate the management of pregnancy. The issue of pregnancy risk and preventive measures should be discussed with women with Down's syndrome and their caregivers (Class I-C, ACC/AHA guidelines on GUCH 2008). The recurrence risk of congenital defects is up to 11%, and genetic counselling is necessary.[7]

References

1. Webb G, *et al.* Atrial septal defects in the adult: recent progress and overview. *Circulation.* 2006;**114**:1645–53.
2. Lindsey JB, *et al.* Clinical update: atrial septal defect in adults. *Lancet.* 2007;**369**:1244–6.
3. Warnes CA, *et al.* Task force 1: the changing profile of congenital heart disease in adult life. *J Am Coll Cardiol.* 2001;**37**:1170–5.
4. Brickner ME, *et al.* Congenital heart disease in adults. Second of two parts. *N Engl J Med.* 2000;**342**:334–42.
5. Sommer RJ, *et al.* Pathophysiology of congenital heart disease in the adult: part i: shunt lesions. *Circulation.* 2008;**117**:1090–9.
6. Warnes CA, *et al.* ACC/AHA 2008 guidelines for the management of adults with congenital heart disease: a report of the American College of Cardiology/American Heart Association Task Force on practice guidelines (writing committee to develop guidelines on the management of adults with congenital heart disease). Developed in collaboration with the American Society of Echocardiography, Heart Rhythm Society, International Society for Adult Congenital Heart Disease, Society for Cardiovascular Angiography and Interventions, and Society of Thoracic Surgeons. *J Am Coll Cardiol.* 2008;**52**:e143–263.
7. Baumgartner H, *et al.* ESC guidelines for the management of grown-up congenital heart disease (new version 2010). *Eur Heart J.* 2010;**31**:2915–57.

Chapter 4

Atrial septal defects

Ostium secundum ASD

Epidemiology

Secundum ASDs account for approximately 7% of all congenital malformations. Females predominate (70%). Secundum ASD is the most common cardiac manifestation of Holt–Oram syndrome (triphalangeal thumbs, ASD, or VSD) due to mutation of TBX5. Familial forms associated with gene mutations are rare and usually coexist with conduction disturbances.

Pathophysiology

The pathophysiology of ASD is complex and multifactorial.[1] Conventionally, an ASD must be at least 10 mm in diameter for a significant left-to-right shunt (although most ASDs are not circular). A left-to-right atrial shunt is considered significant when the Qp/Qs ratio is greater than 1.5 or if it causes dilation of the right heart chambers. The RV is more compliant than the LV and, as a result, left atrial blood is shunted to the right atrium, causing increased pulmonary blood flow and dilatation of the pulmonary arteries. However, as opposed to VSD, pulmonary hypertension is uncommon, even with large defects, although, when it develops, it results in pulmonary pressures that approach systemic levels. It has been suggested that the ASD may be an associated marker of pulmonary hypertension but not necessarily causative. Once a patient has reached adulthood with normal PA pressures he seldom develops pulmonary hypertension later. Left ventricular hypertrophy and mitral stenosis increase left-to-right shunting, whereas pulmonary stenosis, tricuspid stenosis, and pulmonary hypertension reduce a left-to-right shunt and may also cause a right-to-left shunt.

Presentation

Patients with small defects are asymptomatic. Patients with moderate/large ASDs often have no symptoms until the third of fifth decade of life despite substantial left-to-right shunting. The age at which symptoms appear is variable and not exclusively related to the size of the shunt. SOBOE is the most common initial presenting symptom. Atrial fibrillation or flutter due to atrial dilatation occurs at >40 years of age and is symptomatic. Eisenmenger syndrome occurs rarely in adults with ASD (<10%, predominantly in females).[2] Occasionally, a paradoxical embolus or transient ischaemic attack may be the first clue to the presence of an ASD. Rarely, cyanosis may be seen, especially with inferior sinus venosus defects. Patients with unexplained RV volume overload should be investigated to rule out obscure ASD, partial anomalous venous connection, or coronary sinoseptal defect (ACC/AHA guidelines on GUCH 2008, I-C).

Physical examination

- The absence of clinical signs does not necessarily exclude a haemodynamically important ASD.
- **Dilated pulmonary artery** may be palpable in the second left interspace.
- **Right ventricular lift** may be felt on held expiration or in the subxiphoid area on deep inspiration.
- **Soft systolic ejection murmur** is heard at the upper left sternal border (pulmonary flow).
- **Wide and fixed split of S_2**, the auscultatory hallmark of an ASD, is not always present.
- **Tricuspid diastolic rumble** heard at the lower left sternal border reflects a large shunt.
- **Loud P_2** and **tricuspid regurgitation** may be heard with pulmonary hypertension.

Investigations

- **ECG** SR, AF, or atrial flutter with right axis deviation and RV hypertrophy (incomplete RBBB). Inverted P waves in the inferior leads suggest an absent or deficient sinus node, as may be seen in a sinus venosus defect. First-degree heart block suggests a primum ASD but may be seen in older patients with a secundum ASD.
- **Chest radiography** May be normal, even with significant ASD. The central pulmonary arteries may also be characteristically enlarged, with pulmonary plethora and peripheral vascular pattern of shunt vascularity (well-visualized small pulmonary arteries in the periphery of both lungs).
- **Transthoracic echocardiography** The functional importance of the defect can be estimated by the size of the right atrium and ventricle, the presence/absence of paradoxical septal motion (right ventricular volume overload), ventricular septal orientation in diastole (volume overload) and systole (pressure overload), and an estimation of the shunt ratio. Pulmonary artery systolic pressures may be estimated from the Doppler velocity of tricuspid regurgitation.
- **Transoesophageal echocardiography** may be needed to confirm the type of ASD and to delineate the pulmonary venous return, and to guide device closure.

- **Cardiac magnetic resonance** is the gold standard for the assessment of right ventricular size and function and pulmonary venous return. In patients who cannot have an MRI, computed tomographic scanning and angiography can offer similar information.
- **Cardiac catheterization** Not necessary any more, unless to test vasoreactivity in pulmonary hypertension. Oximetry is now rarely used for shunt detection and Qp/Qs calculation. Coronary angiography is needed preoperatively in patients >40 years old.
- **Maximal exercise testing** may be useful to document exercise capacity in patients with symptoms that are discrepant with clinical findings or to document changes in oxygen saturation in patients with mild or moderate PAH (ACC/AHA 2008, IIa-C).

Therapy

Small defects (<1 cm) may be left alone, but some patients develop right heart dilation later in life due to increased LVEDP and left-to-right shunting. Efforts should be made to maintain SR (Table 4.1).

Closure indications

Indications for ostium secundum ASDs are presented in Tables 4.1 and 4.2.[3,4] Main indications for closure are:

- Qp/Qs >1.5
- RA/RV enlargement
- Paradoxical embolism.

Device closure of significant secundum ASDs is beneficial regardless of age.[5]

Closure contraindications

- Irreversible pulmonary arterial hypertension (see VSD). There have been case reports of such patients being managed with intravenous epoprostenol or oral bosentan in a way that ASD closure subsequently became possible.[6]
- Severe left ventricular dysfunction.

Table 4.1 ACC/AHA 2008 GL on GUCH. Management of ASD

Recommendations for medical therapy	
Cardioversion after appropriate anticoagulation to attempt restoration of SR if AF occurs.	I-A
Rate control and anticoagulation if SR cannot be maintained by medical or interventional means.	I-A
Recommendations for interventional and surgical therapy	
Percutaneous or surgical ASD closure for right atrial and RV enlargement with or without symptoms.	I-B
A sinus venosus, coronary sinus, or primum ASD should be repaired surgically rather than by percutaneous closure	I-B
Surgeons with training and expertise in CHD should perform operations for various ASD closures.	I-C
Surgical closure of secundum ASD when concomitant surgical repair/replacement of a tricuspid valve is considered or when the anatomy of the defect precludes the use of a percutaneous device.	IIa-C
Percutaneous or surgical ASD closure for paradoxical embolism.	IIa-C
Percutaneous or surgical ASD closure for documented platypnoea orthodeoxia.	IIa-B
Percutaneous or surgical ASD closure with net left-to-right shunting and PA pressure <2/3 systemic levels, PVR <2/3 SVR, or when responsive to either pulmonary vasodilator therapy or test occlusion.	IIb-C
Concomitant Maze procedure may be considered for atrial tachyarrhythmias.	IIb-C
Ireversible PAH and no evidence of a left-to-right shunt.	III-B
Recommendations for post-intervention follow-up	
Early post-operative symptoms of undue fever, fatigue, vomiting, chest pain, or abdominal pain may represent post-pericardiotomy syndrome with tamponade and should prompt immediate evaluation with echocardiography.	I-C
Annual clinical follow-up is recommended for patients post-operatively if their ASD was repaired as an adult and the following conditions persist or develop:	I-C
a. Pulmonary arterial hypertension.	
b. Atrial arrhythmias.	
c. RV or LV dysfunction.	
d. Coexisting valvular or other cardiac lesions.	
Evaluation for possible device migration, erosion, or other complications is recommended for patients 3 months to 1 year after device closure and periodically thereafter.	I-C
Device erosion, which may present with chest pain or syncope, should warrant urgent evaluation.	I-C

ACC/AHA 2008 guidelines for the management of adults with congenital heart disease. *J Am Coll Cardiol* 2008;**52**:e1–e121.

Table 4.2 ESC 2010 GL on GUCH

Indications for intervention in ASD	
ASD closure, regardless of symptoms in significant shunt (signs of RV volume overload) and PVR <5 WU.	I-B
Device closure for secundum ASD closure when applicable.	I-C
Intervention for ASDs, regardless of size in patients with suspicion of paradoxical embolism (exclusion of other causes).	IIa-C
Intervention for patients with PVR ≥5 WU, but <2/3 SVR or PAP <2/3 systemic pressure (baseline or when challenged with vasodilators, preferably nitric oxide, or after targeted PAH therapy), and evidence of net L–R shunt (Qp/Qs >1.5).	IIb-C
ASD closure in patients with Eisenmenger physiology.	III-C

ESC Guidelines for the management of grown-up congenital heart disease (new version 2010). *Eur Heart J.* 2010;**31**:2915–57.

Device closure is the treatment of choice for secundum ASDs.[3, 4] Unsuitable anatomy includes inadequate atrial septal rims to allow stable device deployment (<5 mm), proximity of the defect to the AV valves, the coronary sinus, or the vena cavae, and very large secundum ASD (>35 mm). Complications are device embolization (<1%) and cardiac perforation (<0.1%). Small residual shunts seen on transoesophageal echocardiography after the end of the procedure are of no clinical significance. Late complications, such as mitral valve dysfunction, obstruction of the pulmonary veins, and erosion or perforation of the atrial wall or aorta, are very rare. However, arrhythmia and neurologic events remain long-term risks after ASD closure (device or surgical), especially if the patient had pre-existing arrhythmia.[7] After closure, aspirin and clopidogrel are prescribed for 6 to 12 months. Device erosion, which may present with chest pain or syncope, should warrant urgent evaluation (Table 4.1).

Surgical closure is required for patients with secundum ASD, whose anatomy is unsuitable for device closure. Perioperative mortality is <1%. Surgical repair, particularly before the age of 25 years, has been shown to result in normal long-term survival and reduce the incidence of arrhythmias, such as atrial flutter and fibrillation and RV failure and stroke.[8] Patients over the age of 40 remain at risk of atrial arrhythmias and systemic thromboembolism despite complete closure of the ASD, but surgery is also preferable to medical treatment.[9, 10] Age and pre-procedure arrhythmia are risk factors for late arrhythmia.[7]

Endocarditis prophylaxis

It is not recommended for unrepaired ASDs. Revised indications are discussed in Chpater 1 and Chapter 79 on endocarditis.

Pregnancy

It is well tolerated in the absence of severe pulmonary arterial hypertension, with a small risk of paradoxical embolus and stroke, arrhythmia, and heart failure (see Chapter 1). Thus, in ASD diagnosed during pregnancy, closure can be deferred for 6 months after delivery. For a secundum defect, catheter device closure can be performed during pregnancy, if necessary, with transoesophageal or intracardiac echocardiographic guidance. The recurrence rate in offspring is estimated in 6–10%.[3]

Sinus venosus defect

Partial anomalous pulmonary venous return to the SVC or the right atrium is very common with **superior sinus venosus defect** (5–10% of all ASDs). Diagnosis is often more difficult than for other forms of ASD, and catheter closure is not possible. The **inferior sinus venosus defect** near the IVC is very rare. **Surgical closure** is required for patients with sinus venosus ASD. Indications for closure are presented in Table 4.1.[3, 4]

Patent foramen ovale

The prevalence of a patent foramen ovale (PFO) ranges from 15–25% in autopsy studies to 20–40% with transoesophageal echocardiography in patients with a history of cerebral events. The average PFO size ranges from 1 to 19 mm but increases with each decade of life; the mean diameter in the first decade is 3.4 mm and in the tenth decade 5.8 mm.[11] A common association is **atrial septal aneurysm** where part, or all, of the atrial septum shows aneurysmal dilatation, protruding into either atria (prevalence 1–5%) for, at least, 15 mm during the cardiorespiratory cycle. Under normal physiological conditions, the left atrial pressure is higher than the right one and pushes the thin septum primum against the septum secundum and, except for very brief periods in each cardiac cycle, seals the potential opening of the PFO. Actions, such as the release of a Valsalva manoeuvre, can transiently reverse the normal left-to-right pressure gradient and cause an exaggerated transient leftward shift of the free edge of the septum primum, with apparent enlargement of the orifice of the PFO. Transoesophageal echocardiography can diagnose PFO by injecting saline contrast, preferably in the femoral vein than the upper extremities, and detect microbubbles in the left atrium immediately after arriving in the right atrium. If bubbles appear in the left atrium before or >5 beats after they appear in the right atrium, then the possibility of an anomalous venous connection to the left atrium or pulmonary arteriovenous malformations must be considered.[11] PFO is a potential risk factor for several clinical syndromes, including paradoxic systemic embolism, such as ischaemic stroke, myocardial infarction, decompression sickness in divers, and possibly migraine or Alzheimer's disease.[11]

PFO and cryptogenic stroke

Approximately 25% to 50% of strokes are cryptogenic, and there is evidence for association between a PFO and cryptogenic stroke.[11–13] The size of the PFO and interatrial shunt, the presence of an atrial septal aneurysm and Chiari strands (congenital remnants of the right valve of the sinus venosus), as well as the Eustachian valve that virtually extends the vena cava to the foramen ovale, may all contribute to the relative risk for stroke. Cryptogenic stroke due to tiny emboli (a few millimeters in size) can form anywhere in the venous system and occur with increasing frequency after 50 years of age. Paradoxical embolism does not necessarily require clinically apparent deep vein thrombosis since thrombi may emerge from the inferior vena cava. Still, however, a definitive causal relationship between PFO and cryptogenic stroke has not been convincingly established for the majority of affected patients, and concurrent aetiologies are identified for more than one-third of recurrent ischaemic events in patients with cryptogenic stroke.[14, 15] The annual risk of recurrent cryptogenic stroke, with or without PFO, is estimated to be 6–8% without any treatment. With either medical treatment or PFO closure, the annual risk decreases to approximately 2–4%.[11] Atrial septal aneurysm is found in 7–15% of stroke patients, and the association also remains debatable.

PFO and migraine

There is accumulating evidence that migraine headaches improve in selected patients who are subjected to PFO closure. However, the only randomized trial to test this hypothesis has failed to confirm it, and other studies have found no association between migraine headaches and the presence of PFO (MIST).[16] Thus, closure of a PFO for migraine is not yet considered standard medical practice.

Indications for PFO closure

The optimal therapy for prevention of recurrent stroke or transient ischaemic attack in patients with cryptogenic stroke and patent foramen ovale remains controversial (Table 4.3). Treatment choices include medical therapy with antiplatelet agents or vitamin K antagonists or percutaneous device closure. Percutaneous device closure is now easy, and the simplest technique is with the Amplatzer occluder. Complications include cardiac perforation or air embolization during implantation, induced atrial fibrillation, non-specific malaise attributed to nickel allergy, and puncture site problems. However, existing data do not support a recommendation for PFO closure in patients with cryptogenic stroke or TIA and PFO. CLOSURE I, the first randomized trial, has failed to detect any benefit by PFO closure in these patients.[17] A recent observational study demonstrated a significant reduction of a composite outcome of TIA, stroke, and peripheral embolism,[18] and a meta-analysis indicated potential benefits, especially in the elderly, patients with atrial septal aneurysm, and patients with thrombophilia, following paradoxical embolism.[19] It is not known whether failures of the CLOSURE I and MIST trials can be attributed to failures of some of the devices used.[20] Recently, results of two RCTs were reported. In the RESPECT trial of 980 patients with prior cryptogenic stroke, the intent-to-treat analysis did not achieve statistical significance (risk reduction 51%, $p = 0.08$), but the per-protocol (risk reduction 63%, $p = 0.03$) and as-treated (risk reduction 73%, $p = 0.007$) analyses did reach significance.[21] In the PC trial, closing the PFO did not significantly reduce the primary composite endpoint of death from any cause, non-fatal stroke, transient ischaemic attack (TIA), and peripheral embolism (risk reduction 37%, $p = 0.34$) in 414 patients with prior cryptogenic stroke compared with standard medical therapy.[22]

Currently, the labelled indication for PFO device closure is recurrent stroke in patients who had an event despite treatment, or are not candidates for anticoagulation.[23, 24] Closure is also recommended in the platypnoea orthodeoxia syndrome [dyspnoea (platypnoea) and arterial desaturation in the upright position with improvement in the supine position (orthodeoxia)] and, probably, in divers for prevention of decompression illness.[1] The potential role of PFO in fat embolism following long bone fracture is also investigated; the potential value of preoperative closure in these patients remains to be determined.[25]

Table 4.3 AHA/ASA 2011 GL. Recommendations for patients with PFO

Antiplatelet therapy for patients with an ischemic stroke or TIA and a PFO.	IIa-B
Insufficient data to establish whether anticoagulation is equivalent or superior to aspirin for secondary stroke prevention in patients with PFO.	IIb-B
Insufficient data to make a recommendation regarding PFO closure in patients with stroke and PFO.	IIb-C

Guidelines for the Prevention of Stroke in Patients With Stroke or Transient Ischemic Attack: a guideline for healthcare professionals from the American Heart Association/American Stroke Association. *Stroke*. 2011;**42**:227–276.

References

1. Sommer RJ, *et al.* Pathophysiology of congenital heart disease in the adult: part i: shunt lesions. *Circulation*. 2008;**117**: 1090–9.
2. Brickner ME, *et al.* Congenital heart disease in adults. Second of two parts. *N Engl J Med*. 2000;**342**:334–42.
3. Baumgartner H, *et al.* ESC guidelines for the management of grown-up congenital heart disease (new version 2010). *Eur Heart J*. 2010;**31**:2915–57.
4. Warnes CA, *et al.* ACC/AHA 2008 guidelines for the management of adults with congenital heart disease: a report of the American College of Cardiology/American Heart Association

Task Force on practice guidelines (writing committee to develop guidelines on the management of adults with congenital heart disease). Developed in collaboration with the American Society of Echocardiography, Heart Rhythm Society, International Society for Adult Congenital Heart Disease, Society for Cardiovascular Angiography and Interventions, and Society of Thoracic Surgeons. *J Am Coll Cardiol.* 2008;**52**:e143–263.
5. Humenberger M, *et al.* Benefit of atrial septal defect closure in adults: impact of age. *Eur Heart J.* 2011;**32**:553–60.
6. Webb G, *et al.* Atrial septal defects in the adult: recent progress and overview. *Circulation.* 2006;**114**:1645–53.
7. Kutty S, *et al.* Long-term (5- to 20-year) outcomes after transcatheter or surgical treatment of hemodynamically significant isolated secundum atrial septal defect. *Am J Cardiol.* 2012;**109**:1348–52.
8. Murphy JG, *et al.* Long-term outcome after surgical repair of isolated atrial septal defect. Follow-up at 27 to 32 years. *N Engl J Med.* 1990;**323**:1645–50.
9. Attie F, *et al.* Surgical treatment for secundum atrial septal defects in patients >40 years old. A randomized clinical trial. *J Am Coll Cardiol.* 2001;**38**:2035–42.
10. Konstantinides S, *et al.* A comparison of surgical and medical therapy for atrial septal defect in adults. *N Engl J Med.* 1995;**333**:469–73.
11. Kutty S, *et al.* Patent foramen ovale: the known and the to be known. *J Am Coll Cardiol.* 2012;**59**:1665–71.
12. Handke M, *et al.* Patent foramen ovale and cryptogenic stroke in older patients. *N Engl J Med.* 2007;**357**:2262–68.
13. Maron BA, *et al.* Paradoxical embolism. *Circulation.* 2010;**122**:1968–72.
14. Messe SR, *et al.* Practice parameter: recurrent stroke with patent foramen ovale and atrial septal aneurysm: report of the quality standards subcommittee of the American Academy of Neurology. *Neurology.* 2004;**62**:1042–50.
15. Mono ML, *et al.* Patent foramen ovale may be causal for the first stroke but unrelated to subsequent ischemic events. *Stroke.* 2011;**42**:2891–5.
16. Dowson A, *et al.* Migraine intervention with starflex technology (MIST) trial: a prospective, multicenter, double-blind, sham-controlled trial to evaluate the effectiveness of patent foramen ovale closure with starflex septal repair implant to resolve refractory migraine headache. *Circulation.* 2008;**117**:1397–404.
17. Furlan AJ, *et al.* Closure or medical therapy for cryptogenic stroke with patent foramen ovale. *N Engl J Med.* 2012;**366**:991–9.
18. Wahl A, *et al.* Long-term propensity score-matched comparison of percutaneous closure of patent foramen ovale with medical treatment after paradoxical embolism. *Circulation.* 2012;**125**:803–12.
19. Agarwal S, *et al.* Meta-analysis of transcatheter closure versus medical therapy for patent foramen ovale in prevention of recurrent neurological events after presumed paradoxical embolism. *JACC Cardiovasc Interv.* 2012;**5**:777–89.
20. Tobis J, *et al.* Percutaneous treatment of patent foramen ovale and atrial septal defects. *J Am Coll Cardiol.* 2012;**60**:1722–32.
21. Carroll JD, *et al.*, for the RESPECT Investigators. Closure of patent foramen ovale versus medical therapy after cryptogenic stroke. *N Engl J Med.* 2013;**368**:1092–1100.
22. Meier B, *et al.*, for the PC Trial Investigators. Percutaneous closure of patent foramen ovale in cryptogenic embolism. *N Engl J Med.* 2013;**368**:1083–91.
23. Guidelines for management of ischaemic stroke and transient ischaemic attack 2008. *Cerebrovasc Dis.* 2008;**25**: 457–507.
24. Sacco RL, *et al.* Guidelines for prevention of stroke in patients with ischemic stroke or transient ischemic attack: a statement for healthcare professionals from the American Heart Association/American Stroke Association Council on Stroke: co-sponsored by the Council on Cardiovascular Radiology and Intervention: the American Academy of Neurology affirms the value of this guideline. *Circulation.* 2006;**113**:e409–49.
25. Forteza AM, *et al.* Transcranial doppler detection of cerebral fat emboli and relation to paradoxical embolism: a pilot study. *Circulation.* 2011;**123**:1947–52.

Chapter 5

Patent ductus arteriosus

Definition

The patent ductus arteriosus (PDA) connects the proximal descending aorta to the roof of the main pulmonary artery near the origin of the left pulmonary artery.[1] This fetal structure normally closes spontaneously within the first days after birth. It rarely closes after infancy.

Epidemiology

PDA accounts for approximately 10% of all congenital heart disease in the adult with a 2:1 female to male ratio.

Aetiology

PDA occurs in genetic syndromes with chromosomal aberrations (such as trisomy 21 and 4p syndrome), single-gene mutations (such as Carpenter's syndrome and Holt–Oram syndrome), and X-linked mutations (such as incontinentia pigmenti). Although most cases of PDA are seemingly sporadic, many may be due to multifactorial inheritance. In a family having one sibling with a PDA, there is a 3% chance of a PDA in a subsequent offspring. Rubella infection during the first trimester of pregnancy, children born in high altitude, and prematurity are associated with a high incidence of PDA.[1]

Pathophysiology and natural history

The shunt flow depends on the ductal resistance and the pressure gradient between the aorta and the pulmonary artery. Left-to-right shunting through the ductus arteriosus results in increased pulmonary fluid volume and left atrial and ventricular volume overload. If the ductus is large enough, the diastolic run-off may result in 'steal' phenomenon with impaired coronary perfusion. When pulmonary vascular resistance approaches and exceeds systemic vascular resistance, ductal shunting reverses and becomes right-to-left, with eventual development of Eisenmenger syndrome.[2] Patients with Eisenmenger syndrome are cyanotic and typically have differential cyanosis (cyanosis and clubbing of the toes, but not the fingers, because the right-to-left ductal shunting is distal to the subclavian arteries). Cyanosis may be more profound when systemic vascular resistance is elevated, such as in hot weather or after exercise. Infective endarteritis and aneurysm of ductus arteriosus are the most common complications. Rarely, the ductus arteriosus aneurysm may rupture or present with symptoms of a thoracic mass, including hoarseness due to left vocal cord paralysis from recurrent left laryngeal nerve impingement and left bronchial obstruction. In previous series, one-third of patients with unrepaired PDA died of heart failure, pulmonary hypertension, or endarteritis by the age of 40 years, and two-thirds died by the age of 60 years.[3]

Presentation

The clinical significance of the PDA depends on its size. Patients may be completely asymptomatic with a heart murmur or present due to exercise intolerance, endovascular infection, or atrial fibrillation. Although most patients compensate well, even with a moderate left-to-right shunt, and remain asymptomatic during childhood, they may develop congestive heart failure or Eisenmenger syndrome in adulthood.

Physical examination

Patients with **very small** patent ductus have no abnormal physical findings. A continuous murmur may be heard.

In **moderate** or **large** ductus:

- **Machinery murmur** Continuous murmur in upper left sternal border below the left clavicle. It is louder in systole and may radiate into the back, and a thrill may be present. **S_2** may be inaudible.
- **LV apex** prominent and collapsing **peripheral pulses.**
- **Pulmonary ejection click** and **pulmonary regurgitation** appear as pulmonary hypertension (PAH) develops.

Investigations

- **Chest radiograph** may be normal or display cardiomegaly (LA and LV enlargement) with increased pulmonary vascular markings. The main pulmonary artery is enlarged, and, in older adults with pulmonary hypertension, calcification of the ductus may be evident.
- **ECG** Normal or AF, LV hypertrophy, and LA enlargement in patients with moderate or large ductus shunts.
- **Echocardiography** Colour Doppler is used for detecting the presence of a PDA and estimating the degree of ductal shunting (Table 5.1). In patients with high pulmonary vascular resistance and PDA with low velocity or right-to-left flow, the ductus arteriosus may be very difficult to demonstrate. Findings, such as septal flattening, unexplained right ventricular hypertrophy, and high-velocity pulmonary regurgitation, should prompt a thorough investigation for a PDA. **Contrast echocardiography** may be helpful.
- **Cardiac magnetic resonance** useful in patients with unusual PDA geometry and associated abnormalities of the aortic arch. **Computed tomography** can assess the degree of calcification which may be important if surgical therapy is considered.
- **Cardiac catheterization** Diagnostic cardiac catheterization for uncomplicated PDA with adequate non-invasive imaging, is not indicated (ACC/AHA 2008 III-B). Detailed assessment of the ductal anatomy by angiography is essential for the selection of the proper device size for transcatheter closure. In patients with elevated pulmonary artery pressure, assessment of pulmonary vascular resistance and its response to vasodilating agents may be helpful in determining the possibility of ductus closure.

Therapy

PDA is associated with various complications of prematurity, and cyclo-oxygenase inhibitors, such as high-dose ibuprofen, are the first-line intervention for closure of the PDA.[4]

Indications for closure of PDA are presented in Tables 5.1 and 5.2. Routine closure of even small PDAs is now recommended by most experts. The rationale is that endarteritis of clinically silent PDA has been reported, and device closure is now effective and safe.[5,6] Patients with PDA and pulmonary vascular disease, who are considered unacceptable candidates for definitive closure, may be managed with pulmonary vasodilating agents, such as chronic oxygen, PGI_2, calcium channel blockers, endothelin antagonists, and phosphodiesterase inhibitors. One strategy in such patients is to accomplish partial closure of the ductus by

Table 5.1 ACC/AHA 2008 GL on GUCH

Recommendations for medical therapy	
Routine follow-up is recommended for patients with a small PDA without evidence of left-sided heart volume overload. Follow-up is recommended every 3 to 5 years for patients with a small PDA without evidence of left-heart volume overload.	I-C
Endocarditis prophylaxis is not recommended for those with a repaired PDA without residual shunt.	III-C
Recommendations for closure of patent ductus arteriosus	
Closure of a PDA, either percutaneously or surgically, for:	
a. Left atrial and/or LV enlargement or if PAH is present, or in the presence of net left-to-right shunting.	I-C
b. Prior endarteritis.	I-C
Careful evaluation and consultation with ACHD interventional cardiologists is recommended before surgical closure is selected as the method of repair for patients with a calcified PDA.	I-C
3. Surgical repair, by a surgeon experienced in CHD surgery, is recommended when:	
a. The PDA is too large for device closure.	I-C
b. Distorted ductal anatomy precludes device closure (e.g. aneurysm or endarteritis).	I-B
Closure of asymptomatic small PDA by catheter device.	IIa-C
PDA closure in PAH with a net left-to-right shunt.	IIa-C
PDA closure in PAH and net right-to-left shunt.	III-C

ACC/AHA 2008 guidelines for the management of adults with congenital heart disease. *J Am Coll Cardiol* 2008;**52**:e1–e121.

Table 5.2 ESC 2010 GL on GUCH

Indications for intervention in PDA	
PDA closure in patients with signs of LV volume overload.	I-C
PDA closure in patients with pulmonary arterial hypertension (PAH) but PAP <2/3 of systemic pressure or PVR <2/3 of SVR.	I-C
Device closure is the method of choice where technically suitable.	I-C
PDA closure in patients with PAH and PAP >2/3 of systemic pressure or PVR >2/3 of SVR but still net L–R shunt (Qp/Qs >1.5) or when testing (preferably with nitric oxide) or treatment demonstrates pulmonary vascular reactivity.	IIa-C
Device closure of small PDAs with continuous murmur (normal LV and PA pressure).	IIa-C
PDA closure should be avoided in silent duct (very small, no murmur).	III-C
PDA closure in PDA Eisenmenger and patients with exercise-induced lower limb desaturation.	III-C

ESC Guidelines for the management of grown-up congenital heart disease (new version 2010). *Eur Heart J.* 2010;**31**:2915–57.

surgery or transcatheter techniques to make it 'restrictive', but not completely closed, followed by long-term therapy with pulmonary vasodilating agents. If, in follow-up, the pulmonary vascular resistance decreases, then complete closure may be considered.[1] Routine follow-up is recommended for patients with a small PDA without evidence of left-sided heart volume overload. Follow-up is recommended every 3 to 5 years for patients with a small PDA without evidence of left heart volume overload. (ACC/AHA guidelines on GUCH 2008, I-C).

Transcatheter closure has become the treatment of choice in children and adults, especially in cases of calcified ductus arteriosus with increased pulmonary vascular resistance. The most commonly used occluders are the Nit-Occlud coil occlusion system and the Amplatzer duct occluder. Complications of transcatheter closure, such as device embolization of the patent ductus, are rare. Other rare complications are flow disturbance in the proximal left pulmonary artery or descending aorta from a protruding device, haemolysis from high-velocity residual shunting, and infection.

Surgical repair remains the treatment of choice for the rare very large ductus.

Infective endocarditis prophylaxis is not recommended any more for unrepaired PDAs. For closed PDAs, prophylaxis is recommended for 6 months after the procedure (see also Chapter 1).[7,8]

References

1. Schneider DJ, *et al.* Patent ductus arteriosus. *Circulation.* 2006;**114**:1873–82
2. Sommer RJ, *et al.* Pathophysiology of congenital heart disease in the adult: part i: shunt lesions. *Circulation.* 2008;**117**: 1090–9
3. Brickner ME, *et al.* Congenital heart disease in adults. First of two parts. *N Engl J Med.* 2000;**342**:256–63
4. Meissner U, *et al.* Improved closure of patent ductus arteriosus with high doses of ibuprofen. *Pediatr Cardiol.* 2012;**33**:586–90
5. Harrison DA, *et al.* Percutaneous catheter closure of the persistently patent ductus arteriosus in the adult. *Am J Cardiol.* 1996;**77**:1094–7
6. Hosking MC, *et al.* Transcatheter occlusion of the persistently patent ductus arteriosus. Forty-month follow-up and prevalence of residual shunting. *Circulation.* 1991;**84**: 2313–17
7. Baumgartner H, *et al.* ESC guidelines for the management of grown-up congenital heart disease (new version 2010). *Eur Heart J.* 2010;**31**:2915–57
8. Warnes CA, *et al.* ACC/AHA 2008 guidelines for the management of adults with congenital heart disease: a report of the American College of Cardiology/American Heart Association Task Force on practice guidelines (writing committee to develop guidelines on the management of adults with congenital heart disease). Developed in collaboration with the American Society of Echocardiography, Heart Rhythm Society, International Society for Adult Congenital Heart Disease, Society for Cardiovascular Angiography and Interventions, and Society of Thoracic Surgeons. *J Am Coll Cardiol.* 2008;**52**:e143–263

Chapter 6

Right ventricular outflow tract obstruction

Definitions and classification of RVOT obstruction

Obstruction to the right ventricular outflow tract (RVOT) in the adult patient can be either congenital or acquired. Congenital obstruction can be at the pulmonary valve, below the pulmonary valve, or above the valve. Below the pulmonary valve, obstruction can be either at the infundibular (as happens in Fallot) or the subinfundibular level. Congenital pulmonary stenosis constitutes 10% of the cases of congenital heart disease in adults.[1]

Valvular pulmonary stenosis

Obstruction of the RV outflow tract is valvular in 90% of patients. Valvar pulmonary stenosis may be an isolated abnormality or in association with a VSD or Noonan's syndrome (dysplastic pulmonary valve, facial dysmorphism, cardiac defects, and variable cognitive deficits). The leaflets are thin and pliant. In 10–15% of patients, the valve is dysplastic and the leaflets thickened and immobile, composed of myxomatous tissue.[1,2]

Presentation

Adults may be asymptomatic. With severe stenosis, exercise intolerance, SOBOE, anginal pain, and syncope may occur. Gradients >30 mmHg may deteriorate with ageing and result in RV hypertrophy and eventually right heart failure (elevated JVP, hepatic congestion, ascites, and peripheral oedema).

Physical examination

- **RV heave and thrill** may be present in moderate/severe PS
- **S_2 widely split** but moves normally with respiration
- **Pulmonary ejection click**
- **Crescendo-decrescendo murmur** increased by inspiration.

Investigations

ECG may show right axis deviation and RV hypertrophy.
Chest radiography may show post-stenotic dilatation of the main PA and diminished vascular markings.
Echocardiography reveals RV hypertrophy and paradoxical septal motion. Doppler mean gradients are considered (Table 6.1).[3]

Table 6.1 Severity of PS

PV	Area	Peak gradient	RV SP
Mild	>1 cm^2	<50 mmHg	<75 mmHg
Moderate	0.5–2 cm^2	50–80 mmHg	75–100 mmHg
Severe	<0.5 cm^2	>80 mmHg	>100 mmHg

Brickner ME, *et al*. Congenital heart disease in adults. First of two parts. *N Engl J Med*. 2000;**342**:256–63.

Cardiac catheterization is not necessary for diagnosis. It may be used for accurate gradient assessment in patients with echo peak gradients >36 mmHg for consideration of balloon valvotomy (Class I-C, ACC/AHA 2008 on valve disease).

Therapy

Asymptomatic patients with mild stenosis do not need intervention (Tables 6.2 and 6.3) (see also Chapter 15 on valve disease).[4,5] Balloon valvotomy is the treatment of choice for symptomatic patients with less than moderate PR and peak gradient >50 mmHg (mean >30 mmHg) or asymptomatic patients with peak gradient >60 mmHg (mean >40 mmHg). Surgical valvotomy or replacement with a bioprosthetic valve is reserved for patients with significant pulmonary regurgitation (PR) (an ominous prognostic sign for subsequent RV dilation and failure) or dysplastic valves unsuitable for balloon valvuloplasty. Rare complications of balloon valvotomy are PR, pulmonary oedema, cardiac perforation, AV block, and transient reactive RVOT obstruction.

Subvalvular pulmonary stenosis

Usually occurs in association with tetralogy of Fallot (before or after surgery) or double-chambered RV.[2] In double-chambered RV, a muscular band divides the RV into a high-pressure proximal inflow portion and a low-pressure distal outflow chamber. VSD or membranous subaortic stenosis may also be present. When the obstruction is mild, these patients may present with exercise intolerance and a harsh systolic murmur as young adults. With more severe obstruction and hypertrophy, ventricular arrhythmia, syncope, and sudden cardiac death may be the first presenting sign. Surgical muscle resection, with or without patching of the outflow tract, is indicated in symptomatic patients with peak Doppler gradient >60 mmHg (mean 40 mmHg).[5]

Table 6.2 ACC/AHA 2008 GL on GUCH*

Recommendations for intervention in patients with valvular pulmonary stenosis	
Balloon valvotomy for asymptomatic patients with a domed pulmonary valve and a peak instantaneous Doppler gradient >60 mmHg or a mean Doppler gradient >40 mmHg (in association with less than moderate PR).	I-B
Balloon valvotomy for symptomatic patients with a domed pulmonary valve and a peak instantaneous Doppler gradient >50 mmHg or a mean Doppler gradient >30 mmHg (in association with less than moderate PR).	I-C
Surgical therapy in severe PS and an associated hypoplastic pulmonary annulus, severe pulmonary regurgitation, subvalvular PS, or supravalvular PS. Surgery is also preferred for most dysplastic pulmonary valves and when there is associated severe TR or the need for a surgical Maze procedure.	I-C
Surgeons with training and expertise in CHD should perform operations for the RVOT and pulmonary valve.	I-B
Balloon valvotomy in asymptomatic patients with a dysplastic pulmonary valve and a peak instantaneous gradient by Doppler >60 mmHg or a mean Doppler gradient >40 mmHg.	IIb-C
Balloon valvotomy in selected symptomatic patients with a dysplastic pulmonary valve and peak instantaneous gradient by Doppler >50 mmHg or a mean Doppler gradient >30 mmHg.	IIb-C
Balloon valvotomy for asymptomatic patients with a peak instantaneous gradient by Doppler <30 mmHg or <50 mmHg and normal cardiac output.	III-C
Balloon valvotomy is not recommended for symptomatic patients with PS and severe PR.	III-C

* The ACC/AHA 2008 Guidelines on valve disease recommend balloon valvotomy in adolescent and young adult patients with pulmonic stenosis who have, at catheterization, an RV-to-pulmonary artery peak-to-peak gradient >40 mmHg or >30 mmHg in the presence of exertional dyspnoea, angina, syncope, or presyncope (I-C).
ACC/AHA 2008 guidelines for the management of adults with congenital heart disease. *J Am Coll Cardiol.* 2008;**52**:e1–e121.

Supravalvar pulmonary stenosis

Supravalvar pulmonary stenosis can occur as an isolated abnormality or in association with complex cardiac malformations, such as Williams syndrome (infantile hypercalcaemia, elfin facies, and mental retardation), tetralogy of Fallot, Noonan's syndrome, and rubella or toxoplasmosis infection during the first trimester of pregnancy.[1] It may also be the result of surgical scarring from operations, such as pulmonary artery banding or arterial switch. Patients with exercise intolerance or significant gradients are referred for surgery. Stent-based valve implants are experimental.

Branch pulmonary artery stenosis

They may be isolated or multiple, as happens in Williams and Noonan's syndromes, congenital rubella, and Alagille (intrahepatic cholestasis) and Keutel (cartilage calcification and brachytelephalangia) syndromes.[1] Although uncommon, the diagnosis of branch PA stenosis should always be considered in patients with a history of congenital heart disease who present with symptoms of pulmonary embolism, such as dyspnoea, fatigability, and segmental lung ventilation-perfusion mismatches. Balloon and stent angioplasty are used in isolated stenoses with >50% diameter stenosis and RVSP >50 mmHg (Table 6.4).[5]

Double-chambered RV and **RV to PA conduits** may also result in RVOT obstruction (Tables 6.5 to 6.7).

Table 6.3 ESC 2010 GL on GUCH

Indications for intervention in RVOT obstruction	
Repair of RVOTO at any level, regardless of symptoms, when Doppler peak gradient is >64 mmHg (peak velocity >4m/s), provided that RV function is normal and no valve substitute is required.	I-C
In valvular PS, balloon valvotomy should be the intervention of choice.	I-C
In asymptomatic patients in whom balloon valvotomy is ineffective and surgical valve replacement is the only option, surgery should be performed in the presence of a systolic RVP >80 mmHg (TR velocity >4.3 m/s).	I-C
Intervention in patients with gradient <64 mmHg in the presence of:	IIa-C
• Symptoms related to PS, or	
• Decreased RV function, or	
• Double-chambered RV (which is usually progressive), or	
• Important arrhythmias, or	
• Right-to-left shunting via an ASD or VSD.	
Repair in peripheral PS, regardless of symptoms, if >50% diameter narrowing and RV systolic pressure >50 mmHg and/or lung perfusion abnormalities are present.	IIa-C

ESC Guidelines for the management of grown-up congenital heart disease (new version 2010). *Eur Heart J.* 2010;**31**:2915–57.

Table 6.4 ACC/AHA 2008 GL on GUCH

Recommendations for interventional therapy in the management of branch and peripheral pulmonary stenosis	
Percutaneous interventional therapy for the management of appropriate focal branch and/or peripheral pulmonary artery stenosis with >50% diameter narrowing, elevated RV systolic pressure >50 mmHg, and/or symptoms.	I-B
Surgeons with training and expertise in CHD should perform operations for management of branch pulmonary artery stenosis not anatomically amenable to percutaneous interventional therapy.	I-B

ACC/AHA 2008 guidelines for the management of adults with congenital heart disease. *J Am Coll Cardiol.* 2008;**52**:e1–e121.

Table 6.5 ACC/AHA 2008 GL on GUCH

Recommendations for reintervention in patients with right ventricular-pulmonary artery conduit or bioprosthetic pulmonary valve stenosis	
Surgeons with training and expertise in CHD should perform operations for patients with severe pulmonary prosthetic valve stenosis (peak gradient >50 mmHg) or conduit regurgitation and any of the following:	I-C
a. Decreased exercise capacity.	
b. Depressed RV function.	
c. At least moderately enlarged RV end-diastolic size.	
d. At least moderate TR.	
Surgical or percutaneous therapy in symptomatic patients with discrete with discrete RV-pulmonary artery conduit obstructive lesions with >50% diameter narrowing or when a bioprosthetic pulmonary valve has a peak gradient by Doppler > 50mmHg or a mean gradient >30 mmHg.	IIa-C
Surgical or percutaneous therapy in asymptomatic patients when a pulmonary bioprosthetic valve has a peak Doppler gradient >50 mmHg.	IIa-C
Surgical intervention preferable to percutaneous catheter intervention when an associated Maze procedure is being considered.	IIb-C

ACC/AHA 2008 guidelines for the management of adults with congenital heart disease. *J Am Coll Cardiol.* 2008;**52**:e1–e121.

Table 6.6 ACC/AHA 2008 GL on GUCH

Recommendations for intervention in patients with double-chambered right ventricle	
Surgery for patients with a peak mid-ventricular gradient by Doppler >60 mmHg or a mean Doppler gradient >40 mmHg, regardless of symptoms.	I-B
Symptomatic patients with a peak mid-ventricular gradient by Doppler >50 mmHg or a mean Doppler gradient > 30mmHg may be considered for surgical resection if no other cause of symptoms can be discerned.	IIb-C

ACC/AHA 2008 guidelines for the management of adults with congenital heart disease. *J Am Coll Cardiol.* 2008;**52**:e1–e121.

Table 6.7 ESC 2010 GL on GUCH

Indications for intervention in patients with right ventricular to pulmonary artery conduits	
Surgery for symptomatic patients with RV systolic pressure >60 mmHg (TR velocity >3.5 m/s; may be lower in case of reduced flow) and/or moderate/severe PR	I-C
Surgery for asymptomatic patients with severe RVOTO and/or severe when at least one of the following criteria is present:	IIa-C
• Decrease in exercise capacity (CPET).	
• Progressive RV dilation.	
• Progressive RV systolic dysfunction.	
• Progressive TR (at least moderate).	
• RV systolic pressure >80 mmHg (TR velocity >4.3 m/s).	
• Sustained atrial/ventricular arrhythmias.	

ESC Guidelines for the management of grown-up congenital heart disease (new version 2010). *Eur Heart J.* 2010;**31**:2915–57.

References

1. Brickner ME, *et al.* Congenital heart disease in adults. First of two parts. *N Engl J Med.* 2000;**342**:256–63
2. Rhodes JF, *et al.* Pathophysiology of congenital heart disease in the adult, part ii. Simple obstructive lesions. *Circulation.* 2008;**117**:1228–37
3. Silvilairat S, *et al.* Outpatient echocardiographic assessment of complex pulmonary outflow stenosis: Doppler mean gradient is superior to the maximum instantaneous gradient. *J Am Soc Echocardiogr.* 2005;**18**:1143–8
4. Baumgartner H, *et al.* ESC guidelines for the management of grown-up congenital heart disease (new version 2010). *Eur Heart J.* 2010;**31**:2915–57
5. Warnes CA, *et al.* ACC/AHA 2008 guidelines for the management of adults with congenital heart disease: a report of the American College of Cardiology/American Heart Association Task Force on practice guidelines (writing committee to develop guidelines on the management of adults with congenital heart disease). Developed in collaboration with the American Society of Echocardiography, Heart Rhythm Society, International Society for Adult Congenital Heart Disease, Society for Cardiovascular Angiography and Interventions, and Society of Thoracic Surgeons. *J Am Coll Cardiol.* 2008;**52**:e143–263

Chapter 7

Left ventricular outflow tract obstruction

Definitions and classification of LVOT obstruction

Left ventricular outflow tract (LVOT) obstruction syndromes include subvalvar AS, valvular AS, and supravalvular AS.[1] Aortic coarctation is also considered a form of LVOT obstruction.[2] Obstruction can occur singly or at multiple levels, as an isolated lesion, or in combination with septal defects or conotruncal anomalies. LVOTOs are congenital in the vast majority of individuals younger than 50 years, although some variants of subaortic obstruction do exist. For recommendations for the evaluation and management of these patients, see also Chapter 15 on valve disease.

Valvular aortic stenosis (bicuspid aortic valve)

Epidemiology

Bicuspid aortic valve (BAV) is the most common congenital heart defect, with a prevalence estimated between 0.5% and 2%.[3] There is a male predominance of approximately 3:1. In patients with symptomatic AS, younger than 65 years of age, a bicuspid valve is the most common pathological finding.[4] Although BAV is more likely due to mutations in different genes with dissimilar patterns of inheritance, clinical studies have reported a 9% prevalence of BAV in first-degree relatives of patients and echocardiographic screening in first-degree relatives is recommended.[5,6] Associated abnormalities (20% of patients with bicuspid valves) are coarctation and PDA. Aortic root dilatation is also common. In addition, BAV is found in several genetic syndromes involving left-sided obstructive lesions, such as Shone's syndrome (multiple left-sided lesions of inflow and outflow obstruction, and parachute mitral valve), Williams syndrome with supravalvular stenosis, and Turner's syndrome with coarctation of the aorta.

Pathophysiology

The morphologic patterns of the bileaflet valve vary according to which commissures have fused, with the most common pattern involving fusion of the right and left cusps. Dilatation of the thoracic aorta is associated with a bicuspid valve and is attributed to structural abnormalities of the medial layer of the aortic (and the pulmonary) wall, such as decreased fibrillin, elastin fragmentation, and apoptosis, rather than to pure post-stenotic dilation. The bicuspid valve is not stenotic at birth, but it is subjected to haemodynamic stress that leads to thickening and calcification of the leaflets.

Presentation and natural history

Symptoms usually develop in adulthood due to haemodynamically induced calcification of the valve. By the age of 50 years, 25–49% of patients will require surgery or suffer a major cardiac event.[7,8] AS, AR, aortic aneurysm or dissection, and endocarditis may occur.

Physical examination

Ejection click followed by **murmur of AS** and possibly **AR.**

Investigations

Echocardiography The main task is to establish the diagnosis and exclude a tricuspid valve. The valve must be visualized in systole in the short-axis view since, during diastole, the raphe can make the valve appear trileaflet. In diastole, the orifice has a characteristic 'fish-mouthed' appearance. Evidence of aortic dilation should be always looked for in patients with a bicuspid valve. In asymptomatic adolescents and young adults with a mean Doppler gradient >30 mmHg or peak instantaneous gradient >50 mmHg, yearly echocardiographic assessment is recommended (Class I-B, ACC/AHA 2008). All patients with a bicuspid aortic valve should have both the aortic root and ascending thoracic aorta evaluated for evidence of aortic dilatation (Class I-B, ACC/AHA 2010 on aortic disease).[5]

Transoesophageal echocardiography or cardiac magnetic resonance may be needed in case of uncertainty.

Exercise stress testing is useful in patients with a mean Doppler gradient >30 mmHg or peak Doppler gradient >50 mmHg if the patient is interested in athletic participation or if clinical findings differ from non-invasive measurements (Class IIa-C, ACC/AHA 2008).

Dobutamine stress testing may be used in the evaluation of a mild aortic valve gradient in the face of low LV ejection fraction and reduced cardiac output.

First-degree relatives of patients with a bicuspid aortic valve should be evaluated for the presence of a bicuspid aortic valve and asymptomatic thoracic aortic disease (Class I-B, ACC/AHA 2008).

Therapy

Beta blockers in aortic root dilatation and ACE/ARB in hypertension are useful. Statins may also be used to slow the degenerative process (Table 7.1). Patients with moderate AS (mean gradient at least 25 mmHg or peak at least 40 mmHg) should be restricted from competitive sports.[9] Intervention is usually recommended in asymptomatic

Table 7.1 ACC/AHA 2008 GL on GUCH. Medical therapy and intervention in AS

Recommendations for medical therapy	
Treat systemic hypertension in patients with AS while monitoring diastolic blood pressure to avoid reducing coronary perfusion.	IIa-C
Beta blockers in patients with BAV and aortic root dilatation.	IIa-C
Long-term vasodilator therapy in patients with AR and systemic hypertension while carefully monitoring diastolic blood pressure to avoid reducing coronary perfusion.	IIa-C
Statins in patients with risk factors for atherosclerosis with statins for slowing down degenerative changes in the aortic valve and preventing atherosclerosis.	IIb-C
Vasodilator therapy is not indicated for long-term therapy in AR for the following:	
a. The asymptomatic patient with only mild to moderate AR and normal LV function.	III-B
b. The asymptomatic patient with LV systolic dysfunction who is a candidate for AVR.	III-B
c. The asymptomatic patient with either LV systolic function or mild to moderate LV diastolic dysfunction who is a candidate for AVR.	III-C
Recommendations for catheter interventions for adults with valvular aortic stenosis	
Aortic balloon valvotomy in young adults without calcified aortic valves and no AR in:	I-C
a. Angina, syncope, dyspnoea on exertion, and peak-to-peak gradients at catheterization >50 mmHg.	
b. ST or T wave abnormalities in the left precordial leads on ECG at rest or with exercise and a peak-to-peak catheter gradient >60 mmHg.	
Aortic balloon valvotomy in asymptomatic adolescents or young adults with a peak-to-peak gradient on catheterization >50 mmHg when the patient is interested in playing competitive sports or becoming pregnant.	IIa-C
Aortic balloon valvotomy may as a bridge to surgery in haemodynamically unstable adults or at high risk for AVR, or when AVR cannot be performed due to co-morbidities.	IIb-C
In older adults, aortic balloon valvotomy is not recommended as an alternative to AVR (younger patients may be an exception).	III-B
Aortic balloon valvotomy in adolescents and young adults with a peak-to-peak gradient <40 mmHg without symptoms or ECG changes.	III-B
Recommendations for aortic valve repair/replacement and aortic root replacement (see also Chapter 19 on AR and Chapters 70 and 71 on aortic diseases)	
Aortic valvuloplasty, AVR, or Ross repair in patients with severe AS or chronic severe AR while they undergo cardiac surgery.	I-C
AVR for patients with severe AS and LV dysfunction (LVEF <50%).	I-C
AVR in adolescents or young adults with severe AR and:	
a. Development of symptoms.	I-C
b. Development of persistent LV dysfunction (LVEF <50%) or progressive LV dilatation (LV end-diastolic diameter—4 standard deviations above normal).	I-C
Surgery to repair or replace the ascending aorta in a patient with a BAV when the ascending aorta diameter is ≥5.0 cm or when there is progressive dilation at a rate ≥5 mm per year.	I-B
AVR for asymptomatic patients with severe AR and normal systolic function (LVEF >50%) but with severe LV dilatation (LV end-diastolic diameter >75 mm or end-systolic dimension >55 mm*).	IIa-B
Surgical aortic valve repair or replacement in patients with moderate AS undergoing other cardiac or aortic root surgery.	IIa-B
AVR for asymptomatic patients with any of the following indications:	IIb-C
a. Severe AS and abnormal response to exercise.	
b. Evidence of rapid progression of AS or AR.	
c. Mild AS while undergoing other cardiac surgery and evidence of a calcific aortic valve.	
d. Extremely severe AS (aortic valve area <0.6 cm and/or mean Doppler systolic AV gradient >60 mmHg).	
e. Moderate AR undergoing other cardiac surgery.	
f. Severe AR with rapidly progressive LV dilation, end-diastolic dimension 70 mm or end-systolic dimension 50 mm, with declining exercise tolerance or with abnormal haemodynamic response to exercise.	
Surgical repair in adults with AS or AR and concomitant ascending aortic dilatation (ascending aorta diameter >4.5 cm) coexisting with AS or AR.	IIb-B
Early surgical repair in adults with the following indications:	IIb-C
a. AS and a progressive increase in ascending aortic size.	
b. Mild AR if valve-sparing aortic root replacement is being considered.	
AVR for prevention of sudden death in asymptomatic adults with AS and without Class IIa/IIb indications for intervention.	III-B
AVR in asymptomatic patients with AR and normal LV size and function.	III-B

* Consider lower threshold values for patients of small stature of either gender.

ACC/AHA 2008 guidelines for the management of adults with congenital heart disease. *J Am Coll Cardiol.* 2008;**52**:e1–e121.

Table 7.2 ESC 2010 GL on GUCH

Indications for intervention in AS	
Valve replacement in severe AS and any valve-related symptoms (AP, dyspnoea, syncope).	I-B
Valve replacement for asymptomatic patients with severe AS when they develop symptoms during exercise testing.	I-C
Valve replacement regardless of symptoms, when systolic LV dysfunction is present in severe AS (LVEF <50%), unless it is due to other causes.	I-C
Valve replacement regardless of symptoms, when patients with severe AS undergo surgery of the ascending aorta or of another valve, or CABG.	I-C
Valve replacement regardless of symptoms, if the ascending aorta is >50 mm (27.5 mm/m^2 BSA) and no other indications for cardiac surgery are present.	IIa-C
Valve replacement in asymptomatic patients with severe AS when they present with a fall in blood pressure below baseline during exercise testing.	IIa-C
Valve replacement in asymptomatic patients with severe AS and moderate to severe calcification and a rate of peak velocity progression of ≥0.3 m/s/year	IIa-C
Additional valve replacement in patients with moderate AS undergoing CABG or surgery of the ascending aorta or another valve.	IIa-C
Valve replacement for severe AS with low gradient (<40 mmHg) and LV dysfunction with contractile reserve.	IIa-C
Valve replacement in severe AS with low gradient (<40 mmHg) and LV dysfunction without contractile reserve.	IIb-C
Valve replacement in asymptomatic patients with severe AS and excessive LV hypertrophy (≥15 mm), unless this is due to hypertension.	IIb-C

ESC Guidelines for the management of grown-up congenital heart disease (new version 2010). *Eur Heart J*. 2010;**31**:2915–57.

patients with peak-to-peak gradients >60 mmHg at catheterization or symptomatic patients with peak-to-peak catheter gradients >50 mmHg. Valvuloplasty is the treatment of choice in children and perhaps young adults with BAV. Following successful valvuloplasty, sudden death is extremely rare and exercise restriction is not recommended.[10] The aortic root size should be taken into account: aortic root size >5 cm indicates AVR and root replacement, and changes in root size >0.5 cm/year are an indication for root replacement (ACC/AHA 2008 GL on valve disease, I-C). If the patient is undergoing surgery for aortic valve disease, repair of the aortic root or replacement of the ascending aorta is indicated if the diameter of the aortic root or ascending aorta is greater than 4.5 cm (ACC/AHA 2008 GL on valve disease, I-C). The ACC/AHA and ESC recommendations for management are presented in Tables 7.1 and 7.2.[1,6] For recommendations on bicuspid aortic valve, see also Chapter 18 on AS and Chapter 19 on AR.

Subvalvular aortic stenosis

Subvalvular aortic stenosis comprises a spectrum of obstructive processes in the LV outflow tract that ranges from a discrete subaortic membranous obstruction to a fibromuscular tunnel-type obstruction to hypertrophic cardiomyopathy.[11] In patients with **membranous obstruction**, a thin fibrous membrane of variable thickness and with a central lumen stretches across the LV outflow tract from the septal surface to the anterior leaflet of the mitral valve. In adults, as opposed to children, progression of the obstruction and development of AR is slow over time. With the **tunnel-type obstruction**, a thick fibromuscular tubular narrowing diffusely reduces the diameter of the outflow tract. This condition has to be differentiated from hypertrophic cardiomyopathy. Aortic regurgitation is present in 30–80% of patients and thought to develop secondary to aortic valve damage caused by the high-velocity subvalvular jet.[12] Surgery is offered when symptoms, in the context of a peak gradient >50 mmHg or LV hypertrophy with reduced systolic function, develop (Tables 7.3 and 7.4). Survival is excellent after surgery for discrete subaortic stenosis, but over time the LVOT gradient slowly increases, mild AR is common, and reoperation for recurrent discrete subaortic stenosis may be needed.[13] Myectomy does not show additional advantages, and because it is associated with an increased risk of complete heart block, it should not be performed routinely.[13] Stress testing to determine exercise capability, symptoms, ECG changes or arrhythmias, or increase in LVOT gradient is reasonable in the presence of otherwise

Table 7.3 ACC/AHA 2008 GL on GUCH

Recommendations for surgical intervention in subaortic stenosis	
Surgical intervention in subAS and a peak instantaneous gradient of 50 mmHg or a mean gradient of 30 mmHg on echocardiography-Doppler.	I-C
Surgical intervention in subAS with <50 mmHg peak or <30 mmHg mean gradient and progressive AR and an LV end-systolic diameter of 50 mm or LVEF <55%.	I-C
Surgical resection in patients with a mean gradient of 30 mmHg, but careful follow-up is required to detect progression of stenosis or AR.	IIb-C
Surgical resection may be considered for patients with <50 mmHg peak gradient or <30 mmHg mean gradient in the following situations:	IIb-C
a. When LV hypertrophy is present.	
b. When pregnancy is being planned.	
c. When the patient plans to engage in strenuous/competitive sports.	
Surgical intervention to prevent AR for patients with subAS and trivial LVOT obstruction or trivial to mild AR.	III-C

ACC/AHA 2008 guidelines for the management of adults with congenital heart disease. *J Am Coll Cardiol*. 2008;**52**:e1–e121.

Table 7.4 ESC 2010 GL on GUCH

Indications for intervention in subaortic stenosis	
Surgery for symptomatic patients (spontaneous or on exercise test) with a mean Doppler gradient ≥50 mmHg or severe AR.	I-C
Surgery in asymptomatic patients when:	
• LVEF is <50% (gradient may be <50 mmHg due to low flow).	IIa-C
• AR is severe and LVESD >50mm (or 25 mm/mÇ BSA) and/or EF <50%.	IIa-C
• Mean Doppler gradient is ≥50 mmHg and LVH marked.	IIa-C
• Mean Doppler gradient is ≥50 mmHg* and blood pressure response is abnormal on exercise testing.	IIb-C
• Mean Doppler gradient is ≥50 mmHg, LV normal, exercise testing normal, and surgical risk low.	IIb-C
• Progression of AR is documented, and AR becomes more than mild (to prevent further progression).	IIb-C

* Doppler-derived gradients may overestimate the obstruction and may need confirmation by cardiac catheterization.

ESC Guidelines for the management of grown-up congenital heart disease (new version 2010). *Eur Heart J*. 2010;**31**:2915–57.

equivocal indications for intervention (Class IIa-C, ACC/AHA 2008). Lifelong cardiology follow-up is recommended in all patients with subaortic stenosis. Patients without operation should be subjected to yearly echocardiograms. Discrete subaortic stenosis progresses very slowly in adulthood, but patients with associated congenital lesions, particularly a VSD, are at risk for faster disease progression and should be monitored cautiously.[12] In patients with isolated thin discrete subaortic stenosis, transluminal balloon tearing of the membrane is another option with good long-term results.[14]

Supravalvular aortic stenosis

Rare condition usually associated with the Williams–Beuren syndrome (neurodevelopmental disorder characterized by connective tissue and central nervous system abnormalities).[11] Isolated supravalvar aortic stenosis occurs at the level of the sinotubular junction in 70% of patients with cardiovascular manifestations. The supravalvar lesion may involve the entire aortic root, the coronary arteries, and/or the aortic valve. In children, it is felt to be a progressive disease, perhaps related to an inadequate growth of the supravalvar aortic root and the sinotubular junction. However, progression of subvalvular AS in adulthood is rare.[15] Diffuse hypoplasia and PA stenosis, coarctation of the aorta, and septal defects are other associated conditions. TTE and/or TOE and either MRI or CT should be performed to assess the anatomy of the LVOT, aortic and mitral valve, the ascending aorta, and main and branch pulmonary artery anatomy. Adults with a history or presence of supraAS should be screened periodically for myocardial ischaemia (Class I- C, ACC/AHA 2008). Due to the potential of regression, surgery is recommended in the case of symptoms in the context of a peak gradient >70 mmHg or LV dysfunction (Tables 7.5 and 7.6).

Supravalvar AS, whether associated with Williams syndrome or non-syndromic, has a strong likelihood of being an inherited disorder. Undetected family members may be at risk for hypertension, coronary disease, or stroke; therefore, all available relatives should be screened (Class I- C,

Table 7.5 ACC/AHA 2008 GL on GUCH

Recommendations for interventional and surgical therapy in supravalvar aortic stenosis	
Operative intervention in supravalvular LVOT obstruction (discrete or diffuse) with symptoms (i.e. angina, dyspnoea, or syncope) and/or mean gradient >50 mmHg or peak instantaneous gradient by Doppler echocardiography >70 mmHg.	I-B
Surgical repair in lesser degrees of supravalvular LVOT obstruction and the following indications:	
a. Symptoms (i.e. angina, dyspnoea, or syncope).	I-B
b. LV hypertrophy.	I-C
c. Desire for greater degrees of exercise or a planned pregnancy.	I-C
d. LV systolic dysfunction.	I-C
Interventions for coronary artery obstruction in patients with supraAS should be performed in ACHD centres with demonstrated expertise.	I-C

ACC/AHA 2008 guidelines for the management of adults with congenital heart disease. *J Am Coll Cardiol*. 2008;**52**:e1–e121.

Table 7.6 ESC 2010 GL on GUCH

Indications for intervention in supravalvar aortic stenosis	
Surgery for patients with symptoms (spontaneous or on exercise test) and mean Doppler gradient ≥50 mmHg.	I-C
Surgery for patients with mean Doppler gradient <50 mmHg when they have:	
• Symptoms attributable to obstruction (exertional dyspnoea, angina, syncope), and/or	I-C
• LV systolic dysfunction (without other explanation),	I-C
• Severe LVH, attributable to obstruction (not related to hypertension),	I-C
• When surgery for significant coronary artery disease is required.	I-C
Repair in patients with mean Doppler gradient ≥50 mmHg* but without symptoms, LV systolic dysfunction, LVH, or abnormal exercise test when the surgical risk is low.	IIb-C

* Doppler-derived gradients may overestimate the obstruction and may need confirmation by cardiac catheterization.

ESC Guidelines for the management of grown-up congenital heart disease (new version 2010). *Eur Heart J*. 2010;**31**:2915–57.

ACC/AHA 2008). Patients with significant obstruction, coronary involvement, or aortic disease should be counselled against pregnancy (Class I- C, ACC/AHA 2008).

References

1. Baumgartner H, *et al.* ESC guidelines for the management of grown-up congenital heart disease (new version 2010). *Eur Heart J.* 2010;**31**:2915–57
2. Aboulhosn J, *et al.* Left ventricular outflow obstruction: subaortic stenosis, bicuspid aortic valve, supravalvar aortic stenosis, and coarctation of the aorta. *Circulation.* 2006;**114**:2412–22
3. Siu SC, *et al.* Bicuspid aortic valve disease. *J Am Coll Cardiol.* 2010;**55**:2789–800
4. Brickner ME, *et al.* Congenital heart disease in adults. First of two parts. *N Engl J Med.* 2000;**342**:256–63
5. Hiratzka LF, *et al.* 2010 CCF/AHA/AATS/ACR/ASA/SCA/SCAI/SIR/STS/SVM guidelines for the diagnosis and management of patients with thoracic aortic disease. a report of the American College of Cardiology Foundation/American Heart Association Task Force on practice guidelines, American Association for Thoracic Surgery, American College of Radiology, American Stroke Association, Society of Cardiovascular Anesthesiologists, Society for Cardiovascular Angiography and Interventions, Society of Interventional Radiology, Society of Thoracic Surgeons, and Society for Vascular Medicine. *J Am Coll Cardiol.* 2010;**55**:e27–129
6. Warnes CA, *et al.* ACC/AHA 2008 guidelines for the management of adults with congenital heart disease: a report of the American College of Cardiology/American Heart Association Task Force on practice guidelines (writing committee to develop guidelines on the management of adults with congenital heart disease). Developed in collaboration with the American Society of Echocardiography, Heart Rhythm Society, International Society for Adult Congenital Heart Disease, Society for Cardiovascular Angiography and Interventions, and Society of Thoracic Surgeons. *J Am Coll Cardiol.* 2008;**52**:e143–263
7. Michelena HI, *et al.* Natural history of asymptomatic patients with normally functioning or minimally dysfunctional bicuspid aortic valve in the community. *Circulation.* 2008;**117**:2776–84
8. Tzemos N, *et al.* Outcomes in adults with bicuspid aortic valves. *JAMA.* 2008;**300**:1317–25
9. Graham TP, Jr., *et al.* Task Force 2: congenital heart disease. *J Am Coll Cardiol.* 2005;**45**:1326–33
10. Brown DW, *et al.* Sudden unexpected death after balloon valvuloplasty for congenital aortic stenosis. *J Am Coll Cardiol.* 2010;**56**:1939–46
11. Rhodes JF, *et al.* Pathophysiology of congenital heart disease in the adult, part ii. Simple obstructive lesions. *Circulation.* 2008;**117**:1228–37
12. van der Linde D *et al.* Natural history of discrete subaortic stenosis in adults: A multicentre study. *Eur Heart J.* 2013;**34**:1548–1556
13. van der Linde D, *et al.* Surgical outcome of discrete subaortic stenosis in adults. A multicenter study. *Circulation.* 2013;**127**:1184–91
14. de Lezo JS, *et al.* Long-term outcome of patients with isolated thin discrete subaortic stenosis treated by balloon dilation: a 25-year study. *Circulation.* 2011;**124**:1461–68
15. Greutmann M, *et al.* Cardiac outcomes in adults with supravalvar aortic stenosis. *Eur Heart J.* 2012;**33**:2442–50

Chapter 8

Coarctation of the aorta

Definitions

Aortic arch obstruction may be due to:

- **Coarctation of the aorta (CoA)**, i.e. a discrete obstructive lesion located just distal to the origin of the left subclavian artery where the fetal ductus arteriosus inserted into the aorta
- **Tubular hypoplasia** of some part of the aorta
- **Aortic arch interruption.**

Epidemiology

CoA is found in about 5–8% of patients with congenital heart disease and is 2–5 times more common in males. Although most cases of CoA are sporadic, there is clearly a genetic component with congenital heart disease, occurring in, at least, 4% of offspring of women with CoA. Linkage analysis studies suggest a genetic susceptibility locus on chromosomes 2p23, 10q21, and 16p12. CoA is also present in 12–17% of patients with Turner's syndrome who are at high risk of aortic dissection.[1]

Pathophysiology and natural history

Obstruction of the aorta reduces flow to the juxtaglomerular apparatus in the kidneys, with resultant increase in vascular tone and intravascular volume. Thus, significant hypertension in the upper body occurs, and collateral circulation develops in the form of **intracranial** (circle of Willis) and **intercostal artery aneurysms.** In adults, a **bicuspid aortic valve** has been reported in 25–75% of patients with CoA.

In children, **VSD, PDA,** and **mitral valve abnormalities** are also common. The average survival of the adult with unrepaired coarctation is 35 years of age, with a 25% survival rate beyond 50 years of age.[2] Although the main cause of death in patients with corrected coarctation is coronary artery disease, coarctation itself does not predict for the development of coronary artery disease after adjustment for other risk factors, such as ageing, associated hypertension, hypercholesterolaemia, and diabetes mellitus.[3]

Presentation

In early age, CoA may lead to heart failure, but the adult is usually asymptomatic. Rarely, headache, epistaxis, dizziness, palpitations, and claudication are reported. Diagnosis is suspected when hypertension is associated with diminished or absent femoral pulses.

Physical examination

Patients with systemic arterial hypertension should have the brachial and femoral pulses palpated simultaneously to assess timing and amplitude evaluation to search for the 'brachial-femoral delay' of significant aortic coarctation. Supine bilateral arm (brachial artery) blood pressures and prone right or left supine leg (popliteal artery) blood pressures should be measured to search for **differential pressure.** There is differential systolic blood pressure (brachial-popliteal >10 mmHg) and radial-femoral pulse delay, unless significant AR coexists. The **diastolic** pressure is similar in arms and legs and, therefore, a widened pulse is felt in the arms.

Auscultation may reveal:

- **Interscapular systolic murmur**
- **Widespread crescendo-decrescendo systolic murmur** due to intercostal collaterals.

There may be also **'corkscrew' tortuosity** of retinal arteries.

Investigations

Chest radiography may be normal. Rib notching (unilateral or bilateral) in 50% of cases. The typical 'figure 3' configuration of the aorta may also be seen in the PA projection.
ECG may show LVH.
Echocardiography is useful, but **MRA** is the modality of choice, particularly for post-intervention surveillance. Every patient with coarctation (repaired or not) should have cardiovascular MRI or CT scan for complete evaluation of the thoracic aorta and intracranial vessels (Class I-B, ACC/AHA 2008).

Therapy

The natural history of unrepaired CoA includes the development of systemic hypertension. Most untreated patients will die before 50 years of age, and the condition should be diagnosed at a young age before hypertension develops. Early detection and treatment of CoA is associated with the best outcomes, although some patients will develop hypertension despite repair.

Table 8.1 ACC/AHA 2008 GL on GUCH

Recommendations for interventional and surgical treatment of coarctation of the aorta in adults	
Intervention for coarctation in:	I-C
a. Peak-to-peak coarctation gradient ≥ 20 mmHg.	
b. Peak-to-peak coarctation gradient <20 mmHg in the presence of anatomic imaging evidence of significant coarctation with radiological evidence of significant collateral flow.	
Choice of percutaneous catheter intervention versus surgical repair of native discrete coarctation should be determined by consultation with a team of ACHD cardiologists, interventionalists, and surgeons at an ACHD centre.	I-C
Percutaneous catheter intervention is indicated for recurrent, discrete coarctation and a peak-to-peak gradient ≥20 mmHg.	I-B
Surgeons with training and expertise in CHD should perform operations for previously repaired coarctation and the following indications:	I-B
a. Long recoarctation segment.	
b. Concomitant hypoplasia of the aortic arch.	
Stent placement for long-segment coarctation (usefulness not well established, and long-term efficacy and safety unknown).	IIb-C

ACC/AHA 2008 guidelines for the management of adults with congenital heart disease. *J Am Coll Cardiol*. 2008;**52**:e1–e121.

Table 8.2 ESC 2010 GL on GUCH

Indications for intervention in coarctation of the aorta	
Intervention in all patients with a non-invasive pressure difference >20 mmHg between upper and lower limbs, regardless of symptoms, but with upper limb hypertension (>140/90 mmHg in adults), pathological blood pressure response during exercise, or significant LVH.	I-C
Intervention independent of the pressure gradient, in hypertensive patients with ≥50% aortic narrowing relative to the aortic diameter at the diaphragm level (on CMR, CT, or invasive angiography).	IIa-C
Intervention independent of the pressure gradient and presence of hypertension, in patients with ≥50% aortic narrowing relative to the aortic diameter at the diaphragm level (on CMR, CT, or invasive angiography).	IIb-C

ESC Guidelines for the management of grown-up congenital heart disease (new version 2010). *Eur Heart J*. 2010;**31**:2915–57.

Surgical or endovascular repair indications

Indications for repair are presented in Tables 8.1 and 8.2. Main indications are:

- CoA gradient >20 mmHg
- Non-invasive pressure difference >20 mmHg between upper and lower limb, with upper limb hypertension (>140/90 mmHg)

- Anatomic imaging evidence of significant coarctation with collaterals.

Surgical repair

The surgical risk in simple CoA is <1%, but it increases significantly beyond the age of 30–40 years and carries the risk of spinal cord injury. **Recoarctation, aneurysms, or pseudoaneurysms** may occur in 10% of cases. When repair of CoA is performed between the ages of 20 and 40 years, the 25-year survival is 75%; in patients over 40 years old, the 15-year survival is only 50%.[1]

Endovascular repair

Covered stent deployment is increasingly the treatment of choice for adults with comparable results with surgery,[4] but long-term results are missing. Stenting appears to offer lower acute complications compared with surgery patients or balloon angioplasty but is more likely to require a planned re-intervention.[5] Percutaneous intervention (balloon or stent) is particularly recommended for recoarctation.[6] Systemic hypertension can occur after both surgical and endovascular repair and may be due to residual or recurrent coarctation, but even patients with a successful repair may develop hypertension. Risk factors for subsequent hypertension include an older age at the time of repair and higher blood pressure before the time of repair. The pathophysiology of hypertension that occurs after repair of coarctation of the aorta is not fully known. Anatomical and functional changes in the arterial tree, such as impaired elasticity and compliance and aortic stiffness, may be involved. Post-repair surveillance for **hypertension, endocarditis or arteritis, and rupture of berry or thoracic aneurysms** is necessary. Even if the coarctation repair appears to be satisfactory, late post-operative thoracic aortic imaging should be performed to assess for aortic dilatation or aneurysm formation. Thus, lifelong cardiology follow-up is recommended for all patients with aortic coarctation (repaired or not).

Pregnancy

It is allowed after repair. In unrepaired coarctation, residual significant hypertension, or aortic aneurysms, there is an increased risk of aortic rupture.[7]

References

1. Brickner ME, *et al.* Congenital heart disease in adults. First of two parts. *N Engl J Med.* 2000;**342**:256–63
2. Cohen M, *et al.* Coarctation of the aorta. Long-term follow-up and prediction of outcome after surgical correction. *Circulation.* 1989;**80**:840–5
3. Roifman I, *et al.* Coarctation of the aorta and coronary artery disease: fact or fiction? *Circulation.* 2012;**126**:16–21
4. Tanous D, *et al.* Coarctation of the aorta: evaluation and management. *Curr Opin Cardiol.* 2009;**24**:509–15
5. Forbes TJ, *et al.* Comparison of surgical, stent, and balloon angioplasty treatment of native coarctation of the aorta: an observational study by the CCISC (Congenital Cardiovascular Interventional Study Consortium). *J Am Coll Cardiol.* 2011;**58**:2664–74
6. Warnes CA, *et al.* ACC/AHA 2008 guidelines for the management of adults with congenital heart disease: a report of the American College of Cardiology/American Heart Association Task Force on practice guidelines (writing committee to develop guidelines on the management of adults with congenital heart disease). Developed in collaboration with the American Society of Echocardiography, Heart Rhythm Society, International Society for Adult Congenital Heart Disease, Society for Cardiovascular Angiography and Interventions, and Society of Thoracic Surgeons. *J Am Coll Cardiol.* 2008;**52**:e143–263
7. Regitz-Zagrosek V, *et al.* ESC guidelines on the management of cardiovascular diseases during pregnancy: the Task Force on the management of cardiovascular diseases during pregnancy of the European Society of Cardiology (ESC). *Eur Heart J.* 2011;**32**:3147–97

Chapter 9

Tetralogy of Fallot

Definition

Tetralogy of Fallot denotes a group of conditions characterized by ventricular septal defect, overriding of the aorta, right ventricular outflow obstruction, and right ventricular hypertrophy.[1] It is the most common form of cyanotic congenital heart disease. Despite the basically similar anatomy, these conditions are variable in terms of pulmonary artery anatomy and associated abnormalities.

Epidemiology

About 3.5% of all infants born with a congenital heart disease have tetralogy of Fallot, with males and females being affected equally.[1] The risk of recurrence in siblings is about 2–3% if there are no other affected first-degree relatives.

Aetiology

Approximately 15% of patients with Fallot have a deletion of the q11 region of chromosome 22 (di George syndrome) that has been associated with late-onset neuropsychiatric disorders. Screening for 22q11 deletion should be offered to all patients with Fallot since this mutation raises the risk of recurrence in offspring to 50%. Right aortic arch (25%), ASD (10%), and coronary artery anomalies (10%) are associated abnormalities.[2]

Pathophysiology

The ventricular septal defect is almost always large, ensuring that the pressure is equal in the two ventricles. Since the resistance to flow across the RV outflow tract is relatively fixed, changes in systemic vascular resistance affect the magnitude of right-to-left shunting. Most patients develop increasing cyanosis during the first few weeks and months of life. Severe cyanosis, recurrent hypercyanotic spells, and squatting for reduction of cyanosis, through increase in pulmonary flow and reduction of the shunt, are nowadays rare because usually infants undergo surgery at age of 3–6 months. Due to recent advances in the diagnosis and surgical treatment, almost all those born with tetralogy of Fallot are now expected to survive to adulthood.

Presentation

Survival to adult life is rare without palliation or correction, and only 11% reach 20 years of life.[2] These patients are cyanotic with marked clubbing. Usually, patients with repaired tetralogy are seen. Approximately 85% of patients with a previous repair remain asymptomatic but with reduced exercise ability and life expectancy (85% vs 92% 35-year survival, respectively).

Physical examination

- **Unoperated patients**
  - RV heave and palpable thrill
  - RVOT systolic ejection murmur (intensity and duration inversely related to obstruction severity)
  - Single A2 and diastolic murmur due to AR
- **Patients with palliative surgery** with systemic-to-pulmonary arterial shunts
  - Cyanosis with worsening of RVOT obstruction and/or aortopulmonary shunt stenosis. Progressive dilation of the aortic root may also occur.
- **Patients with anatomic repair**
  - PR or RVOT systolic ejection murmur
  - Progressive dilation of the aortic root with aortic ejection click and AR.

Investigations

- **Chest radiography** Normal-sized boot-shaped heart (coeur en sabot) with prominence of the right heart and and the apex lifted off the hemidiaphragm. Lung fields are oligaemic, and the aortic arch may be on the right side.
- **ECG** Right axis deviation with RV and RA hypertophy and RBBB, especially after anatomic repair. QRS width (to >180 ms) reflects RV dilatation and is a risk factor for VT.
- **BNP** levels correlate with end-diastolic RV dimensions and PR severity.[3]
- **Echocardiography** is adequate for diagnosis before or after operation, but the ideal method for assessing PR is cardiac **MRI**.
- **Cardiac catheterization** may be useful in cases of **pulmonary atresia**, with **major aortopulmonary collaterals** to delineate arterial supply to lungs or to delineate **coronary artery anatomy** before reoperation (Class I-B, ACC/AHA 2008).

Therapy

Anatomical repair is traditionally aimed at VSD closure and relief of RVOT obstruction (with resection of the infundibulum and pulmonary valvotomy and, if needed, RVOT or transannular patches). A modern approach is preservation of the pulmonary valve and avoidance of ventriculotomy at the expense of an accepted degree of RVOT obstruction.[1] **Palliative** systemic-to-pulmonary arterial shunts, such as **Blalock–Taussig** (either subclavian to respective PA), **Waterston** (back of ascending aorta to PA), or **Potts** (descending aorta to left PA), are associated with long-term complications, such as LV volume overload and pulmonary hypertension and distortion of pulmonary artery branches. They may still be offered today in the context of a staged procedure.

Clinical problems of adults with repaired tetralogy

Ventricular tachycardia, atrial macro re-entrant tachycardia, and atrial fibrillation are frequent (14–20%) and appear to be influenced more by left- than right-sided ventricular function.[4] Ventricular arrhythmias can be detected with Holter monitoring in up to 50% of patients with repaired tetralogy of Fallot. The incidence of sudden death in the adult population with Fallot is approximately 2.5% per decade of follow-up.[5] Patients with tetralogy of Fallot are the largest subgroup of implantable cardioverter defibrillator recipients with congenital heart disease. Significant PR (main predictor), QRS >180 ms, NSVT on Holter, and inducible VT at EPS, and older age repair have been identified as risk markers for sudden death.[5–8] Currently, ICDs are indicated for secondary prevention (previous cardiac arrest or sustained VT). Both RV and biventricular pacing might improve the intraventricular dyssynchrony of right ventricular contraction.

Pulmonary regurgitation The degree of residual PR has been related to the most severe adverse outcomes of progressive exercise intolerance, right heart failure, ventricular arrhythmia, and sudden death. Indications for surgery are new-onset symptomatic sustained ventricular tachycardia, exercise intolerance, and right heart failure. Pulmonary valve replacement in adults with palliated Fallot is a safe procedure, with a 93% 10-year survival.[9] It leads to stabilization of QRS duration and, in conjunction with intraoperative cryoablation, to a decrease in the incidence of pre-existing atrial and ventricular tachyarrhythmia.[10]

Percutaneous pulmonary valve replacement is now possible with no periprocedural mortality and low late mortality.[11] Care must be taken during deployment to avoid compression of coronary arteries, which might be adjacent to the right ventricular outflow tract. Valve failure occurs but usually can be treated by implantation of a second valve. The major limitation of the technique is that it is unsuitable for most patients with patch reconstruction of the right ventricular outflow tract and those with a grossly dilated native outflow tract.

Residual RVOT obstruction may require surgery, and **branch pulmonary stenosis**, especially in the setting of free pulmonary regurgitation, is treated by balloon dilation with or without stent.

Aortic root dilation is an increasingly recognized feature of late post-operative tetralogy of Fallot and can lead to significant AR. Progressive AR and aortic root dilation >55 mm are indications for surgery. However, although nearly one-third of adults with repaired TOF have an aortic root diameter ≥40 mm, the prevalence of a dilated aortic root, when defined by an indexed ratio of observed to expected values, is low, and moderate or severe AR is uncommon.[12]

Table 9.1 ACC/AHA 2008 GL on GUCH. Tetralogy of Fallot

Recommendations for surgery for adults with previous repair of tetralogy of Fallot	
Surgeons with training and expertise in CHD should perform operations in adults with previous repair of tetralogy of Fallot.	I-C
Pulmonary valve replacement is indicated for severe PR and symptoms of decreased exercise tolerance.	I-B
The possibility of an anomalous LAD across the RVOT should be ascertained before operative intervention.	I-C
Pulmonary valve replacement in adults with previous tetralogy of Fallot, severe PR, and any of the following:	
a. Moderate to severe RV dysfunction.	IIa-B
b. Moderate to severe RV enlargement.	IIa-B
c. Development of symptomatic or sustained atrial and/or ventricular arrhythmias.	IIa-C
d. Moderate to severe TR.	IIa-C
Collaboration between ACHD surgeons and ACHD interventional cardiologists to determine the most feasible treatment for pulmonary artery stenosis.	IIa-C
Surgery in adults with prior repair of tetralogy of Fallot and residual RVOT obstruction (valvular or subvalvular) and any of the following indications:	
a. Residual RVOT obstruction (valvular or subvalvular) with peak instantaneous echocardiography gradient >50 mmHg.	IIa-C
b. Residual RVOT obstruction (valvular or subvalvular) with RV/LV pressure ratio >0.7.	IIa-C
c. Residual RVOT obstruction (valvular or subvalvular) with progressive and/or severe dilatation of the right ventricle with dysfunction.	IIa-C
d. Residual VSD with a left-to-right shunt >1.5:1.	IIa-B
e. Severe AR with associated symptoms or more than mild LV dysfunction.	IIa-C
f. A combination of multiple residual lesions (e.g. VSD and RVOT obstruction), leading to RV enlargement or reduced RV function.	IIa-C

ACC/AHA 2008 guidelines for the management of adults with congenital heart disease. *J Am Coll Cardiol.* 2008;**52**:e1–e121.

Indications for intervention after repair

They are presented in Tables 9.1 and 9.2. Main indications are:

- Severe symptomatic PR or PS
- Residual RVOT obstruction with gradient >50 mmHg or RV/LV pressure ratio >0.7
- AR with LV dysfunction.

Participation in exercise

Full exercise activity should be encouraged for patients with only minimal residual abnormalities. Sports should be avoided by individuals with exercise-induced life-threatening arrhythmias. In patients with high right ventricular pressure (>50% of systemic values), severe pulmonary regurgitation with right ventricular dilatation, or rhythm disturbances, restriction to low dynamic and low static sport activities is advised.

Pregnancy

Before pregnancy, consultation with a geneticist is advisable. The risk is low in patients without substantial residual obstruction across the right ventricular outflow tract, severe pulmonary regurgitation, tricuspid regurgitation, and right and left ventricular dysfunction.[1, 13] The right ventricle is already compromised from previous surgery, and pregnancy in these patients is associated with persisting midterm dilatation of the subpulmonary ventricle. Thus, patients with repaired tetralogy of Fallot and severe pulmonary regurgitation should be considered for pulmonary valve replacement before becoming pregnant. Vaginal delivery is

Table 9.2 ESC 2010 GL on GUCH

Indications for intervention after repair of tetralogy of Fallot	
Aortic valve replacement in patients with severe AR with symptoms or signs of LV dysfunction.	I-C
PV replacement in symptomatic patients with severe PR and/or stenosis (RVsystolic pressure >60 mmHg, TR velocity >3.5 m/s).	I-C
PV replacement in asymptomatic patients with severe PR and/ or PS when at least one of the following criteria is present:	IIa-C
• Decrease in objective exercise capacity.	
• Progressive RV dilation.	
• Progressive RV systolic dysfunction.	
• Progressive TR (at least moderate).	
• RVOTO with RV systolic pressure >80 mmHg (TR velocity >4.3 m/s).	
• Sustained atrial/ventricular arrhythmias.	
VSD closure in patients with residual VSD and significant LV volume overload or if the patient is undergoing pulmonary valve surgery	IIa-C

ESC Guidelines for the management of grown-up congenital heart disease (new version 2010). *Eur Heart J*. 2010;**31**:2915–57.

the recommended mode of delivery for most women with tetralogy of Fallot. If right ventricular failure occurs during pregnancy, delivery should be considered before term. The estimated recurrence rate in the offspring is 3%.[6]

References

1. Apitz C WG, Redington AN. Tetralogy of Fallot. *Lancet*. 2009;**374**:1462–71
2. Brickner ME, *et al*. Congenital heart disease in adults. Second of two parts. *N Engl J Med*. 2000;**342**:334–42
3. Eindhoven JA, *et al*. The usefulness of brain natriuretic peptide in complex congenital heart disease: a systematic review. *J Am Coll Cardiol*. 2012;**60**:2140–9
4. Khairy P, *et al*. Arrhythmia burden in adults with surgically repaired tetralogy of Fallot: a multi-institutional study. *Circulation*. 2010;**122**:868–75
5. Warnes CA, *et al*. ACC/AHA 2008 guidelines for the management of adults with congenital heart disease: a report of the American College of Cardiology/American Heart Association Task Force on practice guidelines (writing committee to develop guidelines on the management of adults with congenital heart disease). Developed in collaboration with the American Society of Echocardiography, Heart Rhythm Society, International Society for Adult Congenital Heart Disease, Society for Cardiovascular Angiography and Interventions, and Society of Thoracic Surgeons. *J Am Coll Cardiol*. 2008;**52**:e143–263
6. Baumgartner H, *et al*. ESC guidelines for the management of grown-up congenital heart disease (new version 2010). *Eur Heart J*. 2010;**31**:2915–57
7. Gatzoulis MA, *et al*. Risk factors for arrhythmia and sudden cardiac death late after repair of tetralogy of Fallot: a multicentre study. *Lancet*. 2000;**356**:975–81
8. Khairy P, *et al*. Value of programmed ventricular stimulation after tetralogy of Fallot repair: a multicenter study. *Circulation*. 2004;**109**:1994–2000
9. Jain A, *et al*. Risk factors associated with morbidity and mortality after pulmonary valve replacement in adult patients with previously corrected tetralogy of Fallot. *Pediatr Cardiol*. 2012;**33**:601–6
10. Therrien J, *et al*. Impact of pulmonary valve replacement on arrhythmia propensity late after repair of tetralogy of Fallot. *Circulation*. 2001;**103**:2489–94
11. Momenah TS, *et al*. Extended application of percutaneous pulmonary valve implantation. *J Am Coll Cardiol*. 2009;**53**:1859–63
12. Mongeon FP, *et al*. Aortic root dilatation in adults with surgically repaired tetralogy of Fallot: a multicenter cross-sectional study. *Circulation*. 2013;**127**:172–9
13. Regitz-Zagrosek V, *et al*. ESC guidelines on the management of cardiovascular diseases during pregnancy: the Task Force on the management of cardiovascular diseases during pregnancy of the European Society of Cardiology (ESC). *Eur Heart J*. 2011;**32**:3147–97

Chapter 10

Transposition of great arteries

Definitions and classification of TGA

Morphological right and left ventricles refer to the anatomic characteristics of the chambers and not their positions.[1]

Atrioventricular discordance Inappropriate connections of the morphological right atrium to the morphological left ventricle and morphological left atrium to right ventricle.

Ventriculoarterial discordance The pulmonary artery arises from a morphological left ventricle, and the aorta arises from a morphological right ventricle.

Complete or d-transposition of great arteries (TGA) denotes that the aorta arises from the morphological right ventricle, and the pulmonary artery arises from the morphological left ventricle (i.e. there is ventriculoarterial discordance).

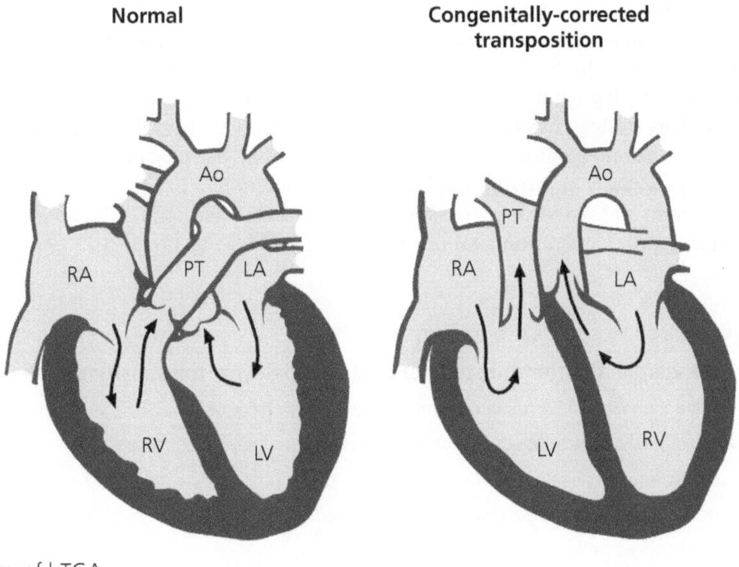

Figure 10.1 Anatomy of l-TGA.

Warnes CA. Transposition of the great arteries. *Circulation*. 2006;**114**:2699–709.

In **congenitally 'corrected' or l-TGA**, there are inappropriate connections of the morphological right atrium to the morphological left ventricle and morphological left atrium to right ventricle (atrioventricular discordance and ventriculoarterial discordance) (Figure 10.1).

Complete TGA (d-TGA)

Anatomy and pathophysiology

d-TGA refers to the normal rightward (dextro) bend of the embryonic heart tube and indicates that the inflow portion of the right ventricle is to the right of the morphological left ventricle. The aorta arises from the morphological right ventricle, and the pulmonary artery arises from the morphological left ventricle. The aorta also tends to be on the right and anterior, and the great arteries are parallel, rather than crossing as they do in the normal heart. Because the systemic and pulmonary circulations run in parallel, there has to be a communication between them, such as VSD, ASD, or PDA. Without intervention, the mortality rate is 90% by 6 months of age.[1]

Epidemiology

d-TGA accounts for 5% of all forms of congenital heart disease and is one of the most common cyanotic defects.[2]

Clinical problems and therapy in adults

Adult patients with TGA have survived due to previous repair. Their condition depends on the mode of operation performed.

Atrial switch (Senning and Mustard operations)

Atrial switch or atrial baffle procedures are the Senning (creation of an atrial baffle from autologous tissue to direct the venous return to the contralateral atrioventricular (AV) valve and ventricle) or Mustard (excision of the atrial septum and creation of the baffle with synthetic material) operations. These operations leave the morphological RV to support the systemic circulation, and **RV failure** and **TR** are common. **Atrial arrhythmias** (a marker of sudden death), **sinus nodal dysfunction**, **pulmonary hypertension**, and **atrial baffle obstruction** are problems encountered in adulthood.

Rastelli operation

When d-TGA coexists with a large subaortic VSD and PS, the Rastelli procedure may be used. A patch is placed to direct flow from the LV to the aorta through the VSD; the PV is oversewn, and continuity between RV and PV is established through a valve conduit. This operation has the advantage that the LV supports systemic circulation, but **conduit degeneration** and **atrial arrhythmias** are common and **sudden death** may occur.

Arterial switch

The modern surgical approach is arterial switch that restores normal anatomy of circulation. Arterial switch involves transection of the great arteries above the sinuses and restoration of their anatomic sites (i.e. the aorta to LV outflow tract if normal, and the pulmonary artery anterior to the aorta to the morphological right ventricle).[3] This operation is performed in the first weeks of life or later as a two-stage procedure with PA banding, in the absence of PV stenosis, to 'train' the LV in higher pressures. Late arterial switch after 'training' of the LV with a PV band can also be performed in young patients with previous atrial switch operations and failing RV. This strategy has the theoretical advantage of relieving the haemodynamic burden on the RV and tricuspid valve, potentially improving surgical results and longevity. Long-term and arrhythmia-free survival is excellent after arterial switch operation, and most patients maintain normal systolic function and exercise capacity.[4] Complications include **chronotropic incompetence**, and **dilatation of the neoaortic root with AR**, **branch pulmonary stenosis**, **PR**, and **coronary stenoses**. The effect of ACE inhibitors on RV function is debated, but they may be indicated in symptomatic patients with RV dysfunction.[5]

The ACC/AHA and ESC recommendations are presented in Tables 10.1 to 10.3.

Table 10.1 ACC/AHA 2008 GL on GUCH. Dextro-transposition

Recommendations for interventional catheterization for adults with dextro-transposition of the great arteries	
Interventional catheterization of the adult with d-TGA can be performed in centres with expertise.	I-C
For adults with d-TGA after atrial baffle procedure (Mustard or Senning), interventional catheterization to assist in:	IIa-B
a. Occlusion of baffle leak.	
b. Dilation or stenting of superior vena cava or inferior vena cava pathway obstruction.	
c. Dilation or stenting of pulmonary venous pathway obstruction.	
For adults with d-TGA after ASO, interventional catheterization to assist in dilation or stenting of supravalvular and branch pulmonary artery stenosis.	IIa-B
For adults with d-TGA, VSD, and PS, after Rastelli type repair, interventional catheterization to assist in:	IIa-C
a. Dilation with or without stent implantation of conduit obstruction (RV pressure >50% of systemic levels or peak-to-peak gradient >30 mmHg (these indications may be lessened in the setting of RV dysfunction).	
b. Device closure of residual VSD.	
Recommendations for surgical interventions after atrial baffle procedure (Mustard, Senning)	
Surgeons with training and expertise in CHD should perform operations in patients with d-TGA and:	I-B
a. Moderate to severe systemic (morphological tricuspid) AV valve regurgitation without significant ventricular dysfunction.	
b. Baffle leak with left-to-right shunt >1.5:1, right-to-left shunt with arterial desaturation at rest or with exercise, symptoms, and progressive ventricular enlargement that is not amenable to device intervention.	
c. Superior vena cava or inferior vena cava obstruction not amenable to percutaneous treatment.	
d. Pulmonary venous pathway obstruction not amenable to percutaneous intervention.	
e. Symptomatic severe subpulmonary stenosis.	
Recommendations for surgical interventions after arterial switch operation	
Surgery in patients after arterial switch operation (ASO) with the following indications:	I-C
a. RVOT obstruction peak-to-peak gradient >50 mmHg or right ventricle/left ventricle pressure ratio >0.7, not amenable or responsive to percutaneous treatment; lesser degrees of obstruction if pregnancy is planned, greater degrees of exercise are desired, or concomitant severe pulmonary regurgitation is present.	
b. Coronary artery abnormality with myocardial ischaemia not amenable to percutaneous intervention.	
c. Severe neoaortic valve regurgitation.	
d. Severe neoaortic root dilatation (>55 mm) after ASO.	
Recommendations for surgical interventions after Rastelli procedure	
Reoperation for conduit and/or valve replacement after Rastelli repair of d-TGA with:	I-C
a. Conduit obstruction peak-to-peak gradient >50 mmHg.	
b. RV/LV pressure ratio >0.7 (level of evidence: C).	
c. Lesser degrees of conduit obstruction if pregnancy is being planned or greater degrees of exercise are desired.	
d. Subaortic (baffle) obstruction (mean gradient >50 mmHg).	
e. Lesser degrees of subaortic baffle obstruction if LV hypertrophy is present, pregnancy is being planned, or greater degrees of exercise are desired.	

(continued)

Table 10.1 (continued)

f. Presence of concomitant severe AR.	
Reoperation for conduit regurgitation after Rastelli repair of d-TGA in patients with severe conduit regurgitation and:	I-C
a. Symptoms or declining exercise tolerance.	
b. Severely depressed RV function.	
c. Severe RV enlargement.	
d. Development/progression of atrial or ventricular arrhythmias.	
e. More than moderate TR.	
Collaboration between surgeons and interventional cardiologists, which may include preoperative stenting, intraoperative stenting, or intraoperative patch angioplasty, with or without conduit replacements, to determine the most feasible treatment for pulmonary artery stenosis.	I-C
Surgical closure of residual VSD in adults after Rastelli repair of d-TGA with:	
a. Qp/Qs >1.5:1.	I-B
b. Systolic pulmonary artery pressure >50 mmHg.	I-B
c. Increasing LV size from volume overload.	I-C
d. Decreasing RV function from pressure overload.	I-C
e. RVOT obstruction (peak instantaneous gradient >50 mmHg).	I-B
Pulmonary artery pressure <2/3 of systemic pressure or PVR <2/3 of systemic vascular resistance, with a net left-to-right shunt of 1.5:1, or a decrease in pulmonary artery pressure with pulmonary vasodilators (oxygen, nitric oxide, or prostaglandins).	I-B
Surgery after Rastelli repair of d-TGA in adults with branch pulmonary artery stenosis not amenable to percutaneous treatment.	I-C
In the presence of a residual intracardiac shunt or significant systemic venous obstruction, permanent pacing, if indicated, should be performed with epicardial leads.	I-B
Concomitant Maze procedure for atrial tachyarrhythmias in adults with d-TGA requiring reoperation for any reason.	IIa-C

ACC/AHA 2008 guidelines for the management of adults with congenital heart disease. *J Am Coll Cardiol.* 2008;**52**:e1–e121.

Table 10.2 ESC 2010 GL on GUCH. Indications for intervention in transposition of the great arteries after atrial switch

Indications for surgical intervention	
Valve repair or replacement in patients with severe symptomatic systemic (tricuspid) AV valve regurgitation without significant ventricular dysfunction (RVEF ≥45%).	I-C
Significant systemic ventricular dysfunction, with or without TR, should be treated conservatively or, eventually, with cardiac transplantation.	I-C
Surgery for LVOTO if symptomatic or if LV function deteriorates.	I-C
Surgical repair in symptomatic pulmonary venous obstruction (catheter intervention rarely possible).	I-C
Surgery for symptomatic patients with baffle stenosis not amenable to catheter intervention.	I-C
Surgery for symptomatic patients with baffle leaks not amenable to stenting.	I-C
Valve repair or replacement for severe asymptomatic systemic (tricuspid) AV valve regurgitation without significant ventricular dysfunction (RVEF ≥45%).	IIa-C
Pulmonary artery banding in adult patients to create septal shift, or as left ventricular training with subsequent arterial switch, is currently experimental and should be avoided.	III-C
Indications for catheter intervention	
Stenting in symptomatic patients with baffle stenosis.	I-C
Stenting (covered) or device closure in symptomatic patients with baffle leaks and substantial cyanosis at rest or during exercise.	I-C
Stenting (covered) or device closure in patients with baffle leaks and symptoms due to L–R shunt.	I-C
Stenting (covered) or device closure in asymptomatic patients with baffle leaks with substantial ventricular volume overload due to L–R shunt.	IIa-C
Stenting in asymptomatic patients with baffle stenosis who require a pacemaker.	IIa-C
Stenting in other asymptomatic patients with baffle stenosis.	IIb-C

ESC Guidelines for the management of grown-up congenital heart disease (new version 2010). *Eur Heart J.* 2010;**31**:2915–57.

Table 10.3 ESC 2010 GL on GUCH

Indications for intervention in transposition of the great arteries after arterial switch	
Stenting or surgery (depending on substrate) for coronary artery stenosis causing ischaemia.	I-C
Surgical repair of RVOTO in symptomatic patients with RV systolic pressure >60 mmHg (TR velocity >3.5 m/s).	I-C
Surgical repair of RVOTO, regardless of symptoms, when RV dysfunction develops (RVP may then be lower).	I-C
Surgical repair in asymptomatic patients with RVOTO and systolic RVP >80 mmHg (TR velocity >4.3 m/s).	IIa-C
Aortic root surgery when the (neo-) aortic root is >55 mm, providing average adult stature.	IIa-C
Stenting or surgery (depending on substrate) for peripheral PS, regardless of symptoms, if >50% diameter narrowing and RV systolic pressure >50 mmHg and/or lung perfusion abnormalities are present.	IIa-C

ESC Guidelines for the management of grown-up congenital heart disease (new version 2010). *Eur Heart J*. 2010;**31**:2915–57.

Pregnancy

Pregnancy can be tolerated by successfully operated patients in the presence of reasonable RV function, but it carries a risk of heart failure. The risk of congenital heart defect in the offspring is <5%. Most patients need endocarditis prophylaxis, unless they have had an arterial switch procedure and have no residual valve dysfunction or outflow tract disturbance.[2, 6]

Congenitally corrected transposition (l-TGA)

Anatomy and pathophysiology

There are inappropriate connections of the morphological right atrium to the morphological left ventricle and morphological left atrium to right ventricle. The right atrium enters the left ventricle, which gives rise to the pulmonary artery, and the left atrium enters the right ventricle, which gives rise to the aorta. The aorta is usually anterior and to the left, and the tricuspid valve always enters a morphological RV. Thus, the circulation continues in the appropriate direction but flows through the wrong ventricles. It is also called l-TGA since the morphological right ventricle is on the left of the morphological left ventricle.[1]

Associated anomalies

A **VSD** occurs in 70% of patients, usually in the perimembranous location.

Pulmonary stenosis occurs in 40% of patients and is commonly subvalvular, either due to an aneurysm of the membranous septum or due to fibrous tissue or ring in the subvalvular area. Associated valvar pulmonary stenosis also occurs.

Abnormalities of the TV, especially inferior displacement resembling Ebstein's anomaly, occur in up to 70% of patients.

Due to the displacement of the AV node and His bundle, **complete AV block** occurs at 2% per year. Tricuspid valve or VSD surgery may also precipitate heart block.

Epidemiology

l-TGA is a rare anomaly and comprises <1% of all forms of congenital heart disease.

Presentation

Patients may present for the first time in adulthood, and the diagnosis is often overlooked. Some patients may be relatively normal from a functional standpoint, and survival to the eighth decade has been reported in the absence of associated anomalies. Failure of the systemic ventricle is much more common earlier in life, usually with concomitant tricuspid regurgitation.

Physical findings

Physical signs are those of:

- **Systemic ventricular (RV) failure**
- **Left AV valve regurgitation**
- **Complete AV block** and **SVT** or **AF**.

The cause of systemic ventricular failure is not established. Perfusion of the systemic ventricle by a single coronary artery (RCA) as well as systemic AV valve regurgitation are probably responsible.

Investigations

Chest radiograph With mesocardia or levocardia, the diagnosis may be suspected from the chest radiograph (Figure 10.2). The vascular pedicle appears abnormally straight because the normal arterial relationships are lost. The ascending aorta is not visible on the right side, and the convexities from the descending aortic knob and pulmonary artery are absent on the left side. l-TGA is one of the most common anomalies associated with dextrocardia and should be suspected when there is abdominal situs solitus (gastric bubble on the left) and dextrocardia (Figure 10.2).

ECG The ECG may resemble inferior myocardial infarction, with Q waves in the right precordial leads and absent Q waves in the left precordial leads. Various degrees of AV block may be present.

Echocardiography can be difficult, particularly with mesocardia or dextrocardia. Subcostal imaging facilitates detection of atrial situs and position of the cardiac apex and thus determines the presence or absence of dextrocardia or mesocardia. The morphological RV is on the patient's left (l-loop) and has prominent trabeculations. A high parasternal short-axis view may show the abnormal

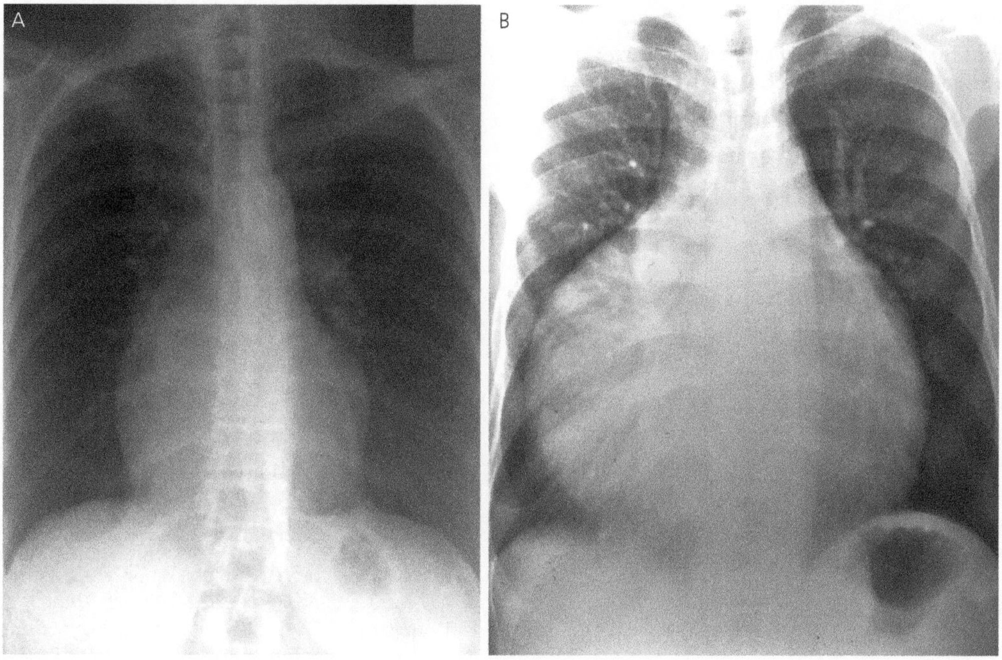

Figure 10.2 Chest X-rays in l-TGA.
Warnes CA. Transposition of the great arteries. *Circulation*. 2006;**114**:2699–709.

arterial relationships, with the aorta usually anterior and to the left of the pulmonary artery.

Therapy

ACE inhibitors may be beneficial in symptomatic only patients with RV dysfunction.[5]

Surgical repair

Various procedures have been used in adult patients but with rather disappointing results (up to 67% 10-year survival).[7] The current approach is a double switch, i.e. a two-stage procedure with PA banding, in the absence of PV stenosis, to 'train' the LV in higher pressures. A venous switch (either Mustard or Senning) and, in those with normal LVOT, an arterial switch can be performed later. If a large VSD is present, the Rastelli procedure may be used. Concomitant tricuspid valve surgery can also be performed, if necessary. LV failure, AR, and atrial arrhythmias are common problems with this approach, the long-term results of which are unknown. Patients with corrected transposition should be scrutinized for the presence of systemic atrioventricular valve regurgitation. Valve replacement should be considered before systemic ventricular EF falls below 40% or the subpulmonary ventricular systolic pressure exceeds 50 mmHg (Tables 10.4 and 10.5).[2,8,9]

Table 10.4 ACC/AHA 2008 GL on GUCH

Patients with congenitally corrected transposition of the great arteries: recommendations for surgical intervention	
Surgeons with training and expertise in CHD should perform operations for patients with CCTGA for:	I-B
a. Unrepaired CCTGA and severe AV valve regurgitation.	
b. Anatomic repair with atrial and arterial level switch/ Rastelli repair in cases in which the left ventricle is functioning at systemic pressures.	
c. Simple VSD closure when the VSD is not favourable for left ventricle-to-aorta baffling or is restrictive.	
d. LV-to-pulmonary artery conduit in rare cases with LV dysfunction and severe LV outflow obstruction.	
e. Evidence of moderate or progressive systemic AV valve regurgitation.	
f. Conduit obstruction with systemic or nearly systemic RV pressures and/or RV dysfunction after anatomic repair.	
g. Conduit obstruction and systemic or suprasystemic LV pressures in a patient with non-anatomic correction.	
h. Moderate or severe AR/neo-AR and onset of ventricular dysfunction or progressive ventricular dilatation.	

ACC/AHA 2008 guidelines for the management of adults with congenital heart disease. *J Am Coll Cardiol.* 2008;**52**:e1–e121.

Table 10.5 ESC 2010 GL on GUCH

Indications for intervention in congenitaly corrected transposition of the great arteries	
Systemic AV valve (tricuspid valve) surgery for severe regurgitation before systemic (subaortic) ventricular function deteriorates (before RVEF <45%).	IIa-C
Anatomic repair (atrial switch + arterial switch or Rastelli when feasible in case of non-restrictive VSD) may be considered when LV is functioning at systemic pressure.	IIb-C

ESC Guidelines for the management of grown-up congenital heart disease (new version 2010). *Eur Heart J.* 2010;**31**:2915–57.

Pregnancy

Systemic ventricular ejection fraction <40% or significant systemic AV valve regurgitation are contraindications for pregnancy. Otherwise, pregnancy can be tolerated in most women with l-TGA, but careful evaluation is mandatory. Most patients require endocarditis prophylaxis, unless they have no valvular dysfunction, outflow obstruction, or VSD.[2,6]

References

1. Warnes CA. Transposition of the great arteries. *Circulation.* 2006;**114**:2699–709
2. Warnes CA, *et al.* ACC/AHA 2008 guidelines for the management of adults with congenital heart disease: a report of the American College of Cardiology/American Heart Association Task Force on practice guidelines (writing committee to develop guidelines on the management of adults with congenital heart disease). Developed in collaboration with the American Society of Echocardiography, Heart Rhythm Society, International Society for Adult Congenital Heart Disease, Society for Cardiovascular Angiography and Interventions, and Society of Thoracic Surgeons. *J Am Coll Cardiol.* 2008;**52**:e143–263
3. Jatene AD, *et al.* Successful anatomic correction of transposition of the great vessels. A preliminary report. *Arq Bras Cardiol.* 1975;**28**:461–4
4. Khairy P, *et al.* Cardiovascular outcomes after the arterial switch operation for D-transposition of the great arteries. *Circulation.* 2013;**127**:331–9
5. van der Bom T *et al.* . Effect of valsartan on systemic right ventricular function: a double-blind, randomized, placebo-controlled pilot trial. *Circulation.* 2013;**127**: 322–30
6. Regitz-Zagrosek V, *et al.* ESC guidelines on the management of cardiovascular diseases during pregnancy: the Task Force on the management of cardiovascular diseases during pregnancy of the European Society of Cardiology (ESC). *Eur Heart J.* 2011;**32**:3147–97
7. Hraska V, *et al.* Long-term outcome of surgically treated patients with corrected transposition of the great arteries. *J Thorac Cardiovasc Surg.* 2005;**129**:182–91
8. Baumgartner H, *et al.* ESC guidelines for the management of grown-up congenital heart disease (new version 2010). *Eur Heart J.* 2010;**31**:2915–57
9. Mongeon FP, *et al.* Congenitally corrected transposition of the great arteries ventricular function at the time of systemic atrioventricular valve replacement predicts long-term ventricular function. *J Am Coll Cardiol.* 2011;**57**:2008–17.

Chapter 11

Ebstein's anomaly

Definition

Ebstein's anomaly is a malformation of the tricuspid valve, with apical displacement of the septal and posterior leaflets from the atrioventricular ring, resulting in a reduction in size of the right ventricle.[1,2] There are no cords to suspend the leaflets, so they arise from the cavity of the ventricle and are attached to its wall. The anomaly results in right ventricular dysplasia, with dilatation and dyskinesis of the atrialized right ventricle. Thus, the disease is characterized by:[2]

- Adherence of the septal and posterior leaflets to the underlying myocardium
- Downward (apical) displacement of the functional annulus
- Dilation of the 'atrialized' portion of the right ventricle, with various degrees of hypertrophy and thinning of the wall
- Redundancy, fenestrations, and tethering of the anterior leaflet
- Dilation of the right atrioventricular junction (true tricuspid annulus).

Epidemiology

It represents 1% of all congenital heart disease. Associated cardiac malformations are ASD (80%), left ventricular fibrosis, and ventricular non-compaction.

Presentation

Ebstein's anomaly has an extremely variable natural history and prognosis. Adults usually present with exercise intolerance and varying degrees of dyspnoea and cyanosis and/or supraventricular tachycardia. Paradoxical embolization, brain abscess, and sudden death may occur. Patients with Ebstein's anomaly who reach late adolescence and adulthood often have a good outcome.[3]

Physical examination

- S_1 and S_2 are widely split
- S_3 or S_4 usually present
- **Systolic murmur** of TR
- **Hepatomegaly** due to right heart failure may be present.

Investigations

The **ECG** shows enlarged P waves, prolonged PR interval, and complete or incomplete RBBB. The QRS duration is a marker of RV enlargement and dysfunction. QRS fractionation is associated with a greater atrialized RV volume. A preserved surface ECG identifies a subset of patients with Ebstein anomaly with mild morphological and functional abnormalities and better clinical profile. [4] Arrhythmias are very common and represent AVRT (6–30% of patients have right lateral or posteroseptal accessory pathways), intra-atrial reentry, atrial flutter, or AVNRT.[5] Wolff–Parkinson–White syndrome with overt ventricular pre-excitation is seen in 60% of patients presenting with arrhythmias. In patients without pre-excitation, the absence of RBBB is a strong predictor of accessory pathways.

Chest radiography reveals cardiomegaly in severe cases. A cardiothoracic ratio >0.65 carries a poor prognosis.[2]

Two-dimensional echocardiography is essential to establish the diagnosis and guide management (Figure 11.1).

Three-dimensional echocardiography and **magnetic resonance imaging** also provide precise anatomical and functional assessment of the tricuspid valves and the right ventricle.

Therapy

Anticoagulation with warfarin is recommended for patients with Ebstein's anomaly with a history of paradoxical embolus or AF (Class I-C, ACC/AHA 2008). Surgery is recommended in symptomatic patients or in

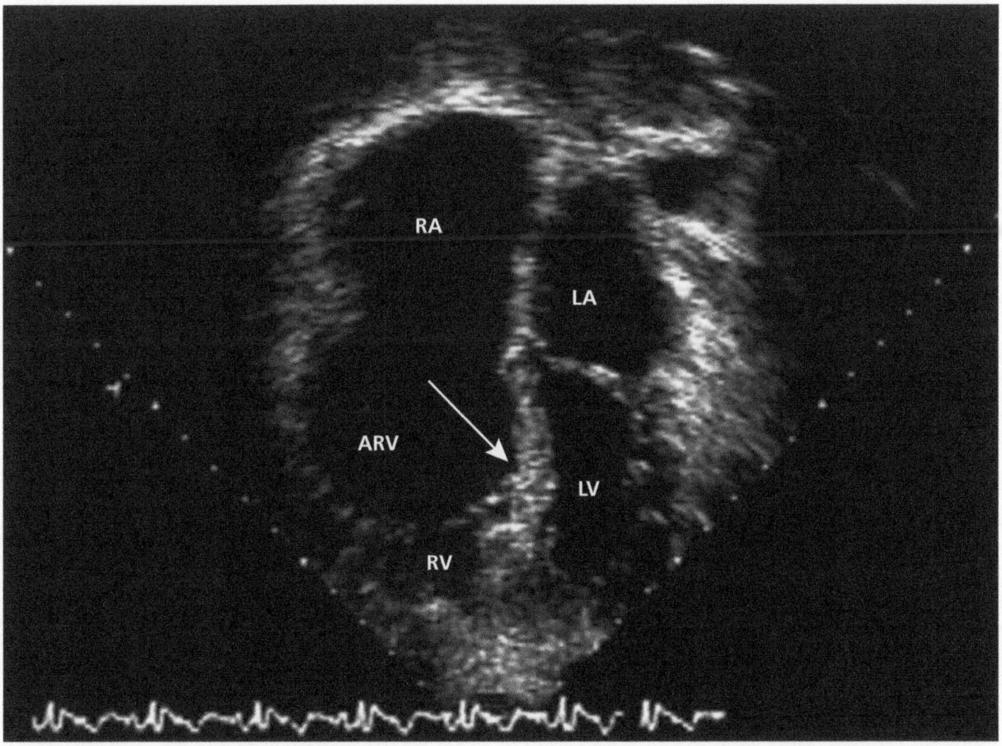

Figure 11.1 Ebstein's anomaly. Example of an echocardiogram (4-chamber view, apex down) of a patient with severe Ebstein's anomaly, showing a grossly displaced septal leaflet (arrow). The anterior leaflet is severely tethered and nearly immobile. The functional right ventricle (RV) is small.

ARV indicates atrialized right ventricle; LA, left atrium; LV, left ventricle; and RA, right atrium. Attenhofer Jost CH, *et al*. Ebstein's anomaly. *Circulation*. 2007;**115**:277–85.

Table 11.1 ACC/AHA 2008 GL on GUCH. Ebstein's anomaly

Recommendations for surgical interventions	
Surgeons with training and expertise in CHD should perform tricuspid valve repair or replacement with concomitant closure of an ASD, when present, for patients with Ebstein's anomaly and: a. Symptoms or deteriorating exercise capacity. b. Cyanosis (oxygen saturation <90%). c. Paradoxical embolism. d. Progressive cardiomegaly on chest X-ray. e. Progressive RV dilation or reduction of RV systolic function.	I-B
Surgeons with training and expertise in CHD should perform concomitant arrhythmia surgery in patients with Ebstein's anomaly and: a. Appearance/progression of atrial and/or ventricular arrhythmias not amenable to percutaneous treatment. b. Ventricular pre-excitation not successfully treated in the electrophysiology laboratory.	I-B
Surgical repair or replacement of the tricuspid valve in adults with Ebstein's anomaly with: a. Symptoms, deteriorating exercise capacity, or NYHA III or IV. b. Severe TR after repair with progressive RV dilation, reduction of RV systolic function, or appearance/progression of atrial and/or ventricular arrhythmias. c. Bioprosthetic tricuspid valve dysfunction with significant mixed regurgitation and stenosis. d. Predominant bioprosthetic valve stenosis (mean gradient >12–15 mmHg). e. Operation can be considered earlier with lesser degrees of bioprosthetic stenosis, with symptoms or decreased exercise tolerance.	I-B

ACC/AHA 2008 guidelines for the management of adults with congenital heart disease. *J Am Coll Cardiol.* 2008;**52**:e1–e121.

Table 11.2 ESC 2010 GL on GUCH

Indications for interventions in Ebstein's anomaly	
Surgical repair in patients with more than moderate TR and symptoms (NYHA class >II or arrhythmias) or deteriorating exercise capacity measured by cardiopulmonary exercise testing.	I-C
Surgical ASD/PFO closure at the time of valve repair if tricuspid valve surgery is indicated.	I-C
Surgical repair, regardless of symptoms, in patients with progressive right heart dilation or reduction of RV systolic function and/or progressive cardiomegaly on chest X-ray.	IIa-C
Indications for catheter intervention	
Patients with relevant arrhythmias should undergo electrophysiologic testing, followed by ablation therapy, if feasible, or surgical treatment of the arrhythmias in the case of planned heart surgery.	I-C
Isolated device closure of ASD/PFO in the case of documented systemic embolism, probably caused by paradoxical embolism.	IIa-C
If cyanosis (oxygen saturation at rest <90%) is the leading problem, isolated device closure of ASD/PFO may be considered but requires careful evaluation before intervention.	IIb-C

ESC Guidelines for the management of grown-up congenital heart disease (new version 2010). *Eur Heart J.* 2010;**31**:2915–57.

the presence of cyanosis (O_2 saturation <90%), progressive RV dilatation, severe TR, or paradoxical embolism (Tables 11.1 and 11.2).[6, 7] Surgical treatment is now feasible at specializing centers, with biventricular or univentricular tricuspid repair or tricuspid valve replacement with a bioprosthesis. Mortality is now <2.5%, with late death rate over 7 years of 7.6%.[2, 8] Catheter ablation of accessory pathways is difficult, with 80% success rate and up to 40% recurrence rate,[5] and surgical ablation may be needed. Intra-atrial reentry and cavotricuspid isthmus flutter may also occur.

Pregnancy

Acyanotic patients with good RV tolerate pregnancy well, although there is an increased risk of RV failure, arrhythmia, and pardoxical embolism.

References

1. Attenhofer Jost CH, *et al.* Ebstein's anomaly. *Circulation.* 2007;**115**:277–85
2. Paranon S, *et al.* Ebstein's anomaly of the tricuspid valve: from fetus to adult: congenital heart disease. *Heart.* 2008;**94**: 237–43
3. Celermajer DS, *et al.* Ebstein's anomaly: presentation and outcome from fetus to adult. *J Am Coll Cardiol.* 1994;**23**:170–6
4. Egidy Assenza G VA, *et al.* QRS duration and QRS fractionation on surface electrocardiogram are markers of right ventricular dysfunction and atrialization in patients with Ebstein anomaly. *Eur Heart J.* 2013;**34**:191–200
5. Roten L, *et al.* Catheter ablation of arrhythmias in Ebstein's anomaly: a multicenter study. *J Cardiovasc Electrophysiol.* 2011;**22**:1391–6
6. Baumgartner H, *et al.* ESC guidelines for the management of grown-up congenital heart disease (new version 2010). *Eur Heart J.* 2010;**31**:2915–57
7. Warnes CA, *et al.* ACC/AHA 2008 guidelines for the management of adults with congenital heart disease: a report of the American College of Cardiology/American Heart Association Task Force on practice guidelines (writing committee to develop guidelines on the management of adults with congenital heart disease). Developed in collaboration with the American Society of Echocardiography, Heart Rhythm Society, International Society for Adult Congenital Heart Disease, Society for Cardiovascular Angiography and Interventions, and Society of Thoracic Surgeons. *J Am Coll Cardiol.* 2008;**52**:e143–263
8. Boston US, *et al.* Tricuspid valve repair for Ebstein's anomaly in young children: a 30-year experience. *Ann Thorac Surg.* 2006;**81**:690–5; discussion 695–6

Chapter 12

Anomalous PV connections, AV malformations, coronary and LV abnormalities

Total anomalous pulmonary venous connection (TAPVC)

In TAPVC, all four pulmonary veins drain into systemic veins or the right atrium, with or without pulmonary venous obstruction. Systemic and pulmonary venous blood mix in the right atrium. A VSD or an ASD allows flow to the left atrium, and a PDA may be present. Diagnosis of most patients occurs in early infancy.

Connections have been classified into **supracardiac** (the four pulmonary veins drain via a common vein into the right superior vena cava, left superior vena cava, or their tributaries), **cardiac** (the pulmonary veins connect directly to the right heart, e.g. coronary sinus or directly to the right atrium), **infradiaphragmatic** (the common pulmonary vein is anterior to the oesophagus through the diaphragm to connect to the portal venous system), and **mixed** (the right and left pulmonary veins drain to different sites, e.g. left pulmonary veins into the left vertical vein to the left innominate, right pulmonary veins directly into the right atrium or coronary sinus). The degree of cyanosis in the neonate depends on the degree of venous obstruction and the size of the ASD.

Without surgery, up to 90% of patients die within the first year of life. Surgical mortality in experienced centres is <10%, and 3-year survival exceeds 85%.[1] Most patients survive surgery without late cardiovascular problem manifestations. An increased incidence of neurodevelopmental difficulties has been reported, and there is a risk for recurrent pulmonary vein stenosis or anastomosis at the anastomosis site between the common pulmonary vein and the left atrium. Post-operative pulmonary vein obstruction may occur in patients with hypoplastic/stenotic pulmonary veins.[1]

Partial anomalous pulmonary venous connection (PAPVC)

Part, or all, of one lung drains into systemic veins or the right atrium. Sinus venosus defects have PAPVC from the right upper and middle lobe pulmonary veins to the SVC. PAPVC to the IVC (**scimitar syndrome**) may be associated with a hypoplastic right lung, pulmonary sequestration, and ASD. Signs and symptoms resemble those of a secundum ASD. Surgical correction is indicated in the presence of RV overload.[2]

Pulmonary arteriovenous malformations

They are abnormal connections between branches of the pulmonary arterial and pulmonary venous system. They are usually part of the hereditary haemorrhagic telangiectasia syndrome, an autosomal dominant disorder, but may also occur as isolated or multiple defects secondary to trauma or infection.[3] They may create a pulmonary right-to-left shunt because the desaturated blood bypasses the oxygenation mechanisms at the alveolar level. In the presence of clinical cyanosis, transcatheter embolization is the treatment of choice. Surgical lung resections are rarely required.

Congenital coronary anomalies

Congenital anomalous origin of the coronary arteries may occur in 1–5% of all coronary angiograms performed, with 0.15% of them having the highest-risk lesions of the left coronary artery arising from the right sinus of Valsalva.[3] Anomalous origination of the left coronary artery from the right sinus is consistently related to sudden death (59% of cases), which follows exercise in 81% of events. Coronary anomalies account for approximately 15% of sudden cardiac deaths in athletes (potentially due to torsion or compression of the proximal coronary artery, exercise-induced compression, vasospasm, or ischaemic or scar-induced ventricular arrhythmia).[4] In 80% of autopsies in athletes with sudden cardiac death and anomalous coronary artery origins, the affected coronary artery coursed between the aorta and the pulmonary artery.[3,4] Treatment is necessary in these high-risk cases as described in Table 12.1. Myocardial bridges (intramyocardial course of the coronary) with systolic compression occurs in 1% of coronary angiograms and requires treatment when causing ischaemia.[3] CABG is the treatment of choice, although stents have also been successfully tried.

Coronary fistulas

Communications between the coronary arteries and the cardiac chambers (coronary-cameral fistulas) or low-pressure veins (coronary arteriovenous malformations) are, most often, congenital in nature (usually to RV, RA, or

Table 12.1 ACC/AHA 2008 on GUCH

Recommendations for congenital coronary anomalies of ectopic arterial origin	
The evaluation of unexplained aborted sudden cardiac death or unexplained life-threatening arrhythmia, coronary ischaemic symptoms, or LV dysfunction should include assessment of coronary artery origins and course.	I-B
CT or magnetic resonance angiography as the initial screening method.	I-B
Surgical coronary revascularization with: a. Anomalous left main coronary artery coursing between the aorta and pulmonary artery.* b. Documented coronary ischaemia due to coronary compression (when coursing between the great arteries or in intramural fashion). c. Anomalous origin of the right coronary artery between aorta and pulmonary artery with evidence of ischaemia.*	I-B
Surgical coronary revascularization in documented vascular wall hypoplasia, coronary compression, or documented obstruction to coronary flow, regardless of inability to document coronary ischaemia.	IIa-C
Delineation of potential mechanisms of flow restriction via intravascular ultrasound in patients with documented anomalous coronary artery origin from the opposite sinus.	IIa-C
Surgical coronary revascularization in anomalous LAD coursing between the aorta and pulmonary artery.*	IIb-C
Recommendations for anomalous left coronary artery from the pulmonary artery	
Reconstruction of a dual coronary artery supply should be performed by surgeons with training and expertise in CHD.	I-C
For adult survivors of ALCAPA repair, clinical evaluation with echocardiography and non-invasive stress testing is indicated every 3 to 5 years.	I-C

* These recommendations for surgery in adults have also been adopted by the ACCF/AHA/SCAI 2011 Guidelines on CABG.
ACC/AHA 2008 guidelines for the management of adults with congenital heart disease. *J Am Coll Cardiol*. 2008; **52**:e1–e121.

Table 12.2 ACC/AHA 2008 on GUCH

Recommendations for coronary arteriovenous fistula	
The origin of a continuous murmur should be defined by echocardiography, MRI, CT angiography, or cardiac catheterization.	I-C
A large coronary arteriovenous fistula (CAVF), regardless of symptomatology, should be closed via either a transcatheter or surgical route after delineation of its course and its potential to fully obliterate the fistula.	I-C
A small to moderate CAVF, in the presence of documented myocardial ischaemia, arrhythmia, otherwise unexplained ventricular systolic or diastolic dysfunction or enlargement, or endarteritis, should be closed via either a transcatheter or surgical approach after delineation of its course and its potential to fully obliterate the fistula.	I-C
Clinical follow-up with echocardiography every 3 to 5 years for patients with small, asymptomatic CAVF to exclude development of symptoms or arrhythmias or progression of size or chamber enlargement.	IIa-C
Patients with small, asymptomatic CAVF should not undergo closure of CAVF.	III-C
Recommendations for management strategies of coronary arteriovenous fistula	
Surgeons with training and expertise in CHD should perform operations for management of patients with CAVF.	I-C
Transcatheter closure of CAVF should be performed only in centres with expertise in such procedures.	I-C
Transcatheter delineation of CAVF course and access to distal drainage should be performed in all patients with audible continuous murmur and recognition of CAVF.	I-C

ACC/AHA 2008 guidelines for the management of adults with congenital heart disease. *J Am Coll Cardiol*. 2008;**52**:e1–e121.

PAs).[5] They also may be acquired secondary to trauma or from invasive cardiac procedures, such as pacemaker implantation, endomyocardial biopsy, coronary artery bypass grafting, or coronary angiography. With larger fistulas, a diastolic run-off may occur, drawing blood away from the normal coronary pathway with a widened pulse pressure and a coronary steal, thus creating a left-to-right or left-to-left shunt. Most coronary artery fistulas are small, and patients are asymptomatic. A continuous murmur may be audible at the left lower sternal border. Small coronary fistulas in children tend to grow with age and may cause clinical symptoms, such as angina or congestive heart failure, and, rarely, endocarditis or fistula rupture in up to 60% of older patients. Large, haemodynamically significant fistulas can be closed electively, either by surgery on a beating heart from the epicardial surface or through transcatheter occlusion techniques (Table 12.2).

Left ventricular protrusions

Congenital left ventricular outpouchings include diverticula, aneurysms, and hernias and can be seen in up to 0.8% of patients undergoing cardiac catheterization and found to have normal coronary arteries.[6] Diverticula have a thick wall, made up of histologically normal heart wall tissue, and are connected to the main left ventricular chamber through a narrow neck, whereas aneurysms are thin-walled, fibrotic, and non-contractile and have a wide communication with the main chamber. Cardiac hernias are defined as myocardium protruding through a pericardial defect. Left ventricular protrusions can be a source of embolic stroke.

References

1. Seale AN, *et al.* Total anomalous pulmonary venous connection: morphology and outcome from an international population-based study. *Circulation.* 2010;**122**:2718–26
2. Warnes CA, *et al.* ACC/AHA 2008 guidelines for the management of adults with congenital heart disease: a report of the American College of Cardiology/American Heart Association Task Force on practice guidelines (writing committee to develop guidelines on the management of adults with congenital heart disease). Developed in collaboration with the American Society of Echocardiography, Heart Rhythm Society, International Society for Adult Congenital Heart Disease, Society for Cardiovascular Angiography and Interventions, and Society of Thoracic Surgeons. *J Am Coll Cardiol.* 2008;**52**:e143–263
3. Angelini P, *et al.* Coronary anomalies: incidence, pathophysiology, and clinical relevance. *Circulation.* 2002;**105**:2449–54
4. Maron BJ, *et al.* Sudden death in young competitive athletes. Clinical, demographic, and pathological profiles. *JAMA.* 1996;**276**:199–204
5. Sommer RJ, *et al.* Pathophysiology of congenital heart disease in the adult: part iii: complex congenital heart disease. *Circulation.* 2008;**117**:1340–50
6. Megevand P, *et al.* A palpable source of stroke. *Circulation.* 2011;**124**:e232–3

Chapter 13

The Fontan patient

Definition

The Fontan operation is a generic term for a group of operations that redirect the systemic venous return to the pulmonary arteries without passing through a subpulmonary ventricle.[1, 2] The classic Fontan consisted of a valved conduit between the right atrium and pulmonary artery. It was subsequently modified to a direct anastomosis of the right atrium to a divided pulmonary artery (Figure 13.1A). The intracardiac lateral tunnel consists of an end-to-side anastomosis of the superior vena cava to the undivided right pulmonary artery and a composite intra-atrial tunnel that uses the right atrial lateral wall and prosthetic material to channel inferior vena caval flow to the pulmonary artery (Figure 13.1B). The 'extracardiac' variant of the total cavopulmonary connection Fontan consists of directing inferior vena caval flow to the pulmonary artery by means of an external conduit (Figure 13.1C).[3]

Pathophysiology

Fontan is usually offered to patients with single-ventricle physiology, i.e. a functionally single ventricle, or when biventricular repair is not feasible. The following conditions are treated with a Fontan: **tricuspid atresia**, **hypoplastic left heart syndrome**, **double-inlet ventricle**, and **isomerism** (complex abnormalities of visceral and atrial situs). Thus, nowadays, the so-called Fontan physiology consists of staged approaches that eventually end up in a single functional ventricle that maintains both the systemic and the passive pulmonary circulation. Symptoms develop when the single functional ventricle fails. The 12-year survival after various types of operation is 70%.[1] Extracardiac conduit total cavopulmonary connection and lack of clinical arrhythmia or right heart failure are good prognostic signs, whereas exercise intolerance is not associated with long-term mortality.[4] Considerable mortality is still observed during the first years of life among patients with single ventricle. In patients with a functionally univentricular heart undergoing the Fontan procedure, RV dominance is the most important risk factor for death but only before bidirectional superior cavopulmonary anastomosis.[5]

Clinical problems

Patients present with classic right heart failure. There is a **non-pulsatile high JVP** (10 cm), with **single S2** and a **murmur** only if subaortic obstruction or significant systemic AV valve regurgitation. Oedema and ascites may be seen as a sign of **protein-losing enteropathy**. Other problems are: **Arrhythmias** due to post-op atrial scarring: intra-atrial reentrant tachycardia, atrial flutter, and fibrillation. The most frequent of these is intra-atrial reentrant tachycardia, particularly seen with atrio-pulmonary connections. With modern techniques, its incidence has been reduced to 7%.[6] **Sick sinus syndrome** and **AV block**, **thromboembolic complications**, and progressive **AV valve deterioration** may also occur. **Obstruction of the Fontan connection or the pulmonary artery branches** are being dealt with by stent-based transcatheter pulmonary valve implantation. These patients need attention in experienced GUCH centres.[7, 8]

Therapy

Recommendations are presented in Tables 13.1 and 13.2.

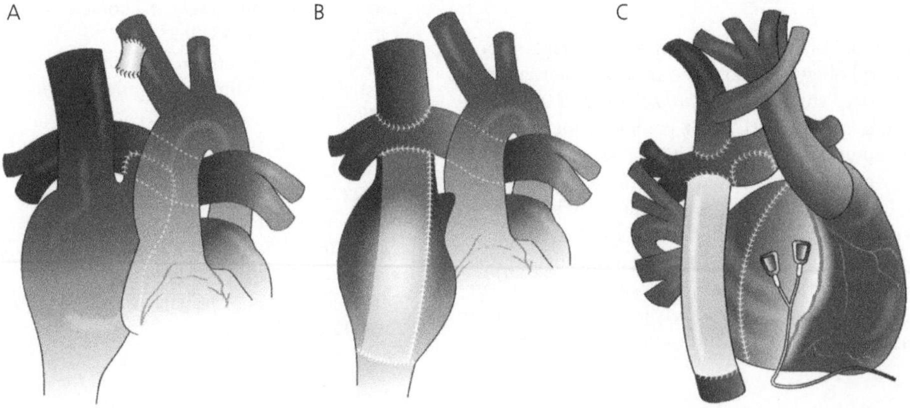

Figure 13.1 Variations of Fontan surgery. A, The modified classic Fontan. B, The intracardiac lateral tunnel Fontan. C, The extracardiac.

Khairy P, Poirier N. Is the extracardiac conduit the preferred fontan approach for patients with univentricular hearts?: the extracardiac conduit is not the preferred fontan approach for patients with univentricular hearts. *Circulation*. 2012;**126**:2516–25

Table 13.1 ESC 2010 GL on GUCH

Special considerations and indications for intervention in univentricular hearts	
Only well-selected patients after careful evaluation (low pulmonary vascular resistances, adequate function of the AV valve(s), preserved ventricular function) should be considered candidates for a Fontan operation.	IIa-C
PA banding or tightening of a previously placed band in patients with increased pulmonary blood flow (unlikely at adult age).	IIa-C
Bidirectional Glenn shunt in patients with severe cyanosis, with decreased pulmonary blood flow without elevated PVR.	IIa-C
Heart transplantation and heart-lung transplantation when there is no conventional surgical option in patients with poor clinical status.	IIa-C

ESC Guidelines for the management of grown-up congenital heart disease (new version 2010). *Eur Heart J*. 2010;**31**:2915–57.

Table 13.2 ACC/AHA 2008 GL on GUCH. Recommendations for patients with prior Fontan repair

Recommendations for medical therapy	
Warfarin with a documented atrial shunt, atrial thrombus, atrial arrhythmias, or a thromboembolic event.	I-C
ACE inhibitors and diuretics for SV dysfunction.	IIa-C
Recommendations for surgery for adults with prior Fontan repair	
Surgeons with training and expertise in CHD should perform operations on patients with prior Fontan repair for single-ventricle physiology.	I-C
Reoperation after Fontan is indicated for : a. Unintended residual ASD that results in right-to-left shunt with symptoms and/or cyanosis not amenable to transcatheter closure. b. Haemodynamically significant residual systemic artery-to-pulmonary artery shunt, residual surgical shunt, or residual ventricle-to-pulmonary artery connection not amenable to transcatheter closure. c. Moderate to severe systemic AV valve regurgitation. d. Significant (>30 mmHg peak-to-peak) subaortic obstruction. e. Fontan pathway obstruction. f. Development of venous collateral channels or pulmonary arteriovenous malformation not amenable to transcatheter management. g. Pulmonary venous obstruction. h. Rhythm abnormalities, such as complete AV block or sick sinus syndrome, that require epicardial pacemaker insertion. i. Creation or closure of a fenestration not amenable to transcatheter intervention.	I-C

(continued)

Table 13.2 (continued)

Recommendations for evaluation and follow-up after Fontan procedure	
Reoperation for Fontan conversion (i.e. revision of an atriopulmonary connection to an intracardiac lateral tunnel, intra-atrial conduit, or extracardiac conduit) for recurrent AF or flutter without haemodynamically significant anatomic abnormalities. A concomitant Maze procedure should also be performed.	IIa-C
Heart transplantation for severe SV dysfunction or protein-losing enteropathy.	IIb-C
Recommendations for electrophysiology testing/pacing issues in single-ventricle physiology and fter Fontan procedure	
Electrophysiological studies in adults with Fontan physiology should be performed at centres with expertise in the management of such patients.	I-C
New-onset atrial tachyarrhythmias should prompt a comprehensive non-invasive imaging evaluation to identify associated atrial/baffle thrombus, anatomic abnormalities of the Fontan pathway, or ventricular dysfunction.	I-C
There is high risk of symptomatic intra-atrial reentrant tachycardia (IART) in adult patients. This can cause serious haemodynamic compromise and contribute to atrial thrombus formation. Treatment is often difficult, and consultation with an electrophysiologist who is experienced with CHD is recommended.	I-C

ACC/AHA 2008 guidelines for the management of adults with congenital heart disease. *J Am Coll Cardiol.* 2008;**52**:e1–e121.

References

1. Fontan F, *et al.* Outcome after a 'perfect' Fontan operation. *Circulation.* 1990;**81**:1520–36
2. Sommer RJ, *et al.* Pathophysiology of congenital heart disease in the adult: part iii: complex congenital heart disease. *Circulation.* 2008;**117**:1340–50
3. Khairy P, *et al.* Is the extracardiac conduit the preferred Fontan approach for patients with univentricular hearts? The extracardiac conduit is not the preferred Fontan approach for patients with univentricular hearts. *Circulation.* 2012;**126**:2516–25; discussion 2525
4. Diller GP, *et al.* Predictors of morbidity and mortality in contemporary Fontan patients: results from a multicenter study including cardiopulmonary exercise testing in 321 patients. *Eur Heart J.* 2010;**31**:3073–83
5. d'Udekem Y, *et al.* Predictors of survival after single-ventricle palliation: the impact of right ventricular dominance. *J Am Coll Cardiol.* 2012;**59**:1178–85
6. Stephenson EA, *et al.* Arrhythmias in a contemporary Fontan cohort: prevalence and clinical associations in a multicenter cross-sectional study. *J Am Coll Cardiol.* 2010;**56**:890–6
7. Baumgartner H, et al. ESC guidelines for the management of grown-up congenital heart disease (new version 2010). *Eur Heart J.* 2010;**31**:2915–57
8. Warnes CA, et al. ACC/AHA 2008 guidelines for the management of adults with congenital heart disease: a report of the American College of Cardiology/American Heart Association Task Force on practice guidelines (writing committee to develop guidelines on the management of adults with congenital heart disease). Developed in collaboration with the American Society of Echocardiography, Heart Rhythm Society, International Society for Adult Congenital Heart Disease, Society for Cardiovascular Angiography and Interventions, and Society of Thoracic Surgeons. *J Am Coll Cardiol.* 2008;**52**:e143–263

Chapter 14

Eisenmenger syndrome

Definition

Eisenmenger syndrome results when elevated pulmonary vascular resistance becomes irreversible and leads to a reversal of shunt, desaturation, cyanosis, and secondary erythrocytosis.[1]

Pathophysiology

With long-standing left-to-right shunting, exposure of the pulmonary artery system to high pressure and increased flow leads to progressive arteriolar medial hypertrophy, intimal proliferation and fibrosis, and obliteration of pulmonary arterioles and capillaries. These changes are reversible, but more advanced morphologic changes, such as occlusion of small arterioles, plexiform lesions, and necrotizing arteritis, are irreversible. The precise pathophysiological mechanisms for this are not completely understood, but there is evidence that microvascular injury stimulates production of growth factors and enzymes that result in intimal proliferation and medial hypertrophy. Endothelial dysfunction and platelet activation may also play a role in

Table 14.1 ACC/AHA 2008 GL on GUCH

Recommendations for medical therapy of Eisenmenger physiology	
Avoidance of :	
a. Pregnancy.	I-B
b. Dehydration.	I-C
c. Moderate and severe strenuous exercise, particularly isometric exercise.	I-C
d. Acute exposure to excessive heat (e.g. hot tub or sauna).	I-C
e. Chronic high altitude exposure, (particularly at an elevation >5000 feet above sea level).	I-C
f. Iron deficiency.	I-B
Prompt therapy for arrhythmias and infections.	I-C
Haemoglobin, platelet count, iron stores, creatinine, and uric acid should be assessed at least yearly.	I-C
Assessment of digital oximetry, both with and without supplemental oxygen therapy, at least yearly. The presence of oxygen-responsive hypoxaemia should be investigated further.	I-C
Exclusion of air bubbles in intravenous tubing during treatment.	I-C
Non-cardiac surgery and cardiac catheterization should be performed only in centres with expertise. In emergent situations, consultation with designated caregivers should be performed.	I-C
All medications should undergo rigorous review for the potential to change systemic blood pressure, loading conditions, intravascular shunting, and renal or hepatic flow or function.	IIa-C
Pulmonary vasodilator therapy can be beneficial because of the potential for improved quality of life.	IIa-C
Recommendations for reproduction	
Patients and their partners should be counseled about the absolute avoidance of pregnancy and educated regarding safe and appropriate methods of contraception.	I-B
Women with CHD and pulmonary hypertension (CHD-PAH) who become pregnant should: a. Receive individualized counselling from cardiovascular and obstetric experts. b. Undergo the earliest possible pregnancy termination.	I-C
Surgical sterilization carries some operative risk for women with CHD-PAH but is a safer option than pregnancy.	I-C
Pregnancy termination in the last two trimesters of pregnancy poses a high risk to the mother. It may be reasonable, however, after the risks of termination are balanced against the risks of continuation of the pregnancy.	IIb-C
Pregnancy in women with CHD-PAH, especially those with Eisenmenger physiology, should be absolutely avoided in view of the high risk of maternal mortality.	III-B
The use of single barrier contraception alone in women with CHD-PAH is not recommended, owing to the frequency of failure.	III-C
Oestrogen-containing contraceptives should be avoided.	III-C

ACC/AHA 2008 guidelines for the management of adults with congenital heart disease. *J Am Coll Cardiol.* 2008;**52**:e1–e121.

the obliteration of pulmonary arterioles. When pulmonary vascular resistance approaches and exceeds systemic vascular resistance, shunting reverses and becomes right-to-left and cyanosis appears.

Clinical problems

Adult patients with Eisenmenger syndrome have a better haemodynamic profile and life expectancy compared to patients with idiopathic pulmonary arterial hypertension but poorer quality of life. Patients present with fatigue, SOBOE, palpitations. Symptoms of **hyperviscosity** (headaches, visual disturbances, dizziness, paraesthesiae), **secondary polycythaemia** and **iron deficiency**, **gallstones**, and **gouty arthritis** develop, and patients are at risk for both bleeding and thrombosis. **Symptomatic hypertrophic osteoarthropathy**, **haemoptysis**, **cerebrovascular accidents**, **pulmonary artery thrombosis**, **and brain abscess** may also be seen. Death is sudden due to arrhythmias or heart failure, but some patients die of massive haemoptysis, brain abscess, or stroke.

Physical examination

Patients are cyanotic with clubbing, but there may be no murmur during systole or diastole because shunting may be minimal.

- **V waves in JVP**
- **RV parasternal heave**
  - **S_4 and loud P_2**
  - **High-frequency diastolic decrescendo murmur of PR**

- **Holosystolic murmur of TR**
- **Peripheral oedema** may be present late in the course of disease when right ventricular dysfunction is present.

Investigations

ECG shows RV hypertophy.
Chest radiography reveals prominent central PAs with decreased vascular markings (pruning) of the peripheral vessels. Cardiomegaly may be seen in patients with ASD.
Echocardiography reveals RV pressure overload and pulmonary hypertension. Demonstration of shunting may be difficult with Doppler imaging because of the low velocity of the jet and often requires contrast echocardiography. RV dysfunction, as measured by tricuspid annular plane systolic excursion, and right atrial area and pressure are associated with worse outcomes in patients with Eisenmenger syndrome.[2,3]
Cardiac catheterization is mandatory for assessing the severity and potential reversibility of pulmonary vascular disease. PA pressure >2/3 of Ao pressure or PVR >2/3 of SVR (approximately 7 Wood units) that do not respond to vasodilators, such as oxygen, nitric oxide, adenosine, or epoprostenol, indicate irreversible pulmonary damage that does not allow intervention. The value of lung biopsy is not proven.

Therapy

The patient with Eisenmenger syndrome needs care in specialized centres. In general, intense exercise and acute heat exposure, as in hot tubs or saunas, are avoided. Annual influenza vaccination and Pneumovax every 5 years are recommended. Pregnancy in patients with Eisenmenger syndrome is not recommended, owing to excessive maternal and fetal mortality, and should be strongly discouraged.

Long-term oxygen administration for 12–15 h/day may improve symptoms but not survival. **Diuretics** should be used with caution to avoid dehydration. **Calcium channel blockers** may increase the right-to-left shunt. The use of **anticoagulation** is controversial and should be considered only if additional indications exist. **Phlebotomy** with isovolumic replacement should be reserved for moderate to severe hyperviscosity syndromes (haematocrit >65%). Vasodilator therapy is an important adjunct to management and can provide functional improvement. The dual endothelin receptor antagonist **bosentan** has been shown to improve haemodynamics and exercise capacity, and perhaps survival, and is currently recommended to all patients by the ESC guidelines. The phosphodiesterase type V inhibitor **sildenafil** that raises cGMP levels may improve functional class, oxygen saturation, and haemodynamics.

Table 14.2 ESC 2010 GL on GUCH

Recommendations for targeted pulmonary hypertension therapy in congenital heart disease	
Targeted PAH therapy in CHD should only be performed in specialized centres.	I-C
The endothelin receptor antagonist (ERA) bosentan should be initiated in WHO functional class III* patients with Eisenmenger syndrome.	I-B
Other ERAs, phosphodiesterase type 5 inhibitors, and prostanoids in WHO functional class III* patients with Eisenmenger syndrome.	IIa-C
Combination therapy may be considered in WHO functional class IIIc patients with Eisenmenger syndrome.	IIb-C
The use of calcium channel blockers should be avoided in patients with Eisenmenger syndrome.	III-C

* Although recent data support the use of ERAs, such as bosentan, also in WHO functional class II in patients with idiopathic PAH and PAH associated with connective tissue diseases, such data are currently not available for Eisenmenger patients. Because of marked differences in the natural history between these groups, the results cannot simply be applied to congenital patients, and further studies are required before recommendations.
ESC Guidelines for the management of grown-up congenital heart disease (new version 2010). *Eur Heart J.* 2010;**31**:2915–57.

Beneficial effects of the single endothelin receptor antagonist **sitaxsentan**, and **prostacyclin** and **prostacyclin analogs** have also been reported. **Heart-lung transplantation** is a therapeutic option. Recommendations for pulmonary hypertension and Eisenmenger syndrome are presented in Tables 14.1 and 14.2.[4,5]

References

1. Beghetti M, *et al.* Eisenmenger syndrome: a clinical perspective in a new therapeutic era of pulmonary arterial hypertension. *J Am Coll Cardiol.* 2009;**53**:733–40
2. Moceri P, *et al.* Echocardiographic predictors of outcome in Eisenmenger syndrome. *Circulation.* 2012;**126**:1461–8
3. Van De Bruaene A, *et al.* Right ventricular function in patients with Eisenmenger syndrome. *Am J Cardiol.* 2012;**109**:1206–11
4. Baumgartner H, *et al.* ESC guidelines for the management of grown-up congenital heart disease (new version 2010). *Eur Heart J.* 2010;**31**:2915–57
5. Warnes CA, *et al.* ACC/AHA 2008 guidelines for the management of adults with congenital heart disease: a report of the American College of Cardiology/American Heart Association Task Force on practice guidelines (writing committee to develop guidelines on the management of adults with congenital heart disease). Developed in collaboration with the American Society of Echocardiography, Heart Rhythm Society, International Society for Adult Congenital Heart Disease, Society for Cardiovascular Angiography and Interventions, and Society of Thoracic Surgeons. *J Am Coll Cardiol.* 2008;**52**:e143–263

Part II

Valve disease

Relevant Guidelines

ACC/AHA 2008 guidelines on valve disease

2008 focused update incorporated into the ACC/AHA 2006 guidelines for the management of patients with valvular heart disease. *J Am Coll Cardiol.* 2008;**52**:e1–142.

ESC 2012 guidelines on valve disease

Guidelines on the management of valvular heart disease (version 2012). The Joint Task Force on the management of valvular heart disease of the European Society of Cardiology (ESC) and the European Association for Cardio-Thoracic Surgery (EACTS) *Eur Heart J.* 2012;**33**:2451–96

ESC 2009 guidelines on infective endocarditis

Guidelines on the prevention, diagnosis, and treatment of infective endocarditis (new version 2009): the Task Force on the prevention, diagnosis, and treatment of infective endocarditis of the European Society of Cardiology (ESC). Endorsed by the European Society of Clinical Microbiology and Infectious Diseases (ESCMID) and the International Society of Chemotherapy (ISC) for Infection and Cancer. *Eur Heart J.* 2009;**30**:2369–413

ESC 2011 guidelines on pregnancy 2011

ESC Guidelines on the management of cardiovascular diseases during pregnancy. *Eur Heart J.* 2011;**32**:3147–97

ACCF/AATS/SCAI/STS 2012 Expert Consensus Document on TAVI 2012

2012 ACCF/AATS/SCAI/STS expert consensus document on transcatheter aortic valve replacement. *J Am Coll Cardiol.* 2012;**59**:1200–54

ACCP 2012 guidelines on antithrombotic therapy

American College of Chest Physicians Antithrombotic Therapy and Prevention of Thrombosis Panel. Executive summary: antithrombotic therapy and prevention of thrombosis, 9th ed: American College of Chest Physicians evidence-based clinical practice guidelines. *Chest.* 2012;**141**(2 Suppl):7S–47S. Erratum in: *Chest.* 2012;**141**:1129

ACCF/AHA 2011 Guideline on CABG 2011

2011 ACCF/AHA Guideline on CABG. *Circulation.* 2011;**124**:2610–42

ESC 2010 guidelines on revascularization

ESC Guidelines on myocardial revascularization. *Eur Heart J.* 2010;**31**:2501–55

ACC/AHA 2008 guidelines on GUCH

ACC/AHA 2008 guidelines for the management of adults with congenital heart disease. *J Am Coll Cardiol.* 2008;**52**:e1–e121

ESC 2010 guidelines on GUCH 2010

ESC Guidelines for the management of grown-up congenital heart disease (new version 2010). *Eur Heart J.* 2010;**31**:2915–57

ESC 2001 Task Force report on aortic dissection

Task Force on aortic dissection, European Society of Cardiology. Diagnosis and management of aortic dissection. *Eur Heart J.* 2001;**22**:1642–81

ACC/AHA 2010 Guidelines on thoracic aortic disease

2010 ACCF/AHA/AATS/ACR/ASA/SCA/SCAI/SIR/STS/SVM Guidelines for the diagnosis and management of patients with thoracic aortic disease. *J Am Coll Cardiol.* 2010;**55**:e27–e129

Chapter 15

General principles

Epidemiology

The prevalence of any valve disease in the general population in the USA is 2.5%, and increases with age, from 0.7% in persons 18-44 year-old to 13.2% in those ≥75years.[1] Data are provided by epidemiological studies such as the CARDIA (Coronary Artery Risk Development in Young Adults), ARIC (Atherosclerosis Risk in Communities), and CHS (Cardiovascular Health Study), as well as the Olmsted County community study. Survival of participants in those studies with valve disease is 79% at 5 years compared with 93% in participants without valve disease.[2] Approximately 0.4% have aortic stenosis (AS), 0.5% aortic regurgitation (AR), 0.1% mitral stenosis (MS), and 1.7% mitral regurgitation (MR).2 In Europe data are collected by the EuroHeart Survey among patients with established valve disease. Prevalence is AS 43%, MR 31.5%, AR 13.3%, and MS 12.1%.[3]

Cardiac auscultation

Heart sounds

First sound (S_1) is due to simultaneous MV and TV closure.

- **Loud:** MS, hyperkinetic states, short PR <160 ms
- **Soft:** long PR (>200 ms), severe MS, LV dysfunction
- **Widely split:** RBBB.

Second sound (S_2) is due to AV followed by PV closure. Splitting normally increases with inspiration. A loud P_2 suggests pulmonary hypertension.

- **Single:** AS or PS
- **Widely split:** RBBB, MR
- **Fixed splitting:** ASD
- **Reversed splitting:** LBBB, AS, hypertrophic cardiomyopathy (HCM), RV pacing.

Third sound (S_3) is pathological over the age of 30 years. Probably due to rapid LV filling. Audible in LV failure, severe MR, VSD. A high-pitched S_3 may be heard in restrictive cardiomyopathy and pericardial constriction.
Fourth sound (S_4) corresponds to atrial contraction and is produced at end-diastole before S_1. It can be heard in conditions with LVH or after acute MI.
Ejection sound Bicuspid AV or PS.
Mid-systolic (non-ejection) click Mitral valve prolapse (MVP).
Opening snap MS, rarely TS, Ebstein's anomaly.

Murmurs

Murmurs are produced by turbulent blood flow, and are described according to their location, intensity, timing, frequency, and radiation (Tables 15.1 to 15.3 and Figure 15.1).
Innocent murmurs are due to pulmonary flow and can be heard in children, pregnancy, and high-flow states, such as hyperthyroidism and anaemia. They are heard over the left sternal edge and are ejection systolic, and there are no added sounds or thrill. The **cervical venous hum** is a continuous murmur, common in children and typically reduced by turning the head laterally or bending the elbows back. The **mammary soufflé** is a continuous murmur that may be heard in pregnancy.
Dynamic auscultation manoeuvres may help bedside diagnosis of systolic murmurs (Table 15.2).[4,5] Murmurs originating within the right-sided chambers of the heart can be differentiated from all other murmurs by augmentation of their intensity with inspiration and diminution with expiration. The murmur of hypertrophic cardiomyopathy is distinguished from all other systolic murmurs by an increase in intensity with the Valsalva manoeuvre and during squatting-to-standing, and by a decrease in intensity during standing-to-squatting action, passive leg elevation, and handgrip. The murmurs of MR and VSD have similar responses but can be differentiated from other systolic murmurs by augmentation of their intensity with handgrip and during transient arterial occlusion.[4]

Table 15.1 Heart murmurs

Systolic	
Early	Acute MR, VSD, TR.
Mid-systolic	AS (valvular, supra- or subvalvular), AR, HCM, PS (valvular, supra- or subvalvular), ASD.
Late systolic	MR due to MVP or chordal rupture, TR.
Pansystolic	MR, TR, VSD.
Diastolic	
Early	AR (valvular or due to dilation of the ring, bicuspid AV), PR (valvular or due to dilation of the ring, congenital).
Mid-diastolic	MS, Carey Coombs, VSD, PDA, ASD, TR, AR.
Late diastolic	Presystolic accentuation of MS, Austin Flint.
Continuous	
Coronary or intercostal AV fistula or anomalous left coronary artery, PDA, ruptured sinus of Valsalva aneurysm, ASD, cervical venous hum, mammary soufflé of pregnancy.	

Table 15.2 ACC/AHA 2008 GL on valve disease

Interventions used to alter the intensity of cardiac murmurs
Respiration
Right-sided murmurs generally increase with inspiration. Left-sided murmurs usually are louder during expiration.
Valsalva manoeuvre
Most murmurs decrease in length and intensity. Two exceptions are the systolic murmur of HCM, which usually becomes much louder, and that of MVP, which becomes longer and often louder. After release of the Valsalva, right-sided murmurs tend to return to baseline intensity earlier than left-sided murmurs.
Exercise
Murmurs caused by blood flow across normal or obstructed valves (e.g. PS and MS) become louder with both isotonic and isometric (handgrip) exercise.
Murmurs of MR, VSD, and AR also increase with handgrip exercise.
Positional changes
With standing, most murmurs diminish, two exceptions being the murmur of HCM, which becomes louder, and that of MVP, which lengthens and often is intensified. With brisk squatting, most murmurs become louder, but those of HCM and MVP usually soften and may disappear. Passive leg raising usually produces the same results as brisk squatting.
Post-ventricular premature beat or atrial fibrillation
Murmurs originating at normal or stenotic semilunar valves increase in intensity during the cardiac cycle after a VPB or in the beat after a long cycle length. In AF, by contrast, systolic murmurs due to atrioventricular valve regurgitation do not change, diminish (papillary muscle dysfunction), or become shorter (MVP).
Pharmacological interventions
During the initial relative hypotension after amyl nitrite inhalation, murmurs of MR, VSD, and AR decrease, whereas murmurs of AS increase because of increased stroke volume. During the later tachycardia phase, murmurs of MS and right-sided lesions also increase. This intervention may thus distinguish the murmur of the Austin Flint phenomenon from that of MS. The response in MVP often is biphasic (softer, then louder than control).
Transient arterial occlusion
Transient external compression of both arms by bilateral cuff inflation to 20 mmHg greater than peak systolic pressure augments the murmurs of MR, VSD, and AR, but not murmurs due to other causes.
AF indicates atrial fibrillation; AR, aortic regurgitation; AS, aortic stenosis; HCM, hypertrophic cardiomyopathy; MR, mitral regurgitation; MS, mitral stenosis; MVP, mitral valve prolapse; PS, pulmonic stenosis; VPB, ventricular premature beat; and VSD, ventricular septal defect.

ACC/AHA guidelines on valve disease 2008 focused update incorporated into the ACC/AHA 2006 guidelines for the management of patients with valvular heart disease. *J Am Coll Cardiol*. 2008;**52**:e1–142.

Table 15.3 ESC 2012 GL on VD. Management of coronary artery disease in patients with valvular heart disease

Diagnosis of coronary artery disease	
Coronary angiography[a] is recommended before valve surgery in patients with severe valvular heart disease and any of the following: • History of coronary artery disease • Suspected myocardial ischaemia[b] • Left ventricular systolic dysfunction • In men aged over 40 years and post-menopausal women • ≥1 cardiovascular risk factor.	I-C
Coronary angiography is recommended in the evaluation of secondary mitral regurgitation.	I-C
Indications for myocardial revascularization	
CABG is recommended in patients with a primary indication for aortic/mitral valve surgery and coronary artery diameter stenosis ≥70%.[c]	I-C
CABG should be considered in patients with a primary indication for aortic/mitral valve surgery and coronary artery diameter stenosis ≥50–70%.	IIa-C

[a] Multi-slice computed tomography may be used to exclude coronary artery disease in patients who are at low risk of atherosclerosis.
[b] Chest pain, abnormal non-invasive testing.
[c] ≥50% can be considered for left main stenosis.
ESC guidelines on the management of valvular heart disease (version 2012). *European Heart Journal* 2012;**33**:2451–2496.

Coronary angiography

Indications are presented in Tables 15.3 and 15.4.[6] They are also discussed in individual chapters (see also Chapter 84).

Endocarditis prophylaxis

Prophylaxis is now indicated only in high-risk patients (i.e. patients with prosthetic cardiac valves or prosthetic material used for cardiac valve repair, patients with previous infective endocarditis, and cardiac transplant recipients with valve regurgitation due to a structurally abnormal valve) and only before dental procedures that involve manipulation of gingival tissue or the periapical region of teeth or perforation of the oral mucosa and before vaginal delivery. Prophylaxis against infective endocarditis is not recommended for non-dental procedures (such as transoesophageal echocardiogram, oesophagogastroduodenoscopy, or colonoscopy) in the absence of active infection. In patients with unoperated valve disease, prophylaxis is not recommended any more for any procedure. For a detailed discussion see Chapter 79 on infective endocarditis.

Pregnancy

Valvular lesions associated with high maternal and/or fetal risk during pregnancy are (see also Chapter 84):[7]

- MS with NYHA functional class II–IV symptoms
- Severe AS with or without symptoms
- AR or MR with NYHA functional class III–IV symptoms
- Severe pulmonary hypertension (pulmonary pressure >2/3 of systemic pressures) or LV dysfunction (LVEF <40%)
- Mechanical prosthetic valve requiring anticoagulation
- Marfan's syndrome with or without aortic regurgitation.

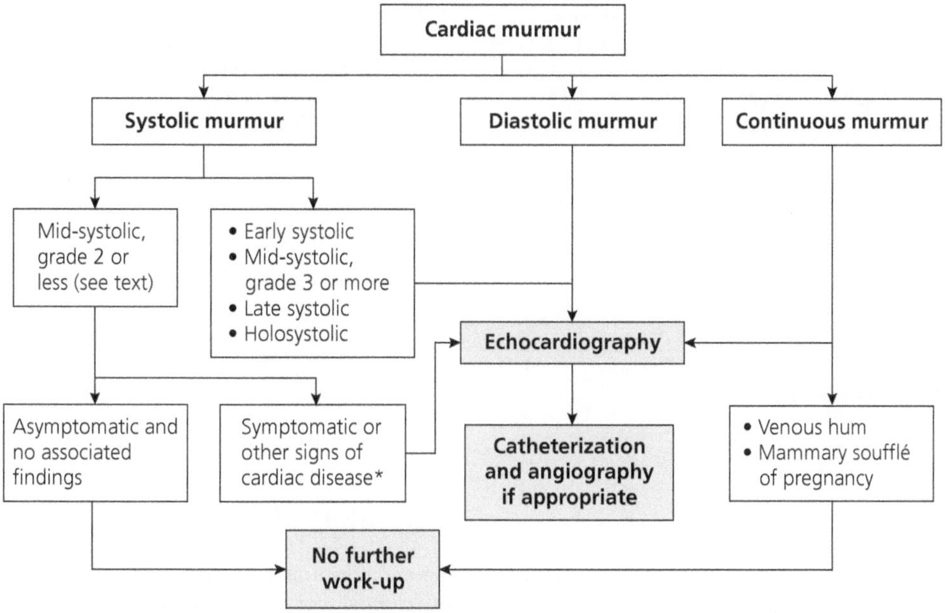

Figure 15.1 ACC/AHA 2008 guidelines on VD. Strategy for evaluating heart murmurs

* If an electrocardiogram or chest X-ray has been obtained and is abnormal, echocardiography is indicated.

ACC/AHA 2008 focused update incorporated into the ACC/AHA 2006 guidelines for the management of patients with valvular heart disease. *J Am Coll Cardiol*. 2008;**52**:e1–142

Table 15.4 ACC/AHA 2008 GL on VD. Diagnosis of coronary artery disease

Coronary angiography before valve surgery (including infective endocarditis) or mitral balloon commissurotomy in patients with chest pain, other objective evidence of ischaemia, decreased LV systolic function, history of CAD, or coronary risk factors (including age). Patients undergoing MBC need not undergo coronary angiography solely on the basis of coronary risk factors.	I-C
Coronary angiography in patients with apparently mild to moderate valvular heart disease but with progressive angina (Canadian Heart Association ≥II), objective evidence of ischaemia, decreased LV systolic function, or overt congestive heart failure.	I-C
Coronary angiography performed before valve surgery in men aged 35 years or older, premenopausal women aged 35 years or older who have coronary risk factors, and post-menopausal women.	I-C
Coronary angiography can be deferred for patients having emergency valve surgery for acute valve regurgitation, aortic root disease, or infective endocarditis.	IIa-C
Coronary angiography for patients undergoing catheterization to confirm the severity of valve lesions before valve surgery without pre-existing evidence of CAD, multiple coronary risk factors, or advanced age.	IIb-C
Coronary angiography in young patients undergoing non-emergency valve surgery when no further haemodynamic assessment by catheterization is deemed necessary and there are no coronary risk factors, history of CAD, or evidence of ischaemia.	III-C
Coronary angiography before valve surgery in severely haemodynamically unstable patients.	III-C

ACC/AHA 2008 focused update incorporated into the ACC/AHA 2006 guidelines for the management of patients with valvular heart disease. *J Am Coll Cardiol*. 2008;**52**:e1–142.

Valve disease in pregnancy is also discussed in chapters on specific valve diseases.

References

1. Nkomo VT, *et al.* Burden of valvular heart diseases: A population-based study. *Lancet*. 2006;**368**:1005–1011
2. Go AS, *et al.* Heart disease and stroke statistics—2013 update: a report from the American Heart Association. *Circulation*. 2013;**127**:e6–245
3. Iung B, *et al.* A prospective survey of patients with valvular heart disease in europe: The euro heart survey on valvular heart disease. *Eur Heart J*. 2003;**24**:1231–43
4. Lembo NJ, *et al.* Bedside diagnosis of systolic murmurs. *N Engl J Med*. 1988;**318**:1572–8
5. Ma I, *et al.* Name that murmur—eponyms for the astute auscultician. *N Engl J Med*. 2010;**363**:2164–8
6. Patel MR, *et al.* ACCF/SCAI/AATS/AHA/ASE/ASNC/HFSA/HRS/SCCM/SCCT/SCMR/STS 2012 appropriate use criteria for diagnostic catheterization: a report of the American College of Cardiology Foundation Appropriate Use Criteria Task Force, Society for Cardiovascular Angiography and Interventions, American Association for Thoracic Surgery, American Heart Association, American Society of Echocardiography, American Society of Nu-

clear Cardiology, Heart Failure Society of America, Heart Rhythm Society, Society of Critical Care Medicine, Society of Cardiovascular Computed Tomography, Society for Cardiovascular Magnetic Resonance, and Society of Thoracic Surgeons. *J Am Coll Cardiol.* 2012;**59**:1995–2027

7. Regitz-Zagrosek V, *et al.* ESC guidelines on the management of cardiovascular diseases during pregnancy: the Task force on the management of cardiovascular diseases during pregnancy of the European Society of Cardiology (ESC). *Eur Heart J.* 2011;**32**:3147–97

Chapter 16

Mitral stenosis

Epidemiology

Mitral stenosis (MS) is highly prevalent in developing countries because of its association with rheumatic fever (6/1000 children in India vs 0.5/1000 in developed countries) but is also seen in developed countries where patients are of increased age.[1,2] In developed countries, the prevalence of MS detected by echocardiography is about 0.1–0.2%.[3] Although the attack rate for rheumatic fever is roughly equal among genders, MS is 2 to 3 times more common in women.

Aetiology

Rheumatic fever is the main cause of MS, although less than 60% of affected patients provide a relevant history.[1,2] The M protein antigen held in common between the heart and group A haemolytic Streptococcus results in an autoimmune attack of the heart in response to streptococcal infection. The rheumatic process leads to inflammation of endocardium, myocardium, and pericardium, but the disease affects mainly the endocardium. Persistent inflammatory valve damage results in gradual progression that is strongly associated with repeated episodes of rheumatic fever. In the western world, symptoms of MS usually appear after 15 to 20 years following the rheumatic fever attack. **Degenerative** causes may be identified in up to 12.5% in developed countries.[4] In 6–8% of patients with severe **mitral annular calcification**, who are often elderly or dialysis-dependent, calcium encroaching into the valve leaflets causes mitral stenosis. Other rare causes are **congenital MS (Lutembacher syndrome when combined with ASD, mucopolysaccharidoses, Fabry's disease, systemic lupus erythematosus, rheumatoid arthritis, anorectic drugs**, and disorders associated with abnormal serotonin metabolism (**carcinoid and methysergide treatment**).[1]

Pathophysiology and natural history

The main features are leaflet thickening and calcification with chordal shortening and fusion.[1,2] Patients usually have a dilated and stiff LA and may develop systolic and diastolic LV dysfunction. Procoagulation abnormalities are common. The normal mitral valve area is 4–5 cm^2, and a gradient is rare, unless the valve is less than 2 cm^2. The valve area narrows gradually by 0.1–0.3 cm^2 per year, and symptoms start when the mitral valve area becomes less than 1.5 cm^2. Pulmonary ooedema may develop with valve areas <1 cm^2 (Table 16.1). Patients with pulmonary ooedema rarely have severe pulmonary arterial hypertension whereas those with severe hypertension (pulmonary vascular resistance >6–8 Wood units) seem to present with right heart failure rather than pulmonary oedema. The 10-year survival of untreated patients presenting with MS is 50–60%, depending on symptoms at presentation. Death in neglected cases is mainly due to heart failure or systemic embolism.

Table 16.1 Classification of MS

ACC/AHA 2008 GL on valve disease. Classification of the severity of mitral valve stenosis in adults

	Mild	Moderate	Severe
Mean gradient (mmHg)	<5	5–10	>10
PA systolic pressure (mmHg)	<30	30–50	>50
Valve area (cm^2)	>1.5	1–1.5	<1

ESC 2012 Guidelines on valve disease. Definition of severe mitral stenosis

Valve area <1 cm^2.

Mean gradient >10 mmHg (in patients with sinus rhythm, to be interpreted according to heart rate).

ACC/AHA 2008 focused update incorporated into the ACC/AHA 2006 guidelines for the management of patients with valvular heart disease. *J Am Coll Cardiol.* 2008;**52**:e1–142.

ESC guidelines on the management of valvular heart disease (version 2012). *European Heart Journal* 2012;**33**:2451–2496

Presentation

Patients usually present with **SOBOE** or **fatigue**. Later symptoms include **haemoptysis** (pulmonary ooedema or bronchial vein rupture), **chest pain**, and **systemic embolism**. The enlarged left atrium may impinge on the left recurrent laryngeal nerve, causing hoarseness (**Ortner's syndrome**). **Atrial fibrillation** occurs in approximately 50% of patients with mitral stenosis, precipitates such symptoms, greatly increases the risk of systemic embolization, and reduces cardiac output and exercise capacity. **Pulmonary arterial hypertension** is reversible and resolves after intervention. Moderate to severe **tricuspid regurgitation** is seen in up to a third of patients with mitral stenosis and may not be improved with valvuloplasty and, if severe, requires ring annuloplasty at time of mitral surgery. It usually results from RV dilation and, if severe, requires ring annuloplasty at time of mitral surgery. **Rheumatic AR** is associated with MS that may blunt the presentation of AR due to reduced cardiac output.

Physical examination

Mitral facies with plethoric bluish cheeks with telangiectases are now rarely seen.

- **A diastolic thrill** may be palpated in the left lateral decubitus position.
- **Increased intensity of the S_1** because the transmitral gradient holds the mitral valve open for all of diastole so that ventricular systole closes the mitral valve from a long moment arm. In advanced disease, S_1 may become soft.
- **Mitral valve opening snap** The distance from S_2 is a measure of MS severity. An S_2 opening snap interval <0.08 s usually indicates severe disease.
- **A low-pitched mitral rumble** follows the opening snap. **Presystolic accentuation** of the murmur audible in normal sinus rhythm or during long RR intervals in atrial fibrillation indicates tight stenosis.
- A high-pitched blowing murmur (**Graham Steell**) may be heard at the cardiac base. Although this murmur is thought to represent the PR of pulmonary hypertension, in reality, it is more often due to concomitant AR.[5]
- **Pulse pressure** may also be reduced in advanced disease.
- **Elevated JVP, TR, hepatomegaly, ascites, and peripheral oedema** may be found in severe pulmonary hypertension and RV failure.
- **P_2** increased in pulmonary hypertension.

Investigations

ECG Left atrial enlargement (P wave >0.12 s in lead II) and RV hypertrophy, often with AF.

Chest radiography Left atrial enlargement and, in longstanding MS, pulmonary congestion and pulmonary arterial hypertension. Interstitial oedema is manifested as Kerley A lines (dense, short, horizontal lines at the costophrenic angles) or Kerley B lines (straight, dense lines towards the hilum).

Echocardiography is used to exclude conditions that mimic mitral stenosis (atrial myxoma, tricuspid stenosis, ball-valve thrombus, or ASD), calculate valve area, assess mitral regurgitation, and provide information about suitability for percutaneous balloon valvuloplasty (PBV).

Stenosis severity is determined by:

Planimetry The most reliable method to calculate valve area is planimetry with 2D or 3D echocardiography. 2D echocardiography underestimates the severity of mitral stenosis, especially moderate to severe disease and underestimates the extent of commissural splitting by PBV.

Doppler-derived pressure half-time Valve area is given by the empirical formula 220/PHT (Figures 16.1 and 16.2). This method is affected by left ventricular chamber compliance and heart rate.

Transoesophageal echocardiography provides an improved image of the commissural anatomy and calcification and allows detection of left atrial appendage thrombus and calculation of the echo score (Table 16.2).

Exercise or dobutamine stress echocardiography is needed for patients with inconclusive symptoms or haemodynamics.

Cardiac catheterization is rarely needed, with imaging methods now available (echo, cardiac CT and MRI). It is indicated when the non-invasive tests are inconclusive to resolve the issue of stenosis severity and evaluate MR (Table 16.3). Cardiac output and transvalvular gradient measurements are used to calculate valve area with the Gorlin formula to reassess stenosis severity (Figure 16.3). It may also be used to assess the response of PA and LA pressures to exercise or to assess the cause of pulmonary arterial hypertension when it is inproportional to MS severity.[6]

Coronary angiography is indicated only in patients with evidence of myocardial ischaemia (Tables 15.3 and 15.4 in Chapter 15 on general principles).

Therapy

Medical

Diuretics and beta blockers or rate-slowing calcium channel blockers (e.g. diltiazem) are the mainstay for control of heart rate. The role of statins in slowing progression of MS is under investigation.

Anticoagulation is indicated in AF or prior embolic event or left atrial thrombus (Table 16.4).[6]

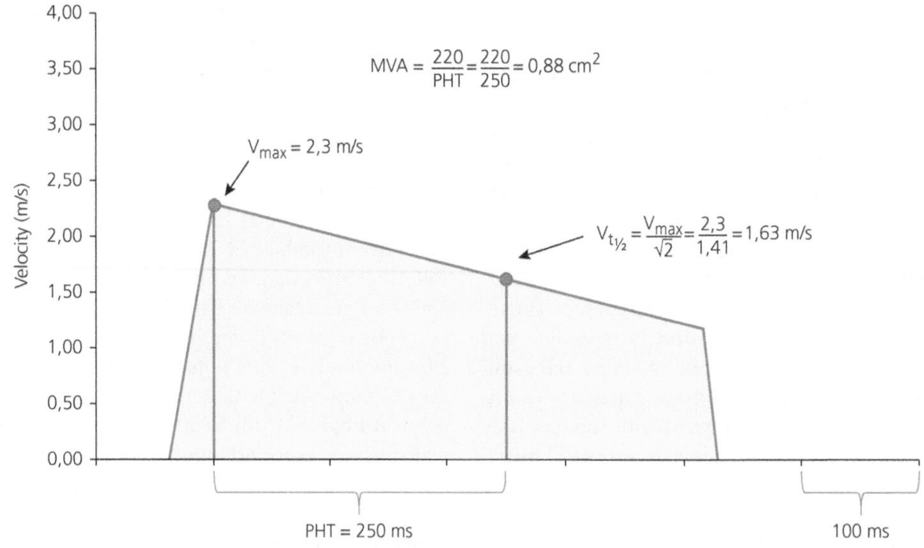

Figure 16.1 Pressure half-time is the time taken for the pressure to halve from the peak value. It is the same as the time for peak velocity to decrease to a velocity equal to the peak velocity divided by the square root of 2 (= 1.4).

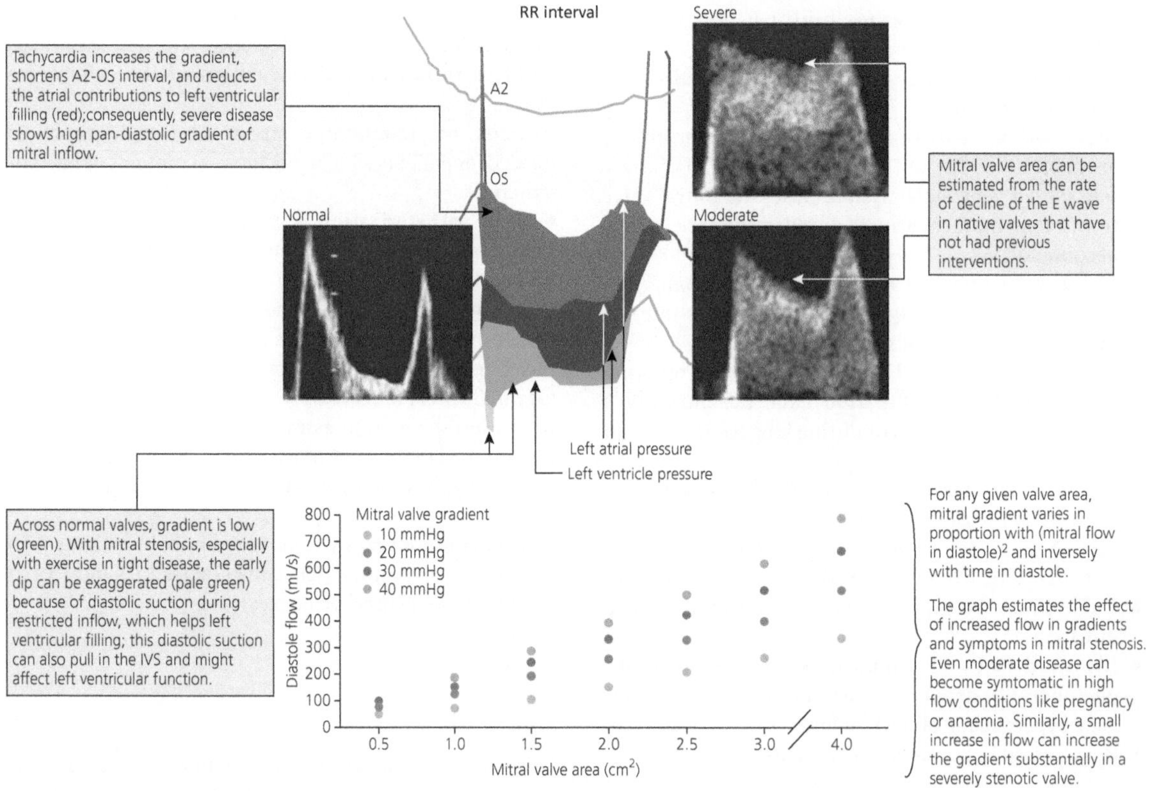

Figure 16.2 Physiology of severity of mitral stenosis. Gradient between left atrium and left ventricle is shown as normal to very low (green), moderate (black), and severe (red). Arrows indicate the extent of gradient towards the end of diastole. A2–OS, A2 to opening snap interval; IVS, interventricular septum.

Chandrashekhar Y, *et al*. Mitral stenosis. *Lancet*. 2009;**374**:1271–83.

Table 16.2 Wilkins echocardiographic mitral valve score

Grade	Mobility	Subvalvular thickening	Thickening	Calcification
1	Highly mobile valve with only leaflet tips restricted	Minimal thickening just below the mitral leaflets	Leaflets near normal in thickness (4 to 5 mm)	A single area of increased echo brightness
2	Leaflet mid- and base portions have normal mobility	Thickening of chordal structures extending up to one-third of the chordal length	Midleaflets normal, considerable thickening of margins (5 to 8 mm)	Scattered areas of brightness confined to leaflet margins
3	Valve continues to move forward in diastole, mainly from the base	Thickening extending to the distal third of the chords	Thickening extending through the entire leaflet (5–8 mm)	Brightness extending into the mid-portions of the leaflets
4	No or minimal forward movement of the leaflets in diastole	Extensive thickening and shortening of all chordal structures extending down to the papillary muscles	Considerable thickening of all leaflet tissue (>8–10 mm)	Extensive brightness throughout much of the leaflet tissue

Wilkins GT, *et al. Br Heart J.* 1988;**60**:299–308.

Table 16.3 ACC AHA 2008 GL on valve disease

Indications for invasive haemodynamic evaluation	
Cardiac catheterization for assessment of severity of MS when non-invasive tests are inconclusive or when there is discrepancy between non-invasive tests and clinical findings regarding severity of MS.	I-C
Catheterization, including left ventriculography (to evaluate severity of MR), for patients with MS is indicated when there is a discrepancy between the Doppler-derived mean gradient and valve area.	I-C
Cardiac catheterization to assess the haemodynamic response of pulmonary artery and left atrial pressures to exercise when clinical symptoms and resting haemodynamics are discordant.	IIa-C
Cardiac catheterization to assess the cause of severe pulmonary arterial hypertension when out of proportion to severity of MS as determined by non-invasive testing.	IIa-C
Diagnostic cardiac catheterization is not recommended to assess the MV haemodynamics when 2D and Doppler echocardiographic data are concordant with clinical findings.	III-C

ACC/AHA 2008 focused update incorporated into the ACC/AHA 2006 guidelines for the management of patients with valvular heart disease. *J Am Coll Cardiol.* 2008;52:e1–142.

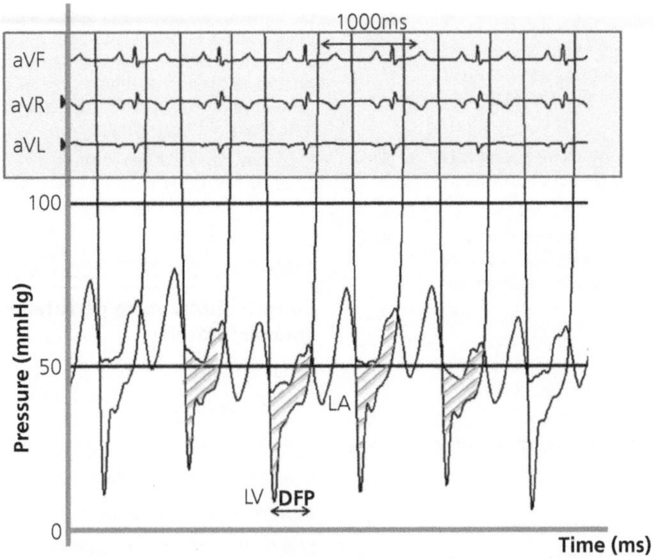

Figure 16.3 Calculation of mitral valve area (MVA) in the catheter laboratory.

MVA = mitral valve flow (mL/s)/31$\sqrt{\text{mean mitral gradient (mmHg)}}$.

Mitral valve flow = angiographic cardiac output (mL/min)/diastolic filling period (s/min). 31 is the Gorlin constant, assuming LVEDP of 5 mmHg.

Systemic embolization may occur in 10–20% of patients with MS, even in the absence of left atrial thrombi. Retrospective studies indicate a 4–15-fold decrease in the incidence of embolic events with anticoagulation.[6]

AF develops in 30–40% of patients and is associated with a poorer prognosis (10-year survival 25% compared to 46% in SR). Pharmaceutical or electrical cardioversion is recommended after transoesophageal exclusion of left appendix thrombi or following 3 weeks of warfarin under IV heparin. Warfarin is continued after cardioversion for, at least, one month or indefinitely, if indicated.

Table 16.4 ACC/AHA 2008 GL on valve disease

Medical therapy: prevention of systemic embolization	
Anticoagulation in patients with MS and AF (paroxysmal, persistent, or permanent).	I-B
Anticoagulation in patients with MS and a prior embolic event, even in sinus rhythm.	I-B
Anticoagulation in patients with MS with left atrial thrombus.	I-B
Anticoagulation for asymptomatic patients with severe MS and left atrial dimension ≥55 mm by echocardiography.	IIb-B
Anticoagulation for patients with severe MS, an enlarged left atrium, and spontaneous contrast on echocardiography.	IIb-C

ACC/AHA 2008 focused update incorporated into the ACC/AHA 2006 guidelines for the management of patients with valvular heart disease. *J Am Coll Cardiol*. 2008;**52**:e1–142.

Table 16.5 ACC/AHA 2008 GL on valve disease

Indications for percutaneous mitral balloon valvotomy (PMBV)	
Symptomatic patients (NYHA II, III, or IV), with moderate or severe MS and valve morphology favourable for percutaneous mitral balloon valvotomy in the absence of left atrial thrombus or moderate to severe MR.	I-A
Asymptomatic patients with moderate or severe MS and valve morphology that is favourable for PMBV, who have pulmonary hypertension (PA systolic pressure >50 mmHg at rest or >60 mmHg with exercise) in the absence of left atrial thrombus or moderate to severe MR.	I-C
Patients with moderate or severe MS who have a non-pliable calcified valve, are in NYHA III–IV, and are not candidates or at high risk for surgery.	IIa-C
Asymptomatic patients with moderate or severe MS and valve morphology favourable for PMBV who have new onset of AF in the absence of left atrial thrombus or moderate to severe MR.	IIb-C
Symptomatic patients (NYHA II, III, or IV) with MV area >1.5 cm^2 and evidence of significant MS (PA systolic pressure >60 mmHg, PA wedge pressure ≥25 mmHg, or mean MV gradient >15 mmHg during exercise).	IIb-C
PMBV as an alternative to surgery for patients with moderate or severe MS who have a non-pliable calcified valve and are in NYHA III–IV.	IIb-C
Patients with mild MS.	III-C
Patients with moderate to severe MR or left atrial thrombus.	III-C

ACC/AHA 2008 focused update incorporated into the ACC/AHA 2006 guidelines for the management of patients with valvular heart disease. *J Am Coll Cardiol*. 2008;**52**:e1–142.

Interventional/surgical

As with all valvular heart disease, no randomized trials have been performed to ascertain the best timing of intervention. Recommendations are based on observational data.[6,7]

Percutaneous mitral balloon valvotomy (PMBV), or commisurotomy (PMC) improves survival, especially in patients with NYHA class III or IV (Tables 16.5 to 16.7, and Figures 16.4 to 16.7). The technique is as effective as open valvotomy and more effective than closed valvotomy.[8] Nearly half of all patients who undergo percutaneous

Table 16.6 ESC 2012 GL on valve disease

Indications for percutaneous mitral commissurotomy (PMC) in mitral stenosis with valve area ≤1.5 cm^2	
Symptomatic patients with favourable characteristics* for PMC.	I-B
Symptomatic patients with contraindication or high risk for surgery.	I-C
As initial treatment in symptomatic patients with unfavourable anatomy but favourable clinical characteristics.	IIa-C
Asymptomatic patients without unfavourable characteristics and:	IIa-C
High thromboembolic risk (previous history of embolism), dense spontaneous contrast in the left atrium, recent or paroxysmal AF, and/or high risk of haemodynamic decompensation (systolic pulmonary pressure >50 mmHg at rest, need for major non-cardiac surgery, desire of pregnancy	

* Unfavourable characteristics for percutaneous mitral commissurotomy can be defined by the presence of several of the following characteristics:
Clinical characteristics: old age, history of commissurotomy, NYHA class IV, permanent atrial fibrillation, severe pulmonary hypertension.
Anatomical characteristics: echo score >8, Cormier score 3 (calcification of mitral valve of any extent, as assessed by fluoroscopy), very small mitral valve area, severe tricuspid regurgitation.

ESC Guidelines on the management of valvular heart disease (version 2012). *European Heart Journal* 2012;**33**:2451–2496.

Table 16.7 ESC 2012 GL on valve disease

Contraindications to percutaneous mitral commissurotomy
Mitral valve area >1.5 cm^2.
Left atrial thrombus.
More than mild MR.
Severe or bicommissural calcification.
Absence of commissural fusion.
Severe concomitant aortic valve disease or severe combined TS and TR.
Concomitant coronary artery disease requiring bypass surgery.

ESC Guidelines on the management of valvular heart disease (version 2012). *European Heart Journal* 2012;**33**:2451–2496.

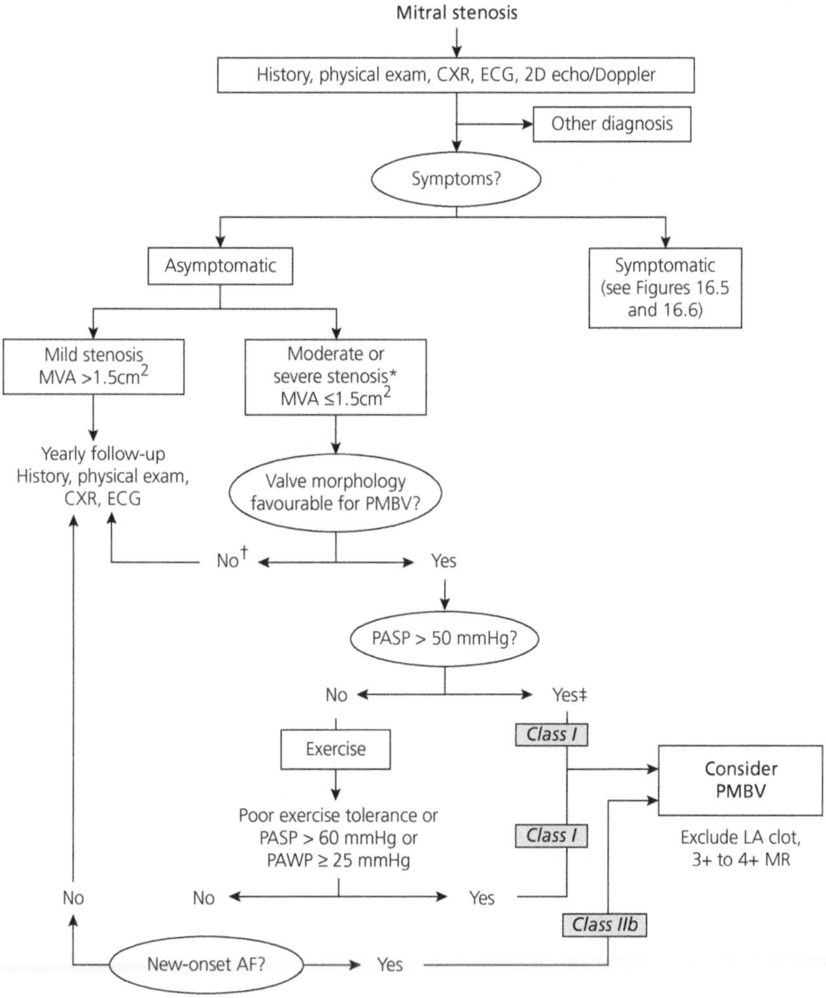

Figure 16.4 ACC/AHA 2008 GL on valve disease. Management strategy for patients with mitral stenosis.

* There may be variability in the measurement of mitral valve area (MVA), and the mean transmitral gradients, pulmonary artery wedge pressure (PAWP), and pulmonary artery systolic pressure (PP) should also be taken into consideration.

† There is controversy as to whether patients with severe mitral stenosis (MVA <1.0 cm^2) and severe pulmonary hypertension (pulmonary artery pressure >60 mmHg) should undergo percutaneous mitral balloon valvotomy (PMBV) or mitral valve replacement to prevent right ventricular failure.

‡ Assuming no other cause for pulmonary hypertension is present.

AF indicates atrial fibrillation; CXR, chest X-ray; ECG, electrocardiogram; echo, echocardiography; LA, left atrial; MR, mitral regurgitation; and 2D, two-dimensional.

ACC/AHA 2008 focused update incorporated into the ACC/AHA 2006 guidelines for the management of patients with valvular heart disease. *J Am Coll Cardiol.* 2008;**52**:e1–142

mitral commissurotomy remain free from cardiovascular death or surgery at 20 years, and 25% of them need a repeat preocedure.[9] Successful PMBV is usually defined as a post-procedure mitral valve area of >1.5 cm^2 with no more than moderate mitral regurgitation. Suitability for PMBV is determined by valve morphology and the amount of mitral regurgitation present. The Wilkins score (Table 16.2) is the most widely used echo score and gives a rough guide to the suitability of the valve morphology for PMBV. This scoring system assigns a point value from 1 to 4 for each of (1) valve calcification, (2) leaflet mobility, (3) leaflet thickening, and (4) disease of the subvalvular apparatus. In general, patients with a score of <8–9, with no calcification and less than moderate mitral regurgitation, have the best outcomes, although many patients have benefited from PMBV despite higher valve scores. Patients with favourable morphology have more than 90% procedural success, very low occurrence of complications (<2%), and acceptably low frequency of re-stenosis on follow-up. Procedural mortality is nowadays <1% and is mainly due to

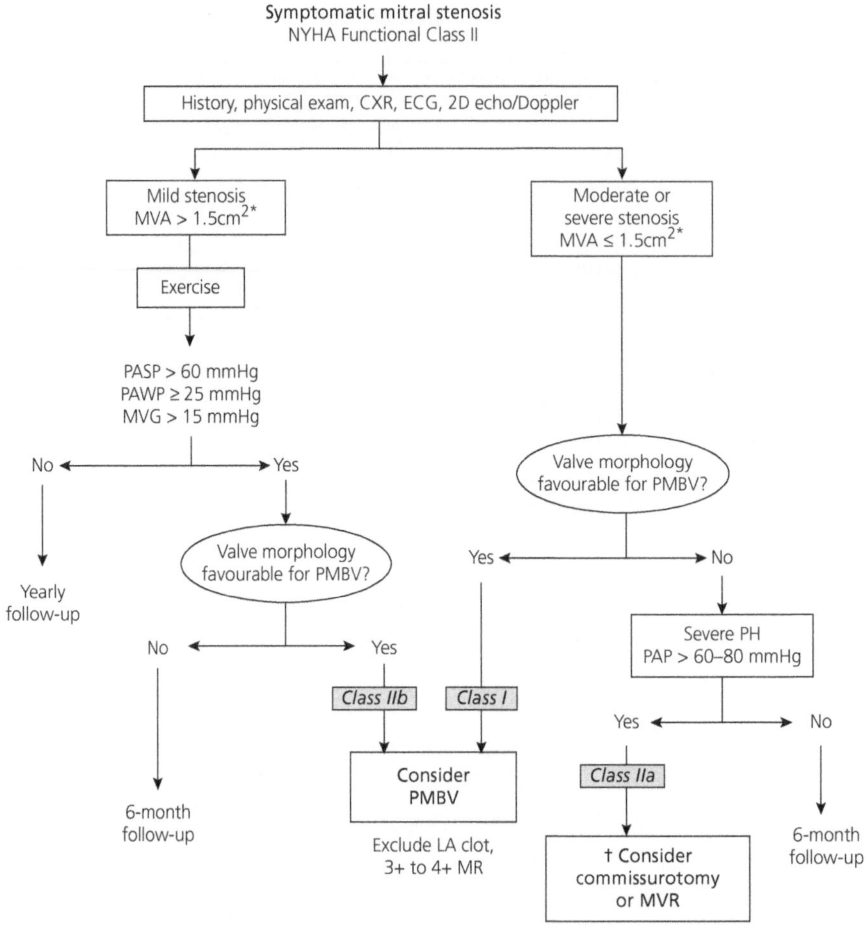

Figure 16.5 ACC/AHA 2008 GL on valve disease. Management strategy for patients with mitral stenosis and mild symptoms.

* There may be variability in the measurement of mitral valve area (MVA), and the mean transmitral gradient, pulmonary artery wedge pressure (PAWP), and pulmonary artery systolic pressure (PP) should also be taken into consideration.

† There is controversy as to whether patients with severe mitral stenosis (MVA <1.0 cm^2) and severe pulmonary hypertension (PH; PP >60–80 mmHg) should undergo percutaneous mitral balloon valvotomy (PMBV) or mitral valve replacement to prevent right ventricular failure.

CXR indicates chest X-ray; ECG, electrocardiogram; echo, echocardiography; LA, left atrial; MR, mitral regurgitation; MVG, mean mitral valve pressure gradient; NYHA, New York Heart Association; PAP, pulmonary artery pressure; and 2D, two-dimensional.

ACC/AHA 2008 focused update incorporated into the ACC/AHA 2006 guidelines for the management of patients with valvular heart disease. *J Am Coll Cardiol*. 2008;**52**:e1–142

tamponade or severe mitral regurgitation. Complications include severe mitral regurgitation (2–10%, although 25% of patients increase severity by one grade), most often due to non-commissural tear, urgent surgery (<1%), haemopericardium (0.5–12%), embolism (0.5–5%), and residual ASD (<5%). Re-stenosis can often be treated with repeat PMBV, but results are poorer than those after the first intervention. Recently, a benefit of PMBV was demonstrated in asymptomatic patients with moderate MS (<1.5 m^2) and suitable morphology, even in the absence of other conventional indication for intervention.[10]

Open valvotomy is attractive in cases unsuitable for PMBV; it allows conservation of the native valve and allows controlled reconstruction of the valves and simultaneous tricuspid valve repair or mitral valve replacement, if necessary. The risk of surgery is 1–3%.[6] Patients with mitral stenosis and severe tricuspid regurgitation do better with surgical repair than with PMBV.

Mitral valve replacement with preservation of the subvalvar apparatus is the treatment of choice in elderly patients with anatomy that is unfavourable for other options (Table 16.8). Patient prosthesis mismatch and prosthesis

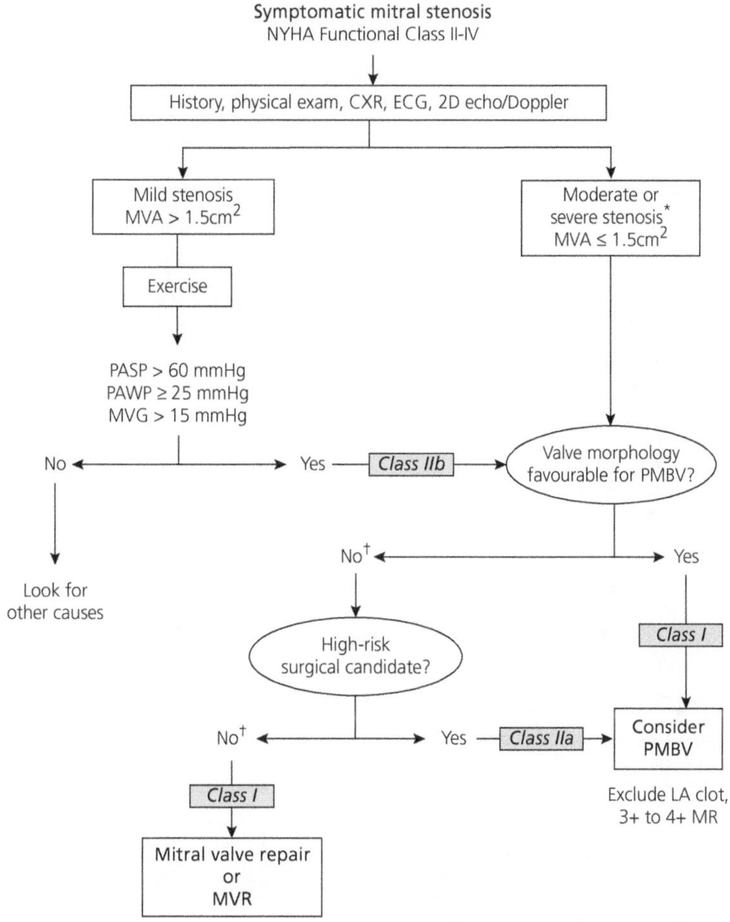

Figure 16.6 ACC/AHA 2008 GL on valve disease. Management strategy for patients with mitral stenosis and moderate to severe symptoms.

* There may be variability in the measurement of mitral valve area (MVA), and the mean transmitral gradient, pulmonary artery wedge pressure (PAWP), and pulmonary artery systolic pressure (PP) should also be taken into consideration.

† It is controversial as to which patients with less favourable valve morphology should undergo percutaneous mitral balloon valvotomy (PMBV) rather than mitral valve surgery (see text).

CXR, chest X-ray; ECG, electrocardiography;echo, echocardiography; LA, left atrial; MR, mitral regurgitation; MVG, mean mitral valve pressure gradient; MVR, mitral valve replacement; NYHA, New York Heart Association; and 2D, two-dimensional.

ACC/AHA guidelines on valve disease 2008 focused update incorporated into the ACC/AHA 2006 guidelines for the management of patients with valvular heart disease. *J Am Coll Cardiol*. 2008;**52**:e1–142.

stenosis due to ingrowth of pannus are the main problems. The operative risk is <5% in the absence of other co-morbidities but may reach 20% in the elderly with pulmonary hypertension.[6] The choice of prosthesis is based on patient age and the risk of anticoagulation (see Chapter 22 on prosthetic valves). **Congenital MS** is rare. Surgery is indicated with a mean MV gradient >10 mmHg in the presence of symptoms or a PA pressure >50 mmHg (Table 16.9). Concomitant surgical ablation with a modification of the MAZE or alternative procedures may be needed in the case of drug-refractory AF.[11]

Transcatheter transapical mitral valve-in-valve implantation for dysfunctional biological mitral prosthesis is also a recent possibility.[12]

Non-cardiac surgery

In asymptomatic patients with significant MS and a systolic pulmonary artery pressure <50 mmHg, non-cardiac surgery can be performed safely.[7] In symptomatic patients or in patients with systolic pulmonary artery pressure >50 mmHg, percutaneous mitral commissurotomy should

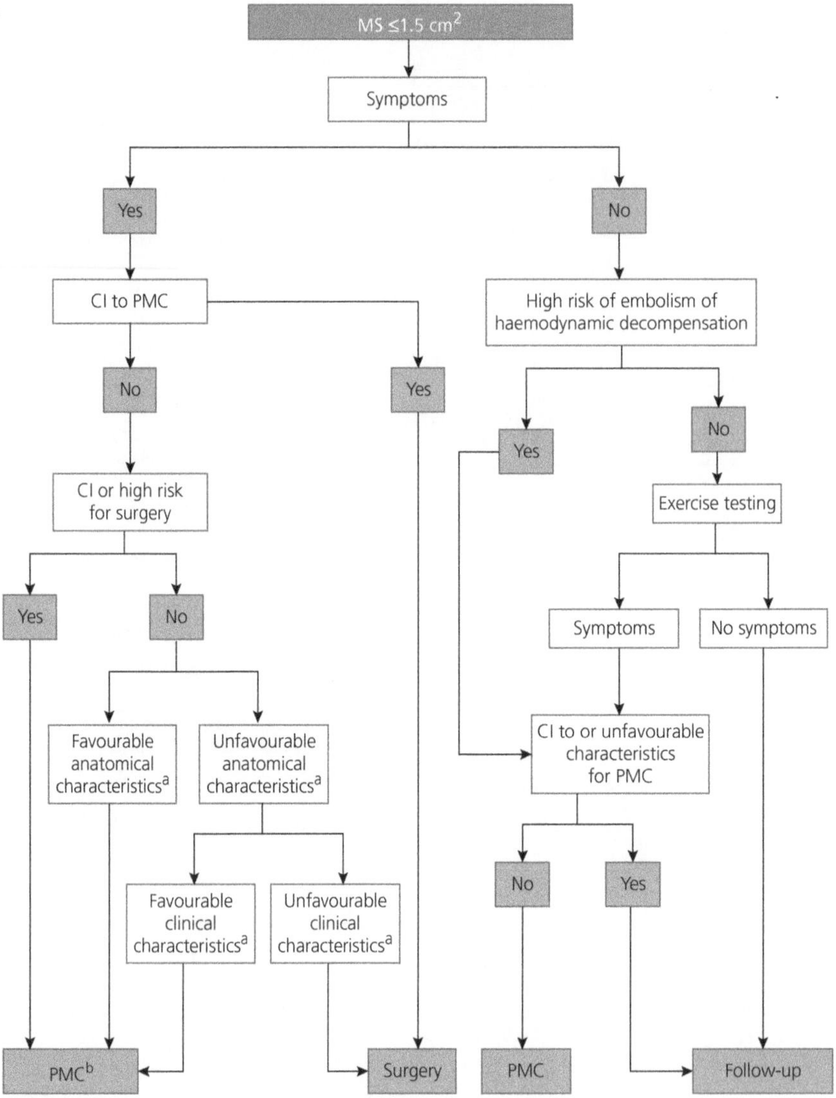

Figure 16.7 ESC 2012 GL on valve disease. Management of clinically significant mitral stenosis.

CI, contraindication; MS, mitral stenosis; PMC, percutaneous mitral commissurotomy.

a: See Table 16.6.

b: Surgical commissurotomy may be considered by experienced surgical teams or in patients with contraindications to percutaneous mitral commissurotomy.

ESC Guidelines on the management of valvular heart disease (version 2012). *European Heart Journal* 2012;**33**:2451–2496.

be attempted before non-cardiac surgery if it is high-risk. If valve replacement is needed, the decision should be individualized.

Pregnancy

Mitral stenosis in pregnancy is associated with substantial morbidity (including pulmonary oedema), even in asymptomatic or minimally symptomatic patients with mild to moderate disease (mitral valve area 1–1·5 cm^2). Indications for intervention are the occurrence of severe symptoms (NYHA class III/IV or pulmonary oedema) that are refractory to medical treatment. PBV is the treatment of choice (IIa-C, ESC 2011 GL on pregnancy).[13] Beta blockers can be given for pulmonary hypertension and diuretics can be added if symptoms persist (I-C, ESC 2011 GL on

Table 16.8 ACC/AHA 2008 GL on valve disease

Indications for surgery for mitral stenosis	
MV surgery (repair if possible) in patients with symptomatic (NYHA III–IV) moderate or severe MS when:	I-B
1) Percutaneous mitral balloon valvotomy (PMBV) is unavailable,	
2) PMBV is contraindicated because of left atrial thrombus despite anticoagulation or because concomitant moderate to severe MR is present, or	
3) The valve morphology is not favourable for PMBV in a patient with acceptable operative risk.	
Symptomatic patients with moderate to severe MS, who also have moderate to severe MR, should receive MV replacement, unless valve repair is possible at the time of surgery.	I-C
MV replacement for patients with severe MS and severe pulmonary hypertension (PA systolic pressure >60 mmHg) with NYHA I–II symptoms who are not considered candidates for percutaneous mitral balloon valvotomy or surgical MV repair.	IIa-C
MV repair for asymptomatic patients with moderate or severe MS who have had recurrent embolic events while receiving adequate anticoagulation and who have valve morphology favourable for repair.	IIb-C
MV repair for MS in patients with mild MS.	III-C
Closed commissurotomy in patients undergoing MV repair (open commissurotomy is the preferred approach).	III-C

ACC/AHA 2008 focused update incorporated into the ACC/AHA 2006 guidelines for the management of patients with valvular heart disease. *J Am Coll Cardiol*. 2008;**52**:e1–142.

Table 16.9 ACC/AHA 2008 GL on valve disease

Indications for surgery in congenital mitral stenosis	
Adolescent or young adult with congenital MS, and:	
Symptoms (NYHA III or IV) and mean MV gradient >10 mmHg on Doppler echocardiography.	I-C
Mild symptoms (NYHA II) and mean MV gradient >10 mmHg on Doppler.	IIa-C
PA systolic pressure ≥50 mmHg and a mean MV gradient ≥10 mmHg.	IIa-C
New-onset AF or multiple systemic emboli while receiving adequate anticoagulation.	IIb-C

ACC/AHA 2008 focused update incorporated into the ACC/AHA 2006 guidelines for the management of patients with valvular heart disease. *J Am Coll Cardiol*. 2008;**52**:e1–142.

pregnancy). Therapeutic anticoagulation is recommended in the case of atrial fibrillation, left atrial thrombosis, or prior embolism (I-C, ESC 2011 GL on preganancy).

References

1. Chandrashekhar Y, *et al.* Mitral stenosis. *Lancet*. 2009;**374**:1271–83
2. Maganti K, *et al.* Valvular heart disease: diagnosis and management. *Mayo Clin Proc*. 2010;**85**: 483–500
3. Nkomo VT, *et al.* Burden of valvular heart diseases: a population-based study. *Lancet*. 2006;**368**:1005–1011
4. Iung B, *et al.* A prospective survey of patients with valvular heart disease in Europe: the Euro Heart Survey on valvular heart disease. *Eur Heart J*. 2003;**24**:1231–43
5. Carabello BA. Modern management of mitral stenosis. *Circulation*. 2005;**112**:432–7
6. Bonow RO, *et al.* 2008 focused update incorporated into the ACC/AHA 2006 guidelines for the management of patients with valvular heart disease: a report of the American College of Cardiology/American Heart Association Task Force on practice guidelines (writing committee to revise the 1998 guidelines for the management of patients with valvular heart disease). Endorsed by the Society of Cardiovascular Anesthesiologists, Society for Cardiovascular Angiography and Interventions, and Society of Thoracic Surgeons. *J Am Coll Cardiol*. 2008;**52**:e1–42
7. Vahanian A, *et al.* Guidelines on the management of valvular heart disease (version 2012). *Eur Heart J*. 2012;**33**:2451–96
8. Iung B, *et al.* Immediate results of percutaneous mitral commissurotomy. A predictive model on a series of 1514 patients. *Circulation*. 1996;**94**:2124–30
9. Bouleti CIB, *et al.* Reinterventions after percutaneous mitral commissurotomy during long-term follow-up, up to 20 years: The role of repeat percutaneous mitral commissurotomy. *Eur Heart J*. 2013 Mar 20. [Epub ahead of print].
10. Kang DH, *et al.* Early percutaneous mitral commissurotomy vs conventional management in asymptomatic moderate mitral stenosis. *Eur Heart J*. 2012;**33**:1511–17
11. Fragakis N, *et al.* Surgical ablation for atrial fibrillation. *Europace*. 2012;**14**:1545–52
12. Cheung A, *et al.* Five-year experience with transcatheter transapical mitral valve-in-valve implantation for bioprosthetic valve dysfunction online first. *J Am Coll Cardiol*. 2013; doi:10.1016/j.jacc.2013.1001.1058
13. de Souza JA, *et al.* Percutaneous balloon mitral valvuloplasty in comparison with open mitral valve commissurotomy for mitral stenosis during pregnancy. *J Am Coll Cardiol*. 2001;**37**:900–3

Chapter 17

Mitral regurgitation

Classification

Mechanisms of MR are classified as functional (mitral valve is structurally normal, and disease results from valve deformation caused by ventricular or atrial remodelling) or organic (intrinsic valve lesions) (Table 17.1).[1]

Epidemiology

Although a trivial form of this valve disease is often seen in healthy people, moderate or severe MR is the most frequent valve disease in the USA and is the second most common form of valvular heart disease (after aortic stenosis) needing surgery in Europe.[2-4] Degenerative changes and prolapse might be non-familial or genetically transmitted as an autosomal trait or X chromosome-linked. The prevalence of moderate or severe MR in the general population in the USA is estimated 1.6% (0.5% in age 18–44 years to 9.3% in ≥75 years).[2] The prevalence of mitral valve prolapse is approximately 2.4% and half of them have maximal leaflet thickness of at least 5 mm.[5]

Aetiology

Mitral regurgitation (MR) may result from disorders of the valve leaflets or the mitral apparatus. The main causes in the western world are **degenerative disease** (60–70% of cases) and **ischaemic** mitral regurgitation (20%) usually due to an inferior infarction involving the inferolateral and the posteromedial papillary muscle.[1] Degenerative disease is rarely due to annular calcification. **Mitral valve prolapse**, is defined on echocardiography as systolic atrial displacement of the mitral valve such that it extends above a saddle-shaped annulus by a minimum of 2 mm. It is the most common functional abnormality associated with degenerative mitral valve disease, resulting from both leaflet redundancy and chordal elongation, and often overdiagnosed. Patients with typical **Barlow's syndrome** (initial description of mitral valve prolapse) have diffuse, generalized thickening and billowing of the leaflets whereas in those with **fibroelastic dysplasia**, the disease is localized to isolated regions of the valve.[6,7] The chordae tendineae may be elongated and prone to rupture. Mitral valve prolapse may be detected in 2% of the population and can be an inheritable condition, linked to a marker on chromosome 16.[8] Less common causes are **rheumatic disease** (2–5% in western countries but the leading cause in developing countries), **endocarditis** (2–5%), **cardiomyopathies, congenital anomalies, carcinoid disease, systemic lupus erythematosus (Libman–Sacks), anorectic drugs**, and **atrial fibrillation**. Acute MI (45% of acute MR cases), endocarditis (28%), chordal or papillary muscle rupture (26%) or dysfunction due to ischaemia, acute rheumatic carditis, myocarditis, Takotsubo cardiomyopathy, and prosthetic valve dysfunction may lead to **acute MR.**[9]

Pathophysiology and natural history

In **acute MR**, the unprepared left atrium and left ventricle cannot accommodate the regurgitant volume, which causes large v waves in the left atrium and results in pulmonary congestion. Patients with chronic MR and preserved LV function may tolerate the marked increase in volume better, whereas patients with impaired ventricular function may quickly decompensate with acute worsening of MR.

In **chronic** cases, the adaptive changes to volume overload include LV dilatation and eccentric hypertrophy and left atrial

Table 17.1 Types of MR according to Carpentier classification

	Organic		**Functional**	
	Type I*	**Type II†**	**Type IIIa‡**	**Type I*/Type IIIb‡**
Non-ischaemic	Endocarditis (perforation); degenerative (annular calcification), congenital (cleft leaflet)	Degenerative (billowing/ flail leaflets); endocarditis (ruptured chordae); traumatic (ruptured chord/PM); rheumatic (acute RH)	Rheumatic (chronic RF); iatrogenic (radiation/ drug); inflammatory (lupus/ anticardiolipin, eosinophilic endocardial disease, endomyocardial fibrosis)	Cardiomyopathy; myocarditis; left ventricular; dysfunction (any cause)
Ischaemic		Ruptured PM	–	Functional ischaemic

MR, mitral regurgitation; PM, papillary muscle; RF, rheumatic fever.* Mechanism involves normal leaflet movement. † Mechanism involves excessive valve movement. ‡ Restricted valve movement, IIIa in diastole, IIIb in systole.

Carpentier A. Cardiac valve surgery—the "French Correction". *J Thor Cardiovasc Surg.* 1983; **86**: 323–37.

enlargement that allows accommodation of the regurgitant volume at a lower pressure. Regurgitant fractions <40% may be tolerated indefinitely. The LV ejection fraction in chronic MR is usually greater than normal because of the increase in preload and the afterload-reducing effect of ejection into the low-impedance left atrium. Thus, LV dysfunction in severe MR is defined as LVEF ≤60% or an elevated end-systolic dimension (>40 mm by ACC/AHA and >45 mm by ESC). Advanced myocardial dysfunction may occur while LV ejection fraction appears normal. Ventricular dysfunction should be suspected when end-systolic dimensions are large but is often masked by a large ejection volume and is revealed after surgical elimination of mitral regurgitation, with a post-operative average immediate ejection fraction drop of about 10%. In patients with organic mitral regurgitation, RV function impairment is frequent (30%), constitutes a predictor of post-operative cardiovascular survival, and depends weakly on pulmonary artery systolic pressure but mainly on left ventricular remodeling and septal function.[10] Thus, biventricular impairment is a powerful predictor of both cardiovascular and overall survival. The risk of AF and heart failure increases with severity of MR. Patients with severe MR usually develop symptoms within the next 6 to 10 years and have an increased risk for sudden death. The rate of death from cardiovascular causes among asymptomatic patients with, at least, moderate mitral regurgitation or an LVEF <50% exceeds 3% per year.[11–13] Patients with severe MR and flail leaflets have an annual mortality of 6–7%, and, in 10 years, 90% of them are dead or require MV operation.

The prognosis of **mitral valve prolapse** is benign in the absence of moderate to severe MR, LVEF <50%, and thickened mitral leaflets (>5 mm), with survival similar to that of people without prolapse.[6,7] Infective endocarditis (100 cases per 100 000 patient-years of follow-up), spontaneous chordal rupture, and sudden death are higher than in the general population. In the presence of flail leaflets, the rate of infective endocarditis is 1.5% per year and that of sudden death 1.8% per year.[7] Fibrin emboli, as well as the increased incidence of mitral valve prolapse in Von Willebrand's disease and other coagulopathies, are responsible for visual symptoms with involvement of the ophthalmic or posterior cerebral circulation. MR of mitral valve prolapse that is purely mid-late systolic has more benign consequences and outcomes than holosystolic MR.[14] Recently, a subset of patients with prolapse who experienced life threatening ventricular arrhythmias was desdcribed. This phenotype is characterized by bileaflet MVP, female sex, and frequent complex ventricular ectopy including PVC of outflow tract alternating with papillary muscle/fascicular origin.[15]

Presentation

Acute MR Patients who develop acute severe MR usually present with symptomatic heart failure because their ventricles are ill prepared to accept the sudden increase in volume load. Some patients may present solely with new-onset dyspnoea, without evidence of impending cardiovascular collapse, and may be misdiagnosed.

Chronic MR The patient may be entirely asymptomatic, even during vigorous exercise, or present with dyspnoea.

Physical examination

Acute MR Physical examination of the precordium may be misleading because a normal-sized left ventricle does not produce a hyperdynamic apical impulse.

- The **systolic murmur** of MR may not be holosystolic and may even be absent.
- A **third heart sound** or **early diastolic flow rumble** may be the only abnormal physical finding.

Chronic MR

- **Displaced apical impulse** in severe MR
- **Soft S_1** and **widely split S_2**
- **Late systolic murmur** in MVP or papillary muscle dysfunction
- **Mid-systolic click** and perhaps **TR** in the presence of MVP
- **Holosystolic murmur** in chordal rupture and flail leaflet. The radiation of the murmur follows the direction of the regurgitant jet. With a flail posterior leaflet, the murmur radiates anteriorly and may mimic aortic stenosis whereas a murmur associated with a flail anterior leaflet radiates to the back.
- A **diastolic rumble and S_3** may be present and does not necessarily indicate LV dysfunction.
- **Loud P_2** due to pulmonary venous hypertension indicates advanced disease.

Investigations

Chest radiography Cardiomegaly due to LV and left atrial enlargement in chronic MR. Kerley B lines and interstitial oedema can be seen in acute MR or progressive LV failure. Predominant MS is suggested by mild cardiomegaly and significant changes in the lung fields. A unilateral pattern that is found in 2% of cases of pulmonary oedema, usually of the right upper lobe, is always associated with severe functional or organic MR.[16] This entity should be differentiated from lobar pneumonia.

Electrocardiography Left atrial enlargement and atrial fibrillation. Left ventricular enlargement in approximately 30% of patients and RV hypertrophy in 15%. AF is associated with increased mortality.[17]

Transthoracic echocardiography demonstrates the disruption of the MV but may underestimate lesion severity by inadequate imaging of the colour flow jet. Thus, if there is normal or hyperdynamic systolic function of the left ventricle on echocardiography in a patient with acute heart failure, the suspicion of severe MR should be raised. Quantitative assessment of regurgitation is feasible by quantitative Doppler, based on mitral and aortic stroke volumes, or quantitative 2D echo, based on left ventricular volumes, or flow convergence analysis with colour flow imaging proximal to the regurgitant orifice (PISA, proximal isovelocity surface area method) (Tables 17.2 and 17.3, and Figure 17.1). Measures of effective regurgitant orifice area (ERO) and regurgitant volume can be inaccurate in acute MR, particularly in the context of tachycardia. Assessment of mid- or late MR in the context of mitral leaflet prolapse may also be misleading because jet area and ERO by flow convergence appear similar to those of holosystolic MR. 3D measurement of vena contracta area and regurgitant volume is superior to 2D methods.[18] 3-D analysis of the annular shape has also been shown prognostically significant; flattening of the annular saddle (normal) shape is associated with progressive leaflet billowing and increased chordal rupture.[19]

Transoesophageal echocardiography can more accurately assess the colour flow jet and direct successful surgical repair (Class I-B, ACC/AHA guidelines on valve disease 2008), particularly in acute MR.

Exercise testing, with or without Doppler assessment, before and after exercise in symptomatic patients in whom there is a discrepancy between symptoms and resting measures of LV function and pulmonary artery pressure. It is very helpful in identifying patients who develop pulmonary hypertension (>60 mmHg) with exercise.

Cardiac catheterization is indicated when the non-invasive tests are inconclusive to resolve the severity of MR (Table 17.4).

Coronary angiography is necessary before surgery in the haemodynamically stable patient over 40 years of age or with risk factors or clinical suspicion of coronary artery disease (Tables 15.3 and 15.4 in Chapter 15 on general principles). LV angiography at the RAO projection allows visualization and quantification of the regurgitant jet, but the method depends on the amount of contrast injected and the size of the LA.

Cardiac magnetic resonance provides accurate measurement of regurgitant flow and LV volumes and is an emerging modality of increasing significance.

Biomarkers, such as B-natriuretic peptide, are related to functional class, but their value for risk stratification is limited.

Therapy

Anticoagulation for the symptomatic patients with **mitral valve prolapse** is presented in Table 17.5.

Table 17.2 ACC/AHA 2008 GL on valve disease. Criteria for severity of MR

	Mild	Moderate	Severe
Specific signs			
Angiographic grade	1+	2+	3–4+
Colour Doppler jet area	Small, central jet (<4 cm² or <20% LA area)	Signs of MR greater than mild but less than severe MR	Vena contracta width >0.7 cm, with large central MR jet (area >40% of LA area) or with a wall-impinging jet of any size, swirling in LA
Doppler vena contracta width (cm)	<0.3	0.3–0.69	≥0.70
Quantitative (cath or echo)			
RVol (mL per beat)	<30	30–59	≥60
RF (%)	<30	30–49	≥50
ERO (cm²)	<0.20	0.20–0.39	≥0.40
Additional essential criteria			
LA size			Enlarged
LV size			Enlarged

RVol, regurgitant volume; RF, regurgitant fraction; ERO, effective regurgitant orifice area; CW, continuous wave.

Colour flow jets are composed of three distinct segments: the proximal flow convergence zone (the area of flow acceleration into the orifice), the vena contracta (the narrowest and highest velocity central flow region of the jet), and the jet itself distal to the orifice.

Jet and vena contracta estimations at a Nyquist limit of 50–60 cm/s.

Large flow convergence defined as flow convergence radius >0.9 cm for central jets, with a baseline shift at a Nyquist of 40 cm/s. Cut-offs for eccentric jets are higher and should be angled correctly.

ACC/AHA 2008 focused update incorporated into the ACC/AHA 2006 guidelines for the management of patients with valvular heart disease. *J Am Coll Cardiol*. 2008;**52**:e1–142.

Table 17.3 ESC 2012 GL on VD. Echocardiographic criteria for definition of severe MR

Qualitative		
Valve morphology	Flail leaflet/ruptured papillary muscle/large coaptation defect	
Colour flow regurgitant jet	Very large central jet or eccentric jet adhering, swirling, and reaching the posterior wall of the left atrium	
CW signal of regurgitant jet	Dense/triangular	
Other	Large flow convergence zone[a]	
Semi-quantitative		
Vena contracta width (mm)	≥7 (>8 for biplane)[b]	
Upstream vein flow[c]	Systolic pulmonary vein flow reversal	
Inflow	E wave dominant ≥1.5 m/s[d]	
Other	TVI mitral/TVI aortic >1.4	
Quantitative		
	Primary	**Secondary**[e]
EROA (mm^2)	≥40	≥20
RVol (mL/beat)	≥60	≥30
+ enlargement of cardiac chambers/vessels	LV, LA	

a: At a Nyquist limit of 50–60 cm/s.
b: For average between apical four- and two-chamber views.
c: Unless other reasons for systolic blunting (atrial fibrillation, elevated atrial pressure).
d: In the absence of other causes of elevated left atrial pressure and of mitral stenosis.
e: Different thresholds are used in secondary MR where an EROA >20mm² and regurgitant volume >30 mL identify a subset of patients at increased risk of cardiac events.
ESC guidelines on the management of valvular heart disease (version 2012). *European Heart Journal* 2012;**33**:2451–2496.

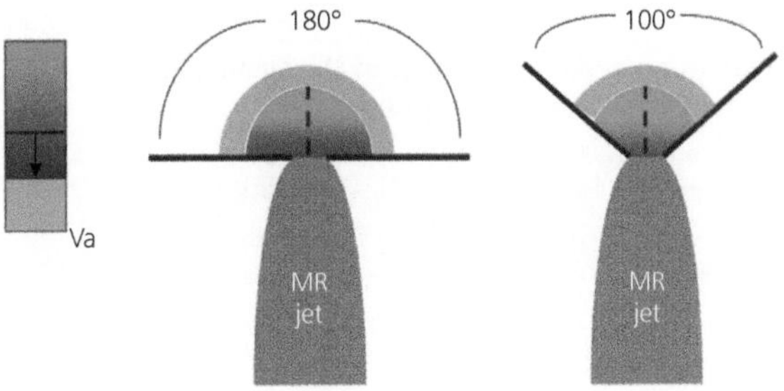

Peak MR flow rate = $2\pi r^2 \times Va \times (angle/180°)$
EROA = peak MR flow rate/peak velocity of MR Jet

Figure 17.1 Schematic example of the proximal isovelocity surface area (PISA) method. Left, the colour Doppler baseline is shifted downward (in the direction of the mitral regurgitation (MR) jet) until the proximal convergence zone (middle) appears hemispheric. The aliasing velocity (Va) is used to calculate peak regurgitant flow rate from the formula, where r is the radius from the blue-red alias line to the orifice. Note that this formula assumes that peak flow rate from the PISA radius occurs at the same time as peak velocity of the MR jet by continuous wave Doppler. If the proximal flow convergence does not occur over a flat (180°) plane, angle correction must be used (right). It is important to shift the baseline in the direction of the MR jet, not to merely lower the aliasing velocity. It is also important to turn off variance, which makes the red-blue alias line easier to identify.

EROA indicates effective regurgitant orifice area.
Grayburn PA,*et al*. Quantitation of mitral regurgitation. *Circulation*. 2012;**126**:2005–17.

Acute MR

Medical therapy is aimed at stabilizing haemodynamics in preparation for surgical repair or MV replacement (usually with endocarditis). Nitroprusside in the normotensive patient and dopamine with or without nitroprusside in hypotension are administered. Aortic balloon counterpulsation increases forward output and mean arterial pressure while diminishing regurgitant volume and LV filling pressure and can also be used. MV repair or replacement, combined with CABG for papillary muscle rupture-induced MR, can now be offered, with <10% mortality.[9] Surgical mortality for endocarditis-induced acute MR is 10–20%. The prognosis of patients with ischaemic cardiogenic shock is inversely related to the degree of MR and also argues for aggressive revascularization when feasible.[20]

Table 17.4 ACC/AHA 2008 GL on VD

Indications for cardiac catheterization	
Left ventriculography and haemodynamic measurements when non-invasive tests are inconclusive regarding severity of MR, LV function, or the need for surgery.	I-C
Haemodynamic measurements when pulmonary artery pressure is out of proportion to the severity of MR, as assessed by non-invasive testing, or when there is a discrepancy between clinical and non-invasive findings regarding severity of MR.	I-C
Coronary angiography is indicated before MV repair or MV replacement in patients at risk for CAD.	I-C
Left ventriculography and haemodynamic measurements are not indicated in patients in whom valve surgery is not contemplated.	III-C

ACC/AHA 2008 focused update incorporated into the ACC/AHA 2006 guidelines for the management of patients with valvular heart disease. *J Am Coll Cardiol*. 2008;**52**:e1–142.

Table 17.5 ACC/AHA 2008 GL on VD

Evaluation and management of the symptomatic patient with mitral valve prolapse	
Aspirin therapy (75–325 mg/day) for symptomatic patients who experience cerebral transient ischaemic attacks.	I-C
In AF, warfarin therapy for patients aged >65 or those with hypertension, MR murmur, or a history of heart failure.	I-C
Aspirin therapy (75–325 mg/day) for patients with AF who are <65 years old and have no history of MR, hypertension, or heart failure.	I-C
In patients with a history of stroke, warfarin for patients with MR, AF, or left atrial thrombus.	I-C
Warfarin for patients with a history of stroke who do not have MR, AF, or left atrial thrombus if there is echocardiographic evidence of thickening (≥5 mm) and/or redundancy of the valve leaflets.	IIa-C
In patients with a history of stroke, aspirin if there is no MR, AF, left atrial thrombus, or echocardiographic evidence of thickening (≥5 mm) or redundancy of the valve leaflets.	IIa-C
Warfarin for patients with transient ischaemic attacks despite aspirin therapy.	IIa-C
Aspirin (75–325 mg/day) for patients with a history of stroke who have contraindications to anticoagulants.	IIa-B
Aspirin (75–325 mg/day) for patients in sinus rhythm with echocardiographic evidence of high-risk MVP.	IIb-C

ACC/AHA 2008 focused update incorporated into the ACC/AHA 2006 guidelines for the management of patients with valvular heart disease. *J Am Coll Cardiol*. 2008;**52**:e1–142.

Table 17.6 ACC/AHA 2008 GL on VD

Indications for mitral valve operation	
Symptomatic patient with acute severe MR.	I-B
Patients with chronic severe MR and NYHA II, III, or IV symptoms in the absence of severe LV dysfunction (LVEF <30%) and/or end-systolic dimension >55 mm).	I-B
Asymptomatic patients with chronic severe MR and mild to moderate LV dysfunction, LVEF 30–60%, and/or end-systolic dimension ≥40 mm.	I-B
MV repair preferable to replacement and patients should be referred to surgical centres experienced in MV repair.	I-C
MV repair in experienced centres for asymptomatic patients with chronic severe MR with preserved LV function (LVEF >60% and end-systolic dimension <40 mm) in whom the likelihood of successful repair without residual MR is greater than 90%.	IIa-B
MV surgery for asymptomatic patients with chronic severe MR, preserved LV function, and new-onset AF.	IIa-C
MV surgery for asymptomatic patients with chronic severe MR, preserved LV function, and pulmonary hypertension (PA systolic pressure >50 mmHg at rest or >60 mmHg with exercise).	IIa-C
MV surgery for patients with chronic severe MR due to a primary abnormality of the mitral apparatus and NYHA III–IV symptoms and severe LV dysfunction (LVEF <30%) and/or end-systolic dimension >55 mm) in whom MV repair is highly likely.	IIa-C
MV repair for patients with chronic severe secondary MR due to severe LV dysfunction (LVEF <30%) who have persistent NYHA III–IV symptoms despite optimal therapy for heart failure, including biventricular pacing.	IIb-C
MV surgery for asymptomatic patients with MR and preserved LV function (LVEF >60% and end-systolic dimension <40 mm) in whom significant doubt about the feasibility of repair exists.	III-C
Isolated MV for patients with mild or moderate MR.	III-C

ACC/AHA 2008 focused update incorporated into the ACC/AHA 2006 guidelines for the management of patients with valvular heart disease. *J Am Coll Cardiol*. 2008;**52**:e1–142.

Table 17.7 ESC 2012 GL on valve disaese

Indications for surgery in severe primary mitral regurgitation	
Mitral repair is preferred when expected to be durable.	I-C
Symptomatic patients with LVEF >30% and ESD <55 mm.	I-B
Asymptomatic patients with LV dysfunction (ESD ≥45 mm and/or LVEF ≤60%).	I-C
Asymptomatic patients with preserved LV function and new-onset AF or pulmonary hypertension (systolic pulmonary artery pressure >50 mmHg at rest).	IIa-C
Asymptomatic patients with preserved LV function, high likelihood of durable repair, and low risk for surgery and flail leaflet, and LVESD ≥40 mm.	IIa-C
Patients with severe LV dysfunction (LVEF <30% and/or LVESD >55 mm) and/or refractory to medical therapy with high likelihood of durable repair and low co-morbidity.	IIa-C
Patients with severe LV dysfunction (LVEF <30% and/or ESD >55 mm) refractory to medical therapy with low likelihood of repair and low co-morbidity.	IIb-C
Asymptomatic patients with preserved LV function, high likelihood of durable repair, low surgical risk and:	IIb-C
Left atrial dilatation (volume index ≥60mL/m² BSA) and sinus rhythm, or Pulmonary hypertension on exercise (systolic PA pressure ≥60 mmHg at exercise).	

* Lower values can be considered for patients of small stature.
ESC guidelines on the management of valvular heart disease (version 2012). *European Heart Journal* 2012;**33**:2451–2496.

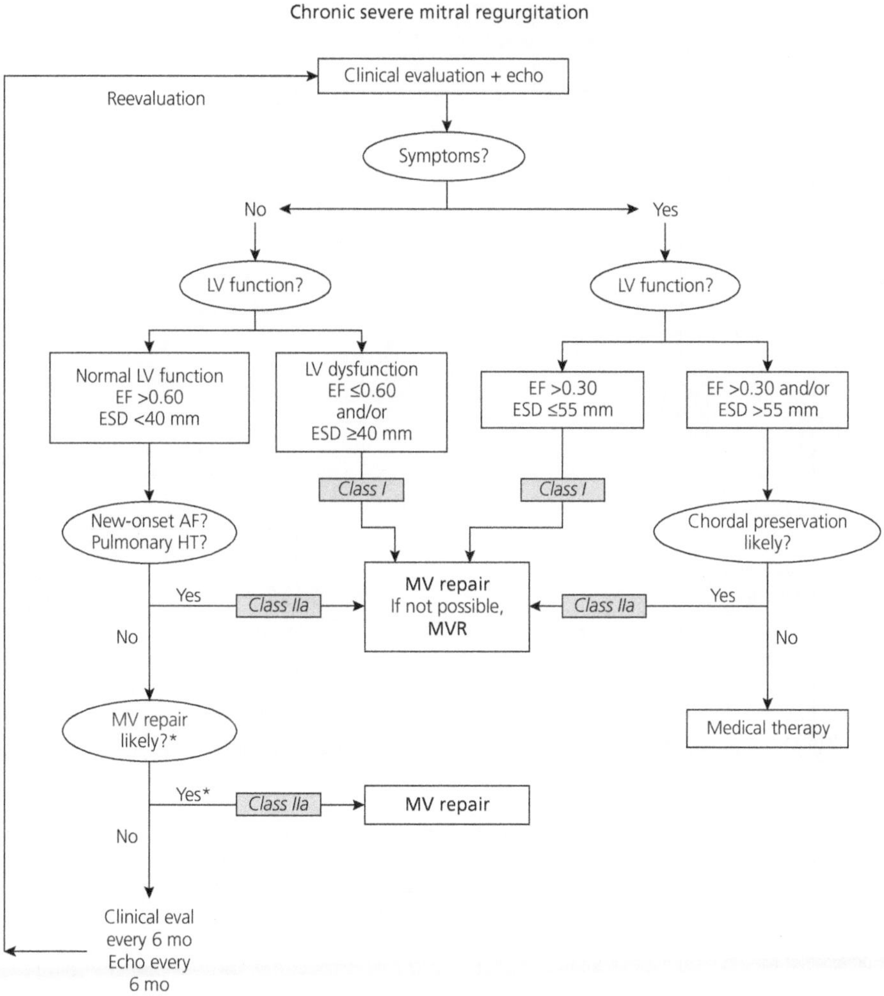

Figure 17.2 ACC/AHA 2008 Management strategy for patients with chronic severe mitral regurgitation.

* Mitral valve (MV) repair may be performed in asymptomatic patients with normal left ventricular (LV) function if performed by an experienced surgical team and if the likelihood of successful MV repair is greater than 90%.

AF indicates atrial fibrillation; echo, echocardiography; EF, ejection fraction; ESD, end-systolic dimension; eval, evaluation; HT, hypertension; and MVR, mitral valve replacement.

ACC/AHA 2008 focused update incorporated into the ACC/AHA 2006 guidelines for the management of patients with valvular heart disease. *J Am Coll Cardiol*. 2008;**52**:e1–142

Chronic MR

Medical therapy is aimed at reducing the afterload and pulmonary congestion with ACE/ARB and diuretics. Beta blockers in MR may increase LVEDD and were thought to be contraindicated, but recent evidence indicated beneficial reverse remodeling, especially in functional MR but also in degenerative disease.[21] They are also recommended in patients with MVP, no severe MR, and palpitations. Aspirin (75–325 mg od) or warfarin in non-responders is recommended for patients with MVP and TIAs.[22]

Surgery is mainly recommended for (Tables 17.6 and 17.7, and Figures 17.2 and 17.3):[22,23]

- Symptomatic patients with severe MR and preserved LV function (i.e. LVEF >30% and LVEDD <55 mm)
- Asymptomatic patients with severe MR and mild to moderate LV dysfunction (LVEF 30–60% and/or LVESD ≥40–45 mm) or development of AF or PA hypertension (>50 mmHg)
- Mitral valve repair is also recommended for asymptomatic patients with severe MR and well-preserved LV function (LVEF >60% and LVESD <40 mm) and/or pulmonary hypertension

Concomitant coronary artery disease should be treated with CABG at time of MV operation (I-A for stenosis

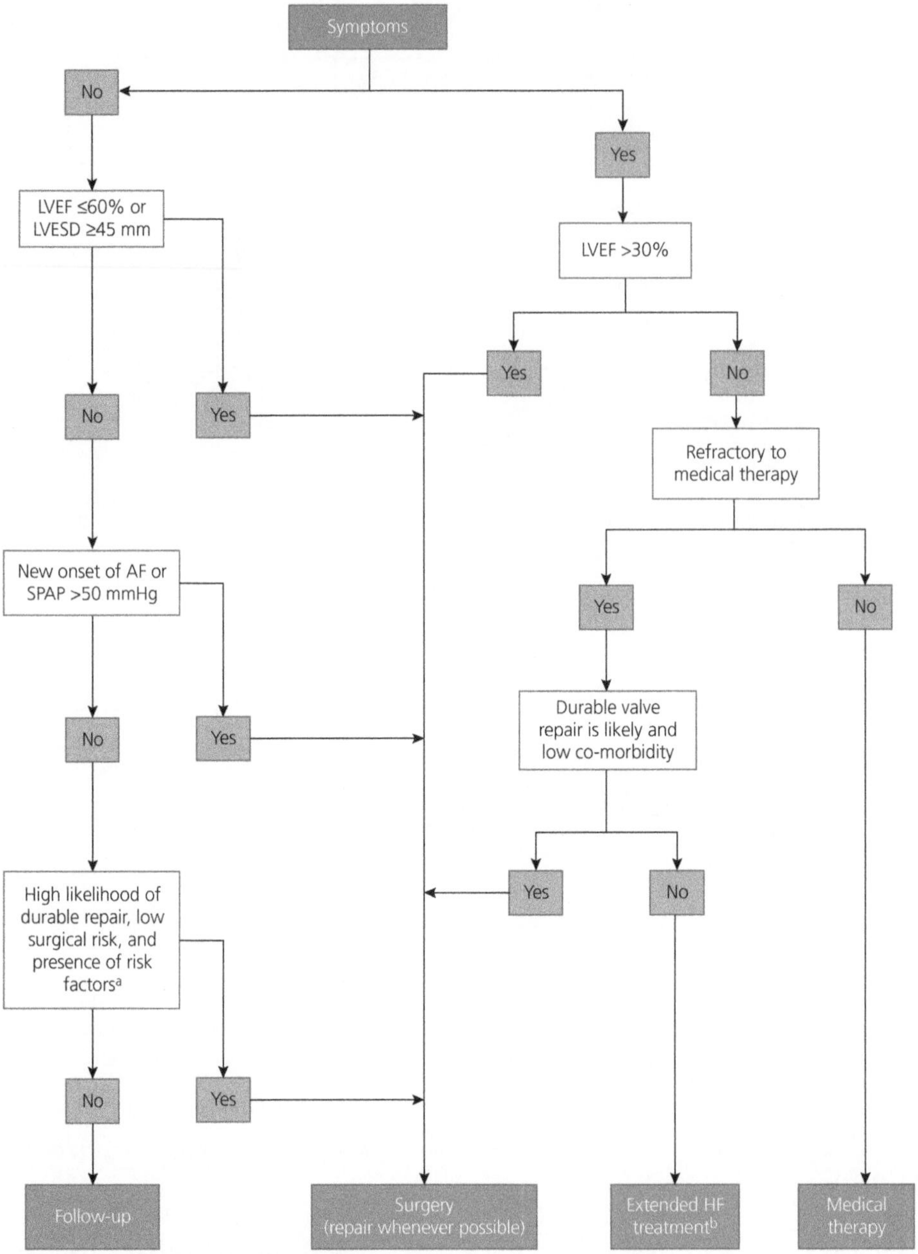

Figure 17.3 ESC 2012 Management of severe organic MR.

BSA, body surface area; SPAP, systolic pulmonary arterial pressure.

a: When there is a high likelihood of durable valve repair at a low risk, valve repair should be considered (IIaC) in patients with flail leaflet and LVESD ≥40 mm; valve repair may be considered (IIbC) if one of the following is present: LA volume ≥60 mL/mÇ BSA and sinus rhythm or pulmonary hypertension on exercise (SPAP ≥60 mmHg).

b: Extended HF management includes the following: cardiac resynchronization therapy: ventricular assist devices; cardiac restraint devices; heart transplantation.

ESC guidelines on the management of valvular heart disease (version 2012). *European Heart Journal* 2012;**33**:2451–2496

>70% or IIa-C for stenosis 50–70%, ESC 2010 guideline on revascularization).

Although the issue is controversial,[24] most retrospective studies support early repair, particularly in the context of organic MR[25,26] and before the establishment of pulmonary hypertension.[27] These patients should be referred to centres with known expertise and a greater than 90% likelihood of successful repair. A watchful waiting approach should probably be preferred if the likelihood of a high-quality repair is low and in the presence of high surgical risk and/or low probability of a durable repair, which is typically the case in elderly patients with relevant co-morbidities and/or complex valve lesions.[28]

However, in a recent analysis of the Medicare database, elderly patients (≥75 years) who underwent repair had a life expectancy similar to that of the age- and sex-matched US population.[29] Operative mortality for patients who underwent repair was 3.9% compared with 8.9% for replacement. Thus, an approach of earlier identification and surgical referral than that recommended by current guidelines should be probably considered regardless of age.

MV repair is recommended over **MV replacement** (Table 17.8).[30,31] Calcified mitral annulus, rheumatic disease, and involvement of the anterior leaflet diminish the likelihood of repair. In experienced centres, reoperation after 10 years is necessary in 5% of patients with repaired posterior leaflet prolapse and 10% of those with anterior leaflet repair. MV repair for degenerative MR restores life span to normal except in patients with symptoms at rest and impaired left ventricular function. Advanced age and complex mitral valve pathologies increased the risk of late recurrent MR.[32] When repair is not feasible, **MV replacement** with preservation of the subvalvar apparatus is preferred. The choice of prosthesis is based on patient age and the risk of anticoagulation (see Chapter 22 on prosthetic valves). Concomitant coronary artery disease should be treated with CABG at time of mitral valve operation (I-A for stenosis >70% or IIa-C for stenosis 50–70%–ESC 2010 GL on revascularization).

Functional MR

Functional is defined as secondary MR due to cardiomyopathies or chronic ischaemic heart disease. The prognosis of these patients is worse than other kinds of MR, and the role of surgery is controversial.[33] Recently, an analysis of the STICH trial cohort suggested potentially improved survival when MV repair with an annuloplasty ring was added to CABG in ischaemic patients with LVEF ≤35% and moderate to severe MR.[34] Two small RCTs have addressed this issue and detected improved exercise capacity and LV remodelling but no change in 1-year[35] or 5-year[36] mortality. Although CABG may improve MR in some patients,[37] moderate ischaemic mitral regurgitation does not reliably resolve,[38] and development of significant MR may be actually seen following isolated CABG.[39] Cardiac resynchronization therapy is a potential therapeutic option in heart failure patients with moderate-severe functional MR and high risk for surgery.[40] Recommendations for surgery are given in Table 17.9.

Table 17.8 ACC/AHA 2008 GL on VD

Recommendations for myxomatous mitral valve	
MV repair when anatomically possible for patients with severe degenerative MR. Patients should be referred to surgeons who are expert in repair.	I-B
Patients who have undergone successful MV repair should:	
Continue to receive antibiotics as indicated for endocarditis prophylaxis.	I-C
Continue to receive long-term anticoagulation with warfarin.	I-B
Undergo 2D and Doppler echocardiography before discharge or at the first post-operative outpatient visit.	I-C
Tricuspid valve repair is beneficial for severe TR in patients with MV disease that requires MV surgery.	I-B
Oral anticoagulation for the first 3 months after MV repair.	IIa-C
Long-term treatment with low-dose aspirin (75–100 mg per day) in patients who have undergone successful MV repair and remain in sinus rhythm.	IIa-C
Tricuspid annuloplasty for mild TR in patients undergoing MV repair when there is pulmonary hypertension or tricuspid annular dilatation.	IIa-C
Maze procedure may be considered at the time of M repair in patients with a history of AF.	IIb-B

ACC/AHA 2008 focused update incorporated into the ACC/AHA 2006 guidelines for the management of patients with valvular heart disease. *J Am Coll Cardiol*. 2008;**52**:e1–142.

Table 17.9 Surgery in functional MR

ESC 2012 GL on valve disease. Indications for surgery in chronic secondary mitral regurgitation	
Patients with severe MR,[1] undergoing CABG, and LVEF >30%.	I-C
Patients with moderate MR undergoing CABG.[2]	IIa-C
Symptomatic patients with severe MR, LVEF <30%, option for revascularization, and evidence for viability.	IIa-C
Patients with severe MR, LVEF >30%, refractory to medical therapy (including CRT if indicated), and low co-morbidity, when revascularization is not indicated.	IIb-C

1: The thresholds for severity (EROA ≥20 mm²; RVol >30 mL) differ from that of primary MR and are based on the prognostic value of these thresholds to predict poor outcome.
2: When exercise echocardiography is feasible, the development of dyspnoea and increased severity of MR associated with pulmonary hypertension are further incentives to surgery.

ESC guidelines on the management of valvular heart disease (version 2012). *European Heart Journal* 2012;**33**:2451–2496.

ACCF/AHA 2011 on CABG. Indications for surgery in chronic ischaemic mitral regurgitation	
Concomitant mitral valve repair or replacement at the time of CABG. In patients undergoing CABG who have severe ischaemic mitral valve regurgitation not likely to resolve with revascularization.	I-B
Concomitant mitral valve repair or replacement at the time of CABG, in patients undergoing CABG who have moderate ischaemic mitral valve regurgitation not likely to resolve with revascularization.	IIa-B

Recommendations for surgery in (rare) **congenital MR** are given in Table 17.10.

Percutaneous techniques for MR, such as edge-to-edge anterior and posterior leaflet attachment with a clip and coronary sinus cinching, are under investigation.[41–43] The EVEREST II randomized controlled trial failed to show convincing benefits of the Mitraclip technique in comparison with surgical repair in all-comers with severe MR. However, subsequent analysis of outcomes in higher risk subjects (predicted surgical mortality >12%) within the trial compared with registry controls receiving medical therapy alone suggested a possible role for percutaneous treatment.[44]

Transcatheter transapical mitral valve-in-valve implantation for dysfunctional biological mitral prosthesis is also a recent possibility.[45]

Table 17.10 ACCF/AHA 2008 on VD

Indications for surgery in severe congenital MR	
MV surgery in symptomatic adolescent or young adult with severe congenital MR and NYHA III or IV symptoms or LV systolic dysfunction (EF <0.60).	I-C
MV repair in experienced surgical centres in the asymptomatic adolescent or young adult with severe congenital MR with preserved LV systolic function if the likelihood of successful repair without residual MR is >90%.	IIa-B
The effectiveness of MV surgery is not well established in asymptomatic adolescent or young adult patients with severe congenital MR and preserved LV systolic function in whom valve replacement is highly likely.	IIb-C

ACC/AHA 2008 focused update incorporated into the ACC/AHA 2006 guidelines for the management of patients with valvular heart disease. *J Am Coll Cardiol*. 2008;**52**:e1–142.

Non-cardiac surgery

In patients with AR or MR, if LV dysfunction is severe (EF <30%), non-cardiac surgery should only be performed, if strictly necessary, after optimization of medical therapy for HF.[22]

Pregnancy

Patients with severe mitral regurgitation and symptoms or impaired ventricular function or ventricular dilatation should be treated surgically pre-pregnancy (I-C, ESC 2011 GL on pregnancy).

References

1. Enriquez-Sarano M, *et al.* Mitral regurgitation. *Lancet*. 2009;**373**:1382–94
2. Go AS, *et al.* Heart disease and stroke statistics—2013 update: a report from the American Heart Association. *Circulation*. 2013; **127**:e6–245
3. Iung B, *et al.* A prospective survey of patients with valvular heart disease in Europe: the Euro Heart Survey on valvular heart disease. *Eur Heart J*. 2003;**24**:1231–43
4. Nkomo VT, *et al.* Burden of valvular heart diseases: a population-based study. *Lancet*. 2006;**368**:1005–11
5. Freed LA, *et al.* Prevalence and clinical outcome of mitral valve prolapse. *N Engl J Med*. 1999;**341**:1–7
6. Foster E. Clinical practice. Mitral regurgitation due to degenerative mitral valve disease. *N Engl J Med*. 2010;**363**:156–65
7. Guy TS, *et al.* Mitral valve prolapse. *Ann Rev Med*. 2012;**63**:277–292
8. Disse S, *et al.* Mapping of a first locus for autosomal dominant myxomatous mitral valve prolapse to chromosome 16p11.2-p12.1. *Am J Hum Genet*. 1999;**65**:1242–51
9. Stout KK, *et al.* Acute valvular regurgitation. *Circulation*. 2009;**119**:3232–41
10. Le Tourneau TDG, *et al.* Right ventricular systolic function in organic mitral regurgitation: Impact of biventricular impairment. *Circulation*. 2013;**127**:1597–608
11. Avierinos JF, *et al.* Natural history of asymptomatic mitral valve prolapse in the community. *Circulation*. 2002;**106**: 1355–61
12. Enriquez-Sarano M, *et al.* Quantitative determinants of the outcome of asymptomatic mitral regurgitation. *N Engl J Med*. 2005;**352**:875–83
13. Rosenhek R, *et al.* Outcome of watchful waiting in asymptomatic severe mitral regurgitation. *Circulation*. 2006;**113**: 2238–44
14. Topilsky Y, *et al.* Mitral valve prolapse with mid-late systolic mitral regurgitation: pitfalls of evaluation and clinical outcome compared with holosystolic regurgitation. *Circulation*. 2012;**125**:1643–51
15. Sriram CS, *et al.* Malignant bileaflet mitral valve prolapse syndrome in patients with otherwise idiopathic out of hospital cardiac arrest. *J Am Coll Cardiol*. 2013; doi: 10.1016/j.jacc.2013.1002.1060
16. Attias D, *et al.* Prevalence, characteristics, and outcomes of patients presenting with cardiogenic unilateral pulmonary oedema. *Circulation*. 2010;**122**:1109–15
17. Grigioni F, *et al.* Atrial fibrillation complicating the course of degenerative mitral regurgitation: determinants and long-term outcome. *J Am Coll Cardiol*. 2002;**40**:84–92
18. Grayburn PA, *et al.* Quantitation of mitral regurgitation. *Circulation*. 2012;**126**:2005–17
19. Lee A P-W, *et al.* Quantitative analysis of mitral valve morphology in mitral valve prolapse with real-time 3-dimensional echocardiography: Importance of annular saddle shape in the pathogenesis of mitral regurgitation. *Circulation*. 2013;**127**:832–41
20. Hochman JS, *et al.* Early revascularization in acute myocardial infarction complicated by cardiogenic shock. SHOCK Investigators. Should We Emergently Revascularize Occluded Coronaries for Cardiogenic Shock. *N Engl J Med*. 1999;**341**:625–34
21. Ahmed MI, *et al.* A randomized controlled phase iib trial of beta(1)-receptor blockade for chronic degenerative mitral regurgitation. *J Am Coll Cardiol*. 2012;**60**:833–8
22. Bonow RO, *et al.* 2008 focused update incorporated into the ACC/AHA 2006 guidelines for the management of patients with valvular heart disease: a report of the American College of Cardiology/American Heart Association Task Force on practice guidelines (writing committee to revise the 1998 guidelines for the management of patients with valvular

heart disease). Endorsed by the Society of Cardiovascular Anesthesiologists, Society for Cardiovascular Angiography and Interventions, and Society of Thoracic Surgeons. *J Am Coll Cardiol.* 2008;**52**:e1–42
23. Vahanian A, *et al.* Guidelines on the management of valvular heart disease (version 2012). *Eur Heart J.* 2012;**33**:2451–96
24. Gillam LD, *et al.* Primum non nocere: the case for watchful waiting in asymptomatic 'severe' degenerative mitral regurgitation. *Circulation.* 2010;**121**:813–21
25. Enriquez-Sarano M, *et al.* Early surgery is recommended for mitral regurgitation. *Circulation.* 2010;**121**:804–11
26. Grigioni F, *et al.* Outcomes in mitral regurgitation due to flail leaflets: a multicentre European study. *JACC Cardiovasc Imaging.* 2008;**1**:133–41
27. Barbieri A, *et al.* Prognostic and therapeutic implications of pulmonary hypertension complicating degenerative mitral regurgitation due to flail leaflet: a multicentre long-term international study. *Eur Heart J.* 2011;**32**:751–9
28. De Bonis M, *et al.* Mitral valve surgery: wait and see vs early operation. *Eur Heart J.* 2013;**34**:13–19
29. Vassileva CM, *et al.* Long-term survival of patients undergoing mitral valve repair and replacement: A longitudinal analysis of medicare fee-for-service beneficiaries. *Circulation.* 2013;**127**:1870–6
30. Glower DD. Surgical approaches to mitral regurgitation. *J Am Coll Cardiol.* 2012;**60**:1315–22
31. Vassileva CM, *et al.* Meta-analysis of short-term and long-term survival following repair versus replacement for ischaemic mitral regurgitation. *Eur J Cardiothorac Surg.* 2011;**39**:295–303
32. David TE, *et al.* Late outcomes of mitral valve repair for mitral regurgitation due to degenerative disease. *Circulation.* 2013;**127**:1485–92
33. Bonow RO. Chronic mitral regurgitation and aortic regurgitation: have indications for surgery changed? *J Am Coll Cardiol.* 2013;61:693–701
34. Deja MA, *et al.* Influence of mitral regurgitation repair on survival in the surgical treatment for ischaemic heart failure trial. *Circulation.* 2012;**125**:2639–48
35. Chan KM, *et al.* Coronary artery bypass surgery with or without mitral valve annuloplasty in moderate functional ischaemic mitral regurgitation: final results of the randomized ischaemic mitral evaluation (RIME) trial. *Circulation.* 2012;**126**:2502–10
36. Fattouch K, *et al.* POINT: efficacy of adding mitral valve restrictive annuloplasty to coronary artery bypass grafting in patients with moderate ischaemic mitral valve regurgitation: a randomized trial. *J Thorac Cardiovasc Surg.* 2009;**138**:278–285
37. Penicka M, *et al.* Predictors of improvement of unrepaired moderate ischaemic mitral regurgitation in patients undergoing elective isolated coronary artery bypass graft surgery. *Circulation.* 2009;**120**:1474–81
38. Lam BK, *et al.* Importance of moderate ischaemic mitral regurgitation. *Ann Thorac Surg.* 2005;**79**:462–70; discussion 462–70
39. Campwala SZ, *et al.* Mitral regurgitation progression following isolated coronary artery bypass surgery: frequency, risk factors, and potential prevention strategies. *Eur J Cardiothorac Surg.* 2006;**29**:348–53
40. van Bommel RJ, *et al.* Cardiac resynchronization therapy as a therapeutic option in patients with moderate-severe functional mitral regurgitation and high operative risk. *Circulation.* 2011;**124**:912–19
41. Chiam PT, *et al.* Percutaneous transcatheter mitral valve repair: a classification of the technology. *JACC Cardiovasc Interv.* 2011;**4**:1–13
42. Feldman T, *et al.* Percutaneous repair or surgery for mitral regurgitation. *N Engl J Med.* 2011;**364**:1395–406
43. Van Mieghaem NM, *et al.* Anatomy of the mitral valvular complex and its implications for transcatheter interventions for mitral regurgitation. *J Am Coll Cardiol.* 2010;**56**:617–26
44. Whitlow PL, *et al.* Acute and 12-month results with catheter-based mitral valve leaflet repair: The EVEREST II (endovascular valve edge-to-edge repair) high risk study. *J Am Coll Cardiol.* 2012;**59**:30–139
45. Cheung A, *et al.* Five-year experience with transcatheter transapical mitral valve-in-valve implantation for bioprosthetic valve dysfunction online first. *J Am Coll Cardiol.* 2013; doi:10.1016/j.jacc.2013.1001.1058

Chapter 18

Aortic stenosis

Epidemiology

Aortic stenosis (AS) is the most prevalent form of cardiovascular disease in the western world after hypertension, coronary artery disease, and mitral valve disease.[1,2] It is the most common form of valvular heart disease needing surgery in Europe.[2] Aortic sclerosis, defined as irregular valve thickening without obstruction to LV outflow, is present in about 25% of adults over 65 years of age and is associated with clinical factors, such as age, sex, hypertension, smoking, serum low-density lipoprotein and lipoprotein(a) levels, and diabetes mellitus.[3,4] The prevalence of moderate or severe aortic stenosis in patients ≥7% years old is 2.8%.[1]

Aetiology

The most common cause of AS in adults is calcification of a normal trileaflet or congenital bicuspid valve.[3] The disease process is characterized by lipid accumulation, inflammation, and calcification, with many similarities to atherosclerosis.[4] However, the pathophysiological processes in calcific AS are locally determined and regulated.[5] Rheumatic AS, due to fusion of the commissures with scarring and eventual calcification of the cusps, is less common in developed countries and is invariably accompanied by mitral valve disease. In the young, AS is due to congenital malformations, such as bicuspid aortic valve, discrete subvalvular obstruction, or supravalvular stenosis (see Chapter 7). Calcific valvular disease is known to cluster within families, and recently the CHARGE Extracoronary Calcium Working Group reported one single nucleotide polymorphism in the lipoprotein(a) locus that is associated with aortic valve calcification.[6]

Pathophysiology and natural history

Inflammation, fibrosis, and calcification contribute to the development of AS.[4] Metabolic syndrome is an independent predictor of AS progression, especially in younger patients.[7] The calcific disease progresses gradually over many years from the base of the cusps to the leaflets, eventually causing a reduction in leaflet motion and effective valve area without commissural fusion. The LV adapts to the obstruction by increasing wall thickness while maintaining normal chamber size. The consequent concentric hypertrophy is a compensatory mechanism to normalize the LV wall stress. As a result of increased wall thickness and diminished compliance of the chamber, LV end-diastolic pressure increases without chamber dilatation. LV systolic function is usually preserved, and cardiac output is maintained for many years. If LV systolic dysfunction is present, it usually improves after aortic valve replacement (AVR). Irreversible LV dysfunction is possible but cannot be easily diagnosed by preoperative imaging. Once even moderate stenosis is present (jet velocity >3.0 m/s), the average rate of progression is an increase in mean pressure gradient of 7 mmHg per year, and a decrease in valve area of 0.1 cm^2 per year.[8] Most patients with AV velocity of 4 m/s become symptomatic within the next 5 years and carry a 1% risk of sudden death per year.[9] Asymptomatic patients with very severe aortic stenosis (jet velocity >5 m/s) have a poor prognosis, with a high event rate (75% at 3 years have AVR or die) and a risk of rapid functional deterioration.[10] Impaired platelet function and decreased levels of Von Willebrand factor develop with severe disease and predispose to epistaxis and ecchymosis.[7]

Severe aortic stenosis is defined as an effective orifice area (valve area) ≤1cm^2 (0.6 cm^2/m^2 BSA) in the context of a mean transvalvular gradient ≥40 mmHg (Table 18.1). However, gradients are a squared function of flow as expressed by the stroke volume, and even a modest decrease of flow may lead to an important reduction in gradient, even in the presence of a severe stenosis. Thus, there has been a tendency to characterize severe aortic stenosis in terms of flow and gradient.[11]

Low-flow/low-gradient severe AS is defined as orifice area <1 cm^2 and mean gradient <40 mmHg, in the context of a reduced stroke volume (indexed stroke volume <35 mL/m^2) probably due to reduced systemic arterial compliance and intrinsic myocardial dysfunction.[12,13] This pattern is seen in 5–10% of patients with severe AS, and 20–30% of them have pseudosevere AS.

Pseudosevere AS is defined as a final aortic valve area ≥1.2 cm^2, mean transaortic pressure gradient <40 mmHg, and ≥20% increase in stroke volume (flow or contractile reserve) at peak dobutamine infusion (see Diagnosis).[12,13] Most of these patients have a depressed LV function and a dilated LV due to afterload mismatch and/or ischaemic heart disease.

Low-flow, low-gradient severe AS with normal LVEF or **paradoxical low-flow, low-gradient severe AS** is characterized by an orifice area <1 cm^2, a mean aortic pressure gradient <40 mmHg, an indexed LV stroke volume <35 mL/m^2, but a preserved LVEF (≥50%).[11-14] This pattern is seen in at least 10% of patients with severe AS, and the discrepancy between LVEF and stroke volume is attributed to high global afterload and restricted physiology with pronounced concentric remodelling and myocardial fibrosis that are mainly reflected in impaired longitudinal function.

Presentation

Patients, even with severe AS, may be asymptomatic. Usually with progression of stenosis severity, SOBOE or heart failure (50%), angina (35%), and syncope (15%) appear. Once symptoms develop, AVR is needed because the average survival is only 2 to 3 years, with an increased risk of sudden death. Table 18.1 presents the differential diagnosis of LVOT obstruction.

Physical examination

- **Slow arterial pulse** (pulsus parvus et tardus) in severe AS. May not be present with AR, in hypertension, or in the elderly due to rigid vasculature.
- Prominent **a waves** in JVP in severe AS (reduced RV compliance due to hypertrophy of the interventricular septum. The **v wave** may be prominent if there is RV failure.
- **Soft S_1** and **single S_2** (late or absent A_2)
- **S_4** (vigorous atrial contraction) indicates severe AS.

Table 18.1 ACC/AHA 2008 GL on valve disease. Factors that differentiate the various causes of left ventricular outflow tract obstruction

Factor	Valvular	Supravalvular	Discrete subvalvular	Obstructive HCM
Valve calcification	Common after age 40 y	No	No	No
Dilated ascending aorta	Common after age 40 y	Rare	Rare	Rare
PP after VPB	Increased	Increased	Increased	Decreased
Valsalva effect on SM	Decreased	Decreased	Decreased	Increased
Murmur of AR	Common after age 40 y	Rare	Sometimes	No
Fourth heart sound (S_4)	If severe	Uncommon	Uncommon	Common
Paradoxical splitting	Sometimes*	No	No	Rather common*
Ejection click	Most (unless valve calcified)	No	No	Uncommon or none
Maximal thrill and murmur	2nd RIS	1st RIS	2nd RIS	4th LIS
Carotid pulse	Normal to anacrotic* (parvus et tardus)	Unequal	Normal to anacrotic	Brisk, jerky, systolic rebound

* Depends on severity.

AR indicates aortic regurgitation; HCM, hypertrophic cardiomyopathy; LIS, left intercostal space; PP, pulse pressure; RIS, right intercostal space; SM, systolic murmur; and VPB, ventricular premature beat.

ACC/AHA 2008 focused update incorporated into the ACC/AHA 2006 guidelines for the management of patients with valvular heart disease. *J Am Coll Cardiol*. 2008;**52**:e1–142.

- A **thrill** may be present.
- Hyperdynamic LV suggests concomitant MR or AR.
- **Crescendo-decrescendo systolic murmur** along the left sternal border that radiates to the upper right sternal border and the carotids. It may also radiate to the LV apex (the Gallavardin phenomenon) and may be mistaken for MR.
- The intensity of the murmur does not correspond to the severity of AS.
- **Diastolic murmur** if AR is also present.
- **Systolic ejection click** in young patients with bicuspid valve.

Investigations

ECG LV hypertrophy. Left atrial enlargement in severe AS and AF in <15% of patients. Various degrees of AV and intraventricular block may be seen.

Chest radiography Usually normal. Cardiomegaly is a late feature in AS, and calcification is a universal finding, but rarely visible on chest X-ray. The proximal ascending aorta may be dilated, particularly in patients with bicuspid valves.

Echocardiography is the standard imaging procedure. Two-dimensional echocardiography puts the diagnosis and usually identifies a bicuspid valve. Doming of the aortic leaflets due to asymmetry and restriction is often seen in young patients with bicuspid aortic valves. Doppler echocardiography allows quantification of jet velocity, pressure gradient derived as 4 × (jet velocity)^2, and valve area (Table 18.2). An annual increase in jet velocity >0.3 m/s or a decrease in valve area >0.1 cm^2 indicates rapid hemodynamic progression.[15] All patients with mean gradients >30 mmHg or peak >50 mm Hg should be followed with yearly echocardiograms (Class I-C, ACC/AHA guidelines on valve disease 2008). In patients with mixed AS and AR, peak aortic jet velocity reflects both stenosis and regurgitation and represents a useful predictive parameter.[16]

Doppler-derived gradients tend to be higher and effective orifice area lower compared to those derived by cardiac catheterization. This is because the blood flow contracts to pass through the stenotic orifice, and a portion of the potential energy of the blood (i.e. pressure) is converted into kinetic energy (i.e. velocity), thus resulting in a pressure drop and acceleration of flow. Downstream of the vena contracta (i.e. the effective orifice area), a large part of the kinetic energy is irreversibly dissipated as heat because of flow turbulences. The remaining portion of the kinetic energy that is reconverted back to potential energy represents the so-called 'pressure recovery' (Figure 18.1).[17] This can be accounted for by calculating the Energy Loss Index (**ELI**). (ELI=[EOA × A_A / A_A- EOA]/BSA, where EOA=effective orifice area by conventional echocardiography, A_A = the cross sectional area of the aorta measured at 1cm downstrteam of the sinotunular junction, and BSA the body surface area). In asymptomatic patients with inconsistent grading of stenosis andobtained by catherization, and provides additional prognostic information independently of aortic gradient.[18]

Aortic sclerosis is characterized by focal areas of valve thickening, typically located in the leaflet centre, with commissural sparing and normal leaflet mobility. Jet velocity

Table 18.2 Classification of AS

ACC/AHA 2008 GL on valve disease. Severity of AS			
AV	**Area (cm²)**	**Mean gradient (mmHg)**	**Jet velocity (m/s)**
Mild	<1.5	<25	<3
Moderate	1–1.5	25–40	3–4
Severe	<1 (<0.6 cm²/m²)	>40	>4
ESC 2012 GL on valve disease. Definition of severe AS			
Valve area (cm²)	<1.0		
Indexed valve area (cm²/m² BSA)	<0.6		
Mean gradient (mmHg) (in patients with normal cardiac output/transvalvular flow)	>40		
Maximum jet velocity (m/s) (in patients with normal cardiac output/transvalvular flow)	>4.0		
Velocity ratio	<0.25		

ACC/AHA 2008 focused update incorporated into the ACC/AHA 2006 guidelines for the management of patients with valvular heart disease. *J Am Coll Cardiol*. 2008;**52**:e1–142.
ESC guidelines on the management of valvular heart disease (version 2012). *European Heart Journal*. 2012;**33**:2451–2496

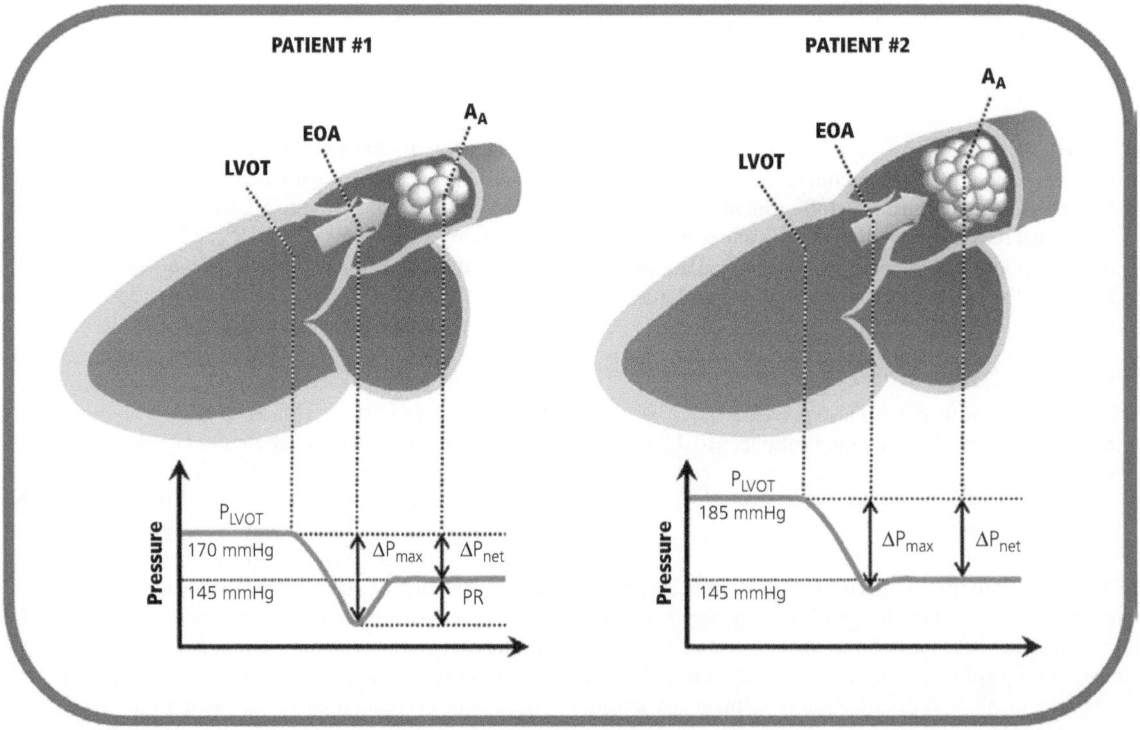

Figure 18.1 The phenomenon of pressure recovery in aortic stenosis. Schematic representation of flow and blood pressure across the left ventricular outflow tract (PLVOT), aortic valve, and ascending aorta (AA) during systole in two theoretical patients having the same stroke volume (80 mL) and valve effective orifice area (EOA; 0.9 cm²) but different sizes of ascending aorta (2.0 cm diameter in patient 1 vs 4.0 cm in patient 2). The maximum pressure gradient recorded at vena contracta (ΔPmax, i.e. the mean gradient measured by Doppler) is the same in the two patients, but patient 1, with the small aorta, has a large amount of pressure recovery (PR) downstream of the valve whereas patient 2 has minimal pressure recovery. Consequently, the net 'irreversible' gradient (ΔPnet, i.e. measured by catheter), and thus the left ventricular systolic pressure, is significantly higher in patient 2 than in patient 1.

LVOT indicates left ventricular outflow tract.

Pibarot P, *et al*. Energy Loss Index in Aortic Stenosis: Fluid Mechanics Concept to Clinical Application. *Circulation*. 2013;**127**:1101–1104 in aortic sclerosis is <2.5 m/s. Diffuse leaflet thickening is not seen in aortic sclerosis, being suggestive of normal ageing changes, significant AS, or imaging artefact. In AS, the aortic valve is usually thickened and calcified, with limited excursion and a reduced aortic valve area.

Low-dose dobutamine haemodynamic measurements or **exercise echocardiography** is useful in cases of **low-flow/low-gradient severe AS** in order to differentiate patients with anatomically severe AS from those with pseudosevere AS (ACC/AHA guidelines on valve disease 2008, IIa-C/B). Dobutamine (5–20 microgram/kg/min) in AS with LV dysfunction and gradient <40 mmHg produces an increment in stroke volume (>20%) and valve area (>1 cm^2 and/or an increase ≥0.3 cm^2) but no change in gradient, in haemodynamically non-significant stenosis (pseudosevere AS). In significant AS, the valve area remains unchanged (or increases <0.2 cm^2 but remains <1 cm^2) whereas the gradient and stroke volume increase (mean gradient >40 mmHg). In ambiguous response, calculation of the projected orifice area that would have occurred at a standardized flow rate of 250 mL/s may be useful (TOPAS trial).[19] Patients who fail to show at least 20% stroke volume increase with dobutamine (lack of the so-called contractile or, more accurately, **flow reserve**) have a poor prognosis with either medical or surgical therapy,[12] but this finding may not necessarily preclude consideration of AVR or TAVI.[13]

In **paradoxical low-flow, low-gradient severe AS**, detailed echocardiographic examination to avoid miscalculation of the stroke volume, evaluation of the systemic arterial compliance and valvuloarterial impedance (Z_{VA}), and interpretation of findings in the context of peripheral blood pressure are recommended.[20] Impaired longitudinal function, i.e. lower basal longitudinal strain and tissue velocities and mitral plane excursion, is assessed by speckle-tracking echocardiography.[21] Reduced stroke volume index (<35 mL/m^2) and impaired longitudinal strain and lower tissue velocities and mitral plane excursion are markers of worse prognosis.

Plasma BNP A high value (>550 pg/mL) is a powerful predictor of mortality in patients with low-flow/low-gradient AS, regardless of medical or surgical treatment or the presence and/or absence of flow reserve.[22]

Treadmill exercise testing (closely supervised) is no longer contraindicated in asymptomatic AS[23] and may be considered to elicit exercise-induced symptoms and abnormal blood pressure responses (ACC/AHA guidelines on valve disease 2008, IIb-B). Development of symptoms or a hypotensive response are predictors of sudden death and indicate the need of valve replacement. Exercise testing is contraindicated in symptomatic AS. Truly severe AS shows only small changes in valve area (increase <0.2 cm^2 and remaining <1 cm^2), with increasing flow rate but a significant increase in gradients (mean gradient >40 mmHg), whereas pseudosevere AS shows a marked increase in valve area but only minor changes in gradients. In addition, this test may detect the presence of flow reserve, which has favourable prognostic implications.

Table 18.3 ACC/AHA 2008 GL on valve disease

Indications for cardiac catheterization	
Coronary angiography before AVR in patients with AS at risk for CAD.	I-B
Cardiac catheterization for assessment of severity of AS in symptomatic patients when non-invasive tests are inconclusive or when there is a discrepancy between non-invasive tests and clinical findings regarding severity of AS.	I-C
Coronary angiography before AVR in patients with AS for whom a pulmonary autograft (Ross procedure) is contemplated and if the origin of the coronary arteries was not identified by non-invasive technique.	I-C
Cardiac catheterization for haemodynamic measurements is not recommended for the assessment of severity of AS before AVR when non-invasive tests are adequate and concordant with clinical findings or for the assessment of LV function and severity of AS in asymptomatic patients.	III-C

ACC/AHA 2008 focused update incorporated into the ACC/AHA 2006 guidelines for the management of patients with valvular heart disease. *J Am Coll Cardiol*. 2008;**52**:e1–142.

Computed tomography is useful for the assessment of aortic root dilatation. In addition, it can be used in 'low-flow/low-gradient' AS. A calcium score of >1651 U has been found 93% sensitive and 75% specific in the identification of patients with truly severe AS.[24]

Cardiac magnetic resonance allows anatomic measurement of the valve area and estimation of jet velocity and stroke volume (especially in paradoxical low-flow, low-gradient AS).

Cardiac catheterization may be necessary for assessment of the gradient in the case of inconclusive non-invasive tests results (Table 18.3). Dobutamine can also be used to identify low-flow/low-gradient AS.

Coronary angiography is necessary before surgery in patients with risk factors or clinical suspicion of coronary artery disease (Table 18.3 and Tables 15.3 and 15.4 in Chapter 15) and occasionally before a Ross procedure to identify the origins of the coronaries.

Therapy

Medical therapy consists of exercise restriction and cautious use of diuretics and ACE/ARB that may delay progression of AS.[25] Vasodilators can cause an increase in cardiac output that helps offset the drop in systemic vascular resistance, even in severe AS.[26] Initial evidence about the beneficial effect of statins in reducing progression of AS has not been verified.[27] Osteoporotic and antifibrotic therapies are also under consideration.[4]

AVR is indicated in symptomatic patients with severe AS, even in the presence of LVEF <35%, unless this is due to previous myocardial infarctions (Tables 18.4 and 18.5, Figures 18.2 to 18.4).[8,28] Recent evidence suggests that AVR may be advisable in asymptomatic patients with severe AS.[10,28]

Surgical risk can be estimated by online risk calculators from the Society of Thoracic Surgeons (http://www.sts.org/quality-research-patient-safety/quality/risk-calculator-and-models/risk-calculator) or the European System for Cardiac Operative Risk Evaluation (EuroSCORE; http://www.euroscore.org). The STS score tends to underestimate risk for AVR whereas the logistic EuroSCORE overestimates risk for isolated valve surgery.[29] According to the STS National Database, the operative mortality for isolated AVR has declined from 3.4% in 2002 to 2.6% today in the USA (http://www.sts.org/sites/default/files/documents/2011 2ndHarvestExecutiveSummary.pdf).

Long-term survival after surgical aortic valve replacement in the elderly is excellent, although patients with a high (≥10) STS perioperative risk of mortality and those with certain co-morbidities (lung disease and renal failure, particularly dialysis-dependent renal failure) carry a particularly poor long-term prognosis.[30]

Patients with **low-flow/low-gradient severe AS** have poor prognosis, with medical therapy (survival rates <50% at 3-year follow-up).[13] Operative risk is 22–33% in those with no flow reserve (increase in stroke volume <20% with dobutamine) but 5–8% in the presence of preserved flow reserve.[13] The role of TAVI in these patients is under investigation.

Patients with **low-flow/low-gradient pseudosevere AS** have a 5-year survival under medical therapy better than patients with true severe AS.[31]

The prognosis of patients with **paradoxical low-flow, low-gradient severe AS** is controversial. It has been reported to be worse than those with high-gradient se-

Table 18.4 ACC/AHA 2008GL on valve disease

Indications for aortic valve replacement	
Symptomatic patients with severe AS.	I-B
Patients with severe AS undergoing cardiac surgery	I-C
Severe AS and LV systolic dysfunction (LVEF <0.50).	I-C
Patients with moderate AS undergoing CABG or surgery on the aorta or other heart valves.	IIa-B
Asymptomatic patients with severe AS and abnormal response to exercise (e.g. development of symptoms or asymptomatic hypotension).	IIb-C
Severe asymptomatic AS if there is a high likelihood of rapid progression (age, calcification, and CAD) or if surgery might be delayed at the time of symptom onset.	IIb-C
Patients undergoing CABG who have mild AS when there is evidence, such as moderate to severe valve calcification, that progression may be rapid.	IIb-C
Asymptomatic patients with extremely severe AS (aortic valve area <0.6 cm², mean gradient >60mmHg, and jet velocity >5.0 m/s) when the patient's expected operative mortality is ≤1%.	IIb-C
AVR for prevention of sudden death in asymptomatic patients with AS who have none of the findings listed under Class IIa/IIb.	III-B

ACC/AHA 2008 focused update incorporated into the ACC/AHA 2006 guidelines for the management of patients with valvular heart disease. *J Am Coll Cardiol*. 2008;**52**:e1–142.

Table 18.5 ESC 2012 GL on valve disease

Indications for aortic valve replacement in aortic stenosis	
Patients with severe AS and symptoms related to AS.	I-B
Patients with severe AS undergoing coronary artery bypass surgery, surgery of the ascending aorta or on another valve.	I-C
Asymptomatic patients with severe AS and systolic LV dysfunction (LVEF <50%) not due to other cause.	I-C
Asymptomatic patients with severe AS and abnormal exercise test showing symptoms on exercise related to AS	I-C
AVR in high-risk patients with severe symptomatic AS who are suitable for TAVI but in whom surgery is favoured by a 'heart team', based on the individual risk profile and anatomic suitability.	IIa-B
Asymptomatic patients with severe AS and abnormal exercise test showing fall in blood pressure below baseline.	IIa-C
Patients with moderate AS* undergoing coronary artery bypass surgery, surgery of the ascending aorta or another valve.	IIa-C
Symptomatic patients with low-flow, low-gradient (<40 mmHg) AS with normal EF only after careful confirmation of severe AS.**	IIa-C
Symptomatic patients with severe AS, low-flow, low-gradient with reduced EF, and evidence of flow (contractile) reserve.	IIa-C
Asymptomatic patients, with normal EF and none of the above mentioned exercise test abnormalities, if the surgical risk is low, and one or more of the following findings is present: • Very severe AS defined by a peak transvalvular velocity >5.5 m/s or, • Severe valve calcification and a rate of peak transvalvular velocity progression ≥0.3 m/s per year.	IIa-C
Symptomatic patients with severe AS low-flow, low-gradient and LV dysfunction without flow (contractile) reserve.	IIb-C
Asymptomatic patients with severe AS, normal EF, and none of the above mentioned exercise test abnormalities, if surgical risk is low, and one or more of the following findings is present: • Markedly elevated natriuretic peptide levels confirmed by repeated measurements and without other explanations • Increase of mean pressure gradient with exercise by >20 mmHg • Excessive LV hypertrophy in the absence of hypertension.	IIb-C

* Moderate AS is defined as valve area 1.0–1.5 cm² (0.6 cm²/m²–0.9 cm²/m² BSA) or mean aortic gradient 25–40 mmHg in the presence of normal flow conditions. However, clinical judgement is required.

** Patients with a small valve area, but low gradient despite preserved LVEF, explanations for this finding (other than the presence of severe AS) are frequent and must be carefully excluded.

ESC guidelines on the management of valvular heart disease (version 2012). *European Heart Journal* 2012;**33**:2451–2496.

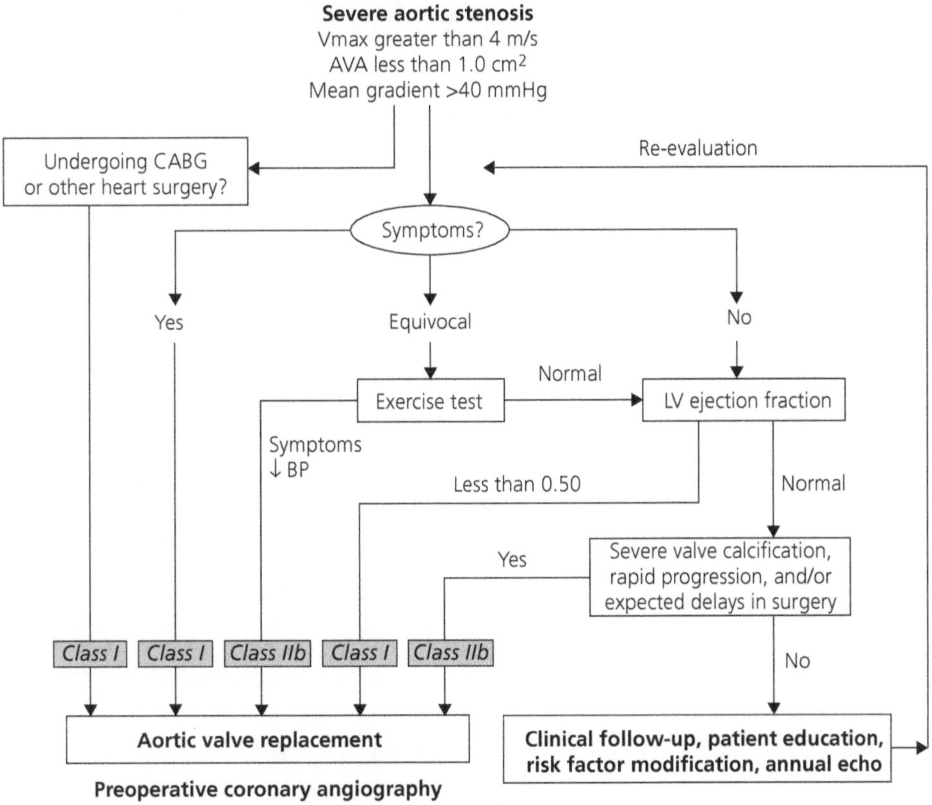

Figure 18.2 ACC/AHA 2008 GL on valve disease. Management of severe AS.

ACC/AHA 2008 focused update incorporated into the ACC/AHA 2006 guidelines for the management of patients with valvular heart disease. *J Am Coll Cardiol*. 2008;**52**:e1–142

vere AS or those with moderate AS and improve with surgery,[32] but, in the SEAS study, outcome was similar to that of patients with moderate stenosis.[33] Patients with paradoxical low-flow/low-gradient severe AS can be managed medically with serial (6–12 months) clinical and echocardiographic evaluations. Patients who develop symptoms on exercise, and particularly those with stroke volume index <35mL/m², should be referred for surgery.[33] A proposed management scheme of patients with low-gradient severe AS is presented in Figure 18.5.[34]

The **choice of prosthesis** is based on patient age and the risk of anticoagulation (see Chapter 22 on prosthetic valves). Indications for **concomitant CABG** are presented in Tables 18.6 and 18.7. Recommendations of ACC/AHA for congenital AS are presented in Table 18.8 (see also Chapter 7 on LVOT obstruction). Concomitant coronary artery disease should be treated with CABG at time of aortic valve operation (I-A for stenosis >70% or IIa-C for stenosis 50–70%; ESC 2010 Guideline on revascularization).

TAVI

Percutaneous implantation of bioprosthetic valves is evolving fast, with very promising results in selected inoperable patients.[35–39] Inoperable patients were initially defined as those with STS score>10 or logistic EuroSCORE>20%, and now as judged by a team of surgeons and cardiologists. The Edwards SAPIEN valve system (Edwards Lifesciences Inc, Irvine, CA) is a trileaflet bovine pericardial valve mounted on a cobalt chromium stent frame (Figure 18.6). The CoreValve system (Medtronic, Minneapolis, MN) is a trileaflet porcine pericardial valve mounted in a self-expanding nitinol stent (Figure 18.6). Other devices are also under study (Portico by St Jude). The devices are usually implanted by a transfemoral retrograde approach; the alternatives are a subclavian or trans-aortic approach. The transapical approach is also an option but carries a high complication rate.[40] Procedural complications, including death (6–7% with overall 30-day mortality of approximately 9%), stroke (1–3%), renal failure (2.5–5%), coronary occlusion (1%), and valve embolization (1%), are not significantly different between Sapien and CoreValve).[35,41–43] Significant AR

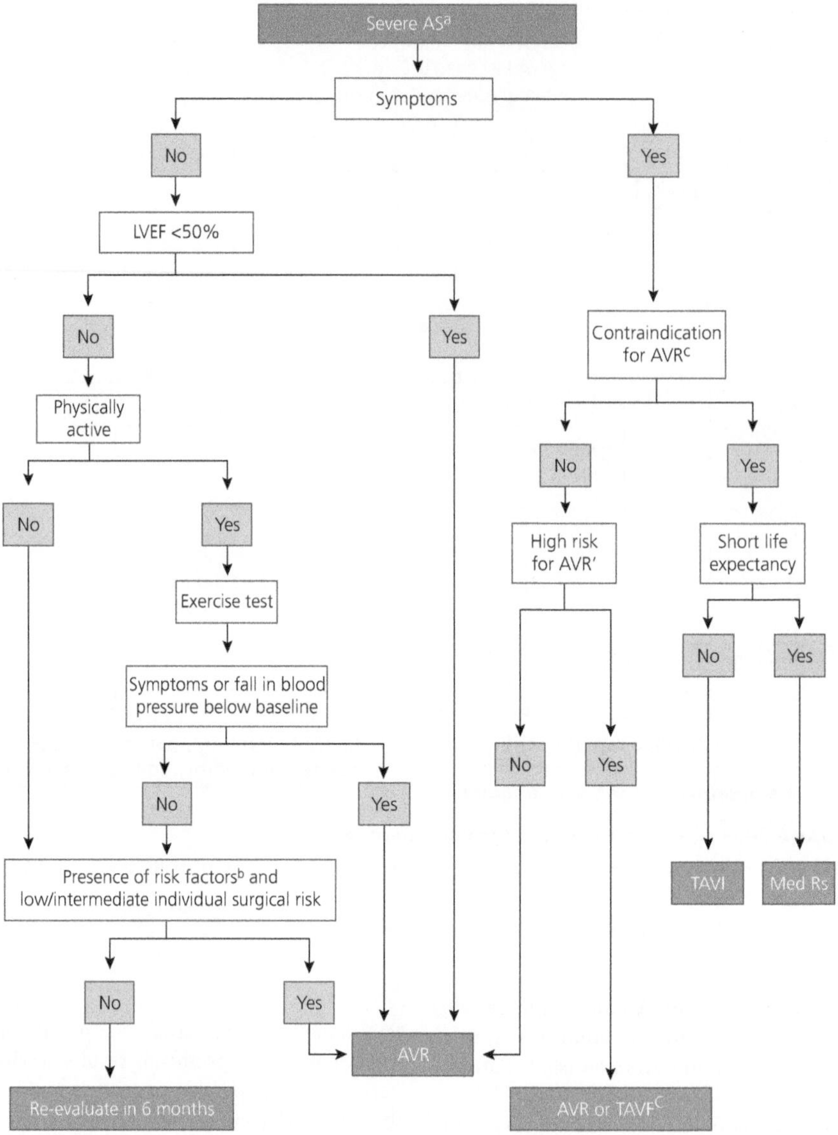

Figure 18.3 ESC 2012 GL on valve disease. Management of severe AS.

AS = aortic stenosis; AVR = aortic valve replacement; BSA = body surface area; LVEF = left ventricular ejection fraction; Med Rx = medical therapy; TAVI = transcatheter aortic valve implantation. a: See Table 18.2 for definition of severe AS. b: Surgery should be considered (IIaC) if one of the following is present: peak velocity >5.5m/s; severe valve calcification + peak velocity progression ≥0.3 m/s/year. Surgery may be considered (IIbC) if one of the following is present: markedly elevated natriuretic peptide levels; mean gradient increase with exercise >20 mmHg; excessive LV hypertrophy. c: The decision should be made by the 'heart team' according to individual clinical characteristics and anatomy.

ESC guidelines on the management of valvular heart disease (version 2012). *European Heart Journal* 2012;**33**:2451–2496

(grade ≥3) occurs in 5% but moderate regurgitation may be seen in up to 24% of patients.[44] Vascular complications are higher with the Sapien valves that required 22 or 24 French delivery systems (22% vs 11%).[43] There is a higher incidence of the need for permanent pacing with the CoreValve (25% vs 5%), and probably LBBB that may occur in up to 40% of patients.[41–43,45] The prognostic significance of LBBB following surgical valve replacement is adverse, but controversial after TAVI. It has been identified as an independent predictor of mortality following SAPIEN (51% vs 12%),[46] but not CoreValve implantation.[45] The reported 1-year mortality in TAVI patients is 20%, similar to that of high-risk patients subjected to surgical AVR (18%).[30,35,41–43] Two-year mortality is probably similar (33.9 vs 35%)[37], and long-term (5 years) results have detected a valve failure rate of 3.4%.[39]

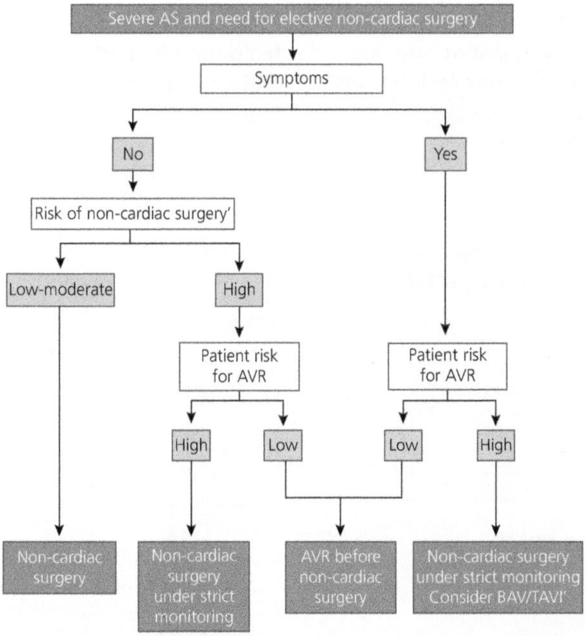

Figure 18.4 ESC 2012 GL on valve disease. Management of severe aortic stenosis and elective non-cardiac surgery according to patient characteristics and the type of surgery.

AS = aortic stenosis; AVR = aortic valve replacement; BAV = balloon aortic valvuloplasty; TAVI = transcatheter aortic valve implantation. a: Classification into three groups according to the risk of cardiac complications (30-day death and myocardial infarction) for non-cardiac surgery (high risk >5%; intermediate risk 1–5%; low risk <1%) b: Non-cardiac surgery performed only if strictly needed. The choice between balloon aortic valvuloplasty and transcatheter aortic valve implantation should take into account patient life expectancy.

ESC guidelines on the management of valvular heart disease (version 2012). *European Heart Journal* 2012;**33**:2451–2496

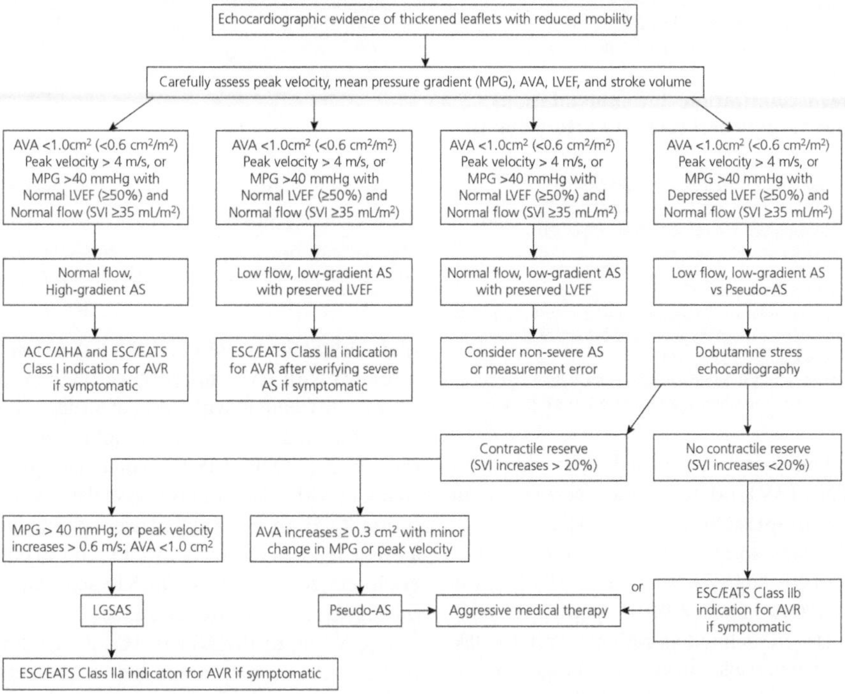

Figure 18.5 A proposed management scheme for patients with low gradient severe AS.

Tandon A, *et al*. Imaging of low-gradient severe aortic stenosis. *J Am Coll Cardiol Img.* 2013;**6**:184–195

Table 18.6 CABG at time of AVR

ACC/AHA GL on valve disease. Treatment of coronary artery disease at the time of aortic valve replacement*	
CABG for patients undergoing AVR with significant stenosis of major coronary arteries. (≥70% reduction in luminal diameter).	I-C
Use of the LIMA for LAD stenosis ≥50–70% during AVR.	IIa-C
CABG in patients undergoing AVR with moderate coronary stenosis (50–70% reduction in luminal diameter).	IIa-C
ESC 2010 GL on revascularization. Recommendations for combined valve surgery and coronary artery bypass grafting	
CABG in patients with a primary indication for aortic/mitral valve surgery and coronary artery diameter stenosis >70%.	I-C
CABG in patients with a primary indication for aortic/mitral valve surgery and coronary artery diameter stenosis 50–70%.	IIa-C

* Also adopted by ACCF/AHA 2011 on CABG.

ACC/AHA 2008 focused update incorporated into the ACC/AHA 2006 guidelines for the management of patients with valvular heart disease. *J Am Coll Cardiol*. 2008;**52**:e1–142.

ESC/EACTS Guidelines on myocardial revascularization. The Task Force on ESC Guidelines on myocardial revascularization. *Eur Heart J*. 2010;**31**:2501–55

Table 18.7 AVR at time of CABG

ACC/AHA 2008 GL on valve disease. Aortic valve replacement in patients undergoing coronary artery bypass surgery*	
AVR during CABG in patients with severe AS who meet the criteria for valve replacement.	I-C
AVR in patients undergoing CABG who have moderate AS (mean gradient 30–50 mmHg or Doppler velocity 3–4m/s).	IIa-B
AVR in patients undergoing CABG who have mild AS (mean gradient <30 mmHg or Doppler velocity <3 m/s) when there is evidence, such as moderate-severe valve calcification, that progression may be rapid.	IIb-C
ESC 2010 GL on revascularization. Recommendations for combined valve surgery and coronary artery bypass grafting	
Aortic valve surgery in patients with a primary indication for CABG and moderate aortic stenosis (mean gradient 30–50 mmHg or Doppler velocity 3–4 m/s or heavily calcified aortic valve, even when Doppler velocity 2.5–3 m/s).	IIa-C

* Also adopted by ACCF/AHA 2011 on CABG.

ACC/AHA guidelines on valve disease 2008 focused update incorporated into the ACC/AHA 2006 guidelines for the management of patients with valvular heart disease. *J Am Coll Cardiol*. 2008;**52**:e1–142.

ESC/EACTS Guidelines on myocardial revascularization The Task Force ESC Guidelines on myocardial revascularization. *Eur Heart J*. 2010;**31**:2501–55

In the only randomized trial published so far and which used the SAPIEN, TAVI offered better survival than medical therapy in **inoperable** patients (PARTNER B).[38] Two-year mortality was 43.3% vs 68%, P <001, albeit at an increased risk of stroke (6.7% vs 1.7%, P = 0.02 in the first 30 days and 2.2% vs 0.6%, P = 0.16 beyond 30 days).[38] Inoperable patients were defined as patients with a ≥50% risk of mortality or irreversible morbidity as judged by two surgeons and one cardiologist. The STS score was 11.2 ± 5.8, but other factors, such as porcelain aorta, chest wall deformities, COPD, and frailty, were also considered. In

Table 18.8 ACC/AHA 2008 GL on valve disease

Indications for aortic balloon valvotomy in adolescents and young adults with congenital (usually bicuspid) AS (see also LVOT obstruction in GUCH)	
Adolescent or young adult patient with angina, syncope, or dyspnoea on exertion and a catheterization peak LV to peak aortic gradient ≥50 mmHg without a heavily calcified valve.* Asymptomatic adolescent or young adult patient with:	I-C
Catheterization peak LV to peak aortic gradient >60 mmHg.*	I-C
ST or T wave changes over the left precordium at rest or with exercise and a catheterization peak LV to aortic gradient >50 mmHg.*	I-C
Catheterization peak LV to peak aortic gradient >50 mmHg, and the patient wants to play competitive sports or desires to become pregnant.*	IIa-C
Catheterization peak LV to peak aortic gradient <40 mmHg without symptoms or ECG changes.*	III-C
In the adolescent or young adult patient with AS, aortic balloon valvotomy, performed in experienced centres, is preferred to valve surgery.	IIa-C

* Gradients are usually obtained with patients sedated. If general anaesthesia is used, the gradients may be somewhat lower.

ACC/AHA 2008 focused update incorporated into the ACC/AHA 2006 guidelines for the management of patients with valvular heart disease. *J Am Coll Cardiol*. 2008;**52**:e1–142.

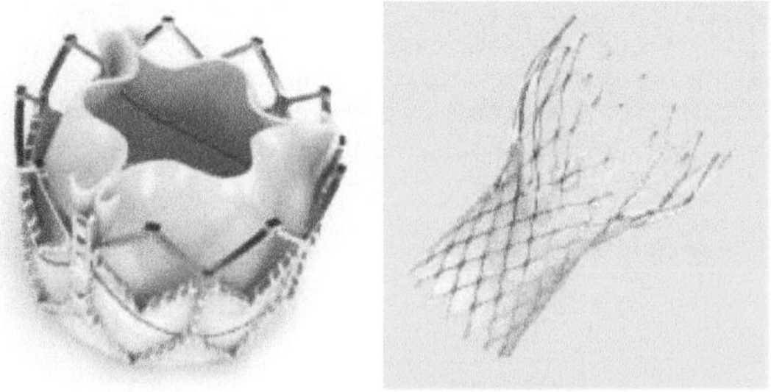

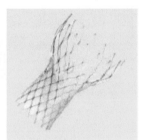

Figure 18.6 Sapien (Edwards Lifesciences) left, and CoreValve (Medtronic) right.

Webb JG, *et al*. Current status of transcatheter aortic valve replacement. *J Am Coll Cardiol*. 2012 Aug 7;**60**(6):483–92

high-risk patients (PARTNER A), there was similar 2-year mortality with TAVI and surgery (33.9% vs 35%).[37] Strokes were more frequent with TAVI at 30 days (4.6% vs 2.4%, P = 0.12), but, at 2 years, they did not differ significantly with the two approaches. Perivalvular regurgitation was more frequent with TAVI and was associated with increased late mortality. High-risk patients were defined as patients with a predicted risk of mortality ≥15% by 30 days after the operation by two surgeons. The STS score was 11.8 ± 3.3, and the logistic EuroSCORE29.3 ± 16.

According to the recent ACCF/STS consensus document, TAVI is recommended in patients with severe, symptomatic, calcific stenosis of a trileaflet aortic valve who have aortic and vascular anatomy suitable for TAVI and a predicted survival >12 months and who have a

Table 18.9 2012 ACCF/AATS/SCAI/STS expert consensus document on transcatheter aortic valve replacement

Patient selection: inclusion and exclusion criteria in clinical trials
Inclusion criteria
1. Patient has calcific aortic valve stenosis with echocardiographically derived criteria: mean gradient >40 mmHg or jet velocity >4.0 m/s and an initial AVA of <0.8 cm^2 or indexed EOA <0.5 cm^2/m^2. Qualifying AVA baseline measurement must be within 45 days of the date of the procedure.
2. A cardiac interventionalist and two experienced cardiothoracic surgeons agree that medical factors either preclude operation or are high risk for surgical AVR, based on a conclusion that the probability of death or serious, irreversible morbidity exceeds the probability of meaningful improvement. The surgeons' consult notes shall specify the medical or anatomic factors leading to that conclusion and include a printout of the calculation of the STS score to additionally identify the risks in the patient. At least one of the cardiac surgeon assessors must have physically evaluated the patient.
3. Patient is deemed to be symptomatic from his/her aortic valve stenosis, as differentiated from symptoms related to co-morbid conditions and as demonstrated by NYHA functional class II or greater.
Exclusion criteria (candidates will be excluded if any of the following conditions are present)
1. Evidence of an acute myocardial infarction ≤1 month (30 days) before the intended treatment (defined as: Q wave MI, or non-Q wave MI with total CK elevation of CK-MB ≥ twice normal in the presence of MB elevation and/or troponin level elevation [WHO definition]).
2. Aortic valve is a congenital unicuspid or congenital bicuspid valve or is non-calcified.
3. Mixed aortic valve disease (aortic stenosis and aortic regurgitation with predominant aortic regurgitation >3+).
4. Haemodynamic or respiratory instability requiring inotropic support, mechanical ventilation, or mechanical heart assistance within 30 days of screening evaluation.
5. Need for emergency surgery for any reason.
6. Hypertrophic cardiomyopathy with or without obstruction.
7. Severe left ventricular dysfunction with LVEF <20%.
8. Severe pulmonary hypertension and RV dysfunction.
9. Echocardiographic evidence of intracardiac mass, thrombus, or vegetation.
10. A known contraindication or hypersensitivity to all anticoagulation regimens or inability to be anticoagulated for the study procedure.
11. Native aortic annulus size <18 mm or >25 mm as measured by echocardiogram.*
12. MRI confirmed CVA or TIA within 6 months (180 days) of the procedure.
13. Renal insufficiency (creatinine >3.0 mg/dL) and/or end-stage renal disease requiring chronic dialysis at the time of screening.
14. Estimated life expectancy <12 months (365 days) due to non-cardiac co-morbid conditions.
15. Severe incapacitating dementia.
16. Significant aortic disease, including abdominal aortic or thoracic ancurysm defined as maximal luminal diameter 5 cm or greater; marked tortuosity (hyperacute bend), aortic arch atheroma (especially if thick [>5 mm], protruding, or ulcerated) or narrowing (especially with calcification and surface irregularities) of the abdominal or thoracic aorta, severe 'unfolding' and tortuosity of the thoracic aorta.
17. Severe mitral regurgitation.

AVA, aortic valve area; AVR, aortic valve replacement; CK, creatine kinase; CVA, cerebrovascular accident; EOA, effective orifice area; LVEF, left ventricular ejection fraction;
MB, MB isoenzyme; MI, myocardial infarction; MRI, magnetic resonance imaging; NYHA, New York Heart Association; RV, right ventricular; STS, Society of Thoracic Surgeons;
TIA, transient ischaemic attack; WHO, World Health Organization. *The boundaries of annulus size will continue to change in concert with changing device size.
2012 ACCF/AATS/SCAI/STS Expert Consensus Document on Transcatheter Aortic Valve Replacement. *J Am Coll Cardiol*. 2012 Jan 30. [Epub ahead of print] PubMed PMID: 22300974.

prohibitive surgical risk as defined by an estimated 50% or greater risk of mortality or irreversible morbidity at 30 days or other factors, such as frailty, prior radiation therapy, porcelain aorta, and severe hepatic or pulmonary disease (Table 18.9).[36] PCI, if indicated, may be performed before TAVI to improve procedural safety of TAVI. Risk factors are LVEF ≤30% and a STS ≥10).[47] TAVI may also be used in patients with degenerated stenotic or regurgitant bioprosthetic valves.[48] Operators and institutions performing TAVI should fulfill several requirements.[49,50] The 2012 ESC guidelines on valve disease recommendations for TAVI are presented in Tables 18.10 and 18.11.

Balloon valvotomy has only a palliative role or as a bridge for surgery in adults with tricuspid stenotic aortic valve. It may be the treatment of choice in **congenital (bicuspid or unicuspid) AS** as described in Table 18.10 (see also Chapter 7 on LVOT obstruction).

Non-cardiac surgery

In patients with severe AS needing elective non-cardiac surgery, the management depends mainly on the presence of symptoms and the type of surgery (Figure 18.3).

Table 18.10 ESC 2012 on VD

Recommendations for the use of transcatheter aortic valve implantation (TAVI)	
TAVI should only be undertaken with a multidisciplinary 'heart team', including cardiologists and cardiac surgeons and other specialists if necessary.	I-C
TAVI should only be performed in hospitals with cardiac surgery on-site.	I-C
TAVI is indicated in patients with severe symptomatic AS who are not suitable for AVR, as assessed by a 'heart team', and who are likely to gain improvement in their quality of life and to have a life expectancy of more than 1 year after consideration of their co-morbidities.	I-B
TAVI should be considered in high-risk patients with severe symptomatic AS who may still be suitable for surgery but in whom TAVI is favoured by a 'heart team' based on the individual risk profile and anatomic suitability.	IIa-B

ESC guidelines on the management of valvular heart disease (version 2012). The Joint Task Force on the Management of Valvular Heart Disease of the European Society of Cardiology (ESC) and the European Association for Cardio-Thoracic Surgery (EACTS) *European Heart Journal* 2012;**33**:2451–2496.

Table 18.11 ESC 2012 on VD. Contraindications for transcatheter aortic valve implantation (TAVI)

Absolute contraindications
Absence of a 'heart team' and no cardiac surgery on the site
Appropriateness of TAVI as an alternative to AVR not confirmed by a 'heart team'
Clinical
Estimated life expectancy <1 year
Improvement of quality of life by TAVI unlikely because of co-morbidities
Severe primary associated disease of other valves with major contribution to the patient's symptoms that can be treated only by surgery
Anatomical
Inadequate annulus size (<18 mm, >29 mm*)
Thrombus in the left ventricle
Active endocarditis
Elevated risk of coronary ostium obstruction (asymmetric valve calcification, short distance between annulus and coronary ostium, small aortic sinuses)
Plaques with mobile thrombi in the ascending aorta or arch
For transfemoral/subclavian approach: inadequate vascular access (vessel size, calcification, tortuosity)
Relative contraindications
Bicuspid or non-calcified valves
Untreated coronary artery disease requiring revascularization
Haemodynamic instability
LVEF <20%
For transapical approach: severe pulmonary disease, LV apex not accessible

* Contraindication when using the current devices.
ESC guidelines on valve disease 2012. Guidelines on the management of valvular heart disease (version 2012). The Joint Task Force on the Management of Valvular Heart Disease of the European Society of Cardiology (ESC) and the European Association for Cardio-Thoracic Surgery (EACTS) *European Heart Journal* 2012;**33**:2451–2496.

The management of patients with congenital AS is described in Chapter 1 on GUCH. The management of patients with AS subjected to non-cardiac surgery is presented in Figure 18.3.

Pregnancy

Patients with severe AS should undergo intervention pre-pregnancy in the presence of symptoms (I-C), LV dysfunction (LVEF <50%, I-C), when they when they develop symptoms (I-C) or a fall in blood pressure below baseline during exercise testing (IIa-C, ESC 2011 GL on pregnancy).

References

1. Go AS, *et al.* Heart disease and stroke statistics—2013 update: a report from the American Heart Association. *Circulation.* 2013;**127**:e6–e245
2. Iung B, *et al.* A prospective survey of patients with valvular heart disease in Europe: The Euro Heart Survey on valvular heart disease. *Eur Heart J.* 2003;**24**:1231–43
3. Maganti K, *et al.* Valvular heart disease: diagnosis and management. *Mayo Clin Proc.* 2010;**85**:483–500
4. Dweck MR, *et al.* Calcific aortic stenosis: a disease of the valve and the myocardium. *J Am Coll Cardiol.* 2012;**60**:1854–63
5. van der Linde D, *et al.* Natural history of discrete subaortic stenosis in adults: A multicentre study. *Eur Heart J.* 2013;**34**:1548–1556

6. Thanassoulis GCC, *et al.* Genetic associations with valvular calcification and aortic stenosis. *N Engl J Med.* 2013;**368**:503–12
7. Capoulade R, *et al.* Impact of metabolic syndrome on progression of aortic stenosis: influence of age and statin therapy. *J Am Coll Cardiol.* 2012;**60**:216–23
8. Bonow RO, *et al.* 2008 focused update incorporated into the ACC/AHA 2006 guidelines for the management of patients with valvular heart disease: a report of the American College of Cardiology/American Heart Association Task Force on practice guidelines (writing committee to revise the 1998 guidelines for the management of patients with valvular heart disease). Endorsed by the Society of Cardiovascular Anesthesiologists, Society for Cardiovascular Angiography and Interventions, and Society of Thoracic Surgeons. *J Am Coll Cardiol.* 2008;**52**:e1–42
9. Pellikka PA, *et al.* Outcome of 622 adults with asymptomatic, haemodynamically significant aortic stenosis during prolonged follow-up. *Circulation.* 2005;**111**:3290–5
10. Rosenhek R, *et al.* Natural history of very severe aortic stenosis. *Circulation.* 2010;**121**:151–6
11. Lancellotti P, *et al.* Clinical outcome in asymptomatic severe aortic stenosis: insights from the new proposed aortic stenosis grading classification. *J Am Coll Cardiol.* 2012;**59**:235–43
12. Awtry E, *et al.* Low-flow/low-gradient aortic stenosis. *Circulation.* 2011;**124**:e739–41
13. Pibarot P, *et al.* Low-flow, low-gradient aortic stenosis with normal and depressed left ventricular ejection fraction. *J Am Coll Cardiol.* 2012;**60**:1845–53
14. Lauten J, *et al.* Invasive hemodynamic characteristics of low gradient severe aortic stenosis despite preserved ejection fraction. *J Am Coll Cardiol.* 2013; doi: 10.1016/j.jacc.2013.1002.1009
15. Bates ER. Treatment options in severe aortic stenosis. *Circulation.* 2011;**124**:355–9
16. Zilberszac R. Outcome of combined stenotic and regurgitant aortic valve disease. *J Am Coll Cardiol.* 2013; doi:10.1016/j.jacc.2012.1011.1070
17. Pibarot P, *et al.* Improving assessment of aortic stenosis. *J Am Coll Cardiol.* 2012;**60**:169–80
18. Bahlmann E, *et al.* Prognostic value of energy loss index in asymptomatic aortic stenosis. *Circulation.* 2013;**127**:1149–56
19. Blais C, *et al.* Projected valve area at normal flow rate improves the assessment of stenosis severity in patients with low-flow, low-gradient aortic stenosis: the multicentre topas (truly or pseudosevere aortic stenosis) study. *Circulation.* 2006;**113**:711–21
20. Dumesnil JG, *et al.* Paradoxical low-flow and/or low-gradient severe aortic stenosis despite preserved left ventricular ejection fraction: implications for diagnosis and treatment. *Eur Heart J.* 2010;**31**:281–9
21. Adda J, *et al.* Low-flow, low-gradient severe aortic stenosis despite normal ejection fraction is associated with severe left ventricular dysfunction as assessed by speckle-tracking echocardiography: a multicentre study. *Circ Cardiovasc Imaging.* 2012;**5**:27–35
22. Bergler-Klein J, *et al.* B-type natriuretic peptide in low-flow, low-gradient aortic stenosis: relationship to haemodynamics and clinical outcome: results from the multicentre truly or pseudosevere aortic stenosis (TOPAS) study. *Circulation.* 2007;**115**:2848–55
23. Picano E, *et al.* The emerging role of exercise testing and stress echocardiography in valvular heart disease. *J Am Coll Cardiol.* 2009;**54**:2251–60
24. Cueff C, *et al.* Measurement of aortic valve calcification using multislice computed tomography: correlation with haemodynamic severity of aortic stenosis and clinical implication for patients with low ejection fraction. *Heart.* 2011;**97**:721–6
25. Sverdlov AL, *et al.* Determinants of aortic sclerosis progression: implications regarding impairment of nitric oxide signalling and potential therapeutics. *Eur Heart J.* 2012;**33**:2419–25
26. Carabello BA. Georg ohm and the changing character of aortic stenosis: it's not your grandfather's oldsmobile. *Circulation.* 2012;**125**:2295–7
27. Chan KL, *et al.* Effect of lipid lowering with rosuvastatin on progression of aortic stenosis: results of the aortic stenosis progression observation: measuring effects of rosuvastatin (ASTRONOMER) trial. *Circulation.* 2010;**121**:306–14
28. Vahanian A, *et al.* Guidelines on the management of valvular heart disease (version 2012). *Eur Heart J.* 2012;**33**:2451–96
29. Osswald BR, *et al.* Overestimation of aortic valve replacement risk by EuroSCORE: implications for percutaneous valve replacement. *Eur Heart J.* 2009;**30**:74–80
30. Brennan JM, *et al.* Long-term survival after aortic valve replacement among high-risk elderly patients in the United States: insights from the Society of Thoracic Surgeons Adult Cardiac Surgery Database, 1991 to 2007. *Circulation.* 2012;**126**:1621–9
31. Fougeres E, *et al.* Outcomes of pseudosevere aortic stenosis under conservative treatment. *Eur Heart J.* 2012;**33**:2426–33
32. Clavel MA, *et al.* Outcome of patients with aortic stenosis, small valve area, and low-flow, low-gradient despite preserved left ventricular ejection fraction. *J Am Coll Cardiol.* 2012;**60**:1259–67
33. Jander N, *et al.* Outcome of patients with low-gradient 'severe' aortic stenosis and preserved ejection fraction. *Circulation.* 2011;**123**:887–95
34. Tandon AGP. Imaging of low-gradient severe aortic stenosis. *J Am Coll Cardiol Img.* 2013;**6**:184–95
35. Genereux P, *et al.* Clinical outcomes after transcatheter aortic valve replacement using valve academic research consortium definitions: a weighted meta-analysis of 3,519 patients from 16 studies. *J Am Coll Cardiol.* 2012;**59**:2317–26
36. Holmes DR, Jr., *et al.* 2012 ACCF/AATS/SCAI/STS Expert Consensus document on transcatheter aortic valve replacement. *J Am Coll Cardiol.* 2012;**59**:1200–54
37. Kodali SK, *et al.* Two-year outcomes after transcatheter or surgical aortic-valve replacement. *N Engl J Med.* 2012;**366**:1686–95
38. Makkar RR, *et al.* Transcatheter aortic-valve replacement for inoperable severe aortic stenosis. *N Engl J Med.* 2012;**366**:1696–704
39. Toggweiler S, *et al.* 5-year outcome after transcatheter aortic valve implantation. *J Am Coll Cardiol.* 2013;**61**:413–19

40. Nielsen HH KK, *et al.* A prospective, randomised trial of transapical transcatheter aortic valve implantation vs. Surgical aortic valve replacement in operable elderly patients with aortic stenosis: The staccato trial. *EuroIntervention.* 2012;**8**:383–9
41. Chieffo A BG, Van Mieghem NM, *et al.* Transcatheter aortic valve implantation with the Edwards SAPIEN versus the Medtronic CoreValve Revalving system devices: a multicentre collaborative study: the PRAGMATIC Plus Initiative (Pooled-RotterdAm-Milano-Toulouse In Collaboration). *J Am Coll Cardiol.* 2013;**61**:830–6
42. Jilaihawi H, *et al.* Meta-analysis of complications in aortic valve replacement: comparison of Medtronic-CoreValve, Edwards SAPIEN and surgical aortic valve replacement in 8,536 patients. *Catheter Cardiovasc Interv.* 2012;**80**:128–38
43. Khatri PJWJ, *et al.* Adverse effects associated with transcatheter aortic valve implantation: A meta-analysis of contemporary studies. *Ann Intern Med.* 2013;**158**:35–46
44. Generaux P, *et al.* Paravalvular leak after transcatheter aortic valve replacement: The new achilles' heel? A comprehensive review of the literature. *J Am Coll Cardiol.* 2013 [ePub ahead of print]
45. Testa L, *et al.* Clinical impact of persistent left bundle-branch block after transcatheter aortic valve implantation with corevalve revalving system. *Circulation.* 2013;**127**:1300–7
46. Houthuizen P, *et al.* Left bundle-branch block induced by transcatheter aortic valve implantation increases risk of death. *Circulation.* 2012;**126**:720–8
47. Goel SS, *et al.* Percutaneous coronary intervention in patients with severe aortic stenosis: implications for transcatheter aortic valve replacement. *Circulation.* 2012;**125**: 1005–13
48. Dvir D, *et al.* Transcatheter aortic valve replacement for degenerative bioprosthetic surgical valves: results from the Global Valve-in-Valve Registry. *Circulation.* 2012;**126**:2335–44
49. Kappetein AP, *et al.* Updated standardized endpoint definitions for transcatheter aortic valve implantation: the valve academic research consortium-2 consensus document. *J Am Coll Cardiol.* 2012;**60**:1438–54
50. Tommaso CL, *et al.* Multisociety (AATS, ACCF, SCAI, and STS) Expert Consensus statement: operator and institutional requirements for transcatheter valve repair and replacement, part 1: transcatheter aortic valve replacement. *J Am Coll Cardiol.* 2012;**59**:2028–42

Chapter 19

Aortic regurgitation

Epidemiology

The prevalence of aortic regurgitation in the western world ranges from 0.1% in subjects 45–54 year-old to 2% in those ≥75 years.[1]

Aetiology

Aortic regurgitation (AR) results from abnormalities of the aortic leaflets or the aortic root and annulus (Table 19.1). Degenerative and congenital conditions are the most prevalent causes of **chronic AR** in the western world, although no cause can be identified in certain occasions. Rheumatic heart disease is the most common cause worldwide.[2,3] **Acute AR** is most commonly caused by endocarditis, aortic dissection, ruptured fenestration of an aortic leaflet, chest trauma, or prosthetic valve dysfunction.[4] Hypertension is associated with aortic root dilation rather than AR itself. Bicuspid aortic valve is discussed in Chapter 1 on GUCH.

Pathophysiology and natural history

Acute AR leads to rapid decompensation due to low forward cardiac output and pulmonary congestion. There is no time for compensatory LV dilation to occur, and there is marked increase in end-diastolic pressure. Although there is some degree of compensation by the Frank–Starling mechanism, the ventricle is functioning on a steep pressure-volume curve because of the lack of chamber dilation. Thus, severe hypotension with a narrow pulse pressure occurs rather than the systolic hypertension and widened pulse pressure that are characteristics of chronic severe AR. Mitral regurgitation in acute AR may occur either in diastole or in systole (when LVEDP exceeds LA pressure). Diastolic MR results in increased LA pressure and pulmonary oedema and is a specific indicator of acute severe AR.[5]

Chronic AR results in combined volume and pressure overload of the LV that is related to the severity of the

Table 19.1 Aetiology of AR

Diseases that primarily affect the leaflets
Congenital AV abnormalities (mainly bicuspid aortic valve, jet lesion due to subaortic stenosis)
Rheumatic heart disease
Myxomatous degeneration
Atherosclerotic degeneration
Infective endocarditis
VSD
Connective tissue or inflammatory diseases (ankylosing spondylitis, systemic lupus erythymatosus, giant cell arteritis, Takayasu's arteritis, Whipple's disease, Crohn's disease)
Antiphospholipid syndrome
Trauma
Anorectic drugs
Diseases that primarily affect the annulus or aortic root
Congenital abnormalities (bicuspid aortic valve, Marfan's)
Idiopathic aortic root dilation
Ehlers–Danlos syndrome
Osteogenesis imperfecta
Aortic dissection
Syphilitic aortitis
Connective tissue diseases (ankylosing spondylitis, psoriatic arhtitis, giant cell arteritis, Behcet's syndrome, relapsing polychonditis, Reiter's syndrome)
Ulcerative colitis

regurgitant flow (Table 19.2). Systolic hypertension can contribute to progressive dilation of the aortic root and subsequent worsening of AR. In early, compensated severe AR, the LV adapts to the volume overload by eccentric hypertrophy with replication of sarcomeres in series and elongation of myofibres. Over time, progressive LV dilation and systolic hypertension increase wall stress and the volume/mass ratio that eventually leads to overt LV systolic dysfunction. In decompensated severe AR, LV systolic dysfunction is accompanied by decreased LV diastolic compliance as a result of hypertrophy and fibrosis, leading to high filling pressures and heart failure symptoms. Asymptomatic patients with AR and normal LV function may develop LV dysfunction (<3.5%/year) or symptoms (<6%/year) and carry a risk of sudden death (<0.2%/year). Asymptomatic patients with LV systolic dysfunction develop symptoms at a rate >25%/year. Symptomatic patients have a 10% yearly mortality rate.[6]

Presentation

Acute AR is usually catastrophic, and the patient may present in cardiogenic shock.

In **chronic AR**, exertional dyspnoea is the most common manifestation, but angina can also occur because of a reduction in coronary flow reserve with predominantly systolic coronary flow.

Physical examination

In **acute AR**, auscultation can be confusing due to the difficulty in distinguishing diastole from systole, and the diastolic murmur may be absent because of rapid equilibration of aortic and LV diastolic pressures. The only clue may be an **absent S_2** in the setting of tachycardia, hypotension, and pulmonary oedema. S_1 may be soft due to early MV closure that is an ominous prognostic sign calling for urgent surgery.

In **chronic AR**, physical findings are related to increased stroke volume and widened blood pressure:

- Bounding carotid pulse (**Corrigan's pulse**), head bobbing (**de Musset's sign**), pulsation of the uvula (**Muller's sign**), pistol shot sounds over the femoral artery with compression (**Traube's sign**), and capillary pulsations on the fingernail during compression with a glass slide (**Quincke's sign**) have been described with severe AR.
- Diffuse, **hyperdynamic apical impulse** and perhaps **systolic thrill** may be present.
- Soft or absent or paradoxically splitted S_2
- S_3 may be present that does not necessarily indicates a failing LV.
- **Decrescendo diastolic murmur** at the aortic area or the left sternal border with the patient leaning forward in expiration.
- Mid-diastolic apical rumble (**Austin Flint murmur**), possibly due to restriction of the MV opening by the high-pressure AR jet or to vibrations of the anterior mitral leaflet by a posteriorly directed AR jet.
- **Systolic ejection murmur** due to high ejection volume.
- **Ejection click** with bicuspid aortic valve.

Investigations

ECG Normal or LV hypertrophy. With early volume overload, there may be prominent Q waves in leads I, aVL, and V_3 to V_6. With progressive disease, the Q waves decrease, but the total QRS amplitude increases.

Chest radiography Usually normal. Cardiomegaly is a late feature in AS, and calcification is a universal finding but rarely visible on chest X-ray. The proximal ascending aorta may be dilated, particularly in patients with bicuspid valves.

Echocardiography is the standard imaging procedure for assessment of the leaflets and the aortic root and quantitation of the severity of AR. M-mode echo is also very useful in demonstrating premature mitral valve closure. Doppler

Table 19.2 ACC/AHA 2008 GL on valve disease

Criteria for classification of AR

	Mild	Moderate	Severe
Specific signs			
Angiographic grade	1+	2+	3–4+
Colour Doppler jet area	Central jet, width <25% of LVOT	Greater than mild but no signs of severe AR	Central jet, width greater than 65% LVOT
Doppler vena contracta width (cm)	<0.3	0.3–0.6	≥0.60
Quantitative (cath or echo)			
RVol (mL per beat)	<30	30–59	≥60
RF (%)	<30	30–49	≥50
ERO (cm^2)	<0.10	0.10–0.29	≥0.30
Additional essential criteria			
LV size			Increased

RVol, regurgitant volume; RF, regurgitant fraction; ERO, effective regurgitant orifice area.
Colour flow jets are composed of three distinct segments: the proximal flow convergence zone (the area of flow acceleration into the orifice), the vena contracta (the narrowest and highest velocity central flow region of the jet), and the jet itself distal to the orifice. Jet and vena contracta estimations at a Nyquist limit of 50–60 cm/s.
ACC/AHA 2008 focused update incorporated into the ACC/AHA 2006 guidelines for the management of patients with valvular heart disease. *J Am Coll Cardiol*. 2008;**52**:e1–142.

colour flow mapping is used for quantification of AR (Tables 19.2 and 19.3). Vena contracta imaging and assessment of jet eccentricity are used whereas PISA is less reliable than in MR. Volumetric LV measures and regurgitant fraction are superior to linear diameters in identifying patients at higher risk.[7] In patients with mixed AS and AR, peak aortic jet velocity reflects both stenosis and regurgitation and represents a useful predictive parameter.[8] Transoesophageal echocardiography may be necessary for accurate assessment and particularly when dissection is suspected.

Computed tomography is useful for the assessment of aortic root dilatation.

Cardiac magnetic resonance is a very promising technique for LV volumes, EF, and regurgitant fraction assessment.[9]

Cardiac catheterization Aortography allows visualization and quantification of the regurgitant jet (Table 19.4). Grade 1 AR is contrast appearing in the LV but clearing with each beat. Grade 2 AR is faint opacification of the entire LV over several cardiac cycles. Grade 3 AR is opacification of the entire LV with the same intensity as in the aorta. Grade 4 AR is opacification of the entire LV on the first heart beat with an intensity higher than in the aorta. This method is subjective and depends on the amount of contrast injected and the size of the LV, particularly in significant AR.

Coronary angiography is necessary before surgery in patients with risk factors or clinical suspicion of coronary artery disease (see Tables 15.3 and 15.4 in Chapter 15 on general principles).

Therapy

Acute AR

Vasodilation with sodium nitroprusside is used as a bridge to emergency surgery. Aortic balloon counterpulsation is absolutely contraindicated. Beta blockers prolong diastole and may worsen AR.

Chronic AR

Medical therapy is aimed at reducing systolic hypertension, and thereby wall stress, and improve LV function. Two randomized studies have shown improvement of LV function with hydralazine and nifedipine, respectively.[10,11] Theoretically, vasodilation with ACE/ARB should also be beneficial. Significant reduction of the regurgitant volume cannot be achieved with medical therapy because the regurgitant orifice area is fixed and the diastolic blood pressure already low. Thus, vasodilator therapy is recommended either in inoperable patients (ACC/AHA 2008, I-B) or as a bridge to surgery (IIa-C) or in asymptomatic patients who have LV dilation but normal LVEF (IIb-B).

Surgery for AVR is indicated in patients with severe AR and symptoms or signs of reduced LV function (Tables 19.5 and 19.6; Figures 19.1 and 19.2). A detailed history for detection of symptoms is, therefore, essential.[12] AVR should also be considered with progressive increases in LV volume or decreases in LVEF in serial studies. Mortality rates are presented in Table 22.1 in Chapter 22 on prosthetic heart valves. Recommendations for patients with **congenital AR** are presented in Table 19.7.

Table 19.3 ESC 2012 GL on valve disease

Echocardiographic criteria for definition of severe AR	
Qualitative	
Valve morphology	Abnormal/flail/large coaptation defect
Colour flow regurgitant jet	Large in central jets, variable in eccentric jets[a]
CW signal of regurgitant jet	Dense
Other	Holodiastolic flow reversal in descending aorta (EDV >20 cm/s)
Semi-quantitative	
Vena contracta width (mm)	>6
Upstream vein flow[b]	–
Inflow	–
Other	Pressure half-time <200 ms[c]
Quantitative	
EROA (mm^2)	≥30
RVol (mL/beat)	≥60
+ enlargement of cardiac chambers/vessels	LV

a: At a Nyquist limit of 50–60 cm/s.
b: Unless other reasons for systolic blunting (atrial fibrillation, elevated atrial pressure).
c: Pressure half-time is shortened with increasing left ventricular diastolic pressure, vasodilator therapy, and in patients with a dilated compliant aorta or lengthened in chronic aortic regurgitation.
ESC guidelines on the management of valvular heart disease (version 2012). *European Heart Journal* 2012;**33**:2451–2496.

Table 19.4 ACC/AHA 2008 GL on valve disease

Indications for cardiac catheterization	
Cardiac catheterization with aortic root angiography and measurement of LV pressure for assessment of severity of regurgitation, LV function, or aortic root size when non-invasive tests are inconclusive or discordant with clinical findings.	I-B
Coronary angiography before AVR in patients at risk for CAD.	I-C
Cardiac catheterization with aortic root angiography and measurement of LV pressure is not indicated for assessment of LV function, aortic root size, or severity of regurgitation before AVR when non-invasive tests are adequate and concordant with clinical findings and coronary angiography is not needed, or in asymptomatic patients when non-invasive tests are adequate.	III-C

ACC/AHA 2008 focused update incorporated into the ACC/AHA 2006 guidelines for the management of patients with valvular heart disease. *J Am Coll Cardiol*. 2008;**52**:e1–142.

Table 19.5 ACC/AHA 2008 GL on valve disease

AVR in AR	
Symptomatic patients with severe AR, irrespective of LV systolic function.	I-B
Asymptomatic patients with chronic severe AR and LV systolic dysfunction (LVEF ≤50%) at rest.	I-B
Patients with chronic severe AR while undergoing cardiac surgery.	I-C
Asymptomatic patients with severe AR with normal LV systolic function (LVEF ≥50%) but with severe LV dilatation (end-diastolic dimension >75 mm or end-systolic dimension >55 mm).*	IIa-B
Patients with moderate AR while undergoing CABG or surgery on the ascending aorta.	IIb-C
Asymptomatic patients with severe AR and normal LV systolic function at rest (LVEF >50%) when LV end-diastolic dimension is >70 mm or end-systolic dimension >50 mm, when there is evidence of progressive LV dilatation, declining exercise tolerance, or abnormal haemodynamic responses to exercise.*	IIb-C
Asymptomatic patients with mild, moderate, or severe AR and normal LV systolic function at rest (LVEF >50%) when degree of dilatation is not moderate or severe (end-diastolic dimension <70 mm, end-systolic dimension <50 mm).*	III-B

* Consider lower threshold values for patients of small stature of either gender.
ACC/AHA 2008 focused update incorporated into the ACC/AHA 2006 guidelines for the management of patients with valvular heart disease. *J Am Coll Cardiol*. 2008;**52**:e1–142.

Table 19.6 ESC 2012 GL on valve disease. AVR in AR

Severe AR	
Symptomatic patients.	I-B
Asymptomatic patients with resting LVEF ≤50%.	I-B
Patients undergoing CABG or surgery of ascending aorta or on another valve.	I-C
Asymptomatic patients with resting LVEF >50% with severe LV dilatation:	
End-diastolic dimension >70 mm, or	IIa-C
ESD >50 mm (or >25 mm/m^2 BSA)[1]	IIa-C
Aortic root disease (whatever the severity of AR)	
Patients who have aortic root disease with maximal aortic diameter:[2]	
≥50 mm for patients with Marfan's syndrome.	I-C
≥45 mm for patients with Marfan's syndrome with risk factors.[3]	IIa-C
≥50 mm for patients with bicuspid valves with risk factors.[4]	IIa-C
≥55 mm for other patients.	IIa-C

1: Changes in sequential measurements should be taken into account.
2: Decision should take into account the shape of the different parts of the aorta. Lower thresholds can be used for combining surgery on the ascending aorta for patients who have an indication for surgery on the aortic valve.
3: Family history of aortic dissection and/or aortic size increase >2 mm/year (on repeated measurements using the same imaging technique, measured at the same aorta level with side-by-side comparison and confirmed by another technique), severe AR or mitral regurgitation, desire of pregnancy.
4: Coarctation of the aorta, systemic hypertension, family history of dissection, or increase in aortic diameter >2 mm/year (on repeated measurements using the same imaging technique, measured at the same aorta level with side-by-side comparison and confirmed by another technique).
ESC guidelines on the management of valvular heart disease (version 2012). *European Heart Journal* 2012;**33**:2451–2496.

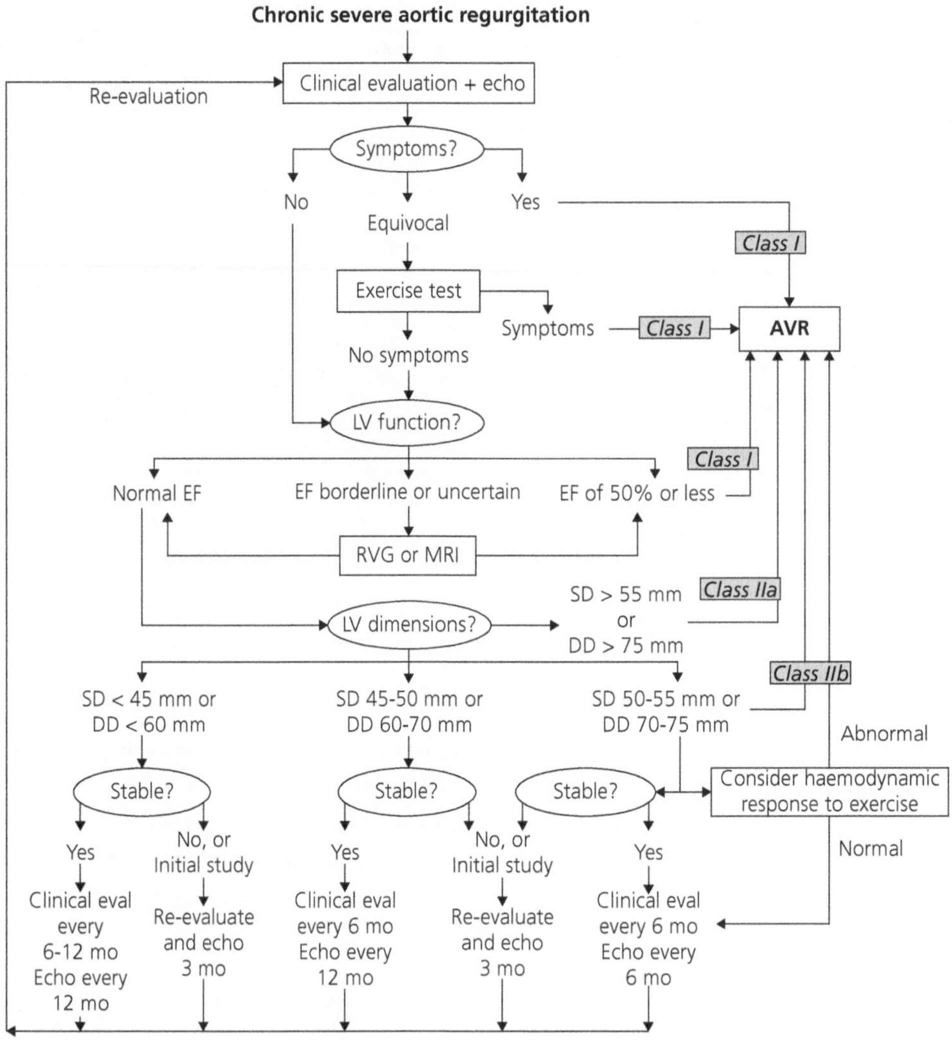

Figure 19.1 ACC/AHA 2008 GL on valve disease. Management strategy for patients with chronic severe aortic regurgitation.

Preoperative coronary angiography should be performed routinely as determined by age, symptoms, and coronary risk factors. Cardiac catheterization and angiography may also be helpful when there is discordance between clinical findings and echocardiography. 'Stable' refers to stable echocardiographic measurements. In some centres, serial follow-up may be performed with radionuclide ventriculography (RVG) or magnetic resonance imaging (MRI) rather than echocardiography (echo) to assess left ventricular (LV) volume and systolic function.

AVR indicates aortic valve replacement; DD, end-diastolic dimension; EF, ejection fraction; eval, evaluation; and SD, end-systolic dimension.
ACC/AHA 2008 focused update incorporated into the ACC/AHA 2006 guidelines for the management of patients with valvular heart disease. *J Am Coll Cardiol.* 2008;**52**:e1–142

Indications for surgery in patients with bicuspid aortic valves or aortic root aneurysms are also presented in Chapter 7 on left ventricular outflow tract obstruction and Chapter 71 on aortic aneurysms. The choice of prosthesis is based on patient age and the risk of anticoagulation (see Chapter 22 on prosthetic valves). As with other valve diseases, optimum management of patients is hampered by the lack of definitive prospective clinical trials. TAVR may also be an option in inoperable patients, but the possibility of requiring 2 valves and leaving residual aortic regurgitation remain important considerations.[13]

Non-cardiac surgery

In patients with AR, if LV dysfunction is severe (EF <30%), non-cardiac surgery should only be performed if strictly necessary, after optimization of medical therapy for HF.[14]

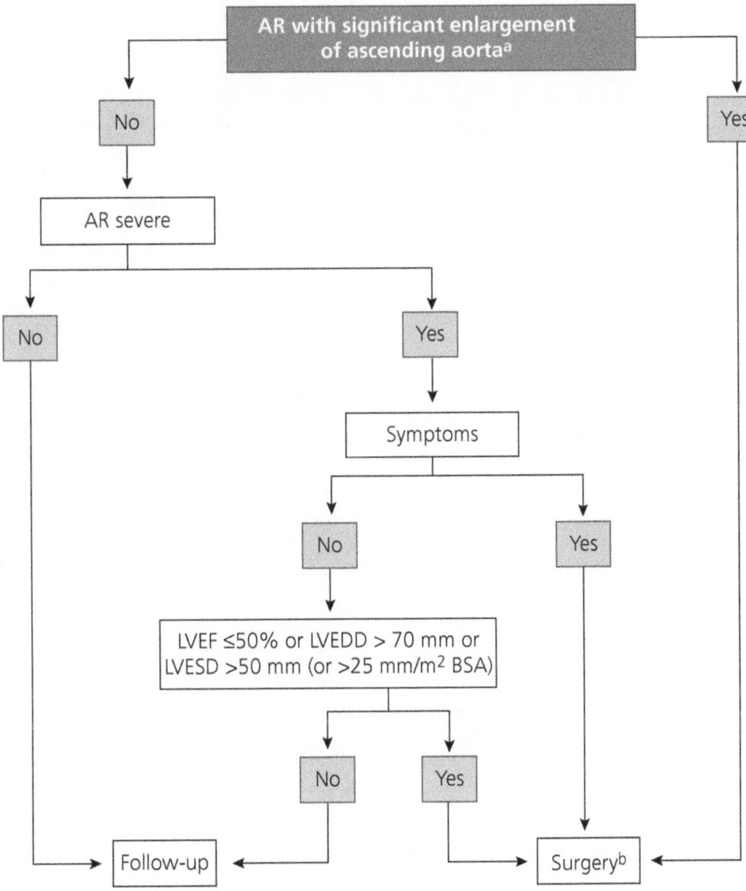

Figure 19.2 ESC GL 2012 Management of AR.

a: See Table 19.6 for definition. b: Surgery must also be considered if significant changes in LV or aortic size occur during follow-up.
ESC guidelines on the management of valvular heart disease (version 2012). *European Heart Journal* 2012;**33**:2451–2496

Table 19.7 ACC/AHA 2008 GL on valve disease. Surgery in congenital AR

Aortic valve repair or replacement in adolescent or young adult with chronic severe AR and:	
Onset of symptoms of angina, syncope, or dyspnoea on exertion.	I-C
LVEF <0.50 on serial studies 1–3 months apart.	I-C
Progressive LV enlargement (EDD >4 standard deviations above normal).	I-C
Moderate AS (peak LV to peak aortic gradient >40 mmHg at cardiac catheterization).	IIb-C
Onset of ST depression or T wave inversion over the left precordium on ECG at rest.	IIb-C
Coronary angiography before AVR in adolescent or young adult patients with AR in whom a pulmonary autograft (Ross operation) is contemplated when the origin of the coronary arteries has not been identified by non-invasive techniques.	I-C

ACC/AHA 2008 focused update incorporated into the ACC/AHA 2006 guidelines for the management of patients with valvular heart disease. *J Am Coll Cardiol*. 2008;**52**:e1–142.

Pregnancy

Patients with severe aortic regurgitation and symptoms or impaired ventricular function or ventricular dilatation should be treated surgically pre-pregnancy (I-C, ESC 2011 GL on pregnancy).

References

1. Nkomo VT, *et al.* Burden of valvular heart diseases: A population-based study. *Lancet.* 2006;**368**:1005–1011
2. Bekeredjian R, *et al.* Valvular heart disease: aortic regurgitation. *Circulation.* 2005;**112**:125–34
3. Maganti K, *et al.* Valvular heart disease: diagnosis and management. *Mayo Clin Proc.* 2010;**85**:483–500
4. Stout KK, *et al.* Acute valvular regurgitation. *Circulation.* 2009;**119**:3232–41
5. Hamirani YS, *et al.* Acute aortic regurgitation. *Circulation.* 2012;**126**:1121–6
6. Bonow RO, *et al.* 2008 focused update incorporated into the ACC/AHA 2006 guidelines for the management of patients with valvular heart disease: a report of the American College of Cardiology/American Heart Association Task Force on practice guidelines (writing committee to revise the 1998 guidelines for the management of patients with valvular heart disease). Endorsed by the Society of Cardiovascular Anesthesiologists, Society for Cardiovascular Angiography and Interventions, and Society of Thoracic Surgeons. *J Am Coll Cardiol.* 2008;**52**:e1–42
7. Detaint D, *et al.* Quantitative echocardiographic determinants of clinical outcome in asymptomatic patients with aortic regurgitation: a prospective study. *JACC Cardiovasc Imaging.* 2008;**1**:1–11
8. Zilberszac R, *et al.* Outcome of combined stenotic and regurgitant aortic valve disease. *J Am Coll Cardiol.* 2013;**61**:doi:10.1016/j.jacc.2012.1011.1070
9. Myerson SG, *et al.* Aortic regurgitation quantification using cardiovascular magnetic resonance: association with clinical outcome. *Circulation.* 2012;**126**:1452–60
10. Greenberg B, *et al.* Long-term vasodilator therapy of chronic aortic insufficiency. A randomized double-blinded, placebo-controlled clinical trial. *Circulation.* 1988;**78**:92–103
11. Scognamiglio R, *et al.* Nifedipine in asymptomatic patients with severe aortic regurgitation and normal left ventricular function. *N Engl J Med.* 1994;**331**:689–94
12. Bonow RO. Chronic mitral regurgitation and aortic regurgitation: Have indications for surgery changed? *J Am Coll Cardiol.* 2013;**61**:693–701
13. Roy DA, *et al.* Transcatheter aortic valve implantation for pure severe native aortic valve regurgitation. *J Am Coll Cardiol.* 2012
14. Vahanian A, *et al.* Guidelines on the management of valvular heart disease (version 2012). *Eur Heart J.* 2012;**33**:2451–96

Chapter 20

Tricuspid valve disease

Tricuspid regurgitation

Epidemiology

Tricuspid regurgitation (TR) may affect as much as 0.8% of the general population in the USA (with an estimate of 1.6% for moderate to severe MR).[1] Approximately 30% of patients with severe MR may also have severe TR, and up to 80% of patients referred for echocardiography have some degree of TR.[2]

Aetiology

TR is usually (>75% of cases) functional, i.e. secondary to other disease process causing right ventricular (RV) dilatation, distortion of the subvalvular apparatus, or tricuspid annular dilatation and papillary muscle displacement (Table 20.1). Main cause is pulmonary hypertension secondary to MV disease. Congenital TR is usually due to Ebstein's anomaly. Pacemaker, and especially ICD lead placement, has been reported to result in

Table 20.1 Causes of TV regurgitation

Functional (morphologically normal leaflets with annular dilatation)
LV dysfunction or valve disease, resulting in pulmonary hypertension Pulmonary hypertension (primary or secondary)
RV dysplasia, infarction
Idiopathic tricuspid annular dilatation Endomyocardial fibrosis
Structural
Acquired
Rheumatic heart disease Endocarditis
Traumatic
Carcinoid heart disease
Endomyocardial fibrosis
Iatrogenic (PPM/ICD lead, radiation, drugs, RV biopsy)
Congenital
Ebstein's anomaly
TV dysplasia, hypoplasia, double-orifice TV

worsening of TR in up to 25% of patients.[3] However, in a recent study, device lead implantation in patients with a bioprosthetic tricuspid valve was not associated with an increased incidence of significant prosthetic TR.[4]

Pathophysiology and natural history

The tricuspid valve apparatus consists of the annulus, the septal, anterior, and posterior (or inferior) leaflets, chordae, and papillary muscles.[5] Most of the TV annulus lies on the atrioventricular junction; thus, its size depends on RV volume. When TR develops, there is a prolonged period of progressive RV and RA volume overload that engenders additional TR until right heart failure develops. PA pressure in functional TR is >55 mmHg. RV failure with severe TR or constrictive pericarditis are possible causes of cardiac cirrhosis due to ischaemic hepatopathy. The 1-year survival of patients with severe, moderate, or no TR is 64%, 79%, and 92%, respectively.[6]

Presentation

Symptoms of TR are often non-specific, and patients with severe TR may be asymptomatic. Symptoms are usually of fatigue and decreased exercise tolerance as a result of low cardiac output. Elevated right atrial (RA) pressure leads to atrial arrhythmias (mainly AF), peripheral oedema, and hepatic congestion, with decreased appetite and abdominal fullness. Eventually, right heart failure with ascites and anasarca develops.

Physical findings

- **Elevated JVP** with a prominent v wave in 35% to 75% of patients with severe TR.
- **Hepatomegaly** is present in 90%, but pulsating liver is noted inconsistently.
- The **holosystolic murmur** of TR is heard along the sternal border, increasing in intensity with inspiration as a result of increased systemic venous return (it is heard in <20% of patients with severe TR due to equalization of pressures between the RA and RV).

Investigations

Haemodynamic catheterization is rarely required to confirm the diagnosis of severe TR, and right ventriculography is not helpful because the catheter may induce TR. Echocardiography (2D or preferably 3D) is the main diagnostic tool (Table 20.2).[1,5] Vena contracta width (indirectly reflects the effective regurgitant orifice area) >0.7 cm, large flow convergence (PISA radius >0.9 cm at Nyquist limit of 40 cm/s), and systolic flow reversal in hepatic veins are specific signs of severe TR.[7] Additional supportive signs are a dense 'dagger-shaped', triangular, early-peaking systolic continuous wave Doppler signal, inferior vena cava dilatation and respiratory diameter variation ≤50%, a prominent E wave, and RA/RV dilatation. There is major respiratory variation of TR and RV shape, and echocardiographic as-

Table 20.2 ESC 2012 on valve disease. Echocardiographic criteria for definition of severe TR

Qualitative	
Valve morphology	Abnormal/flail/large coaptation defect
Colour flow regurgitant jet	Very large central jet or eccentric wall impinging jet[1]
CW signal of regurgitant jet	Dense/triangular with early peaking (peak <2 m/s in massive TR)
Other	–
Semi-quantitative	
Vena contracta width (mm)	≥7[a]
Upstream vein flow	Systolic hepatic vein flow reversal
Inflow	E wave dominant ≥1 m/s[b]
Other	PISA radius >9 mm[c]
Quantitative	
EROA (mm^2)	≥40
RVol (mL/beat)	≥45
+ enlargement of cardiac chambers/vessels	RV, RA, inferior vena cava

a: At a Nyquist limit of 50–60 cm/s.
b: In the absence of other causes of elevated left atrial pressure and of mitral stenosis.
c: Baseline Nyquist limit shift of 28 cm/s.
ESC guidelines on the management of valvular heart disease (version 2012). *European Heart Journal* 2012;**33**:2451–2496.

sessment requires multiplying measurements throughout the cardiac cycle in order to appropriately assess TR and right ventricular pressure.[8]

Therapy

Diuretics is the only proven therapy for symptomatic relief but, when excessive, may decrease cardiac output.

TV repair or replacement is the only effective treatment for symptomatic TR, and, recently, there has been evidence in favour of a more aggressive surgical approach to secondary TR.[8] Consequently, indications for TV surgery in patients with severe TR are (Tables 20.3 and 20.4):[7,10]

- Symptomatic RV failure
- Progressive RV enlargement
- Surgery for MV or other valve disease (even with moderate TR)
- Traumatic TV flail (early surgery is recommended)
- Carcinoid heart disease (high-risk group).

Operative mortality for concomitant TV surgery is doubled (up to 4.5%) compared to that for isolated MV surgery but avoids the usual post-operative deterioration of existing TR and results in better mid-term survival.

In patients with both primary and functional TV disease, **TV repair** is associated with better survival than TV replacement. Ring annuloplasty is preferable to purse-string annuloplasty (De Vega).[1,2]

TV replacement is indicated for patients whose valves are not amenable to repair. No difference has been found in survival among patients with mechanical versus biological TV prostheses, but a bioprosthesis is preferred due to the low incidence of thromboembolic complications. Right-sided bioprostheses have superior durability compared with left-sided bioprostheses. Pericardial bioprostheses are generally avoided in the tricuspid position because of leaflet stiffness and risk of obstruction.[3]

Transcatheter TV implantation is also a new option under investigation,[11] and novel percutaneous procedures are being developed as an alternative to surgery for high-risk patients.[8]

When severe symptomatic TR is secondary to leaflet perforation or lead impingement from a **pacemaker lead**, removal or repositioning of the lead may decrease the degree of TR. Recently, however, it was shown that lead implantation in patients with a bioprosthetic tricuspid valve was not associated with an increased incidence of significant prosthetic TR.[4]

Asymptomatic patients with severe **carcinoid heart disease** may require valve replacement, enabling partial hepatic resection or liver transplantation. Carcinoid heart disease patients represent a high-risk surgical subgroup primarily because of perioperative haemodynamic lability (carcinoid crisis), characterized by peripheral vasodilatation and hypotension that requires IV octreotide administration.[5]

In patients with **pulmonary hypertension** and severe TR secondary to pulmonary thromboembolic disease, pulmonary thromboendarterectomy alone has been shown to reduce pulmonary hypertension and usually reduces TR severity without the need for concomitant tricuspid annuloplasty. TR secondary to severe primary pulmonary hypertension is usually treated with pulmonary vasodilator

Table 20.3 ACC/AHA 2008 GL on valve disease

Management of TR	
Tricuspid valve repair for severe TR in patients with MV disease requiring MV surgery.	I-B
Tricuspid valve replacement or annuloplasty for severe primary TR when symptomatic.	IIa-C
Tricuspid valve replacement for severe TR secondary to diseased/abnormal tricuspid valve leaflets not amenable to annuloplasty or repair.	IIa-C
Tricuspid annuloplasty for less than severe TR in patients undergoing MV surgery when there is pulmonary hypertension or tricuspid annular dilatation.	IIb-C
Tricuspid valve replacement or annuloplasty in asymptomatic patients with TR whose PA systolic pressure is <60 mmHg in the presence of a normal MV.	III-C
Tricuspid valve replacement or annuloplasty in patients with mild primary TR.	III-C

ACC/AHA 2008 focused update incorporated into the ACC/AHA 2006 guidelines for the management of patients with valvular heart disease. *J Am Coll Cardiol*. 2008;**52**:e1–142.

Table 20.4 ESC 2012 GL on valve disease

Indications for tricuspid valve surgery	
Symptomatic patients with severe TS.[a]	I-C
Severe TS undergoing left-sided valve intervention.[b]	I-C
Severe primary or secondary TR undergoing left-sided valve surgery.	I-C
Symptomatic patients with severe isolated primary TR without severe RV dysfunction.	I-C
Moderate primary TR undergoing left-sided valve surgery.	IIa-C
Mild or moderate secondary TR with dilated annulus (≥40 mm or >21 mm/m^2) undergoing left-sided valve surgery.	IIa-C
Asymptomatic or mildly symptomatic patients with severe isolated primary TR and progressive RV dilatation or deterioration of RV function.	IIa-C
After left-sided valve surgery, surgery should be considered in patients with severe TR who are symptomatic or have progressive RV dilatation/dysfunction, in the absence of left-sided valve dysfunction, severe RV or LV dysfunction, and severe pulmonary vascular disease.	IIa-C

a: Percutaneous balloon valvuloplasty can be attempted as a first approach if TS is isolated.

b: Percutaneous balloon valvuloplasty can be attempted if PMC can be performed on the mitral valve.

ESC guidelines on the management of valvular heart disease (version 2012). *European Heart Journal* 2012;**33**:2451–2496.

and diuretic therapy alone because of the risk of cardiac surgical intervention and overall poor prognosis.

Although **percutaneous balloon mitral valvuloplasty** may result in less TR, TV repair, combined with mitral valve replacement, is better than mitral balloon valvuloplasty alone in patients with severe functional TR, especially if atrial fibrillation or RV enlargement is present.[1]

The management of **congenital TR** is described in Table 20.5.

Recommendations on **pregnancy** are presented in Chapter 84 on cardiovascular disease in pregnancy.

Tricuspid stenosis

Epidemiology and aetiology

Tricuspid stenosis (TS) is a very rare condition in developed countries. It is mainly due to rheumatic disease, but only 3% to 5% with rheumatic mitral valve disease have concurrent TS. Other causes are congenital TS, carcinoid, endomyocardial fibrosis, and right atrial tumours.[1,7]

Physical findings and diagnosis

Due to the usual coexistence of mitral valve disease, it is difficult to separate symptoms and signs specific to TS:

Table 20.5 ACC/AHA 2008 GL on valve disease

Indications for intervention in congenital tricuspid	
Surgery for severe TR for adolescent and young adult patients with:	
Deteriorating exercise capacity (NYHA III or IV).	I-C
Progressive cyanosis and arterial saturation <80% at rest or with exercise.	I-C
NYHA II symptoms if the valve appears to be repairable.	IIa-C
AF.	IIa-C
Increasing heart size and a cardiothoracic ratio >65%.	IIb-C
Stable heart size and an arterial saturation <85% when the tricuspid valve appears repairable.	IIb-C
Interventional catheterization closure of the atrial communication for the adolescent or young adult with TR who is hypoxaemic at rest and with exercise intolerance due to increasing hypoxaemia with exercise, when the tricuspid valve appears difficult to repair surgically.	I-C
Catheter closure of the atrial communication in adolescent and young adult patients with TR who are mildly cyanotic at rest but who become very hypoxaemic with exercise, when the valve does not appear amenable to repair.	IIb-C
Preoperative electrophysiological study to identify accessory pathways if surgery for Ebstein's anomaly is planned in adolescents and young adult patients (tricuspid valve repair or replacement). If present, these may be considered for mapping and ablation, either preoperatively or at the time of surgery.	IIb-C

ACC/AHA 2008 focused update incorporated into the ACC/AHA 2006 guidelines for the management of patients with valvular heart disease. *J Am Coll Cardiol.* 2008;**52**:e1–142.

- SOBOE and peripheral oedema
- Elevated JVP with a prominent a wave and slow y descent
- Opening snap, followed by a diastolic rumbling murmur at the right sternal border that varies with respiration.

As with TR, physical findings may be subtle and the murmur often inaudible.

Diagnosis is made by echocardiography. TS is considered severe when the valve area is <1.0 cm^2 (ACC/AHA 2008), but the accuracy of echocardiography is less than with MS. The 2012 ESC Guideline on VD define severe TS as a valve with mean gradient ≥5 mmHg.[7]

Therapy

Valve replacement is the only treatment. Tricuspid balloon valvotomy may result in severe TR. Management in pregnancy is described in Chapter 84.

References

1. Chan KM, *et al.* Tricuspid valve disease: pathophysiology and optimal management. *Prog Cardiovasc Dis.* 2009;**51**:482–6
2. Bruce CJ, *et al.* Right-sided valve disease deserves a little more respect. *Circulation.* 2009;**119**:2726–34
3. Kim JB SD, *et al.* The effect of transvenous pacemaker and implantable cardioverter defibrillator lead placement on tricuspid valve function: An observational study. *J Am Soc Echocardiogr.* 2008;**21**:284–287
4. Eleid MF, *et al.* Bioprosthetic tricuspid valve regurgitation associated with pacemaker or defibrillator lead implantation. *J Am Coll Cardiol.* 2012;**59**:813–18
5. Rogers JH, *et al.* The tricuspid valve: current perspective and evolving management of tricuspid regurgitation. *Circulation.* 2009;**119**:2718–25
6. Nath J, *et al.* Impact of tricuspid regurgitation on long-term survival. *J Am Coll Cardiol.* 2004;**43**:405–9
7. Vahanian A, *et al.* Guidelines on the management of valvular heart disease (version 2012). *Eur Heart J.* 2012;**33**:2451–96
8. Topilsky Y, *et al.* Pathophysiology of tricuspid regurgitation: quantitative Doppler echocardiographic assessment of respiratory dependence. *Circulation.* 2010;**122**:1505–13
9. Taramasso M, *et al.* The growing clinical importance of secondary tricuspid regurgitation. *J Am Coll Cardiol.* 2012;**59**:703–10
10. Bonow RO, *et al.* 2008 focused update incorporated into the ACC/AHA 2006 guidelines for the management of patients with valvular heart disease: a report of the American College of Cardiology/American Heart Association Task Force on practice guidelines (writing committee to revise the 1998 guidelines for the management of patients with valvular heart disease). Endorsed by the Society of Cardiovascular Anesthesiologists, Society for Cardiovascular Angiography and Interventions, and Society of Thoracic Surgeons. *J Am Coll Cardiol.* 2008;**52**:e1–42
11. Lauten A, *et al.* Heterotopic transcatheter tricuspid valve implantation: first-in-man application of a novel approach to tricuspid regurgitation. *Eur Heart J.* 2011;**32**:1207–13

Chapter 21

Pulmonary valve disease

Pulmonary valve regurgitation

Aetiology

Mild pulmonary regurgitation (PR) may be a normal finding on Doppler echocardiography. The most common causes of pathologic PR in adults are prior interventions for congential heart disease, such as tetralogy of Fallot repair, or surgical valvotomy for congenital pulmonary stenosis. Other rare causes of PR are congenital pulmonary annular dilation, pulmonary hypertension, rheumatic or carcinoid heart disease, endocarditis, and trauma.[1,2]

Pathophysiology

Long-standing severe PR results in progressive RV dilation and reduced RV function. RV dilatation is reflected on QRS duration and is associated with ventricular arrhythmias and sudden death. This mechanical-electrical association has been described in patients with repaired tetralogy of Fallot. Significant PR is the main predictor of sudden death in these patients (see Chapter 2 on VSD).

Physical examination

- **RV parasternal heave** in severe PR with enlarged RV
- **Systolic ejection murmur** increased by inspiration
- Soft, **diastolic, decrescendo murmur** best heard in the left upper sternal border. An increase in intensity of the murmur may be noted during inspiration.

- **ECG** findings are non-specific or reflect RV enlargement.

Chest radiography may demonstrate cardiomegaly and pulmonary artery enlargement.

The diagnosis is made by **echocardiography**. Severe PR is indicated by a colour jet filling the outflow tract and a dense continuous wave Doppler signal with a steep deceleration slope.[1] **Cardiac magnetic resonance** is the imaging modality of choice to assess RV size and function in asymptomatic patients and guide therapy.

Therapy

Medical therapy is not effective in reducing the degree of PR or affecting the impact of PR on the RV. PV replacement is recommended in symptomatic patients (NYHA II or III) and severe PR. The management of asymptomatic patients is controversial. Most would agree that PVR is indicated in: decreased RV systolic function (ejection fraction <40% by cardiac magnetic resonance imaging), progressive RV dilation (cardiac magnetic resonance imaging RV end-diastolic volume 160 mL/m^2 or 82 mL/m^2 for RV end-systolic volume) or TR related to progressive annular dilatation, severe PR in a patient requiring another cardiac operation, and QRS duration 180 ms or QRS duration increase >3.5 ms/y).[2]

Pulmonary valve stenosis

The majority (>95%) of pulmonary stenosis cases are related to congenital or genetic disorders and are discussed in Chapter 1 on GUCH. Carcinoid syndrome and rheumatic valve disease may cause pulmonary stenosis but essentially always occur in conjunction with other valve disease.

References

1. Bonow RO, *et al.* 2008 focused update incorporated into the ACC/AHA 2006 guidelines for the management of patients with valvular heart disease: a report of the American College of Cardiology/American Heart Association Task Force on practice guidelines (writing committee to revise the 1998 guidelines for the management of patients with valvular heart disease). Endorsed by the Society of Cardiovascular Anesthesiologists, Society for Cardiovascular Angiography and Interventions, and Society of Thoracic Surgeons. *J Am Coll Cardiol.* 2008;**52**:e1–42
2. Bruce CJ, *et al.* Right-sided valve disease deserves a little more respect. *Circulation.* 2009;**119**:2726–2734

Chapter 22

Prosthetic heart valves

Risk stratification for surgery

The EuroSCORE (http://www.euroscore.org/calc.html) and the US Society of Thoracic Surgeons (http://www.sts.org) have provided algorithms for risk calculation of patients subjected to cardiac surgery. Table 22.1 presents reported mortality in valve disease surgery. Current risk scores (including EuroSCORE, STS, and Ambler score) are useful but may not always provide a reliable estimate of operative mortality, regardless of other patient characteristics.[1]

Prosthetic heart valves (PHV) are either mechanical or bioprostheses (tissue valves). Tissue engineering is also employed for the creation of tissues analogous to a native human heart valve.[2]

Mechanical valves

- **Ball-cage** (Starr–Edwards)
- **Tilting disc** (Medtronic-Hall, Omniscience, and the old Lillihei-Kaster and Bjork–Shiley valves)
- **Bileaflet** (St Jude and CarboMedics).

Randomized and observational long-term studies have shown good and comparable outcomes with FDA-approved mechanical valves, such as the Starr–Edwards valve, the Medtronic-Hall valve, and the St Jude Medical valve for AVR and MVR.[3] However, the bileaflet valves are the most commonly implanted due to low bulk and better haemodynamics and lower thrombogenicity in the mitral position. The Starr–Edwards, although the most durable valve, has a higher risk of haemolysis and thrombogenicity and is not suiTable for MVR.

Tissue valves (bioprostheses)

- **Porcine stented xenografts (heterografts)** (Hancock, Carpentier–Edwards Perimount, Medtronic Intact).
- **Porcine stentless xenografts** (Medtronic Freestyle, Edwards Prima, St Jude) are recently developed and are supposed to offer better haemodynamics.
- **Pericardial bovine xenografts** are fabricated valves (Carpentier–Edwards, Sorin Pericarbon).
- **Homograft** (allograft) aortic valves harvested from cadavers.
- **Autograft** aortic valves. Fabricated from the patients' own pericardium or pulmonary autografts (Ross principle).

Mechanical valves have less structural deterioration beyond 10 years, and especially in the young, but require anticoagulation for life and patients are at an increased risk of haemorrhagic complications. They are preferred in patients <60 years of age for AVR and 65 years for MVR and in surgery for infective endocarditis. In older patients, in patients on chronic haemodialysis, and in patients in need of anticoagulation for AF or thromboembolic situations, a mechanical valve is preferred (Tables 22.2 to 22.4).[3–5] A mechanical valve is also recommended in patients on chronic haemodialysis, based on the concern of accelerated calcification of bioprosthetic valves in patients with end-stage renal disease, but no significant difference in survival of dialysis patients after cardiac valve replacement with tissue versus mechanical valves has been demonstrated.[6,7] Patients who receive bioprostheses do not need chronic anticoagulation and are less likely to develop valve-related

Table 22.1 ESC 2012 GL on valve disease. Operative mortality after surgery for valvular heart disease

	EACTS (2010)	STS (2010)	UK (2004–2008)	Germany (2009)
Aortic valve replacement, no CABG (%)	2.9 (40 662)	3.7 (25 515)	2.8 (17 636)	2.9 (11 981)
Aortic valve replacement + CABG (%)	5.5 (24 890)	4.5 (18 227)	5.3 (12 491)	6.1 (9113)
Mitral valve repair, no CABG (%)	2.1 (3231)	1.6 (7293)	2 (3283)	2 (3335)
Mitral valve replacement, no CABG (%)	4.3 (6838)	6.0 (5448)	6.1 (3614)	7.8 (1855)
Mitral valve repair/replacement + CABG (%)	6.8/11.4 (2515/1612)	4.6/11.1 (4721/2427)	8.3/11.1 (2021/1337)	6.5/14.5 (1785/837)

( ): number of patients; EACTS: European Association for Cardiothoracic Surgery;
STS: Society of Thoracic Surgeons (USA). Mortality for STS includes first and redo interventions.
ESC guidelines on the management of valvular heart disease (version 2012). *European Heart Journal* 2012;**33**:2451–2496.

Table 22.2 ESC 2012 GL on valve disease. Choice of the aortic/mitral prosthesis

In favour of a mechanical prosthesis	
Desire of the informed patient and no contraindications for long-term anticoagulation.[1]	I-C
Patients at risk of accelerated structural valve deterioration.[2]	I-C
Patients already on anticoagulation due to a mechanical prosthesis in another valve position.	I-C
Patients aged <60 years for prostheses in the aortic position and <65 years for prostheses in the mitral position.[3]	IIa-C
Patients with a reasonable life expectancy[4] for whom future redo valve surgery would be at high risk.	IIa-C
Patients already on long-term anticoagulation due to high risk of thromboembolism.[5]	IIb-C
In favour of a bioprosthesis	
Desire of the informed patient.	I-C
Good quality anticoagulation is unlikely (compliance problems; not readily available) or contraindicated because of high bleeding risk (prior major bleed; co-morbidities; unwillingness; compliance problems; lifestyle; occupation).	I-C
For reoperation for mechanical valve thrombosis despite good long-term anticoagulant control.	I-C
Patients for whom future redo valve surgery would be at low risk.	IIa-C
Young women contemplating pregnancy.	IIa-C
Patients aged >65 years for prosthesis in aortic position or >70 years in mitral position or those with life expectancy[6] lower than the presumed durability of the bioprosthesis.[7]	IIa-C

1: Increased bleeding risk because of co-morbidities, compliance concerns, geographic, lifestyle and occupational conditions.
2: Young age (<40 years), hyperparathyroidism.
3: In patients aged 60–65 years who should receive an aortic prosthesis and those between 65 and 70 years in the case of mitral prosthesis, both valves are acceptable and the choice requires careful analysis of other factors than age.
4: Life expectancy should be estimated >10 years, according to age, gender, co-morbidities, and country-specific life expectancy.
5: Risk factors for thromboembolism are atrial fibrillation, previous thromboembolism, hypercoagulable state, severe left ventricular systolic dysfunction.
6: Life expectancy should be estimated according to age, gender, co-morbidities, and country-specific life expectancy.
7: In patients aged 60–65 years who should receive an aortic prosthesis and those 65–70 years in the case of mitral prosthesis, both valves are acceptable and the choice requires careful analysis of factors other than age.
ESC guidelines on the management of valvular heart disease (version 2012). *European Heart Journal* 2012;**33**:2451–2496.

complications, especially in the aortic position.[6] A recent report from the STS National Database found that among AVR patients, long-term mortality rates were similar for bioprosthetic versus mechanical valve patients. Bioprostheses were associated with a higher long-term risk of reoperation and endocarditis, but a lower risk of stroke and hemorrhage.[8]

Table 22.3 ACC/AHA 2008 GL on valve disease

Major criteria for aortic valve selection	
Mechanical prosthesis for AVR in patients with a mechanical valve in the mitral or tricuspid position.	I-C
Bioprosthesis for AVR in patients of any age who will not take warfarin or who have major medical contraindications to warfarin therapy.	I-C
Patient preference is a reasonable consideration in the selection of aortic valve operation and valve prosthesis. A mechanical prosthesis is reasonable for AVR in patients <65 years of age who do not have a contraindication to anticoagulation. A bioprosthesis is reasonable for AVR in patients <65 years who elect to receive this valve for lifestyle considerations versus the likelihood that a second AVR may be necessary in the future.	IIa-C
Bioprosthesis for AVR in patients aged ≥65 years without risk factors for thromboembolism.	IIa-C
Aortic valve re-replacement with a homograft for patients with active prosthetic valve endocarditis.	IIa-C
Bioprosthesis for AVR in a woman of childbearing age.	IIb-C

ACC/AHA 2008 focused update incorporated into the ACC/AHA 2006 guidelines for the management of patients with valvular heart disease. *J Am Coll Cardiol*. 2008;**52**:e1–142.

Table 22.4 ACC/AHA 2008 GL on valve disease

Selection of a mitral valve prosthesis	
Bioprosthesis in a patient who will not take warfarin, is incapable of taking warfarin, or has a clear contraindication to warfarin therapy.	I-C
Mechanical prosthesis for MV replacement in patients <65 years with long-standing AF.	IIa-C
Bioprosthesis for MV replacement in patients ≥65 years.	IIa-C
Bioprosthesis for MV replacement in patients <65 years in sinus rhythm who accept the risks of anticoagulation versus the likelihood that a second MV replacement may be necessary in the future.	IIa-C

ACC/AHA 2008 focused update incorporated into the ACC/AHA 2006 guidelines for the management of patients with valvular heart disease. *J Am Coll Cardiol*. 2008;**52**:e1–142.

The Ross procedure is performed for aortic valve disease. The patient's own PV and adjacent main pulmonary artery are removed and used to replace the AV and, if necessary, the aortic root with reimplantation of the coronary arteries into the graft. A human pulmonary or aortic homograft is inserted in the pulmonary position. However, reoperations after the Ross procedure, when required, may be complex, frequently involving multiple structures, and carry significant morbidity.[8] The value of this approach, particularly in adults with rheumatic heart disease or AR, is questionable.

Anticoagulation

Target INR for mechanical prostheses is presented in Tables 22.5 and 22.6. As a general rule, for mechanical

Table 22.5 ESC GL 2012 GL on valve disease

Target INR in patients with mechanical prosthetic valves

Prosthesis thrombogenicity[a]	Patient-related risk factors[b]	
	No risk factor	Risk factor ≥1
Low	2.5	3.0
Medium	3.0	3.5
High	3.5	4.0

a: Prosthesis thrombogenicity:
Low: Carbomedics, Medtronic-Hall, St Jude Medical, ON-X
Medium: other bileaflet valves
High: Lillehei–Kaster, Omniscience, Starr–Edwards, Bjork–Shiley, and other tilting-disc valves.
b: Patient-related risk factors: mitral or tricuspid valve replacement; previous thromboembolism; atrial fibrillation; left atrial diameter >50 mm; mitral stenosis of any degree, LVEF <35%.
ESC guidelines on the management of valvular heart disease (version 2012). *European Heart Journal* 2012;**33**:2451–2496.

prostheses in aortic position, an INR of 2–3 is indicated for bileaflet and Medtronic-Hall valves and 2.5–3.5 for the others. For MVR, an INR of 2.5–3.5 is targeted. Bioprostheses (and MV repair) require anticoagulation for 3 months post-operatively according to current guidelines; however, continuation of warfarin for up to 6 months resulted in reduced cardiovascular mortality in a recent large registry.[10] Low-dose aspirin is recommended in all patients receiving warfarin. If INR >5, warfarin is withheld, and the INR is determined after 24 h. The American College of Chest Physicians (ACCP) guidelines recommend oral vitamin K (phytonadione, 1–2.5 mg) only when INR is >10 in the absence of bleeding.[11] In major bleeding, four-factor prothrombin complex concentrate is preferred to fresh frozen plasma since >1500 mL of fresh frozen plasma are needed to achieve a meaningful increase in coagulation factor levels.[12] Intravenous vitamin K (1–10 mg) may also be given, although, at 24h, oral vitamin K produces similar results. Dose is 2.5 mg po or 1–2 mg of the IV preparation in a cup of orange juice. Dabigatran should not be used for anticoagulation in the presence of mechanical prosthetic valves (FDA alert December 2012). The RE-ALIGN trial was prematurely stopped due to increased incidence of thrombotic events with dabigatran compared to warfarin. No data exist for bioprosthetic valves in this respect.

Bridging to non-cardiac surgery

The risk of thromboembolism without anticoagulation in the presence of a mechanical prosthesis is 0.03 to 0.05 per day. In a recent meta-analysis, heparin bridging in patients

Table 22.6 Antithrombotic therapy with prosthetic valves

ACC/AHA 2008 GL on valve disease. Antithrombotic therapy with prosthetic valves	
After AVR with bileaflet mechanical or Medtronic-Hall prostheses, in patients with no risk factors,* warfarin to achieve an INR 2.0–3.0. If the patient has risk factors, warfarin to achieve INR 2.5–3.5.	I-B
After AVR with Starr–Edwards valves or mechanical disc valves (other than Medtronic-Hall prostheses), in patients with no risk factors,* warfarin to achieve INR 2.5–3.5.	I-B
After MV replacement with any mechanical valve, warfarin to achieve INR 2.5–3.5.	I-C
After AVR or MV replacement with a bioprosthesis and no risk factors,* aspirin at 75–100 mg/day.	I-C
After AVR with a bioprosthesis and risk factors,* warfarin to achieve INR 2.0–3.0.	I-C
After MV replacement with a bioprosthesis and risk factors,* warfarin to achieve INR 2.0–3.0.	I-C
Aspirin 75–325 mg/day for patients unable to take warfarin after MV replacement or AVR.	I-B
Addition of aspirin at 75–100 mg/day to therapeutic warfarin for all patients with mechanical heart valves and those patients with biological valves who have risk factors.*	I-B
Warfarin to achieve INR 2.5–3.5 during the first 3 months after AVR with a mechanical prosthesis.	IIa-C
Warfarin to achieve an INR 2.0–3.0 during the first 3 months after AVR or MV replacement with a bioprosthesis in patients with no risk factors.*	IIa-C
Clopidogrel (75 mg per day) or warfarin to achieve INR 3.5–4.5 in high-risk patients with prosthetic heart valves in whom aspirin cannot be used.	IIb-C
* Risk factors include atrial fibrillation, previous thromboembolism, LV dysfunction, and hypercoagulable condition.	
ESC 2012 GL on valve disease. Indications for antithrombotic therapy after valvular surgery	
Lifelong oral anticoagulation for all patients with a mechanical prosthesis.	I-B
Lifelong oral anticoagulation patients with bioprostheses who have other indications for anticoagulation.[1]	I-C
Addition of low-dose aspirin in patients with a mechanical prosthesis and concomitant atherosclerotic disease.	IIa-C
Addition of low-dose aspirin should in patients with a mechanical prosthesis after thromboembolism despite adequate INR.	IIa-C
Oral anticoagulation for the first 3 months after implantation of a mitral or tricuspid bioprosthesis.	IIa-C
Oral anticoagulation for the first 3 months after mitral valve repair.	IIa-C
Low-dose aspirin for the first 3 months after implantation of an aortic bioprosthesis.	IIa-C
Oral anticoagulation for the first 3 months after implantation of an aortic bioprosthesis.	IIb-C

1: Atrial fibrillation, venous thromboembolism, hypercoagulable state, or, with a lesser degree of evidence, severely impaired left ventricular dysfunction (ejection fraction <35%).
ACC/AHA 2008 focused update incorporated into the ACC/AHA 2006 guidelines for the management of patients with valvular heart disease. *J Am Coll Cardiol.* 2008;**52**:e1–142.
ESC guidelines on the management of valvular heart disease (version 2012). *Eur Heart J.* 2012;**33**:2451–2496.

receiving vitamin K antagonists for AF, PHV, or VTE conferred a >5-fold increased risk for bleeding whereas the risk of thromboembolic events was not significantly different between bridged and non-bridged patients.[13] The use of therapeutic dose LMWH was associated with an increased risk of bleeding compared with prophylactic or intermediate dose.[13] Minor procedures, such as dental extraction, do not require interruption of anticoagulation. Alternatively, warfarin may be stopped 2–3 days before the procedure or a prohaemostatic agent (i.e. tranexamic acid as a 5 mL oral dose, 5–10 min before the dental procedure, and 3–4 times daily for 1–2 days after the procedure) may be given with continuation of warfarin.[14] Patients with bileaflet mechanical aortic valves in sinus rhythm and no previous thromboembolism are low risk, and no bridging is required for interruption of warfarin.[15] Implantation of pacemakers or defibrillators in patients with moderate to high thromboembolic risk does not necessitate interruption of warfarin (INR 2–3.5) since heparin use is associated with more pocket haematomas.[16] SC LMWH is convenient, but, in patients with stage IV renal failure, anti-Xa monitoring is required while, in stage V, IV UFH is recommended.[17] For major surgical procedures, the ACC/AHA and ACCP guidelines are presented in Table 22.7.

MRI

Magnetic resonance imaging can be performed safely in patients with prosthetic heart valves, except those with a Pre 6000 Starr–Edwards caged-ball prosthesis.[17]

Thrombosis of prosthetic valves

Prosthetic valve thrombosis in the current era has a reported incidence of 0.03 to 0.13% per patient-year,[18] although it used to be up to 8% with the initial mechanical valves. The major contributing factors are inadequate anticoagulant therapy and mitral location of the prosthesis. Obstruction of prosthetic valves may be caused by thrombus formation, pannus ingrowth, or both. If the prosthesis is obstructed by pannus, the valve needs to be replaced. Emergency surgery is recommended for a thrombosed left-sided prosthetic valve and NYHA III–IV symptoms or a large clot (>10 mm) or peripheral embolism (Table 22.8, and Figures 22.1 and 22.2). Fibrinolytic therapy for a left-sided prosthetic valve obstructed by thrombus may be considered for small thrombi <10 mm as determined by transoesophageal echocardiography in sTable or inoperable patients. Fibrinolysis should be also considered in critically ill patients unlikely to survive surgery, situations in which surgery is not immediately available, and in thrombosis of tricuspid or pulmonary valve replacements,

Table 22.7 Bridging therapy to non-cardiac surgery

ACC/AHA 2008 GL on valve disease. Bridging therapy in patients with mechanical valves who require interruption of warfarin therapy for non-cardiac surgery, invasive procedures, or dental care	
In patients at low risk of thrombosis (i.e. bileaflet mechanical AVR with no risk factors), warfarin should be stopped 48–72 h before the procedure (so INR falls to <1.5) and restarted within 24 h after the procedure. Heparin is usually unnecessary.	I-B
In patients at high risk of thrombosis (i.e. any mechanical MV replacement or a mechanical AVR with any risk factor), therapeutic doses of IV UFH should be started when INR falls <2.0 (typically 48 h before surgery), stopped 4–6 h before the procedure, restarted as early after surgery as bleeding stability allows, and continued until the INR is again therapeutic with warfarin therapy.	I-B
Fresh frozen plasma to patients with mechanical valves who require interruption of warfarin for emergency non-cardiac surgery, invasive procedures, or dental care. Fresh frozen plasma is preferable to high-dose vitamin K1.	IIa-B
In patients at high risk of thrombosis, therapeutic doses of subcutaneous UFH (15 000 U every 12 h) or LMWH (100 U per kg every 12 h) may be considered during the period of a subtherapeutic INR.	IIb-B
In patients with mechanical valves who require interruption of warfarin therapy for non-cardiac surgery, invasive procedures, or dental care, high-dose vitamin K1 should not be given routinely because this may create a hypercoagulable condition.	III-B
ACCP 2012 GL on antithrombotic therapy. Perioperative management of antithrombotic therapy	
Stopping VKAs approximately 5 days before surgery.	Grade 1C
Resuming of VKA 12–24h after surgery.	Grade 2C
Bridging anticoagulation in patients with a mechanical heart valve, AF, or VTE at high risk for thromboembolism but no bridging in low-risk patients.	Grade 2C
In minor dental procedures, continuing VKAs with co-administration of an oral prohaemostatic agent or stopping VKAs 2–3 days before the procedure.	Grade 2C
In minor dermatologic procedures,continuing VKAs around the time of the procedure and optimizing local haemostasis.	Grade 2C
In cataract surgery, continuing VKAs around the time of the surgery.	Grade 2C
Stopping of bridging UFH 4– 6 h before surgery.	Grade 2C
Stopping of bridging SC LMWH and administering the last preoperative dose approximately 24 h before surgery.	Grade 2C
In patients undergoing high bleeding risk surgery, resumption of therapeutic dose LMWH 48–72 h after surgery.	Grade 2C

1C: strong recommendation, low-quality evidence
2C: weak recommendation, low-quality evidence
ACC/AHA guidelines on valve disease 2008 focused update incorporated into the ACC/AHA 2006 guidelines for the management of patients with valvular heart disease. *J Am Coll Cardiol*. 2008;**52**:e1–142.
ACCP 2012 guidelines on antithrombotic therapy. *Chest*. 2012;**141**(2 Suppl):7S–47S. Erratum in: *Chest*. 2012;**141**:1129

Table 22.8 ACC/AHA 2008 GL on valve disease

Thrombosis of prosthetic heart valves	
Transthoracic and Doppler echocardiography in patients with suspected prosthetic valve thrombosis to assess haemodynamic severity.	I-B
Transoesophageal echocardiography and/or fluoroscopy in patients with suspected valve thrombosis to assess valve motion and clot burden.	I-B
Emergency operation for patients with a thrombosed left-sided prosthetic valve and NYHA III–IV symptoms.	IIa-C
Emergency operation for patients with a thrombosed left-sided prosthetic valve and a large clot burden.	IIa-C
Fibrinolysis for thrombosed right-sided prosthetic heart valves with NYHA III–IV symptoms or a large clot burden.	IIa-C
Fibrinolysis as a first-line therapy for patients with a thrombosed left-sided prosthetic valve, NYHA functional class I–II symptoms, and a small clot burden.	IIb-B
Fibrinolysis as a first-line therapy for patients with a thrombosed left-sided prosthetic valve, NYHA III–IV symptoms, and a small clot burden if surgery is high-risk or not available.	IIb-B
Fibrinolysis for patients with an obstructed, thrombosed left-sided prosthetic valve who have NYHA functional class II–IV symptoms and a large clot burden if emergency surgery is high risk or not available.	IIb-C
IV UFH as an alternative to fibrinolytic therapy for patients with a thrombosed valve who are in NYHA functional class I–II and have a small clot burden.	IIb-C

ACC/AHA 2008 focused update incorporated into the ACC/AHA 2006 guidelines for the management of patients with valvular heart disease. *J Am Coll Cardiol*. 2008;**52**:e1–142.

because of the higher success rate and low risk of systemic embolism.[5] It is recommended as the first-line treatment for obstructive valve thrombosis, independent of NYHA class and thrombus size if there are no contraindications, by the Society for Heart Valve Disease.[19] Fibrinolysis is less likely to be successful in mitral prostheses in chronic thrombosis. In case of haemodynamic instability a short protocol is recommended, using either intravenous recombinant tissue plasminogen activator 10mg bolus+90mg in 90 minutes with UFH, or streptokinase 1 500 000 U in 60 minutes without UFH. Longer durations of infusions can be used in sTable patients.[5] If fibrinolytic therapy is successful, it should be followed by intravenous UFH until warfarin achieves an INR of 3.5 for aortic and 4 for mitral prosthetic valves. Low-dose aspirin is also given. If partially successful, subcutaneous UFH twice daily (to achieve an aPTT of 55–80 s) is added to warfarin for 3 months (ACC/AHA guidelines on valve disease 2008). It is unlikely to be successful in mitral prostheses, chronic thrombosis, or in the presence of pannus that may be difficult to distinguish from thrombus. Fibrinolysis is associated with a risk of cerebral embolism, 12–15% depending on the size of the clot (odds ratio of 2.41 per 1 cm^2 increment).[20]

Haemolysis

Subclinical intravascular haemolysis is noted in most patients with a normally functioning mechanical prosthetic valve; severe haemolytic anemia is uncommon and suggests paravalvular leakage due to partial dehiscence of the valve or infection. Diagnosis of valve-induced haemolysis is made by increased serum lactate dehydrogenase concentrations, decreased serum haptoglobin concentrations, and reticulocytosis.[21]

Paravalvular leaks

Paravalvular regurgitation affects 5–17% of all surgically implanted prosthetic heart valves and mainly the mitral valve. Patients may be asymptomatic or present with haemolysis or heart failure. Reoperation is associated with increased morbidity and is not always successful because of underlying tissue friability, inflammation, or calcification. Percutaneous closure should be considered for closure of clinically symptomatic paravalvular leaks, and, in experienced centres, it is successful in up to 90% of the cases, with <10% complications rate (obstruction of the tilting valve leaflet, embolization of the device, coronary artery obstruction, or stroke).[22]

Annual follow-up with echocardiography is recommended for patients with bioprosthetic valves after the first 5 years (Class I-C, ACC/AHA guidelines on valve disease 2008).

Pregnancy

Maternal mortality is estimated to be between 1% and 4% in women with mechanical valves.[5]

In pregnant women with mechanical valves, anticoagulation management is not established.

According to the ACC/AHA 2008 guidelines on valve disease (Table 22.9):

1. Between weeks 6 and 12 (highest risk of fetal defects), warfarin may be replaced by:
   Subcutaneous unfractionated heparin (UFH) in high doses, up to 20 000/12h to maintain an aPTT twice the control value 4 h after administration, or
   Subcutaneous low molecular weight heparin (LMWH) twice daily to maintain an anti-Xa level between 0.7 and 1.2 U/mL 4 h after administration. It is also important to consider both peak and trough levels of anti-Xa activiy.[23]

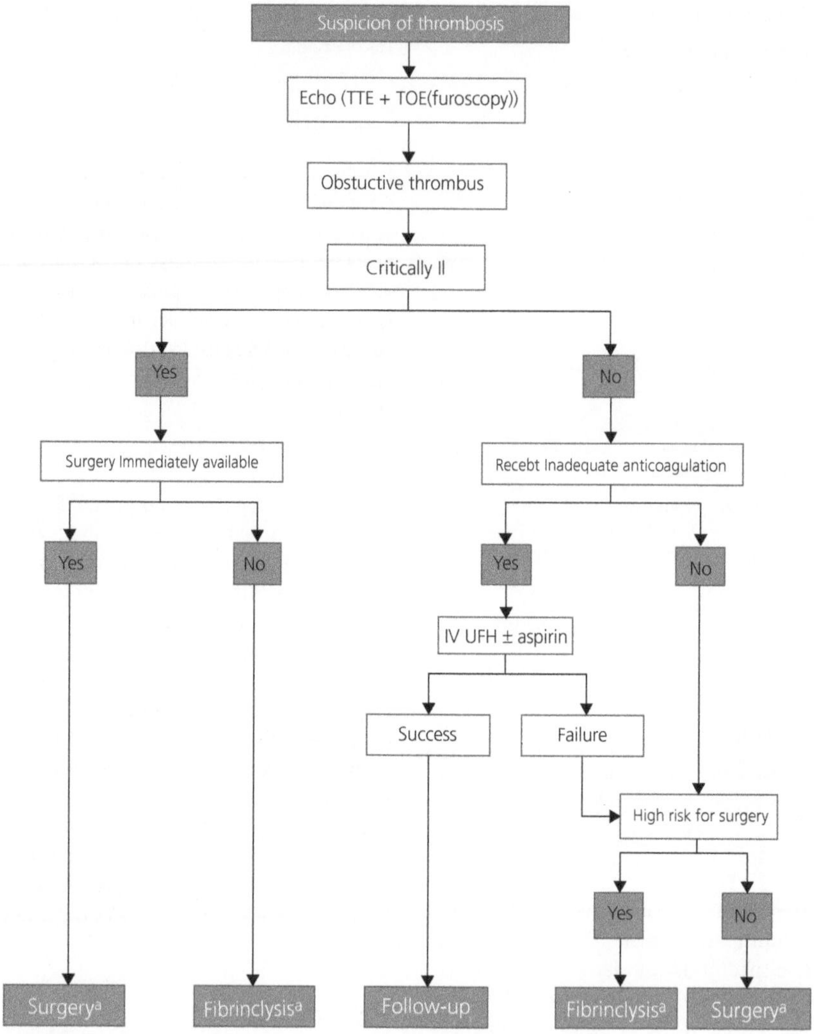

Figure 22.1 ESC 2012 on VD. Management of left-sided obstructive prosthetic thrombosis.

IV UFH, intravenous unfractionated heparin; TOE, transoesophageal echocardiography; TTE, transthoracic echocardiography. a: Risk and benefits of both treatments should be individualized. The presence of a first-generation prosthesis is an incentive to surgery.
ESC guidelines on the management of valvular heart disease (version 2012). *European Heart Journal* 2012;**33**:2451–2496.

2. At week 36, continuous IV UFH heparin is administered.
3. For the rest of pregnancy period, either warfarin (INR 2.5–3.5) or UFH or LMWH can be used. IV UHF carries a lower risk for the fetus but higher maternal risk of prosthetic valve thrombosis, systemic embolization, osteoporosis, and heparin-induced thrombocytopenia.
4. In women with mechanical prosthetic valves, aspirin (75–100 mg/day) may be added to warfarin or heparin.

The new ESC guidelines on pregnancy also provide the option of warfarin between weeks 6 and 12, provided that the necessary dose is <5 mg/day (Table 22.10).[24] See also Chapter 84 on cardiovascular disease in pregnancy in Miscellaneous topics.

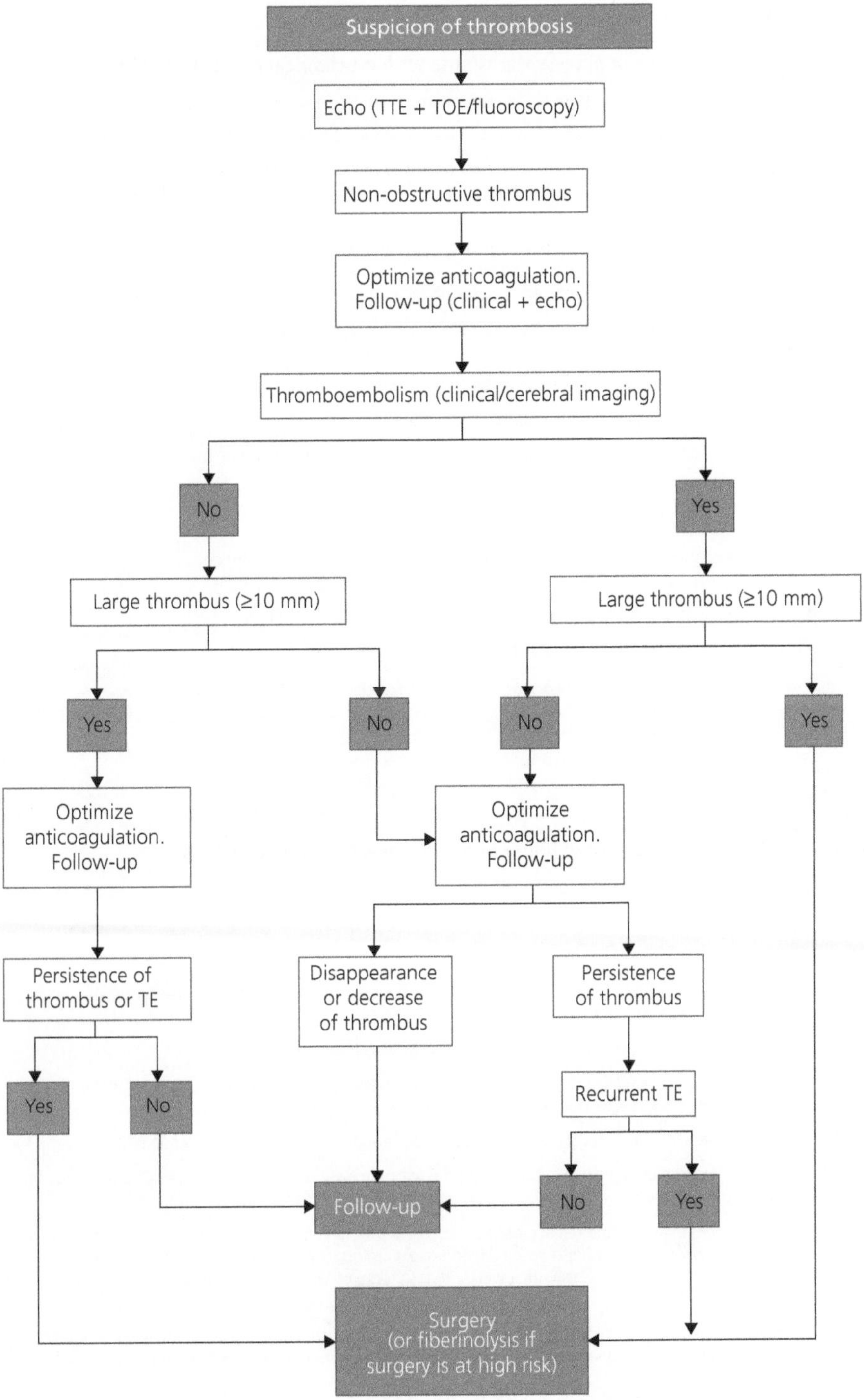

Figure 22.2 ESC 2012 on VD. Management of left-sided non-obstructive prosthetic thrombosis.

ESC guidelines on the management of valvular heart disease (version 2012). *European Heart Journal* 2012;**33**:2451–2496

Table 22.9 ACC/AHA 2008 GL on valve disease

Selection of anticoagulation regimen in pregnant patients with mechanical prosthetic valves	
All patients must receive continuous therapeutic anticoagulation with frequent monitoring.	I-B
Pregnancy tests should be monitored with discussions about subsequent anticoagulation therapy, so that anticoagulation can be continued uninterrupted when pregnancy is achieved.	I-C
Patients who elect to stop warfarin between weeks 6 and 12 of gestation should receive continuous IV UFH, dose-adjusted UFH, or dose-adjusted subcutaneous LMWH.	I-C
For patients up to 36 weeks of gestation, the therapeutic choice of continuous IV or dose-adjusted SC UFH, dose-adjusted LMWH, or warfarin should be discussed fully. If continuous IV UFH is used, the fetal risk is lower, but the maternal risks of prosthetic valve thrombosis, systemic embolization, infection, osteoporosis, and heparin-induced thrombocytopenia are relatively higher.	I-C
In patients who receive dose-adjusted LMWH, the LMWH should be administered twice daily SC to maintain the anti-Xa level between 0.7 and 1.2 U per ml 4 h after administration.	I-C
In patients who receive dose-adjusted UFH, the aPTT should be at least twice control.	I-C
In patients who receive warfarin, the INR goal should be 3.0 (range 2.5 to 3.5).	I-C
Warfarin should be discontinued and continuous IV UFH given starting 2 to 3 weeks before planned delivery.	I-C
Avoid warfarin between weeks 6 and 12 of gestation owing to the high risk of fetal defects.	IIa-C
Resume UFH 4 to 6 h after delivery and begin oral warfarin in the absence of significant bleeding.	IIa-C
Low-dose aspirin (75 to 100 mg od) in the second and third trimesters of pregnancy in addition to anticoagulation with warfarin or heparin.	IIa-C
LMWH should not be administered unless anti-Xa levels are monitored 4 to 6 h after administration.	III-C
Dipyridamole should not be used instead of aspirin because of its harmful effects on the fetus.	III-B

aPTT, activated partial thromboplastin time; UFH, unfractionated heparin; LMWH, low molecular weight heparin; IV, intravenous; SC, subcutaneous.
ACC/AHA 2008 focused update incorporated into the ACC/AHA 2006 guidelines for the management of patients with valvular heart disease. *J Am Coll Cardiol*. 2008;**52**:e1–142.

Table 22.10 ESC 2011 GL on pregnancy

Recommendations for the management of valvular heart disease. Mechanical valves	
OACs are recommended during the second and third trimesters until the 36th week.	I-C
Change of anticoagulation regimen during pregnancy should be implemented in hospital.	I-C
If delivery starts while on OACs, caesarean delivery is indicated.	I-C
OAC should be discontinued and dose-adjusted UFH (a PTT ≥2 x control) or adjusted-dose LMWH (target anti-Xa level 4–6 hours post-dose 0.8–1.2 U/mL) started at the 36th week of gestation.	I-C
In pregnant women managed with LMWH, the post-dose anti-Xa level should be assessed weekly.	I-C
LMWH should be replaced by intravenous UFH at least 36 hours before planned delivery. UFH should be continued until 4–6 hours before planned delivery and restarted 4–6 hours after delivery if there are no bleeding complications.	I-C
Immediate echocardiography is indicated in women with mechanical valves presenting with dyspnoea and/or an embolic event.	I-C
Continuation of OACs should be considered during the first trimester if the warfarin dose required for therapeutic anticoagulation is <5 mg/day (or phenprocoumon <3 mg/day or acenocoumarol <2 mg/day), after patient information and consent.	IIa-C
Discontinuation of OAC between weeks 6 and 12 and replacement by adjusted-dose UFH (a PTT ≥2 x control; in high risk patients applied as intravenous infusion) or LMWH twice daily (with dose adjustment according to weight and target anti-Xa level 4–6 hours post-dose 0.8–1.2 U/mL) should be considered in patients with a warfarin dose required of >5 mg/day (or phenprocoumon >3 mg/day or acenocoumarol >2mg/day).	IIa-C
Discontinuation of OACs between weeks 6 and 12 and replacement by UFH or LMWH under strict dose control (as described above) may be considered on an individual basis in patients with warfarin dose required for therapeutic anticoagulation <5 mg/day (or phenprocoumon <3 mg/day or acenocoumarol <2 mg/day).	IIb-C
Continuation of OACs may be considered between weeks 6 and 12 in patients with a warfarin dose required for therapeutic anticoagulation >5 mg/day (or phenprocoumon >3 mg/day or acenocoumarol >2 mg/day).	IIb-C
LMWH should be avoided, unless anti-Xa levels are monitored.	III-C

OACs, oral anticoagulants.
ESC Guidelines on the management of cardiovascular diseases during pregnancy. *Eur Heart J*. 2011;**32**:3147–97

References

1. Rosenhek R, *et al.* ESC working group on valvular heart disease position paper: Assessing the risk of interventions in patients with valvular heart disease. *Eur Heart J.* 2012;**33**:822–8, 828a, 828b
2. Rippel RA GH, Seifalian AM. Tissue-engineered heart valve: Future of cardiac surgery. *World J Surg.* 2012;**36**:1581–1591
3. Rahimtoola SH. Choice of prosthetic heart valve in adults: an update. *J Am Coll Cardiol.* 2010;**55**:2413–26
4. Bonow RO, *et al.* 2008 focused update incorporated into the ACC/AHA 2006 guidelines for the management of patients with valvular heart disease: a report of the American College of Cardiology/American Heart Association Task Force on practice guidelines (writing committee to revise the 1998 guidelines for the management of patients with valvular heart disease). Endorsed by the Society of Cardiovascular Anesthesiologists, Society for Cardiovascular Angiography and Interventions, and Society of Thoracic Surgeons. *J Am Coll Cardiol.* 2008;**52**:e1–42
5. Vahanian A, *et al.* Guidelines on the management of valvular heart disease (version 2012). *Eur Heart J.* 2012;**33**:2451–96
6. Boning A, *et al.* Heart valve prosthesis selection in patients with end-stage renal disease requiring dialysis: a systematic review and meta-analysis. *Heart.* 2012;**98**:99
7. Herzog CA, *et al.* Long-term survival of dialysis patients in the United States with prosthetic heart valves: should ACC/AHA practice guidelines on valve selection be modified? *Circulation.* 2002;**105**:1336–41
8. Brennan JMEF, *et al.* on behalf of the DEcIDE AVR Research Team. Long-term safety and effectiveness of mechanical versus biologic aortic valve prostheses in older patients: Results from the Society of Thoracic Surgeons (STS) adult cardiac surgery national database. *Circulation* 2013, Mar 28 [Epub ahead of print].
9. Stulak JM, *et al.* Spectrum and outcome of reoperations after the Ross procedure. *Circulation.* 2010;**122**:1153–8
10. Merie C, *et al.* Association of warfarin therapy duration after bioprosthetic aortic valve replacement with risk of mortality, thromboembolic complications, and bleeding. *JAMA.* 2012;**308**:2118–25
11. Guyatt GH, *et al.* Executive summary: antithrombotic therapy and prevention of thrombosis, 9th ed: American College of Chest Physicians evidence-based clinical practice guidelines. *Chest.* 2012;**141**:7S–47S
12. Garcia DA, *et al.* Reversal of warfarin: case-based practice recommendations. *Circulation.* 2012;**125**:2944–7
13. Siegal D, *et al.* Periprocedural heparin bridging in patients receiving vitamin K antagonists: systematic review and meta-analysis of bleeding and thromboembolic rates. *Circulation.* 2012;**126**:1630–9
14. Douketis JD, *et al.* Perioperative management of antithrombotic therapy: antithrombotic therapy and prevention of thrombosis, 9th ed: American College of Chest Physicians evidence-based clinical practice guidelines. *Chest.* 2012;**141**:e326S-50S
15. Wysokinski WE, *et al.* Periprocedural bridging management of anticoagulation. *Circulation.* 2012;**126**: 486–90
16. Ahmed I, *et al.* Continuing warfarin therapy is superior to interrupting warfarin with or without bridging anticoagulation therapy in patients undergoing pacemaker and defibrillator implantation. *Heart Rhythm.* 2010;**7**:745–9
17. Randall PA, *et al.* Magnetic resonance imaging of prosthetic cardiac valves *in vitro* and *in vivo*. *Am J Cardiol.* 1988;**62**:973–6
18. Hammermeister KSG, *et al.* Outcomes 15 years after valve replacement with a mechanical versus a bioprosthetic valve: Final report of the veterans affairs randomized trial. *J Am Coll Cardiol.* 2000;**36**:1152–8
19. Lengyel MHD, *et al.* Working Group Infection. Recommendations for the management of prosthetic valve thrombosis. *J Heart Valve Dis.* 2005;**14**:567–75
20. Tong AT, *et al.* Transoesophageal echocardiography improves risk assessment of thrombolysis of prosthetic valve thrombosis: results of the International PRO-TEE registry. *J Am Coll Cardiol.* 2004;**43**:77–84
21. Vongpatanasin W, *et al.* Prosthetic heart valves. *N Engl J Med.* 1996;**335**:407–16
22. Rihal CS, *et al.* Principles of percutaneous paravalvular leak closure. *JACC Cardiovasc Interv.* 2012;**5**:121–30
23. Elkayam U, *et al.* The search for a safe and effective anticoagulation regimen in pregnant women with mechanical prosthetic heart valves. *J Am Coll Cardiol.* 2012;**59**:1116–18
24. Regitz-Zagrosek V, *et al.* ESC guidelines on the management of cardiovascular diseases during pregnancy: the Task Force on the management of cardiovascular diseases during pregnancy of the European Society of Cardiology (ESC). *Eur Heart J.* 2011;**32**:3147–97

Part III

Systemic hypertension

Relevant guidelines

AHA 2005 recommendations for blood pressure measurements

Recommendations for blood pressure measurement in humans and experimental animals: part 1: blood pressure measurement in humans: a statement for professionals from the Subcommittee of Professional and Public Education of the American Heart Association Council on High Blood Pressure Research. *Circulation.* 2005;**111**:697–716.

ACCF/AHA 2013 guideline on peripheral artery disease

Management of patients with peripheral artery disease (compilation of 2005 and 2011 ACCF/AHA guideline recommendations). *J Am Coll Cardiol.* 2013;**61**.

ESH/ESC 2013 guidelines on hypertension

2013 ESH/ESC Guidelines for the management of arterial hypertension. *Eur Heart J.* 2013. doi:10. 1093/eurheartj/eht151.

ESC 2011 guidelines on pregnancy

ESC Guidelines on the management of cardiovascular diseases during pregnancy. *Eur Heart J.* 2011;**32**:3147–97.

ACCF/AHA 2011 expert consensus document on hypertension in the elderly

ACCF/AHA 2011 expert consensus document on hypertension in the elderly. *J Am Coll Cardiol.* 2011;**57**:2037–114.

ESC 2012 guidelines on cardiovascular disease prevention

European Guidelines on cardiovascular disease prevention in clinical practice (version 2012). *Eur Heart J.* 2012;**33**:1635–701.

ESC 2012 guidelines on heart failure

ESC Guidelines for the diagnosis and treatment of acute and chronic heart failure 2012. *Eur Heart J.* 2012;**33**:1787–847.

Chapter 23

Classification and pathophysiology of hypertension

Definition

Hypertension in adults aged 18 or older is defined as blood pressure (BP) ≥140/90 mmHg, based on the average of ≥2 seated blood pressure measurements, properly measured with well-maintained equipment, at each of ≥2 visits to the office or clinic.[1] Hypertension has been divided into stages by JNC 7 and ESC, as shown in Table 23.1.[1, 2] Home blood pressures are consistently lower than clinic pressures in most hypertensive patients, and the American Society of Hypertension recommends 135/85 mmHg as the upper limit of normal for home blood pressure.[3] Threshold values for office and home normal values, as well as for ambulatory blood pressure measurements,[4] are presented in Table 23.2.

Epidemiology

Hypertension is an increasingly important public health issue, affecting approximately 25% of the overall population.[5, 6] Its prevalence increases with advancing age. In the USA, the National Health and Nutrition Examination Survey estimates that more than 50% of people aged 60 to 69 years old and approximately 75% of those aged 70 years and older are affected.[6] According to data from the Framingham Heart Study, the lifetime risk of hypertension is approximately 90% for men and women who were not hypertensive at 55 or 65 years old and survived to age 80 to 85. Even after adjusting for competing mortality, the remaining lifetime risks of hypertension were 86 to 90% in women and 81 to 83% in men.[7] Suboptimal BP control is the most common attributable risk for death worldwide, being responsible for 62% of cerebrovascular disease and 49% of ischaemic heart disease, as well as an estimated 7.1 million deaths a year.[8] In most cases (>90%), no underlying pathology can be identified (primary or essential hypertension). Blood pressure is a complex genetic trait with heritability estimates of 30–50%, but the intrinsic origin of essential hypertension remains obscure although many environmental factors are known[9]. Single nucleotide polymorphisms have also been identified as risk factors for hypertension and coronary artery disease.[10]

Pathophysiology

Systolic pressure within the aorta is a composite of two items: (1) the outgoing pressure wave, generated by ventricular contraction; and (2) pressure wave reflection from the periphery. Since the pulse wave is amplified in transit from the heart to the brachial artery, central aortic systolic pressure is usually lower than brachial pressure. The magnitude of amplification is greatest in people with healthy compliant arteries and diminishes with age.

Established hypertension exposes the arterial tree to increased pulsatile stress, but, paradoxically, major complications are thrombotic, rather than haemorrhagic, referred to as the so-called thrombotic paradox of hypertension. Blood flow abnormalities, endothelial damage or dysfunction, and a hypercoagulable state are consequences of long-standing hypertension.[11] The prothrombotic state could be the result of chronic low-grade inflammation and damage and remodelling of the vascular endothelium due to elevated shear stress. The mechanisms leading to endothelial dysfunction are multifactorial, and include decreased activity of vasodilator agents and increased activity (or sensitivity) to vasoconstrictor agents. Enhanced activity of the renin-angiotensin system and kallikrein-kinin system has opposite effects, resulting in vasoconstriction and vasodilation, respectively, but, with respect to coagulation, they both cause a hypercoagulable state.[12] Thus, hypertension not only confers a hypercoagulable state (vulnerable blood) but also gives rise to left ventricular hypertrophy, ventricular and atrial arrhythmias, increased aortic stiffness, and impaired coronary reserve (vulnerable myocardium), thereby fulfilling all criteria for a vulnerable patient. In enhancing the coagulation fibrinolysis balance, antihypertensive treatment can decrease the frequency of thrombotic events, independent of blood pressure.

Target organ disease due to essential hypertension comprises damage of the heart, brain, and kidneys. Left ventricular hypertrophy, coronary artery disease, atrial fibrillation, and ventricular arrhythmias are consequences of long-standing hypertension. Hypertension is the most common cause of atrial fibrillation and congestive heart failure. Typically, hypertension leads to LV hypertrophy that progresses to dilated cardiac failure. However, recent evidence indicates that patients with hypertension may progress directly to dilated cardiac failure in the absence of myocardial infarction or antecedent concentric hypertrophy.[13] Microalbuminuria, proteinuria and elevated creatinine levels, and reduced glomerular filtration rate are signs of progressive renal impairment. Retinopathy, Binswanger lesions (subcortical vascular dementia), transient ischaemic attacks, and, eventually, stroke and dementia are manifestations of brain damage.

Table 23.1 Classification of hypertension schemes

Classification of hypertension (JNC-7)

BP classification	Systolic BP mmHg	Diastolic BP mmHg
Normal	<120	<80
Prehypertensive	120–139	80–89
Stage 1 hypertension	140–159	90–99
Stage 2 hypertension	≥160	≥100

Seventh report of the Joint National Committee on Prevention, Detection, Evaluation, and Treatment of High Blood Pressure. *Hypertension*. 2003;**42**:1206–52.

Definitions and classification of blood pressure levels (mmHg)*

ESH/ESC 2013 GL on hypertension

Category	Systolic	Diastolic
Optimal	<120, and	<80
Normal	120–129, and/or	80–84
High normal	130–139, and/or	85–89
Grade 1 hypertension	140–159, and/or	90–99
Grade 2 hypertension	160–179, and/or	100–109
Grade 3 hypertension	≥180, and/or	≥110
Isolated systolic hypertension	≥140, and	<90

*: The blood pressure (BP) category is defined by the highest level of BP, whether systolic or diastolic. Isolated systolic hypertension should be graded 1, 2, or 3 according to systolic BP values in the ranges indicated.

Table 23.2 Normal values

ESH/ESC 2013 GL on hypertension. Blood pressure thresholds (mmHg) for definition of hypertension with different types of measurement

Category	Systolic BP (mmHg)		Diastolic BP (mmHg)
Office blood pressure	≥140	and/or	≥90
Ambulatory blood pressure			
Daytime (or awake)	≥135	and/or	≥85
Night time (or asleep)	≥120	and/or	≥70
24-h	≥130	and/or	≥80
Home blood pressure	≥135	and/or	≥85

2013 ESH/ESC Guidelines for the management of arterial hypertension. *Eur Heart J*. 2013. doi:10.1093/eurheartj/eht151.

Diagnostic thresholds for ambulatory blood pressure measurements (mmHg)

	24-hour	Daytime	Night time
Optimal	<115/75	<120/80	<100/65
Normal	<125/75	<130/85	<110/70
Ambulatory hypertension	≥130/80	≥140/85	≥120/70

Kikuya M, *et al*; International Database on Ambulatory blood pressure monitoring in relation to Cardiovascular Outcomes Investigators. Diagnostic thresholds for ambulatory blood pressure monitoring based on 10-year cardiovascular risk. *Circulation*. 2007;**115**:2145–52.

Subtypes of hypertension

Prehypertension

The term prehypertension (systolic BP 120–139 mmHg, diastolic BP 80–89 mmHg) reflects the fact that health risks attributable to increasing blood pressure in adults are continuous, beginning at 115/75 mmHg.[14] These patients may develop established hypertension later, and blockade of the renin-angiotensin axis has been found to decrease this risk.[15, 16] However, drug therapy for this population is highly debated due to complications and cost considerations.[17] Lifestyle modification by means of low salt diet, weight loss, exercise, and alcohol restriction are the best way for treating these patients.[18–21]

Isolated systolic hypertension

With increasing age, systolic blood pressure, unlike diastolic brood pressure, tends to rise in response to increasing arterial stiffness and losses in arterial compliance, particularly after the age of 40. Isolated systolic hypertension is a common condition in individuals aged older than 60 years.[3] In the young, isolated systolic hypertension has been thought to result from an amplification of the pressure wave between the aorta and the brachial artery due to very elastic arteries in the context of normal aortic systolic pressure. Recent evidence suggests that isolated systolic hypertension in the young is a heterogeneous condition and may result from an increased stroke volume and/or aortic stiffness whereas the major haemodynamic abnormality underlying essential hypertension is an increased peripheral vascular resistance.[22] The prevalence of isolated systolic hypertension has nearly doubled among young adults during the last decade and is associated with obesity, smoking, and low socio-economic status.[23]

Isolated diastolic hypertension

Although diastolic pressure is generally thought to be the best predictor of risk in patients younger than 50, some prospective studies of isolated diastolic hypertension have indicated that the prognosis may be relatively benign, and the topic remains controversial.[3]

Pulse pressure

In older hypertensive patients, increased pulse pressure (systolic-diastolic) is the major determinant of cardiovascular risk.[24]

White coat hypertension

Differences between office and home measurements are present in the majority of hypertensive patients. White coat, or isolated office, hypertension is defined as a persistently elevated average office blood pressure of >140/90 and an average awake ambulatory reading of <135/85 mmHg,[3] or as at least three separate measurements of >140/90 mmHg at the doctor's office and at least two non office-based measurements of <140/90 mmHg. Whether subjects with white-coat hypertension have a higher cardiovascular risk than normotensive individuals is an issue still under debate, with both affirmative and negative results having been reported.[25–27] Risk of patients with white coat hypertension is probably higher than in normotensive individuals but distinctly lower than in people with sustained hypertension. These patients are very likely to develop sustained hypertension later. However, the value of therapy is not proven in patients without established hypertension,[28] and ambulatory blood pressure or repeat (>5) pressure measurements at home are superior to office blood pressure measurements in predicting treatment-induced regression of left ventricular hypertrophy.[29]

Masked hypertension

Normal blood pressure measurements at the office, but elevated values elsewhere, may be due to alcohol abuse or smoking. Target organ damage (as LV hypertrophy or renal impairment) is related to the more prolonged elevations in pressure, and its presence can assist the diagnosis. There is evidence that such patients are at increased risk.[3] Masked hypertension may also occur with severe peripheral arterial disease.

Pseudohypertension

May be seen with stiff, calcified vessels in the elderly and patients with long-standing diabetes or chronic renal failure that are difficult to compress. The Osler manoeuvre (palpable radial pulse despite occlusive cuff pressure) is not a sensitive, or specific, sign of pseudohypertension. Intra-arterial radial pressure measurement may be necessary for correct diagnosis.

Orthostatic hypotension

It is defined by a fall >20 mmHg systolic and/or >10 mmHg diastolic in response to standing from the supine position within 3 minutes or during head-up tilt at 60 degrees. It is usually a sign of dysautonomic syndromes, diabetes, Parkinsons's disease, multiple myeloma, or multiple system atrophy but may also be seen in patients with vasovagal syncope. The major therapeutic problem is inability to control the level of blood pressure in patients with orthostatic hypotension who concomitantly have supine hypertension.

Blood pressure during exercise

BP increases during dynamic and static exercise, and the increase is more pronounced for systolic than for diastolic BP. There is currently no consensus on normal BP response during dynamic exercise testing. A SBP of ≥210 mmHg for men and ≥190 mmHg for women has been termed 'exercise hypertension'.[2] The results on the independent relationships of the blood pressure response to physical and mental stressors, future hypertension, and target organ damage are not consistent, and exercise testing to predict future hypertension is not recommended.[2] However, an exercise test may provide some additional prognostic information, at least in subjects with mild blood pressure elevation. The 21-year follow-up study of 1999, apparently healthy, men disclosed independently predictive information on cardiovascular death, of both supine systolic BP and 6-minute exercise systolic BP taken at an early moderate workload but not of maximal systolic BP during exercise.[30]

Blood pressure differential

At the first visit, BP should be checked in both arms. Differences between the two arms >15 mmHg may be seen in up to 12–15% of patients with hypertension and is an independent predictor of cardiovascular disease and death.[31] These patients may deserve further investigations for peripheral and coronary artery disease. Differences >20 mmHg may be seen in subclavian artery stenosis, severe supravalvular AS, coarctation, Ao dissection, or as a normal variant. Leg BP is up to 20 mmHg higher than in the arms.

Blood pressure measurement

Measured with the patient seated with the back supported or supine and the arm at heart level. The patient should have refrained from smoking or drinking coffee for at least 30 min, and allowed to sit for 3–5 min (Table 23.3).

Patient position

Diastolic pressure measured while sitting is higher than when measured supine (by 5 mmHg), although there is less agreement about systolic pressure. When the arm position is adjusted so that the cuff is at the level of the right atrium in both positions, the systolic pressure has been reported to be 8 mmHg higher in the supine than the upright position. If the back is not supported (as when the patient is seated on an examination table as opposed to a chair), the diastolic pressure may be increased by 6 mmHg. Crossing the legs may raise systolic pressure by 2 to 8 mmHg. In the supine position, the arm should be supported with a pillow. In the sitting position, the right atrium level is the midpoint of the sternum or the fourth intercostal space; it is preferred in diabetics due to increased possibility of postural hypotension.

Cuff size

The cuff should be held at the heart level, whatever the position of the patient. The length and width of the cuff should be 80%/40% of the arm circumference, 1–2 cm above the antecubital fossa. Too small cuffs overestimate BP whereas too large ones underestimate it.

The recommended cuff sizes are:[3]

- For arm circumference of 22 to 26 cm, the cuff should be 'small adult' size: 12 × 22 cm
- For arm circumference of 27 to 34 cm, the cuff should be 'adult' size: 16 × 30 cm
- For arm circumference of 35 to 44 cm, the cuff should be 'large adult' size: 16 × 36 cm
- For arm circumference of 45 to 52 cm, the cuff should be 'adult thigh' size: 16 × 42 cm.

Cuff should be deflated at 2–3 mmHg/s, with neither the patient nor the doctor talking. Traditionally, the Korotkoff sounds have been classified into five phases: phase I, appearance of clear tapping sounds, corresponding to the appearance of a palpable pulse; phase II, sounds become softer and longer; phase III, sounds become crisper and louder; phase IV, sounds become muffled and softer; and phase V, sounds disappear completely. The fifth phase is thus recorded as the last audible sound. The onset of phase I

Table 23.3 ESH/ESC 2013 GL on Hypertension

Office blood pressure measurement
◆ To allow the patients to sit for 3–5 minutes before beginning BP measurements.
◆ To take at least two BP measurements, in the sitting position, spaced 1–2 min apart, and dditional measurements if the rst two are quite different. Consider the average BP if deemed appropriate.
◆ To take repeated measurements of BP to improve accuracy in in patienst with arrhythmia such as AF.
◆ To use a standard bladder (12–13 cm wide and 35 cm long), but have a larger and a smaller bladder available for large (arm circumference >32 cm) and thin arms, respectively.
◆ To have the cuff at the heart level, whatever the position of the patient.
◆ When adopting the auscultatory method, use phase I and V (disappearance) Korotkoff sounds to identify systolic and diastolic BP, respectively.
◆ To measure BP in both arms at first visit to detect possible differences. In this instance, take the arm with the higher value as the reference.
◆ To measure at the first visit, BP 1 and 3 min after assumption of the standing position in elderly subjects, diabetic patients, and in other conditions in which orthostatic hypotension may be frequent or suspected.
◆ To measure, in case of conventional BP measurement, heart rate by pulse palpation (at least 30 s) after the second measurement in the sitting position.

corresponds to systolic pressure but tends to underestimate the systolic pressure recorded by direct intra-arterial measurement whereas the disappearance of sounds (phase V) corresponds to diastolic pressure but tends to occur before diastolic pressure determined by direct intra-arterial measurement.[3] Early disappearance and recurrence of sounds (**auscillatory gap**) may occur in the elderly. The auscultatory gap often can be eliminated by elevating the arm over head for 30 seconds before inflating the cuff and then bringing the arm to the usual position to continue in the measurement. This manoeuvre reduces vascular volume in the limb and improves inflow to enhance the Korotkoff sounds. In severe AR or large AV fistulas and, rarely, in pregnancy, Korotkoff sounds may be heard until complete deflation of the cuff. In these cases, the phase IV pressure should be noted.[3] At least three measurements should be taken.[29] The Korotkoff sound method tends to give values for systolic pressure that are lower than the true intra-arterial pressure, and diastolic values that are higher.

Sphygmomanometers

All devices may be inaccurate due to technical problems and need frequent calibration. Mercury sphygmomanometers are perhaps the most reliable despite concerns about mercury toxicity. **Oscillometric automated monitors** that provide read-outs of systolic and diastolic pressure should be subjected by independent investigators to formal validation protocols, such as those developed by the Association for the Advancement of Medical Instrumentation and the British Hypertension Society.[3] **Mercury sphygmomanometers** should be examined by checking that the upper curve of the meniscus of the mercury column is at 0 mmHg, that the column is free of dirt, and that it rises and falls freely during cuff inflation and deflation. **Aneroid devices** or other non-mercury devices should be checked by connecting the manometer to a mercury column or an electronic testing device with a Y-tube. The needle should rest at the zero point before the cuff is inflated and should register a reading that is within 4 mmHg of the mercury column when the cuff is inflated to pressures of 100 and 200 mmHg. The needle should return to zero after deflation.[3]

Ambulatory and home BP measurements

Ambulatory BP

Although office BP should be used as reference, ambulatory BP may improve prediction of cardiovascular risk in untreated and treated patients. 24-hour systolic BP is associated with the progression of cerebrovascular disease and cognitive decline in the elderly much better than office measurements.[32] Ambulatory BP monitoring should also be considered when there is a marked discrepancy between BP values measured in the office and at home, resistance to drug treatment or hypotensive episodes are suspected, particularly in elderly and diabetic patients, and office BP is elevated in pregnant women and pre-eclampsia is suspected.

Home BP

Self-measurement of BP at home is of clinical value, and its prognostic significance is now demonstrated. These measurements should be encouraged in order to provide more information on the BP-lowering effect of treatment at trough and thus on therapeutic coverage throughout the dose-to-dose time interval (ESC 2007).

Normal values are different for office, ambulatory, and home BP (Table 23.2).

Blood pressure variability

Despite initial evidence about the adverse prognostic significance of visit-to-visit blood pressure variability in the ASCOT and MRC trials,[33] only the average BP levels were found important in the recent ELSA trial.[34]

References

1. Chobanian AV, *et al.* Seventh report of the Joint National Committee on Prevention, Detection, Evaluation, and Treatment of High Blood Pressure. *Hypertension*. 2003;**42**:1206–52
2. 2013 ESH/ESC Guidelines for the management of arterial hypertension. *Eur Heart J*. 2013. doi:10.1093/eurheartj/eht151
3. Pickering TG, *et al.* Recommendations for blood pressure measurement in humans and experimental animals: part 1: blood pressure measurement in humans: a statement for professionals from the Subcommittee of Professional and Public Education of the American Heart Association Council on High Blood Pressure Research. *Circulation*. 2005;**111**:697–716
4. Kikuya M, *et al.* Diagnostic thresholds for ambulatory blood pressure monitoring based on 10-year cardiovascular risk. *Circulation*. 2007;**115**:2145–52
5. Burt VL, *et al.* Prevalence of hypertension in the US adult population. Results from the Third National Health and Nutrition Examination Survey, 1988–1991. *Hypertension*. 1995;**25**:305–13
6. Wolf-Maier K, *et al.* Hypertension prevalence and blood pressure levels in 6 European countries, Canada, and the United States. *JAMA*. 2003;**289**:2363–9
7. Vasan RS, *et al.* Residual lifetime risk for developing hypertension in middle-aged women and men: The Framingham Heart Study. *JAMA*. 2002;**287**:1003–10
8. WHO. *World Health Report 2002: reducing risks, promoting healthy life*. Geneva, Switzerland: World Health Organization. 2002
9. Ehret GBCM. Genes for blood pressure: An opportunity to understand hypertension. *Eur Heart J*. 2013;**34**:951–61
10. Roberts R, *et al.* Genes and coronary artery disease: where are we? *J Am Coll Cardiol*. 2012;**60**:1715–21
11. Messerli FH, *et al.* Essential hypertension. *Lancet*. 2007;**370**:591–603

12. Dielis AW, *et al.* The prothrombotic paradox of hypertension: role of the renin-angiotensin and kallikrein-kinin systems. *Hypertension*. 2005;**46**:1236–42
13. Drazner MH. The progression of hypertensive heart disease. *Circulation*. 2011;**123**:327–34
14. Lewington S, *et al.* Age-specific relevance of usual blood pressure to vascular mortality: a meta-analysis of individual data for one million adults in 61 prospective studies. *Lancet*. 2002;**360**:1903–13
15. Julius S, *et al.* Feasibility of treating prehypertension with an angiotensin-receptor blocker. *N Engl J Med*. 2006; **354**:1685–97
16. Luders S, *et al.* The PHARAO study: prevention of hypertension with the angiotensin-converting enzyme inhibitor ramipril in patients with high-normal blood pressure: a prospective, randomized, controlled prevention trial of the German Hypertension League. *J Hypertens*. 2008;**26**:1487–96
17. Mitka M. Drug therapy for prehypertension questioned. *JAMA*. 2006;**296**:2787–8
18. Cutler JA, *et al.* Randomized trials of sodium reduction: an overview. *Am J Clin Nutr*. 1997;**65**:643S-651S
19. Whelton PK, *et al.* Effects of oral potassium on blood pressure. Meta-analysis of randomized controlled clinical trials. *JAMA*. 1997;**277**:1624–32
20. Whelton SP, *et al.* Effect of aerobic exercise on blood pressure: a meta-analysis of randomized, controlled trials. *Ann Intern Med*. 2002;**136**:493–503
21. Xin X, *et al.* Effects of alcohol reduction on blood pressure: a meta-analysis of randomized controlled trials. *Hypertension*. 2001;**38**:1112–17
22. McEniery CM, *et al.* Increased stroke volume and aortic stiffness contribute to isolated systolic hypertension in young adults. *Hypertension*. 2005;**46**:221–6
23. Grebla RC, *et al.* Prevalence and determinants of isolated systolic hypertension among young adults: the 1999–2004 US National Health And Nutrition Examination Survey. *J Hypertens*. 2010;**28**:15–23
24. Blacher J, *et al.* Pulse pressure not mean pressure determines cardiovascular risk in older hypertensive patients. *Arch Intern Med*. 2000;**160**:1085–9
25. Franklin SS, *et al.* Significance of white-coat hypertension in older persons with isolated systolic hypertension: a meta-analysis using the international database on ambulatory blood pressure monitoring in relation to cardiovascular outcomes population. *Hypertension*. 2012;**59**: 564–571
26. Mancia G, *et al.* Long-term risk of mortality associated with selective and combined elevation in office, home and ambulatory blood pressure. *Hypertension*. 2006;**47**: 846–853
27. Pierdomenico SD, *et al.* Prognostic value of white-coat and masked hypertension diagnosed by ambulatory monitoring in initially untreated subjects: an updated meta analysis. *Am J Hypertens*. 2011;**24**:52–58
28. Fagard RH, *et al.* Response to antihypertensive therapy in older patients with sustained and nonsustained systolic hypertension. Systolic Hypertension in Europe (Syst-Eur) Trial Investigators. *Circulation*. 2000;**102**:1139–44
29. Powers BJ, *et al.* Measuring blood pressure for decision making and quality reporting: where and how many measures? *Ann Intern Med*. 2011;**154**:781–8, W-289–790
30. Kjeldsen SE, *et al.* Supine and exercise systolic blood pressure predict cardiovascular death in middle-aged men. *J Hypertens*. 2001;**19**:1343–8
31. Clark CE, *et al.* Association of a difference in systolic blood pressure between arms with vascular disease and mortality: a systematic review and meta-analysis. *Lancet*. 2012;**379**:905–14
32. White WB, *et al.* Average daily blood pressure, not office blood pressure, is associated with progression of cerebrovascular disease and cognitive decline in older people. *Circulation*. 2011;**124**:2312–9
33. Rothwell PM, *et al.* Effects of beta blockers and calcium-channel blockers on within-individual variability in blood pressure and risk of stroke. *Lancet Neurol*. 2010;**9**:469–80
34. Mancia G, *et al.* Visit-to-visit blood pressure variability, carotid atherosclerosis, and cardiovascular events in the European Lacidipine Study on Atherosclerosis. *Circulation*. 2012;**126**:569–78

Chapter 24

Primary (essential) hypertension

Risk stratification

Investigations in hypertensive patients are aimed at establishing risk factors, subclinical or overt organ damage, and, when suspected, diagnosis of causes of secondary hypertension. For risk stratification, the Framingham and SCORE models are mainly used.[1,2]

Risk factors

BP ≥180 mmHg systolic and/or ≥110 mmHg, diabetes mellitus, cardiovascular or renal disease, and evidence of subclinical organ damage denote high-risk subjects.[3] Factors influencing prognosis are presented in Table 24.1 and Figure 24.1.

Prediabetes is defined as:

- Fasting blood glucose 6.1 mM–6.9 mM (110–125 mg/dL) according to WHO, or 100–125 mg/dL (5.6 mM to 6.9 mM) according to American Diabetes Association (ADA), or
- 140–199 mg/dL (7.8–11.0 mM) 2-h after 75 gm glucose solution (glucose tolerance test) (ADA), or
- HbA1c 5.7–6.4% (ADA).

Values above these define clinical diabetes.

Metabolic syndrome is defined as the occurrence of, at least, three out of the following five risk factors: abdominal obesity, BP >130/85 mmHg, borderline or abnormal fasting glucose, low HDL, and high triglycerides. Increased body mass index [body weight (kg)/height (m)^2] is overweight ≥25 kg/m^2 and obesity ≥30 kg/m^2.

Abdominal obesity (waist circumference: men >102 cm, women >88 cm). However, in patients with hypertension and coronary artery disease, overweight and obesity is associated with a decreased mortality risk compared with normal weight (obesity paradox).[4]

Family history of premature cardiovascular disease (men <55 years, women <65 years).

Absence of a family history of hypertension suggests secondary hypertension.

Age (men >55 years, women >65 years).

Physical examination

History and physical examination should enquire about cardiovascular risk, organ damage and secondary hypertension (Table 24.2).

Table 24.1 ESC 2013 GL on hypertension

Factors—other than office BP—influencing prognosis
Risk factors
Male sex
Age (men ≥55 years; women ≥65 years)
Smoking
Dyslipidaemia
Total cholesterol >4.9 mmol/L (190 mg/dL), and/or
Low-density lipoprotein cholesterol >3.0 mmol/L (115 mg/dL), and/or
High-density lipoprotein cholesterol: men <1.0 mmol/L (40 mg/dL), women <1.2 mmol/L (46 mg/dL), and/or
Triglycerides >1.7 mmol/L (150 mg/dL)
Fasting plasma glucose 5.6–6.9 mmol/L (102–125 mg/dL)
Abnormal glucose tolerance test
Obesity [BMI ≥30 kg/m^2 (height^2)]
Abdominal obesity (waits circumference: men ≥102 cm; women ≥88 cm) (in Caucasians)
Family history of premature CVD (men aged <55 years; women aged <65 years)
Asymptomatic organ damage
Pulse pressure (in the elderly) ≥60 mmHg
Electrocardiographic LVH (Sokolow–Lyon index >3.5 mV; RaVL >1.1mV; Cornell voltage duration product >244 ,V*ms), or
Electrocardiographic LVH [LVM index: men >115 g/m^2; women >95 g/m^2 (BSA)][a]
Carotid wall thickening (IMT >0.9 mm) or plaque
Carotid-femoral PWV >10 m/s
Ankle-brachial index <0.9
CKD with eGFR 30–60 ml/min/1.73 m^2 (BSA)
Microalbuminuria (30–300 mg/24 h), or albumin–creatinine ratio (30–300 mg/g; 3.4–34 mg/mmol) (preferentially on morning spot urine)

(Continued)

Table 24.1 (Continued)

Factors—other than office BP—influencing prognosis
Diabetes mellitus
Fasting plasma glucose ≥7.0 mmol/L (126 mg/dL) on two repeated measurements, and/or
HBA_{1c} >7% (53 mmol/mol), and/or
Post-load plasma glucose >11.0 mmol/L (198 mg/dL)
Established CV or renal disease
Cerebrovascular disease: ischaemic stroke; cerebral haemorrhage; transient ischaemic attack
CHD: myocardial infarction; angina; myocardial revascularization with PCI or CABG
Heart failure, including heart failure with preserved EF
Symptomatic lower extremities peripheral artery disease
CKD with eGFR <30 mL/min/1.73m^2 (BSA); proteinuria (>300 mg/24 h)
Advanced retinopathy: haemorrhages or exudates, papilloedema

BMI: body mass index; BP: blood pressure; BSA: body surface area; CABG: coronary artery bypass graft; CHD: coronary heart disease; CKD: chronic kidney disease; CV: cardiovascular; CVD: cardiovascular disease; EF: ejection fraction; eGFR: estimated glomerular filtration rate; HbA1c: glycated haemoglobin; IMT: intima-media thickness; LVH: left ventricular hypertrophy; LVM: left ventricular mass; PCI: percutaneous coronary intervention; PWV: pulse wave velocity.
A Risk maximal for concentric LVH: increased LVM index with a wall thickness/radius ratio of>0.42

Total cardiovascular risk assessment	
In asymptomatic subjects with hypertension but free of CVD, CKD, and diabetes, using the SCORE model is recommended as a minimal requirement.	I-B
OD predicts CV death independently of SCORE, and search for OD should be considered, particularly in individuals at moderate risk.	IIa-B
Decisions on treatment strategies should depend on the initial level of total CV risk.	I-B

CKD, chronic kidney disease; CV, cardiovascular; CVD, cardiovascular disease; OD, organ damage; SCORE, Systematic COronary Risk Evaluation.
2013 ESH/ESC Guidelines for the management of arterial hypertension. *Eur Heart J*. 2013. doi:10.1093/eurheartj/eht151

Other risk factors, asymptomatic organ damage or disease	Blood Pressure (mmHg)			
	High normal SBP 130–139 or DBP 85–89	Grade 1 HT SBP 140–159 or DBP 90–99	Grade 2 HT SBP 160–179 or DBP 100–109	Grade 3 HT SBP ≥180 or DBP ≥110
No other RF	• No BP intervention	• Lifestyle changes for several months • Then add BP drugs targeting <140/90	• Lifestyle changes for several weeks • Then add BP drugs targeting <140/90	• Lifestyle changes • Immediate BP drugs targeting <140/90
1–2 RF	• Lifestyle changes • No BP intervention	• Lifestyle changes for several weeks • Then add BP drugs targeting <140/90	• Lifestyle changes for several weeks • Then add BP drugs targeting <140/90	• Lifestyle changes • Immediate BP drugs targeting <140/90
≥3 RF	• Lifestyle changes • No BP intervention	• Lifestyle changes for several weeks • Then add BP drugs targeting <140/90	• Lifestyle changes • BP drugs targeting <140/90	• Lifestyle changes • Immediate BP drugs targeting <140/90
OD, CKD stage 3 or diabetes	• Lifestyle changes • No BP intervention	• Lifestyle changes • BP drugs targeting <140/90	• Lifestyle changes • BP drugs targeting <140/90	• Lifestyle changes • Immediate BP drugs targeting <140/90
Symptomatic CKD, CKD stage ≥4 or diabetes with OD/RFs	• Lifestyle changes • No BP intervention	• Lifestyle changes • BP drugs targeting <140/90	• Lifestyle changes • BP drugs targeting <140/90	• Lifestyle changes • Immediate BP drugs targeting <140/90

Figure 24.1 ESC 2013 GL on hypertension. Initiation of lifestyle changes and antihypertensive drug treatment. Targets of treatment are also indicated. Colours indicate risk, with red the highest. In patients with diabetes, the optimal DBP target is between 80 and 85 mmHg. In the high normal BP range, drug treatment should be considered in the presence of a raised out-of-office BP (masked hypertension).

Table 24.2 ESC 2013 GL on hypertension

Blood pressure measurement, history, and physical examination	
Comprehensive medical history and physical examination to verify the diagnosis, detect causes of secondary hypertension, record CV risk factors, and to identify OD and other CVDs.	I-C
Family history to investigate familial predisposition to hypertension and CVDs.	I-B
Office BP for screening and diagnosis of hypertension.	I-B
The diagnosis of hypertension should be based on at least two BP measurements per visit and on at least two visits	I-C
All hypertensive patients should undergo palpation of the pulse at rest to determine heart rate and to search for arrhythmias, especially atrial fibrillation	I-B
Out-of-office BP to confirm the diagnosis of hypertension, identify the type of hypertension, detect hypotensive episodes, and maximize prediction of CV risk	IIa-B
For out-of-office BP measurements, ABPM or HBPM may be considered depending on indicaton, availability, ease, cost of use and, if appropriate, patient preference	IIb-C

ABPM: ambulatory blood pressure monitoring; BP: blood pressure; CV: cardiovascular; CVD: cardiovascular disease; HBPM: home blood pressure monitoring; OD: organ damage.

Physical examination for secondary hypertension, organ damage and obesity
Signs suggesting secondary hypertension
Features of Cushing syndrome
Skin stigmata of neurofibromatosis (phaeochromocytoma)
Palpation of enlarged kidneys (polycystic kidney)
Auscultation of abdominal murmurs (renovascular hypertension)
Auscultation of precordial or chest murmurs (aortic coarctation; aortic disease; upper extremity artery disease)
Diminished and delayed femoral pulses and reduced femoral blood pressure compared to simultaneous arm BP (aortic coarctation; aortic disease; lower extremity artery disease)
Left–right arm BP difference (aortic coarctation; subclavian artery stenosis)
Signs of organ damage
Brain: motor or sensory defects
Retina: fundoscopic abnormalities
Heart: heart rate, 3rd or 4th heart sound, heart murmurs, arrhythmias, location of apical impulse, pulmonary rales, peripheral oedema
Peripheral arteries: absence, reduction, or asymmetry of pulses, cold extremities, ischaemic skin lesions
Carotid arteries: systolic murmurs
Evidence of obesity
Weight and height
Calculate BMI: body weight/height^2 (kg/m^2)
Waist circumference measured in the standing position, at a level midway between the lower border of the costal margin (the lowest rib) and uppermost border of the iliac crest

BP: blood pressure; BMI: body mass index
2013 ESH/ESC Guidelines for the management of arterial hypertension. *Eur Heart J*. 2013. doi:10.1093/eurheartj/eht151

Investigations

Laboratory tests recommended by the ESC are presented in Table 24.3.

Therapy

General principles

- **Low-salt diet** (<100 mmol/day, i.e. 2.4 g Na or 6 g NaCl), weight loss, exercise, and alcohol restriction (up to two drinks a day, i.e. 1 oz, or 28 g of alcohol for men and one drink for women) are the best way for small, but significant, blood pressure reductions[5–8] and are recommended in all hypertensive patients, regardless of drug therapy (Table 24.4). Visceral adiposity, a feature of metabolic syndrome, is related to hypertension. Although systolic blood pressure temporarily raises after coffee, chronic caffeine consumption is not associated with increased risk of hypertension.[9] **Smoking** increases BP by 10–20 mmHg with each cigarette, thus increasing the risk of hypertension with habitual smoking. High-risk patients with hypertension should also receive a **statin and low-dose aspirin.**[10] Drug-induced hypertension should be considered. **Non-steroidal anti-inflammatory** agents are the main cause, but **paracetamol** use also increases blood pressure in patients with coronary artery disease.[11] The ESC recommendations for initiation of drug therapy are presented in Table 24.5.
- **Target values** are <140/90 mmHg, unless the patient is diabetic or has renal disease (target is <130/80 mmHg)

Table 24.3 ESC 2013 GL on hypertension

Laboratory investigations

Routine tests

Haemoglobin and/or haematocrit
Fasting plasma glucose
Serum total cholesterol, low-density lipoprotein cholesterol, high-density lipoprotein cholesterol
Fasting serum triglycerides
Serum potassium and sodium
Serum uric acid
Serum creatinine (with estimation of GFR)
Urine analysis: microscopic examination; urinary protein by dipstick test; test for microalbuminuria
12-lead ECG

Additional tests, based on history, physical examination, and findings from routine laboratory tests

Haemoglobin A_{1c} (if fasting plasma glucose is >5.6 mmol/L (102 mg/dL) or previous diagnosis of diabetes)
Quantitative proteinuria (if dipstick test is positive); urinary potassium and sodium concentration and their ratio
Home and 24-h ambulatory BP monitoring
Echocardiogram
Holter monitoring in case of arrhythmias

Carotid ultrasound
Peripheral artery/abdominal ultrasound
Pulse wave velocity
Ankle-brachial index
Fundoscopy

Extended evaluation (mostly domain of the specialist)

Further search for cerebral, cardiac, renal, and vascular damage, mandatory in resistant and complicated hypertension
Search for secondary hypertension when suggested by history, physical examination, or routine and additional tests

BP: blood pressure; ECG: electrocardiogram; GFR: glomerular filtration rate.

Cut-off values for parameters used in the assessment of LV remodelling and diastolic function in patients with hypertension

Parameter	Abnormal if
LV mass index (g/m²)	>95 (women) >115 (men)
Relative wall thickness (RWT)	>0.42
Diastolic function: Septal e' velocity (cm/sec) Lateral e' velocity (cm/sec) LA volume index (mL/m²)	 <8 <10 ≥34
LV filling pressures: E/e' (averaged) ratio	≥13

LA: left atrium; LV: left ventricle; RWT: relative wall thickness

Search for asymptomatic organ damage, cardiovascular disease, and chronic kidney disease

Heart	
An ECG to detect LVH, left atrial dilatation, arrhythmias, or concomitant heart disease	I-B
A stress ECH test in all patients with a history or physical examination suggestive or major arrhythmias, long-term ECG monitoring, and, in case of suspected exercise-induced arrhythmias	IIa-C
An echocardiogram to refine CV risk, and confirm ECG diagnosis of LVG, left atrial dilatation or suspected concomitant heart disease, when these are suspected	IIa-B
Whenever history suggests myocardial ischaemia, a stress ECG test is recommended, and, if positive or ambiguous, an imaging stress test (stress echocardiography, stress cardiac magnetic resonance or nuclear scintigraphy) is recommended	I-C
Arteries	
Ultrasound scanning of carotid arteries to detect vascular hypertrophy or asymptomatic atherosclerosis, particularly in the elderly	IIa-B
Carotid–femoral PWV to detect large artery stiffening	IIa-B
Ankle–brachial index to detect PAD	IIa-B

(Continued)

Table 24.3 (Continued)

Search for asymptomatic organ damage, cardiovascular disease, and chronic kidney disease	
Kidney	
Measurement of serum creatinine and estimation of GFR in all hypertensive patients[a]	I-B
Assessment of urinary protein in all hypertensive patients by dipstick	I-B
Assessment of microalbuminuria in spot urine and related to urine creatinine excretion	I-B
Fundoscopy	
Examination of the retina in difficult to control or resistant hypertensive patients to detect haemorrhages, exudates, papilloedema, which are associated with increased CV risk	IIa-C
Examination of the retina is not recommended in mild-to-moderate hypertensive patients without diabetes, expect in young patients	III-C
Brain	
In hypertensive patients with cognitive decline, brain magnetic resonance imaging or computed tomography for detecting silent brain infarctions, lacunar infarctions, microbleeds, and white matter lesions	IIb-C

CV, cardiovascular; ECG, electrocardiogram; GFR, glomerural filtration rate; LVH, left ventricular hypertrophy; MRI, magnetic resonance imaging; PAD, peripheral artery disease; PWV, pulse wave velocity

[a] The MDRD formula is currently recommended but new methods such as the CKD-EPI method aim to improve the accuracy of the measurement.

2013 ESH/ESC Guidelines for the management of arterial hypertension. *Eur Heart J*. 2013. doi:10.1093/eurheartj/eht151

Table 24.4 Lifestyle changes

ACCF/AHA 2011 Expert Consensus Document on Hypertension in the Elderly
Lifestyle Modifications to Manage Hypertension

Modification	Recommendation	Approximate systolic BP reduction, range
Weight reduction	Maintain normal body weight (BMI 18.5–24.9 kg/m^2)	5–20 mmHg/10 kg weight loss
Adopt DASH eating plan	Consume a diet rich in fruits, vegetables, and low-fat dairy products with areduced content of saturated and total fat	8–14 mmHg
Dietary sodium reduction	Reduce dietary sodium intake to no more than 100 mEq/L (2.4 g sodium or 6 g sodium chloride)	2–8 mmHg
Physical activity	Engage in regular aerobic physical activity, such as brisk walking (at least 30 min/d, most days of the week)	4–9 mmHg
Moderation of alcohol consumption	Limit consumption to no more than 2 drinks/d (1 oz or 30 mL ethanol [e.g. 24 oz beer, 10 oz wine, or 3 oz 80-proof whisky]) in most men and no more than 1 drink/d in women and lighter weight persons	2–4 mmHg

For overall cardiovascular risk reduction, stop smoking. The effects of implementing these modifications are dose and time dependent and could be higher for some individuals.

BMI indicates body mass index calculated as weight in kilograms divided by the square of height in meters; BP, blood pressure; and DASH, Dietary Approaches to Stop Hypertension.

ESC 2013 GL on hypertension. Adoption of lifestyle changes	
Salt restriction to 5–6 g per day	I-A/B
Alcohol consumption ≤ 20–30 g of ethanol per day in men and ≤ 10–20 g of ethanol per day in women	I-A/B
Increased consumption of vegetables, fruits, and low-fat dairy products	I-A/B
Reduction of weight to BMI of 25 kg/m^2 and of waist circumference to <102 cm in men and <88 cm in women is unless contraindicated	I-A/B
Regular exercise, i.e. at least 30 min of moderate dynamic exercise on 5 to 7 days per week	I-A/B
Give all smokers advice to quit smoking and offer assistance	I-A/B

ESC 2013 GL on hypertension

Summary of recommendations on treatment of risk factors associated with hypertension	
Statins in hypertensive patients:	
at moderate to high CV risk, targeting a low-density lipoprotein cholesterol value <3.0 mmol/L (115 mg/dL)	I-A
when overt CHD is present, targeting low-density lipoprotein cholesterol levels <1.8 mmol/L (70 mg/dL)	I-A
Antiplatelet therapy, in particular low-dose aspirin, in hypertensive patients with previous CV events	I-A
Aspirin in hypertensive patients with reduced renal function or a high CV risk, provided that BP is well controlled	IIa-B
Aspirin is not recommended in low-moderate risk hypertensive patients, in whom absolute benefit and harm are equivalent	III-A
In hypertensive patients with diabetes, a HbA1c target of <7.0% with antidiabetic treatment	I-B
HbA1c target of <7.5–8.0% in more fragile elderly patients with a longer diabetes duration, more comorbidities and at high risk	IIa-C

BP, blood pressure; CHD, coronary heart disease; CV, cardiovascular; HbA1c, glycated haemoglobin

2013 ESH/ESC Guidelines for the management of arterial hypertension. *Eur Heart J*. 2013. doi:10.1093/eurheartj/eht151

Table 24.5 ESC 2013 GL on hypertension

Initiation of antihypertensive drug treatment	
Prompt initiation of drug treatment in individuals with grade 2 and 3 hypertension with any level of CV risk, a few weeks after or simultaneously with initation of lifestyle changes	I-A
Lowering BP with drugs when total CV risk is high because of OD, diabetes, CVD or CKD, even when hypertension is in the grade I range	I-B
Initiation of antihypertensive drug treatment in grade I hypertensive patients at low to moderate risk, when BP is within this range at several repeated visits or elevated by ambulatory BP criteria, and remains within this range despite a reasonable period of time with lifestyle measures	IIa-B
In elderly hypertensive patients drug treatment when SBP is ≥160 mmHg	I-A
Antihypertensive drug treatment in the elderly (at least when younger than 80 years) when SBP is in the 140–159 mmHg range, provided that antihypertensive treatment is well tolerated	IIb-C
Unless the necessary evidence is obtained it is not recommended to initiate antihypertensive drug therapy at high normal BP	III-A
Lack of evidence does not allow recommending to initiate antihypertensive drug therapy in young individuals with isolated elevation of brachial SBP, but these individuals should be followed closely with lifestyle recommendations	III-A

BP, blood pressure; CKD, chronic kidney disease; CV, cardiovascular; CVD, cardiovascular disease; OD, organ damage; SBP, systolic blood pressure.

Treatment strategies and choice of drugs	
Diuretics (thiazides, chlorthalidone and indapamide), beta-blockers, calcium antagonists, ACE inhibitors, and angiotensin receptor blockers are all suitable and recommended for the initiation and maintenance of antihypertensive treatment, either as monotherapy or in some combinations with each other	I-A
Some agents should be considered as the preferential choice in specific conditions because used in trials in those conditions or because of greater effectiveness in specific types of OD	IIa-C
Initiation of antihypertensive therapy with a two-drug combination may be considered in patients with markedly high baseline BP or at high CV risk	IIb-C
The combination of two antagonists of the RAS is not recommended and should be discouraged	III-A
Other drug combinations should be considered and probably are beneficial in proportion to the extent of BP reduction. However, combinations that have been successfully used in trials may be prefereable	IIa-C
Combinations of two antihypertensive drugs at fixed doses in a single tablet may be recommended and favoured, because reducing the number of daily pills improves adherence, which is low in patients with hypertension	IIb-B

ACE, angiotensin-converting enzyme; BP, blood pressure; CV, cardiovascular; OD, organ damage; RAS, renin-angiotensin system.
2013 ESH/ESC Guidelines for the management of arterial hypertension. *Eur Heart J*. 2013. doi:10.1093/eurheartj/eht151

or heart failure (<120/80mm Hg) (Table 24.6).[12] The J-curve phenomenon refers to increase in cardiac events, but not stroke, with very low diastolic blood pressures achieved by therapy.[13] A probable association of a diastolic BP ≤70 mmHg with cerebral atrophy has been reported,[14] and these low values should be avoided, especially in the presence of concomitant coronary heart disease.[15] The BP lowering effect should last 24 hours, and drugs which exert their antihypertensive effect over 24 hours with a once-a-day administration should be preferred.

- In patients with **type 2 diabetes**, an angiotensin enzyme converting (ACE) inhibitor or angiotensin receptor blocker (ARB) is necessary, particularly in diabetic nephropathy with proteinuria. An ARB combined with a calcium channel blocker (CCB) slows progression of nephropathy to a greater extent than when combined with a thiazide.[16] Thiazides are associated with increased risk for new-onset diabetes, but in established diabetics their use is not precluded since they are usually necessary in combination therapies for control of hypertension. Treatment strategies should consider an intervention against all cardiovascular risk factors, including a statin. Because of the greater chance of postural hypotension, blood pressure should also be measured in the erect posture. In patients with the **metabolic syndrome**, drug treatment should start with a blocker of the renin-angiotensin system, followed, if needed, by the addition of a calcium antagonist or a low-dose thiazide diuretic. Statins should be given to all diabetics with hypertension above the age of 40 years according to American Diabetes Association recommendations.[17] Recently, the Canadian Diabetes Association recommended that all diabetics should take statins when >40 years, and antihypertensive drugs when >55 years even in the absence of hypertension or other risk factors.[18] Recommendations of the ESC for patients with diabetes or metabolic syndrome are presented in Table 24.7.
- In patients with **renal impairment**, strict blood pressure control (probably systolic BP<130 mm Hg if proteinuria is >1 g/day) is indicated. An angi-

Table 24.6 ESC 2013 GL on hypertension

Blood pressure goals in hypertensive patients	
A SBP goal <140 mmHG:	
a) in patients at low–moderate CV risk	I-B
b) in patients with diabetes;	I-A
c) in patients with previous stroke or TIA;	IIa-B
d) in patients with CHD;	IIa-B
e) in patients with diabetic or non-diabetic CKD	IIa-B
In elderly hypertensives less than 80 years old with SBP ≥160 mmHg there is solid evidence to recommend reducing SBP to between 150 and 140 mmHg	I-A
In fit elderly patients less than 80 years old SBP values <140 mmHg may be considered, whereas in the fragile elderly population SBP goals should be adapted to individual tolerability	IIb-C
In individuals older than 80 years and with initial SBP ≥160 mmHg, it is recommended to reduce SBP to between 150 and 140 mmHg provided they are in good physical and mental conditions	I-B
A DBP target of <90 mmHg is always recommended, except in patients with diabetes, in whom values <85 mmHg are recommended. It should nevertheless be considered that DBP values between 80 and 85 mmHg are safe and well tolerated	I-A

CHD, coronary heart disease; CKD, chronic kidney disease; CV, cardiovascular; DBP, diastolic blood pressure; SBP, systolic blood pressure; TIA, transient ischaemic attack
2013 ESH/ESC Guidelines for the management of arterial hypertension. *Eur Heart J.* 2013. doi:10.1093/eurheartj/eht151

Table 24.7 ESC 2013 GL on hypertension

Treatment strategies in patients with diabetes	
While initiation of antihypertensive drug treatment in diabetic patients whose SBP is ≥160 mmHg is mandatory, it is strongly recommended to start drug treatment also when SBP is ≥140 mmHg	I-A
A SBP goal <140 mmHg is recommended in patients with diabetes	I-A
The DBP target in patients with diabetes is recommended to be <85 mmHg	I-A
All classes of antihypertensive agents are recommended and can be used in patients with diabetes; RAS blockers may be preferred, especially in the presence of proteinuria or microalbuminuria	I-A
It is recommended that individual drug choice takes comorbidities into account	I-C
Simultaneous administration of two blockers of the RAS is not recommended and should be avoided in patients with diabetes	III-B

DBP, diastolic blood pressure; RAS, renin–angiotensin system; SBP, systolic blood pressure

Treatment strategies in hypertensive patients with metabolic syndrome	
Lifestyle changes, particularly weight loss and physical exercise, are to be recommended to all individuals with the metabolic syndrome. These interventions improve not only BP, but the metabolic components of the syndrome and delay diabetes onset	I-B
As the metabolic syndrome can be considered a 'pre-diabetic' state, antihypertensive agents potentially improving or at least not worsening insulin sensitivity, such as RAS blockers and calcium antagonists, should be considered as the preferred drugs. Beta-blockers (with the exception of vasodilating beta-blockers) and diuretics should be considered only as additional drugs, preferably in association with a potassium-sparing agent	IIa-C
Prescribe antihypertensive drugs with particular care in hypertensive patients with metabolic disturbances when BP is ≥140/90 mmHg after a suitable period of lifestyle changes, and to maintain BP <140/90 mmHg	I-B
BP lowering drugs are not recommended in individuals with metabolic syndrome and high normal BP	III-A

BP, blood pressure; RAS, renin–angiotensin system.
2013 ESH/ESC Guidelines for the management of arterial hypertension. *Eur Heart J.* 2013. doi:10.1093/eurheartj/eht151

otensin receptor blocker or an ACE inhibitor (but not the combination of both), often with loop diuretics are required (Table 24.8). All antihypertensive drugs except diuretics can be used in the haemodialysis patients, with doses determined by the haemodynamic instability and the ability of the drug to be dialysed.[3] An integrated therapeutic intervention (antihypertensive, statin, and antiplatelet therapy) has to be considered in patients with renal damage. When NSAIDs are prescribed, concomitant administration of an ACE (or ARB) and a duretic may be associated with increased risk of kidney injury.[19]

- Hypertension is a major risk factor for **coronary artery disease** (see Chapter 26). Recommendations for patients with coronary artery disease and heart failure are presented in Table 24.9.

Table 24.8 ESC 2013 GL on hypertension

Therapeutic strategies in hypertensive patients with nephropathy	
Lowering SBP to <140 mmHG should be considered	IIa-B
When overt proteinuria is present, SBP values <130 mmHg may be considered, provided that changes in eGFR are monitored	IIb-B
RAS blockers are more effective in reducing albuminuria than other antihypertensive agents, and are indicated in hypertensive patients in the presence of microalbuminuria or overt proteinuria	I-A
Reaching BP goals usually requires combination therapy, and it is recommended to combine RAS blockers with other antihypertensive agents	I-A
Combination of two RAS blockers, though potentially more effective in reducing proteinuria, is not recommended	III-A
Aldosterone antagonists cannot be recommended in CKD, especially in combination with a RAS blocker, because of the risk of excessive reduction in renal function and of hyperkalaemia	III-C

BP, blood pressure; CKD, chronic kidney disease; eGFR, estimated glomerular filtration rate; RAS, renin–angiotensin system; SBP, systolic blood pressure.
2013 ESH/ESC Guidelines for the management of arterial hypertension. *Eur Heart J*. 2013. doi:10.1093/eurheartj/eht151

Table 24.9 Therapy of hypertension in patients with heart disease

ESC 2013 GL on hypertension. Therapeutic strategies in hypertensive patients with heart disease	
In hypertensive patients with CHD, a SBP goal <140 mmHg should be considered	IIa-B
In hypertensive patients with a recent myocardial infarction beta-blockers are recommended. In case of other CHD all antihypertensive agents can be used, but beta-blockers and calcium antagonists are to be preferred, for symptomatic reasons (angina)	I-A
Diuretics, beta-blockers, ACE inhibitors, angiotensin receptor blockers, and/or mineralocorticoid receptor antagonists are recommended in patients with heart failure or severe LV dysfunction to reduce mortality and hospitalization	I-A
In patients with heart failure and preserved EF, there is no evidence that antihypertensive therapy per se or any particular drug, is beneficial. However, in these patients, as well as in patients with hypertension and systolic dysfunction, lowering SBP to around 140 mmHg should be considered. Treatment guided by relief of symptoms (congestion with diuretic, high heart rate with beta-blockers, etc.) should also be considered	IIa-C
ACE inhibitors and angiotensin receptor blockers (and beta-blockers and mineralocorticoid receptor antagonists if heart failure coexists) should be considered as antihypertensive agents in patients at risk of new or recurrent atrial fibrillation	IIa-C
It is recommended that all patients with LVH receive antihypertensive agents	I-B
In patients with LVH, initiation of treatment with one of the agents that have shown a greater ability to regress LVH should be considered, i.e. ACE inhibitors, angiotensin receptor blockers and calcium antagonists	IIa-B

BP, blood pressure; CKD, chronic kidney disease; eGFR, estimated glomerular filtration rate; RAS, renin–angiotensin system; SBP, systolic blood pressure.
2013 ESH/ESC Guidelines for the management of arterial hypertension. *Eur Heart J*. 2013. doi:10.1093/eurheartj/eht151

ESC 2012 GL on heart failure. Recommendations for the treatment of hypertension in patients with symptomatic HF (NYHA functional class II–IV) and LV systolic dysfunction	
Step 1	
One or more of an ACE inhibitor (or ARB), beta blocker, and MRA as first-, second-, and third-line therapy (reducing the risk of HF hospitalization and reducing the risk of premature death).	I-A
Step 2	
A thiazide diuretic (or, if the patient is treated with a thiazide diuretic, switching to a loop diuretic) is when hypertension persists despite treatment with a combination of as many as possible of an ACE inhibitor (or ARB), beta blocker, and MRA.	I-C
Step 3	
When hypertension persists despite treatment with a combination of as many as possible of an ACE inhibitor (or ARB), beta blocker, MRA, and diuretic.	
Amlodipine	I-A
Hydralazine	I-A
Felodipine	IIa-B
Moxonidine is NOT recommended (increased mortality)	III-B
Alpha-adrenoceptor antagonists are NOT recommended (neurohumoral activation, fluid retention, worsening HF)	III-A

ACE: angiotensin-converting enzyme; ARB: angiotensin receptor blocker; HF: heart failure; LV: left ventricular; LVEF: left ventricular ejection fraction; MRA: mineralocorticoid receptor antagonist.
ESC Guidelines for the diagnosis and treatment of acute and chronic heart failure 2012. *Eur Heart J*. doi:10.1093/eurheartj/ehs104.

- In patients with a history of **stroke or TIAs**, antihypertensive treatment has markedly reduced the incidence of stroke recurrence in almost all large RCTs, using different drug regimens. Although target values <130/80 mmHg have been recommended, hard evidence on this issue is lacking, and diastolic values <70 mmHg should be probably avoided.[14] Calcium channel blockers may have a slightly greater efficacy in stroke prevention (see below), but in clinical practice, all regimens are acceptable for stroke prevention.[3] Recommendations for patients with cerebrovascular disease and atherosclerotic disease in general are provided in Table 24.10.
- Reduction of blood pressure produces benefits in the **elderly**, and there is no age threshold beyond which hypertension treatment cannot be justified.[20,21] Hypertension raises the risk for dementia, and antihypertensive therapy reduces the risk of dementia of both the vascular and Alzheimer's type,[22] although aggressive lowering may have opposite effects in the elderly due to cerebral hypoperfusion.[23,24] ARBs, calcium channel blockers, and thiazides reduce the risk of stroke more than other antihypertensive drugs,[25,26] and ARBs, ACE inhibitors, and calcium channel blockers are the drugs that have been associated with a beneficial effect on cognitive function beyond blood pressure reduction.[27] However, for patients older than age 55 years as well as in blacks, thiazides or calcium channel blockers are more effective than ACE inhibitors and ARBs in achieving desirable blood pressure reduction (low renin group).[28] Octogenarians should be seen frequently with the medical history updated at each visit. Standing BP should always be checked for excessive orthostatic decline. BP values below which vital organ perfusion is impaired in octogenarians are not known, but systolic BP <130 and diastolic BP <65 mm Hg should be avoided.[29] The systolic BP target recently recommended by the ESC for people >80 years is <150 mmHg (Table 24.11).[3]
- In **young patients** BP should be reduced to <140/90 mmHg. The case may be different for young individuals with isolated systolic hypertension (diastolic BP<90 mmHg). These individuals may have a normal central systolic BP, and can be followed with lifestyle measures only.[3] Compared with older antihypertensive drugs, newer agents (ARBs, ACE inhibitors, calcium antagonists and vasodilating beta-blockers) have neutral or even beneficial effects on **erectile function.**[3] Phospho-diesterase-5 inhibitors may be safely administered to hypertensives, even those on multiple drug regimens (with the possible exception of alpha-blockers and in absence of nitrate administration).[3]
- Use of oral contraceptives is associated with some small but significant increases in BP. Recommendations for therapy of hypertension in **women** as well as during pregnancy are discussed later (Hypertension in pregnancy).
- The management of "**white-coat**" hypertension depends on the underlying cardiovascular risk of the patient (Table 24.12).

Table 24.10 ESC 2013 GL on hypertension

Therapeutic strategies in hypertensive patients with cerebrovascular disease	
It is not recommended to intervene with BP-lowering therapy during the first week after acute stroke ireespective of BP level, although clinical judgement should be used in the face of very high SBP values	III-B
Antihypertensive treatment in hypertensive patients with a history of stroke or TIA, even when initial SBP is in the 140–159 mmHg range	I-B
In hypertensive patients with a history of stroke or TIA, a SBP goal of <140 mmHg should be considered	IIa-B
In elderly hypertensives with previous stroke or TIA, SBP values for intervention and goal may be considered to be somewhat higher	IIb-B
All drug regimens are recommended for stroke prevention, provided that BP is effectively reduced	I-A

BP, blood pressure; SBP, systolic blood pressure; TIA, transient ischaemic attack.

Therapeutic strategies in hypertensive patients with atherosclerosis, arteriosclerosis, and peripheral artery disease	
In the presence of carotid atherosclerosis, prescription of calcium antagonists and ACE inhibitors should be considered as these agents have shown a greater efficacy in delaying atherosclerosis progression than diuretics and beta-blockers	IIa-B
In hypertensive patients with a PWV above 10 m/s all antihypertensive drugs should be considered provided that a BP reduction to <140/90 mmHg is consistently achieved	IIa-B
Antihypertensive therapy is recommended in hypertensive patients with PAD to achieve a goal of <140/90 mmHg, because of their high risk of myocardial infarction, stroke, heart failure, and CV death	I-A
Though a careful follow up is necessary, beta-blockers may be considered for the treatment of arterial hypertension in patients with PAD, since their use does not appear to be associated with exacerbation of PAD symptoms	IIb-A

ACE, angiotensin-converting enzyme; BP, blood pressure; CV, cardiovascular; PAD, peripheral artery disease; PWV, pulse wave velocity.
2013 ESH/ESC Guidelines for the management of arterial hypertension. *Eur Heart J*. 2013. doi:10.1093/eurheartj/eht151

Table 24.11 Hypertension in the elderly

ACCF/AHA 2011 Expert Consensus Document on Hypertension in the Elderly
Recommendations for Prevention and Management of Ischemic Heart Disease: Blood Pressure Targets

Patient type	Goal BP (mm Hg)
Left ventricular dysfunction	<120/80
Diabetes mellitus	<130/80
Chronic renal disease	<130/80
CAD or CAD risk equivalents*	<130/80
Carotid artery disease	<130/80
Peripheral arterial disease	<130/80
Abdominal aortic aneurysm	<130/80
High-risk (10-y FRS ≥10%)	<130/80
Uncomplicated hypertension (none of above)	<140/80

*CAD risk equivalents include diabetes mellitus, peripheral arterial disease, carotid arterial disease, and abdominal aortic aneurysm.
BP indicates blood pressure; CAD, coronary artery disease; and FRS, Framingham Risk Score.

ACCF/AHA 2011 Expert Consensus Document on Hypertension in the Elderly
Treatment of hypertension in the elderly

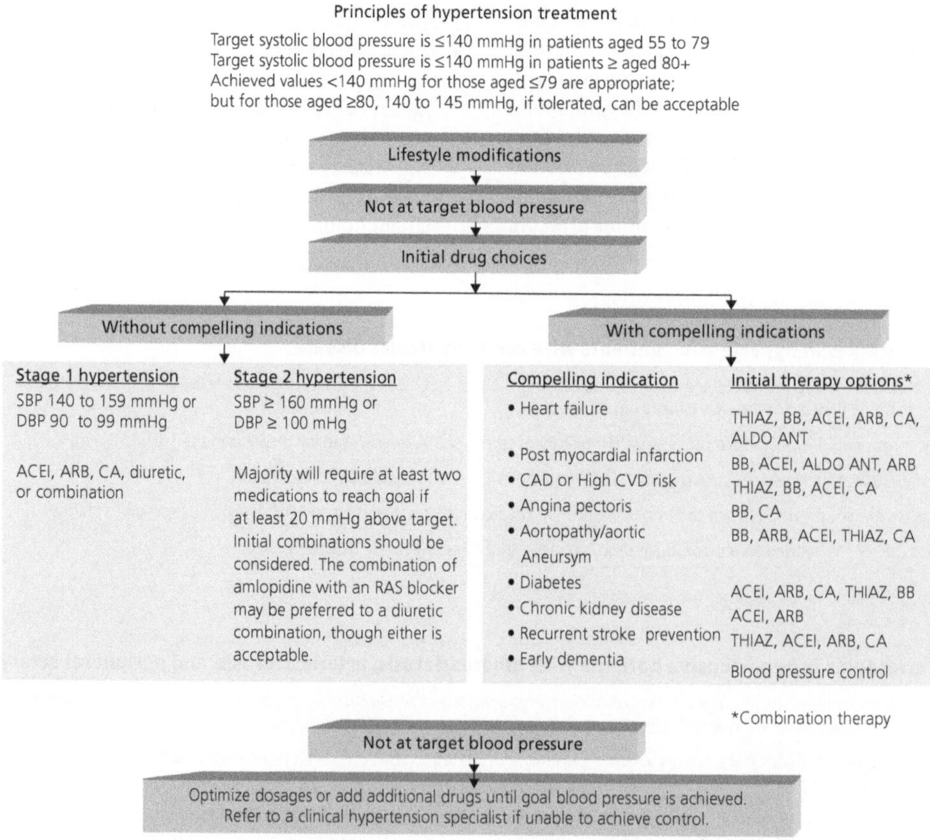

ACEI indicates angiotensin-converting enzyme inhibitor; ALDO ANT, aldosterone antagonist; ARB, aldosterone receptor blocker; BB, beta blocker; CA, calcium antagonist; CAD, coronary artery disease; CVD, cardiovascular disease; DBP, diastolic blood pressure; RAS, renin-angiotensin system; SBP, systolic blood pressure; and THIAZ, thiazide diuretic.
ACCF/AHA 2011 Expert Consensus Document on Hypertension in the Elderly. *J Am Coll Cardiol*. 2011;**57**:2037–114.

Table 24.11 (Continued)

ESC 2013 GL on hypertension **Antihypertensive treatment strategies in the elderly**	
In elderly hypertensives with SBP ≥160 mmHg there is solid evidence to recommend reducing SBP to between 150 and 140 mmHg	I-A
In fit elderly patients <80 years old antihypertensive treatment may be considered at SBP values ≥140 mmHg with a target SBP <140 mmHg if treatment is well tolerated	IIb-C
In individuals older than 80 years with an initial SBP ≥160 mmHg, reduce SBP to between 150 and 140 mmHg, provided they are in good physical and mental conditions	I-B
In frail elderly patients, leave decisions on antihypertensive therapy to the treating physician, and based on monitoring of the clinical effects of treatment	I-C
Continuation of well-tolerated antihypertensive treatment when a treated individual becomes octogenarian	IIa-C
All hypertensive agents are recommended and can be used in the elderly, although diuretics and calcium antagonists may be preferred in isolated systolic hypertension	I-A

SBP = systolic blood pressure
2013 ESH/ESC Guidelines for the management of arterial hypertension. *Eur Heart J*. 2013. doi:10.1093/eurheartj/eht151

Table 24.12 ESC 2013 GL on hypertension

Treatment strategies in white-coat and masked hypertension	
In white-coat hypertensives without additional risk factors, therapeutic intervention should be considered to be limited to lifestyle changes only, but this decision should be accompanied by a close follow-up	IIa-C
In white-coat hypertensives with a higher CV risk because of metabolic derangements or asymptomatic OD, drug treatment may be considered in addition to lifestyle changes	IIb-C
In masked hypertension, both lifestyle measures and antihypertensive drug treatment should be considered, because this type of hypertension has been consistently found to have a CV risk very close to that of in- and out-of-office hypertension	IIa-C

CV = cardiovascular; OD = organ damage
2013 ESH/ESC Guidelines for the management of arterial hypertension. *Eur Heart J*. 2013. doi:10.1093/eurheartj/eht151

- **Sleep apnoea** stimulates atrial natriuretic peptide release, with resultant nocturnal diuresis and sympathetic nerve activity; thus, beta blockers are more efficacious than thiazides, but ACE inhibitors and ARBs have been equally effective in some studies.[30] Patients with treatment-resistant hypertension usually have a good antihypertensive response to spironolactone.[28] Sleep apnoea is mainly associated with hypertension in patients <60 years old.[29,30]
- A satisfactory blood pressure response is rarely reached with **monotherapy** alone. Useful combinations are: ACE inhibitor or ARB with a diuretic or a CCB, and a beta blocker with a diuretic or a dihydropyridine.[31] A subanalysis of the ACCOMPLISH trial suggested that diuretic-based regimens are beneficial in **obese patients** in whom there is usually an excess volume. In lean patients, calcium channel blockers may be preferable.[32]
- Specific recommendations and criteria for drug choice in Table 24.13. Doses of drugs are presented in Table 24.14.

Drugs

Renin-angiotensin inhibitors

ACE inhibitors and ARBs are first-choice therapy in most instances, and especially in young people who generally have a more active renin-angiotensin system (Table 24.8). Adherence to medication is better with ARB, followed by ACE inhibitors, CCBs, diuretics, and beta blockers in descending order.[33]

ARBs have a considerably lower incidence of cough.[34] They may prevent stroke and the development of dementia in hypertensives better than ACE inhibitors due to angiotensin II type 1 (AT1) receptor blockade and AT2 stmulation by increased production of angiotensin II and IV.[35] AT2 receptors reduce focal cerebral ischaemia by vasodilation and antioxidant activities. Such an advantage of ARBs over ACE inhibitors, however, has not been apparent in clinical trials.[36]

Initial suggestions that ARBs (such as telmisartan) are associated with a modestly increased risk of new cancer diagnosis,[37,38] were subsequently refuted by recent re-analyses.[39–41] In a meta-analysis of 32 trials, the FDA (2 June 2011) has concluded that treatment with an ARB medication does not increase a patient's risk of developing cancer.[42]

The combined use of ACE inhibitors and ARBs is no longer recommended for the treatment of hypertension.[43,44]

Since ARBs and ACE inhibitors both increase plasma renin activity, a drug class, such as the direct renin inhibitor **aliskiren** (150–300 mg od), has the potential to be more beneficial. It has been shown to have comparable

Table 24.13 Criteria for antihypertensive drugs selection

ESC 2013 GL on hypertension
Compelling and possible contra-indications to the use of antihypertensive drugs

Drug	Compelling	Possible
Diuretics (thiazides)	Gout	Metabolic syndrome Glucose intolerance Pregnancy Hypercalcaemia Hypokalaemia
Beta-blockers	Asthma A–V block (grade 2 or 3)	Metabolic syndrome Glucose intolerance Athletes and physically active patients Chronic obstructive pulmonary disease (except for vasodilator beta-blockers)
Calcium antagonists (dihydropyridines)		Tachyarrhythmia Heart failure
Calcium antagonists (verapamil, diltiazem)	A–V block (grade 2 or 3, trifascicular block) Severe LV dysfunction Heart failure	
ACE inhibitors	Pregnancy Angioneurotic oedema Hyperkalaemia Bilateral renal artery stensosis	Women with child bearing potential
Angiotensin receptor blockers	Pregnancy Hyperkalaemia Bilateral renal artery stenosis	Women with child bearing potential
Mineralocorticoid receptor antagonists	Acute or severe renal failure (eGFR <30 mL/min) Hyperkalaemia	

A-V, atrio-ventricular; eGFR, estimated glomerular filtration rate; LV, left ventricular.

Drugs to be preferred in specific conditions

Condition	Drug
Asymptomatic organ damage	
LVH	ACE inhibitor, calcium antagonist, ARB
Asymptomatic atherosclerosis	Calcium antagonist, ACE inhibitor
Microalbuminuria	ACE inhibitor, ARB
Renal dysfunction	ACE inhibitor, ARB
Clinical CV event	
Previous stroke	Any aent effectively lowering BP
Previous myocardial infarction	BB, ACE inhibitor, ARB
Angina pectoris	BB, calcium antagonist
Heart failure	Diuretic, BB, ACE inhibitor, ARB, mineralocorticoid receptor antagonists
Aotric aneurysm	BB
Atrial fibrillation, prevention	Consider ARB, ACE inhibitor, BB or mineralocorticoid receptor antagonist
Atrial fibrillation, ventricular rate control	BB, non-dihydropyridine calcium antagonist
ESRD/proteinuria	ACE inhibitor, ARB
Peripheral artery disease	ACE inhibitor, calcium antagonist
Other	
ISH (elderly)	Diuretic, calcium antagonist
Metabolic syndrome	ACE inhibitor, ARB, calcium antagonist
Diabetes mellitus	ACE inhibitor, ARB
Pregnancy	Methyldopa, BB, calcium antagonist
Blacks	Diuretic, calcium antagonist

ACE, angiotensin-converting enzyme; ARB, angiotensin receptor blocker; BB, beta-blocker; BP, blood pressure; CV, cardiovascular; ESRD, end-stage renal disease; ISH, isolated systolic hypertension; LVH, left ventricular hypertrophy.
2013 ESH/ESC Guidelines for the management of arterial hypertension. *Eur Heart J*. 2013. doi:10.1093/eurheartj/eht151

Table 24.14 Dosages of drugs for hypertension (in mg)

ACEI	
Captopril	12.5–25 bd
Enalapril	2.5–10 bd
Lisinopril	10–40 od
Perindopril	4–8 od
Ramipril	2.5–10 od
Trandolapril	0.5–4 bd
ARB	
Valsartan	8–320 od
Irbesartan	150–300 od
Telmisartan	40–80 od
Calcium channel blockers	
Nifedipine (slow release)	30–90 od
Amlodipine	5–10 od
Felodipine	5–10 od
Lacidipine	2–6 od
Verapamil slow release	240–480 od
Diltiazem slow release	120–360 od
Aldosterone antagonists	
Eplerenone	25–50 od
Spironolactone	25–50 od
Other potassium-sparing diuretics	
Amiloride	2.5–5 od
Loop diuretics	
Furosemide	10–40 bd
Bumetanide	0.5 to 1.0 bd (not licensed for hypertension in the USA)
Torsemide	5–10 od
Thiazide diuretics	
Hydrochlorothiazide	12.5 od
Bendrofluazide	1.25 od
Thiazide-like	
Metolazone	2.5–5 mg od
Indapamide	1.25 mg od
Chlorthalidone	12.5–15 od
Beta blockers	
Carvedilol	6.25–25 bd
Nebivolol	2.5–10 od

efficacy and side effects with ARBs.[45] Combinations of aliskiren with valsartan or amlodipine have been more effective than either drug alone.[46, 47] However, aliskiren should not be used with an ACE inhibitor or ARB in patients with type 2 diabetes and renal impairment (the ALTITUDE trial was stopped in December 2011 due to an increased incidence of non-fatal stroke, renal complications, hyperkalaemia, and hypotension with this combination).[48]

Calcium channel blockers

Both long-acting dihydropyridines and non-dihydropyridine calcium channel blockers have been studied in hypertension and are now considered first-choice drugs together with ACE inhibitors/ARBs.

CCBs may offer protection against dementia due to a reduction of excess intracellular free calcium in neurons, which seems to happen in patients with dementia of the Alzheimer's type.[22, 35] **Diltiazem** and **verapamil** cause less peripheral oedema than dihydropyridines and no tachycardia, and are better tolerated (particularly diltiazem; verapamil may cause constipation). They can be added to a scheme containing a dihydropyridine in resistant cases. They are especially useful in patients with chronic renal disease and renal transplantation,[49, 50] but care is needed because diltiazem may interfere with cyclosporine levels. The combination of CCBs with renin-angiotensin system blockers reduce the risk of CCB-associated peripheral oedema, and ACE inhibitors might be more efficacious than ARBs in this respect.[51] However, there is evidence that patients with hypertension, and especially diabetics, treated with CCBs have increased incident HF,[52] and, as monotherapy, CCBs are inferior to ACE inhibitors, ARBs, and diuretics for reducing the risk of acute myocardial infarction, congestive heart failure, and major cardiovascular events.[53] All CCBs are contraindicated in heart failure, and diltiazem and verapamil in sick sinus syndrome, AV nodal conduction disease, and concomitant use of high doses of beta blockers.

Thiazide diuretics

Thiazides exert their action by reducing extracellular fluid and plasma volume, leading to decreased cardiac preload. They also reduce systemic vascular resistance, but the exact mechanisms are unclear. Secondary activation of the renin-aldosterone axis makes their combination with ACE inhibitors/ARB attractive. They are particularly indicated in **low-renin or salt-sensitive hypertension (elderly, obese, blacks)** and in **resistant hypertension.**

Thiazides effectively reduce blood pressure and the risk of cardiovascular events but at a risk of an excess of 3–4% of new cases of diabetes over several years compared to other antihypertensive medications.[54] Patients with hypertension have a higher risk of developing **new-onset diabetes** in general, and that risk appears to be small with diuretics. However, the odds ratio of developing it with diuretics almost doubles compared to ARB (odds ratio for ARB 0.57, ACE inhibitor 0.67, CCB 0.75, placebo 0.77, beta blocker 0.90 with diuretics as reference).[55] In the ALLHAT study, the largest randomized trial performed to date, **chlorthalidone** (12.5–25 mg daily) was more effective in reducing systolic blood pressure and cardiovascular complications than lisinopril (10–40 mg daily) or amlodipine (2.5–10 mg daily) but at an increased risk of diabetes.[56] Chlorthalidone is a thiazide-like diuretic that binds to erythrocyte carbonic hydrase and has a longer half-life than hydrochlorothiazide. It is twice as potent as hydrochlorothiazide,[57] but whether this translates into better clinical outcome is not known.[58] Chlorthalidone has been shown to produce more pronounced hypokalemia in the elderly than hydrochlorothiazide.[59] Recently, a meta-analysis of 14 studies showed that **hydrochlorothiazide** in doses 12.5–25 mg was significantly less effective as monotherapy in reducing blood pressure compared to ARB, ACE inhibitors, beta blockers, and calcium channel blockers.[60] Whether this also applies to other thiazides is not known. Thiazides are a reasonable choice in obese patients with excess volume, but they are less protective than calcium channel blockers against cardiovascular events in lean patients.[61] **Indapamide** is a non-thiazide sulphonamide that also possesses Vaughan-Williams class III activity and may prolong the QT.

Thiazides are considered ineffective when the **glomerular filtration rate** decreases below 30–40 mL/min/1.73 m^2 of BSA, since the reduced glomerular filtration rate limits the overall filtered sodium load reaching the distal tubule, and reabsorption in the distal tubule is only modestly effective as compared with that in the thick ascending limb, although direct evidence is lacking. However, thiazides can elicit an antihypertensive response in patients with chronic kidney disease.[54]

Hypokalaemia and **hypomagnesaemia** are common, especially with hydroxyclorothiazide or chlorthalidone doses exceeding 25 mg daily. Hydrochlorothiazide appears safer than chlorothalidone in the elderly, in this respect.[59] Hypokalaemia is managed by salt restriction, hypomagnesaemia correction, and addition of an ARB/ACE inhibitor or a potassium-sparing diuretic (preferred to supplemental KCl). These should also be considered from the beginning of therapy if baseline potassium levels are <3.8 mmol/L. Potassium homeostasis is important in view of the evidence that hypokalemia is implicated in thiazide-induced dysglycemia and the development of coronary events.[62] **Dilutional hyponatraemia** may also occur, especially with combinations with loop diuretics. SSRIs and excessive water intake should be avoided. Correction of hypokalaemia may also reduce night **muscle cramps**. Alternatively, calcium channel blockers, such as diltiazem, vitamin B complex, and naftidrofuryl oxalate (a drug that may enhance utilization of oxygen and glucose in peripheral vascular disease and protection of brain parenchyma during anoxia), may be tried for muscle cramps.[63] Quinine derivatives are better avoided for routine use because of the potential of toxicity.

Thiazides reduce the excretion of calcium and uric acid, and exacerbations of **gout** may require discontinuation of the thiazide during the acute attack if uric acid levels are significantly elevated. Reduced uric acid excretion is also accentuated by low-dose aspirin administration. Uricosuric prophylaxis may be needed in the long term.

Thiazides may increase **total cholesterol and LDL** by 5–7% in the first year of therapy.[54]

Concerns had also been raised about a possible association between long-term use of diuretics and **renal carcinoma**, but hypertension itself increases the risk of malignant disease.[64]

Loop diuretics, aldosterone antagonists, and potassium-sparing agents

Loop diuretics are less effective in reducing blood pressure than thiazides.[54] Usually, **furosemide** (40–80 mg twice daily) is used in diuretic tolerance (see Chapter 31 on CCF) or renal failure (glomerular filtration rate <40 mL/min/1.73 m^2 of BSA, usually, but not invariably, corresponding to a creatinine >2.5 mg/dL). **Bumetanide** (1 mg od, more powerful diuretic) and **torsemide** (10 mg od, longer action than furosemide, can be used once daily) may be used in patients not responsive to furosemide.

Aldosterone antagonists. Eplerenone (25–50 mg od) is a selective aldosterone antagonist that, combined with enalapril, decreases proteinuria and LVH beyond what is achieved by either drug alone.[65,66] Renal function and serum potassium levels must be closely monitored due to the risk of hyperkalaemia, especially when these agents are used together with an ACE inhibitor or ARB. **Spironolactone** (25–50 mg od) is also effective but may cause painful gynaecomastia in men (antagonist of aldosterone and androgen and progesterone receptors). Aldosterone antagonists have been found particularly effective in patients who are obese or have sleep apnoea.[30] They should not be used in the presence of hyperkalaemia (K >5 mmol/L) or creatinine >2.5 mg/dL.

Potassium-sparing agents are amiloride and triamterene. **Amiloride** (2.5–5 mg od) is an epithelial sodium channel blocker that is more effective than spironolactone in blacks with drug-resistant hypertension.[67] It is combined with thiazides for correction of hypokalaemia.

Beta blockers

In patients with uncomplicated hypertension, beta blockers exert a relatively weak effect in reducing stroke; they do not have any protective effect with regard to coronary artery disease and may increase the risk for new-onset diabetes.[68–71] In contrast to patients with myocardial infarction and heart failure, beta blocker-associated reduction in heart rate might increase the risk of cardiovascular events and death for hypertensive patients.[72] These effects has been attributed to suboptimal effect in lowering blood pressure compared to other drugs, their 'pseudoantihypertensive' efficacy (failure to lower central aortic pressure), lack of an effect on regression of left ventricular hypertrophy and endothelial dysfunction, and unfavourable metabolic effects. However, much of the unfavourable data were collected from studies involving traditional beta blockers, such as atenolol. Vasodilatory third-generation beta blockers (i.e. carvedilol and nebivolol) reduce blood pressure, in large part through reducing systemic vascular resistance rather than by decreasing cardiac output, and have less effects on metabolic and lipid parameters. **Carvedilol** is a very slightly β_1-selective beta blocker that becomes non-selective at higher doses. In addition, it possesses alpha 1-blocking (vasodilatory) and antioxidant properties.[73] **Nebivolol** is the most β_1-selective beta blocker (3-fold that of bisoprolol and more than 4-fold that of metoprolol) at doses <10 mg. It does not have sympathomimetic activity, but it is an agonist of β_2 and β_3 receptors and can cause relatively less bronchoconstriction or sexual dysfunction. It also improves endothelial dysfunction via stimulation of endothelial nitric oxide synthase and antioxidant properties.[74] According to published evidence, beta blockers, in general, are indicated in hypertensive patients with prior myocardial infarction (metoprolol), heart failure (carvedilol, metoprolol, bisoprolol, and nebivolol in the elderly), arrhythmias (propranolol, carvedilol, metoprolol, bisoprolol), patients <60 years old with increased sympathetic activity (metoprolol, bisoprolol, carvedilol, nebivolol). In phaeochromocytoma, labetalol, a beta and alpha blocker, is preferred to avoid unopposed alpha-mediated vasoconstriction.

Device-based therapy

Various methods for therapeutic modulation of the sympathetic nervous system, via radiofrequency ablation (mainly) and baroreceptor stimulation within the renal arteries, are under study.[75–77] Renal denervation in particular is useful in cases of resistant hypertension.[78]

Follow-up

Titration to BP control requires regular visits, followed by 6-month follow-up after establishment of normal values. Therapy is usually needed for life, unless lifestyle modifications are successful.

Resistant hypertension

Resistant hypertension is defined (JNC 7) as failure to achieve goal blood pressure (BP) <140/90 mmHg for the overall population and <130/80 mmHg for those with diabetes mellitus or chronic kidney disease, when a patient adheres to maximum tolerated doses of three antihypertensive drugs, including a diuretic.[79] However, there is no consensus on a uniform definition for resistant hypertension, and its exact prevalence is not known, with reported values ranging from 13 to 30%.[79,80] Refractory hypertension can be either true (Table 24.15) or apparent, i.e. pseudohypertension, bad measuring technique, or due to non-adherence to treatment. According to the largest published studies so far (NHANES, ACOT, ALLHAT, ACCOMPLISH), up to one-third of hypertensive patients remain uncontrolled on two antihypertensive agents while, among patients with incident hypertension and treatment with ≥3 antihypertensive agents, 2% will develop resistant

Table 24.15 True resistant hypertension

Poor adherence to therapeutic plan
Associated condition
Diabetes mellitus or metabolic syndrome
Excess alcohol intake
Obesity (visceral obesity)
Obstructive sleep apnoea
Anxiety-induced hyperventilation or panic attacks
Pain
Unsuspected secondary cause
Irreversible or scarcely reversible organ damage
Volume overload
Excessive dietary sodium intake
Inadequate diuretic treatment
Reduced renal function
Hyperaldosteronism
Compensatory response to vasodilatory drugs
Drug-induced
Non-steroidal anti-inflammatory drugs (including COX2 inhibitors and paracetamol)
Sympathicomimetics (nasal drops, appetite suppressants)
Cocaine, amphetamines
Oral contraceptives
Glucocorticoids/mineralocorticoids
Liquorice
Herbal drugs (ginseng, yohimbin, ma huang, bitter orange)
Erythropoietin, cyclosporin, tacrolimus, carbenoxolone
Antiangiogenic and anti–vascular endothelial growth factor (VEGF) chemotherapy agents (bevacizumab, sorafenib, sunitinib, pazopanib)
Causes of spurious resistant hypertension
Isolated office (white coat) hypertension
Failure to use large cuff on large arm
Pseudohypertension

hypertension and will have an increased risk of cardiovascular events.[81] Since volume overload is the commonest cause of resistant hypertension, diuretics are essential.[82] Hyperaldosteronism is also common in patients with resistant hypertension.[83, 84]

The management of resistant hypertension (Table 24.16) can be improved by evaluating whether the failure of blood pressure control results from sodium-volume excess (**low plasma renin activity**), insufficiently blocked renin levels (**high plasma renin activity**), or a combination of both (**medium plasma renin activity**) and adjusting therapy accordingly.[85, 86] Low plasma renin activity indicates a diuretic, and high plasma renin activity an ACE inhibitor or ARB or a direct renin inhibitor, such as aliskiren, and, if this fails, addition of a vasodilating beta blocker. In patients with normal plasma renin activity who are already on triple therapy of ACE inhibitor/ARB, diuretic, and calcium channel blockers, an aldosterone antagonist, if the patient is obese or has sleep apnoea, may be beneficial. If BP control is still not achieved with full doses of a four-drug combination, the use of other agents, such as alpha blockers (**doxazosin** 4–8 mg od),[87] the imidazoline I_1-receptor agonist **moxonidine** (0.2–0.4 mg od) that has favourable effects on the insulin resistance syndrome, drugs with central action on the sympathetic system (alpha agonists, such as **methyldopa** (250–750 mg bd) and **clonidine**), or vasodilators, such as **hydralazine**, may be needed. These agents are effective for lowering BP but have poor tolerability and lack of positive outcome data. Novel drugs, such as endothelin receptor antagonists (**darusentan**), aldosterone synthetase inhibitors, and gene therapies are under study.[88]

Renal denervation is now recommended by the ESC (but not yet approved by the FDA) when the following criteria are fulfilled:[78]

- Office-based systolic BP ≥ 160 mmHg (≥150 mmHg diabetes type 2)
- ≥3 antihypertensive drugs in adequate dosage and combination (incl. diuretic)
- Lifestyle modification
- Exclusion of secondary hypertension
- Exclusion of pseudo-resistance using ambulatory BP monitoring (average BP > 130 mmHg or mean daytime BP > 135 mmHg)
- Preserved renal function (GFR ≥45 ml/min/1.73 m^2)
- Eligible renal arteries: no polar or accessory arteries, no renal artery stenosis, no prior revascularization

Hypertensive crisis

Hypertensive emergencies are presented in Table 24.17. Hypertension with a diastolic BP >140 mmHg consists of an emergency. Care should be taken that extremely rapid falls in blood pressure may not be associated with complications, such as underperfusion of the brain and cerebral infarction or damage to the myocardium and kidneys. Excessive or rapid reductions in blood pressure should be avoided in acute stroke.

Therapy

Less severe cases: sublingual captopril 125–25 mg
Urgent reduction: nitroprusside (0.25–10 micrograms/kg/min IV)
LV failure: nitroglycerine (5–100 micrograms/min IV) with furosemide (boluses of 20–40 mg IV).
Ischaemia and tachycardia: Esmolol (200–500 mg/kg for 4 min, then 50–300 micrograms/kg/min IV), or labetalol (20–80 mg IV every 10 min or 2 mg/min or infusion 2.5–30 micrograms/kg/min IV)

Table 24.16 ESC 2013 on hypertension

Therapeutic strategies in patients with resistant hypertension	
In resistant hypertensive patients it is recommended that physicians check whether the drugs included in the existing multiple drug regimen have any BP lowering effect, and withdraw them if their effect is absent or minimal	I-C
Mineralocorticoid receptor antagonists, amiloride, and the alpha-1-blocker doxazosin should be considered, if no contraindication exists	IIa-B
In case off ineffectiveness of drug treatment invasive procedures such as renal denervation and baroreceptor stimulation may be considered	IIb-C
Until more evidence is available on the long-term efficacy and safety of renal denervation and baroreceptor stimulation, it is recommended that these procedures remain in the hands of experienced operators and diagnosis and follow-up restricted to hypertension centers	I-C
It is recommended that the invasive approaches are considered only for truly resistant hypertensive patients, with clinic values ≥160 mmHg SBP or ≥110 mmHg DBP and with BP elevation confirmed by ABPM	I-C

ABPM . ambulatory blood pressure monitoring; BP, blood pressure; DBP, diastolic blood pressure; SBP, systolic blood pressure.
2013 ESH/ESC Guidelines for the management of arterial hypertension. *Eur Heart J*. 2013. doi:10.1093/eurheartj/eht151

Table 24.17 Hypertensive emergencies

Hypertensive encephalopathy
Hypertensive left ventricular failure
Hypertension with myocardial infarction
Hypertension with unstable angina
Hypertension and dissection of the aorta
Severe hypertension associated with subarachnoid haemorrhage or cerebrovascular accident
Crisis associated with phaeochromocytoma
Use of recreational drugs, such as amphetamines, LSD, cocaine, or ecstasy
Hypertension perioperatively
Severe pre-eclampsia or eclampsia

Severe hypertension with renal failure: fenoldopam (0.2–0.5 micrograms/kg/min).
Phaeochromocytoma: labetalol or phentolamine 1–3 mg boluses.
No cardiac complications: Nicardipine (5–15 mg/h IV) or labetalol, together with furosemide (boluses of 20–40 mg IV, unless volume depletion). Alternatively, esmolol (200–500 mg/kg for 4 min, then 50–300 micrograms/kg/min IV).

Nitroprusside is the most effective agent, but it lowers venous return and cardiac output and may increase intracranial pressure. Liquid or sublingual nifedipine may result in ischaemic complications due to too rapid reduction of blood pressure and is no longer recommended.[89] Treatment of pre-eclampsia and phaechromocytoma are discussed in the relevant sections.

Hypertension in pregnancy

In pregnancy, hypertension is defined on absolute values >140/90 mmHg.[90]

Pre-existing hypertension complicates 1–5% of pregnancies, and either precedes pregnancy or develops before 20 weeks of gestation. Hypertension usually persists >42 days post-partum. It may be associated with proteinuria. Undiagnosed hypertensive women may appear normotensive in early pregnancy because of the physiological BP fall commencing in the first trimester.

Gestational hypertension is pregnancy-induced hypertension and complicates 6–7% of pregnancies. Gestational hypertension develops after 20 weeks gestation and resolves in most cases within 42 days post-partum. Gestational hypertension needs close attention since 50% of patients will develop pre-eclampsia.

Pre-eclampsia is a pregnancy-specific syndrome that occurs after mid-gestation, defined by the *de novo* appearance of hypertension, accompanied by new onset of significant proteinuria (≥0.3 g/day in a 24 h urine collection or ≥30 mg/mmol urinary creatinine in a spot random urine sample).

Pre-eclampsia complicates 5–7% of pregnancies but increases to 25% in women with pre-existing hypertension. Pre-eclampsia occurs more frequently during the first pregnancy, in multiple fetuses, hydatidiform mole, or diabetes and is one of the most common causes of prematurity.

Symptoms and signs of severe pre-eclampsia include right upper quadrant/epigastric pain (liver oedema), headache, occipital lobe blindness, hyperflexia and convulsions (cerebral oedema), and HELLP syndrome (haemolysis, elevated liver enzymes, low platelet count). Women with no proteinuria, but who have these features and fetal compromise, are likely to have pre-eclampsia, even if proteinuria is absent.[91] Elevated blood pressure during pregnancy, regardless of type and even without known risk factors, indicates high risk of later cardiovascular disease, chronic kidney disease, and diabetes mellitus.[92]

Therapy

Non-pharmacological management (including close supervision and restriction of activities) should be considered for pregnant women with systolic BP 140–149 mmHg or diastolic BP 90–95 mmHg. Systolic BP levels ≥170 or diastolic BP ≥110 mmHg should be considered an emergency requiring hospitalization (Table 24.18). Labetalol (100–1200 mg bd), oral methyldopa (250–1250 mg tds), nifedipine (long-acting), and possibly other beta blockers (but not atenolol) are drugs of choice.[87, 89] No association with low weight for gestational age has been found for labetalol (started after the 6th week of gestation) as opposed to atenolol. Hydrochlorothiazide may also be used since previous concerns about increased risk are not supported by recent data.[93] In pre-eclampsia with pulmonary oedema, nitroglycerine is the drug of choice; diuretic therapy is inappropriate because plasma volume is reduced. As emergency, intravenous labetalol,[94] oral methyldopa, and oral nifedipine are indicated. Intravenous infusion of sodium nitroprusside is useful in hypertensive crises, but prolonged administration should be avoided.

Calcium channel blockers, diuretics, and angiotensin-converting enzyme inhibitors pose little risk to **breastfed infants**. Beta blockers, especially those not secreted by the kidneys, may be given under supervison of the baby.[95] Detailed comments on the drug use in pregnancy are presented in Appendix 3.

Table 24.18 ESC 2013 on hypertension

Treatment strategies in hypertensive women	
Hormone therapy and selective oestrogen receptor modulators are not recommended and should not be used for primary or secondary prevention of CVD. If treatment of younger perimenopausal women is considered for severe menopausal symptoms, the benefits should be weighed against potential risks	III-A
Drug treatment of severe hypertension in pregnancy (SBP >160 mmHg or DBP >110 mmHg) is recommended	I-C
Drug treatment may also be considered in pregnanct women with persistent elevation of BP ≥150/95 mmHg, and in those with BP ≥140/90 mmHg in the presence of gestational hypertension, sublinical OD or symptoms	IIb-C
In women at high risk of pre-eclampsia, provided they are at low risk of gastrointestinal haemorrhage, treatment with low dose aspirin from 12 weeks until delivery may be considered	IIb-B
In women with child-bearing potential RAS blockers are not recommended and should be avoided	III-C
Methyldopa, labetolol and nifedipine should be considered preferential antihypertensive drugs in pregnancy. Intravenous labetolol or infusion of nitroprusside should be considered in case of emergency (pre-eclampsia)	IIa-B

BP, blood pressure; CVD, cardiovascular disease; DBP, diastolic blood pressure; OD = organ damage; RAS, renin–angiotensin system; SBP, systolic blood pressure.
2013 ESH/ESC Guidelines for the management of arterial hypertension. *Eur Heart J*. 2013. doi:10.1093/eurheartj/eht151

References

1. Conroy RM, *et al.* Estimation of ten-year risk of fatal cardiovascular disease in Europe: the SCORE project. *Eur Heart J*. 2003;**24**:987–1003
2. D'Agostino RB, Sr., *et al.* Validation of the Framingham coronary heart disease prediction scores: results of a multiple ethnic groups investigation. *JAMA*. 2001;**286**:180–7
3. 2013 ESH/ESC Guidelines for the management of arterial hypertension. *Eur Heart J*. 2013.doi:10.1093/eurheartj/eht151
4. Uretsky SMF, *et al.* Obesity paradox in patients with hypertension and coronary artery disease. *Am J Med*. 2007;**120**:863–70
5. Cutler JA, *et al.* Randomized trials of sodium reduction: an overview. *Am J Clin Nutr*. 1997;**65**:643S–51S
6. Whelton PK, *et al.* Effects of oral potassium on blood pressure. Meta-analysis of randomized controlled clinical trials. *JAMA*. 1997;**277**:1624–32
7. Whelton SP, *et al.* Effect of aerobic exercise on blood pressure: a meta-analysis of randomized, controlled trials. *Ann Intern Med*. 2002;**136**:493–503
8. Xin X, *et al.* Effects of alcohol reduction on blood pressure: a meta-analysis of randomized controlled trials. *Hypertension*. 2001;**38**:1112–17
9. Winkelmayer WC, *et al.* Habitual caffeine intake and the risk of hypertension in women. *JAMA*. 2005;**294**:2330–5
10. European guidelines on cardiovascular disease prevention in clinical practice (version 2012). *Eur Heart J*. 2012;**33**:1635–1701
11. Sudano I, *et al.* Acetaminophen increases blood pressure in patients with coronary artery disease. *Circulation*. 2010;**122**:1789–96
12. Zhang Y, *et al.* Is a systolic blood pressure target <140 mmHg indicated in all hypertensives? Subgroup analyses of findings from the randomized FEVER trial. *Eur Heart J*. 2011;**32**:1500–8
13. Bangalore S, *et al.* J-curve revisited: an analysis of blood pressure and cardiovascular events in the Treating to New Targets (TNT) trial. *Eur Heart J*. 2010;**31**:2897–08
14. Jochemsen H, *et al.* Blood pressure and progression of brain atrophy: The smart-mr study. *JAMA Neurology.*. 2013;DOI: 10.1001/jamaneurol.2013.1217
15. Fagard RH, *et al.* On-treatment diastolic blood pressure and prognosis in systolic hypertension. *Arch Intern Med*. 2007;**167**:1884–91
16. Bakris GL, *et al.* Renal outcomes with different fixed-dose combination therapies in patients with hypertension at high risk for cardiovascular events (ACCOMPLISH): a prespecified secondary analysis of a randomised controlled trial. *Lancet*. 2010;**375**:1173–81
17. Association Ad. Executive summary: Standards of medical care in diabetes - 2013. *Diabetes Care*. 2013;**36**:S4–10.
18. Cheng A, *et al.* CDA clinical practice guidelines. *2013*.
19. Lapi F AL, Yin H, Nessim SJ, Suissa S. Concurrent use of diuretics, angiotensin converting enzyme inhibitors, and angiotensin receptor blockers with non-steroidal anti-inflammatory drugs and risk of acute kidney injury: Nested case-control study. *BMJ*. 2013;**346**:e8525.
20. Beckett NS, *et al.* Treatment of hypertension in patients 80 years of age or older. *N Engl J Med*. 2008;**358**:1887–1898
21. Blood Pressure Lowering Treatment Trialists' Collaboration, Neal TF, *et al.* Effects of different regimens to lower blood pressure on major cardiovascular events in older and younger adults: Meta-analysis of randomised trials. *BMJ*. 2008;**336**:1121–1123
22. Duron E, *et al.* Effects of antihypertensive therapy onw cognitive decline in Alzheimer's disease. *Am J Hypertens*. 2009;**22**:1020–4
23. Glynn RJ, *et al.* Current and remote blood pressure and cognitive decline. *JAMA*. 1999;**281**:438–45
24. Guo Z, *et al.* Low blood pressure and dementia in elderly people: the KUNGSHOLMEN project. *BMJ*. 1996;**312**:805–8
25. Boutitie F, *et al.* Does a change in angiotensin II formation caused by antihypertensive drugs affect the risk of stroke? A meta-analysis of trials according to treatment with potentially different effects on angiotensin II. *J Hypertens*. 2007;**25**:1543–53
26. Schrader J, *et al.* Morbidity and mortality after stroke, eprosartan compared with nitrendipine for secondary prevention: principal results of a prospective randomized controlled study (MOSES). *Stroke*. 2005;**36**:1218–26
27. Duron E, *et al.* Antihypertensive treatments, cognitive decline, and dementia. *J Alzheimers Dis*. 2010;**20**:903–14

28. Messerli FH, *et al.* Essential hypertension. *Lancet.* 2007; **370**:591–603
29. Aronow WS, *et al.* ACCF/AHA 2011 expert consensus document on hypertension in the elderly: a report of the American College of Cardiology Foundation Task Force on clinical expert consensus documents developed in collaboration with the American Academy of Neurology, American Geriatrics Society, American Society for Preventive Cardiology, American Society of Hypertension, American Society of Nephrology, Association of Black Cardiologists, and European Society of Hypertension. *J Am Coll Cardiol.* 2011; **57**:2037–114
30. Ziegler MG, *et al.* Antihypertensive therapy for patients with obstructive sleep apnea. *Curr Opin Nephrol Hypertens.* 2011;**20**:50–5
31. Sever PS, *et al.* Hypertension management 2011: Optimal combination therapy. *Eur Heart J.* 2011;**32**:2499–506
32. Weber MA, *et al.* Effects of body size and hypertension treatments on cardiovascular event rates: subanalysis of the ACCOMPLISH randomised controlled trial. *Lancet.* 2013;**381**:537–45
33. Kronish IM, *et al.* Meta-analysis: impact of drug class on adherence to antihypertensives. *Circulation.* 2011;**123**: 1611–21
34. Matchar DB, *et al.* Systematic review: comparative effectiveness of angiotensin-converting enzyme inhibitors and angiotensin II receptor blockers for treating essential hypertension. *Ann Intern Med.* 2008;**148**:16–29
35. Fournier A, *et al.* Prevention of dementia by antihypertensive drugs: how AT1-receptor-blockers and dihydropyridines better prevent dementia in hypertensive patients than thiazides and ACE-inhibitors. *Expert Rev Neurother.* 2009;**9**:1413–31
36. Anderson C, *et al.* Renin-angiotensin system blockade and cognitive function in patients at high risk of cardiovascular disease: analysis of data from the ONTARGET and TRANSCEND studies. *Lancet Neurol.* 2011;**10**:43–53
37. Benson SC, *et al.* Inhibition of cardiovascular cell proliferation by angiotensin receptor blockers: are all molecules the same? *J Hypertens.* 2008;**26**:973–80
38. Sipahi I, *et al.* Angiotensin-receptor blockade and risk of cancer: meta-analysis of randomised controlled trials. *Lancet Oncol.* 2010;**11**:627–36
39. Bangalore S, *et al.* Antihypertensive drugs and risk of cancer: network meta-analyses and trial sequential analyses of 324,168 participants from randomised trials. *Lancet Oncol.* 2011;**12**:65–82
40. Collaboration. TAT. Effects of telmisartan, irbesartan, valsartan, candesartan, and losartan on cancers in 15 trials enrolling 138 769 individuals. *J Hypertens.* 2011;**29**:623–635.
41. Pasternak B, *et al.* Use of angiotensin receptor blockers and the risk of cancer. . *Circulation.* 2011;**123**:1729–36.
42. USFDA. FDA drug safety communication: No increase in risk of cancer with certain blood pressure drugs—angiotensin receptor blockers (ARBS). 2 June 2011.
43. Mann JF, *et al.* Renal outcomes with telmisartan, ramipril, or both, in people at high vascular risk (the ONTARGET study): a multicentre, randomised, double-blind, controlled trial. *Lancet.* 2008;**372**:547–53
44. Messerli FH, *et al.* Of fads, fashion, surrogate endpoints and dual ras blockade. *Eur Heart J.* 2010;**31**:2205–8
45. Gao D, *et al.* Aliskiren vs angiotensin receptor blockers in hypertension: meta-analysis of randomized controlled trials. *Am J Hypertens.* 2011;**24**:613–21
46. Brown MJ, *et al.* Aliskiren and the calcium channel blocker amlodipine combination as an initial treatment strategy for hypertension control (ACCELERATE): a randomised, parallel-group trial. *Lancet.* 2011;**377**:312–20
47. Oparil S, *et al.* Efficacy and safety of combined use of aliskiren and valsartan in patients with hypertension: a randomised, double-blind trial. *Lancet.* 2007;**370**:221–9
48. Parving HH, *et al.* Cardiorenal end points in a trial of aliskiren for type 2 diabetes. *N Engl J Med.* 2012;**367**:2204–13
49. Gashti CN, *et al.* The role of calcium antagonists in chronic kidney disease. *Curr Opin Nephrol Hypertens.* 2004;**13**:155–61
50. Mangray M, *et al.* Hypertension after kidney transplant. *Am J Kidney Dis.* 2011;**57**:331–41
51. Makani H, *et al.* Effect of renin-angiotensin system blockade on calcium channel blocker-associated peripheral oedema. *Am J Med.* 2011;**124**:128–35
52. Shibata MC, *et al.* Do calcium channel blockers increase the diagnosis of heart failure in patients with hypertension? *Am J Cardiol.* 2010;**106**:228–35
53. Pahor M, *et al.* Health outcomes associated with calcium antagonists compared with other first-line antihypertensive therapies: a meta-analysis of randomised controlled trials. *Lancet.* 2000;**356**:1949–54
54. Ernst ME, *et al.* Use of diuretics in patients with hypertension. *N Engl J Med.* 2009;**361**:2153–64
55. Elliott WJ MPI. Incident diabetes in clinical trials of antihypertensive drugs: a network meta-analysis. *Lancet.* 2007;**369**:201–7
56. Major outcomes in high-risk hypertensive patients randomized to angiotensin-converting enzyme inhibitor or calcium channel blocker vs diuretic: the Antihypertensive and Lipid-Lowering Treatment to Prevent Heart Attack Trial (ALLHAT). *JAMA.* 2002;**288**:2981–97
57. Ernst ME, *et al.* Meta-analysis of dose-response characteristics of hydrochlorothiazide and chlorthalidone: effects on systolic blood pressure and potassium. *Am J Hypertens.* 2010;**23**:440–6
58. Psaty BM, *et al.* Meta-analysis of health outcomes of chlorthalidone-based vs nonchlorthalidone-based low-dose diuretic therapies. *JAMA.* 2004;**292**:43–4
59. Dhalla IA, *et al.* Chlorthalidone versus hydrochlorothiazide for the treatment of hypertension in older adults: A population-based cohort study. *Ann Intern Med.* 2013; **158**:447–55
60. Messerli FH, *et al.* Antihypertensive efficacy of hydrochlorothiazide as evaluated by ambulatory blood pressure monitoring: a meta-analysis of randomized trials. *J Am Coll Cardiol.* 2011;**57**:590–600
61. Weber MA JK, *et al.* Effects of body size and hypertension treatments on cardiovascular event rates: Subanalysis of the accomplish randomised controlled trial. *Lancet.* 2013;**381**:537–45
62. Carter BL, *et al.* Thiazide-induced dysglycemia: call for research from a working group from the National Heart, Lung, and Blood Institute. *Hypertension.* 2008;**52**:30–6

63. Katzberg HD, *et al.* Assessment: symptomatic treatment for muscle cramps (an evidence-based review): report of the Therapeutics and Technology Assessment Subcommittee of the American Academy of Neurology. *Neurology*. 2010; **74**:691–6
64. Grossman E, *et al.* Antihypertensive therapy and the risk of malignancies. *Eur Heart J*. 2001;**22**:1343–52
65. Williams GH, *et al.* Efficacy of eplerenone versus enalapril as monotherapy in systemic hypertension. *Am J Cardiol*. 2004;**93**:990–6
66. Pitt B, *et al.* Effects of eplerenone, enalapril, and eplerenone/enalapril in patients with essential hypertension and left ventricular hypertrophy: The 4e-left ventricular hypertrophy study. *Circulation*. 2003;**108**:1831–8
67. Saha C, *et al.* Improvement in blood pressure with inhibition of the epithelial sodium channel in blacks with hypertension. *Hypertension*. 2005;**46**:481–7
68. Bradley HA, *et al.* How strong is the evidence for use of beta blockers as first-line therapy for hypertension? Systematic review and meta-analysis. *J Hypertens*. 2006;**24**:2131–41
69. Dahlof B, *et al.* Cardiovascular morbidity and mortality in the Losartan Intervention for Endpoint Reduction in Hypertension Study (LIFE): a randomised trial against atenolol. *Lancet*. 2002;**359**:995–1003
70. Dahlof B, *et al.* Prevention of cardiovascular events with an antihypertensive regimen of amlodipine adding perindopril as required versus atenolol adding bendroflumethiazide as required, in the Anglo-Scandinavian Cardiac Outcomes Trial-Blood Pressure Lowering Arm (ASCOT-BPLA): a multicentre randomised controlled trial. *Lancet*. 2005;**366**:895–906
71. Lindholm LH, *et al.* Should beta blockers remain first choice in the treatment of primary hypertension? A meta-analysis. *Lancet*. 2005;**366**:1545–53
72. Bangalore S, *et al.* Relation of beta blocker-induced heart rate lowering and cardioprotection in hypertension. *J Am Coll Cardiol*. 2008;**52**:1482–9
73. Yaoita H, *et al.* Different effects of carvedilol, metoprolol, and propranolol on left ventricular remodeling after coronary stenosis or after permanent coronary occlusion in rats. *Circulation*. 2002;**105**:975–80
74. Munzel T, *et al.* Nebivolol: The somewhat-different beta-adrenergic receptor blocker. *J Am Coll Cardiol*. 2009; **54**:1491–9
75. Bisognano JD, *et al.* Baroreflex activation therapy lowers blood pressure in patients with resistant hypertension: Results from the double-blind, randomized, placebo-controlled rheos pivotal trial. *J Am Coll Cardiol*. 2011;**58**:765–73
76. Krum H, *et al.* Device-based antihypertensive therapy: therapeutic modulation of the autonomic nervous system. *Circulation*. 2011;**123**:209–15
77. Esler MD, *et al.* Renal sympathetic denervation in patients with treatment-resistant hypertension (The Symplicity HTN-2 Trial): a randomised controlled trial. *Lancet*. 2010;**376**:1903–9
78. Mahfoud F, *et al.* Expert consensus document fromthe european society of cardiology on catheter-based renal denervation. *Eur Heart J*. 2013; doi:10.1093/eurheartj/eht1154
79. Chobanian AV, *et al.* Seventh report of the Joint National Committee on prevention, detection, evaluation, and treatment of high blood pressure. *Hypertension*. 2003;**42**: 1206–52
80. Calhoun DAJD, *et al.* Resistant hypertension: Diagnosis, evaluation, and treatment: A scientific statement from the american heart association professional education committee of the council for high blood pressure research. *Circulation*. 2008;**117**:e510–26
81. Daugherty SL, *et al.* Incidence and prognosis of resistant hypertension in hypertensive patients. *Circulation*. 2012;**125**:1635–42
82. Sarafidis PA, *et al.* Resistant hypertension: an overview of evaluation and treatment. *J Am Coll Cardiol*. 2008;**52**:1749–57
83. Calhoun DA, *et al.* Hyperaldosteronism among black and white subjects with resistant hypertension. *Hypertension*. 2002;**40**:892–6
84. Eide IK, *et al.* Low-renin status in therapy-resistant hypertension: a clue to efficient treatment. *J Hypertens*. 2004;**22**:2217–26
85. Alderman MH, *et al.* Pressor responses to antihypertensive drug types. *Am J Hypertens*. 2010;**23**:1031–7
86. Turner ST, *et al.* Plasma renin activity predicts blood pressure responses to beta blocker and thiazide diuretic as monotherapy and add-on therapy for hypertension. *Am J Hypertens*. 2010;**23**:1014–22
87. Chapman N, *et al.* Effect of doxazosin gastrointestinal therapeutic system as third-line antihypertensive therapy on blood pressure and lipids in the Anglo-Scandinavian Cardiac Outcomes Trial. *Circulation*. 2008;**118**:42–8
88. Unger T, *et al.* Therapeutic perspectives in hypertension: novel means for renin-angiotensin-aldosterone system modulation and emerging device-based approaches. *Eur Heart J*. 2011;**32**:2739–47
89. Kaplan N. Systemic hypertension: therapy. In: Libby P. Bonow RO, Mann DL, Zipes DP (Eds). *Braunwald's heart disease*. pp.1047–70, Saunders, [CITY] 2008.
90. Regitz-Zagrosek V, *et al.* ESC guidelines on the management of cardiovascular diseases during pregnancy: the Task Force on the management of cardiovascular diseases during pregnancy of the European Society of Sardiology (ESC). *Eur Heart J*. 2011;**32**:3147–97
91. Higgins JR, *et al.* Blood-pressure measurement and classification in pregnancy. *Lancet*. 2001;**357**:131–5
92. Männistö T, *et al.* Elevated blood pressure in pregnancy and subsequent chronic disease risk. *Circulation*. 2013;**127**:681–90
93. Seely EW, *et al.* Clinical practice. Chronic hypertension in pregnancy. *N Engl J Med*. 2011;**365**:439–46
94. Magee LA, *et al.* Risks and benefits of beta-receptor blockers for pregnancy hypertension: overview of the randomized trials. *Eur J Obstet Gynecol Reprod Biol*. 2000;**88**:15–26
95. Ito S. Drug therapy for breastfeeding women. *N Engl J Med*. 2000;**343**:118–26

Chapter 25

Secondary hypertension

Introduction

Specific causes of hypertension can be diagnosed in less than 10% of patients with established hypertension (Table 25.1).

Renal parenchymal disease

This is the most common cause of secondary hypertension (2–5%). It is due to diabetic nephropathy, hypertensive nephrosclerosis that, by itself, further increases blood pressure, polycystic kidney disease, and chronic glomerulonephritis. **Kidney ultrasound** (for kidney size, cortical thickness, urinary tract obstruction, and cysts or masses), assessment of **serum creatinine** and **electrolytes**, and **urinalysis** for red and white blood cells and proteinuria, are essential initial tests in all patients with established hypertension. In haemodialysis patients (lack of renin activity), hypertension is labile and sensitive to changes in fluid volumes.

Acute renal disease, such as acute glomerulonephritis or urinary tract obstruction, may also result in hypertension.

Renovascular hypertension

This is the second most common cause of secondary hypertension (2%). However, renal artery stenosis is difficult to prove to be the cause of hypertension.[1, 2] Clinical clues for such an association are:

- Resistant hypertension
- Sudden onset of hypertension before 50 years of age
- Negative family history for hypertension
- Generalized atherosclerosis
- Hypokalaemia
- Deterioration of renal function with ACEI/ARB.

Aetiology

Two forms of renal artery stenosis are described in adults.

Fibromuscular dysplasia, involving the distal two-thirds of the main renal artery, accounts for 10–15% of cases and responds to ACE inhibitors/ARBs and angioplasty. Fibromuscular dysplasia is a non-atherosclerotic, non-inflammatory vascular disease that primarily affects women in the prime of their life. It most commonly affects the renal, carotid, and vertebral arteries but may occur in virtually every artery of the body. It is the second most frequent cause of renovascular hypertension. An angiographic classification of renal artery fibromuscular dysplasia lesions into a unifocal and a multifocal subtype has been recently proposed.[3] A cerebrovascular event, including transient ischaemic attack, stroke, and/or amaurosis fugax, occurs in 25% of patients.[4] The presence of a carotid bruit in a patient under 60 or an epigastric bruit in a patient with hypertension should alert the clinician to the possible diagnosis of the condition.

Atherosclerotic disease (85–90%), involving the proximal one-third of the main renal artery, is usually seen in old men. ACE inhibitors and ARBs are effective in these patients, but the loss of renal mass and reduction in transcapillary filtration pressure can produce acute or chronic renal insufficiency, especially if renal artery stenosis affects both kidneys or the sole functional kidney. Medical therapy consists of diuretics, CCBs, ACEI/ARBs (in the absence of bilateral stenosis), and statins.

Rare causes are **aortic dissection** with renal artery involvement, **acute renal artery occlusion** (thrombosis, embolism, or trauma), **Takayasu** or **giant cell arteritis**, **congenital mid-aortic syndrome**, and **antiphospholipid antibodies syndrome**.

Pathophysiology

A decrease in renal perfusion pressure activates the renin-angiotensin system, which leads to the release of renin and the production of angiotensin II, has direct effects on sodium excretion, sympathetic nerve activity, intrarenal prostaglandin concentrations, and nitric oxide production, and causes renovascular hypertension. When hypertension is sustained, plasma renin activity decreases, partially explaining the limitations of renin measurements for identifying patients with renovascular hypertension.[2]

Diagnosis

Kidney ultrasonography may show a difference of more than 1.5 cm in length between the two kidneys in 60–70% of the patients with renovascular hypertension and is diagnostic for renal artery stenosis (Table 25.1). **Doppler ultrasonography** is capable of detecting stenosis, particularly when localized proximally, but **gadolinium-enhanced MRI** is considered the diagnostic procedure of choice,[5] but is contraindicated in the presence of GFR <30mL/min.

Significant renal artery stenosis is defined as ≥50% diameter stenosis, associated with peak translesional gradient

Table 25.1 ESC 2013 GL on hypertension

Clinical indications and diagnostics of secondary hypertension					
	Clinical indications			**Diagnostics**	
Common causes	**Clinical history**	**Physical examination**	**Laboratory investigations**	**First-line test(s)**	**Additional/ confirmatory test(s)**
Renal parenchymal disease	History of urinary tract infection or obstruction, haematuria, analgesic abuse; family history of polycystic kidney disease	Abdominal masses (in case of polycystic kidney disease)	Presence of protein, erythrocytes, or leucocytes in the urine, decreased GFP	Renal ultrasound	Detailed work-up for kidney disease
Renal artery stenosis	Fibromuscular dysplasia: early onset hypertension (especially in women). Atherosclerotic stenosis: hypertension of abrupt onset, worsening or increasingly difficult to treat; flash pulmonary oedema	Abdominal bruit	Difference of >1.5 cm in length between the two kidneys (renal ultrasound), rapid deterioration in renal function (spontaneous or in response to RAA blockers)	Renal Duplex Doppler ultrasonography	Magentic resonance angiography, spiral computed tomography, intra-arterial digial subtraction angiography
Primary aldosteronism	Muscle weakness; family history of early onset hypertension and cerebrovascular events at age <40 years	Arrhythmias (in case of severe hypokalaemia)	Hypokalaemia (spontaneous or diuretic-induced); incidental discovery of adrenal masses	Aldosterone–renin ratio under standardized conditions (correction of hypokalaemia and withdrawal of drugs affecting RAA system)	Confirmatory tests (oral sodium loading, saline infusion, fludrocortisone suppression, or captopril test); adrenal CT scan; adrenal vein sampling
Uncommon causes					
Phaeochromocytoma	Paroxysmal hypertension or a crisis superimposed to sustained hypertension; headache, sweating, palpitations and pallor; positive family history of phaeochromocytoma	Skin stigmata of neurofibromatosis (café-au-lait spots, neurofibromas)	Incidental discovery of adrenal (or in some cases, extra-adrenal) masses	Measurement of urinary fractionated metanephrines or plasma-free metanephrines	CT or MRI of the abdomen and pelvis; 123 I-labelled meta-iodobenzyl-guanidine scalling; genetic scanning for pathogenic mutations
Cushing's syndrome	Rapid weight gain, polyuria, polydipsia, psychological disturbances	Typical body habitus (central obesity, moon-face, buffalo hump, red striae, hirsutism)	Hyperglycaemia	24-h urinary cortisol exretion	Dexamethasone-suppression tests

CT, computed tomography; GFR, glomerular filtration rate; MRI, magnetic resonance imaging; RAA, renin–angiotensin–aldosterone.
2013 ESH/ESC Guidelines for the management of arterial hypertension. *Eur Heart J*. 2013. doi:10.1093/eurheartj/eht151

≥20 mmHg, or a mean gradient ≥10 mmHg.[1] However, both arteriography and Doppler measurements overestimate renal artery stenosis as defined by the detection of a distal renal to aortic pressure ratio of <0.9.[6]

Therapy

Angioplasty with stenting has a modest, but significant, effect on blood pressure and may be considered for patients with atherosclerotic renal artery stenosis and poorly controlled hypertension, although it does not improve or preserve renal function and its value has been questioned.[7, 8] Surgical revascularization carries a higher mortality.[2]

Angioplasty or surgical revascularization has also yielded moderate benefits in patients with fibromuscular dysplasia renal artery stenosis.[9]

Thus, intervention is not recommended if renal function has remained stable over the past 6–12 months and if hypertension can be controlled with an acceptable medical regimen (Table 25.2).[9] Anatomically relevant renal artery stenosis >70% should be verified by functional measurements as systolic pressure gradient ≥21 mmHg or Pd/Pa pressure ratio <0.9.[6] The best evidence supporting intervention may be for bilateral stenosis with 'flash' pulmonary oedema unrelated to acute coronary syndrome (Pickering syndrome).[10]

Primary aldosteronism

The prevalence of primary aldosteronism in patienst with hypertension varies among reported studies because of

Table 25.2 ACCF/AHA 2013 guideline on peripheral artery disease

Treatment of renovascular disease (RAS)	
Medical treatment	
ACE inhibitors for hypertension associated with unilateral RAS.	I-A
Angiotensin receptor blockers for hypertension associated with unilateral RAS.	I-B
Calcium-channel blockers for hypertension associated with unilateral RAS.	I-A
Beta blockers for hypertension associated with RAS.	I-A
Indications for revascularization	
ASYMPTOMATIC STENOSIS	
Percutaneous revascularization for treatment of an asymptomatic bilateral or solitary viable kidney with a hemodynamically significant RAS.	IIb-C
The usefulness of percutaneous revascularization of an asymptomatic unilateral hemodynamically significant RAS in a viable kidney is not well established and is presently clinically unproven.	IIb-C
HYPERTENSION	
Percutaneous revascularization for patients with hemodynamically significant RAS and accelerated hypertension, resistant hypertension, malignant hypertension, hypertension with an unexplained unilateral small kidney, and hypertension with intolerance to medication.	IIa-B
PRESERVATION OF RENAL FUNCTION	
Percutaneous revascularization for patients with RAS and progressive chronic kidney disease with bilateral RAS or a RAS to a solitary functioning kidney.	IIa-B
Percutaneous revascularization for patients with RAS and chronic renal insufficiency with unilateral RAS.	IIb-C
IMPACT OF RAS ON CONGESTIVE HEART FAILURE AND UNSTABLE ANGINA	
Percutaneous revascularization is indicated for hemodynamically significant RAS and recurrent, unexplained congestive heart failure or sudden, unexplained pulmonary edema.	I-B
Percutaneous revascularization for hemodynamically significant RAS and unstable angina.	IIa-B
Endovascular treatment for RAS	
Renal stent placement is indicated for ostial atherosclerotic RAS lesions that meet the clinical criteria for intervention.	I-B
Balloon angioplasty with bailout stent placement if necessary is recommended for fibromuscular dysplasia lesions.	I-B
Surgery for RAS	
Vascular surgical reconstruction for fibromuscular dysplastic RAS with clinical indications for interventions (same angioplasty), especially those exhibiting complex disease that extends into the segmental arteries and those having macroaneurysms.as for percutaneous transluminal.	I-B
Vascular surgical reconstruction for atherosclerotic RAS and clinical indications for intervention, especially those with multiple small renal arteries or early primary branching of the main renal artery.	I-B
Vascular surgical reconstruction for atherosclerotic RAS in combination with pararenal aortic reconstructions (in treatment of aortic aneurysms or severe aortoiliac occlusive disease).	I-C

the unreliability of the renin/aldosterone ratio test; it is, most probably, approximately 5%.[11–13] Adrenal adenomas account for 30% of cases and are usually small (less than 2 cm in diameter) and benign; 70% are caused by adrenal hyperplasia (considered by some a variant of essential hypertension).[11, 14] There are also rare cases of adrenal carcinoma and the autosomal dominant condition of glucocorticoid-remediable aldosteronism.

Diagnosis

The condition should be suspected in resistant hypertension and in unprovoked hypokalaemia, but only a small number of patients will have hypokalaemia at an early stage in their disease. Increased **urinary excretion of potassium** (>30 mmol/day in the presence of hypokalaemia and in the absence of extra potassium intake) points to aldosteronism. It can be confirmed by the overnight **dexamethasone (1 mg) suppression test** and measurement of aldosterone, and renin under standardized conditions. The usefulness of the **aldosterone-to-renin** ratio is controversial.[14] Aldosterone can be high or renin low in elderly people or black patients. Also, a high aldosterone-to-renin ratio is seen in chronic renal disease where high potassium stimulates aldosterone release and, in the case of rare genetic mutations, leading to increased aldosterone levels.[15] **CT, magnetic resonance imaging**, or **isotopic techniques** using radiolabelled cholesterol are used for imaging of the adrenals. Adrenal venous sampling is necessary to avoid false positive results that could provoke unnecessary adrenalectomy for non-functioning tumours.[15]

Therapy

Includes medical therapy with mineralocorticoid receptor antagonists and laparoscopic adrenalectomy for patients with unilateral adenomas.

Phaeochromocytoma

It is a very rare cause of secondary hypertension (0.2–0.4%), inherited or acquired, with an estimated annual incidence of 2–8/million population.[16] Phaeochromocytomas are mostly benign catecholamine-producing tumours of chromaffin cells of the adrenal medulla or of a paraganglion. Typical clinical manifestations are sustained or paroxysmal hypertension, severe headaches, palpitations, and sweating. However, their presentation is highly variable (hypertension occurs in about 70% of all cases of phaeochromocytoma) and can mimic many other diseases. If remaining unrecognized or untreated, they can be a life-threatening condition.

Diagnosis

The test with the highest sensitivity is the measurement of **plasma free metanephrines**, together with **urinary fractionated metanephrines.** However, because measurement of plasma free metanephrines is not widely available for routine diagnosis, measurement of 24-hour urinary fractionated metanephrines and **urinary catecholamines** remains the diagnostic test of choice.[5] Stimulation or suppression tests with glucagon or clonidine, respectively, are less often used nowadays. Phaeochromocytomas are localized by a **computed tomography** scan and **magnetic resonance imaging** of the adrenal glands and abdomen. Complementary **^{123}I-metaiodobenzylguanidine scintigraphy** and **^{18}F-dihydroxyphenylalanine-positron emission tomography** may also be useful. Because approximately 25% of phaeochromocytomas are hereditary (multiple endocrine neoplasia type 2 **(MEN2)**, von Hippel–Lindau disease **(VHL)**, neurofibromatosis type 1, and familial paragangliomas), screening for genetic alterations is important. To date, mutations in five genes have been described leading to familial disorders associated with phaeochromocytomas.[5]

Therapy

Laparoscopic and adrenal-sparing surgical intervention following preoperative alpha blockade (prazosin, phenoxybenzamine or labetalol) and fluid expansion are the treatment of choice and usually curative. In malignant phaeochromocytomas, radiotherapy and chemotherapy are palliative treatment options.

Adrenal 'incidentaloma'

An adrenal 'incidentaloma' is an adrenal mass, generally 1 cm or more in diameter, that is discovered serendipitously during a radiologic examination performed for indications other than an evaluation for adrenal disease.[18]

The majority of adrenal incidentalomas are clinically non-hypersecreting, benign adrenocortical adenomas. Other diagnoses include cortisol-secreting adrenocortical adenoma (5%), phaeochromocytoma (5%), adrenocortical carcinoma (5%), metastatic carcinoma (2.5%), and aldosterone-secreting adenoma (1%). When adrenal masses occur bilaterally (15% of patients with adrenal incidentaloma), the most likely diagnoses are metastatic disease, congenital adrenal hyperplasia, bilateral cortical adenomas, and infiltrative disease of the adrenal glands. Hormone production is determined by overnight dexamethasone suppression and blood or 24-h fractionated metanephrines and catecholamines, and a CT scan is performed. Laparoscopic adrenalectomy is indicated if the adrenal mass is ≥4 cm in diameter and if the mass enlarges by 1 cm or more during a period of 4 years with 6-monthly examinations; if evidence of autonomous hormonal secretion develops, laparoscopic adrenalectomy is considered.[16, 18]

Other causes of hypertension

Cushing's syndrome, coarctation of the aorta, hypo- and hyperthyroidism, intracranial tumours, and **drug-induced hypertension** are also causes of secondary hypertension. Although non-steroidal anti-inflammatory agents are the most common cause of drug-induced hypertension, other drugs, as described in Table 24.15 in Chapter 24 on primary hypertension, should be also considered. Antiangiogenic and anti-vascular endothelial growth factor (VEGF) chemotherapy agents that are currently used for the treatment of various forms of cancer are a common cause of secondary hypertension.[19]

References

1. Baumgartner I, *et al.* Renovascular hypertension: screening and modern management. *Eur Heart J.* 2011;**32**:1590–8
2. Safian RD, *et al.* Renal artery stenosis. *N Engl J Med.* 2001;**344**:431–42
3. Savard S, *et al.* Association between 2 angiographic subtypes of renal artery fibromuscular dysplasia and clinical characteristics. *Circulation.* 2012;**126**:3062–9
4. Olin JW, *et al.* The United States registry for fibromuscular dysplasia: results in the first 447 patients. *Circulation.* 2012;**125**:3182–90

5. Drieghe B, *et al.* Assessment of renal artery stenosis: side-by-side comparison of angiography and duplex ultrasound with pressure gradient measurements. *Eur Heart J.* 2008;**29**:517–24
6. Nordmann AJ, *et al.* Balloon angioplasty or medical therapy for hypertensive patients with atherosclerotic renal artery stenosis? A meta-analysis of randomized controlled trials. *Am J Med.* 2003;**114**:44–50
7. Wheatley K, *et al.* Revascularization versus medical therapy for renal artery stenosis. *N Engl J Med.* 2009;**361**:1953–62
8. Trinquart L, *et al.* Efficacy of revascularization for renal artery stenosis caused by fibromuscular dysplasia: a systematic review and meta-analysis. *Hypertension.* 2010;**56**:525–32
9. Anderson JLHJ, *et al.* Management of patients with peripheral artery disease (compilation of 2005 and 2011 ACCF/AHA guideline recommendations): A report of the American College of Cardiology Foundation/American Heart Association task force on practice guidelines. *Circulation.* 2013; [Epub ahead of print]
10. Messerli FH, *et al.* Flash pulmonary oedema and bilateral renal artery stenosis: the Pickering syndrome. *Eur Heart J.* 2011;**32**:2231–5
11. Ganguly A. Primary aldosteronism. *N Engl J Med.* 1998;**339**: 1828–34
12. Kaplan N. Systemic hypertension: Therapy. In: Libby P, Bonow RR, Mann DL, Zipes DP (Eds). Braunwald's Heart Disease. pp.1047–70, Saunders, [CITY] 2008.
13. Rossi GP, *et al.* A prospective study of the prevalence of primary aldosteronism in 1,125 hypertensive patients. *J Am Coll Cardiol.* 2006;**48**:2293–300
14. Kaplan NM. The current epidemic of primary aldosteronism: causes and consequences. *J Hypertens.* 2004;**22**: 863–9
15. Mancia G, *et al.* 2007 guidelines for the management of arterial hypertension: the Task Force for the management of arterial hypertension of the European Society of Hypertension (ESH) and of the European Society of Cardiology (ESC). *Eur Heart J.* 2007;**28**:1462–536
16. Reisch N, *et al.* Phaeochromocytoma: presentation, diagnosis and treatment. *J Hypertens.* 2006;**24**:2331–9
17. Galan SR, Kann PH. Genetics and molecular pathogenesis of pheochromocytoma and paraganglioma. *Clin Endocrinol (Oxf).* 2013;**78**:165–75
18. Young WF, Jr. Clinical practice. The incidentally discovered adrenal mass. *N Engl J Med.* 2007;**356**:601–10
19. Nazer B, *et al.* Effects of novel angiogenesis inhibitors for the treatment of cancer on the cardiovascular system: focus on hypertension. *Circulation.* 2011;**124**:1687–91

Part IV

Coronary artery disease

Relevant guidelines

Unstable Angina-NSTEMI

ACCF/AHA 2012 guidelines on UA-NSTEMI

2012 ACCF/AHA focused update incorporated into the ACCF/AHA 2007 Guidelines for the management of patients with unstable angina/non–ST-elevation myocardial infarction. *J Am Coll Cardiol.* 2013;**61**:e179–347.

ESC 2011 guidelines on UA-NSTEMI

ESC guidelines for the management of acute coronary syndromes in patients presenting without persistent ST-segment elevation. *Eur Heart J.* 2011;**32**:2999–3054.

ESC 2011 guidelines on pregnancy

ESC Guidelines on the management of cardiovascular diseases during pregnancy. *Eur Heart J.* 2011;**32**:3147–97.

STEMI

ACC/AHA 2013 guidelines on STEMI

2013 ACCF/AHA guideline for the management of ST-elevation myocardial infarction. *J Am Coll Cardiol.* 2013;**61**:e78–140.

ESC 2012 guidelines on STEMI

ESC Guidelines for the management of acute myocardial infarction in patients presenting with ST-segment elevation. *Eur Heart J.* 2012;**33**:2501–2.

ESC 2011 guidelines on pregnancy

ESC Guidelines on the management of cardiovascular diseases during pregnancy. *Eur Heart J.* 2011;**32**:3147–97.

Stable CAD

ACC/AHA 2012 guideline on stable IHD

2012 ACCF/AHA/ACP/AATS/PCNA/SCAI/STS Guideline for the diagnosis and management of patients with stable ischemic heart disease. *J Am Coll Cardiol.* 2012;**60**:e44–e164.

ACCF/AHA guidelines on PCI 2011 and on CABG 2011

2011 ACCF/AHA/SCAI Guideline on percutaneous coronary intervention. *J Am Coll Cardiol.* 2011;**58**:e44–122.

2011 ACCF/AHA Guideline on CABG. *Circulation.* 2011;**124**: 2610–42.

ACC/AHA 2009 guidelines on perioperative cardiovascular evaluation

2009 ACCF/AHA focused update on perioperative beta-blockade incorporated into the ACC/AHA 2007 guidelines on perioperative cardiovascular evaluation and care for non-cardiac surgery. *J Am Coll Cardiol.* 2009;**54**:e13–e118.

AHA/ACCF 2011 guidelines on secondary prevention and risk reduction

AHA/ACCF secondary prevention and risk reduction therapy for patients with coronary and other atherosclerotic vascular disease: 2011 update. *Circulation.* 2011;**124**:2458–73.

AHA 2012 scientific statement on sexual activity and cardiovascular disease

Sexual activity and cardiovascular disease: a scientific statement from the American Heart Association. *Circulation.* 2012;**125**:1058–72.

AHA/ACCF 2012 cardiac disease evaluation and management in kidney and liver transplantation candidates

Cardiac disease evaluation and management among kidney and liver transplantation candidates: a scientific statement from the American Heart Association and the American College of Cardiology Foundation. *J Am Coll Cardiol.* 2012;**60**:434–80.

ESC 2006 guidelines on stable CAD

Guidelines on the management of stable angina pectoris: executive summary: the Task Force on the management of stable angina pectoris of the European Society of Cardiology. *Eur Heart J.* 2006;**27**:1341–81.

ESC 2010 guidelines on revascularization

ESC Guidelines on myocardial revascularization. *Eur Heart J.* 2010;**31**:2501–55.

ESC 2011 guidelines on pregnancy

ESC Guidelines on the management of cardiovascular diseases during pregnancy. *Eur Heart J.* 2011;**32**:3147–97.

ESC 2011 guidelines on dyslipidaemias

ESC/EAS Guidelines for the management of dyslipidaemias: the Task Force for the management of dyslipidaemias of the European Society of Cardiology (ESC) and the European Atherosclerosis Society (EAS). *Eur Heart J.* 2011;**32**: 1769–818.

ESC 2012 on cardiovascular disease prevention

European Guidelines on cardiovascular disease prevention in clinical practice (version 2012). *Eur Heart J.* 2012;**33**:1635–701.

ESC 2012 on heart failure

ESC Guidelines for the diagnosis and treatment of acute and chronic heart failure 2012. *Eur Heart J.* **33**:1787–847.

Chapter 26

Epidemiology and pathophysiology of coronary artery disease

Definitions and classification

Persons with asymptomatic coronary artery atherosclerosis may present with angina pectoris on effort or develop an acute coronary syndrome (ACS). Chronic stable angina is the initial manifestation of CAD in approximately 50% of all patients with CAD. **Stable coronary artery disease** may be detected following a diagnostic ischaemia test or diagnosed after presentation with an acute coronary syndrome. **ACS** refers to an acute imbalance of myocardial oxygen supply and demand due to progressive or abrupt flow-limiting coronary stenosis and/or high-output or increased afterload states. ACS includes unstable angina (UA), non-ST elevation myocardial infarction (NSTEMI), and ST elevation MI (STEMI). **Unstable angina**, with or without enzyme rise but without ST elevation, refers to UA/NSTEMI.[1] **STEMI** refers to myocardial infarction with ST segment elevation. The spectrum of ischaemic heart disease is presented in Figure 26.1.

Epidemiology

Coronary artery disease (CAD) is the single most common cause of death in the developed world, responsible for about one in every six deaths.[2,3] In 2010, out of 52.7 million deaths worldwide, approximately 15.6 million were due to cardiovascular disease (as compared with approximately 3.8 million due to tuberculosis, human immunodeficiency virus, and malaria combined).[2] Mortality from cardiovascular disease, in general, is estimated to reach 23.4 million in 2030.[4] Coronary artery disease is responsible for about half of these cardiovascular deaths. In 2009, 386 324 Americans died of coronary heart disease, and the 2009 overall rate of death attributable to cardiovascular disease (International Classification of Diseases, 10th Revision, codes I00–I99) was 236.1 per 100 000.[3] From 1999 to 2009, the relative rate of death attributable to cardiovascular disease declined by 32.7%. Yet, in 2009, cardiovascular disease still accounted for 32.3% (787 931) of all 2 437 163 deaths, or one of every three deaths in the USA. It is estimated that one in three adults in the USA (about 71 million) has some form of cardiovascular disease, including >13 million with coronary heart disease and nearly 9 million with angina pectoris. Among persons 60 to 79 years of age, approximately 23% of men and 15% of women have prevalent IHD, and these figures rise to 33% and 22% among men and women ≥80 years of age, respectively.[4] The costs of caring for patients with IHD are enormous, estimated at exceeding $150 billion in the USA. More than one half of direct costs are related to hospitalization.[5]

Each year in the USA, approximately 1 100 000 patients are admitted for **ACS**, of which 813 000 have a myocardial infarction and the remainder UA. Approximately two-thirds of patients with myocardial infarction have NSTEMI, and the rest have STEMI.[3] Thus, overall 38–47% of all patients with an ACS have a STEMI.[1] Worldwide, more than 3 million people each year are estimated to have a STEMI, and more than 4 million have an NSTEMI.[6] Hospital mortality is higher in patients with STEMI, but, in the long-term, mortality is higher in patients with non-ST elevation acute coronary syndrome (NSTEACS).[7] MI that occurs in the community still carries a 25% mortality risk whereas in-hospital mortality without fibrinolysis approaches 15%. Current pharmacological and mechanical therapeutic approaches have reduced this risk to 3–4%.[3,8]

Stable CAD was estimated to affect 16.8 million people in the USA in 2008.[9] In patients with stable CAD, the annual mortality rate is approximately 2%, and the annual rate of major events, such as death, myocardial infarction, and stroke, is 4.5%.[10]

Aetiology

More than 90% of myocardial infarctions are attributable to modifiable risk factors, such as smoking, dyslipidaemia, hypertension, diabetes, abdominal obesity, and exposure to traffic air pollution (PM_{10}, $PM_{2.5}$, NO_2, and ozone), psychosocial factors, and insomnia.[11–16] Consumption of fruits, vegetables and alcohol, as well as regular physical activity have a protective effect. Thus, the ten-year risk (National Cholesterol Education Program [NCEP] global risk) of developing symptomatic coronary artery disease should be calculated for all patients who have 2 or more major risk factors to assess the need for primary prevention strategies (Class I-C, ACCF/AHA 2012 GL on UA/NSTEMI).[17] Women who use oral contraceptives containing ethinyl estradiol are at dose-dependent increased risk for thrombotic stroke and myocardial infarction compared to women using progestin alone.[17] These cardiovascular risk factors induce oxidative stress that causes endothelial

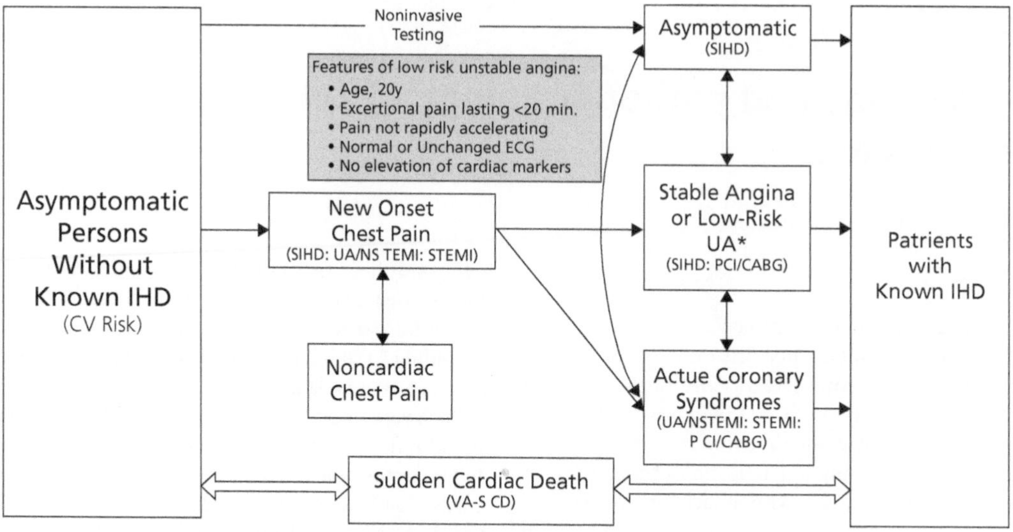

Figure 26.1 ACC/AHA 2012 on stable IHD: spectrum of IHD. Guidelines relevant to the spectrum of IHD are in parentheses.

CABG indicates coronary artery bypass graft; CV, cardiovascular; ECG, electrocardiogram; IHD, ischaemic heart disease; PCI, percutaneous coronary intervention; SCD, sudden cardiac death; SIHD, stable ischaemic heart disease; STEMI, ST elevation myocardial infarction; UA, unstable angina; UA/NSTEMI, unstable angina/non–ST elevation myocardial infarction; and VA, ventricular arrhythmia. 2012 ACCF/AHA/ACP/AATS/PCNA/SCAI/STS Guideline for the diagnosis and management of patients with stable ischemic heart disease. *J Am Coll Cardiol*, 2012; **60**:e44–e164.

inflammation and damage. Stillbirths and miscarriages are associated with increased rates of myocardial infarction, cerebral infarction, and renovascular hypertension.[19] This has been attributed to either shared etiology or the initiation of pathological processes by a pregnancy loss leading to atherosclerosis. Premature coronary artery disease may been seen in 3% of patients with HIV/AIDS.[20] **Secondary unstable angina** is due to additional conditions in the presence of coronary stenoses, such as tachycardia, fever, thyrotoxicosis, anaemia, aortic stenosis, hypertension or hypotension, and hyperviscosity states. Rare, non-atherosclerotic causes of MI are presented in Table 28.2 in Chapter 28 on MI. Distinct morphological characteristics, such as left main or proximal disease, display a high heritability,[21] and epidemiological studies have shown that genetic predisposition accounts for 40–60% of the risk for coronary artery disease.[22] Genome-wide association studies have led to the discovery of more than 33 single nucleotide polymorphisms as genetic risk variants for coronary artery disease.[22–26] Approximately ten of them are associated with hypertension or hyperlipidaemia, and the rest of them (including 9p21.3) mediate their risks through unknown mechanisms. The strongest genetic effect on the risk of coronary artery disease and myocardial infarction is that of single nucleotide polymorphisms at chromosome **9p21.3**, that is also a significant risk factor for abdominal aortic aneurysm, stroke, and Alzheimer's disease.[25] The 9p21 locus shows association with greater burden of CAD, but not with MI, in the presence of underlying CAD, thus supporting the hypothesis that it primarily mediates an atherosclerotic phenotype.[26] The 9p21.3 risk allele is carried by 75% of the European population and confers risk of coronary atherosclerosis in a dose-dependent way (by means of allele copies). The identification of the **ABO blood group** locus as a risk factor for myocardial infarction might provide an explanation on why blood group O offers protection from myocardial infarction compared to blood groups A and B.[27] Recently, the presence of a common **Y chromosome** variant haplogroup I was found to increase coronary risk by 50%.[28] This might explain the higher prevalence of CAD in men. All these genetic variants are not yet ready for routine testing.

Pathophysiology

ACS

The most frequent mechanism of an ACS is a reduction of the myocardial oxygen supply due to rupture or erosion of a vulnerable atherosclerotic plaque, which results in endothelial injury and associated thrombosis and dynamic vasoconstriction. **Vulnerable plaques** likely to rupture or erode have evidence of inflammation with macrophages, and T-cell infiltrates.[29,30] Histologically, vulnerable plaques have thin fibrous caps (<55 μm) with large lipid cores.[29–33] Usually, plaque rupture occurs within usually in an environment of low shear stress. Intraplaque haemorrhage also plays an important triggering role.[34] Plaque haemorrhage may occur from plaque rupture (fissure) or from neovascularization (angiogenesis). Plaque fissure or rupture exposes the highly thrombogenic subendothelium (collagen and tissue factor) to circulating platelets and white blood cells. The resultant platelet adhesion leads to platelet activation. Activated platelets release are also activated by vasoconstrictors, such as thromboxane A2 and adenosine diphosphate (ADP) that binds to $P2Y_{12}$ receptors, and cause increased expression of glycoprotein IIb/IIIa that binds fibrinogen or von Willebrand factor. Thus, platelet aggregation and creation of the **white clot** occurs. The platelet-derived mediators, together with other potent vasoconstrictors, such as activated thrombin, oxygen-derived free radicals, and endothelin, result in dynamic vasoconstriction and transient thrombosis. The coagulation cascade may be activated, and factor X leads to the generation of thrombin that converts fibrinogen to fibrin (**red clot**).[35] If the ischaemia is prolonged and severe enough to cause limited myocardial necrosis, the diagnosis of NSTEMI is put; further damage, usually due to the formation of a red thrombus that causes ST elevation, produces the clinical picture of STEMI. However, erosion or rupture of the coronary atherosclerotic plaque is typically required for an event to happen, but, only when coinciding with a prothrombotic state at the site of plaque rupture or erosion, it leads to an event. In the majority of cases, plaque ruptures or erosions take place in the absence of symptoms and commonly lead to healing and progression of coronary arterial narrowing.[36] Vulnerable plaques, intact or ruptured, may be found along the coronary tree, and the true culprit lesion can be difficult to define. The term 'calcified nodule' is used for a rare type of coronary thrombosis not caused by plaque rupture but related to disruptive nodular calcifications protruding into the lumen, usually tortuous heavily calcified arteries in older individuals.[30]

Additional causes of UA/NSTEMI are **coronary spasm, emboli, coronary arterial inflammation**, or **spontaneous dissection** of the coronary artery in the absence of occlusive atherosclerosis in 10–15% of patients with NSTEMI.[37] Similar proportions of male patients and up to 30% of women with NSTEACS have angiographically normal coronary arteries despite elevated troponins and myocardial infarctions detected by MRI.[31] Vasospasm and embolism without evident plaque disruption are particularly common in women in this setting.[38]

Rupture of vulnerable coronary plaques with subsequent thrombosis and occlusion of the coronary artery is the commonest cause of myocardial infarction.[39,40] Angiography at the acute phase reveals an occluded coronary artery in 90% of cases, although the converse is not the case due to the possible presence of collaterals. Intracoronary thrombi are mainly composed of fibrin (increased content with increased ischaemic time), platelets, erythrocytes, and few cholesterol crystals and leukocytes.[41] Coronary spasm, emboli, or spontaneous dissection of the coronary artery are causes of infarction in the absence of occlusive atherosclerosis and are reported in 5–10% of patients with STEMI.[35] There is a circadian periodicity with most events, occurring between 6 a.m. and noon. Platelet hyper-reactivity and pro-coagulant states contribute to the thrombotic process that diminishes microcirculatory perfusion by reduced coronary artery flow through epicardial stenoses as well as by distal embolization of thrombus. MIs have been shown to frequently occur at sites of mild to moderate stenosis.[42–44] Post-mortem examinations, however, have also demonstrated that ruptured plaques, leading to thrombosis, more likely occur within the segment of significant (>50%) stenoses.[45–47] Angiographic data also indicate that the majority of coronary events occur in patients with complex lesions and significant stenosis.[48–50] In the PROSPECT trial on patients with acute coronary syndromes treated by coronary intervention, 3-year recurrence rates were 20%. Half of them occurred in angiographically mild (<70% stenosis), non-culprit lesions. However, predictors of recurrent events were both a luminal area ≤4 mm^2 and the presence of thin-cap fibroatheroma.[51] An analysis of the data from the COURAGE trial has shown that MIs are not more likely to occur from mild coronary lesions compared with moderate or severe ones; the number of non-revascularized lesions ≥50% was the only angiographic predictor of an acute coronary syndrome.[52] When intravascular imaging information is available, the lesions with <85μm thick cap and >75% cross-sectional luminal area stenosis are the most probable to rupture.[32] **Coronary spasm** is a well-reported cause of cardiac arrest. It occurs commonly in the absence of severe coronary disease and can present with or without anginal pain. Minor coronary disease in the absence of other causes of cardiac arrest might suggest the diagnosis, particularly in a male smoker.[53] Spontaneous **coronary artery dissection** affects predominantly young women with a mean age of 42 years. Postpartum status, cocaine use, Ehlers–Danlos syndrome, hormonal therapy, vasculitis, and extreme physical exertion are conditions that have been associated with spontaneous coronary dissection.[54]

Histochemical stains can identify **zones of necrosis** 2–3 hours after the onset of necrosis while gross pathology changes can be identified 6–12 hours following occlusion. Eight to 10 days after infarction, the thickness of the affected ventricular wall is reduced, as necrotic muscle is removed by mononuclear cells, and, over the next 2–3 months, a firm scar develops. Infarct expansion (disruption and tissue loss not explained by additional necrosis) and ventricular dilation may also occur and determine ventricular remodelling.

Stunned myocardium refers to depressed contractility, ie reduced perfusion with maintained metabolism, due to ischaemic insults of short duration. ***Hibernating myocardium*** is dysfunctional and viable myocardium but with more severe cellular structural changes. Stunned myocardium is more likely to recover than hibernating myocardium.[55]

Stable CAD

The underlying mechanism of chronic CAD is the chronic limited ability to increase oxygen supply to the myocardium in the setting of increased oxygen demand, usually caused by the obstruction of, at least, one large epicardial coronary artery by atheromatous plaque. Because myocytes already extract about 75% of the oxygen in coronary blood at rest, a higher demand is primarily met by increasing coronary blood flow. Myocardial ischaemia results in hypoxia that activates cellular anaerobic pathways; produced mediators, such as lactate, are responsible for the sensation of pain. Originally thought to be dominantly a lipid storage disease, our current understanding of the pathogenesis of atherosclerosis implicates endothelial injury and inflammation. Additional chemical and mechanical factors that may trigger endothelial injury are altered sheer stress, high oxidative stress, smoking, and insulin resistance.[56] Several genetic loci (more than 33) that affect the risk of development of coronary artery disease have also been identified (see Aetiology above).

References

1. Braunwald E *et al.* Unstable angina: Is it time for a requiem? *Circulation.* 2013;**127**:2452–2457
2. Lozano R, *et al.* Global and regional mortality from 235 causes of death for 20 age groups in 1990 and 2010: a systematic analysis for the global burden of disease study 2010. *Lancet.* 2013;**380**:2095–128
3. Go AS, *et al.* Heart disease and stroke statistics—2013 update: a report from the American Heart Association. *Circulation.* 2013;**127**:e6–245
4. Cassar A, *et al.* Chronic coronary artery disease: diagnosis and management. *Mayo Clin Proc.* 2009;**84**:1130–46
5. Fihn SD, *et al.* 2012 ACCF/AHA/ACP/AATS/PCNA/SCAI/STS guideline for the diagnosis and management of patients with stable ischaemic heart disease: a report of the American College of Cardiology Foundation/American Heart Association Task Force on practice guidelines and the American College of Physicians, American Association for Thoracic Surgery, Preventive Cardiovascular Nurses Association, Society for Cardiovascular Angiography and Interventions, and Society of Thoracic Surgeons. *Circulation.* 2012;**126**:e354–471
6. White HD, *et al.* Acute myocardial infarction. *Lancet.* 2008;**372**:570–84
7. Terkelsen CJ, *et al.* Mortality rates in patients with ST elevation vs non-ST elevation acute myocardial infarction: observations from an unselected cohort. *Eur Heart J.* 2005;**26**:18–26
8. Tunstall-Pedoe H, *et al.* Contribution of trends in survival and coronary event rates to changes in coronary heart disease mortality: 10-year results from 37 WHO MONICA project populations. Monitoring trends and determinants in cardiovascular disease. *Lancet.* 1999;**353**:1547–57
9. Roger VL, *et al.* Executive summary: heart disease and stroke statistics—2012 update: a report from the American Heart Association. *Circulation.* 2012;**125**:188–97
10. Steg PG, *et al.* One-year cardiovascular event rates in outpatients with atherothrombosis. *JAMA.* 2007;**297**:1197–206
11. Laugsand LE, *et al.* Insomnia and the risk of acute myocardial infarction: a population study. *Circulation.* 2011;**124**: 2073–81
12. Nawrot TS, *et al.* Public health importance of triggers of myocardial infarction: a comparative risk assessment. *Lancet.* 2011;**377**:732–40
13. Yusuf S, *et al.* Effect of potentially modifiable risk factors associated with myocardial infarction in 52 countries (the INTERHEART study): case-control study. *Lancet.* 2004;**364**:937–52
14. Breton CV, *et al.* Childhood air pollutant exposure and carotid artery intima-media thickness in young adults. *Circulation.* 2012;**126**:1614–20
15. Gold DR, *et al.* New insights into pollution and the cardiovascular system: 2010 to 2012. *Circulation.* 2013;**127**:1903–13
16. Tonne CWP, *et al.* Long-term exposure to air pollution is associated with survival following acute coronary syndrome. *Eur Heart J.* 2013;**34**:1306–11
17. 2012 ACCF/AHA focused update incorporated into the ACCF/AHA 2007 guidelines for the management of patients with unstable angina/non–ST-elevation myocardial infarction. *JACC* 2013:doi.org/10.1016/j.jacc.2013.1001.1014
18. Lidegaard O, *et al.* Thrombotic stroke and myocardial infarction with hormonal contraception. *N Engl J Med.* 2012;**366**:2257–66
19. Ranthe MF, *et al.* Pregnancy loss and later risk of atherosclerotic disease. *Circulation.* 2013;**127**:1775–82
20. Sliwa K, *et al.* Contribution of the human immunodeficiency virus/acquired immunodeficiency syndrome epidemic to *de novo* presentations of heart disease in the Heart of Soweto Study cohort. *Eur Heart J.* 2012;**33**:866–74
21. Fischer M, *et al.* Distinct heritable patterns of angiographic coronary artery disease in families with myocardial infarction. *Circulation.* 2005;**111**:855–62
22. Schunkert H, *et al.* Large-scale association analysis identifies 13 new susceptibility loci for coronary artery disease. *Nat Genet.* 2011;**43**:333–8
23. Harrison SC, *et al.* Association of a sequence variant in dab2ip with coronary heart disease. *Eur Heart J.* 2012;**33**:881–8
24. O'Donnell CJ, *et al.* Genome-wide association study for coronary artery calcification with follow-up in myocardial infarction. *Circulation.* 2011;**124**:2855–64
25. Roberts R, *et al.* Genes and coronary artery disease: where are we? *J Am Coll Cardiol.* 2012;**60**:1715–21
26. Chan K PR, Newcombe P, *et al.* Association between the chromosome 9p21 locus and angiographic coronary artery disease burden: title and subtitle break. A collaborative meta-analysis. *J Am Coll Cardiol.* 2013;**61**:957–70
27. Reilly MP, *et al.* Identification of ADAMTS7 as a novel locus for coronary atherosclerosis and association of ABO with myocardial infarction in the presence of coronary atherosclerosis: two genome-wide association studies. *Lancet.* 2011;**377**:383–92
28. Charchar FJ, *et al.* Inheritance of coronary artery disease in men: an analysis of the role of the y chromosome. *Lancet.* 2012;**379**:915–22

29. Crea F, *et al.* Pathogenesis of acute coronary syndromes. *J Am Coll Cardiol.*2013;**61**:1–11
30. LibbyPL. Mechanisms of acute coronary syndromes and their implications for therapy. *N Engl J Med.* 2013;**268**:2004–13
31. Falk E, *et al.* Update on acute coronary syndromes: The pathologists' view. *European Heart Journal.* 2013;**34**:719–28
32. Narula J, *et al.* Histopathologic characteristics of atherosclerotic coronary disease and implications of the findings for the invasive and noninvasive detection of vulnerable plaques. *J Am Coll Cardiol.* 2013;**61**:1–11
33. Crea F, *et al.* Pathogenesis of acute coronary syndromes. *J Am Coll Cardiol.* 2013;**61**:1–11
34. Michel JB, *et al.* Intraplaque haemorrhages as the trigger of plaque vulnerability. *Eur Heart J.* 2011;**32**:1977–85, 1985a, 1985b, 1985c
35. Mizuno K, *et al.* Angioscopic evaluation of coronary artery thrombi in acute coronary syndromes. *N Engl J Med.* 1992;**326**:287–91
36. Arbab-Zadeh A, *et al.* Acute coronary events. *Circulation.* 2012;**125**:1147–56
37. Casscells W, *et al.* Vulnerable atherosclerotic plaque: a multifocal disease. *Circulation.* 2003;**107**:2072–5
38. Reynolds HR, *et al.* Mechanisms of myocardial infarction in women without angiographically obstructive coronary artery disease. *Circulation.* 2011;**124**:1414–25
39. DeWood MA, *et al.* Prevalence of total coronary occlusion during the early hours of transmural myocardial infarction. *N Engl J Med.* 1980;**303**:897–902
40. Vancraeynest D, *et al.* Imaging the vulnerable plaque. *J Am Coll Cardiol.* 2011;**57**:1961–79
41. Silvain J, *et al.* Composition of coronary thrombus in acute myocardial infarction. *J Am Coll Cardiol.* 2011;**57**:1359–67
42. Ambrose JA, *et al.* Angiographic progression of coronary artery disease and the development of myocardial infarction. *J Am Coll Cardiol.* 1988;**12**:56–62
43. Giroud D, *et al.* Relation of the site of acute myocardial infarction to the most severe coronary arterial stenosis at prior angiography. *Am J Cardiol.* 1992;**69**:729–2
44. Little WC, *et al.* Can coronary angiography predict the site of a subsequent myocardial infarction in patients with mild to moderate coronary artery disease? *Circulation.* 1988;**78**:1157–66
45. Falk E. Plaque rupture with severe pre-existing stenosis precipitating coronary thrombosis. Characteristics of coronary atherosclerotic plaques underlying fatal occlusive thrombi. *Br Heart J.* 1983;**50**:127–34
46. Finn AV, *et al.* Concept of vulnerable/unstable plaque. *Arterioscler Thromb Vasc Biol.* 2010;**30**:1282–92
47. Qiao JH, *et al.* The severity of coronary atherosclerosis at sites of plaque rupture with occlusive thrombosis. *J Am Coll Cardiol.* 1991;**17**:1138–42
48. Alderman EL, *et al.* Five-year angiographic follow-up of factors associated with progression of coronary artery disease in the Coronary Artery Surgery Study (CASS). CASS participating investigators and staff. *J Am Coll Cardiol.* 1993;**22**:1141–54
49. Hulten EA, *et al.* Prognostic value of cardiac computed tomography angiography: a systematic review and meta-analysis. *J Am Coll Cardiol.* 2011;**57**:1237–47
50. Kaski JC, *et al.* Rapid angiographic progression of coronary artery disease in patients with angina pectoris. The role of complex stenosis morphology. *Circulation.* 1995;**92**: 2058–65
51. Stone GW, *et al.* A prospective natural history study of coronary atherosclerosis. *N Engl J Med.* 2011;**364**:226–35
52. Mancini GB, *et al.* Angiographic disease progression and residual risk of cardiovascular events while on optimal medical therapy: observations from the COURAGE trial. *Circ Cardiovasc Interv.* 2011;**4**:545–52
53. Scirica BM, *et al.* Relationship between non-sustained ventricular tachycardia after non-ST elevation acute coronary syndrome and sudden cardiac death: observations from the metabolic efficiency with ranolazine for less ischaemia in non-ST elevation acute coronary syndrome-thrombolysis in myocardial infarction 36 (MERLIN-TIMI 36) randomized controlled trial. *Circulation.* 2010;**122**:455–62
54. Tweet MSHS, *et al.* Clinical features, management, and prognosis of spontaneous coronary artery dissection. *Circulation.* 2012;**126**:579–88
55. Shah BN, *et al.* The hibernating myocardium: current concepts, diagnostic dilemmas, and clinical challenges in the post-STICH era. *Eur Heart J.* 2013;**34**:1323–36
56. Libby P, *et al.* Pathophysiology of coronary artery disease. *Circulation.* 2005;**111**:3481–8

Chapter 27

Unstable angina and non-ST elevation myocardial infarction

Definition

Unstable angina (UA) presents as rest angina (usually lasting >20 minutes), new-onset (within the past 2 months and, at least, Canadian Cardiovascular Society III in severity), and increasing angina (in severity and frequency). Non-ST elevation myocardial infarction (NSTEMI) occurs when the ischaemia is sufficiently severe and prolonged to cause myocardial damage that results in the release of a biomarker of myocardial necrosis into the circulation (TnT, TnI, or CK-MB).[1–3]

Presentation

Typical symptoms are **chest pain, indigestion or 'heartburn', nausea and/or vomiting, persistent shortness of breath, or dizziness and/or loss of consciousness**, although diabetics and the elderly may have vague symptoms or no symptoms at all. Differential diagnosis of chest pain is discussed in Chapter 29 on stable IHD. Patients at increased risk of ACS, such as those with known coronary artery disease, cerebral or peripheral vascular disease, diabetes mellitus, chronic kidney disease, or a 10-year risk greater than 20% as calculated by Framingham equations, and with symptoms suggestive of an ACS should be evaluated by trained specialists.

Patients with symptoms that may represent an ACS should be instructed to chew 150–325 mg of aspirin (unless already taken or contraindicated) and one dose of nitroglycerin sublingually or by buccal spray (0.4 mg). If symptoms do not respond to medication, emergency transfer to an emergency department with facilities for ECG recording, biomarker determination, and evaluation by a physician is recommended.[1–3] Patients who respond to medication or have chest pain lasting <20 min and in the absence of high-risk features may be seen in an outpatient facility for further evaluation.[1]

Diagnosis

Immediate 12-lead ECG, and then serial ECGs in 15–30 min intervals if the initial ECG is non-diagnostic, are taken. Symptoms of ACS associated with **ST segment depression, T wave inversion, or non-specific ST-T abnormalities** suggest UA/NSTEMI. These findings are present in 30–50% of patients with an ACS. However, apart from assisting in diagnosis, they also carry adverse prognostic significance when present as new findings.[4] New ST segment deviation, even of only 0.05 mV, is an important and specific measure of ischaemia and prognosis. T wave inversion is sensitive for ischaemia but is less specific, unless it is marked (≥0.3 mV).[4,5] Comparison with previous ECGs is valuable for the assessment of ST changes.

Cardiac biomarkers (preferably a cardiac-specific troponin) are measured, and, if negative within 6 h of the onset of symptoms, they are remeasured within 6–12 h after symptom onset. The degree of elevation of troponin is associated with mortality in ACS.[6,7] Biomarkers for risk stratification in patients with established diagnosis of ACS are CRP, white blood cell count, BNP or NT-pro-BNP, and GDF-15, a member of the transforming growth factor family that is released by myocytes during ischaemia and reperfusion.[8–10] A rapid protocol (0 and 3 h) is recommended when highly sensitive troponin tests are available (I–B, ESC 2011). (Figure 27.1). Accelerated diagnostic protocols (2 h), including TIMI score, ECG, and triple marker panels (CK-MB, myoglobin, and troponin), may identify low-risk patients that can be discharged early.[11]

Stress testing and CT coronary angiography In patients with acute chest pain, CT angiography in an experienced centre is faster to obtain than a stress test and improves diagnostic ability albeit at an increased radiation exposure.[12,13]

Risk stratification models, such as TIMI (Thrombolysis In Myocardial Infarction),[14] GRACE (Global Registry of Acute Coronary Event),[15] PURSUIT, or FRISC, are useful for subsequent decision-making (Tables 27.1 to 27.3). Clinical features, ECG, and laboratory findings have been incorporated into these clinical risk scores that stratify patients into risk categories. The most simple, but less accurate, is the TIMI. The TIMI is mainly recommended by the ACCF/AHA 2012,[1] and the GRACE by the ESC 2011 guidelines.[1] Resting myocardial perfusion imaging (MPI) in patients with ongoing chest discomfort and non-diagnostic ECG or biomarker results will also identify active ischaemia. However, MPI cannot distinguish between recent and older infarcts; thus, abnormal MPI is not specific for ACS.[16] CMR can provide substantial information regarding ventricular function, ongoing ischaemia/perfusion, early and late regions of infarction, and coronary anatomy.[17] The greatest benefit of non-invasive CT angiography is to exclude CAD in patients with a low to intermediate probability of ACS.[18]

Therapy

Oxygen Should be administered when the arterial saturation is <90%.

Nitroglycerin Sublingually or as a buccal spray (0.4 mg), can be given for pain relief every 5 min for a total of three doses (Table 27.4). If the pain persists or hypertension or heart failure is present, IV nitroglycerin (initial dose 5–10 micrograms/min, with 10 micrograms/min increases until the systolic BP falls below 100 mmHg) can be given. Contraindicated if sildenafil has been taken within the previous 24 h (or tadalafil in the previous 48 h).

Morphine Is used for pain relief, although there are observational indications that it may increase mortality in ACS.[19]

Antiplatelets

Aspirin

It should be administered as soon as possible and then indefinitely, unless if there is a history of documented allergy or active bleeding. A loading dose of 162–325 mg po (ACC/AHA) or 150–300 mg po (ESC) or 150–300 IV mg, followed by 75–162 mg/day po (ACC/AHA), or 75–100 mg/day po (ESC) should be given indefinitely. Aspirin mainly acts by irreversibly inhibiting platelet

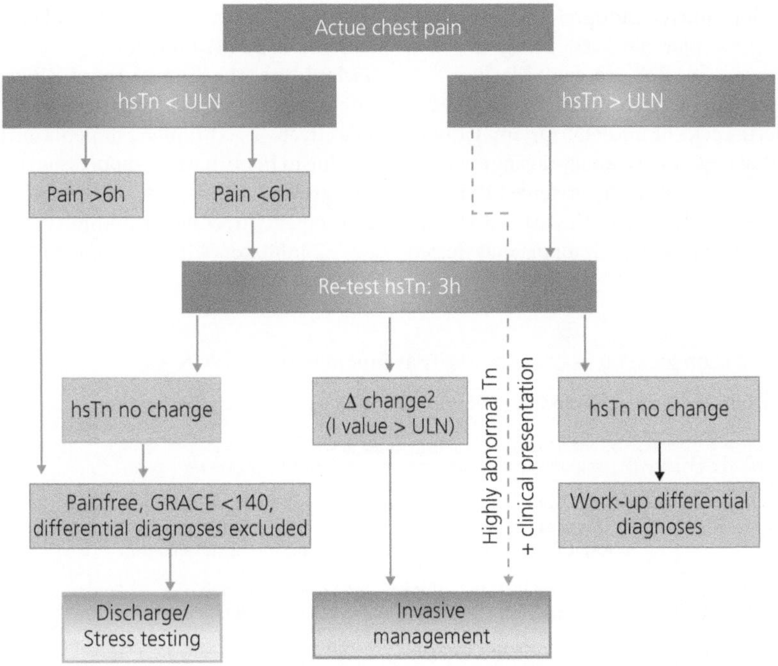

Figure 27.1 ESC 2011. Rapid rule-out of ACS with high-sensitivity troponin.

GRACE: Global Registry of Acute Coronary Events; hsTn: high-sensitivity troponin; ULN: upper limit of normal, 99th percentile of healthy controls. [a]Δ change, dependent on assay. At the end of this step, the decision has to be made whether the patient should go on to cardiac catheterization. ESC guidelines for the management of acute coronary syndromesin patients presenting without persistent ST-segment elevation. *Eur Heart J*. 2011;**32**:2999–3054.

Table 27.1 The TIMI risk score predictor variables

TIMI risk score	All-cause mortality, new or recurrent MI, or severe recurrent ischaemia requiring urgent revascularization through 14 d after randomization (%)
0–1	4.7
2	8.3
3	13.2
4	19.9
5	26.2
6–7	40.9

The TIMI risk score is determined by the sum of the presence of 7 variables at admission; 1 point is given for each of the following variables:

1. Age ≥65 years
2. At least three risk factors for coronary artery disease, including family history, hypertension, hypercholesterolaemia, diabetes, smoking
3. Prior coronary stenosis ≥50%
4. ST segment deviation
5. At least two anginal events in prior 24 hours
6. Use of aspirin in prior 7 days
7. Elevated serum cardiac markers.

Prior coronary stenosis of 50% or more remained relatively insensitive to missing information and remained significant predictor of events.

Antman EM, *et al*. The TIMI risk score for unstable angina/non-ST-elevation MI: method for prognostication and therapeutic decision making. *JAMA* 2000;**284:**835–42.

cyclooxygenase 1 (COX-1) and decreasing the synthesis of thromboxane A_2. The effects of aspirin are only reversed when new unaffected platelets enter the circulation, which occurs every 7 to 14 days. Aspirin also inhibits prostacyclin production in gastric endothelial cells and, therefore, carries a slightly greater risk for gastric ulcer formation than the $P2Y_{12}$ inhibitors. A **proton pump inhibitor (PPI)**, preferably not omeprazole, should be added to patients with a history of duodenal ulcer or GI bleeding, age >65 years, or concurrent use of anticoagulants or steroids. In patients at high risk for gastrointestinal ulceration, the use of prophylactic proton pump inhibition with aspirin is safer than clopidogrel alone without a proton pump inhibitor. Aspirin resistance is extremely rare; pseudoresistance, reflecting delayed and reduced drug absorption, may complicate enteric coated but not immediate release aspirin.[20] The administration of NSAIDs (selective COX-2 or not), with or without aspirin, is contraindicated due to increased risk of infarction and myocardial rupture. Aspirin should not be withheld before elective or non-elective CABG.

$P2Y_{12}$ receptor blockers

Added to aspirin or used instead of it in cases of aspirin allergy.

Thienopyridines (ticlopidine, clopidogrel, and prasugrel) are irreversible $P2Y_{12}$ receptor blockers. **Ticagrelor** is a non-thienopyridine reversible $P2Y_{12}$ receptor blocker.

Clopidogrel and prasugrel are 'pro-drugs' that require activation in the liver via the cytochrome P450 system. Ticagrelor is not a pro–drug but requires twice daily dosing owing to its short half-life. Ticagrelor is now the preferred $P2Y_{12}$ receptor blocker in UA/NSTEMI, both by the ESC (2011) and AACF/AHA (2012) guidelines, especially for patients treated invasively (Tables 27.4 to 27.7 and Figure 27.2). There is no antidote for P2Y12 inhibitors.

Ticlopidine, the first of the ADP receptor blockers, is rarely used in practice because of uncommon, but serious, side effects (e.g. thrombocytopenia purpura and neutropenia due to bone marrow suppression).

Ticagrelor (loading dose 180 mg po, 90 mg twice daily) is a cyclopentyltriazolopyrimidine and a reversibly binding P2Y12 inhibitor, with a plasma half-life of <12 h. It is an

Table 27.2 GRACE prediction score for all-cause mortality at 6 months after an ACS

Risk calculator for 6-month postdischarge mortality after hospitalization for acute coronary syndrome

Record the points for each variable at the bottom left and sum the points to calculate the total risk score. Fine the total score on the x-axis of the nanogram plot. The corresponding probability on the y-axis is the estimated probability of all-cause mortality from hospital discharge to 6 months.

Medical history		Findings at initial hospital presentation		Findings during hospitalization	
① Age in years	Points	④ Resting heart rate, beats/min	Points	⑦ Initial serum creatinline, mg/dL	Points
≤29	0				
30–39	0	≤49.9	1	0–0.39	1
40–49	18	50–69.9	3	0.4–0.79	3
50–59	36	70–89.9	9	0.8–1.19	5
60–69	55	90–109.9	14	1.2–1.59	7
70–79	73	110–149.9	23	1.5–1.99	9
80–89	81	150–199.9	35	2–3.99	15
≥90	100	≥200	43	≥4	20
② History of congestive Heart failure	24	⑤ Systolic blood pressure, mm Hg		⑧ Elevated cardiac enzymes	15
③ History of myocardial infarction	12	≤79.9	24	⑨ No in-hospital Percutaneous Coronary invervention	12
		80–99.9	22		
		100–119.9	16		
		120–139.9	14		
		140–159.9	10		
		160–199.9	4		
		≥200	0		
		⑥ ST-Segment Depression	11		

Points

① ______
② ______
③ ______
④ ______
⑤ ______
⑥ ______
⑦ ______
⑧ ______
⑨ ______

Total risk score ______ (Sum of points)

Mortality risk ______ (From plot)

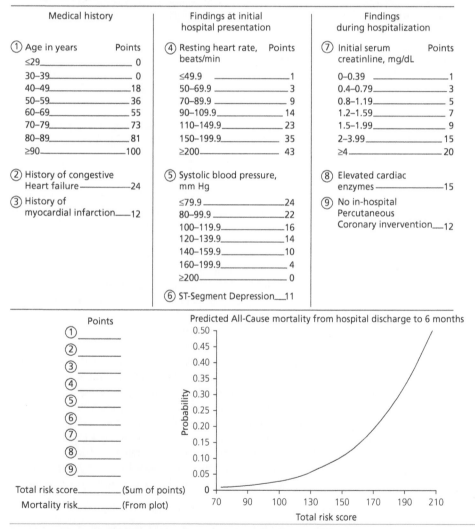

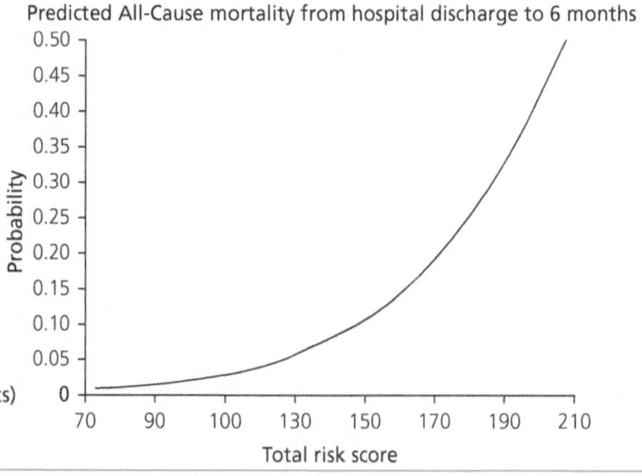

Eagle KA, *et al.* A validated prediction model for all forms of acute coronary syndrome: estimating the risk of 6-month postdischarge death in an international registry. *JAMA* 2004;**291**:2727–33

(Continued)

Table 27.2 (Continued)

ESC GL 2011 GL on UA/NSTEMI. Mortality in hospital and at 6 months in low, intermediate, and high risk categories in registry populations, according to the GRACE risk score.

Rick category (tertile)	GRACE risk score	In-hospital death (%)
Low	≤108	<1
Intermediate	109–140	1–3
High	>140	>3
Risk category (tertile)	**GRACE risk score**	**Post-discharge to 6-month death (%)**
Low	≤88	<3
Intermediate	89–118	3–8
High	>118	>8

Table 27.3 Risk stratification

ACCF/AHA 2012 GL on UA/NSTEMI. Short-term risk of death or non-fatal MI in patients with UA/NSTEMI

	High risk	Intermediate risk	Low risk
Feature	**At least one of the following features must be present:**	**No high-risk features are present, but patient must have one of the following:**	**No high- or intermediate-risk features are present, but patient may have any of the following:**
History	Accelerating tempo of ischaemic symptoms in preceding 48 h	Prior MI, peripheral or cerebrovascular disease, or CABG Prior aspirin use	
Character of pain	Prolonged ongoing (>20 min) rest pain	Prolonged (>20 min) rest angina, now resolved, with moderate or high likelihood of CAD Rest angina (>20 min) or relieved with rest or sublingual NTG Nocturnal angina New-onset or progressive CCS class III or IV angina in previous 2 wk without prolonged (>20 min) rest pain but with intermediate or high likelihood of CAD	Increased angina frequency, severity, or duration Angina provoked at a lower threshold New-onset angina, with onset 2 wk to 2 mo before presentation
Clinical findings	Pulmonary oedema, most likely due to ischaemia New or worsening mitral regurgitation murmur S_3 or new/ worsening rales Hypotension, bradycardia, or tachycardia Age >75 y	Age >70 y	
ECG	Angina at rest with transient ST segment changes >0.5 mm Bundle branch block, new or presumed new Sustained ventricular tachycardia	T wave changes Pathological Q waves or resting ST depression <1 mm in multiple lead groups (anterior, interior, lateral)	Normal or unchanged ECG
Cardiac markers	Elevated cardiac TnT, TnI, or CK-MB (i.e. TnT or TnI >0.1 ng/mL)	Slightly elevated cardiac TnT, TnI, or CK-MB (i.e. TnT >0.01 but <0.1 ng/mL)	Normal

Estimation of the short-term risks of death and non-fatal cardiac ischaemic events in UA or NSTEMI is a complex, multivariable problem that cannot be fully specified in a table such as this. Therefore, the table is meant to offer general guidance and illustration, rather than rigid algorithms.

CABG indicates coronary artery bypass graft; CAD, coronary artery disease; CCS, Canadian Cardiovascular Society; CK-MB, creatine kinase-MB fraction; ECG, electrocardiogram; MI, myocardial infarction; NTG, nitroglycerin; N/A, not available; TnI, troponin I; TnT, troponin T; and UA/NSTEMI, unstable angina/non-ST elevation myocardial infarction.

2012 ACCF/AHA focused update incorporated into the ACCF/AHA 2007 Guidelines for the management of patients with unstable angina/non–ST-elevation myocardial infarction. *J Am Coll Cardiol.* 2013;**61**:e179–347.

(Continued)

Table 27.3 (Continued)

ACCF/AHA 2012 GL on UA/NSTEMI. Recommendations for early risk stratification	
A rapid clinical determination of the likelihood risk of obstructive CAD (i.e., high, intermediate, or low) in all patients with chest discomfort or other symptoms suggestive of an ACS.	I-C
Patients who present with chest discomfort or other ischemic symptoms should undergo early risk stratification for the risk of cardiovascular events (e.g., death or [re] MI) that focuses on history, including anginal symptoms, physical findings, ECG findings, and biomarkers of cardiac injury.	I-C
A 12-lead ECG should be shown to an experienced emergency physician as soon as possible after ED arrival, with a goal of within 10 min of ED arrival for all patients with chest discomfort (or anginal equivalent) or other symptoms suggestive of ACS.	I-B
Serial ECGs, initially at 15- to 30-min intervals to detect the potential for development of ST-segment elevation or depression, if the initial ECG is not diagnostic but the patient remains symptomatic and there is high clinical suspicion for ACS	I-B
Cardiac biomarkers in all patients who present with chest discomfort consistent with ACS	I-B
A cardiac-specific troponin is the preferred marker in all patients who present with chest discomfort consistent with ACS	I-B
Patients with negative cardiac biomarkers within 6 h of the onset of symptoms should have biomarkers remeasured 8 to 12 h after symptom onset.	I-B
The initial evaluation of the patient should include the consideration of noncoronary causes for the development of unexplained symptoms.	I-C
Use of risk-stratification models, such as the Thrombolysis In Myocardial Infarction (TIMI) or Global Registry of Acute Coronary Events (GRACE) risk score or the Platelet Glycoprotein IIb/IIIa in Unstable Angina: Receptor Suppression Using Integrilin Therapy (PURSUIT) risk model, can be useful	IIa-B
Remeasure positive biomarkers at 6-to 8-h intervals 2 to 3 times or until levels have peaked, as an index of infarct size and dynamics of necrosis	IIa-B
Obtain supplemental ECG leads V7 through V9 in patients whose initial ECG is nondiagnostic to rule out MI due to left circumflex occlusion	IIa-B
Continuous 12-lead ECG monitoring as an alternative to serial 12-lead recordings in patients whose initial ECG is nondiagnostic	IIa-B
For patients who present within 6 h of the onset of symptoms suggestive of ACS: assessment of an early marker of cardiac injury (e.g., myoglobin) in conjunction with a late marker (e.g., troponin) delta CK-MB mass in conjunction with 2-h delta troponin myoglobin in conjunction with CK-MB mass or troponin when measured at baseline and 90 min	IIb-B IIb-B IIb-B
Measurement of B-type natriuretic peptide (BNP) or NT-pro- BNP to supplement assessment of global risk in patients with suspected ACS	IIb-B
Total CK (without MB), aspartate aminotransferase (AST, SGOT), alanine transaminase, beta-hydroxybutyric dehydrogenase, and/or lactate dehydrogenase should not be utilized as primary tests for the detection of myocardial injury	III-C

2012 ACCF/AHA focused update incorporated into the ACCF/AHA 2007 Guidelines for the management of patients with unstable angina/non–ST-elevation myocardial infarction. *J Am Coll Cardiol*. 2013;**61**:e179–347.

ESC 2011 GL on UA/NSTEMI. Recommendations for diagnosis and risk stratification	
Diagnosis and short-term ischaemic/bleeding risk stratification should be based on a combination of clinical history, symptoms, physical findings, ECG (repeated or continuous ST monitoring), and biomarkers.	I-A
ACS patients should be admitted preferably to dedicated chest pain units or coronary care units.	I-C
Use established risk scores for prognosis and bleeding (e.g. GRACE, CRUSADE).	I-B
A 12-lead ECG within 10 min after first medical contact and immediately read by an experienced physician. Repeat in the case of recurrence of symptoms and after 6–9 and 24 h, and before hospital discharge.	I-B
Additional ECG leads (V3R, V4R, V7–V9) when routine leads are inconclusive.	I-C
Blood has to be drawn promptly for troponin (cardiac troponin T or I) measurement. The result should be available within 60 min. The test should be repeated 6–9 h after initial assessment if the first measurement is not conclusive. Repeat testing after 12–24 h if the clinical condition is still suggestive of ACS.	I-A
A rapid rule-out protocol (0 and 3 h) is recommended when highly sensitive troponin tests are available. Echocardiogram for all patients to evaluate regional and global LV function and I-C to rule in or rule out differential diagnoses.	I-B
Coronary angiography in patients in whom the extent of CAD or the culprit lesion has to be determined.	I-C
Coronary CT angiography as an alternative to invasive angiography to exclude ACS when there is a low to intermediate likelihood of CAD and when troponin and ECG are inconclusive.	IIa-B
In patients without recurrence of pain, normal ECG findings, negative troponin tests, and a low-risk score, a non-invasive stress test for inducible ischaemia is recommended before deciding on an invasive strategy.	I-A

ESC guidelines for the management of acute coronary syndromes in patients presenting without persistent ST-segment elevation. *Eur Heart J*. 2011;**32**:2999–3054.

Table 27.4 Medical therapy of UA/NSTEMI

ACCF/AHA 2012 GL on UA/NSTEMI. Anti-ischaemic and analgesic therapy	
O_2 (if SaO_2 <90%)	I-B
Bed/chair rest with continuous ECG monitoring	I-C
O_2 (first 6 h)	IIa-C
Nitroglycerin sublingual (0.4 mg evey 5 min, up to three doses)	I-C
Morphine sulfate IV in uncontrolled ischemic chest discomfort despite NTG, provided that additional therapy is used to manage the underlying ischemia	IIa-B
Nitrates IV for persistent ischaemia, heart failure, or hypertension	I-B
Nitrates in SBP <90 mmHg (≥30 mmHg below baseline), <50 bpm, >100 bpm without asymptomatic HF, or RV infarction	III-C
Nitrates within 24 h of sildenafil or 48 h of tadalafil use (time after vardenafil not determined)	III-C
Beta blockers orally if no signs of acute heart failure or a low-output state, increased risk for cardiogenic shock, PR interval >0.24 s, 2nd or 3rd AV block, active asthma, or reactive airway disease	I-B
Beta blockers IV if no signs of acute heart failure or a low-output state, increased risk for cardiogenic shock, PR interval >0.24 s, 2nd or 3rd AV block, active asthma, or reactive airway disease	IIa-B
Beta blockers IV in HF or low-output state, other risk factors for cardiogenic shock or other contraindications	III-A
Non-dihydropyridines calcium channel blockers in recurrent ischaemia, no LV dysfunction, and contraindication of beta blockers	I-B
Non-dihydropyridines calcium channel blockers in recurrent ischaemia, after beta blockers and nitrates have been used.	IIa-C
Extended release non-dihydropyridines calcium channel blockers	IIb-B
Immediate release dihydropyridines calcium channel blockers with beta blockers for ongoing ischaemia or hypertension	IIa-C
Immediate release dihydropyridines calcium channel blockers without beta blockers	III-A
ACEI in LVEF <40% or pulmonary congestion	I-A
ARB in LVEF <40% or pulmonary congestion and ACEI intolerance	I-A
ACEI in all patients	IIA-B
Intravenous ACEI (possible exception patients with refractory hypertension)	III-B
Intra-aortic balloon pump counterpulsation	IIa-C
NSAIDs, whether non-selective or COX-2-selective, should be discontinued	I-C
2012 ACCF/AHA focused update incorporated into the ACCF/AHA 2007 Guidelines for the management of patients with unstable angina/non–ST-elevation myocardial infarction. *J Am Coll Cardiol.* 2013;**61**:e179–347.	
ESC 2011 GL on UA/NSTEMI	
Anti-ischaemic drugs	
Oral or IV nitrates for angina in recurrent angina and/or HF	I-C
Oral beta blockers in LV dysfunction	I-B
Patients on beta blockers should continue unless in Killip class ≥III	I-B
Calcium channel blockers in recurrent ischaemia, despite nitrates and beta blockers (dihydropyridines), or in contraindication of beta blockers (benzothiazepines or phenylethylamines)	I-B
Calcium channel blockers in vasospastic angina	I-B
IV beta blockers if Killip class <III, hypertension, and/or tachycardia	IIa-C
Nifedipine or other dihydropyridines without beta blockers	III-B

(Continued)

Table 27.4 (Continued)

Secondary prevention	
Beta blockers in all patients with LVEF ≤40%	I-A
ACE inhibitors within 24 h in all patients with LVEF ≤40% and in patients with heart failure, diabetes, hypertension, or CKD, unless contraindicated	I-A
ACE inhibitors for all other patients to prevent recurrence of ischaemic events, with preference given to agents and doses of proven efficacy	I-B
ARBs patients who are intolerant to ACE inhibitors, with preference given to agents and doses of proven efficacy	I-B
Aldosterone blockade with eplerenone in patients after MI who are already being treated with ACE inhibitors and beta blockers and who have an LVEF ≤35% and either diabetes or heart failure, without significant renal dysfunction (serum creatinine >221 μmol/L [>2.5 mg/dL] for men and >177 μmol/L [>2.0 mg/dL] for women) or hyperkalaemia	I-A
Statin therapy with target LDL-C levels <1.8 mmol/L (<70 mg/dL) initiated early after admission	I-B

active drug (clopidogrel and prasugrel are pro-active drugs) and has been shown to reduce mortality in ACS compared to clopidogrel without increased bleeding (PLATO trial).[21] Ticagrelor increases levels of drugs metabolized through CYP3A, such as simvastatin, whilst moderate CYP3A inhibitors, such as diltiazem, increase the levels and reduce the speed of offset of the effect of ticagrelor. Ventricular pauses, mostly in the acute phase of ACS due to sinus node suppression, and mild dyspnoea without any adverse effect on cardiac or pulmonary function may be seen and are believed to be adenosine-mediated.[22] They are of no clinical significance,[23] and higher adenosine levels induced by ticagrelor probably contribute to its efficacy. A lack of efficacy among American patients and a probable reduced effect in co-administration with high-dose aspirin (325 mg as opposed to 75 mg, attributed to increased vascular resistance through inhibition of cyclooxygenase within blood vessels) are probably not matters of concern.[24,25] A slightly greater increase in serum creatinine was seen in the PLATO trial with ticagrelor compared with clopidogrel, but the difference was no longer apparent 1 month after cessation of treatment. Rates of gastrointestinal disturbance and rash are similar with ticagrelor compared with clopidogrel.[2] Ticagrelor, compared with clopidogrel, was associated with similar total major bleeding but increased non-procedure-related major bleeding.[26] Patients with acute coronary syndrome with a prior history of ischaemic stroke or TIA have higher rates of adverse cardiac events and stroke, and ticagrelor may be preferable to clopidogrel.[27]

Clopidogrel (loading dose 300–600 mg po followed by 75 mg/day, starting on presentation) is recommended for up to 1 year (CURE trial).[28] A higher dose 150 mg/daily may be used for the first 7 days in patients who had a loading dose of 600 mg for PCI, provided that the risk of bleeding is low.

There is a high degree of clopidogrel response variability related to genetic and non-genetic factors. Binding of metabolized clopidogrel to platelet adenosine diphosphate (ADP) receptors on the platelet surface is catalyzed mainly by the cytochrome enzyme CYP2C19. Loss-of-function polymorphisms in the gene encoding for CYP2C19 are associated with a reduced response to clopidogrel (2–14% of patients) and a potentially increased risk of adverse cardiovascular events.[29,30] However, among patients with acute coronary syndromes or atrial fibrillation, the effect of clopidogrel, as compared with placebo, has been found consistent, irrespective of CYP2C19 loss-of-function carrier status.[31,32] Other genetic variations, such as the ABCB1 3435 TT genotype, may also affect the pharmacokinetics and clinical efficacy of clopidogrel.[32] Platelet function assays can measure the effect of ADP or P2Y12 activation on platelet aggregation, receptor expression, or the level of intracellular molecules (e.g. vasodilator-stimulated phosphoprotein phosphorylation), thereby directly or indirectly measuring the platelet inhibitory effect of clopidogrel. In practice, three categories of tests are commercially available: aggregation-based tests (light transmission or impedance platelet aggregometry), shear-dependent tests, and flow cytometry tests.[33] CYP2C19 genotyping is possible only in specialty laboratories and requires several days to deliver results. There is now insufficient evidence to recommend either routine genetic or platelet function testing at the present time (ACC/AHA 2012 IIb-B/C, ESC 2001 IIb-B). In the ARCTIC trial, bedside platelet reactivity testing with treatment adjustment (additional IV aspirin or adding a IIb/IIIa antagonist) did not improve outcomes compared to standard antiplatelet therapy.[34] Higher clopidogrel maintenance (150 mg) doses have not improved outcome in patients with higher residual platelet reactivity that defined poor response.[35,36] Ticagrelor is probably the alternative in high-risk patients with poor response (i.e. patients with stent thrombosis while taking clopidogrel) since insufficient platelet inhibition may also occur with prasugrel.[37]

Table 27.5 ACCF/AHA 2012 on UA/NSTEMI. Antiplatelet and anticoagulant therapy

All patients	
Aspirin 162–325 mg chewed, as soon as possible and then indefinitely in patients who tolerate it	I-A
A loading dose, followed by daily maintenance dose of clopidogrel, or	I-B
Prasugrel* (in PCI-treated patients), or	I-C
Ticagrelor† in patients who are unable to take aspirin because of hypersensitivity or major GI intolerance despite PPIs	I-C
In patients at low risk for ischaemic events (e.g. TIMI risk score <2) or at high risk of bleeding and who are already receiving aspirin and a P2Y12 receptor inhibitor, upstream GP IIb/IIIa inhibitors are not recommended	III-B
Anticoagulant therapy should be added to antiplatelet therapy as soon as possible	I-A
Initial conservative (i.e. non-invasive) strategy is selected	
Enoxaparin or UHF, or	I-A
Fondaparinux	I-B
Fondaparinux in increased risk of bleeding	I-B
Enoxaparin or fondaparinux preferable to UFH, unless CABG is planned within 24 h	IIa-B
Clopidogrel or ticagrelor† (loading dose, followed by daily maintenance dose) added to aspirin and anticoagulant as soon as possible and for up to 12 months	I-B
In recurrent symptoms/ischaemia, heart failure, or serious arrhythmias	
Diagnostic angiography with	I-A
IV GP IIb/IIIa inhibitor (eptifibatide or tirofiban), or	I-A
Clopidogrel, or	I-B
Ticagrelor†	I-B
Added to aspirin and anticoagulant therapy before angiography (upstream)	I-C
If recurrent ischaemic discomfort with aspirin, a P2Y12 receptor inhibitor (clopidogrel or ticagrelor), and anticoagulant therapy, add IIb/IIIa inhibitor	IIa-C
Omit IIb/IIIa inhibitor if bivalirudin is selected and at least 300 mg of clopidogrel was administered at least 6 hours earlier than planned PCI	IIa-B
Routine addition of eptifibatide or tirofiban to anticoagulant and oral antiplatelet therapy	IIb-B
Abciximab if PCI is not planned	III-A
No subsequent features that necessitate diagnostic angiography	
Stress test should be performed	I-B
High-risk patient:	
Diagnostic angiography	I-A
Low-risk patient or no stress test performed:	
Aspirin indefinitely	I-A
Clopidogrel or ticagrelor† for up to 12 months	I-B
Discontinue IV GP IIb/IIIa inhibitor if started previously	I-A
Continue UFH for 48 hours, or	I-A
Enoxaparin for the duration of hospitalization, up to 8 days, or	I-A
Fondaparinux for the duration of hospitalization, up to 8 days	I-B
All patients:	
LVEF should be measured	I-B
If LVEF is ≤0.40, perform diagnostic angiography	IIa-B
If LVEF is >0.40, perform stress testing	IIa-B
Medical therapy is selected as a management strategy and coronary artery disease was found on angiography	
Continue aspirin	I-A
Loading dose of clopidogrel or ticagrelor* if not given before diagnostic angiography	I-B
Discontinue IV GP IIb/IIIa inhibitor if started previously	I-B
Continue IV UFH for at least 48 hours or until discharge if given before diagnostic angiography**	I-A
Continue enoxaparin for duration of hospitalization, up to 8 days	I-A
Continue fondaparinux for duration of hospitalization, up to 8 days	I-B
Either discontinue bivalirudin or continue at a dose of 0.25 mg/kg per hour for up to 72 hours	I-B
Evidence of coronary atherosclerosis is present (e.g. luminal irregularities or intravascular ultrasound-demonstrated lesions), albeit without flow-limiting stenosis	
Long-term treatment with aspirin and other secondary prevention measures should be prescribed	I-C
Antiplatelet and anticoagulant therapy should be administered at the discretion of the clinician	I-C
Invasive therapy is selected	
Enoxaparin or UHF, or	I-A
Bivalirudin, or	I-B
Fondaparinux (together with UFH or enoxaparin)	I-B
Dual antiplatelet therapy on presentation for patients at medium or high risk	I-A
One of the following should be added to aspirin as early as possible:	
Clopidogrel 600 mg, or	I-B/A
Ticagrelor 180 mg,† or	I-B
IV GP IIb/IIIa inhibitor	I-A
IV eptifibatide and tirofiban are the preferred GP IIb/IIIa inhibitors, or	I-B
Prasugrel 60 mg (at time of definitive PCI and not later than 1 hour)*	I-B
(There are no data for therapy with two concurrent P2Y12 receptor inhibitors, and this is not recommended in the case of aspirin allergy)	

(Continued)

Table 27.5 (Continued)

Omit IIb/IIIa if bivalirudin was used and at least 300 mg clopidogrel were given at least 6 h earlier than angiography or PCI	IIa-B
If PCI is selected postangiography, IV GP IIb/IIIa inhibitor (abciximab, eptifibatide, or tirofiban) if not started before diagnostic angiography, particularly for troponin-positive and/or other high-risk patients	IIa-A
Upstream IIb/IIIa inhibitors in patients already receiving aspirin and a P2Y12 receptor inhibitor (clopidogrel or ticagrelor) and high-risk (elevated troponin levels, diabetes, or significant ST segment depression, and not at high risk for bleeding)	IIb-B
Loading dose of clopidogrel of 600 mg, followed by a higher maintenance dose of 150 mg daily for 6 days, then 75 mg daily if not high-risk for bleeding	IIb-B
Prasugrel* 60 mg before definition of coronary anatomy if both the risk for bleeding is low and the need for CABG is considered unlikely	IIb-C
In patients with prior history of stroke and/or TIA for whom PCI is planned, prasugrel* is potentially harmful as part of a dual antiplatelet therapy regimen	III-B
Post-PCI management	
Continue aspirin indefinitely	I-A
After PCI, 81 mg aspirin dose is preferred to higher doses	IIa-B
Loading dose of a P2Y12 receptor inhibitor if not started before diagnostic angiography	I-A
Either clopidogrel 75 mg od, prasugrel* 10 mg od, or ticagrelor†90 mg bd should be given for at least 12 months after DES and up to 12 months after BMS	I-B
If the risk of morbidity, because of bleeding, outweighs the anticipated benefit of P2Y12 receptor inhibitors, earlier discontinuation should be considered	I-C
Discontinue anticoagulant therapy after PCI for uncomplicated cases	I-B
Omit administration of an IV GP IIb/IIIa inhibitor if bivalirudin was selected as the anticoagulant and at least 300 mg of clopidogrel was administered at least 6 hours earlier	IIa-B
CABG is selected as a post-angiography management strategy	
1. Continue aspirin	I-A
2. P2Y12 receptor inhibitor is discontinued for at least	I-B
5 days for clopidogrel	I-B
5 days for ticagrelor*	I-C
7 days for prasugrel†	I-C
Unless the need for revascularization and/or the net benefit of the P2Y12 receptor inhibitor outweighs the potential risks of excess bleeding	I-C
3. Discontinue IV GP IIb/IIIa inhibitor (eptifibatide or tirofiban) 4 hours before CABG	I-B
Continue UFH 4. Anticoagulant therapy:	I-B
Discontinue enoxaparin 12 to 24 hours before CABG, and dose with UFH per institutional practice	I-B
Discontinue fondaparinux 24 hours before CABG, and dose with UFH per institutional practice	I-B
Discontinue bivalirudin 3 hours before CABG, and dose with UFH per institutional practice	I-B
All patients (and long-term therapy)	
If the risk of morbidity, because of bleeding, outweighs the anticipated benefit of P2Y12 receptor inhibitors, earlier discontinuation should be considered	I-C
Platelet function testing to determine platelet inhibitory response on P2Y12 if results of testing may alter management	IIb-B
Genotyping for a CYP2C19 loss of function variant on P2Y12 if results of testing may alter management	IIb-C
In indication for anticoagulation, warfarin with an INR of 2.0–3.0	IIb-B
Continuation of a P2Y12 receptor inhibitor beyond 12 months in patients following DES placement	IIb-C
Dipyridamole is not recommended as an antiplatelet agent post-UA/NSTEMI	III-B
IV fibrinolytic therapy is not indicated in patients without acute ST segment elevation, a true posterior MI, or a presumed new left bundle branch block	III-A

† The recommended maintenance dose of aspirin to be used with ticagrelor is 81 mg daily. The benefits of ticagrelor were observed, irrespective of prior therapy with clopidogrel. Issues of patient compliance may be especially important. Consideration should be given to the potential, and as yet undetermined, risk of intracranial haemorrhage in patients with prior stroke or TIA.

* Patients weighing <60 kg have an increased exposure to the active metabolite of prasugrel and an increased risk of bleeding on a 10 mg once daily maintenance dose. Consideration should be given to lowering the maintenance dose to 5 mg in patients who weigh <60 kg, although the effectiveness and safety of the 5 mg dose have not been studied prospectively. For post-PCI patients, a daily maintenance dose should be given for at least 12 months for patients receiving DES and up to 12 months for patients receiving BMS, unless the risk of bleeding outweighs the anticipated net benefit afforded by a P2Y12 receptor inhibitor. Do not use prasugrel in patients with active pathological bleeding or a history of TIA or stroke. In patients aged ≥75 y, prasugrel is generally not recommended because of the increased risk of fatal and intracranial bleeding and uncertain benefit, except in high-risk situations (patients with diabetes or a history of prior MI), in which its effect appears to be greater and its use may be considered. Do not start prasugrel in patients likely to undergo urgent CABG. Additional risk factors for bleeding include body weight <60 kg, propensity to bleed, and concomitant use of medications that increase the risk of bleeding (e.g. warfarin, heparin, fibrinolytic therapy, or chronic use of non-steroidal anti-inflammatory drugs).

** There is an increased risk of heparin-induced thrombocytopenia with UFH therapy beyond 48 h.

2012 ACCF/AHA focused update incorporated into the ACCF/AHA 2007 Guidelines for the management of patients with unstable angina/non–ST-elevation myocardial infarction. *J Am Coll Cardiol.* 2013;**61**:e179–347.

Table 27.6 ESC 2011 on UA/NSTEMI

Oral antiplatelet agents	
Aspirin to all patients without contraindications (loading dose of 150–300 mg, followed by 75–100 mg od long-term).	I-A
A P2Y12 inhibitor added to aspirin as soon as possible and maintained over 12 months, unless contraindications, such as excessive risk of bleeding.	I-A
A proton pump inhibitor (preferably not omeprazole), in combination with dual oral antiplatelet therapy (DAPT) in history of gastrointestinal haemorrhage or peptic ulcer or multiple other risk factors (*Helicobacter pylori* infection, age ≥65 years, concurrent use of anticoagulants or steroids).	I-A
Prolonged or permanent withdrawal of $P2Y_{12}$ inhibitors within 12 months is discouraged, unless clinically indicated.	I-C
Ticagrelor (180 mg loading dose, 90 mg bd) in moderate to high risk of ischaemic events (e.g. elevated troponins), regardless of initial treatment strategy and including patients pre-treated with clopidogrel (which should be discontinued when ticagrelor is commenced).	I-B
Prasugrel (60 mg loading dose, 10 mg od) for $P2Y_{12}$ inhibitor-naive patients (especially diabetics) in whom coronary anatomy is known and who are proceeding to PCI, unless there is a high risk of life-threatening bleeding or other contraindications.*	I-B
Clopidogrel (300 mg loading dose, 75 mg od) for patients who cannot receive ticagrelor or prasugrel.	I-A
A 600 mg loading dose of clopidogrel (or a supplementary 300 mg dose at PCI following an initial 300 mg loading dose) for patients scheduled for an invasive strategy when ticagrelor or prasugrel is not an option.	I-B
A maintenance dose of clopidogrel 150 mg daily for the first 7 days in patients managed with PCI and without increased risk of bleeding.	IIa-B
In patients pre-treated with P2Y12 inhibitors who need to undergo non-emergent major surgery (including CABG), surgery for, at least, 5 days after cessation of ticagrelor or clopidogrel and 7 days for prasugrel, if clinically feasible and unless the patient is at high risk of ischaemic events.	IIa-C
Ticagrelor or clopidogrel should be considered to be (re-) started after CABG surgery as soon as considered safe.	IIa-B
Increasing the maintenance dose of clopidogrel based on platelet function testing is not advised as routine but may be considered in selected cases.	IIb-B
Genotyping and/or platelet function testing may be considered in selected cases when clopidogrel is used.	IIb-B
The combination of aspirin with an NSAID (selective COX-2 inhibitors and non-selective NSAID) is not recommended.	III-C
GP IIb/IIIa receptor inhibitors	
The choice of combination of oral antiplatelet agents, a GP IIb/IIIa receptor inhibitor, and anticoagulants should be made in relation to the risk of ischaemic and bleeding events.	I-C
Addition of a GP IIb/IIIa receptor inhibitor to DAPT for high-risk PCI (elevated troponin, visible thrombus) if the risk of bleeding is low.	I-B
Eptifibatide or tirofiban added to aspirin prior to angiography in high-risk patients not preloaded with $P2Y_{12}$ inhibitors.	IIa-C
Eptifibatide or tirofiban prior to early angiography in addition to DAPT in high-risk patients if ongoing ischaemia and low risk of bleeding.	IIb-C
GP IIb/IIIa receptor inhibitors are not recommended routinely before angiography in an invasive treatment strategy.	III-A
GP IIb/IIIa receptor inhibitors are not recommended for patients on DAPT who are treated conservatively.	III-A
Anticoagulants	
Anticoagulation is recommended for all patients in addition to antiplatelet therapy.	I-A
Should be selected according to both ischaemic and bleeding risks and according to the efficacy-safety profile.	I-C
Fondaparinux (2.5 mg SC od) as having the most favourable efficacy-safety profile with respect to anticoagulation.	I-A
If the initial anticoagulant is fondaparinux, a single bolus of UFH (85 IU/kg, adapted to ACT, or 60 IU in the case of IIb/IIIa receptor inhibitors) should be added at the time of PCI.	I-B
Enoxaparin (1 mg/kg bd) when fondaparinux is not available.	I-B
If fondaparinux or enoxaparin are not available, UFH, with a target aPTT of 50–70 s, or other LMWHs at the specific recommended doses are indicated.	I-C
Bivalirudin plus provisional GP IIb/IIIa receptor inhibitors as an alternative to UFH plus GP IIb/IIIa receptor inhibitors in patients with an intended urgent or early invasive strategy, particularly in patients with a high risk of bleeding.	I-B
In a conservative strategy, anticoagulation should be maintained up to hospital discharge.	I-A
Discontinuation of anticoagulation after an invasive procedure, unless otherwise indicated.	IIa-C
Crossover of heparins (UFH and LMWH) is not recommended.	III-B

*: Prasugrel is in the ESC 2010 GL on revascularrization given a IIa recommendation as the overall indication including clopidogrel-pre-treated patients and/or unknown coronary anatomy. The class I recommendation here refers to the specifically defined subgroup.

ESC guidelines for the management of acute coronary syndromes in patients presenting without persistent ST-segment elevation. *Eur Heart J*. 2011;**32**:2999–3054.

Table 27.7 ESC 2011 GL on UA/NSTEMI. Antiplatelet agents

	Clopidogrel	Prasugrel	Ticagrelor
Class	Thienopyridine	Thienopyridine	Triazolopyrimidine
Reversibility	Irreversible	Irreversible	Reversible
Activation	Pro-drug, limited by metabolization	Pro-drug, not limited by metabolization	Active drug
Onset of effect[a]	2–4 h	30 min	30 min
Duration of effect	3–10 days	5–10 days	3–4 days
Withdrawal before major surgery	5 days	7 days	5 days

[a] 50% inhibition of platelet aggregation.
ESC guidelines for the management of acute coronary syndromes in patients presenting without persistent ST-segment elevation. *Eur Heart J.* 2011;**32**:2999–3054.

Checklist of treatments when an ACS diagnosis appears likely

Aspirin	Initial dose of 150–300 mg non-enteric formulation, followed by 75–100 mg/day (IV administration is acceptable)
P2Y12 inhibitor	Loading dose of ticagrelor or clopidogrel[a]
Anticoagulation	Choice between different options depends on strategy: ◆ Fondaparinux 2.5 mg/daily SC ◆ Enoxaparin 1 mg/kg twice daily SC ◆ UFH IV bolus 60–70 IU/kg (maximum 5000 IU), followed by infusion of 12–15 IU/kg/h (maximum 1000 IU/h), titrated to aPTT 1.5–2.5 × control ◆ Bivalirudin is indicated only in patients with a planned invasive strategy
Oral beta blocker	If tachycardic or hypertensive without signs of heart failure

aPTT, activated partial thromboplastin time; IU, international units; IV, intravenous; UFH, unfractionated heparin.
[a] Prasugrel is not mentioned, as it is not approved as medical therapy before invasive strategy, but only after angiography when anatomy is known.
ESC guidelines for the management of acute coronary syndromes in patients presenting without persistent ST-segment elevation. *Eur Heart J.* 2011;**32**:2999–3054.

Checklist of antithrombotic treatments prior to PCI

Aspirin	Confirm loading dose prior to PCI
P2Y12 inhibitor	Confirm loading dose of ticagrelor or clopidogrel prior to PCI. If P2Y12-naive, consider prasugrel (if <75 years age, >60 kg, no prior stroke or TIA)
Anticoagulation	◆ Fondaparinux pre-treated: add UFH for PCI ◆ Enoxaparin pre-treated: add if indicated ◆ UFH pre-treated: titrate to ACT >250 s or switch to bivalirudin (0.1 mg/kg bolus, followed by 0.25 mg/kg/h)
GP IIb/IIIa receptor inhibitor	◆ Consider tirofiban or eptifibatide in patients with high-risk anatomy or troponin elevation ◆ Abciximab only prior to PCI in high-risk patients

ACT, activated clotting time; GP, glycoprotein; PCI, percutaneous coronary intervention; TIA, transient ischaemic attack; UFH, unfractionated heparin.
ESC guidelines for the management of acute coronary syndromes in patients presenting without persistent ST-segment elevation. *Eur Heart J.* 2011;**32**:2999–3054.

Omeprazole (and especially **lansoprazole**) are proton pump inhibitors that also inhibit the cytochrome enzyme CYP2C19. **Pantoprazole**, that inhibits the enzyme less than omeprazole, should lessen the risk when taken 4 h after clopidogrel.[38] However, in clinical trials, the combination of clopidogrel with proton pump inhibitors has not increased cardiac events.[39,40] Thus, the combination of clopidogrel with a proton pump inhibitor is now considered safe and should not be avoided in patients who are at increased risk of gastrointestinal bleeding.[41] PPIs may potentiate VKA-induced anticoagulation, resulting in increased INR values and bleeding risk, most likely due to facilitated gastric absorption of warfarin; thus careful monitoring is required.[41] PPIs may also be with increased risk for adverse cardiovascular outcomes after discharge, regardless of clopidogrel use for myocardial infarction.[42] In a PLATO substudy, a similar association was observed between cardiovascular events and PPI use during ticagrelor treatment as with clopidogrel treatment (see Clopidrogrel). This suggests that PPI use is a marker for, rather than a cause of, higher rates of cardiovascular events in sicker patients who need a PPI.[43] A diminished pharmacodynamic response to clopidogrel has also been observed when co-administered with lipophilic statins and calcium channel blockers, but, in clinical practice, no increased cardiovascular risk has been demonstrated with these combinations.[44–46] Clopidogrel metabolites can inhibit enzymatic activity of cytochrome P4502C9 and lead to increased plasma levels of NSAIDs.

Clopidogrel hypersensitivity is manifested as generalized exanthema and is caused by a lymphocyte-mediated delayed hypersensitivity in most patients. This can be managed with oral steroids (prednisolone 30 mg bd for 5 days, with gradual tapering over the next 15 days, and diphenhydramine 25 mg every 8 h for pruritus) without clopidogrel discontinuation.[47] Allergenic cross-reactivity with ticlopidine, prasugrel, or both is present in a significant number of patients with clopidogrel hypersensitivity.

Although clopidogrel should be stopped ideally 5 days before CABG, if needed, CABG can be performed in patients on clopidogrel.[48]

Prasugrel (60 mg loading dose, then 10 mg od) is more consistent than clopidogrel, with faster onset of action and fewer potential drug interactions. It has been shown to be better than clopidogrel in patients with NSTEACS, particularly in those with diabetes, for reducing adverse cardiac events and late stent thrombosis, but at an increased risk of major bleeding (TRITON-TIMI 38 trial).[49] The rate of other adverse effects in the TRITON study was similar with prasugrel and clopidogrel. Thrombocytopenia occurred at the same frequency in each group (0.3%) while neutropenia was less common with prasugrel (<0.1% vs 0.2%; p = 0.02). In patients who do not undergo revascularization, prasugrel does not significantly reduce mortality and myocardial infarction, as compared with clopidogrel (TRILOGY ACS).[50] Concerns have been raised regarding a possible increased risk of cancer with prasugrel. Platelets inhibit angiogenesis through the activity of platelet factor 4 and facilitate tumour cell adhesion and trapping in capillaries through the expression of P-selectin. Disruption of tumour platelet aggregates by chronic profound oral platelet inhibition may cause extensive dissemination of initially silent tumours. A recent FDA report concluded that cancer risks after prasugrel are higher in women and after 4 months of therapy, at least, for solid, highly metastatic cancers.[51] Further data are needed for certain conclusions. It can be used instead of clopidogrel in patients undergoing PCI in a 60 mg loading dose followed by 10 mg daily or 5 mg if patient has a weight <60 kg. Not recommended in patients >75 years or if the risk of CABG is high. Contraindicated in patients with a history of TIA/stroke. According to the 2012 ACCF/AHA guideline, prasugrel should not be administered routinely to patients with UA/NSTEMI before angiography, such as in an emergency department, or used in patients with UA/NSTEMI who have not undergone PCI.

Cangrelor, is an IV, fast-acting, $P2Y_{12}$ inhibitor (30 μg/kg bolus followed by an infusion of 4 μg/kg for at least 2h) that given before clopidogrel 600 mg, has been found superior to clopoidogrel alone for PCI.[52] Its comparative efficacy to drugs such as prasugrel or ticagrelor is not known.

Cilostazol, a selective inhibitor of 3-type phosphodiesterase, is commonly used in East Asia as an antiplatelet agent but, outside of peripheral arterial disease, has not found wider acceptance in western populations due to side effects, cost considerations, and lack of definitive evidence of its efficacy. It is recommended (100 mg po bd) for the pharmacological treatment of intermittent claudication in patients with peripheral artery disease (Class I-A, ACCF/AHA 2011 GL on peripheral disaese[53]).

Glycoprotein IIb/IIIa antagonists Glycoprotein IIb/IIIa receptor inhibitors block the final common pathway of platelet activation. **Abciximab** is a Fab fragment that targets the glycoprotein IIb/IIIa receptor and may be specifically used in percutaneous coronary intervention. The small molecule inhibitors **eptifibatide** and **tirofiban** are short-acting and require dose adjustment in patients with poor renal function. They are now the recommended agents in UA/NSTEMI when a IIb/IIIa is indicated; abciximab may be used only in high-risk patients undergoing PCI. In elderly patients, lower efficacy and higher rates of bleeding are seen. IIb/IIa anatagonists initiated early after admission reduce death and myocardial infarction but increase the risk of bleeding.[54] Most studies, however, have been conducted without the use of clopidogrel or new $P2Y_{12}$ receptor blockers.

The benefits of GP IIb/IIIa inhibition are probably greater for high-risk patients with elevated troponin, diabetes, and recurrent angina. Patients treated medically and who develop recurrent ischaemia, heart failure, or serious arrhythmias should be referred for urgent coronary angiography. In these patients, IIb/IIA antogonists may be added to dual antiplatelet therapy and heparin. The main risk is bleeding, usually at the site of the arterial puncture. They should be given with caution if urgent CABG is anticipated. Reversibility of action is slow with abciximab (48 h to 1 week) and faster with tirofiban (4–8 h) and eptifibatide (2–4 h).

They may also be used, instead of clopidogrel loading, on presentation or in addition to dual antiplatelet therapy and heparin in:

- High-risk patients with recurrent symptoms despite dual antiplatelet therapy and heparin or elevated troponin or visible thrombus.
- High-risk patients proceeding to angiography.

- ***Eptifibatide dose***: IV bolus 180 micrograms/kg, followed 10 min later by second IV bolus 180 micrograms/kg, and infusion 2.0 micrograms/kg/min, started after first bolus, for 12–18 h; reduce infusion

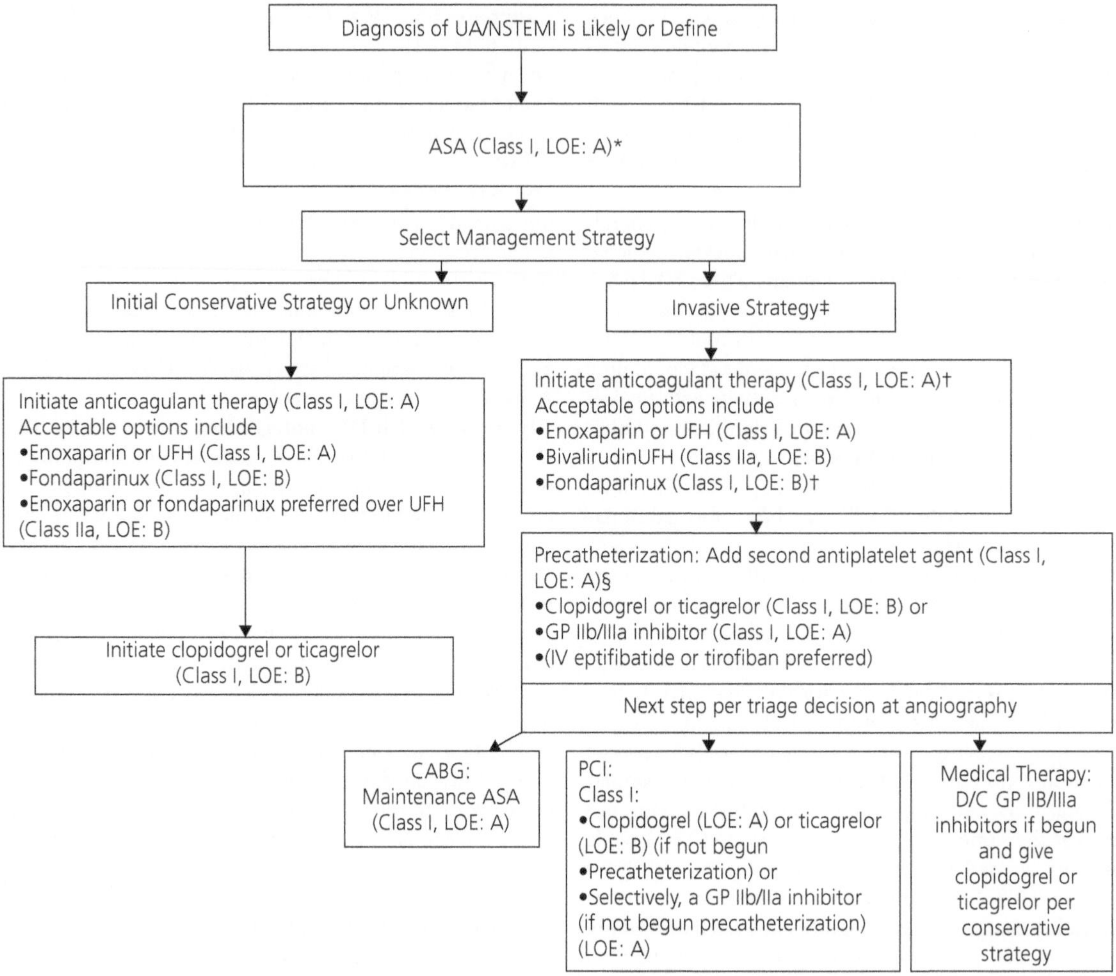

Figure 27.2 ACCF/AHA 2012 GL on UA/NSTEMI. Flowchart for Class I and Class IIa Recommendations for Initial Management of UA/NSTEMI

*A loading dose followed by a daily maintenance dose of either clopidogrel (LOE: B), prasugrel (in PCI-treated patients), or ticagrelor (LOE: C) should be administered to UA/NSTEMI patients who are unable to take ASA because of hypersensitivity or major GI intolerance.
†If fondaparinux is used during PCI (I-B), it must be coadministered with another anticoagulant with Factor IIa activity (i.e., UFH).
‡Timing of invasive strategy generally is assumed to be 4 to 48 h. If immediate angiography is selected, see STEMI guidelines.
§Precatheterization triple antiplatelet therapy (ASA, clopidogrel or ticagrelor, GP inhibitors) is a IIb-B recommendation for selected high-risk patients. Also, note that there are no data for therapy with 2 concurrent P2Y12 receptor inhibitors, and this is not recommended in the case of aspirin allergy.
LOE: level of evidence.
2012 ACCF/AHA focused update incorporated into the ACCF/AHA 2007 Guidelines for the management of patients with unstable angina/non-ST-elevation myocardial infarction. *J Am Coll Cardiol*. 2013;**61**:e179–347.

by 50% in patients with estimated creatinine clearance <50 mL/min. Eptifibatide is contraindicated in patients with CrCl <30 mL/min.

- ***Tirofiban dose***: IV bolus of 25 micrograms/kg, and then infusion of 0.15 micrograms/kg/min for up to 18 h; reduce infusion by 50% in patients with estimated creatinine clearance <30 mL/min.
- ***Abciximab dose***: IV bolus 0.25 mg/kg, followed by infusion 0.125 micrograms/kg/min (max 10 micrograms/min) for 12 h after PCI. There are no specific recommendations for the use of abciximab or for dose adjustment in the case of renal failure. Careful evaluation of haemorrhagic risk is needed before using the drug in the case of renal failure.

Anticoagulants

A low molecular weight heparin (such as enoxaparin) or **unfractionated heparin** is given as soon as possible (Tables 27.5 and 27.6).

Unfractionated heparin (UFH) is a heterogeneous group of negatively charged, sulfated glycosaminoglycans (molecular weight 3000 to 30 000 Da) from animal sources.

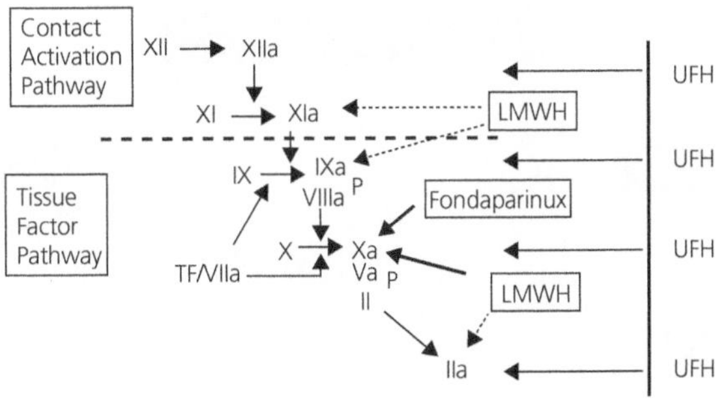

Figure 27.3 Tissue factor pathway: initiation of coagulation is triggered by the tissue factor/factor VIIa complex (TF/VIIa), which activates factor IX (IX) and factor X (X). **Contact activation pathway**: initiation of coagulation is triggered by activation of factor XII (XIIa), which activates factor XI (XIa). Factor XIa activates factor IX, and activated factor IX (IXa) propagates coagulation by activating factor X in a reaction that utilizes activated factor VIII (VIIIa) as a cofactor. Activated factor X (Xa), with activated factor V (Va) as a cofactor, converts prothrombin (II) to thrombin (IIa). Thrombin then converts fibrinogen to fibrin. **UFH** targets steps in both the contact activation pathway (inactivates XIa and XIIa) and tissue factor pathway (inactivates IXa, Xa, and IIa). **Bivalirudin** is cleaved by thrombin, thereby reducing its antithrombotic activity. **Fondaparinux** modulates the tissue factor pathway by inactivating factor Xa. **LMWH** also modulates the tissue factor pathway by inactivating factor Xa and, to a lesser degree, factor IIa. LMWH exerts weak activity against the contact activation pathway. P indicates phospholipid surface; TF, tissue factor.

Hirsh J, et al. Beyond unfractionated heparin and warfarin: current and future advances. *Circulation*. 2007;**116**:552–60

Low molecular weight heparins (LMWHs; molecular weight 2000 to 10 000 Da) are produced from unfractionated heparin by chemical or enzymatic processes. UFH activates antithrombin through the formation of a heparin-antithrombin complex that inhibits other coagulation factors.[55] The protein-binding properties of heparin are mainly responsible for the lack of linear relationship between dose, activated partial thromboplastin time (aPTT), and clinical outcomes. There is a variable therapeutic response, depending on age, weight, and renal function, and also a requirement for aPTT monitoring. Elimination of the drug is mainly by the kidneys (and the reticuloendothelial system) and the half-life is approximately 6 hours.

- ***Dose for conservative therapy***: IV bolus 60 U/kg (max 5000 U), followed by infusion of 12 U/kg/h (max 1000 U/h) to maintain aPTT 1.5–2 times control (50–70 s) for 48 h.
- ***Dose for PCI***: IV bolus of 50–70 U/kg, if not initially given, targeting ACT 250–300 s for HaemoTec (or 300–350 s for Haemochron). If additional IIb/IIIa, IV bolus 50–70 U/kg, targeting ACT 200–250 s. No additional treatment after PCI.

Protamine sulfate is an effective antidote (1mg/100 U heparin IV). Very rarely, allergic shock may occur with its use.

Low molecular weight heparins (LMWH) (enoxaparin, dalteparin, fraxiparin) are specific inhibitors of thrombin and factor Xa with high bioavailability. When given subcutaneously, they provide more consistent anticoagulation, avoiding the need for monitoring, and are associated with a lower risk for heparin-induced thrombocytopenia than unfractionated heparin. Disadvantages are the only partial reversibility by protamine, renal excretion, and reduced efficacy against the contact activation pathway (factors XIa and XIIa) that contributes to thrombosis on catheter tips, stents, and filters (Figures 27.2 and 27.3).[55] Enoxaparin is preferred over UFH by the ESC 2011. Not much data exist about other LMWH, but they might be used if enoxaparin is not available (ESC 2011). **Enoxaparin** reduces death and myocardial infarction compared to unfractionated heparin in NSTEACS.[56] If CABG is planned, LMWH should be discontinued 12–24 h before and replaced with UFH.

- ***Dose for conservative therapy***: IV bolus of 30 mg, followed 15 min later by 1 mg/kg/12 h SC, provided serum creatinine is <2.5 mg/dL in men and <2.0 mg/dL in women, for duration of hospitalization up to 8 days. Therapeutic dosing should achieve an anti-Xa level of 0.6–1 IU/mL, but this is seldom measured. If CrCl <30mL/min, the dose is 1 mg/kg/24 h. For patients >75 years of age, the initial intravenous bolus may be eliminated and the subcutaneous dose reduced to 0.75 mg/kg every 12 hours.
- ***Dose for PCI***: IV bolus of 0.5–0.75 mg/kg or 0.3 mg/kg if the last SC dose was given >8 h. No additional dose if last SC dose was given <8 h. If the procedure is prolonged (>2 h) and an initial dose of 0.5 mg/kg was given, an additional IV dose of 0.25 mg/kg may be given. No additional treatment after PCI.

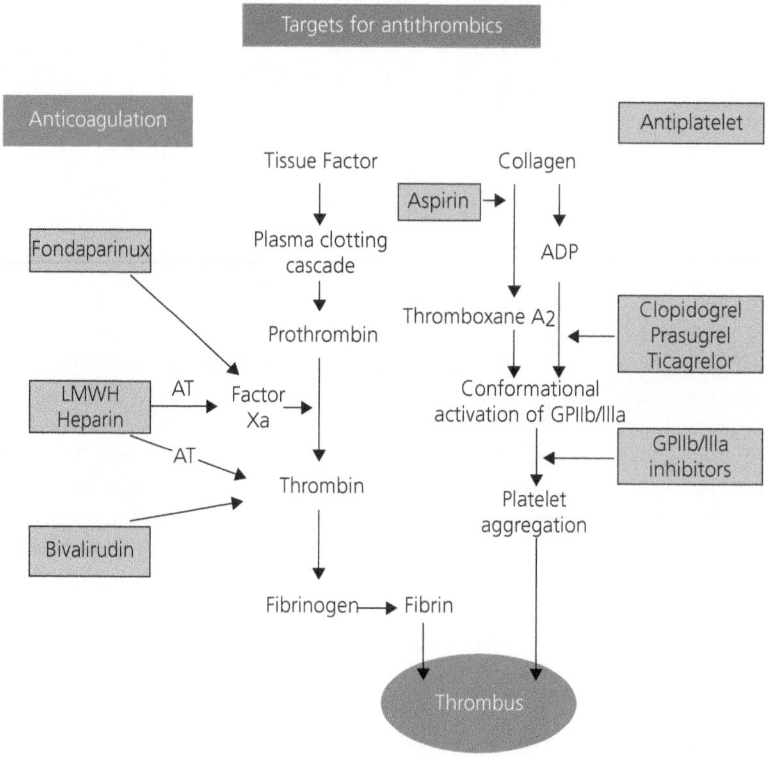

Figure 27.4 ESC 2011 targets for antithrombotic drugs.
AT: antithrombin; GP: glycoprotein; LMWH: low molecular weight heparin. ESC guidelines for the management of acute coronary syndromes in patients presenting without persistent ST-segment elevation. *Eur Heart J.* 2011;**32**:2999–3054.

Direct thrombin inhibitors

Bivalirudin is a reversible direct thrombin inhibitor with additional mild antiplatelet activity. It has a very short half-life and is less likely to accumulate in patients with renal insufficiency. It can be used as an alternative to heparin if an invasive strategy is planned instead of heparin, and plus provisional IIb/IIIa instead of UFH plus IIb/IIa, especially in patients at high risk of bleeding. In moderate- and high-risk patients, bivalirudin alone has similar ischaemic benefit as either unfractionated heparin or enoxaparin with a IIb/IIIa antagonist but with a reduction in major bleeding (ACUITY and ISAR-REACT 4 trials).[57,58] Crossover from UFH or LMWH to bivalirudin at PCI has a protective effect against bleeding. Bivalirudin should be stopped 3 h before CABG and replaced by UFH.

- ***Dose for conservative therapy***: 0.1 mg/kg bolus, 0.25 mg/kg/h infusion for up to 72 h.
- ***Dose for PCI***: 0.75 mg/kg bolus (for patients who have received UFH, wait 30 min), 1.75 mg/kg/h infusion until the end of PCI or up to 4 h later.
- If CrCl <30 mL/min, reduction of the infusion rate to 1.0 mg/kg/h should be considered. If a patient is on haemodialysis, the infusion should be reduced to 0.25 mg/kg/h. No reduction in the bolus dose is needed.

Dabigatran (an oral direct thrombin inhibitor) has not been successful due to increased bleeding risk without reducing ischaemic events (RE-DEEM trial).[59]

Direct factor Xa inhibitors

Fondaparinux reduces major bleeding and improves clinical outcomes compared to enoxaparin with or without a IIb/IIIa (OASIS-5).[60] In patients managed conservatively, it is preferred over heparin, especially when there is high risk of bleeding. If these patients proceed to coronary intervention, a single bolus of UFH (85 IU/kg adapted to ACT, or 60 IU in the case of concomitant use of GP IIb/IIIa receptor inhibitors) should be given. Fondaparinux is the longest acting of the anticoagulants, with a half-life approaching 24 hours through renal clearance. It is contraindicated in patients with creatinine clearance <30 mL/

min, but a much lower risk of bleeding complications were observed in OASIS-5 with fondaparinux when compared with enoxaparin, even in patients with severe renal failure. It is not recommended when an invasive approach is planned. Fondaparinux should be stopped 24 h before CABG and replaced by UFH.

- ***Dose for conservative therapy***: 2.5 mg IV bolus, followed by 2.5 mg SC once daily for duration of hospitalization (up to 8 days).
- If the need for ***PCI*** arises, additional UFH heparin is needed (50–60 U/kg bolus) (risk of catheter thrombosis).

Rivaroxaban (an oral Xa inhibitor) has been used post-discharge. It was shown to reduce the risk of the composite endpoint of death from cardiovascular causes, myocardial infarction, or stroke in patients with a recent acute coronary syndrome, when added to standard therapy (2.5–5 mg bd), but at an increased risk of major bleeding and intracranial haemorrhage (ATLAS 2 trial).[61] The 2.5 mg bd dose also reduced cardiovascular mortality but at the expense of increased intracranial haemorrhage.

Apixaban (oral Xa inhibitor) has also been tried in doses similar to those used in AF (5 mg bd) but did not reduce ischaemic events (APPRAISE 2 trial).[62] Apixaban was also associated with increased major bleeding, including intracranial haemorrhage.

In a recent meta-analysis, addition of a novel anticoagulant to dual antiplatelet therapy reduced cardiovascular events by 13%, but more than doubled the bleeding.[63]

Synopsis of the antiplatelet/anticoagulant therapeutic scheme

All patients should receive:

- **Aspirin**, and
- **$P2Y_{12}$ receptor blocker** (preferably ticagrelor or clopidogrel) or **GP IIa/IIIB receptor inhibitor**, and
- **Heparin** (**LMWH** or **UFH**) or **bivalirudin** (invasive therapy) or **fondaparinux** (conservative therapy).

In stable patients selected for medical therapy, aspirin, ticagrelor or clopidogrel, and enoxaparin or preferably fondaparinux are given. A IIb/IIIa may be given only in patients with recurrent ischaemia or high troponin. If the patient is stable, a stress test should be performed. If, after the test, the patient is classified as low-risk, enoxaparin or fondaparinux are continued for the duration of hospitalization (up to 8 days), and IIb/IIIa, if given, is discontinued. Aspirin is given indefinitely and the $P2Y_{12}$ receptor blocker for at least 1 month and ideally up to 1 year.

In patients selected for PCI, aspirin, a $P2Y_{12}$ receptor blocker, and enoxaparin are continued, and a IIb/IIIa antagonist might be initiated only in high-risk patients. Alternatively, bivalirudin (with or preferably without IIb/IIIa) may be given instead of the combination of enoxaparin and a IIb/IIIA. Enoxaparin or bivalirudin may be discontinued after PCI in stable, uncomplicated cases.

In patients in whom CABG is indicated after angiography, aspirin and UFH are continued. Ticagrelor and clopidogrel should be ideally stopped 5 days and prasugrel 7 days before CABG, if this is possible, although CABG, if needed, can also be performed in patients on clopidogrel. Enoxaparin should be stopped 12–24 h, fondaparinux 24 h, and bivalirudin 3 h before the procedure, respectively, and replaced by UFH. IIb/IIIa (eptifibatide or tirofiban) are discontinued 4 h before surgery (abciximab requires much longer time, at least 48 h).

Other medications

Beta blockers

They should be initiated within the first 24 h for patients who do not have signs of acute heart failure or a low-output state, increased risk for cardiogenic shock, or other relative contraindications to beta blockade (PR interval >0.24 s, second or third degree heart block, active asthma, or reactive airway disease) (Table 27.4). Beta blockers reduce the incidence of recurrent ischaemia and subsequent MI. IV beta blockade may also be considered in the absence of contraindications (mainly patients with Killip class ≥III). Oral therapy should be started and continued indefinitely in patients with reduced LV function. Patients on chronic β-blocker therapy admitted with ACS should be continued on ß-blocker therapy if not in Killip class ≥III.

Calcium channel blockers

In the presence of recurrent symptoms or Prinzmetal variant angina or in patients in whom beta blockers are contraindicated, a non-dihydropyridine calcium channel blocker (e.g. **verapamil** or **diltiazem**) should be given as initial therapy in the absence of clinically significant left ventricular dysfunction or other contraindications. Dihydropyridines are contraindicated in the absence of a beta blocker.

ACE inhibitors (or angiotensin receptor blockers)

Should be administered orally within the first 24 h to patients with pulmonary congestion or LVEF ≤0.40, in the absence of hypotension (systolic blood pressure <100 mmHg or <30 mmHg below baseline) or other contraindications. They may also be used in all patients, provided the systolic blood pressure is >100 mmHg.

Non-steroidal anti-inflammatory drugs (NSAIDs)

Because of the increased risks of mortality, reinfarction, hypertension, HF, and myocardial rupture associated with their use, NSAIDs, except for ASA, whether non-selective or COX-2 selective agents, should be discontinued at the time a patient presents with UA/NSTEMI.

Warfarin

Warfarin, although not specifically indicated for ACS, is often used concurrently for other indications, such as atrial fibrillation, mechanical valves, left ventricular thrombus, or deep venous thrombosis. Warfarin is a racemic mixture of isomers that inhibits synthesis of vitamin K-dependent coagulation factors. The effective dose of warfarin varies significantly among individuals due to genetic variations in its receptor, metabolism via the cytochrome P450 system, and interactions with other drugs, vitamins, and green vegetables. Warfarin use alone increases the risk of bleeding to 13% per year, and risks are highest among new users and the elderly. Combinations of warfarin, aspirin, and clopidogrel carry a substantially higher risk than warfarin monotherapy.[64] The incidence of fatal or non-fatal bleeding per 100 person-years of therapy has been found as 14.2 for triple therapy, 7–10.6 for dual therapy, and 6.6–7 for monotherapy. Preferred INR with triple therapy is 2–3 and 2–2.5 in the elderly and those at increased risk of bleeding. Patients with AF on OAT are often bridged with UFH or LMWH if they need coronary angiography or PCI. Triple therapy with the use of newer anticoagulants (dabigatran, apixaban, and rivaroxaban) is also associated with a substantially increased risk of bleeding.[65]

The following recommendations are useful:[66]

- Observational studies suggest that coronary angiography or PCI can be safely performed without interrupting warfarin and may be associated with a lower rate of complications compared with bridging therapy to heparin. There is no need for additional heparin in patients who undergo PCI while therapeutic on warfarin (INR 2–3). Aspirin and clopidogrel should be administered prior to the procedure when PCI is performed in a patient on warfarin. The use of proton pump inhibitors may help reduce the risk of bleeding.
- The use of platelet glycoprotein IIb/IIIa inhibitors increases the risk of bleeding in patients on warfarin 3- to 13-fold, and the routine use of these agents should be avoided.
- Combinations of aspirin and warfarin does not provide sufficient protection against risk of stent thrombosis. Patients undergoing stent-based PCI should be treated with triple therapy consisting of aspirin, clopidogrel, and warfarin. This combination is associated with an increased risk of bleeding, and use of bare metal stents should be considered in these patients to limit the duration of triple therapy. In patients who need long-term oral anticoagulation, use of drug-eluting stents should be restricted to patients at very high risk of restenosis (long lesions, small vessels, diabetes). Alternatively, omission of aspirin and continuation with warfarin and clopidogrel is an option in patients at high risk for bleeding.[67]
- There are limited data on the safety of cardiac surgery in patients who are on warfarin. Currently, these patients are bridged with heparin prior to surgery. In the need of emergent CABG, fresh frozen plasma and vitamin K may be used to reduce the risk of bleeding.

Invasive vs conservative management

Criteria for an invasive strategy are presented in Tables 27.8 and 27.9.[1,2,68] Thus, current evidence suggests that in **high-risk, unstable patients, intervention within 12–72 hours is preferred** while either an early or a delayed approach may be adopted in other patients. Several (FRISC II, TACTICS-TIMI 18, RITA 3, ISAR-COOL, TIMACS),[69–75] although not all (ICTUS, ELISA, OPTIMA, ABOARD, LIPSIA-NSTEMI),[74–78] randomized trials have provided evidence in favour of an invasive strategy compared to conservative medical therapy in NSTEACS. Overall, the invasive strategy provides better long-term outcomes.[79,80] In addition, 5-year follow-up of patients with non-ST elevation acute coronary syndrome from FRISC II, ICTUS, and RITA-3 Trials 3 trials showed no association between a procedure-related MI and long-term cardiovascular mortality, although there was a substantial increase in long-term mortality after a spontaneous MI.[81] This is particularly true in high-risk patients whereas in low-risk patients, and especially women,[82] a conservative management with a view to intervention, if indicated, can be adopted.[83] The optimal timing of coronary angiography and subsequent intervention, if indicated, i.e. immediately after admission or after pre-treatment with optimal medical therapy, including potent antiplatelet agents, is also debated.[84,85] Delayed catheterization has been thought to allow plaque passivation by pre-treatment with optimal antithrombotic medication and avoidance adverse outcomes, perhaps due to embolic phenomena, by early intervention. However, very early angiography (<14 h) with a view to PCI, if indicated, may be superior to a strategy of preceding anticoagulation and subsequent intervention in patients with NSTEACS, by reducing residual ischaemia and the duration of hospital stay and may also reduce complications, such as bleeding, and major events (death, MI, or stroke).[85] It is particularly beneficial in diabetic patients.[86]

Drug-eluting stents (DES) reduce target lesion revascularization (TLR), but not mortality or the risk of MI, compared to BMS.[87] The rate of recurrent events in patients

Table 27.8 Conservative vs invasive strategies

ACCF/AHA 2012 GL on UA/NSTEMI and 2011 GL on PCI. Selection of initial treatment strategy: invasive versus conservative strategy

Generally preferred strategy	Patient characteristics
Invasive	Recurrent angina or ischemia at rest or with low-level activities despite intensive medical therapy Elevated cardiac biomarkers (TnT or TnI) New or presumably new ST-segment depression Signs or symptoms of OF or new or worsening mitral regurgitation High-risk findings for noninvasive testing Hemodynamic instability Sustained ventricular tachycardia PCI within 6 mo Prior CABG High-risk score (eg, TIMI, GRACE) Mild to moderate renal dysfunction Diabetes mellitus Reduced LV function (LVEF <40%)
Conservative	Low-risk score (eg, TIMI, GRACE) Patient or physician preference in the absence of high-risk features

CABG indicates coronary artery bupass graft; GRACE, Global Registry of Acute Coronary Events; HF, heart failure; LV, left ventricular; LVEF, left ventricular ejection fraction; PCI, percutaneous coronary intervention; TIMII, Thrombolysis in Myocardial Infarction; TnI, troponin I; TNT, troponin T.

ACCF/AHA 2012 GL on UA/NSTEMI and 2011 GL on PCI. Recommendations for initial invasive versus initial conservative strategies

Early invasive strategy (i.e. diagnostic angiography with intent to perform revascularization) in patients without serious co-morbidities or contraindications to such procedures, and:	
a. Refractory angina or haemodynamic or electrical instability.	I-B
b. Stabilized patients who have an elevated risk for clinical events.	I-A
The selection of PCI or CABG for revascularization in ACS is based on the same considerations as in patients without ACS.	I-B
Early invasive strategy (within 12–24 hours of admission) over a delayed invasive strategy for initially stabilized high-risk patients.* For patients not at high risk, a delayed invasive approach is also reasonable.	IIa-B
In initially stabilized patients, an initially conservative (i.e. a selectively invasive) strategy is considered as a treatment strategy for UA/NSTEMI patients who have an elevated risk for clinical events, including those who are troponin positive.	IIb-B
The decision to implement an initial conservative (vs initial invasive) strategy in these patients may be made by considering physician and patient preference.	IIb-C
Early invasive strategy in patients with extensive co-morbidities (e.g. liver or pulmonary failure, cancer), in whom the risks of revascularization and co-morbid conditions are likely to outweigh the benefits of revascularization.	III-C
Early invasive strategy in patients with acute chest pain and a low likelihood of ACS.	III-C
Early invasive strategy in patients who will not consent to revascularization regardless.	III-C

* Immediate catheterization/angiography is recommended for unstable patients.

2012 ACCF/AHA focused update incorporated into the ACCF/AHA 2007 Guidelines for the management of patients with unstable angina/non–ST-elevation myocardial infarction. *J Am Coll Cardiol.* 2013;**61**:e179–347.

Table 27.9 ESC 2011 GL on UA/NSTEMI. Criteria for high risk with indication for invasive management

Criteria for high risk with indication for invasive management
Primary
◆ Relevant rise or fall in troponin[a]
◆ Dynamic ST or T wave changes (symptomatic or silent)
Secondary
◆ Diabetes mellitus
◆ Renal insufficiency (eGFR <60 mL/min/1.73 m^2)

(Continued)

Table 27.9 (Continued)

◆ Reduced LV function (ejection fraction <40%)	
◆ Early post-infarction angina	
◆ Recent PCI	
◆ Prior CABG	
◆ Intermediate to high GRACE risk score (see Table 27.3)	
Recommendations for invasive evaluation and revascularization	
Invasive strategy (within 72 h after first presentation) in patients with, at least, one high-risk criterion or recurrent symptoms.	I-A
Urgent coronary angiography (<2 h) in patients at very high ischaemic risk (refractory angina, with associated heart failure, life-threatening ventricular arrhythmias, or haemodynamic instability).	I-C
Early invasive strategy (<24 h) in patients with a GRACE score >140 or with, at least, one primary high-risk criterion.	I-A
Non-invasive documentation of inducible ischaemia in low-risk patients without recurrent symptoms before deciding for invasive evaluation.	I-A
The revascularization strategy (ad hoc culprit lesion PCI/multivessel PCI/CABG) should be based on the clinical status as well as the disease severity, i.e. distribution and angiographic lesion characteristics (e.g. SYNTAX score), according to the local 'Heart Team' protocol.	I-C
As there are no safety concerns related to the use of DES in ACS, DES are indicated based on an individual basis, taking into account baseline characteristics, coronary anatomy, and bleeding risk.	I-A
PCI of non-significant lesions.	III-C
Routine invasive evaluation of low-risk patients.	III-C

ESC guidelines for the management of acute coronary syndromes in patients presenting without persistent ST-segment elevation. *Eur Heart J.* 2011;**32**:2999–3054.

undergoing PCI is 20% at 3 years. Half of these events are associated with angiographically mild (<70% stenosis), non-culprit lesions. In patients undergoing PCI, the Syntax score is an independent predictor of the 1-year rates of death, cardiac death, MI, and target vessel revascularization.[88] Incomplete revascularization after PCI in ACS, defined as additional stenoses with a diameter percent stenosis 30–70%,[89] or a residual Syntax Score >8.0,[90] is associated with a poor prognosis.

Specific patient groups

Elderly

Patients older than 75 years of age should be investigated at low level of suspicion due to often atypical presentation of ACS. Despite an increased risk for major bleeding, a routine early invasive strategy can significantly improve ischaemic outcomes in elderly patients with unstable angina and non-ST segment elevation MI.[91] Care is needed due to increased risk of bleeding and possibly concurrent renal dysfunction in this group, and drug dosages should be modified accordingly.

Diabetics

All patients with ACS should be screened for diabetes (Table 27.10). Tight glycaemic control to achieve normoglycaemia is no more recommended. Instead, insulin infusion to maintain glucose levels <180 mg/dL, while avoiding hypoglycaemia (>90 mg/dL), is recommended. An early invasive strategy is recommended for diabetic patients with NSTEACS, and DES are preferred to BMS. CABG is preferable to PCI in multivessel disease. Diabetic patients with NSTEACS may receive intravenous GP IIb/IIIa inhibitors as part of the initial medical management which should be continued through the completion of PCI. No more recommended as a routine medication.

Chronic kidney disease

Renal function should be assessed with creatinine clearance (CrCl) estimation in all patients with ACS (Tables 27.11 and 27.12). An invasive strategy, with preparatory hydration and low doses of contrast media, is reasonable in patients with mild (stage II) and moderate (stage III) chronic kidney disease, but no data exist for patients with advanced disease (stages IV and V). Drug dosage adjustments are shown in Table 27.8. Unfractionated heparin adjusted to aPTT is recommended when the CrCl is <30 mL/min or eGFR is <30 mL/min/1.73 m^2.

Pregnancy

Recommendations of the ESC guidelines indicate PCI for STEMI (I-C) or high-risk NSTEMI (IIa-C).[92]

Heart failure

Coronary revascularization, if amenable, is recommended in patients with ACS and LV dysfunction. Patients should be considered, at least, one month after the acute event for device therapy, such as CRT and/or ICD.

Table 27.10 Diabetes mellitus

ACCF/AHA 2012 GL on UA/NSTEMI	
Medical treatment in the acute phase, and decisions on whether to perform stress testing, angiography, and revascularization should be similar in patients with and without diabetes.	I-A
For patients with multivessel disease, CABG with use of the internal mammary arteries can be beneficial over PCI.	IIa-B
PCI is reasonable in patients with single-vessel disease and inducible ischaemia.	IIa-B
Use an insulin-based regimen to achieve and maintain glucose <180 mg/dL while avoiding hypoglycaemia* for hospitalized patients with either a complicated or uncomplicated course.	IIa-B

* There is uncertainty about the ideal target range for glucose necessary to achieve an optimal risk-benefit ratio.

ESC 2011 GL on UA/NSTEMI	
All patients with NSTEACS should be screened for diabetes. Blood glucose levels should be monitored frequently in patients with known diabetes or admission hyperglycaemia.	I-C
Treatment of elevated blood glucose should avoid both excessive hyperglycaemia (10–11 mmol/L [>180–200 mg/dL]) and hypoglycaemia (<5 mmol/L (<90 mg/dL]).	I-B
Antithrombotic treatment is indicated as in non-diabetic patients.	I-C
Renal function should be closely monitored following contrast exposure.	I-C
An early invasive strategy is recommended.	I-A
DES are recommended to reduce rates of repeat revascularization.	I-A
CABG surgery should be favoured over PCI in main stem lesions and/or advanced multivessel disease.	I-B

2012 ACCF/AHA focused update incorporated into the ACCF/AHA 2007 Guidelines for the management of patients with unstable angina/non–ST-elevation myocardial infarction. *J Am Coll Cardiol*. 2013;**61**:e179–347.
ESC guidelines for the management of acute coronary syndromes in patients presenting without persistent ST-segment elevation. *Eur Heart J*. 2011;**32**: 2999–3054

Table 27.11 Chronic kidney disease

ACCF/AHA 2012 GL on UA/NSTEMI	
Creatinine clearance should be estimated, and the doses of renally cleared medications should be adjusted according to the pharmacokinetic data.	I-B
Patients undergoing cardiac catheterization with receipt of contrast media should receive adequate preparatory hydration.	I-B
Calculation of the contrast volume to creatinine clearance ratio to predict the maximum volume of contrast media that can be given.	I-B
An invasive strategy is reasonable in patients with mild (stage 2) and moderate (stage 3) CKD (there are insufficient data on benefit/risk of invasive strategy in UA/NSTEMI patients with advanced CKD [stages 4, 5]).	IIa-B
ESC 2011 GL on UA/NSTEMI	
Kidney function should be assessed by CrCl or eGFR, with special attention to elderly people, women, and patients with low body weight, as near normal serum creatinine levels may be associated with lower than expected CrCl and eGFR levels.	I-C
Patients should receive the same first-line antithrombotic treatment as patients devoid of CKD, with appropriate dose adjustments according to the severity of renal dysfunction.	I-B
Dose adjustment or switch to UFH with fondaparinux, enoxaparin, bivalirudin, and small molecule GP IIb/IIIa receptor inhibitors are indicated.	I-B
UFH infusion, adjusted to aPTT, is recommended when CrCl is <30 mL/min or eGFR is <30 mL/min/1.73 m^2 with most anticoagulants (fondaparinux <20 mL/min).	I-C
In patients considered for invasive strategy, hydration and low- or iso-osmolar contrast medium at low volume (<4 mL/kg) are recommended.	I-B
CABG or PCI is recommended in patients amenable to revascularization after careful assessment of the risk-benefit ratio in relation to the severity of renal dysfunction.	I-B

2012 ACCF/AHA focused update incorporated into the ACCF/AHA 2007 Guidelines for the management of patients with unstable angina/non–ST-elevation myocardial infarction. *J Am Coll Cardiol*. 2013;**61**:e179–347.
ESC guidelines for the management of acute coronary syndromes in patients presenting without persistent ST-segment elevation. *Eur Heart J*. 2011;**32**:2999–3054

Table 27.12 ESC 2011 GL on UA/NSTEMI. Use of drugs in patients with chronic kidney disease

Drug	**Recommendations**
Clopidogrel	No information in patients with renal dysfunction.
Prasugrel	No dose adjustment necessary, including in patients with end-stage disease.
Ticagrelor	No dose reduction required; no information in dialysis patients.
Enoxaparin	Dose reduction to 1 mg/kg once daily in the case of severe renal failure (CrCl <30 mL/min). Consider monitoring of anti-Xa activity.

(Continued)

Table 27.12 (Continued)

Drug	Recommendations
Fondaparinux	Contraindicated in severe renal failure (CrCl <20 mL/min). Drug of choice in patients with moderately reduced renal function (CrCl 30–60 mL/min).
Bivalirudin	Patients with moderate renal impairment (30–59 mL/min) should receive an infusion of 1.75 mg/kg/h. If the creatinine clearance is <30 mL/min, reduction of the infusion rate to 1 mg/kg/h should be considered. No reduction in the bolus dose is needed. If a patient is on haemodialysis, the infusion rate should be reduced to 0.25 mg/kg/h.
Abciximab	No specific recommendations for the use of abciximab or for dose adjustment in the case of renal failure. Careful evaluation of haemorrhagic risk is needed before using the drug in the case of renal failure.
Eptifibatide	The infusion dose should be reduced to 1 microgram/kg/min in patients with CrCl <50 mL/min. The dose of the bolus remains unchanged at 180 micrograms/kg. Eptifibatide is contraindicated in patients with CrCl <30 mL/min.
Tirofiban	Dose adaptation is required in patients with renal failure; 50% of the bolus dose and infusion if CrCl is <30 mL/min.

Recommendations for the use of drugs listed in this table may vary, depending on the exact labelling of each drug in the country where it is used.
CrCl, creatinine clearance.
ESC guidelines for the management of acute coronary syndromes in patients presenting without persistent ST-segment elevation. *Eur Heart J.* 2011;**32**:2999–3054.

Anaemia

Anaemia is a marker of ischaemic and bleeding events, and haemoglobin measurements are mandatory on presentation (ESC 2011, I-B). Blood transfusion is recommended only with Hct <25% or Hb <7g/dL (ESC 2011, I-B).

Complications

Ventricular arrhythmias

In non-ST elevation acute coronary syndromes, NSVT is detected in 18–25% of patients 2 to 9 days after admission, and even short episodes of VT, lasting 4 to 7 beats, are independently associated with the risk of SCD over the subsequent year (MERLIN-TIMI 36 trial).[93] Earlier episodes within 48 hours after admission do not carry the same risk.

Cardiogenic shock

Patients with ACS and evidence of cardiogenic shock benefit from immediate revascularization versus medical therapy.[94]

Bleeding

Bleeding has an ominous prognosis, with mortality increasing as bleeding severity increases.[95–97] Major bleeding is associated with increase in the risk of death (4-fold), MI (5-fold), and stroke (3-fold).[14] Bleeding risk is increased with higher or excessive doses of antithrombotic agents, length of treatment, combinations of several antithrombotic drugs, switch between different anticoagulant drugs, as well as with older age, reduced renal function, low body weight, female gender, baseline haemoglobin, and invasive procedures. Sex-associated factors, such as lower BMI and lower creatinine clearance, and anatomic differences, such as smaller vessel size, may contribute to the excess risk seen in women.[98] Several definitions and classifications of bleeding have been used in trials,[96,99,100] with the simplest one provided by TIMI (Table 27.13).

Minor bleeding should preferably be managed without interruption of active treatments.

Major bleeding requires interruption and/or neutralization of both anticoagulant and antiplatelet therapy and platelet transfusion, unless bleeding can be adequately controlled by specific haemostatic intervention (Table 27.14). The risk of acute thrombotic events after interruption of antithrombotic/antiplatelet agents is maximum after 4–5 days but persists for up to 30 days.[95]

Blood transfusion has been associated with increased risk of MI and death in ACS patients and should be withheld in haemodynamically stable patients with haematocrit >25% or haemoglobin level >7 g/L.[101]

Aspirin and **clopidogrel** are irreversible platelet inhibitors. Their action is slowly reversed by the continuous generation of new platelets (around 10–20% per day), so antiplatelet effects persist for 5–10 days after cessation of treatment. Platelet transfusion is the only possibility to reverse the effects of clopidogrel/aspirin. The recommended minimum dose in adults is 0.5–0.7 x 10^{11} platelets/7 kg of body weight.

Protamine sulfate has less, or no, impact on neutralization of factor Xa activity achieved with **LMWH** or **fondaparinux**. Recombinant factor VII has been recommended but is associated with an increased risk of thrombotic complications.

There is no antidote for **bivalirudin**. Its plasma half-life is 25 min and is partially cleared renally.

Platelet transfusion is needed with **abciximab**. Interruption of **eptifibatide** and **tirofiban** infusion allows platelet function within 4–8 h. In emergencies, fibrinogen supplementation

Table 27.13 TIMI bleeding definitions

Major
Intracranial haemorrhage or clinically overt bleeding (including imaging), with ≥5 g/dL decrease in the haemoglobin concentration
Minor
Clinically overt bleeding (including imaging), with 3 to <5 g/dL decrease in the haemoglobin concentration
Minimal
Clinically overt bleeding (including imaging), with a <3 g/dL decrease in the haemoglobin concentration

All TIMI definitions take into account blood transfusions, such that haemoglobin values are adjusted by 1 g/dL for each unit of packed red blood transfused. Rao AK, *et al*. Thrombolysis in Myocardial Infarction (TIMI) Trial–phase I: haemorrhagic manifestations and changes in plasma fibrinogen and the fibrinolytic system in patients treated with recombinant tissue plasminogen activator and streptokinase. *J Am Coll Cardiol*. 1988;**11**:1–11.

Table 27.14 ESC 2011 GL on UA/NSTEMI

Management of bleeding complications	
Assessment of the individual bleeding risk on the basis of baseline characteristics (by use of risk scores), type, and duration of pharmacotherapy.	I-C
Drugs and non-pharmacological procedures (vascular access) known to carry a reduced risk of bleeding are indicated in high risk of bleeding.	I-B
Interruption and/or neutralization of both anticoagulant and antiplatelet therapies is indicated in case of major bleeding, unless it can be adequately controlled by specific haemostatic measures.	I-C
Proton pump inhibitors are in patients at increased risk of gastrointestinal haemorrhage.	I-B
Minor bleeding should preferably be managed without interruption of active treatments.	I-C
Interruption of antiplatelet drugs and neutralization of their activity with platelet transfusion are recommended, depending on the drugs under consideration and the severity of bleeding.	I-C
Blood transfusion may have deleterious effects on outcome and is indicated only after individual assessment but withheld in haemodynamically stable patients with haematocrit >25% or haemoglobin level >7 g/dL.	I-B
Erythropoietin is not indicated as a treatment for anaemia or blood loss.	III-A

ESC guidelines for the management of acute coronary syndromes in patients presenting without persistent ST-segment elevation. *Eur Heart J*. 2011;**32**:2999–3054.

with fresh frozen plasma or cryoprecipitate with or without platelet transfusion are recommended for immediate reversal of the effects of eptifibatide and tirofiban.

Factors that put patients at higher risk of bleeding are older age, female sex, lower body weight, renal insufficiency.[96]

Additional recommendations to help minimize the risk are:[96]

- Avoid overdosing by adjusting the dose to a patient's weight, age, and renal function.
- Use the shortest possible duration, i.e. 1 month after BMS implantation and 12 months after DES implantation.
- Fondaparinux may be preferred over enoxaparin in NSTEACS, and bivalirudin over unfractionated heparin and a glycoprotein IIb/IIIa inhibitor in STEMI.
- Add a proton pump inhibitor in patients at risk for GI bleed.
- Avoid access site bleeding with the use of small sheaths, closure devices, and radial acccess.
- Prefer BMS over DES in patients on triple therapy for AF.

Heparin-induced thrombocytopenia

Thrombocytopenia is defined as a decrease in platelet count to <100 000/mL or a drop of >50% from baseline platelet count. Thrombocytopenia is considered to be moderate if the platelet count is between 20 000 and 50 000/μL and severe if it is < 10 000/μL.

Non-immune heparin-associated thrombocytopenia is a mild, transient decline in platelet count that occurs 1–4 days after initiating heparin in 10–20% of patients. It rarely leads to a severe reduction in platelet levels and resolves spontaneously despite continuation of UFH.

Pseudothrombocytopenia is a laboratory artefact due to platelet clumping in EDTA-containing tubes and can be avoided by the use of citrate instead of EDTA for blood sampling.

Immune-mediated heparin-induced thrombocytopenia (HIT) is a serious complication that often leads to severe thromboembolic events.[102] It is not dose-dependent, usually causes a severe drop in platelet levels (<50%), and typically appears 5–14 days after the start of UFH treatment but much earlier in patients with recent (within 3 months) UFH exposure. Delayed-onset HIT, occurring several days or weeks after the cessation of UFH treatment, has also been described. HIT is a hypersensitivity reaction to heparin mediated via an IgG antibody to platelet factor 4. This IgG/heparin/platelet factor 4 complex binds to platelets and cross-links their receptors, which causes platelet activation and thrombosis. Bleeding is rare. HIT occurs in 0.5–5% of patients treated with unfractionated heparin (3000 to 30 000 daltons) and <1% with LMWH (less antigenic, 2000 to 9000 daltons).

Thrombocytopenia is very rare with bivalirudin and negligible with fondaparinux[103] despite weak binding to the platelet factor 4 antigen. All patients diagnosed with thrombocytopenia or a thrombotic complication within 4 to 14 days after starting heparin therapy should have heparin discontinued immediately and screening tests performed. It has been reported to occur with abciximab (2.5%) and less with tirofiban (0.5%) or eptifibatide (0.2%).[2] Rarely, it may also occur with clopidogrel.[104]

Diagnosis

The diagnosis of HIT is based on its typical clinical picture of '**4 Ts**'.

- **T**hrombocytopenia: >50% fall or nadir 20–100 × 10^9/L
- **T**iming of platelet fall: days 5 to 10 or ≤1 day if heparin exposure within past 30 days
- **T**hrombosis or other sequelae: proven thrombosis, skin necrosis, or, after heparin bolus, acute systemic reaction
- O**T**her cause for thrombocytopenia: none evident.

Thromboembolic complications are predominantly venous and may be devastating; pulmonary embolism, deep-vein thrombosis, myocardial infarction, and stroke may occur. Associated mortality is 5–10%.[103] Diagnosis is confirmed by circulating heparin-PF4 antibodies that remain detectable for 4 months after the diagnosis of HIT in 10–40% of patients, depending on the assay used. Scoring systems for diagnosis have been developed.[103]

Quinine- or other drug-induced immune thrombocytopenic purpura, as well as glycoprotein IIb/IIIa antagonist-induced thrombocytopenia, typically has more severe thrombocytopenia than that of HIT. Patients with massive, acute venous thromboembolism occasionally develop thrombocytopenia because of platelet consumption on the thrombus surface; their platelet count nadir usually happens within 1 day of heparin initiation. Other causes of repeat thrombotic episodes are the antiphospholipid antibody syndrome, Trousseau's syndrome, cholesterol emboli syndrome, and infective or non-bacterial thrombotic endocarditis. HIT should be also considered if a recently hospitalized patient returns with thromboembolism.

Therapy of HIT

Interruption of heparin (UFH or LMWH) is warranted in the case of documented or suspected HIT. Significant thrombocytopenia (<100 000/mL or >50% drop in platelet count) occurring during treatment with GP IIb/IIIa inhibitors and/or heparin (LMWH or UFH) requires the immediate interruption of these drugs (Table 27.15).

Severe thrombocytopenia (<10 000/mL), induced by GP IIb/IIIa inhibitors, requires platelet transfusion, with or without fibrinogen supplementation, with fresh frozen plasma or cryoprecipitate in the case of bleeding.

In the case of **thrombotic complications**, anticoagulation can be achieved with a direct thrombin inhibitor, such as **bivalirudin**. This is also recommended by the ACCP (2C) for cardiac surgery or coronary intervention.

- Dose for bivalirudin: IV infusion of 0.15–2.0 mg/kg/hour (no bolus) to maintain an APTT of 1.5–2.5 times baseline value.[103] Alternatively, the XA inhibitor **fondaparinux** can be used.
- Dose for fondaparinux: 5.0 mg SC daily for patients <50 kg; 7.5 mg for 50–100 kg; 10.9 mg for >100 kg. No monitoring of anti-Xa activity is necessary.[101]

The direct thrombin inhibitor **argatroban** is approved by the FDA for HIT, and is particularly indicated in renal insufficiency (ACCP 2012–2C). Hypercoagulability may

Table 27.15 ESC 2011 GL on STEMI. Recommendations for thrombocytopenia

Immediate interruption of IIb/IIIa receptor inhibitors and/or heparin (UFH or LMWH) in the case of significant thrombocytopenia (<100 000/μL or >50% drop in platelet count).	I-C
Platelet transfusion, with or without fibrinogen supplementation, with fresh frozen plasma or cryoprecipitate in the case of bleeding and severe thrombocytopenia (<10 000/μL) induced by IIb/IIIa receptor inhibitors.	I-C
Interruption of heparin (UFH or LMWH) is indicated in the case of documented or suspected HIT, to be replaced by a DTI in the case of thrombotic complications.	I-C
Anticoagulants with a low risk of HIT or devoid of risk of HIT (such as fondaparinux or bivalirudin) or brief administration of heparin (UFH or LMWH) is recommended to prevent the occurrence of HIT.	I-C

DTI, direct thrombin inhibitor; HIT, heparin-induced thrombocytopenia.
ESC guidelines for the management of acute coronary syndromes in patients presenting without persistent ST-segment elevation. *Eur Heart J.* 2011;**32**:2999–3054.

occur with discontinuation of the drug, and transition to warfarin may be challenging.

- Dose for argatroban: IV infusion of 2.0 mcg/kg/min; 0.5–1.2 mcg/kg.min in liver disease, critical illness or after cardiac surgery to maintain an APTT of 1.5–3.0 times baseline value (max 10 mcg/kg/min).[103]

The factor Xa inhibitor **danaparoid** and the direct thrombin inhibitor **lepirudin** are also recommended by the ACCP 2012 guidelines (2C).[59,105] Danaparoid is recommended in pregnancy (ACCP 2012–2C).

Platelet glycoprotein IIb/IIIa inhibitors reduce thrombin generation indirectly and inhibit platelet aggregation. However, they lack direct anticoagulant effects and do not inhibit Fc receptor-mediated activation of platelets by HIT antibody.

Platelet transfusions are recommended by the ACCP for invasive procedures (ACCP 2012–2C). They should not be used routinely for prophylaxis of bleeding in HIT because they may exacerbate the hypercoagulable state, leading to additional thrombosis.

Vitamin K inhibitors such as warfarin are started when platelets are >150 x 10^9/L (ACCP 2012–1C). Early introduction should be avoided due to the potential to worsen the prothrombotic state through a rapid reduction of protein C, and an overlap period to allow a therapeutic INR should intervene. Warfarin should be continued for 4–6 weeks, and in patients with thrombosis for 3 months.

Patients with a history of HIT may not invariably have recurrent HIT on heparin re-exposure. In addition, heparin has been tolerated for a brief period, such as during cardiac surgery, in patients in whom heparin-PF4 antibodies have fully waned. Still, it is better to use an alternative anticoagulant.

Risk stratification before discharge

In low- or intermediate-risk patients who have been free of ischaemia at rest or with low-level activity or heart failure for a minimum of 12–24 h, a stress test or an imaging modality are recommended for assessment of ischaemia and risk stratification purposes (Table 27.16). Risk stratification is discussed in detail in the Chapter on Stable CAD. In general, LVEF<=35% at rest and <=50% at exercise, LVEF fall >=10% at stress, fixed or exercise-induced large perfusion defects, and wall-motion score index> 1 on stress echocardiography indicate high risk patients.[1]

Table 27.16 ACCF/AHA 2012 GL UA/NSTEMI. Risk stratification before discharge

Noninvasive stress testing in low- or intermediate-risk patient who have been free of ischemia at rest or with low-level activity and of HF for a minimum of 12 to 24 h.	I-C
Choice of stress test is based on the resting ECG, ability to perform exercise, local expertise, and technologies available. Treadmill exercise is useful in patients able to exercise in whom the ECG is free of baseline ST-segment abnormalities, bundle-branch block, LV hypertrophy, intraventricular conduction defect, paced rhythm, pre-excitation, and digoxin effect.	I-C
An imaging modality should be added in patients with resting ST-segment depression (>= 0.10 mV), LV hypertrophy, bundle-branch block, intraventricular conduction defect, preexcitation, or digoxin who are able to exercise. In patients undergoing a low-level exercise test, an imaging modality can add sensitivity.	I-B
Pharmacological stress testing with imaging when physical limitations (e.g., arthritis, amputation). Severe peripheral vascular disease, severe chronic obstructive pulmonary disease, or general debility) preclude adequate exercise stress.	I-B
Prompt angiography without noninvasive risk stratification for failure of stabilization with intensive medical treatment	I-B
A noninvasive test (echocardiogram or radionuclide angiogram) to evaluate LV function in patients with definite ACS who are not scheduled for coronary angiography and left ventriculography	I-B

Post-hospital discharge care

Aspirin (indefinitely), a P2Y12 inhibitor for 1 year, and a beta blocker are mandatory. In patients receiving a stent (BMS or DES), P2Y12 inhibitors should be given for, at least, 12 months or >15 months with DES use (ACC/AHA 2011 IIb-C). If there is a high risk of bleeding, earlier discontinuation may be considered. Options include clopidogrel 75 mg daily, prasugrel 10 mg daily, and ticagrelor 90 mg twice daily. Rivaroxaban, but not apixaban or dabigatran, has reduced ischaemic events but at an increased risk of bleeding.[59,61,62] Nitrates and calcium channel blockers (other that short-acting dihydropyridines) may also be used for symptomatic relief, especially when beta blockers are contraindicated or ineffective. Patients with LVEF <40%, heart failure, or diabetes should be put on ACE inhibitors or ARBs. In the absence of hyperkalaemia or creatinine clearance <30 mL/min, an aldosterone receptor blocker, such as eplerenone, is also recommended. All patients should be screened for depression, following an ACS (ACC/AHA 2011 on secondary prevention I-A).

Other measures for secondary prevention are discussed in detail in Chapter 29 on stable CAD.

References

1. Anderson JL, *et al.* 2012 ACCF/AHA focused update incorporated into the ACCF/AHA 2007 Guidelines for the management of patients with unstable angina/non–ST-elevation myocardial infarction. *J Am Coll Cardiol.* 2013;**61**:e179–347.
2. Hamm CW, *et al.* ESC guidelines for the management of acute coronary syndromes in patients presenting without persistent ST-segment elevation. *Eur Heart J.* 2011;**32**:2999–3054.
3. Kumar A, *et al.* Acute coronary syndromes: Diagnosis and management, part ii.*Mayo Clin Proc.* 2009;**84**:1021–1036
4. Kumar A, *et al.* Acute coronary syndromes: Diagnosis and management, part i. *Mayo Clin Proc.* 2009;**84**:917–938

5. Savonitto S, *et al.* Prognostic value of the admission electrocardiogram in acute coronary syndromes. *JAMA.* 1999;**281**:707–13
6. Antman EM, *et al.* Cardiac-specific troponin I levels to predict the risk of mortality in patients with acute coronary syndromes. *N Engl J Med.* 1996;**335**:1342–9
7. Newby LK, *et al.* ACCF 2012 expert consensus document on practical clinical considerations in the interpretation of troponin elevations: a report of the American College of Cardiology Foundation Task Force on clinical expert consensus documents. *J Am Coll Cardiol.* 2012;**60**:2427–63
8. Eggers KM, *et al.* Growth differentiation factor-15 for early risk stratification in patients with acute chest pain. *Eur Heart J.* 2008;**29**:2327–35
9. Morrow DA, *et al.* C-reactive protein is a potent predictor of mortality independently of and in combination with troponin T in acute coronary syndromes: a TIMI 11A substudy. Thrombolysis in myocardial infarction. *J Am Coll Cardiol.* 1998;**31**:1460–5
10. Sabatine MS, *et al.* Relationship between baseline white blood cell count and degree of coronary artery disease and mortality in patients with acute coronary syndromes: a TACTICS-TIMI 18 (treat angina with aggrastat and determine cost of therapy with an invasive or conservative strategy-thrombolysis in myocardial infarction 18 trial) substudy. *J Am Coll Cardiol.* 2002;**40**:1761–8
11. Than M, *et al.* A 2-h diagnostic protocol to assess patients with chest pain symptoms in the Asia–Pacific region (aspect): a prospective observational validation study. *Lancet.* 2011;**377**:1077–84
12. Hoffmann U, *et al.* Coronary CT angiography versus standard evaluation in acute chest pain. *N Engl J Med.* 2012;**367**:299–308
13. Litt HI, *et al.* CT angiography for safe discharge of patients with possible acute coronary syndromes. *N Engl J Med.* 2012;**366**:1393–403
14. Antman EM, *et al.* The TIMI risk score for unstable angina/non-ST elevation MI: a method for prognostication and therapeutic decision making. *JAMA.* 2000;**284**:835–42
15. Eagle KA, *et al.* A validated prediction model for all forms of acute coronary syndrome: estimating the risk of 6-month post-discharge death in an international registry. *JAMA.* 2004;**291**:2727–33
16. Udelson JE, *et al.* Myocardial perfusion imaging for evaluation and triage of patients with suspected acute cardiac ischaemia: a randomized controlled trial. *JAMA.* 2002;**288**:2693–700
17. Kwong RY, *et al.* Detecting acute coronary syndrome in the emergency department with cardiac magnetic resonance imaging. *Circulation.* 2003;**107**:531–7
18. Hoffmann U, *et al.* Coronary computed tomography angiography for early triage of patients with acute chest pain: the ROMICAT (rule out myocardial infarction using computer assisted tomography) trial. *J Am Coll Cardiol.* 2009;**53**:1642–50
19. Meine TJ, *et al.* Association of intravenous morphine use and outcomes in acute coronary syndromes: results from the CRUSADE quality improvement initiative. *Am Heart J.* 2005;**149**:1043–9
20. Grosser TFS, *et al.* Drug resistance and pseudoresistance: An unintended consequence of enteric coating aspirin. *Circulation.* 2013;**127**:77–85
21. Wallentin L, *et al.* Ticagrelor versus clopidogrel in patients with acute coronary syndromes. *N Engl J Med.* 2009;**361**:1045–57
22. Storey RF, *et al.* Incidence of dyspnoea and assessment of cardiac and pulmonary function in patients with stable coronary artery disease receiving ticagrelor, clopidogrel, or placebo in the onset/offset study. *J Am Coll Cardiol.* 2010;**56**:185–93
23. Scirica BM, *et al.* The incidence of bradyarrhythmias and clinical bradyarrhythmic events in patients with acute coronary syndromes treated with ticagrelor or clopidogrel in the PLATO (platelet inhibition and patient outcomes) trial: results of the continuous electrocardiographic assessment substudy. *J Am Coll Cardiol.* 2011;**57**:1908–16
24. Gaglia MA, Jr., *et al.* Overview of the 2010 Food and Drug Administration Cardiovascular and Renal Drugs Advisory Committee meeting regarding ticagrelor. *Circulation.* 2011;**123**:451–6
25. Mahaffey KW, *et al.* Ticagrelor compared with clopidogrel by geographic region in the platelet inhibition and patient outcomes (PLATO) trial. *Circulation.* 2011;**124**:544–54
26. Becker RC, *et al.* Bleeding complications with the P2Y12 receptor antagonists clopidogrel and ticagrelor in the platelet inhibition and patient outcomes (PLATO) trial. *Eur Heart J.* 2011;**32**:2933–44
27. James SK, *et al.* Ticagrelor versus clopidogrel in patients with acute coronary syndromes and a history of stroke or transient ischaemic attack. *Circulation.* 2012;**125**:2914–21
28. Yusuf S, *et al.* Effects of clopidogrel in addition to aspirin in patients with acute coronary syndromes without ST segment elevation. *N Engl J Med.* 2001;**345**:494–502
29. Holmes DR, Jr., *et al.* ACCF/AHA clopidogrel clinical alert: approaches to the FDA 'boxed warning': a report of the American College of Cardiology Foundation Task Force on clinical expert consensus documents and the American Heart Association. *Circulation.* 2010;**122**:537–57
30. Mega JL, *et al.* Reduced-function CYP2C19 genotype and risk of adverse clinical outcomes among patients treated with clopidogrel predominantly for PCI: a meta-analysis. *JAMA.* 2010;**304**:1821–30
31. Pare G, *et al.* Effects of CYP2C19 genotype on outcomes of clopidogrel treatment. *N Engl J Med.* 2010;**363**:1704–14
32. Wallentin L, *et al.* Effect of CYP2C19 and ABCB1 single nucleotide polymorphisms on outcomes of treatment with ticagrelor versus clopidogrel for acute coronary syndromes: a genetic substudy of the PLATO trial. *Lancet.* 2010;**376**:1320–8
33. Krishna V, *et al.* Do platelet function testing and genotyping improve outcome in patients treated with antithrombotic agents?: The role of platelet reactivity and genotype testing in the prevention of atherothrombotic cardiovascular events remains unproven. *Circulation.* 2012;**125**:1288–303; discussion 1303
34. Collet JP, *et al.* Bedside monitoring to adjust antiplatelet therapy for coronary stenting. *N Engl J Med.* 2012;**367**:2100–9
35. Parodi G, *et al.* High residual platelet reactivity after clopidogrel loading and long-term cardiovascular events among

patients with acute coronary syndromes undergoing PCI. *JAMA*. 2011;**306**:1215–23
36. Price MJ, *et al.* Standard- vs high-dose clopidogrel based on platelet function testing after percutaneous coronary intervention: the GRAVITAS randomized trial. *JAMA*. 2011;**305**:1097–105
37. Bonello L, *et al.* High on-treatment platelet reactivity after prasugrel loading dose and cardiovascular events after percutaneous coronary intervention in acute coronary syndromes. *J Am Coll Cardiol*. 2011;**58**:467–73
38. Stockl KM, *et al.* Risk of rehospitalization for patients using clopidogrel with a proton pump inhibitor. *Arch Intern Med*. 2010;**170**:704–10
39. Bhatt DL, *et al.* Clopidogrel with or without omeprazole in coronary artery disease. *N Engl J Med*. 2010;**363**:1909–17
40. Simon T, *et al.* Clinical events as a function of proton pump inhibitor use, clopidogrel use, and cytochrome P450 2C19 genotype in a large nationwide cohort of acute myocardial infarction: results from the French registry of acute ST elevation and non-ST elevation myocardial infarction (fast-MI) registry. *Circulation*. 2011;**123**:474–82
41. Agewall S, *et al.* Expert position paper on the use of proton pump inhibitors in patients with cardiovascular disease and antithrombotic therapy. *Eur Heart J*. Feb **20**. [Epub ahead of print] PubMed PMID: 23425521.
42. Charlot M, *et al.* Proton pump inhibitors are associated with increased cardiovascular risk independent of clopidogrel use: a nationwide cohort study. *Ann Intern Med*. 2010;**153**:378–86
43. Goodman SG, *et al.* Association of proton pump inhibitor use on cardiovascular outcomes with clopidogrel and ticagrelor: insights from the platelet inhibition and patient outcomes trial. *Circulation*. 2012;**125**:978–86
44. Good CW, *et al.* Is there a clinically significant interaction between calcium channel antagonists and clopidogrel?: results from the clopidogrel for the reduction of events during observation (CREDO) trial. *Circ Cardiovasc Interv*. 2012;**5**:77–81
45. Olesen JB, *et al.* Calcium channel blockers do not alter the clinical efficacy of clopidogrel after myocardial infarction: a nationwide cohort study. *J Am Coll Cardiol*. 2011;**57**:409–17
46. Saw J, *et al.* Lack of evidence of a clopidogrel-statin interaction in the charisma trial. *J Am Coll Cardiol*. 2007;**50**:291–5
47. Cheema AN, *et al.* Characterization of clopidogrel hypersensitivity reactions and management with oral steroids without clopidogrel discontinuation. *J Am Coll Cardiol*. 2011;**58**:1445–54
48. Nijjer SS, *et al.* Safety of clopidogrel being continued until the time of coronary artery bypass grafting in patients with acute coronary syndrome: a meta-analysis of 34 studies. *Eur Heart J*. 2011;**32**:2970–88
49. Wiviott SD, *et al.* Prasugrel versus clopidogrel in patients with acute coronary syndromes. *N Engl J Med*. 2007;**357**:2001–15
50. Roe MT, *et al.* Prasugrel versus clopidogrel for acute coronary syndromes without revascularization. *N Engl J Med*. 2012;**367**:1297–309
51. Serebruany V, *et al.* Excess of solid cancers after prasugrel: the Food and Drug Administration outlook. *Am J Ther*. 2010 (Epub ahead of print)
52. Bhatt DL, *et al.* for the CHAMPION PHOENIX Investigators. Effect of platelet inhibition with cangrelor during pci on ischemic events. *N Engl J Med*. 2013; doi: 10.1056/NEJMoa1300815
53. Anderson JL, *et al.* Management of patients with peripheral artery disease (compilation of 2005 and 2011 ACCF/AHA guideline recommendations): A report of the american college of cardiology foundation/american heart association task force on practice guidelines. *J Am Coll Cardiol*. 2013; doi: pii: S0735-1097(0713)00177-00170. 00110.01016/j.jacc.02013.00101.00004. 10.1056/NEJMoa1300815
54. Boersma E, *et al.* Platelet glycoprotein IIb/IIIa inhibitors in acute coronary syndromes: a meta-analysis of all major randomised clinical trials. *Lancet*. 2002;**359**:189–98
55. Hirsh J, *et al.* Beyond unfractionated heparin and warfarin: current and future advances. *Circulation*. 2007;**116**:552–60
56. Murphy SA, *et al.* Efficacy and safety of the low molecular weight heparin enoxaparin compared with unfractionated heparin across the acute coronary syndrome spectrum: a meta-analysis. *Eur Heart J*. 2007;**28**:2077–86
57. Kastrati A, *et al.* Abciximab and heparin versus bivalirudin for non-ST elevation myocardial infarction. *N Engl J Med*. 2011;**365**:1980–9
58. Stone GW, *et al.* Bivalirudin for patients with acute coronary syndromes. *N Engl J Med*. 2006;**355**:2203–16
59. Oldgren J, *et al.* Dabigatran vs placebo in patients with acute coronary syndromes on dual antiplatelet therapy: a randomized, double-blind, phase II trial. *Eur Heart J*. 2011;**32**:2781–9
60. Jolly SS, *et al.* Efficacy and safety of fondaparinux versus enoxaparin in patients with acute coronary syndromes treated with glycoprotein IIb/IIIa inhibitors or thienopyridines: results from the OASIS 5 (fifth organization to assess strategies in ischaemic syndromes) trial. *J Am Coll Cardiol*. 2009;**54**:468–76
61. Mega JL, *et al.* Rivaroxaban in patients with a recent acute coronary syndrome. *N Engl J Med*. 2012;**366**:9–19
62. Alexander JH, *et al.* Apixaban with antiplatelet therapy after acute coronary syndrome. *N Engl J Med*. 2011;**365**:699–708
63. Oldgren JWL, *et al.* New oral anticoagulants in addition to single or dual antiplatelet therapy after an acute coronary syndrome: A systematic review and meta-analysis. *Eur Heart J*. 2013.
64. Lamberts M, *et al.* Bleeding after initiation of multiple antithrombotic drugs, including triple therapy, in atrial fibrillation patients following myocardial infarction and coronary intervention: a nationwide cohort study. *Circulation*. 2012;**126**:1185–93
65. Komocsi A, *et al.* Use of new-generation oral anticoagulant agents in patients receiving antiplatelet therapy after an acute coronary syndrome: systematic review and meta-analysis of randomized controlled trials. *Arch Intern Med*. 2012:**172**:1537–45
66. Lip GY, *et al.* Antithrombotic management of atrial fibrillation patients presenting with acute coronary syndrome and/or undergoing coronary stenting: executive summary—a consensus document of the European Society of Cardiology Working Group on thrombosis, endorsed by the European Heart Rhythm Association (EHRA) and the European Association of Percutaneous Cardiovascular Interventions (EAPCI). *Eur Heart J*. 2010;**31**:1311–18

67. Dewilde W. Woest: First randomized trial that compares two different regimens with and without aspirin in patients on oral anticoagulant therapy (OAC) undergoing coronary stent placement (PCI). Presented at: European Society of Cardiology Congress; August 28, 2012; Munich, Germany. 2012
68. Levine GN, *et al.* 2011 ACCF/AHA/SCAI guideline for percutaneous coronary intervention: a report of the American College of Cardiology Foundation/American Heart Association Task Force on practice guidelines and the Society for Cardiovascular Angiography and Interventions. *Circulation.* 2011;**124**:e574–651
69. Invasive compared with non-invasive treatment in unstable coronarymartery disease: FRISC II prospective randomised multicentre study. Fragmin and fast revascularisation during instability in coronary artery disease investigators. *Lancet.* 1999;**354**:708–15
70. Cannon CP, *et al.* Comparison of early invasive and conservative strategies in patients with unstable coronary syndromes treated with the glycoprotein IIb/IIIa inhibitor tirofiban. *N Engl J Med.* 2001;**344**:1879–87
71. Fox KA, *et al.* Interventional versus conservative treatment for patients with unstable angina or non-ST elevation myocardial infarction: the British Heart Foundation RITA 3 randomised trial. Randomized intervention trial of unstable angina. *Lancet.* 2002;**360**:743–51
72. Mehta SR, *et al.* Early versus delayed invasive intervention in acute coronary syndromes. *N Engl J Med.* 2009;**360**:2165–75
73. Neumann FJ, *et al.* Evaluation of prolonged antithrombotic pretreatment ('cooling-off' strategy) before intervention in patients with unstable coronary syndromes: a randomized controlled trial. *JAMA.* 2003;**290**:1593–9
74. de Winter RJ, *et al.* Early invasive versus selectively invasive management for acute coronary syndromes. *N Engl J Med.* 2005;**353**:1095–104
75. van 't Hof AW, *et al.* A comparison of two invasive strategies in patients with non-ST elevation acute coronary syndromes: results of the early or late intervention in unstable angina (ELISA) pilot study. 2B/3A upstream therapy and acute coronary syndromes. *Eur Heart J.* 2003;**24**:1401–5
76. Montalescot G, *et al.* Immediate vs delayed intervention for acute coronary syndromes: a randomized clinical trial. *JAMA.* 2009;**302**:947–54
77. Riezebos RK, *et al.* Immediate versus deferred coronary angioplasty in non-ST segment elevation acute coronary syndromes. *Heart.* 2009;**95**:807–12
78. Thiele H, *et al.* Optimal timing of invasive angiography in stable non-ST elevation myocardial infarction: the Leipzig immediate versus early and late percutaneous coronary intervention trial in NSTEMI (LIPSIA-NSTEMI trial). *Eur Heart J.* 2012;**33**:2035–43
79. Bavry AA, *et al.* Benefit of early invasive therapy in acute coronary syndromes: a meta-analysis of contemporary randomized clinical trials. *J Am Coll Cardiol.* 2006;**48**:1319–25
80. Fox KA, *et al.* Long-term outcome of a routine versus selective invasive strategy in patients with non-ST segment elevation acute coronary syndrome: a meta-analysis of individual patient data. *J Am Coll Cardiol.* 2010;**55**:2435–45
81. Damman P, *et al.* Long-term cardiovascular mortality after procedure-related or spontaneous myocardial infarction in patients with non-ST segment elevation acute coronary syndrome: a collaborative analysis of individual patient data from the FRISC II, ICTUS, and RITA-3 trials (FIR). *Circulation.* 2012;**125**:568–76
82. O'Donoghue M, *et al.* Early invasive vs conservative treatment strategies in women and men with unstable angina and non-ST segment elevation myocardial infarction: A meta-analysis. *JAMA.* 2008;**300**:71–80
83. Patel MR, *et al.* ACCF/SCAI/STS/AATS/AHA/ASNC/HFSA/SCCT 2012 appropriate use criteria for coronary revascularization focused update: a report of the American College of Cardiology Foundation Appropriate Use Criteria Task Force, Society for Cardiovascular Angiography and Interventions, Society of Thoracic Surgeons, American Association for Thoracic Surgery, American Heart Association, American Society of Nuclear Cardiology, and the Society of Cardiovascular Computed Tomography. *J Am Coll Cardiol.* 2012;**59**:857–81
84. Navarese EP GP, *et al.* Optimal timing of coronary invasive strategy in non-st-segment elevation acute coronary syndromes: A systematic review and meta-analysis. *Ann Intern Med.* 2013;**158**:261–70
85. Katritsis DG, *et al.* Optimal timing of coronary angiography and potential intervention in non-ST elevation acute coronary syndromes. *Eur Heart J.* 2011;**32**:32–40
86. O'Donoghue ML, *et al.* An invasive or conservative strategy in patients with diabetes mellitus and non-ST segment elevation acute coronary syndromes: a collaborative meta-analysis of randomized trials. *J Am Coll Cardiol.* 2012;**60**:106–111
87. Greenhalgh J, *et al.* Drug-eluting stents versus bare metal stents for angina or acute coronary syndromes. *Cochrane Database Syst Rev.* 2010;**5**:CD004587
88. Palmerini T, *et al.* Prognostic value of the syntax score in patients with acute coronary syndromes undergoing percutaneous coronary intervention: analysis from the ACUITY (acute catheterization and urgent intervention triage strategy) trial. *J Am Coll Cardiol.* 2011;**57**:2389–97
89. Rosner GF, *et al.* Impact of the presence and extent of incomplete angiographic revascularization after percutaneous coronary intervention in acute coronary syndromes: the acute catheterization and urgent intervention triage strategy (ACUITY) trial. *Circulation.* 2012;**125**:2613–20
90. Généreux PPT, *et al.* Quantification and impact of untreated coronary artery disease after percutaneous coronary intervention: The residual syntax (synergy between pci with taxus and cardiac surgery) score. *J Am Coll Cardiol.* 2012;**59**:2165–74
91. Bach RG, *et al.* The effect of routine, early invasive management on outcome for elderly patients with non-ST segment elevation acute coronary syndromes. *Ann Intern Med.* 2004;**141**:186–95
92. Regitz-Zagrosek V, *et al.* ESC guidelines on the management of cardiovascular diseases during pregnancy: the Task Force on the management of cardiovascular diseases during pregnancy of the European Society of Cardiology (ESC). *Eur Heart J.* 2011;**32**:3147–97
93. Modi S, *et al.* Sudden cardiac arrest without overt heart disease. *Circulation.* 2011;**123**:2994–3008

94. Hochman JS, *et al.* Early revascularization and long-term survival in cardiogenic shock complicating acute myocardial infarction. *JAMA*. 2006;**295**:2511–5
95. Eikelboom JW, *et al.* Adverse impact of bleeding on prognosis in patients with acute coronary syndromes. *Circulation*. 2006;**114**:774–82
96. Steg PG, *et al.* Bleeding in acute coronary syndromes and percutaneous coronary interventions: position paper by the working group on thrombosis of the European Society of Cardiology. *Eur Heart J*. 2011;**32**:1854–64
97. Subherwal S, *et al.* Baseline risk of major bleeding in non-ST segment elevation myocardial infarction: the CRUSADE (can rapid risk stratification of unstable angina patients suppress adverse outcomes with early implementation of the acc/aha guidelines) bleeding score. *Circulation*. 2009;**119**:1873–82
98. Ahmed B and Dauerman HL. Women, bleeding, and coronary intervention. *Circulation*. 2013;**127**:641–9
99. Mehran R, *et al.* Standardized bleeding definitions for cardiovascular clinical trials: a consensus report from the Bleeding Academic Research Consortium. *Circulation*. 2011;**123**:2736–47
100. Rao AK, *et al.* Thrombolysis in myocardial infarction (TIMI) trial—phase I: haemorrhagic manifestations and changes in plasma fibrinogen and the fibrinolytic system in patients treated with recombinant tissue plasminogen activator and streptokinase. *J Am Coll Cardiol*. 1988;**11**:1–11
101. Chatterjee S, *et al.* Association of blood transfusion with increased mortality in myocardial infarction: a meta-analysis and diversity-adjusted study sequential analysis. *JAMA Intern Med*. 2013;**173**;132–9
102. Jang IK, *et al.* When heparins promote thrombosis: review of heparin-induced thrombocytopenia. *Circulation*. 2005;**111**:2671–83
103. Bennett CL, *et al.* Thrombotic thrombocytopenic purpura associated with clopidogrel. *N Engl J Med*. 2000;**342**:1773–7
104. Hirulog and early reperfusion or occlusion (HERO)-2 trial investigators. Thrombin-specific anticoagulation with bivalirudin versus heparin in patients receiving fibrinolytic therapy for acute myocardial infarction: the HERO-2 randomised trial. *Lancet*. 2001;**358**:1855–63.
105. Eikelboom JW, *et al.* Antiplatelet drugs: Antithrombotic therapy and prevention of thrombosis, 9th ed: American College of Chest Physicians evidence-based clinical practice guidelines. *Chest*. 2012;**141**:e89S–119S

Chapter 28

Acute myocardial infarction

Definition

According to the third universal definition of myocardial infarction (MI) from the Joint ESC/ACCF/AHA/WHF Task Force, an MI diagnosis requires a **cardiac troponin (I or T)** level above the 99th percentile of a normal reference population **plus one, or more**, of the following:

- Symptoms of ischaemia
- New significant ST/T wave changes or new LBBB
- Pathologic Q waves on ECG
- Imaging evidence of new loss of viable myocardium or regional wall motion abnormality
- Intracoronary thrombus diagnosed by angiography or autopsy.

A classification of MI is provided in Table 28.1.[1]

The pathophysiology and aetiology of MI are described under ACS section in Chapter 26 on the epidemiology and pathophysiology of coronary artery disease. Non-atherosclerotic causes of MI are presented in Table 28.2.

Presentation

Prodromal symptoms of chest discomfort may be absent, and retrosternal compressing or heaviness-like pain that lasts more than 30 min is typical. They are described with a clenched fist against the sternum (Levine sign). The pain may radiate to both sites of the chest, with a predilection for the left side, the jaw, or the arms and wrists. It may be epigastric, misdiagnosed as indigestion. Diaphoresis, nausea, and vomiting may appear. In up to 25% of cases, the infarction may be silent. Diabetics, the elderly, and heart transplant recipients may not have symptoms. Silent MIs accounted for 25% of all MIs in the Framingham study, and approximately 17% of diabetics have pathological Q waves.[2] In patients with acute chest pain, the prevalence of acute MI is 80% in the presence of ≥1 mm of new ST segment elevation and 20% with new ST segment depression or T wave inversion. In the absence of electrocardiographic changes consistent with the presence of ischaemia, the risk of acute myocardial infarction is 4% among patients with acute chest pain and a history of coronary artery disease and 2% among patients with no such history.[3]

Physical examination

- With uncomplicated MIs, physical examination **may be unremarkable**.
- **Tachycardia** and **elevated respiratory rate** may be present.

Table 28.1 Joint ESC/ACCF/AHA/WHF 2012 universal classification of myocardial infarction

Type 1: spontaneous myocardial infarction
Spontaneous myocardial infarction related to atherosclerotic plaque rupture, ulceration, fissuring, erosion, or dissection, with resulting intraluminal thrombus in one, or more, of the coronary arteries, leading to decreased myocardial blood flow or distal platelet emboli with ensuing myocyte necrosis. The patient may have underlying severe CAD but, on occasion, non-obstructive, or no, CAD.
Type 2: myocardial infarction secondary to an ischaemic imbalance
In instances of myocardial injury with necrosis where a condition other than CAD contributes to an imbalance between myocardial oxygen supply and/or demand, e.g. coronary endothelial dysfunction, coronary artery spasm, coronary embolism, tachy-/bradyarrhythmias, anaemia, respiratory failure, hypotension, and hypertension with or without LVH.
Type 3: myocardial infarction resulting in death when biomarker values are unavailable
Cardiac death with symptoms suggestive of myocardial ischaemia and presumed new ischaemic ECG changes or new LBBB, but death occurring before blood samples could be obtained, before cardiac biomarker could rise, or, in rare cases, when cardiac biomarkers were not collected.
Type 4a: myocardial infarction related to percutaneous coronary intervention (PCI)
Myocardial infarction associated with PCI is arbitrarily defined by elevation of cTn values >5 × 99th percentile of a normal reference population (URL) in patients with normal baseline values (≤99th percentile URL) or a rise of cTn values >20% if the baseline values are elevated and are stable or falling. In addition, either (i) symptoms suggestive of myocardial ischaemia, or (ii) new ischaemic ECG changes or new LBBB, or (iii) angiographic loss of patency of a major coronary artery or a side branch or persistent slow or no-flow or embolization, or (iv) imaging demonstration of new loss of viable myocardium or new regional wall motion abnormality are required.
Type 4b: myocardial infarction related to stent thrombosis
Myocardial infarction associated with stent thrombosis is detected by coronary angiography or autopsy in the setting of myocardial ischaemia and with a rise and/or fall of cardiac biomarkers values with at least one value above the 99th percentile URL.
Type 5: myocardial infarction related to coronary artery bypass grafting (CABG)
Myocardial infarction associated with CABG is arbitrarily defined by elevation of cardiac biomarker values >10 × 99th percentile URL in patients with normal baseline cTn values (≤99th percentile URL). In addition, either (i) new pathological Q waves or new LBBB, or (ii) angiographic documented new graft or new native coronary artery occlusion, or (iii) imaging evidence of new loss of viable myocardium or new regional wall motion abnormality.

ESC/ACCF/AHA/WHF Expert Consensus Document. Third Universal Definition of Myocardial Infarction. *European Heart Journal* 2012;**33**,2551–2567.

- **Fever** may appear between 4 and 48 h and resolves by the fourth day post-MI.
- S_4 is invariably present.
- **Pericardial friction rubs** are common within the first 2–3 days following a transmural infarct.

Diagnosis

ECG changes

They are essential for diagnosis (Table 28.3) but may not be present, depending on the extent and location of myocardial injury and the presence of pre-existing abnormalities (conduction defects, hypertension and ventricular hypertrophy, electrolyte disturbances, and drugs). The typical ECG patterns of MI seen in leads that face the area of damage are appearance of **Q waves** (>0.03 s, loss of forces directed towards the electrode), **ST segment elevation** (upward convexity), and **T wave inversion** (after 4 hours) (Tables 28.4 and 28.5). ST-T changes are not specific; healthy young men may have concave ST segment elevation of 1 to 3 mm in one, or more, precordial leads.[4] Other conditions associated with ST elevation are shown in Table 28.6 and Figure 28.1. However, ST elevation and symptoms of MI are indications for reperfusion therapy (Class I indication), and the number of leads demonstrating ST elevation has been a useful risk marker in MI. The presence of Q

Table 28.2 Non-atherosclerotic causes of myocardial infarction

Embolic
Infective endocarditis
Neoplasms
Prosthetic valves
Arteritis
Syphilitic aortitis
Takayasu's arteritis
Polyarteritis nodosa
Giant cell arteritis
Systemic lupus erythematosus
Kawasaki disease
Vital infections
Prothrombotic states
Polycythaemia vera
Sickle cell disease
Disseminated intravascular coagulation
Thrombocytosis
Thrombocytopenic purpura
Other
Takotsubo cardiomyopathy, severe AS, prolonged hypotension, thyrotoxicosis, carbon monoxide poisoning, chest trauma, mediastinal radiation, spontaneous coronary dissection, cocaine abuse

ESC/ACCF/AHA/WHF Expert Consensus Document. Third Universal Definition of Myocardial Infarction. *European Heart Journal* 2012;**33**,2551–2567.

Table 28.3 ESC 2012 GL on STEMI

Recommendations for initial diagnosis	
A 12-lead ECG must be obtained as soon as possible at the point of FMC, with a target delay of ≤10 min.	I-B
ECG monitoring must be initiated as soon as possible in all patients with suspected STEMI.	I-B
Blood sampling for serum markers routinely in the acute phase, but one should not wait for the results before initiating reperfusion treatment.	I-C
Additional posterior chest wall leads (V_7–V_9 ≥0.05 mV) in patients with high suspicion of inferobasal myocardial infarction (circumflex occlusion).	IIa-C
Echocardiography may assist in making the diagnosis in uncertain cases but should not delay transfer for angiography.	IIb-C

ECG, electrocardiogram; FMC, first medical contact; STEMI, ST segment elevation myocardial infarction.
ESC Guidelines for the management of acute myocardial infarction in patients presenting with ST-segment elevation. *Eur Heart J* 2012;**33**:2501–2502.

Table 28.4 ESC/ACCF/AHA/WHF 2012

ECG manifestations of acute myocardial ischaemia (in absence of LVH and LBBB)
New ST elevation at the J point in two contiguous leads with the cut-points: ≥0.1 mV in all leads other than leads V_2–V_1 where the following cut-points apply: ≥0.2 mV in men ≥40 years; ≥0.25 mV in men <40 years, or ≥0.15 mV in women.
ST depression and T wave changes
New horizontal or downsloping ST depression ≥0.05 mV in two contiguous leads and/or T inversion ≥0.1 mV in two contiguous leads with prominent R wave or R/S ratio >1.

0.1 mV corresponds to 1 mm.
ESC/ACCF/AHA/WHF Expert Consensus Document. Third Universal Definition of Myocardial Infarction. *European Heart Journal* 2012;**33**:2551–2567.

Table 28.5 ESC/ACCF/AHA/WHF 2012

ECG changes associated with prior myocardial infarction
Any Q wave in leads V_2–V_3 ≥0.02 s or QS complex in leads V_2 and V_3.
Q wave ≥0.03 s and ≥0.1 mV deep or QS complex in leads I, II, aVL, aVF, or V_4–V_6 in any two leads of a contiguous lead grouping (I, aVL; V_1–V_6; II, III, aVF).[a]
R wave ≥0.04 s in V_1–V_2 and R/S ≥1 with a concordant positive T wave in absence of conduction defect.

0.04 s corresponds to one small square of the ECG trace.
[a] The same criteria are used for supplemental leads V_7–V_9.
ESC/ACCF/AHA/WHF Expert Consensus Document. Third Universal Definition of Myocardial Infarction. *European Heart Journal* 2012;**33**:2551–2567.

waves does not reliably distinguish between transmural or subendocardial MI. Q-wave regression, however, indicates improved LVEF.[5]

ECG criteria for the identification of the infarct-related artery in anterior and inferior MI are shown in Table 28.7.[4,6]

MI in the presence of LBBB Specific markers of MI are:[7]

- ST segment elevation ≥1 mm that is concordant with the QRS complex (in the same direction as the major QRS vector), or
- ST segment depression ≥1mm in lead V_1, V_2, or V_3.

ST segment elevation ≥5 mm that is discordant with the QRS complex indicates a moderate to high probability of MI.

RV infarction Up to 50% of inferior MIs have involvement of the RV. Suspected when ST elevation in V_1 and inferior leads, with ST elevation in lead III > ST elevation in lead II. The most sensitive electrocardiographic sign of right ventricular infarction is ST segment elevation of more than 1 mm, with an upright T wave in lead V_4R, but this sign is rarely present more than 12 hours after the infarction.

Atrial infarction PR elevation, the hallmark of diagnosis, is seen in 10% of MI, but isolated atrial infarction is diagnosed in 3.5% of autopsies of patients with STEMI.[8]

Enzymatic assays

Creatine kinase (starts rising within 4–8 h and returns to normal within 2–3 days) and **myoglobin** (starts rising 1–4 h, peaks at 6 h, and returns to normal at 24 h) are not specific for myocardial injury. Of the **creatine kinase isoenzymes** (MM in skeletal and heart muscle, BB in brain and kidney), the muscle and brain (CK-MB) isoenzyme is of clinical use by means of immunoassays with anti-MB monoclonal antibodies. It is also present in other tissue (small intestine, tongue, diaphragm, uterus, prostate) and rises after physical exercise. In MI, it usually increases 10–20 times above the upper limit of the reference range. Of the three subunits of the **troponin** complex (C that binds to Ca, I binds to actin, and T binds to tropomyosin), **TnI** and **TnT** are of clinical use. They are also present in skeletal muscle but are encoded by different genes; quantitative assays use antibodies specific for the cardiac form. In MI, troponins may increase 20–50 times above the upper limit of the reference range. Cut-off values should be set by each laboratory, depending on the assay used. Timing parameters are shown in Table 28.8 and Figure 28.2. False positive results may happen with all assays. Other causes of troponin elevations are presented in Table 28.9.[9] New high-sensitivity troponin

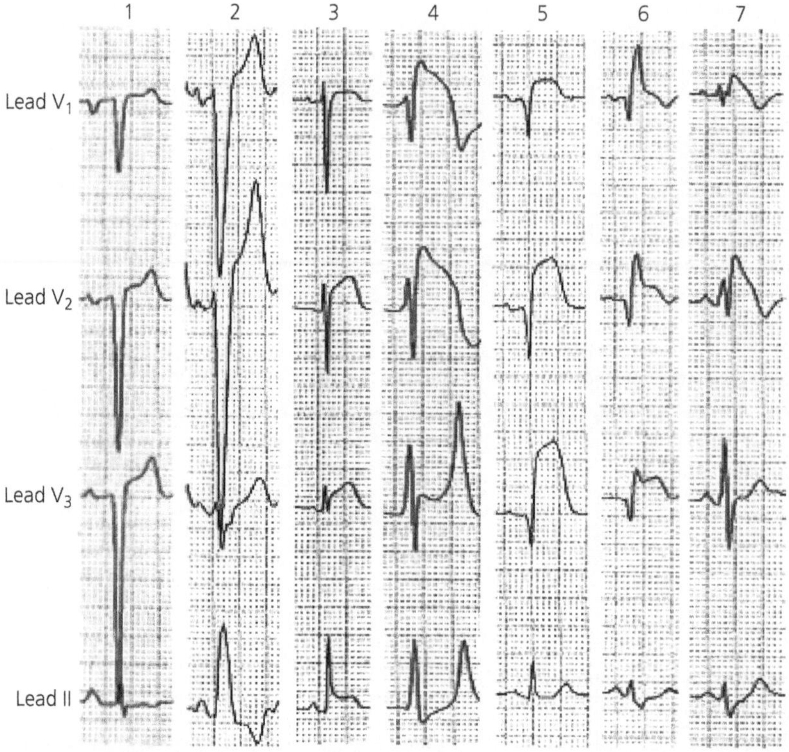

Figure 28.1 ST segment elevation in various conditions. **Tracing 1:** left ventricular hypertrophy. **Tracing 2:** LBBB. **Tracing** 3: acute pericarditis (the only tracing with ST segment elevation in both precordial leads and lead II and PR segment depression). **Tracing 4:** pseudoinfarction pattern in hyperkalaemia. The T wave in V_3 is tall, narrow, pointed, and tented. **Tracing 5**: acute anteroseptal infarction. **Tracing 6**: acute anteroseptal infarction and RBBB (remaining R′ wave and distinct transition between the downstroke of R′ and the beginning of the ST segment). **Tracing 7**: Brugada syndrome type 1 (rSR′ and ST segment elevation limited to V_1 and V_2. The ST segment begins from the top of the R′ and is downsloping).

Wang K, *et al*. ST-segment elevation in conditions other than acute myocardial infarction. *N Engl J Med*. 2003;**349**:2128–35.

Table 28.6 Causes of ST elevation other than myocardial infarction

ST elevation of normal variant	Seen in V_3 through V_5 with inverted T waves
	Short QT, high QRS voltage
Left ventricular hypertrophy	Concave
	Other features of left ventricular hypertrophy
Left bundle branch block	Concave
	ST segment deviation discordant from the QRS
Acute pericarditis	Diffuse ST segment elevation
	Reciprocal ST segment depression in aVR, not in aVL
	Elevation seldom >5 mm
	PR segment depression
Hyperkalaemia	Widened QRS and tall, peaked, tented T waves
	Low-amplitude or absent P waves
	ST segment usually downsloping

(Continued)

Table 28.6 (Continued)

Brugada syndrome (type 1)	rSR' in V_1 and V_2
	ST segment elevation in V_1 and V_2, typically downsloping
Pulmonary embolism	Changes simulating myocardial infarction seen often in both inferior and anteroseptal leads
Cardioversion	Striking ST segment elevation, often >10 mm, but lasting only 1 or 2 min immediately after direct current shock
Prinzmetal's angina	Same as ST segment elevation in infarction but transient
Hiatus hernia and stomach compression	Concave elevation in anterior chest leads without reciprocal inferior ST depression

Modified from Wang K, *et al.* ST segment elevation in conditions other than acute myocardial infarction. *N Engl J Med.* 2003;**349**:2128–35 and Gard JJ, *et al.* Uncommon cause of ST elevation. *Circulation* 2011; **123**:e259–e261.

Table 28.7 ECG criteria for identification of the infarct-related artery in anterior and inferior MI

Anterior MI	
Proximal LAD occlusion	ST elevation in V_1 to V_3 (aVL) and ST depression in II, III, aVF
Proximal LAD occlusion	ST elevation >2.5 mm in V_1 or RBBB with initial Q wave (not sensitive but very specific criteria)
LAD occlusion distal to first diagonal	ST elevation in V_1 to V_3 without ST depression in II, III, aVF
Distal LAD occlusion	ST elevation in V_1 to V_3 (aVL) and ST elevation in II, III, aVF (inferoapical LAD extension)
Inferior MI	
RCA occlusion	ST elevation in III > ST elevation in II, and ST depression in I or aVL
Left Cx occlusion	ST elevation in III not greater than ST elevation in II, and ST elevation or isoelectric in I, aVL, V_5, V_6

Table 28.8 Markers of cardiac damage

	Initial rise	**Peak elevation**	**Return to normal**
CK-MB	3–12 h	24 h	48–72 h
TnT	3–12 h	12–48 h	5–14 d
TnI	3–12 h	24 h	5–10 d

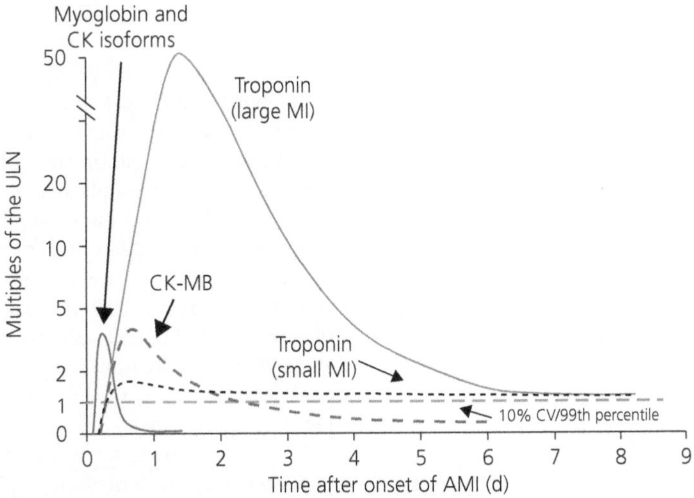

Figure 28.2 Timing of biomarkers after myocardial infarction.

Kumar A, Cannon CP. Acute coronary syndromes: diagnosis and management, part I. *Mayo Clin Proc.* 2009;**84**:917–38.

assays offer a higher negative predictive value (hsTnT <13 pg/mL) for the exclusion of MI.[10] However, the increased sensitivity of these new assays makes it possible to detect low levels of Tn, even in healthy subjects. Thus, they should always be interpreted within the context of clinical situation and repeated in 2–3 hours to confirm myonecrosis by consistent elevation.[11,12] In a recent study, the use of an algorithm enabled ruling MI in or out in 77% of patients within an hour.[13] MI was ruled out when baseline troponin was lower than 12 ng/L, and the level changed less than 3 ng/L in the following hour. MI was diagnosed when baseline troponin was either 52 ng/L, or higher, or when the 1-hour change was 5 ng/L or more. Increases of CK-MB or troponin >20% above the level measured at the time of the recurrent symptoms indicate episodes of reinfarction.[3]

Other investigations

Elevation of **WBC** occurs within the first 2 hours, reaches a peak 2 to 4 days after infarction (12–15 × 10^3/mL), and returns to normal in 1 week. **ESR** rises after the second day and remains elevated for several weeks. **Haemoglobin** powerfully predicts cardiovascular events, with mortality increasing progressively as values fall below 14 mg/dL or increase above 17 mg/dL. Iatrogenic bleeding is associated with a 5-fold increase in mortality. There is a fall of **HDL cholesterol** after 48 h; thus, a lipid profile should be obtained before that time or 8 weeks after the MI.

Table 28.9 Causes of elevated plasma cardiac troponin other than acute coronary syndromes

Cardiac causes	Non-cardiac causes
Cardiac contusion resulting from trauma	Pulmonary embolism
Cardiac surgery	Severe pulmonary hypertension
Cardioversion	Renal failure
Endomyocardial biopsy	Stroke, subarachnoid haemorrhage
Acute and chronic heart failure	Infiltrative diseases, e.g. amyloidosis
Aortic dissection	Cardiotoxic drugs
Aortic valve disease	Critical illness
Hypertrophic cardiomyopathy	Sepsis
Tachyarrhythmia	Extensive burns
Bradyarrhythmia, heart block	Extreme exertion
Apical ballooning syndrome	
Post-percutaneous coronary intervention	
Rhabdomyolysis with myocyte necrosis	
Myocarditis or endocarditis/pericarditis	

Mahajan VS, Jarolim P. How to interpret elevated cardiac troponin levels. *Circulation*. 2011;**124**:2350–4.

Chest radiography Prominent pulmonary vascular markings reflect raised LVEDP. However, up to 12 h can elapse before pulmonary oedema accumulates after the LVEDP has been raised (pulmonary wedge pressure >18 mmHg), and it takes 48 hours to resorb when LV filling pressures become normal. Signs of cardiomegaly may be seen, with previous infarcts and LV dysfunction.

Echocardiography Areas of abnormal regional wall motion are seen almost universally in patients with large MIs at 2D echocardiography. Apical thrombus and flaps of suspect aortic dissection may be seen, and Doppler imaging may reveal MR, TR, or VSD. Small pericardial effusion may be due to myocardial haemorrhage due to anticoagulants, pericarditris, or heart failure. Moderate effusion early after MI should raise the suspicion of free wall rupture.[14]

Exercise testing In patients of low risk and uncertain diagnosis of MI, tests for ischaemia can be undertaken within 6 to 12 h after admission or even immediately.[1]

Cardiac magnetic resonance (CMR) has high sensitivity for detecting small amounts of myonecrosis, assessing the peri-infarction zone and identifying small scars. First-pass perfusion sequences after IV gadolinium administration can also identify myocardial perfusion abnormalities. CMR may detected MI unrecognized by ECG in older individuals, and this is associated by increased mortality risk.[15]

Computed tomographic (CT) scan and CMR are useful for excluding aortic dissection.

Triple-rule-out CT angiography allows simultaneous CT coronary angiography, pulmonary angiography for the exclusion of pulmonary embolism, and ascending aorta angiogram for the exclusion of dissection.[16]

Initial therapy and medication

Initial therapy

Ambulance teams must be trained and equipped to identify STEMI (with the use of ECG recorders and telemetry, as necessary) and administer initial therapy, including thrombolysis, where applicable. **Pre-hospital thrombolysis** may offer survival rates, even higher than that of primary PCI.[17] All hospitals and emergency medical systems participating in the care of patients with STEMI must record and monitor delay times and work to achieve and maintain quality targets, as presented in Tables 28.10 and 28.11. Recommendations for pre-hospital and initial hospital management by the ESC and ACC/AHA are given in Figures 28.3 and 28.4.

In case of resuscitated **cardiac arrest**, therapeutic hypothermia and immediate angiography are indicated (Table 28.12). Although most patients with a cardiac arrest have demonstrable coronary artery disease, only

Table 28.10 ACCF/AHA 2013 on STEMI

Regional systems of STEMI care, reperfusion therapy, and time-to-treatment goals	
All communities should create and maintain a regional system of STEMI care that includes assessment and continuous quality improvement of EMS and hospital-based activities. Performance can be facilitated by participating in programmes, such as Mission: Lifeline and the D2B Alliance.	I-B
Performance of a 12-lead ECG by EMS personnel at the site of first medical contact (FMC) in patients with symptoms consistent with STEMI.	I-B
Reperfusion therapy should be administered to all eligible patients with symptom onset within the prior 12 hours.	I-A
Primary PCI is the recommended method of reperfusion when it can be performed in a timely fashion by experienced operators	I-A
EMS transport directly to a PCI-capable hospital for primary PCI is the recommended triage strategy, with an ideal FMC-to-device time system goal of 90 minutes or less.*	I-B
Immediate transfer to a PCI-capable hospital for primary PCI is the recommended triage strategy for patients with STEMI who initially arrive at, or are transported to, a non-PCI-capable hospital, with an FMC-to-device time system goal of 120 minutes or less.*	I-B
In the absence of contraindications, fibrinolytic therapy should be administered at non-PCI-capable hospitals when the anticipated FMC-to-device time at a PCI capable hospital exceeds 120 minutes.	I-B
When fibrinolytic therapy is indicated or chosen as the primary reperfusion strategy, it should be administered within 30 minutes of hospital arrival.*	I-B
Reperfusion therapy for patients with STEMI and symptom onset within the prior 12 to 24 hours who have clinical and/or ECG evidence of ongoing ischaemia. Primary PCI is the preferred strategy in this population.	IIa-B

* The proposed time windows are system goals. For any individual patient, every effort should be made to provide reperfusion therapy as rapidly as possible.
2013 ACCF/AHA guideline for the management of ST-elevation myocardial infarction. *J Am Coll Cardiol.* 2013;**61**:e78–140.

Table 28.11 ESC 2012 on STEMI

Logistics of pre-hospital care	
Ambulance teams must be trained and equipped to identify STEMI (with use of ECG recorders and telemetry as necessary) and administer initial therapy, including thrombolysis where applicable.	I-B
The pre-hospital management of STEMI patients must be based on regional networks designed to deliver reperfusion therapy expeditiously and effectively, with efforts made to make primary PCI available to as many patients as possible.	I-B
Primary PCI-capable centres must deliver a 24/7 service and be able to start primary PCI as soon as possible but always within 60 min from the initial call.	I-B
All hospitals and EMSs participating in the care of patients with STEMI must record and monitor delay times and work to achieve and maintain the following quality targets:	I-B
◆ First medical contact to first ECG ≤10 min	
◆ First medical contact to reperfusion therapy	
◆ For fibrinolysis ≤30 min	
◆ For primary PCI ≤90 min (≤60 min if the patient presents within 120 min of symptom onset or directly to a PCI-capable hospital).	
All EMSs, emergency departments, and coronary care units must have a written updated STEMI management protocol, preferably shared within geographic networks.	I-C
Patients presenting to a non-PCI-capable hospital and awaiting transportation for primary or rescue PCI must be attended in an appropriately monitored area.	I-C
Patients transferred to a PCI-capable centre for primary PCI should bypass the emergency department and be transferred directly to the catheterization laboratory.	IIa-B

ECG, electrocardiogram; EMS, emergency medical system; PCI, percutaneous coronary intervention; 24/7, 24 hours a day, seven days a week; STEMI, ST segment elevation myocardial infarction.
ESC Guidelines for the management of acute myocardial infarction in patients presenting with ST-segment elevation. *Eur Heart J* 2012; **33**:2501–2502.

38% of cardiac arrest survivors will develop evidence of myocardial infarction, and the use of tenecteplase during advanced life support for out-of-hospital cardiac arrest did not improve outcome.[18] However, approximately 70% of the coronary heart disease deaths annually in the USA occur out of hospital, and, although <30% of them have a shockable initial rhythm (usually VF—see Chapter 67 on SCD), the majority of neurologically intact survivors come from this subgroup.[19] Improved rates of neurologically intact survival can be achieved when comatose patients with out-of-hospital VF or VT cardiac arrest are cooled to 32–34°C for 12 or 24 hours, beginning minutes to hours after the return of spontaneous circulation. Cooling should begin before, or at the time of, cardiac catheterization that is indicated in these patients.[20,21]

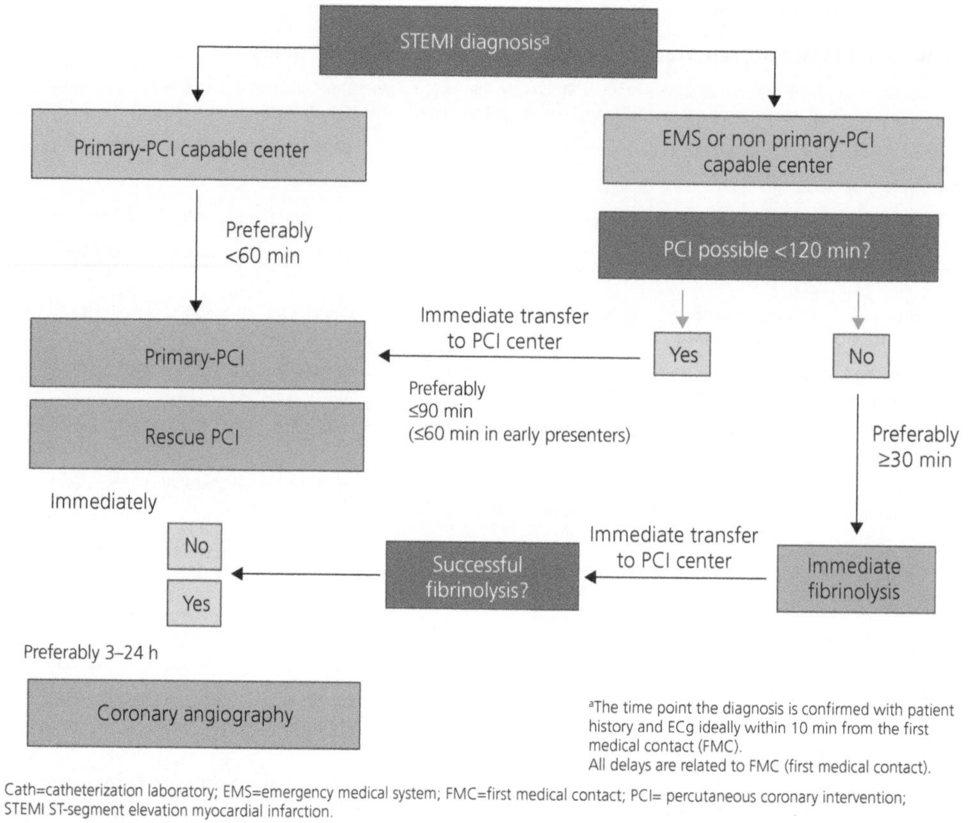

Figure 28.3 ESC 2012 GL on STEMI. Pre-hospital and in-hospital management of MI (first 24 hours).
ESC Guidelines for the management of acute myocardial infarction in patients presenting with ST-segment elevation. *Eur Heart J* 2012;**33**:2501–2502.

Medication

All patients should receive:[19,22]

- **Aspirin** (unless there is true aspirin allergy),
- A **$P2Y_{12}$ inhibitor, such as clopidogrel, ticagrelor (especially for PCI), or prasugrel (especially for PCI)**, and
- An **antithrombin agent (enoxaparin or unfractionated heparin or bivalirudin or fondaparinux)**.

Morphine sulphate

2–8 mg IV, repeated at 5–15 min intervals, or diamorphine (5 mg IV, causes less nausea) are the analgesics of choice in acute MI (Table 28.13). **Oxygen** (4–5 L/min), especially when saturation is <90%.

Aspirin

Chewable, not enteric-coated, aspirin is given: ACC/AHA 162–325 mg and maintenance dose of 81–325 mg, indefinitely; ESC 150–300 mg po or 80–150 mg IV. Higher doses of aspirin are no more recommended following stent implantation. If NSAIDs, non-selective or COX-2 selective, are already given, they are discontinued due to increased risk of re-infarction, heart failure, and myocardial rupture.

$P2Y_{12}$ inhibitors

Clopidogrel, ticagrelor or prasugrel may be used (ACCF/AHA 2013 GL on MI). The ESC (2012 on STEMI) gives preference to ticagrelol and prasugrel over clopidogrel. **Clopidogrel** loading is 300 mg po for fibrinolysis or no reperfusion for patients <75 years old.[23] A dose of 600 mg can be used if initiated 24 h after fibrinolysis (Tables 28.9 and 28.10). For patients >75 years old, the optimum loading dose is not established and much lower doses should be used. Clopidogrel is given for up to 1 year. **For primary PCI**, the loading dose of clopidogrel is 300–600 mg, or preferably 600 mg, and is continued for at least 1 year after stenting, regardless of whether a DES or a BMS was used. Recent evidence suggests that continuation of clopidogrel beyond 12 months in patients treated with PCI may be beneficial.[24] Clopidogrel use been found less efficacious post-MI in diabetic compared to non-diabetic patients.[25]

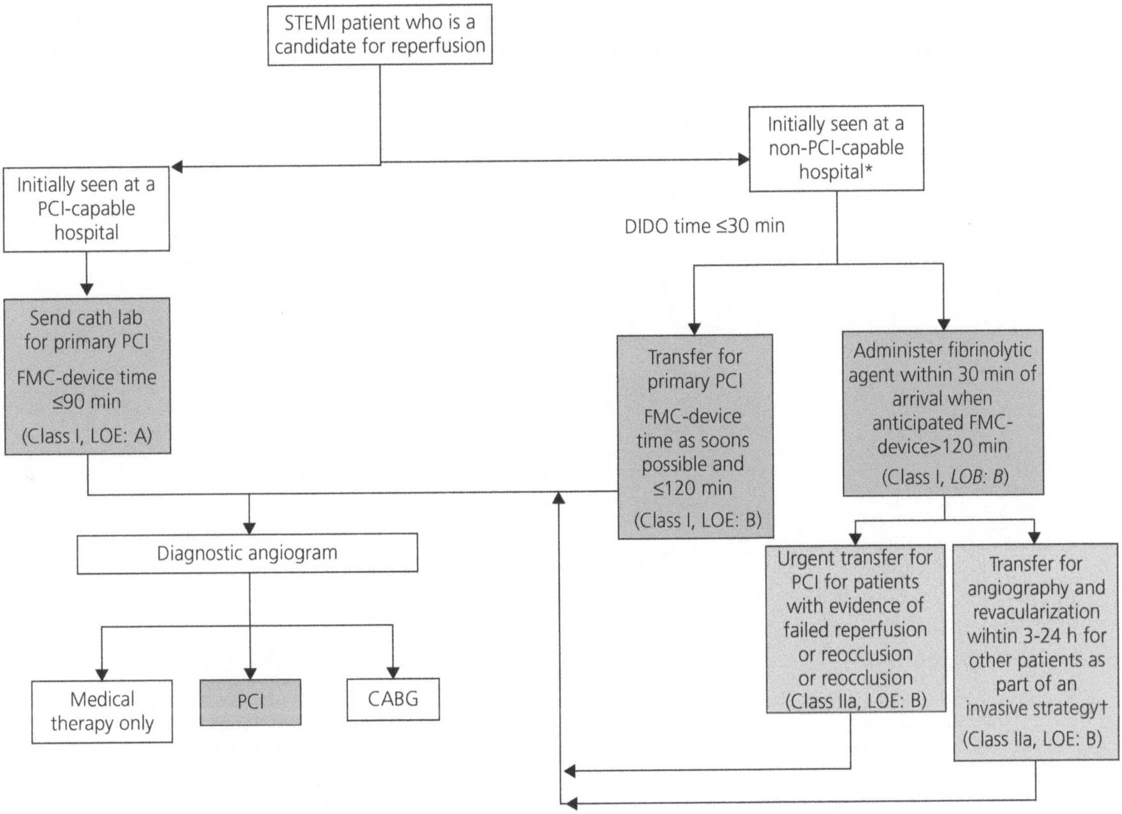

Figure 28.4 ACCF/AHA 2013 GL on STEMI. Reperfusion therapy for patients with STEMI. The bold arrows and boxes are the preferred strategies. Performance of PCI is dictated by an anatomically appropriate culprit stenosis.

* Patients with cardiogenic shock or severe heart failure, initially seen at a non-PCI-capable hospital, should be transferred for cardiac catheterization and revascularization as soon as possible, irrespective of time delay from MI onset (Class I, LOE: B). † Angiography and revascularization should not be performed within the first 2 to 3 hours after administration of fibrinolytic therapy. CABG indicates coronary artery bypass graft; DIDO, door-in-door-out; FMC, first medical contact; LOE, level of evidence; MI, myocardial infarction; PCI, percutaneous coronary intervention; and STEMI, ST elevation myocardial infarction.
2013 ACCF/AHA guideline for the management of ST-elevation myocardial infarction. *J Am Coll Cardiol.* 2013;**61**:e78–140.

Table 28.12 Cardiac arrest

ESC 2012 GL on STEMI. Cardiac arrest	
All medical and paramedical personnel caring for a patient with suspected MI must have access to defibrillation equipment and be trained in cardiac life support.	I-C
ECG monitoring at the point of FMC in all patients with suspected MI.	I-C
Therapeutic hypothermia early after resuscitation of cardiac arrest patients who are comatose or in deep sedation.	I-B
Immediate angiography with a view to primary PCI in patients with resuscitated cardiac arrest whose ECG shows STEMI.	I-B
Immediate angiography with a view to primary PCI in survivors of cardiac arrest without diagnostic ECG ST segment elevation but with a high suspicion of ongoing infarction.	IIa-B
ACCF/AHA 2013 GL on STEMI. Evaluation and management of patients with STEMI and out-of-hospital cardiac arrest	
Therapeutic hypothermia started as soon as possible in comatose patients with STEMI and out-of-hospital cardiac arrest caused by VF or pulseless VT, including patients who undergo primary PCI.	I-B
Immediate angiography and PCI when indicated in resuscitated out-of-hospital cardiac arrest patients whose initial ECG shows STEMI.	I-B

Table 28.13 Initial therapy

ESC 2012 GL on STEMI. Recommendations for relief of pain, breathlessness, and anxiety	
Titrated IV opioids are indicated to relieve pain.	I-C
Oxygen in patients with hypoxia (SaO_2 <95%), breathlessness, or acute heart failure.	I-C
Tranquillizer in very anxious patients.	IIa-C

ESC Guidelines for the management of acute myocardial infarction in patients presenting with ST-segment elevation. *Eur Heart J* 2012; **33**:2501–2502.

ACCF/AHA 2013 GL on STEMI. Selected routine medical therapies

Therapy	Indications	Dose/administration	Avoid/caution
Oxygen	Clinically significant hypoxaemia (oxygen saturation <90%)	2 to 4 L/min via nasal cannula	Caution with chronic obstructive pulmonary disease and CO_2 retention
	HF	Increase rate or change to face mask, as needed	
	Dyspnoea		
Morphine	Pain	4 to 8 mg IV initially, with lower doses in elderly	Lethargic or moribund patient
	Anxiety		Hypotension
	Pulmonary oedema	2 to 8 mg IV every 5 to 15 min if needed	Bradycardia
			Known hypersensitivity
Nitroglycerin	Ongoing chest pain	0.4 mg sublingual every 5 min up to three doses as BP allows	Avoid in suspected RV infarction
	Hypertension and HF		Avoid with SBP <90 mmHg or if SBP >0 mm Hg below baseline. Avoid if recent (24 to 48 h) use of 5-phosphodiestserase inhibitors
	IV dosing to begin at 10 microgram/min	SBP >0 mmHg below baseline, titrate to desired BP effect	Avoid if recent (24 to 48 h) use of 5-phosphodiesterase inhibitors

2013 ACCF/AHA guideline for the management of ST-elevation myocardial infarction. *J Am Coll Cardiol.* 2013;**61**:e78–140.

Ticagrelor is given in a loading dose 180 mg po, followed by 90 mg twice daily.[26] For primary PCI, **prasugrel** 60 mg po loading dose followed by 10 mg od (5 mg if the patient weighs <60 kg)[27] may also be used in patients less than 75 years old and without a history of previous stroke or TIA or increased bleeding risk. There is an increased bleeding risk with coronary artery bypass grafting within 5 days of taking clopidogrel (7 days with prasugrel), and early initiation needs to be carefully considered in patients where clinical features could suggest the need for early surgical revascularization. Ticagrelor and prasugrel reduce major adverse cardiac effects, cause less stent thrombosis, and decrease mortality without increased risk of bleeding following PCI for STEMI patients.[28]

$P2Y_{12}$ inhibitors are continued for at least one year (ACCF/AHA 2013 GL on STEMI[19]) after stenting, regardless of whether a DES or a BMS was used. Following DES, continuation beyond 12 months is optional. Further continuation may be considered in certain cases (bifurcation stenting, long stents etc) in view of delayed DES thrombosis. The ESC 2012 GL on STEMI,[22] recommend duration of 9–12 months of dual antiplatelet therapy, with a strict minimum time of 1 month after bare metal stent, and 6 months after DES.

Antithrombin agents

The antithrombin agent may be unfractionated heparin or enoxaparin or bivalirudin or fondaparinux.

Unfractionated heparin is given IV for 48 h. Prolonged administration increases the risk of heparin-induced thrombocytopenia, and other anticoagulants are preferred if further anticoagulation is needed. Anticoagulation during hospitalization (up to 8 days) is recommended in non-reperfused patients. **Enoxaparin** has been found superior to UFH after fibrinolysis by reducing the risk of death and MI, although it slightly increases the risk of bleeding.[29] It is superior for primary PCI without any difference in bleeding.[30] Maintenance dosing with enoxaparin should be continued for the duration of the index hospitalization for up to 8 days. Bivalirudin may be used with or without heparin. In primary PCI, **bivalirudin**, a direct thrombin inhibitor, reduced mortality as well as major bleeding from 8.3% to 4.9% (p <0.001), compared with unfractionated heparin with a IIb/IIIa antagonist (HORIZONS-MI).[31]

The infusion (for dosing, see Chapter 27 on UA/MSTEMI) is terminated at the end of the procedure or up to 4 h later. **Fondaparinux**, a synthetic factor Xa inhibitor, has been found to reduce 30-day death or myocardial infarction compared to unfractionated heparin, regardless of administration of fibrinolysis (OASIS-6).[32] In primary PCI, there is no benefit with fondaparinux, with an excess of catheter thrombosis noted. Thus, in the presence of increased bleeding risk, bivalirudin may be preferred when an invasive strategy is planned, and fondaparinux (given until end of hospitalization) when conservative management is anticipated (for dosing, see Chapter 27 on UA/MSTEMI).

Other medications

Glycoprotein IIb/IIIa inhibitors are mainly used for primary PCI (and can be deferred until angiography) or in combination with half-dose fibrinolysis.[33,34] They are used in addition to heparin for PCI, especially in patients without thienopyridine loading or with a large thrombus (Tables 28.10, 28.11). When abciximab is used, it can be given intracoronary (ACC/AHA 2011 on PCI, IIb-B). Routine precatheterization use is not recommended. The use of early **intravenous beta blockers** in acute MI reduces the risks of re-infarction and ventricular fibrillation but increases the risk of cardiogenic shock, especially during the first day or so after admission.[35] There is increased risk of cardiogenic shock with age >70 years, systolic BP <120 mmHg, sinus tachycardia >110, or bradycardia <60 bpm. IV beta blockers can be used in patients without contraindications, with high blood pressure, tachycardia, and no signs of heart failure. **Lidocaine** infusion to supress ventricular ectopy is no more indicated. **Insulin** infusion is used to normalize blood sugar (<180–200 mg/dL, but avoiding hypoglycaemia, i.e. <90 mg/dL). Routine insulin-glucose-potassium infusions are not recommended any more.

No evidence supports the use of **nitrates** or **calcium antagonists** in the acute phase of MI. IV **magnesium** routinely is not indicated, unless a deficit is documented. **NSAIDs** (including selective COX-2 agents) are discontinued due to the increased risk of myocardial rupture and re-infarction. Following MI, NSAIDs (both non-selective and selective COX-2 inhibitors) are associated with a 45% increase of risk of recurrent MI or death, even with only 1 week of treatment.[36] Diclofenac confers the highest risk whereas naproxen is the safest agent.[36]

Reperfusion therapy

Recommendations for selection of reperfusion method are provided in Figures 28.3 and 28.4 and Table 28.14.

Primary PCI

Primary PCI results in 25–30% lower mortality (7% vs 9%) and less re-infarction (3% vs 7%) and stroke (1% vs 2%) than fibrinolysis.[37] The benefit of PCI over fibrinolysis increases with greater delay in presentation, particularly after 120 min

Table 28.14 ESC 2012 on STEMI

Reperfusion therapy	
Reperfusion therapy in all patients with symptoms of <12 h duration and persistent ST segment elevation or (presumed) new LBBB.	I-A
Reperfusion therapy (preferably primary PCI) if there is evidence of ongoing ischaemia, even if symptoms may have started >12 h beforehand or if pain and ECG changes have been stuttering.	I-C
Reperfusion therapy with primary PCI may be in stable patients presenting 12–24 h after symptom onset.	IIb-B
Routine PCI of a totally occluded artery >24 h after symptom onset in stable patients without signs of ischaemia (regardless of whether fibrinolysis was given or not) is not recommended.	III-A

A summary of important delays and treatment goals in the management of acute ST segment elevation myocardial infarction

Delay	**Target**
Preferred for first medical contact (FMC) to ECG and diagnosis	**≤10 min**
Preferred for FMC to fibrinolysis ('FMC-to-needle')	**≤30 min**
Preferred for FMC to primary PCI ('door-to-balloon') in primary PCI hospitals	**≤60 min**
Preferred for FMC to primary PCI	**≤90 min** (≤60 min if early presenter with large area at risk)
Acceptable for primary PCI rather than fibrinolysis	**≤120 min** (≤90 min if early presenter with large area at risk) if this target cannot be met, consider fibrinolysis.
Preferred for successful fibrinolysis to angiography	**3–24 h**

ESC Guidelines for the management of acute myocardial infarction in patients presenting with ST-segment elevation. *Eur Heart J* 2012; **33**:2501–2502.

Table 28.15 Primary PCI in STEMI

ESC 2012 GL on STEMI	
Indications	
Primary PCI is the recommended reperfusion therapy over fibrinolysis if performed by an experienced team within 120 min of first medical contact.	I-A
Primary PCI for patients with severe acute heart failure or cardiogenic shock, unless the expected PCI related delay is excessive and the patient presents early after symptom onset.	I-B
Procedural aspects	
Stenting is recommended (over balloon angioplasty alone) for primary PCI.	I-A
Primary PCI should be limited to the culprit vessel, with the exception of cardiogenic shock and persistent ischaemia after PCI of the supposed culprit lesion.	IIa-B
If performed by an experienced radial operator, radial access should be preferred over femoral access.	IIa-B
If the patient has no contraindications to prolonged DAPT (indication for oral anticoagulation or estimated high long-term bleeding risk) and is likely to be compliant, DES should be preferred over BMS.	IIa-A
Routine thrombus aspiration.	IIa-B
Routine use of distal protection devices is not recommended.	III-C
Routine use of IABP (in patients without shock) is not recommended.	III-A

ESC Guidelines for the management of acute myocardial infarction in patients presenting with ST-segment elevation. *Eur Heart J* 2012; **33**:2501–2502.

ACCF/AHA 2013 GL on STEMI	
Indications	
Ischaemic symptoms <12 h	I-A
Ischaemic symptoms <12 h and contraindications to fibrinolytic therapy, irrespective of time delay from FMC	I-B
Cardiogenic shock or acute severe HF, irrespective of time delay from MI onset	I-B
Evidence of ongoing ischaemia 12 to 24 h after symptom onset	IIa-B
PCI of a non-infarct artery at the time of primary PCI in patients without haemodynamic compromise	III-B (harm)

FMC, first medical contact; HF, heart failure; LOE, level of Evidence; MI, myocardial infarction; PCI, percutaneous coronary intervention; and STEMI, ST elevation myocardial infarction.
2013 ACCF/AHA guideline for the management of ST-elevation myocardial infarction. *J Am Coll Cardiol.* 2013;**61**:e78–140.

Technical aspects for primary PCI in STEMI	
Placement of a stent (bare metal stent [BMS] or drug-eluting stent (DES)).	I-A
BMS† should be used in patients with high bleeding risk, inability to comply with 1 year of dual antiplatelet therapy (DAPT), or anticipated invasive or surgical procedures in the next year.	I-C
Manual aspiration thrombectomy for patients undergoing primary PCI	IIa-B
DES should not be used in primary PCI for patients with STEMI who are unable to tolerate or comply with a prolonged course of DAPT because of the increased risk of stent thrombosis with premature discontinuation of one or both agents.	III-B

† Balloon angioplasty without stent placement may be used in selected patients.
2013 ACCF/AHA Guideline for the Management of ST-Elevation Myocardial Infarction. doi: 10.1161/CIR.0b013e3182742cf6.

Table 28.16 Medical therapy

ESC 2012 GL on STEMI. Periproedural antithrombotic medication in primary percutaneous coronary intervention	
Antiplatelet therapy	
Aspirin oral or IV (if unable to swallow) is recommended.	I-B
An ADP receptor blocker is recommended, in addition to aspirin. Options are:	I-A
◆ Prasugrel in clopidogrel-naive patients, if no history of prior stroke/TIA, age <75 years.	I-B
◆ Ticagrelor.	I-B
◆ Clopidogrel, preferably when prasugrel or ticagrelor are either not available or contraindicated.	I-C

Table 28.16 (Continued)

GP IIb/IIIa inhibitors should be considered for bailout therapy if there is angiographic evidence of massive thrombus, slow or no-reflow, or a thrombotic complication.	IIa-C	
Routine use of a GP IIb/IIIa inhibitor, as an adjunct to primary PCI performed with unfractionated heparin, may be considered in patients without contraindications.	IIb-B	
Upstream use of a GP IIb/IIIa inhibitor (vs in-lab use) may be considered in high-risk patients undergoing transfer for primary PCI.	IIb-B	
Options for GP IIb/IIIa inhibitors are (with LOE for each agent):		
◆ Abciximab.		A
◆ Eptifibatide (with double bolus).		B
◆ Tirofiban (with a high bolus dose).		B
Anticoagulants		
An injectable anticoagulant must be used in primary PCI.	I-C	
Bivalirudin (with use of GP IIb/IIIa blocker restricted to bailout) is recommended over unfractionated heparin and a GP IIb/IIIa blocker.	I-B	
Enoxaparin (with or without routine GP IIb/IIIa blocker) may be preferred over unfractionated heparin.	IIb-B	
Unfractionated heparin (with or without routine GP IIb/IIIa blocker) must be used in patients not receiving bivalirudin or enoxaparin.	I-C	
Fondaparinux is not recommended for primary PCI.	III-B	
The use of fibrinolysis before planned primary PCI is not recommended.	III-A	

ESC 2012 GL on STEMI. Doses of antiplatelet co-therapies

With primary PCI	
Aspirin	Loading dose of 150–300 mg orally or of 80–150 mg IV if oral ingestion is not possible, followed by a maintenance dose of 75–100 mg/day.
Clopidogrel	Loading dose of 600 mg orally, followed by a maintenance dose of 75 mg/day.
Prasugrel	Loading dose of 60 mg orally, followed by a maintenance dose of 10 mg/day. In patients with body weight <60 kg, a maintenance dose of 5 mg is recommended. In patients >75 years, prasugrel is generally not recommended, but a dose of 5 mg should be used if treatment is deemed necessary.
Ticagrelor	Loading dose of 180 mg orally, followed by a maintenance dose of 90 mg bd.
Abciximab	Bolus of 0.25 mg/kg IV and 0.125 micrograms/kg/min infusion (maximum 10 micrograms/min) for 12 h.
Eptifibatide	Double bolus of 180 micrograms/kg IV (given at a 10-minute interval) followed by an infusion of 2.0 micrograms/kg/min for 18 h.
Tirofiban	25 micrograms/kg over 3 min IV, followed by a maintenance infusion of 0.15 micrograms/kg/min for 18 h.
With fibrinolytic therapy	
Aspirin	Starting dose 150–500 mg orally or IV dose of 250 mg if oral ingestion is not possible.
Clopidogrel	Loading dose of 300 mg orally if aged ≤75 years, followed by a maintenance dose of 75 mg/day.
Without reperfusion therapy	
Aspirin	Starting dose 150–500 mg orally.
Clopidogrel	75 mg/day orally.

ESC 2012 GL on STEMI. Doses of antithrombin co-therapies

With primary PCI	
Unfractionated heparin	70–100 U/kg IV bolus when no GP IIb/IIIa inhibitor is planned. 50–60 U/kg IV bolus with GP IIb/IIIa inhibitors.
Enoxaparin	0.5 mg/kg IV bolus.
Bivalirudin	0.75 mg/kg IV bolus, followed by IV infusion of 1.75 mg/kg/h for up to 4 h after the procedure, as clinically warranted. After cessation of the 1.75 mg/kg/h infusion, a reduced infusion dose of 0.25 mg/kg/h may be continued for 4–12 h, as clinically necessary.

(Continued)

Table 28.16 (Continued)

With fibrinolytic therapy	
Unfractionated heparin	60 U/kg IV bolus with a maximum of 4000 U, followed by an IV infusion of 12 U/kg with a maximum of 1000 U/h for 24–48 h. Target aPTT: 50–70 s or 1.5 to 2.0 times that of control to be monitored at 3, 6, 12, and 24 h.
Enoxaparin	In patients <75 years of age: 30 mg IV bolus, followed 15 min later by 1 mg/kg SC every 12 h until hospital discharge for a maximum of 8 days The first two doses should not exceed 100 mg. In patients >75 years of age: no IV bolus; start with first SC dose of 0.75 mg/kg with a maximum of 75 mg for the first two SC doses. In patients with creatinine clearance of <30 mL/min, regardless of age, the SC doses are given once every 24 h.
Fondaparinux	2.5 mg IV bolus followed by a SC dose of 2.5 mg once daily up to 8 days or hospital discharge.
Without reperfusion therapy	
Unfractionated heparin	Same dose as with fibrinolytic therapy.
Enoxaparin	Same dose as with fibrinolytic therapy.
Fondaparinux	Same dose as with fibrinolytic therapy.

ESC Guidelines for the management of acute myocardial infarction in patients presenting with ST-segment elevation. *Eur Heart J* 2012; **33**:2501–2502.

ACCF/AHA 2013 GL on STEMI. Adjunctive antithrombotic therapy to support reperfusion with primary PCI

Antiplatelet therapy	
Aspirin	
162 to 325 mg load before procedure	I-B
81 to 325 mg daily maintenance dose (indefinite)*	I-A
81 mg daily is the preferred maintenance dose*	IIa-B
$P2Y_{12}$ inhibitors	
Loading doses	
Clopidogrel: 600 mg as early as possible or at time of PCI	I-B
Prasugrel: 60 mg as early as possible or at time of PCI	I-B
Ticagrelor: 180 mg as early as possible or at time of PCI	I-B
Maintenance doses and duration of therapy	
DES placed: continue therapy for 1 year with:	
Clopidogrel: 75 mg daily	I-B
Prasugrel: 10 mg daily	I-B
Ticagrelor: 90 mg twice a day*	I-B
BMS† placed: continue therapy for 1 year with:	
Clopidogrel: 75 mg daily	I-B
Prasugrel: 10 mg daily	I-B
Ticagrelor: 90 mg twice a day*	I-B
DES placed:	
Clopidogrel, prasugrel, or ticagrelor* continued beyond 1 year	IIb-C
Patients with STEMI with prior stroke or TIA: prasugrel	III-B (harm)
GP IIb/IIIa receptor antagonists in conjunction with UFH or bivalirudin in selected patients	
Abciximab: 0.25 mg/kg IV bolus, then 0.125 micrograms/kg/min (maximum 10 micrograms/min)	IIa-A
Tirofiban: (high-bolus dose): 25 micrograms/kg IV bolus, then 0.15 micrograms/kg/min In patients with CrCl <30 mL/min, reduce infusion by 50%	IIa-B
Eptifibatide (double bolus): 180 micrograms/kg IV bolus, then 2 micrograms/kg/min; a second 180 micrograms/kg bolus is administered 10 min after the first bolus In patients with CrCl <50 mL/min, reduce infusion by 50% Avoid in patients on haemodialysis	IIa-B

Table 28.16 (Continued)

Pre-catheterization laboratory administration of IV GP IIb/IIIa receptor antagonist	IIb-B
Intracoronary abciximab 0.25 mg/kg bolus	IIb-B
Anticoagulant therapy	
UFH:	I-C
UFH with GP IIb/IIIa receptor antagonist planned: 50 to 70 U/kg IV bolus to achieve therapeutic ACT‡	
UFH with no GP IIb/IIIa receptor antagonist planned: 70 to 100 U/kg bolus to achieve therapeutic ACT§	I-C
Bivalirudin: 0.75 mg/kg IV bolus, then 1.75 mg/kg/h infusion with or without prior treatment with UFH. An additional bolus of 0.3 mg/kg may be given if needed.	I-B
Reduce infusion to 1 mg/kg/h with estimated CrCl <30 mL/min	
Preferred over UFH with GP IIb/IIIa receptor antagonist in patients at high risk of bleeding	IIa-B
Fondaparinux: not recommended as sole anticoagulant for primary PCI	IIIb-B (harm)

* The recommended maintenance dose of aspirin to be used with ticagrelor is 81 mg daily.
† Balloon angioplasty without stent placement may be used in selected patients. It might be reasonable to provide P2Y12 inhibitor therapy to patients with STEMI undergoing balloon angioplasty alone, according to the recommendations listed for BMS (*LOE: C*).
‡ The recommended ACT with planned GP IIb/IIIa receptor antagonist treatment is 200 to 250 s.
§ The recommended ACT with no planned GP IIb/IIIa receptor antagonist treatment is 250 to 300 s (HaemoTec device) or 300 to 350 s (Haemochron device).
ACT indicates activated clotting time; BMS, bare metal stent; CrCl, creatinine clearance; COR, class of recommendation; DES, drug-eluting stent; GP, glycoprotein; IV, intravenous; LOE, level of evidence; N/A, not available; PCI, percutaneous coronary intervention; STEMI, ST elevation myocardial infarction; TIA, transient ischaemic attack; and UFH, unfractionated heparin.
2013 ACCF/AHA guideline for the management of ST-elevation myocardial infarction. *J Am Coll Cardiol.* 2013;**61**:e78–140.

of symptom onset and in patients >65 years of age, but is lost with a relative delay (door-to-balloon time vs door-to-needle time) of more than 114 min.[38,39] Each 30-minute delay in reperfusion results in a 7.5% increase in 1-year mortality. Delays in door-to-balloon time for PCI greater than 1 hour over when thrombolytic reperfusion would have occurred may negate the mortality benefit of PCI (Tables 28.14 to 28.16).

Thus, PCI is preferred over fibrinolysis if:

- Can be performed with a delay <120 minutes of first medical contact-to-balloon time
- Cardiogenic shock or severe heart failure
- Symptoms onset within the prior 12–24 h and ongoing ischaemia
- Contraindications to fibrinolysis or diagnosis of STEMI in doubt.

The greater the baseline patient risk and the availability of in-hospital PCI facilities, the longer the acceptable primary PCI delays.[40] The largest trial comparing PCI to fibrinolysis (DANAMI) has shown that transfer for PCI is indicated when patients with STEMI present within 12 h from onset of symptoms and transfer time is <2 hours.[41] In the STREAM trial, prehospital fibrinolysis with tenecteplace in patients who presented within 3 hours after symptom onset and who were unable to undergo primary PCI within 1 hour, resulted in effective reperfusion compared to late primary PCI (135–230 min), but with a slightly increased risk of intracranial bleeding.[42]

A reasonable policy in places without PCI facilities is to fibrinolyze all patients who present within 12 hours from onset of symptoms using half-dose for patients ≥ 75 years of age, and then perform angiography and PCI, if indicated, 3–24 hours later.

It should also be noted that MI with **RBBB** is frequently caused by the complete occlusion of the infarct-related artery, and in-hospital mortality is highest from all ECG presentations of AMI. Thus, RBBB should be considered as a standard indication for reperfusion therapy in the same way as LBBB.[43]

Primary PCI has been recommended generally for up to 12 h after the onset of symptoms. This time limit may be extended to **24 h** in the presence of ongoing ischaemia, or even in stable patients (Class IIb-B by ESC 2012 on MI and Class IIb-B by the ACC/AHA on PCI 2011). When patients presents >24 hours after symptom onset and with an occluded infarct-related artery, the open artery trial (OAT) showed no benefit of PCI in stable patients and is not recommended by current guidelines,[44] although ventricular remodelling is affected by the presence of a patent artery. PCI is also the treatment of choice in cardiogenic shock. The presence of significant stenosis or total occlusions in non-MI related arteries indicates adverse prognosis.[45]

UFH or enoxaparin may be used, but **enoxaparin** has been found superior to heparin (ATOLL study) by means of reducing ischaemic episodes.[30] In patients undergoing primary PCI, abciximab is associated with a possible reduction of mortality.[34] Small molecule glycoprotein IIb/IIIa inhibitors (tirofiban and eptifibatide) have not been extensively studied, but there is evidence for similar efficacy.[46] They are much cheaper, and their shorter duration of action is an advantage. **IIb/IIa inhibitors** may be indicated in primary PCI, and there has been evidence that intracoronary bolus administration results in improved myocardial perfusion compared to IV (INFUSE-AMI and CICERO trials),[47,48] although this is not a consistent finding (AIDA-STEMI trial).[49] **Bivalirudin** is superior to the combination of UFH/enoxaparin with a IIb/IIIa (ISAR-REACT 4)[50] and can be given if the patient had been previously treated with UFH. Bivalirudin is the preferred anticoagulant for PCI by the ACC/AHA 2013 GL on STEMI.

Thrombus aspiration is recommended, but the evidence on its value is not established.[48,51–53] Embolic protection is not beneficial in reducing mortality, compared with PCI alone, whereas mechanical thrombectomy appears to increase mortality.[54]

The use of **DES**, instead of BMS, is safe and reduces the risk of reintervention.[55]

Non-culprit coronary interventions should not be performed at the time of primary PCI;[56] this is the recommendation of current guidelines. However, multivessel revascularization may be safe compared to culprit artery-only revascularization.[57]

In **pregnant women**, primary PCI is the treatment of choice (ESC GL on pregnancy 2011, I-C).[58]

No-reflow phenomenon

Failure to achieve microvascular flow, as assessed by resolution of ST segment elevation or contrast flow by angiography, is seen in up to 25% patients subjected to primary PCI (Table 28.17). Coronary embolization and ischaemia-induced endothelial swelling and neutrophil and platelet activation are thought responsible. Thrombus aspiration and abciximab 0.25 mg/kg bolus and 0.125 mg/kg/min infusion for 12–24 h may be used for no-reflow. Adenosine, as continuous infusion of 70 microgram/kg/min over 3 hours during and after PCI or intracoronary bolus of 30–60 mg, verapamil, as intracoronary bolus of 0.5–1 mg, and intracoronary nitroprusside may also be used (ACCF/AHA 2011 on PCI).

Facilitated PCI

Facilitated PCI that refers to full or half-dose thrombolysis with or without IIb/IIIa inhibitors, followed by immediate PCI, has resulted in increased incidence of major adverse cardiac events.[59,60] However, routine PCI within 24 h, but later than 3 hours after fibrinolysis, appears to offer reduced rates of re-infarction and composite outcomes of myocardial infarction and death compared to ischaemia-guided PCI.[61–63]

Table 28.17 Grading of coronary flow and myocardial blush

TIMI flow
TIMI 0 There is no antegrade flow beyond the point of occlusion.
TIMI 1 The contrast material passes beyond the area of obstruction but 'hangs up' and fails to opacify the entire coronary bed distal to the obstruction for duration of the cine run.
TIMI 2 The contrast material passes across the obstruction and opacifies the coronary bed distal to the obstruction. However, the rate of entry of contrast material into the vessel distal to the obstruction or its rate of clearance from the distal bed (or both) are perceptibly slower than its entry into or clearance from comparable areas not perfused by the previously occluded vessel, e.g. the opposite coronary artery or the coronary bed proximal to the obstruction.
TIMI 3 Antegrade flow into the bed distal to the obstruction occurs as promptly as antegrade flow into the bed proximal to the obstruction, and clearance of contrast material from the involved bed is as rapid as clearance from an uninvolved bed in the same vessel or the opposite artery.
Sheehan FH, *et al.* The effect of intravenous thrombolytic therapy on left ventricular function: a report on tissue-type plasminogen activator and streptokinase from the Thrombolysis in Myocardial Infarction (TIMI Phase I) trial. *Circulation* 1987;**75**:817–829.
Myocardial blush grade
MBG 0 No myocardial blush or staining of blush (due to leakage of dye into the extravascular space)
MBG 1 Minimal myocardial blush
MBG 2 Moderate myocardial blush, less than that obtained during angiography of a contralateral or ipsilateral non-infarct-related artery
MBG 3 Normal myocardial blush, comparable with that obtained during angiography of a contralateral or ipsilateral non-infarct-related artery
Myocardial blush grade (MBG) is a densitometric, semi-quantitative parameter which depends on the tissue phase of myocardial perfusion that appears as a 'blush' or a 'ground glass' after a sufficiently long, 25 frames/s, X-ray acquisition. MBG is measured on patients with TIMI 3 flow and is based on the principle that a functionally preserved microvascular bed allows the injected contrast to pass easily from the arterial to the venous side of coronary circulation, showing an appreciable 'blush' at the myocardial level.
van 't Hof AW, *et al.* Angiographic assessment of myocardial reperfusion in patients treated with primary angioplasty for acute myocardial infarction: myocardial blush grade. Zwolle Myocardial Infarction Study Group. *Circulation* 1998;**97**:2302–2306.

Fibrinolysis

Fibrinolysis is given **within the next 12 h after the onset of symptoms or the next 24 h in case of ongoing ischaemia** (Tables 28.18 to 28.20 and Figures 28.3 and 28.4). Patients presenting beyond the 12 h limit should receive heparin or fondaparinux, regardless of whether reperfusion is attempted. Despite previous reservations, fibrinolyis is recommended in the elderly (>75 years) when primary PCI is not available.[64] Urgent pharmacological reperfusion with fibrinolysis, either pre-hospital within 30 minutes or after transfer with a door-to-needle time <0 min, remains the principal treatment for improving survival after STEMI, unless an absolute contraindication exists (Table 28.14). In patients presenting <2 hours after

Table 28.18 Contraindications to fibrinolysis

ACC/AHA 2013 on STEMI. Contraindications and cautions for fibrinolytic therapy in STEMI*
Absolute contraindications
Any prior ICH
Known structural cerebral vascular lesion (e.g. arteriovenous malformation)
Known malignant intracranial neoplasm (primary or metastatic)
Ischaemic stroke within 3 mo
EXCEPT acute ischaemic stroke within 4.5 h
Suspected aortic dissection
Active bleeding or bleeding diathesis (excluding menses)
Significant closed-head or facial trauma within 3 mo
Intracranial or intraspinal surgery within 2 mo
Severe uncontrolled hypertension (unresponsive to emergency therapy)
For streptokinase, prior treatment within the previous 6 mo
Relative contraindications
History of chronic, severe, poorly controlled hypertension
Significant hypertension on presentation (SBP >180 mmHg or DBP >110 mmHg)
History of prior ischaemic stroke >3 mo
Dementia
Known intracranial pathology not covered in absolute contraindications
Traumatic or prolonged (>10 min) CPR
Major surgery (<3 wk)
Recent (within 2 to 4 wk) internal bleeding
Non-compressible vascular punctures
Pregnancy
Active peptic ulcer
Oral anticoagulant therapy

* Viewed as advisory for clinical decision-making and may not be all-inclusive or definitive.
CPR indicates cardiopulmonary resuscitation; DBP; diastolic blood pressure; ICH, intracranial haemorrhage; SBP, systolic blood pressure; and STEMI, ST elevation myocardial infarction.
2013 ACCF/AHA guideline for the management of ST-elevation myocardial infarction. *J Am Coll Cardiol.* 2013;**61**:e78–140.

ESC 2012 on STEMI. Condraindications to fibrinolysis
Absolute
Previous intracranial haemorrhage or stroke of unknown origin at any time
Ischaemic stroke in the preceding 6 months
Central nervous system damage or neoplasms or atrioventricular malformation
Recent major trauma/surgery/head injury (within the preceding 3 weeks)
Gastrointestinal bleeding within the past month
Known bleeding disorder (excluding menses)
Aortic dissection
Non-compressible punctures in the past 24 h (e.g. liver biopsy, lumbar puncture)
Relative
Transient ischaemic attack in the preceding 6 months
Oral anticoagulant therapy
Pregnancy or within 1 week post-partum
Refractory hypertension (systolic blood pressure >180 mmHg and/or diastolic blood pressure >110 mmHg)
Advanced liver disease
Infective endocarditis
Active peptic ulcer
Prolonged or traumatic resuscitation

ESC Guidelines for the management of acute myocardial infarction in patients presenting with ST-segment elevation. *Eur Heart J* 2012; **33**:2501–2502.

symptom onset, fibrinolysis can achieve mortality rates of <4%, which are similar to those achieved by primary PCI. The earlier that fibrinolysis, the greater the benefit by means of preservation of left ventricular function and reduction in mortality.[65]

Bolus-only fibrin-specific agents **rateplase (rPA) and tenecteplase (TNK-tPA)** are tissue plasminogen activator (tPA) mutants that achieve greater vessel patency than non-fibrin specific agents (streptokinase and urokinase) and similar mortality benefit but with less systemic bleeding than infusion of tPA.[66,67] In patients receiving fibrin-specific fibrinolytic agents, and perhaps streptokinase, **unfractionated heparin**, or **enoxaparin**, commenced early after fibrinolysis is recommended (Table 28.15). UFH should not be given for more than 48 hours due to the risk of heparin-induced thrombocytopenia. Maintenance dosing with enoxaparin or fondaparinux should be continued for the duration of the index hospitalization, up to 8 days.

Combination of half-dose fibrinolytics and glycoprotein **IIb/IIIa inhibition** for pharmacological reperfusion achieves more rapid ST segment resolution and less recurrent infarction than with standard fibrinolytic therapy but no reduction in mortality.[33] It is contraindicated in patients >75 years old.

Intracranial haemorrhage

The occurrence of a change in neurological status during or after reperfusion therapy, particularly within the first 24 hours after initiation of treatment, is considered to be due to intracranial haemorrhage until proven otherwise. The incidence of intracranial haemorrhage following thrombolysis has been estimated between 0.2 and 2%.[68] Certain patient groups, such as the elderly, women, hypertensive

Table 28.19 Fibrinolysis

ESC 2012 GL on STEMI. Fibrinolytic therapy	
Fibrinolytic therapy is recommended within 12 h of symptom onset in patients without contraindications if primary PCI cannot be performed by an experienced team within 120 min of FMC.	I-A
In patients presenting early (<2 h after symptom onset) with a large infarct and low bleeding risk, fibrinolysis should be considered if time from FMC to balloon inflation is >90 min.	IIa-B
If possible, fibrinolysis should start in the pre-hospital setting.	IIa-A
A fibrin-specific agent (tenecteplase, alteplase, reteplase) is recommended (over non-fibrin specific agents).	I-B
Oral or IV aspirin must be administered.	I-B
Clopidogrel is indicated in addition to aspirin.	I-A
Antithrombin co-therapy with fibrinolysis	
Anticoagulation is recommended in STEMI patients treated with lytics until revascularization (if performed) or for the duration of hospital stay up to 8 days. The anticoagulant can be:	I-A
◆ Enoxaparin IV, followed by SC (using the regimen described below) (preferred over UFH)	I-A
◆ UFH given as a weight-adjusted IV bolus and infusion	I-C
In patients treated with streptokinase, fondaparinux IV bolus, followed by SC dose 24 h later	IIa-B
Transfer to a PCI-capable centre following fibrinolysis	
Is indicated in all patients after fibrinolysis.	I-A
Interventions following fibrinolysis	
Rescue PCI is indicated immediately when fibrinolysis has failed (<50% ST segment resolution at 60 min).	I-A
Emergency PCI is indicated in the case of recurrent ischaemia or evidence of reocclusion after initial successful fibrinolysis.	I-B
Emergency angiography with a view to revascularization is indicated in heart failure/shock patients.	I-A
Angiography with a view to revascularization (of the infarct-related artery) is indicated after successful fibrinolysis.	I-A
Optimal timing of angiography for stable patients after successful lysis: 3–24 h.	IIa-A

ESC Guidelines for the management of acute myocardial infarction in patients presenting with ST-segment elevation. *Eur Heart J* 2012; **33**:2501–2502.

ESC 2012 GL on STEMI. Doses of fibrinolytic agents

	Initial treatment	Specific contraindications
Streptokinase (SK)	1.5 million units over 30–60 min IV	Prior SK or anistreplase
Alteplase (tPA)	15 mg IV bolus 0.75 mg/kg over 30 min (up to 50 mg), then 0.5 mg/kg over 60 min IV (up to 35 mg)	
Reteplase (r-PA)	10 units + 10 units IV bolus, given 30 min apart	
Tenecteplase (TNK–tPA)	Single IV bolus: 30 mg if <60 kg, 35 mg if 60 to <70 kg, 40 mg if 70 to <80 kg, 45 mg if 80 to <090 kg, 50 mg if ≥90 kg	

ESC Guidelines for the management of acute myocardial infarction in patients presenting with ST-segment elevation. *Eur Heart J* 2012; **33**:2501–2502.

ACCF/AHA 2013 GL on STEMI. Indications for fibrinolytic therapy when there is a >120-minute delay from FMC to primary PCI

Ischaemic symptoms <12 h	I-A
Evidence of ongoing ischaemia 12 to 24 h after symptom onset and a large area of myocardium at risk or haemodynamic instability	IIa-C
ST depression, except if true posterior (inferobasal) MI is suspected or when associated with ST elevation in lead aVR	III-B (harm)

FMC, first medical contact; MI, myocardial infarction; N/A, not available; and PCI, percutaneous coronary intervention.
2013 ACCF/AHA guideline for the management of ST-elevation myocardial infarction. *J Am Coll Cardiol.* 2013;**61**:e78–140.

(Continued)

Table 28.19 (Continued)

ACCF/AHA 2013 GL on STEMI. Fibrinolytic agents

Fibrinolytic agent	Dose	Fibrin specificity*	Antigenic	Patency rate (90-minute TIMI 2 or 3 flow)
Fibrin-specific				
Tenecteplase (TNK-tPA)	Single IV weight-based bolus†	++++	No	85%
Reteplase (rPA)	10 U + 10 U IV boluses, given 30 min apart	++	No	84%
Alteplase (tPA)	90-minute weight-based infusion‡	++	No	73% to 84%
Non-fibrin-specific				
Streptokinase§	1.5 million units IV, given over 30–60 min	No	Yes**	60% to 68%

* Strength of fibrin specificity; ++++ is more strong; ++ is less strong.
† 30 mg for weight <60 kg; 35 mg for 60–69 kg; 40 mg for 70–79 kg; 45 mg for 80–89 kg; and 50 mg for ≥90 kg.
‡ Bolus 15 mg, infusion 0.75 mg/kg for 30 min (maximum 50 mg), then 0.5 mg/kg (maximum 35 mg) over the next 60 min; total dose not to exceed 100 mg.
§ Streptokinase is no longer marketed in the United States but is available in other countries.
** Streptokinase is highly antigenic and absolutely contraindicated within 6 mo of previous exposure because of the potential for serious allergic reaction.
IV indicates intravenous; rPA, reteplase plasminogen activator; TIMI, Thrombolysis In Myocardial Infarction; TNK-tPA, tenecteplase tissue-type plasminogen activator; and tPA, tissue-type plasminogen activator.
2013 ACCF/AHA guideline for the management of ST-elevation myocardial infarction. *J Am Coll Cardiol.* 2013;**61**:e78–140.

Table 28.20 ACCF/AHA 2013 GL on STEMI. Adjunctive antithrombotic therapy to support reperfusion with fibrinolytic therapy

Antiplatelet therapy	
Aspirin	
162 to 325 mg loading dose	I-A
81 to 325 mg daily maintenance dose (indefinite)	I-A
81 mg daily is the preferred maintenance dose	IIa-B
P2Y12 receptor inhibitors	
Clopidogrel:	I-A
Age ≤75 y: 300 mg loading dose	
Followed by 75 mg daily for at least 14 d and up to 1 year in absence of bleeding	I-A (14d)/C (up to one year)
Age >75 years: no loading dose, give 75 mg	I-A
Followed by 75 mg daily for at least 14 d and up to 1 year in absence of bleeding	I-A (14d)/C (up to one year)
Anticoagulant therapy	
UFH	I-C
Weight-based IV bolus and infusion adjusted to obtain aPTT of 1.5 to 2.0 times control for 48 h or until revascularization. IV bolus of 60 U/kg (maximum 4000 U), followed by an infusion of 12 U/kg/h (maximum 1000 U) initially, adjusted to maintain aPTT at 1.5 to 2.0 times control (approximately 50 to 70 s) for 48 h or until revascularization	
Enoxaparin	I-A
If age <75 years: 30 mg IV bolus, followed in 15 min by 1 mg/kg subcutaneously every 12 h (maximum 100 mg for the first two doses)	
If age ≥75 years: no bolus, 0.75 mg/kg subcutaneously every 12 h (maximum 75 mg for the first two doses)	
Regardless of age, if CrCl <30 mL/min: 1 mg/kg subcutaneously every 24 h	
Duration: for the index hospitalization, up to 8 d or until revascularization	
Fondaparinux	I-B
Initial dose 2.5 mg IV, then 2.5 mg subcutaneously daily starting the following day, for the index hospitalization up to 8 d or until revascularization	
Contraindicated if CrCl <30 mL/min	

aPTT indicates activated partial thromboplastin time; CrCl, creatinine clearance; IV, intravenous; N/A, not available; and UFH, unfractionated heparin.
2013 ACCF/AHA guideline for the management of ST-elevation myocardial infarction. *J Am Coll Cardiol.* 2013;**61**:e78–140.

patients, and diabetics, are at an increased risk of intracranial haemorrhage when subjected to thrombolysis. Fibrinolytic, antiplatelet, and anticoagulant therapies should be discontinued until brain imaging scan shows no evidence of intracranial haemorrhage. Cryoprecipitates, fresh frozen plasma, protamine, and platelets are given, and intracranial pressure is reduced with mannitol, endotracheal intubation, and hyperventilation. Blood pressure and glucose levels are optimized, and neurosurgical consultation is sought.

Failed reperfusion

Criteria of successful thrombolysis are:

- **ST resolution (>70%) within the first 90 minutes after treatment**
- **T wave invertion <4 hours after treatment**
- **Rapid release of biochemical markers**
- **Accelerated idioventricular rhythm 60–120 bpm (benign rhythm).**

Failed reperfusion is defined as continuing chest pain or failure of ST segment resolution by more than 50% at 90 minutes after fibrinolysis and is seen in 40% of cases with fibrinolysis.

Patients with **recurrent ischaemia** should be considered candidates for coronary arteriography and PCI or CABG. Fibrinolytic therapy (other than streptokinase) may be repeated if PCI is not available within the next 60 minutes.

Rescue PCI

This is better than repeat fibrinolysis after failed reperfusion,[69] and associated with lower rates of heart failure (5% absolute reduction) and re-infarction (4% absolute reduction) by 6 months but a 3% increase in stroke, compared to a conservative strategy with PCI only, for recurrent ischaemia after fibrinolysis.[70] Coronary angiography with intent to perform PCI is also recommended in patients who received thrombolysis and develop cardiogenic shock, pulmonary oedema or heart failure, and haemodynamically compromising ventricular arrhythmias (Table 28.21).

Routine angiography following fibrinolysis

ST recovery is an imperfect discriminator between TIMI grade 2 and TIMI grade 3 flow, with up to 50% of patients with persistent ST elevation having a patent infarct-related artery at the time of angiography (Table 28.17).[71] Thus, routine coronary angiography and, if indicated, PCI may be recommended in all patients after successful thrombolysis. This should be done within the next 24 hours and delayed for at least 3 hours following the fibrinolysis, though the optimal timing remains uncertain.[62,72,73] In stable patients who did not receive reperfusion, routine angiography before discharge is an option (Table 28.22).

CABG

CABG mortality is elevated for the first 3 to 7 days after infarction, and the benefit of revascularization must be balanced against this increased risk. However, emergency surgical revascularization may be necessary and can be undertaken, especially in cases of failed PCI of a large LAD or mechanical complications of the MI (Table 28.23).[74]

Complications of MI

Most deaths in hospitalized patients with STEMI are due to heart failure and mechanical complications.

Heart failure (Killip class II and III)

Oxygen by mask (4–5 L/min), loop diuretics (i.e. furosemide 20–40 mg IV, repeated at 1–4 hourly intervals), ACE inhibitors (or ARBs), and nitrates, if the systolic BP >100 mmHg, are mandatory. Dobutamine (can be given through a peripheral line) or dopamine, if there is hypotension (requires central line), can be considered in refractory cases (Table 28.24).

Hypotension

Rapid volume loading and correction of arrhythmias and conduction disturbances are essential in hypotension. If the patient does not respond, consideration of mechanical complications and vasopressor support and/or intra-aortic balloon counterpulsation may be needed.

Cardiogenic shock

Cardiogenic shock is caused by extensive loss of viable myocardial tissue and is characterized by a systolic pressure <90 mmHg and a central filling pressure (wedge pressure) >20 mmHg or a cardiac index <1.8 L/min/m^2. Shock is also considered present if inotropes and/or an intra-aortic balloon pump are needed to maintain a systolic blood pressure >90 mmHg and a cardiac index >1.8 L/min/m^2. Early revascularization by PCI (one or more coronary arteries)[70], or even CABG if necessary, is the only means to possibly reduce mortality that approaches 60% if left untreated (Table 28.24, see also Chapter 31 on CCF). A haemodynamic support device is recommended in patients who do not stabilize with pharmacologic therapy (ACC/AHA 2011 on PCI, I-B). Although intra-aortic balloon pumping is still recommended, its effectiveness is debated, particularly if revascularization is undertaken (IABP-SHOCK II trial).[76,77]

Right ventricular infarction

Patients with inferior STEMI and haemodynamic compromise should be assessed with a right precordial V_{4R} lead to detect ST segment elevation and an echocardiogram to screen for RV infarction.

Table 28.21 ACCF/AHA 2013 GL on STEMI. PCI after fibrinolysis

Indications for PCI of an infarct artery in patients who were managed with fibrinolytic therapy or who did not receive reperfusion therapy	
Cardiogenic shock or acute severe HF	I-B
Intermediate- or high-risk findings on predischarge non-invasive ischaemia testing	I-C
Spontaneous or easily provoked myocardial ischaemia	I-C
Patients with evidence of failed reperfusion or reocclusion after fibrinolytic therapy (as soon as possible)	IIa-B
Stable* patients after successful fibrinolysis, ideally between 3 and 24 h	IIa-B
Stable* patients >24 h after successful fibrinolysis	IIb-B
Delayed PCI of a totally occluded infarct artery >24 h after STEMI in stable patients	III-B (no benefit)

* Although individual circumstances will vary, clinical stability is defined by the absence of low output, hypotension, persistent tachycardia, apparent shock, high-grade ventricular or symptomatic supraventricular tachyarrhythmias, and spontaneous recurrent ischaemia.
HF, heart failure; PCI, percutaneous coronary intervention; and STEMI, ST elevation myocardial infarction.

Adjunctive antithrombotic therapy to support PCI after fibrinolytic therapy	
Antiplatelet therapy	
Aspirin	
162 to 325 mg loading dose given with fibrinolytic agent (before PCI).	I-A
81 to 325 mg daily maintenance dose after PCI (indefinite)	I-A
81 mg daily is the preferred daily maintenance dose	IIa-B
P2Y12 receptor inhibitors	
Loading doses	
For patients who received a loading dose of clopidogrel with fibrinolytic therapy:	
Continue clopidogrel 75 mg daily without an additional loading dose	I-C
For patients who have not received a loading dose of clopidogrel:	
If PCI is performed ≤24 h after fibrinolytic therapy: clopidogrel 300 mg loading dose before or at the time of PCI	I-C
If PCI is performed >24 h after fibrinolytic therapy: clopidogrel 600 mg loading dose before or at the time of PCI	I-C
If PCI is performed >24 h after treatment with a fibrin-specific agent or >48 h after a non-fibrin-specific agent: prasugrel 60 mg at the time of PCI	IIa-B
For patients with prior stroke/TIA: prasugrel	III-B (harm)
Maintenance doses and duration of therapy	
DES placed: continue therapy for at least 1 year with:	
Clopidogrel: 75 mg daily	I-C
Prasugrel: 10 mg daily	IIa-B
BMS placed: continue therapy for at least 30 d and up to 1 year with:	
Clopidogrel: 75 mg daily	I-c
Prasugrel: 10 mg daily	IIa-B
Anticoagulant therapy	
Continue UFH through PCI, administering additional IV boluses, as needed, to maintain therapeutic ACT, depending on use of GP IIb/IIIa receptor antagonist†	I-C
Continue enoxaparin through PCI:	I-B
No additional drug if last dose was within previous 8 h	
0.3 mg/kg IV bolus if last dose was 8 to 12 h earlier	
Fondaparinux:	III-C (harm)
As sole anticoagulant for PCI	

* Balloon angioplasty without stent placement may be used in selected patients. It might be reasonable to provide P2Y12 inhibitor therapy to patients with STEMI undergoing balloon angioplasty after fibrinolysis alone, according to the recommendations listed for BMS (level of evidence: C).
† The recommended ACT with no planned GP IIb/IIIa receptor antagonist treatment is 250–300 s (HaemoTec device) or 300–350 s (Haemochron device).
ACT indicates activated clotting time; BMS, bare metal stent; DES, drug-eluting stent; GP, glycoprotein; IV, intravenous; PCI, percutaneous coronary intervention; TIA, transient ischaemic attack; and UFH, unfractionated heparin.
2013 ACCF/AHA guideline for the management of ST-elevation myocardial infarction. *J Am Coll Cardiol.* 2013;**61**:e78–140.

Table 28.22 ACCF/AHA 2013 GL on STEMI. Coronary angiography after fibrinolysis

Indications for transfer for angiography after fibrinolytic therapy	
Immediate transfer for cardiogenic shock or severe acute HF, irrespective of time delay from MI onset	I-B
Urgent transfer for failed reperfusion or reocclusion	IIa-B
As part of an invasive strategy in stable* patients with PCI between 3 and 24 h after successful fibrinolysis	IIa-B

* Although individual circumstances will vary, clinical stability is defined by the absence of low output, hypotension, persistent tachycardia, apparent shock, high-grade ventricular or symptomatic supraventricular tachyarrhythmias, and spontaneous recurrent ischaemia.
HF, heart failure; MI, myocardial infarction; and PCI, percutaneous coronary intervention.

Indications for coronary angiography in patients who were managed with fibrinolytic therapy or who did not receive reperfusion therapy	
Cardiogenic shock or acute severe HF that develops after initial presentation	I-B
Intermediate- or high-risk findings on predischarge non-invasive ischaemia testing	I-B
Spontaneous or easily provoked myocardial ischaemia	I-C
Failed reperfusion or reocclusion after fibrinolytic therapy	IIa-B
Stable* patients after successful fibrinolysis before discharge and ideally between 3 and 24 h	IIa-B

* Although individual circumstances will vary, clinical stability is defined by the absence of low output, hypotension, persistent tachycardia, apparent shock, high-grade ventricular or symptomatic supraventricular tachyarrhythmias, and spontaneous recurrent ischaemia.
HF, heart failure.
2013 ACCF/AHA guideline for the management of ST-elevation myocardial infarction. *J Am Coll Cardiol.* 2013;**61**:e78–140.

Table 28.23 ACCF/AHA 2013 GL on STEMI. CABG in STEMI

Urgent CABG in patients with STEMI and coronary anatomy not amenable to PCI who have ongoing or recurrent ischaemia, cardiogenic shock, severe HF, or other high-risk features.	I-B
CABG in patients with STEMI at time of operative repair of mechanical defects.	I-B
Use of mechanical circulatory support in patients with STEMI who are haemodynamically unstable and require urgent CABG.	IIa-C
Emergency CABG within 6 hours of symptom onset in patients with STEMI who do not have cardiogenic shock and are not candidates for PCI or fibrinolytic therapy.	IIb-C
Timing of urgent CABG in patients with STEMI in relation to use of antiplatelet agents	
Aspirin should not be withheld before urgent CABG.	I-C
Clopidogrel or ticagrelor should be discontinued at least 24 hours before urgent on-pump CABG, if possible.	I-B
Short-acting IV GP IIb/IIIa receptor antagonists (eptifibatide, tirofiban) should be discontinued at least 2–4 hours before urgent CABG.	I-B
Abciximab should be discontinued at least 12 hours before urgent CABG.	I-B
Urgent off-pump CABG within 24 hours of clopidogrel or ticagrelor administration might be considered, especially if the benefits of prompt revascularization outweigh the risks of bleeding.	I-B
Urgent CABG within 5 days of clopidogrel or ticagrelor administration or within 7 days of prasugrel administration might be considered, especially if the benefits of prompt revascularization outweigh the risks of bleeding.	I-C

2013 ACCF/AHA guideline for the management of ST-elevation myocardial infarction. *J Am Coll Cardiol.* 2013;**61**:e78–140.

Table 28.24 Heart failure and cardiogenic shock

ESC 2012 GL on STEMI. Treatment of heart failure and left ventricular dysfunction	
Treatment of mild heart failure (Killip class II)	
Oxygen is indicated to maintain a saturation >95%.	I-C
Loop diuretics, e.g. furosemide 20–40 mg IV, are recommended and should be repeated at 1–4 h intervals if necessary.	I-C
IV nitrates or sodium nitroprusside should be considered in patients with elevated systolic blood pressure.	IIa-C
An ACE inhibitor is indicated in all patients with signs or symptoms of heart failure and/or evidence of LV dysfunction in the absence of hypotension, hypovolaemia, or renal failure.	I-A

(Continued)

Table 28.24 (Continued)

An ARB (valsartan) is an alternative to ACE inhibitors, particularly if ACE inhibitors are not tolerated.	I-B
An aldosterone antagonist (epleronone) is recommended in all patients with signs or symptoms of heart failure and/or evidence of LV dysfunction, provided no renal failure or hyperkalaemia.	I-B
Hydralazine and isosorbide dinitrate should be considered if the patient is intolerant to both ACE inhibitors and ARBs.	IIa-C
Treatment of moderate heart failure (Killip class III)	
Oxygen is indicated.	I-C
Ventilatory support should be instituted, according to blood gases.	I-C
Loop diuretics, e.g. furosemide 20–40 mg IV, are recommended and should be repeated at 1–4 h intervals if necessary.	I-C
Morphine is recommended. Respiration should be monitored. Nausea is common, and an antiemetic may be required. Frequent low-dose therapy is advisable.	I-C
Nitrates are recommended if there is no hypotension.	I-C
Inotropic agents: Dopamine	IIa-C
Dobutamine (inotropic)	IIa-C
Levosimendan (inotropic/vasodilator).	IIb-C
An aldosterone antagonist, such as spironolactone or eplerenone, must be used if LVEF ≤40%.	I-B
Ultrafiltration should be considered.	IIa-B
Early revascularization must be considered if the patient has not been previously revascularized.	I-C
Treatment of cardiogenic shock (Killip class IV)	
Oxygen/mechanical respiratory support is indicated, according to blood gases.	I-C
Urgent echocardiography/Doppler must be performed to detect mechanical complications, assess systolic function, and loading conditions.	I-C
High-risk patients must be transferred early to tertiary centres.	I-C
Emergency revascularization, with either PCI or CABG, in suitable patients must be considered.	I-B
Fibrinolysis should be considered if revascularization is unavailable.	IIa-C
Intra-aortic balloon pumping may be considered.	IIb-B
LV assist devices may be considered for circulatory support in patients in refractory shock.	IIb-C
Haemodynamic assessment with balloon floating catheter may be considered.	IIb-B
Inotropic/vasopressor agents should be considered: Dopamine	IIa-C
Dobutamine	IIa-C
Norepinephrine (preferred over dopamine when blood pressure is low).	IIb-B

ESC Guidelines for the management of acute myocardial infarction in patients presenting with ST-segment elevation. *Eur Heart J* 2012; **33**:2501–2502.

ACC/AHA 2013 on STEMI. Treatment of cardiogenic shock

Emergency revascularization, with either PCI or CABG, in suitable patients with cardiogenic shock due to pump failure after STEMI, irrespective of the time delay from MI onset.	I-B
In the absence of contraindications, fibrinolytic therapy should be administered to patients with STEMI and cardiogenic shock who are unsuitable candidates for either PCI or CABG.	I-B
Intra-aortic balloon pump (IABP) counterpulsation for patients with cardiogenic shock after STEMI who do not quickly stabilize with pharmacological therapy.	IIa-B
Alternative LV assist devices for circulatory support may be considered in patients with refractory cardiogenic shock	IIb-C

2013 ACCF/AHA guideline for the management of ST-elevation myocardial infarction. *J Am Coll Cardiol.* 2013;**61**:e78–140.

The following principles apply to therapy:

- Early reperfusion should be achieved, if possible.
- AV synchrony should be achieved, and bradycardia should be corrected.
- RV preload should be optimized, with initial volume challenge in patients with haemodynamic instability, provided the jugular venous pressure is normal or low.
- RV afterload should be optimized, with therapy for concomitant LV dysfunction.
- Inotropic support should be used for haemodynamic instability not responsive to volume challenge.

Finally, it is reasonable to delay CABG surgery for 4 weeks to allow recovery of contractile performance.

Myocardial free wall rupture

More commonly occurs in the elderly with hypertension, after large anterior MI, and particularly following expansion. Usually, it occurs 1 day after infarction (up to 7 days without reperfusion).[78] Incidence is 1–6%, and PCI, but not fibrinolysis, reduces the risk. Acute free wall rupture is associated with haemopericardium and electromechanical dissociation and is fatal. Subacute rupture (25%), i.e. sealing of the rupture with thrombus or adhesions, may lead to a relatively stable haemopericardium that allows time for surgical intervention. Patients with tamponade, but without electromechanical dissociation, may have a good prognosis with pericardiocentesis and conservative management. When pericardial effusion in a parasternal short-axis view exceeds 10 mm, the risk of free wall rupture is high, and pericardial aspiration for measurement of haematocrit in the effusion is useful.[14] Moderate pericardial effusions without tamponade carry the risk of late rupture. Patients with free wall rupture should be considered for urgent cardiac surgical repair, and CABG should be undertaken at the same time as repair of free wall rupture.

Pseudoaneurysm, i.e. false aneurysm of pericardium and thrombus communicating with the ventricle, may also occur.

True LV aneurysm may result in intractable VT and/or pump failure, and, in these cases, surgery with concomitant CABG is indicated.

Ventricular septal rupture

Incidence is 0.2–0.45% (1–3% without reperfusion).[78,79] Patients have multivessel disease and anterior MI (apical rupture) or inferior MI (basal rupture with worse prognosis). They develop shortness of breath and hypotension, and a harsh holosystolic murmur with thrill (50%) may be present. Biventricular failure generally ensues within hours or days, and the murmur and thrill are attenuated. It is often associated with AV block or RBBB. Early surgery for repair through the atrium and with a CABG, if needed, is indicated. Although difficult because of friable tissue for the first 6 weeks post-MI, it improves survival. Percutaneous closure with VSD-specific devices has also been successfully tried in apical ruptures.

Acute mitral regurgitation

This is due to papillary muscle dysfunction or rupture or chordal rupture (see also Chapter 17). Transverse rupture of a papillary muscle is rare and usually fatal. Most commonly, there is rupture of the tip of the muscle or a chorde and is due to a relatively small inferior (RCA or Cx) infarct. Posteromedial papillary muscle rupture may occur in 1% of MI, usually 1–7 days after inferior infarction. Anterolateral papillary muscle rupture is rare. The murmur is usually soft, but the ensuing pulmonary oedema is gross. Surgery with MV repair or replacement is indicated.

Thromboembolic and bleeding complications

Management of anticoagulation therapy in patients with AF who undergo primary PCI is presented in Table 28.25. Patients, with or without acute ischaemic stroke, who have a cardiac source of embolism (atrial fibrillation, mural thrombus, or akinetic segment) should receive moderate-intensity (INR 2 to 3) warfarin therapy (in addition to aspirin). Transfusion may be needed for severe bleeding (haematocrit <25% or haemoglobin <7 g/dL). There has been, however, evidence for a 20% relative risk increase with blood transfusion or a liberal blood transfusion strategy compared with a strategy of no transfusion or restricted transfusion in the setting of STEMI.[80]

Pericarditis

Pericardial effusions are more common after anterior MI and when congestive failure is present. Usually of no prognostic significance, although it may take months to resorb. **Pericarditis** may develop and resolve as late as 6 weeks after MI. The pain typically radiates to either edge of the trapezius ridge and becomes worse with deep inspiration. Anticoagulants are stopped, if not necessary, and aspirin is the treatment of choice (Table 28.26). In non-responders, even to higher doses of aspirin, colchicine 0.6 mg/12 h po, acetaminophen, or narcotic analgesics may be given. NSAIDs and steroids have been associated with increased risk of scar thinning and myocardial rupture. **Dressler syndrome** (fever, leukocytosis, elevated ESR, and pericarditis with effusion due to anti-cardiac antibodies), 1 to 8 weeks after non-reperfused MIs, is now rarely seen.

Tachyarrhythmias

The development of **atrial fibrillation** carries a worse prognosis and predicts increased mortality, regardless of the type of MI, especially when it develops in patients

Table 28.25 ACCF/AHA 2013 on STEMI. Thromboembolic and bleeding complications

Anticoagulation	
Anticoagulant therapy with a vitamin K antagonist to patients with STEMI and AF with CHADS2 score ≥2, mechanical heart valves, venous thromboembolism, or hypercoagulable disorder.	I-C
The duration of triple antithrombotic therapy with a vitamin K antagonist, aspirin, and a P2Y12 receptor inhibitor should be minimized to the extent possible to limit the risk of bleeding.*	I-C
Anticoagulant therapy with a vitamin K antagonist for patients with STEMI and asymptomatic LV mural thrombi.	IIa-C
Anticoagulant therapy for patients with STEMI and anterior apical akinesis or dyskinesis.	IIb-C
Targeting vitamin K antagonist therapy to a lower international normalized ratio (e.g. 2.0 to 2.5 in patients receiving DAPT).	IIb-C
Selected risk factors for bleeding in patients with ACS	
Advanced age (>75 years)	
Female sex	
HF or shock	
Diabetes mellitus	
Body size	
History of GI bleeding	
Presentation with STEMI or NSTEMI (vs UA)	
Severe renal dysfunction (CrCl <30 mL/min)	
Elevated white blood cell count	
Anaemia	
Use of fibrinolytic therapy	
Invasive strategy	
Inappropriate dosing of antithrombotic medications	
Chronic oral anticoagulant therapy	

ACS indicates acute coronary syndrome; CrCl, creatinine clearance; GI, gastrointestinal; HF, heart failure; NSTEMI, non-ST elevation myocardial infarction; STEMI, ST elevation myocardial infarction; and UA, unstable angina.

*Individual circumstances will vary and depend on the indications for triple therapy and the type of stent placed during PCI. After this initial treatment period, consider therapy with a vitamin K antagonist plus a single antiplatelet agent. For patients treated with fibrinolysis, consider triple therapy for 14 days, followed by a vitamin K antagonist plus a single antiplatelet agent.

2013 ACCF/AHA guideline for the management of ST-elevation myocardial infarction. *J Am Coll Cardiol.* 2013;**61**:e78–140.

Table 28.26 ACCF/AHA 2013 GL on STEMI. Management of pericarditis after STEMI

Aspirin	I-B
Acetaminophen, colchicine, or narcotic analgesics if aspirin, even in higher doses, is not effective.	IIb-C
Glucocorticoids and non-steroidal anti-inflammatory drugs are potentially harmful for treatment of pericarditis after STEMI.	III-B

2013 ACCF/AHA guideline for the management of ST-elevation myocardial infarction. *J Am Coll Cardiol.* 2013;**61**:e78–140.

Table 28.27 ESC 2012 GL on STEMI. Management of AF

Rhythm control should be considered in patients with atrial fibrillation secondary to a trigger or substrate that has been corrected (e.g. ischaemia).	IIa-C
Acute rate control of atrial fibrillation	
Intravenous beta blockers or non-dihydropyridine CCB (e.g. diltiazem, verapamil)[c] are indicated if there are no clinical signs of acute heart failure.	I-A
Amiodarone or IV digitalis is indicated in case of rapid ventricular response in the presence of concomitant acute heart failure or hypotension.	I-B
Cardioversion	
Immediate electrical cardioversion is indicated when adequate rate control cannot be achieved promptly with pharmacological agents in patients with atrial fibrillation and ongoing ischaemia, severe haemodynamic compromise, or heart failure.	I-C
Intravenous amiodarone is indicated for conversion to sinus rhythm in stable patients with recent-onset atrial fibrillation and structural heart disease.	I-A
Digoxin (III-A), verapamil, sotalol, metoprolol (III-B) and other beta-blocking agents (III-C) are ineffective in converting recent-onset atrial fibrillation to sinus rhythm and should not be used for rhythm control (although beta blockers or digoxin may be used for rate control).	III-A/B/C

[c] Calcium antagonists should be used cautiously or avoided in patients with heart failure because of their negative inotropic effects.

ESC Guidelines for the management of acute myocardial infarction in patients presenting with ST-segment elevation. *Eur Heart J* 2012; **33**:2501–2502.

without history of AF before MI,[81] or more than 1 month after MI (Table 28.27).[82] In haemodynamic instability, DC cardioversion is indicated. For recurrent episodes or for rate control, IV amiodarone, beta blockade, diltiazem or verapamil, and digoxin (in the presence of LV dysfunction) may be used. Cardiac arrest has been previously discussed.

Ventricular arrhythmias—acute phase management

VPBs are of no prognostic significance and should not be treated with antiarrhythmic drugs. **Accelerated idioventricular rhythm** is a slow form of ventricular tachycardia (<100 bpm) which characteristically follows myocardial infarction. It tends to remain stable, usually does not give rise to ventricular fibrillation, and does not require antiarrhythmic treatment. In acute myocardial infarction, **NSVT** during the first 24 h is frequent (45% in patients without thrombolysis and up to 75% in reperfused patients).[83] NSVT during the first 13[84] to 24 hours[83] after acute MI does not carry a prognostic significance. Ventricular fibrillation may be seen during the acute phase (up to 48 hours) due to ischaemia and does not predict future arrhythmia episodes (Table 28.28, see also Chapter 49 on tachyarrhythmias). Sustained monomorphic VT indicates pre-existing scar.
VF or unstable, sustained VT requires DC cardioversion.
Stable VT or unstable VT/VF refractory to cardioversion:

- IV amiodarone (5 mg/kg bolus) and repeat of cardioversion if unstable VT/VF
- Intubation may be necessary in refractory VF/VT
- IV sotalol, procainamide, and overdrive pacing may be also considered.

Incessant VT or electrical storm:
Urgent revascularization, IV beta blockade, and IV amiodarone (5 mg/kg over 10 minutes, followed, if necessary, by repeat doses or constant infusion; total dose <2.2 g over 24 hours). IV procainamide, may be also considered. In electrical storm, beta blockers are especially indicated.[85] The short-acting esmolol is preferred in the presence of reduced LV function, with close monitoring due to the risk of cardiogenic shock.

Normalization of serum K to >4 mEg/L and Mg >2 mEq/L is also recommended.

Ventricular arrhythmias—chronic phase (>48 hours) management

Compared with the pre-reperfusion era, late ventricular tachyarrhythmias are now less common, but they are still documented in approximately 20% of patients with recent MI and EF <0.40 within the next 2 years.[86] In the era of reperfusion and use of beta blockers, NSVT after MI may not be an independent predictor of mortality, especially after ejection fraction is taken into account.[86–88]

VF may, or may not, respond to revascularization, and reassessment by electrophysiology study is indicated 3 months after the intervention.[89] Monomorphic VT does not respond to revascularization.[90] Sudden unexpected death is highest in the first month after myocardial infarction, but recurrent myocardial infarction or myocardial rupture account for a high proportion of sudden unexpected deaths during this period, whereas arrhythmic death may be more likely subsequently.[91] Perhaps, this is why prophylactic ICD in patients with reduced LVEF did not reduce mortality 6–40 days after MI (DINAMIT and IRIS trials).[92,93] Both DINAMIT and IRIS, however, had excluded patients with sustained ventricular arrhythmias during this period, and sudden cardiac death was reduced, despite no effect on overall mortality in the DINAMIT trial. These patients might benefit from early ICD implantation, especially if sustained monomorphic VT (CL ≥200 ms, lasting more than 10 s) is induced at electrophysiology study.[94] The recent ACC/AHA 2013 GL on STEMI now recommend ICD implantation in patients who develop sustained VT/VF more than 48 hours after STEMI, provided the arrhythmia is not due to transient or reversible ischaemia, re-infarction, or metabolic abnormalities (Table 28.28). Patients with an initially reduced LVEF who are possible candidates for ICD therapy should undergo re-evaluation of LVEF ≥40 days after discharge.

Current indications for ICD implantation are also discussed in Chapter 55 on ventricular arrhythmias and Chapter 31 on heart failure.

Conduction disturbances

The sinus node is supplied by the right coronary (60%) or the left circumflex artery (40%). The atrioventricular node is supplied by the RCA (90%) or the left circumflex artery (10%). The bundle of His is supplied by the atrioventricular nodal branch of the RCA and partially from the septal perforators of the LAD. The right bundle branch receives most of its blood from septal perforators of the left anterior descending artery and may be through collaterals from the RCA and Cx. The left anterior fascicle is supplied by septal perforators from the LAD and is particularly susceptible to ischaemia or infarction. The left posterior fascicle is supplied by the RCA (through the AV nodal artery) and by septals of the LAD.[6]
AV block in the post-MI period is a strong predictor of cardiac death.[86] In the era of primary PCI, high-degree AV block is seen in 3.2% of patients with MI, usually inferior and more often in female patients >65 years of age, and indicates increased mortality.[95] **LBBB** does not suggest isolated LAD occlusion. In patients with LVEF<35%, **RBBB** has been associated with significantly greater scar size than

Table 28.28 ACCF/AHA 2013 GL on STEMI. Arrhythmias and conduction disturbances

ICD therapy before discharge	
Implantable cardioverter-defibrillator (ICD) therapy is indicated before discharge in patients who develop sustained VT/VF more than 48 hours after STEMI, provided the arrhythmia is not due to transient or reversible ischaemia, reinfarction, or metabolic abnormalities.	I-B
Assessment of risk for SCD	
Patients with an initially reduced LVEF who are possible candidates for ICD therapy should undergo re-evaluation of LVEF ≥40 days after discharge.	I-B
Bradycardia, AV block, and intraventricular conduction defects	
Temporary pacing is indicated for symptomatic bradyarrhythmias unresponsive to medical treatment.	I-C

2013 ACCF/AHA guideline for the management of ST-elevation myocardial infarction. *J Am Coll Cardiol*. 2013;**61**:e78–140.

Table 28.29 ESC 2012 GL on STEMI. Management of arrhythmias and conduction disturbances in the acute phase

Direct current cardioversion is indicated for sustained VT and VF.	I-C
Sustained monomorphic VT that is recurrent or refractory to direct current cardioversion: should be considered to be treated with IV amiodarone.[a]	IIa-C
May be treated with IV lidocaine or sotalol.[b]	IIb-C
Transvenous catheter pace termination should be considered if VT is refractory to cardioversion or frequently recurrent despite antiarrhythmic medication.	IIa-C
Repetitive symptomatic salvoes of non-sustained monomorphic VT should be considered for either conservative management (watchful waiting) or treated with IV beta blocker,[b] or sotalol,[b] or amiodarone.[a]	IIa-C
Polymorphic VT	
Must be treated by IV beta blocker, or	I-B
IV amiodarone[a]	I-C
Urgent angiography must be performed when myocardial ischaemia cannot be excluded	I-C
May be treated with IV lidocaine	IIb-C
Must prompt assessment and correction of electrolyte disturbances; consider magnesium	I-C
Should be treated with overdrive pacing using a temporary transvenous right ventricular lead or isoproteneral infusion	IIa-C
In cases of sinus bradycardia associated with hypotension, AV block II (Mobitz 2) or AV block III with bradycardia that causes hypotension or heart	
Intravenous atropine is indicated	I-C
Temporary pacing is indicated in cases of failure to respond to atropine	I-C
Urgent angiography with a view to revascularization is indicated if the patient has not received prior reperfusion therapy	I-C
Management of ventricular arrhythmias and risk evaluation for sudden death on long term	
Specialized electrophysiological evaluation of ICD implantation for secondary prevention of sudden cardiac death is indicated in patients with significant LV dysfunction, who suffer from haemodynamically unstable sustained VT or who are resuscitated from VF occurring beyond the initial acute phase.	I-A
Secondary preventive ICD therapy is indicated to reduce mortality in patients with significant LV dysfunction and haemodynamically unstable sustained VT or survived VF not occurring within the initial acute phase.	I-A
Risk evaluation for sudden cardiac death should be performed to assess indication for primary preventive ICD therapy by assessing LVEF (from echocardiography) at least 40 days after the acute event in patients with LVEF ≤40%.	I-A

[a] QT-prolonging agents should not be used if baseline QT is prolonged.
[b] Intravenous sotalol or other beta blockers should not be given if ejection fraction is low.

LBBB and occlusion of a proximal LAD septal perforator causes RBBB.[96]

Anterior MI PR prolongation is often associated with a wide QRS complex (>0.12 s) with a right bundle branch block pattern. Second-degree atrioventricular block with anterior myocardial infarction is usually Mobitz type II block secondary to block in the His-Purkinje system. Complete heart block may occur abruptly during the first 24 hours after myocardial infarction and is almost always preceded by the development of right bundle branch block with right or left axis deviation and QR pattern in lead V_1.

Inferior MI Sinus bradycardia and various degrees of AV block (including complete) can occur within the first 2 hours, due to increased parasympathetic tone, and resolve within 24 hours. Complete AV block complicating inferior MI is usually at the node level, i.e. with a narrow complex escape rhythm. A wide QRS escape rhythm suggests additional LAD disease. Bradycardia during the first 24 hours responds to atropine. After the first 24 hours, symptomatic conduction disturbances require temporary pacing (Tables 28.8 and 28.9).

Transcutaneous patches are recommended for all old, or new, conduction disturbances, apart from isolated first-degree or fascicular block.

Permanent pacing is considered for disturbances that persist beyond 2 weeks after the MI (see Chapter 64 on bradyarrhythmias).

Special clinical settings

Recommendations for the management of patients with renal failure or diabetes are presented in Tables 28.30 and 29.31.

Discharge

Stable patients can be transferred from the CCU after 12–24h and mobilization is allowed. Uncomplicated MIs may be discharged after 3 days after reperfusion (Table 28.32).[97] Echocardiography for assessment of LVEF is essential. Exercise testing or myocardial perfusion imaging or dobutamine echocardiography with baseline abnormalities that compromise ECG interpretation may be performed as early as 4 days after MI in stable patients (Table 28.33). A positive test as well as diabetes mellitus, LVEF <0.40, CHF, prior revascularization, or life-threatening ventricular arrhythmias are indications for coronary angiography in non-reperfused patients or in patients with fibrinolysis who did not have angiography.

Chronic therapy

Smoking cessation, loss of excessive weight, regular exercise exercise, and cardiac rehabilitation offer sustained mortality benefits (see Chapter 29 on stable CAD). **Aspirin** (75–100 mg) should be continued indefinitely and a **P2Y$_{12}$** for up to 12 months (Table 28.34). In patients unable to tolerate aspirin, clopidogrel is an alternative. Prasugrel is contraindicated in patients with a prior history of stroke or TIA. Gastric protection with a proton pump inhibitor is given to patients at high risk of bleeding. Rivaroxaban at a low dose (2.5 mg bd) may be added in patients at high risk of ischaemic complications but low risk of bleeding. Vorapaxar, a platelet activation inhibitor by antagonizing thrombin-mediated activation of the protease receptor 1, reduces the risk of cardiovascular death when added to aspirin and clopidogrel but at increased risk of bleeding.[98] **Angiotensin-converting enzyme inhibitors** are probably indicated in all patients, regardless of the presence of reduced LV function,[99] and especially in reduced LVEF. **Angiotensin II receptor blockers** are used when

Table 28.30 ESC 2012 GL on STEMI. Initial dosing of antithrombotic agents in patients with chronic kidney disease (estimated creatinine clearance <60 mL/min)

Aspirin	No dose adjustment.
Clopidogrel	No dose adjustment.
Prasugrel	No dose adjustment. No experience with end-stage renal disease/dialysis.
Ticagrelor	No dose adjustment. No experience with end-stage renal disease/dialysis.
Enoxaparin	No adjustment of bolus dose. Following thrombolysis, in patients with creatinine clearance <30 mL/min, the SC doses are given once every 24 h.
Unfractionated heparin	No adjustment of bolus dose.
Fondaparinux	No dose adjustment. No experience in patients with end-stage renal disease or dialysis patients.
Bivalirudin	◆ In patients with moderate renal insufficiency (GFR 30–59 mL/min), a lower initial infusion rate of 1.4 mg/kg/h should be given. The bolus dose should not be changed. ◆ In patients with severe renal insufficiency (GFR <30 mL/min) and in dialysis-dependent patients, bivalirudin is contraindicated.
Abciximab	No specific recommendation. Careful consideration of bleeding risk.
Eptifibatide	◆ In patients with moderate renal insufficiency (GFR ≥30 to <50 mL/min), an IV bolus of 180 micrograms should be administered, followed by a continuous infusion dose of 1.0 micrograms/kg/min for the duration of therapy. ◆ In patients with severe renal insufficiency (GFR <30 mL/min), eptifibatide is contraindicated.
Tirofiban	In patients with severe renal insufficiency (GFR <30 mL/min), the infusion dose should be reduced to 50%.

ESC Guidelines for the management of acute myocardial infarction in patients presenting with ST-segment elevation. *Eur Heart J* 2012; **33**:2501–2502.

Table 28.31 ESC 2012 GL on STEMI. Management of hyperglycaemia in ST segment elevation myocardial infarction

Measurement of glycaemia at initial evaluation in all patients and repeated in patients with known diabetes or hyperglycaemia.	I-C
Plans for optimal outpatient glucose control and secondary prevention before discharge.	I-C
In the acute phase, maintain glucose ≤11.0 mmol/L (200 mg/dL) while avoiding <5 mmol/L (<90 mg/dL).	IIa-B
This may require a dose-adjusted insulin infusion with monitoring of glucose, as long as hypoglycaemia is avoided.	
Fasting glucose and HbA1c and, in some cases, a post-discharge oral glucose tolerance test should be considered in patients with hyperglycaemia but without a history of diabetes.	IIa-B
Routine glucose-insulin potassium infusion is not indicated.	III-A

ESC Guidelines for the management of acute myocardial infarction in patients presenting with ST-segment elevation. *Eur Heart J* 2012;**33**:2501–2502.

Table 28.32 ESC 2012 GL on STEMI. Logistical issues for hospital stay

All hospitals participating in the care of STEMI patients should have a coronary care unit equipped to provide all aspects of care for STEMI patients, including treatment of ischaemia, severe heart failure, arrhythmias, and common co-morbidities.	I-C
Length of stay in the coronary care unit	
Patients undergoing uncomplicated successful reperfusion therapy should be kept in the coronary care unit for a minimum of 24 h, after which they may be moved to a step-down monitored bed for another 24–48 h.	I-C
Transfer back to a referring non-PCI hospital	
Early transfer (same day) may be considered in selected, low-risk patients after successful primary PCI without observed arrhythmia.	IIb-C
Hospital discharge	
Early discharge (after approximately 72 h) is reasonable in selected low-risk patients if early rehabilitation and adequate follow-up are arranged.	IIb-B

ESC Guidelines for the management of acute myocardial infarction in patients presenting with ST-segment elevation. *Eur Heart J* 2012;**33**:2501–2502.

Table 28.33 ACCF/AHA 2013 GL on STEMI. Risk-assessment and post-hospitalization care

Use of non-invasive testing for ischaemia before discharge	
Non-invasive testing for ischaemia before discharge to assess the presence and extent of inducible ischaemia in patients with STEMI who have not had coronary angiography and do not have high-risk clinical features for which coronary angiography would be warranted.	I-B
Non-invasive testing for ischaemia before discharge to evaluate the functional significance of a non-infarct artery stenosis previously identified at angiography.	IIb-C
Non-invasive testing for ischaemia might be considered before discharge to guide the post-discharge exercise prescription.	IIb-C
Post-hospitalization plan of care	
Post-hospital systems of care designed to prevent hospital readmissions should be used to facilitate the transition to effective, coordinated outpatient care for all patients with STEMI.	I-B
Exercise-based cardiac rehabilitation/secondary prevention programmes are recommended for patients with STEMI.	I-B
A clear, detailed, and evidence-based plan of care that promotes medication adherence, timely follow-up with the healthcare team, appropriate dietary and physical activities, and compliance with interventions for secondary prevention should be provided to patients with STEMI.	I-C
Encouragement and advice to stop smoking and to avoid secondhand smoke should be provided to patients with STEMI.	I-A

ACE inhibitors are not tolerated.[100] In the absence of severe renal dysfunction (creatinine >2.5 mg/dL) or hyperkalaemia, post-myocardial infarction patients with an ejection fraction of less than 40% or heart failure should receive an **aldosterone antagonist**,[101] such as eplerenone. Steroids or NSAIDs, given early after MI, can cause tissue thinning and MI expansion. **Statins** provide substantial reductions in mortality as well as in non-fatal ischaemic events.[102] A target LDL value of ≤1.8 mmol/L (70 mg/dL) is recommended. The relative benefit of **beta blockers** after

Table 28.34 Long-term therapy

ACCF/AHA 2013 GL on STEMI. Routine medical therapies	
Beta blockers	
Oral beta blockers in the first 24 h in patients without: signs of heart failure, evidence of a low output state, increased risk for cardiogenic shock,* PR interval >0.24 s, second- or third-degree AV block, active asthma, or reactive airway disease.	I-B
during and after hospitalization in the absence of contraindications.	I-B
Patients with early contraindications within the first 24 hours of STEMI should be re-evaluated for subsequent eligibility.	I-C
Beta blockers IV at presentation to patients without contraindications and with hypertension or ongoing ischaemia.	IIa-B

* Risk factors for cardiogenic shock (the greater the number of risk factors present, the higher the risk of developing cardiogenic shock) are age >70 years, systolic BP <120 mmHg, sinus tachycardia >110 bpm or heart rate <60 bpm, and increased time since onset of symptoms of STEMI.

Renin-angiotensin-aldosterone system inhibitors	
ACE inhibitor within the first 24 hours to all patients with STEMI with anterior location, HF, or LVEF <0.40, unless contraindicated.	I-A
ARB to patients who have indications for, but are intolerant of, ACE inhibitors.	I-B
An aldosterone antagonist to patients with no contraindications who are already receiving an ACE inhibitor and beta blocker and who have LVEF ≤0.40 and either symptomatic HF or have diabetes mellitus.	I-B
ACE inhibitors for all patients with STEMI and no contraindications.	IIa-A
Lipid management	
High-intensity statin therapy should be initiated or continued in all patients with STEMI and no contraindications to its use.	I-B
Obtain a fasting lipid profile in patients with STEMI, preferably within 24 hours of presentation.	I-C

2013 ACCF/AHA guideline for the management of ST-elevation myocardial infarction. *J Am Coll Cardiol.* 2013;**61**:e78–140.

ACCF/AHA GL on STEMI. Selected routine medical therapies

Therapy	Indications	Dose/administration	Avoid/caution
Beta receptor antagonists	◆ Oral: all patients without contraindication ◆ IV: patients with refractory hypertension or ongoing ischaemia without contraindication	Individualize: ◆ Metoprolol tartrate 25–50 mg every 6 to 12 h orally, then transition over next 2 to 3 d to twice daily dosing of metoprolol tartrate or to daily metoprolol succinate; titrate to daily dose of 200 mg as tolerated ◆ Carvedilol 6.25 mg twice daily, titrate to 25 mg twice daily as tolerated ◆ Metoprolol tartrate IV 5 mg every 5 min as tolerated up to three doses; titrate to heart rate and BP	◆ Signs of HF ◆ Low output state ◆ Increased risk of cardiogenic shock ◆ Prolonged first-degree or high-grade AV block ◆ Reactive airways disease
ACE inhibitors	◆ For patients with anterior infarction, post-MI LV systolic dysfunction (EF ≤0.40) or HF ◆ May be given routinely to all patients without contraindication	Individualize: ◆ Lisinopril 2.5–5 mg/d to start; titrate to 10 mg/d, or higher, as tolerated ◆ Captopril 6.25–12.5 mg 3 times/d to start; titrate to 25–50 mg 3 times/d as tolerated ◆ Ramipril 2.5 mg twice daily to start; titrate to 5 mg twice daily as tolerated ◆ Trandolapril test dose 0.5 mg; titrate up to 4 mg daily as tolerated	◆ Hypotension ◆ Renal failure ◆ Hyperkalaemia
ARB	◆ For patients intolerant of ACE inhibitors	◆ Valsartan 20 mg twice daily to start; titrate to 160 mg twice daily as tolerated	◆ Hypotension ◆ Renal failure ◆ Hyperkalaemia
Statins	◆ All patients without contraindications	◆ High-dose atorvastatin 80 mg daily	◆ Caution with drugs metabolized via *CYP3A4*, fibrates ◆ Monitor for myopathy, hepatic toxicity ◆ Combine with diet and lifestyle therapies ◆ Adjust dose as dictated by targets for LDL cholesterol and non–HDL cholesterol reduction

ACE indicates angiotensin-converting enzyme; ARB, angiotensin receptor blocker; AV, atrioventricular; BP, blood pressure; CO_2, carbon dioxide; EF, ejection fraction; HDL, high density lipoprotein; HF, heart failure; IV, intravenous; LDL, low density lipoprotein; LV, left ventricular; MI, myocardial infarction; RV, right ventricular; and SBP, systolic blood pressure.
2013 ACCF/AHA guideline for the management of ST-elevation myocardial infarction. *J Am Coll Cardiol.* 2013;**61**:e78–140.

(*Continued*)

Table 28.34 (Continued)

ESC 2012. GL on STEMI. Routine therapies in the acute, subacute, and long-term phase of ST segment elevation myocardial infarction	
Active smokers with STEMI must receive counselling and be referred to a smoking cessation programme.	I-B
Each hospital participating in the care of STEMI patients must have a smoking cessation protocol.	I-C
Exercise-based rehabilitation	I-B
Antiplatelet therapy with low dose aspirin (75–100 mg) indefinitely after STEMI.	I-A
In patients who are intolerant to aspirin, clopidogrel as an alternative to aspirin.	I-B
DAPT with a combination of aspirin and prasugrel or aspirin and ticagrelor is recommended (over aspirin and clopidogrel) in patients treated with PCI.	I-A
DAPT with aspirin and an oral ADP receptor antagonist must be continued for up to 12 months after STEMI, with a strict minimum of:	I-C
◆ 1 month for patients receiving BMS	I-C
◆ 6 months for patients receiving DES	IIb-B
In patients with left ventricular thrombus, anticoagulation for a minimum of 3 months.	IIa-B
In patients with a clear indication for oral anticoagulation (e.g. atrial fibrillation with CHA_2DS_2-VASc score ≥2 or mechanical valve prosthesis), oral anticoagulation in addition to antiplatelet therapy.	I-C
If patients require triple antithrombotic therapy, combining DAPT and OAC, e.g. because of stent placement and an obligatory indication for OAC, the duration of dual antiplatelet therapy should be minimized to reduce bleeding risk.	I-C
In selected patients who receive aspirin and clopidogrel, low-dose rivaroxaban (2.5 mg twice daily) if the patient is at low bleeding risk.	IIb-B
DAPT should be used up to 1 year in patients with STEMI who did not receive a stent.	IIa-C
Gastric protection with a proton pump inhibitor for the duration of DAPT therapy in patients at high risk of bleeding.	IIa-C
Oral treatment with beta blockers during hospital stay and continued thereafter in all STEMI patients without contraindications.	IIa-B
Oral treatment with beta blockers is indicated in patients with heart failure or LV dysfunction.	I-A
Intravenous beta blockers must be avoided in patients with hypotension or heart failure.	III-B
Intravenous beta blockers at the time of presentation in patients without contraindications, with high blood pressure, tachycardia and no signs of heart failure.	IIa-B
A fasting lipid profile must be obtained in all STEMI patients as soon as possible after presentation.	I-C
Initiate or continue high-dose statins early after admission in all STEMI patients without contraindication or history of intolerance, regardless of initial cholesterol values.	I-A
Reassessment of LDL cholesterol after 4–6 weeks to ensure that a target value of ≤1.8 mmol/L (70 mg/dL) has been reached.	IIa-C
Verapamil for secondary prevention in patients with absolute contraindications to beta blockers and no heart failure.	IIb-B
ACE inhibitors, starting within the first 24 h of STEMI in patients with evidence of heart failure, LV systolic dysfunction, diabetes, or an anterior infarct.	I-A
An ARB, preferably valsartan, is an alternative to ACE inhibitors in patients with heart failure or LV systolic dysfunction, particularly those who are intolerant of ACE inhibitors.	I-B
ACE inhibitors in all patients in the absence of contraindications.	IIa-A
Aldosterone antagonists, e.g. eplerenone, in patients with an ejection fraction ≤40% and heart failure or diabetes, provided no renal failure or hyperkalaemia.	I-B

ESC Guidelines for the management of acute myocardial infarction in patients presenting with ST-segment elevation. *Eur Heart J* 2012; **33**:2501–2502.

myocardial infarction, in the context of more aggressive revascularization, is less clear, but these agents are recommended for indefinite oral therapy when the haemodynamic condition after MI has stabilized. Early trials have indicated that metoprolol, propranolol, and timolol unequivocally reduce mortality after MI.[103] However, they may not confer survival benefit in patients with a remote MI (>1 year).[104]

Non-dihydropyridine calcium antagonists may be use when necessary (contraindications to beta blockers and no heart failure). If oral **anticoagulants** are indicated, they may be combined with aspirin and thienopyridines but at an increased risk of bleeding. In patients with a clear indication for **oral anticoagulation** (e.g. atrial fibrillation with CHA2DS2-VASc score ≥2 or mechanical valve prosthesis), oral anticoagulation must be implemented in addition to antiplatelet therapy (ESC 2012 I-C), but the duration of dual antiplatelet therapy should be minimized to reduce bleeding risk. The lowest efficacious INR (2–2.5) should be targeted. In patients with left ventricular thrombus, anticoagulation should be instituted for a minimum of 3 months. (ESC 2012 IIa-B). In selected patients who receive aspirin and clopidogrel, low-dose **rivaroxaban** (2.5 mg twice daily) may be considered if the patient is at low bleeding risk (ESC IIb-B).[105] It is still not approved by FDA for this purpose. Influenza vaccination should be provided to all patients with CAD. **Chelation** therapy is not recommended (III-C by AVCCF/AHA 2012 on stable CAD). There has been some recent evidence that it may be beneficial in combination with high-dose vitamins in post-MI patients.[106]

The ACC/AHA and ESC recommendations for risk reduction and secondary prevention are discussed in Chapter 29 on stable CAD.

Stem cell transplantation

Since the discovery that the heart is not a post-mitotic organ and myocardial tissue regeneration is possible, human embryonic stem cells, skeletal myoblasts, and adult bone marrow stem cells have been used to limit infarct size. Human embryonic stem cells form heart teratomas and have to be differentiated into cardiac progenitor cells prior to transplantation, and immune rejection must be prevented. Transplanted autologous skeletal myoblasts do not form electromechanical connections with host cardiomyocytes, and thus reentrant ventricular arrhythmias can occur. Autologous bone marrow mononuclear cells that mainly contain haematopoietic, mesenchymal, and endothelial stem cells do not have these side effects, and several trials have used them for myocardial regeneration after myocardial infarction. Increases in LVEF and reduction of infarct size has been shown.[107] Results, however, have been inconsistent, and several questions regarding mechanism of action, optimal timing of transplantation, and type of cells used remain.

References

1. Thygesen K, *et al.* Third universal definition of myocardial infarction. *Eur Heart J.* 2012;**33**:2551–67
2. Davis TM, *et al.*; UK PDS Group. Prognostic significance of silent myocardial infarction in newly diagnosed type 2 diabetes mellitus: United Kingdom Prospective Diabetes Study (UKPDS) 79. Circulation. 2013;127:980–7.
3. Lee TH, *et al.* Evaluation of the patient with acute chest pain. *N Engl J Med.* 2000;**342**:1187–95
4. Wang K, *et al.* ST segment elevation in conditions other than acute myocardial infarction. *N Engl J Med.* 2003;**349**:2128–35
5. Delewi R, *et al.* Pathological Q waves in myocardial infarction in patients treated by primary PCI. *J Am Coll Cardiol Img.* 2013;[Epub ahead of print]
6. Zimetbaum PJ, *et al.* Use of the electrocardiogram in acute myocardial infarction. *N Engl J Med.* 2003;**348**:933–40
7. Sgarbossa EB, *et al.* Electrocardiographic diagnosis of evolving acute myocardial infarction in the presence of left bundle-branch block. GUSTO-1 (Global Utilization of Streptokinase and Tissue Plasminogen Activator for Occluded Coronary Arteries) Investigators. *N Engl J Med.* 1996;**334**:481–7
8. Antman E, *et al.* ST-elevation myocardial infarction: Pathology, pathophysiology and clinical features. In: Libby P, Bonow RO, Mann DL, Zipes DP (Eds): Braunwald's heart disease. 8th edition. [pp. 1207–1231], Saunders, Philadelphia, 2008.
9. Wallace TW, *et al.* Prevalence and determinants of troponin T elevation in the general population. *Circulation.* 2006;**113**:1958–65
10. Januzzi JL, Jr., *et al.* High-sensitivity troponin T concentrations in acute chest pain patients evaluated with cardiac computed tomography. *Circulation.* 2010;**121**:1227–34
11. Mahajan VS, *et al.* How to interpret elevated cardiac troponin levels. *Circulation.* 2011;**124**:2350–4
12. Newby LK, *et al.* ACCF 2012 expert consensus document on practical clinical considerations in the interpretation of troponin elevations: a report of the American College of Cardiology Foundation Task Force on Clinical Expert Consensus Documents. *J Am Coll Cardiol.* 2012;**60**:2427–63
13. Reichlin T, *et al.* One-hour rule-out and rule-in of acute myocardial infarction using high-sensitivity cardiac troponin T *Arch Intern Med.* 2012;**172**:1211–18
14. Figueras J, *et al.* Hospital outcome of moderate to severe pericardial effusion complicating ST-elevation acute myocardial infarction. *Circulation.* 2010;**122**:1902–9
15. Schelbert EB, *et al.* Prevalence and prognosis of unrecognized myocardial infarction determined by cardiac magnetic resonance in older adults. *Circulation.* 2012;**380**:890–6
16. Halpern EJ. Triple-rule-out ct angiography for evaluation of acute chest pain and possible acute coronary syndrome. *Radiology.* 2009;**252**:332–45
17. Westerhout CM, *et al.* The influence of time from symptom onset and reperfusion strategy on 1-year survival in ST-elevation myocardial infarction: a pooled analysis of an early fibrinolytic strategy versus primary percutaneous coronary intervention from CAPTIM and WEST. *Am Heart J.* 2011;**161**:283–90
18. Bottiger BW, *et al.* Thrombolysis during resuscitation for out-of-hospital cardiac arrest. *N Engl J Med.* 2008;**359**:2651–62
19. 2013 ACCF/AHA guideline for the management of ST-elevation myocardial infarction: executive summary: a report of the American College of Cardiology Foundation/American Heart Association Task Force on practice guidelines. *Circulation.* 2013;**127**:529–55
20. Bernard SA, *et al.* Treatment of comatose survivors of out-of-hospital cardiac arrest with induced hypothermia. *N Engl J Med.* 2002;**346**:557–63

21. Mild therapeutic hypothermia to improve the neurologic outcome after cardiac arrest. *N Engl J Med.* 2002;**346**: 549–56
22. Steg PG, *et al.* ESC guidelines for the management of acute myocardial infarction in patients presenting with ST segment elevation. *Eur Heart J.* 2012;**33**:2569–619
23. Chen ZM, *et al.* Addition of clopidogrel to aspirin in 45,852 patients with acute myocardial infarction: randomised placebo-controlled trial. *Lancet.* 2005;**366**:1607–21
24. Charlot M, *et al.* Clopidogrel discontinuation after myocardial infarction and risk of thrombosis: a nationwide cohort study. *Eur Heart J.* 2012;**33**:2527–34
25. Andersson C, *et al.* Association of clopidogrel treatment with risk of mortality and cardiovascular events following myocardial infarction in patients with and without diabetes. *JAMA.* 2012;**308**:882–9
26. Cannon CP, *et al.* Comparison of ticagrelor with clopidogrel in patients with a planned invasive strategy for acute coronary syndromes (PLATO): a randomised double-blind study. *Lancet.* 2010;**375**:283–93
27. Montalescot G, *et al.* Prasugrel compared with clopidogrel in patients undergoing percutaneous coronary intervention for ST-elevation myocardial infarction (TRITON-TIMI 38): double-blind, randomised controlled trial. *Lancet.* 2009;**373**:723–31
28. Bellemain-Appaix A, *et al.* New P2Y12 inhibitors versus clopidogrel in percutaneous coronary intervention: a meta-analysis. *J Am Coll Cardiol.* 2010;**56**:1542–51
29. Murphy SA, *et al.* Efficacy and safety of the low-molecular weight heparin enoxaparin compared with unfractionated heparin across the acute coronary syndrome spectrum: a meta-analysis. *Eur Heart J.* 2007;**28**:2077–86
30. Montalescot G, *et al.* Intravenous enoxaparin or unfractionated heparin in primary percutaneous coronary intervention for ST-elevation myocardial infarction: the international randomised open-label ATOLL trial. *Lancet.* 2011;**378**:693–703
31. Stone GW, *et al.* Bivalirudin during primary PCI in acute myocardial infarction. *N Engl J Med.* 2008;**358**:2218–30
32. Yusuf S, *et al.* Effects of fondaparinux on mortality and reinfarction in patients with acute ST segment elevation myocardial infarction: the OASIS-6 randomized trial. *JAMA.* 2006;**295**:1519–30
33. Lincoff AM, *et al.* Mortality at 1 year with combination platelet glycoprotein IIb/IIIa inhibition and reduced-dose fibrinolytic therapy vs conventional fibrinolytic therapy for acute myocardial infarction: GUSTO v randomized trial. *JAMA.* 2002;**288**:2130–5
34. Montalescot G, *et al.* Abciximab in primary coronary stenting of ST-elevation myocardial infarction: a European meta-analysis on individual patients' data with long-term follow-up. *Eur Heart J.* 2007;**28**:443–9
35. Chen ZM, *et al.* Early intravenous then oral metoprolol in 45,852 patients with acute myocardial infarction: randomised placebo-controlled trial. *Lancet.* 2005;**366**:1622–32
36. Schjerning Olsen AM, *et al.* Duration of treatment with nonsteroidal anti-inflammatory drugs and impact on risk of death and recurrent myocardial infarction in patients with prior myocardial infarction: a nationwide cohort study. *Circulation.* 2011;**123**:2226–35
37. Keeley EC, *et al.* Primary angioplasty versus intravenous thrombolytic therapy for acute myocardial infarction: a quantitative review of 23 randomised trials. *Lancet.* 2003;**361**:13–20
38. Cannon CP, *et al.* Relationship of symptom-onset-to-balloon time and door-to-balloon time with mortality in patients undergoing angioplasty for acute myocardial infarction. *JAMA.* 2000;**283**:2941–7
39. Pinto DS, *et al.* Hospital delays in reperfusion for ST-elevation myocardial infarction: implications when selecting a reperfusion strategy. *Circulation.* 2006;**114**:2019–25
40. Boersma E. Does time matter? A pooled analysis of randomized clinical trials comparing primary percutaneous coronary intervention and in-hospital fibrinolysis in acute myocardial infarction patients. *Eur Heart J.* 2006;**27**:779–88
41. Busk M, *et al.* The Danish multicentre randomized study of fibrinolytic therapy vs. primary angioplasty in acute myocardial infarction (the DANAMI-2 trial): outcome after 3 years follow-up. *Eur Heart J.* 2008;**29**:1259–66
42. Armstrong PW, *et al.*, for the STREAM Investigative Team. Fibrinolysis or primary PCI in ST-segment elevation myocardial infarction. *N Engl J Med.* 2013; **368**:1379–87
43. Widimsky P, *et al.* Primary angioplasty in acute myocardial infarction with right bundle branch block: should new onset right bundle branch block be added to future guidelines as an indication for reperfusion therapy? *Eur Heart J.* 2012;**33**:86–95
44. Menon V, *et al.* Lack of benefit from percutaneous intervention of persistently occluded infarct arteries after the acute phase of myocardial infarction is time independent: insights from occluded artery trial. *Eur Heart J.* 2009;**30**:183–91
45. Claessen BE, *et al.* Prognostic impact of a chronic total occlusion in a non-infarct-related artery in patients with ST segment elevation myocardial infarction: 3-year results from the HORIZONS-AMI trial. *Eur Heart J.* 2012;**33**:768–75
46. De Luca G, *et al.* Benefits from small molecule administration as compared with abciximab among patients with ST segment elevation myocardial infarction treated with primary angioplasty: a meta-analysis. *J Am Coll Cardiol.* 2009;**53**:1668–73
47. Gu YL, *et al.* Intracoronary versus intravenous administration of abciximab in patients with ST segment elevation myocardial infarction undergoing primary percutaneous coronary intervention with thrombus aspiration: the comparison of intracoronary versus intravenous abciximab administration during emergency reperfusion of ST segment elevation myocardial infarction (CICERO) trial. *Circulation.* 2010;**122**:2709–17
48. Stone GW, *et al.* Intracoronary abciximab and aspiration thrombectomy in patients with large anterior myocardial infarction: the INFUSE-AMI randomized trial. *JAMA.* 2012;**307**:1817–26
49. Thiele H, *et al.* Intracoronary versus intravenous bolus abciximab during primary percutaneous coronary intervention in patients with acute ST-elevation myocardial infarction: a randomised trial. *Lancet.* 2012;**379**:923–31
50. Kastrati A, *et al.* Abciximab and heparin versus bivalirudin for non-ST-elevation myocardial infarction. *N Engl J Med.* 2011;**365**:1980–9

51. Noman A, *et al.* Impact of thrombus aspiration during primary percutaneous coronary intervention on mortality in ST segment elevation myocardial infarction. *Eur Heart J.* 2012;**33**:3054–61
52. Vlaar PJ, *et al.* Cardiac death and reinfarction after 1 year in the thrombus aspiration during percutaneous coronary intervention in acute myocardial infarction study (TAPAS): a 1-year follow-up study. *Lancet.* 2008;**371**:1915–20
53. TROFI Investigators. Randomized study to assess the effect of thrombus aspiration on flow area in patients with ST-elevation myocardial infarction: an optical frequency domain imaging study—TROFI trial. *Eur Heart J.* 2013;**34**:1050–60
54. Bavry AA, *et al.* Role of adjunctive thrombectomy and embolic protection devices in acute myocardial infarction: a comprehensive meta-analysis of randomized trials. *Eur Heart J.* 2008;**29**:2989–3001
55. Kastrati A, *et al.* Meta-analysis of randomized trials on drug-eluting stents vs. bare-metal stents in patients with acute myocardial infarction. *Eur Heart J.* 2007;**28**:2706–13
56. Toma M, *et al.* Non-culprit coronary artery percutaneous coronary intervention during acute ST segment elevation myocardial infarction: insights from the APEX-AMI trial. *Eur Heart J.* 2010;**31**:1701–7
57. Bangalore S, *et al.* Meta-analysis of multivessel coronary artery revascularization versus culprit-only revascularization in patients with ST segment elevation myocardial infarction and multivessel disease. *Am J Cardiol.* 2011;**107**:1300–10
58. Regitz-Zagrosek V, *et al.* ESC guidelines on the management of cardiovascular diseases during pregnancy: the Task Force on the management of cardiovascular diseases during pregnancy of the European Society of Cardiology (ESC). *Eur Heart J.* 2011;**32**:3147–97
59. Primary versus tenecteplase-facilitated percutaneous coronary intervention in patients with ST segment elevation acute myocardial infarction (ASSENT-4 PCI): randomised trial. *Lancet.* 2006;**367**:569–78
60. Ellis SG, *et al.* Facilitated PCI in patients with ST-elevation myocardial infarction. *N Engl J Med.* 2008;**358**:2205–17
61. Cantor WJ, *et al.* Routine early angioplasty after fibrinolysis for acute myocardial infarction. *N Engl J Med.* 2009;**360**:2705–18
62. Collet JP, *et al.* Percutaneous coronary intervention after fibrinolysis: a multiple meta-analyses approach according to the type of strategy. *J Am Coll Cardiol.* 2006;**48**:1326–35
63. D'Souza SP, *et al.* Routine early coronary angioplasty versus ischaemia-guided angioplasty after thrombolysis in acute ST-elevation myocardial infarction: a meta-analysis. *Eur Heart J.* 2011;**32**:972–82
64. Bueno H, *et al.* Primary angioplasty vs. fibrinolysis in very old patients with acute myocardial infarction: TRIANA (TRatamiento del Infarto Agudo de miocardio eN Ancianos) randomized trial and pooled analysis with previous studies. *Eur Heart J.* 2011;**32**:51–60
65. Steg PG, *et al.* Impact of time to treatment on mortality after prehospital fibrinolysis or primary angioplasty: data from the CAPTIM randomized clinical trial. *Circulation.* 2003;**108**:2851–56
66. Topol EJ, *et al.* Survival outcomes 1 year after reperfusion therapy with either alteplase or reteplase for acute myocardial infarction: results from the global utilization of streptokinase and t-PA for occluded coronary arteries (GUSTO) III trial. *Circulation.* 2000;**102**:1761–5
67. Van De Werf F, *et al.* Single-bolus tenecteplase compared with front-loaded alteplase in acute myocardial infarction: the ASSENT-2 double-blind randomised trial. *Lancet.* 1999;**354**:716–22
68. Simoons ML, *et al.* Individual risk assessment for intracranial haemorrhage during thrombolytic therapy. *Lancet.* 1993;**342**:1523–28
69. Gershlick AH, *et al.* Rescue angioplasty after failed thrombolytic therapy for acute myocardial infarction. *N Engl J Med.* 2005;**353**:2758–68
70. Wijeysundera HC, *et al.* Rescue angioplasty or repeat fibrinolysis after failed fibrinolytic therapy for ST segment myocardial infarction: a meta-analysis of randomized trials. *J Am Coll Cardiol.* 2007;**49**:422–30
71. van 't Hof AW, *et al.* Angiographic assessment of myocardial reperfusion in patients treated with primary angioplasty for acute myocardial infarction: Myocardial blush grade. Zwolle Myocardial Infarction Study Group. *Circulation.* 1998;**97**:2302–6
72. Di Mario C, *et al.* Immediate angioplasty versus standard therapy with rescue angioplasty after thrombolysis in the combined abciximab reteplase stent study in acute myocardial infarction (CARESS-IN-AMI): an open, prospective, randomised, multicentre trial. *Lancet.* 2008;**371**:559–68
73. Fernandez-Aviles F, *et al.* Routine invasive strategy within 24 hours of thrombolysis versus ischaemia-guided conservative approach for acute myocardial infarction with ST segment elevation (GRACIA-1): a randomised controlled trial. *Lancet.* 2004;**364**:1045–53
74. Hillis LD, *et al.* 2011 ACCF/AHA guideline for coronary artery bypass graft surgery: a report of the American College of Cardiology Foundation/American Heart Association Task Force on practice guidelines. *Circulation.* 2011;**124**:e652–35
75. Patel MR, *et al.* ACCF/SCAI/STS/AATS/AHA/ASNC/HFSA/SCCT 2012 appropriate use criteria for coronary revascularization focused update: a report of the American College of Cardiology Foundation Appropriate Use Criteria Task Force, Society for Cardiovascular Angiography and Interventions, Society of Thoracic Surgeons, American Association for Thoracic Surgery, American Heart Association, American Society of Nuclear Cardiology, and the Society of Cardiovascular Computed Tomography. *J Am Coll Cardiol.* 2012;**59**:857–81
76. Sjauw KD, *et al.* A systematic review and meta-analysis of intra-aortic balloon pump therapy in ST-elevation myocardial infarction: should we change the guidelines? *Eur Heart J.* 2009;**30**:459–68
77. Grosser TFS, *et al.* Drug resistance and pseudoresistance: An unintended consequence of enteric coating aspirin. *Circulation.* 2013;**127**:77–85
78. Lopez-Sendon J, *et al.* Factors related to heart rupture in acute coronary syndromes in the Global Registry of Acute Coronary Events. *Eur Heart J.* 2010;**31**:1449–56
79. Birnbaum Y, *et al.* Ventricular septal rupture after acute myocardial infarction. *N Engl J Med.* 2002;**347**:1426–32
80. Chatterjee S, *et al.* Association of blood transfusion with increased mortality in myocardial infarction: a meta-analysis and diversity-adjusted study sequential analysis. *JAMA Intern Med.* **2013;173**:132–9

81. Jabre P, *et al.* Mortality associated with atrial fibrillation in patients with myocardial infarction: a systematic review and meta-analysis. *Circulation.* 2011;**123**:1587–93
82. Jabre P, *et al.* Atrial fibrillation and death after myocardial infarction: a community study. *Circulation.* 2011;**123**:2094–100
83. Heidbuchel H, *et al.* Significance of arrhythmias during the first 24 hours of acute myocardial infarction treated with alteplase and effect of early administration of a beta blocker or a bradycardiac agent on their incidence. *Circulation.* 1994;**89**:1051–9
84. Cheema AN, *et al.* Nonsustained ventricular tachycardia in the setting of acute myocardial infarction: tachycardia characteristics and their prognostic implications. *Circulation.* 1998;**98**:2030–6
85. Nademanee K, *et al.* Treating electrical storm : sympathetic blockade versus advanced cardiac life support-guided therapy. *Circulation.* 2000;**102**:742–7
86. Bloch Thomsen PE, *et al.* Long-term recording of cardiac arrhythmias with an implantable cardiac monitor in patients with reduced ejection fraction after acute myocardial infarction: the Cardiac Arrhythmias and Risk Stratification After Acute Myocardial Infarction (CARISMA) study. *Circulation.* 2010;**122**:1258–64
87. Hofsten DE, *et al.* Prevalence and prognostic implications of non-sustained ventricular tachycardia in ST segment elevation myocardial infarction after revascularization with either fibrinolysis or primary angioplasty. *Eur Heart J.* 2007;**28**:407–14
88. Huikuri HV, *et al.* Prediction of sudden cardiac death after myocardial infarction in the beta-blocking era. *J Am Coll Cardiol.* 2003;**42**:652–8
89. Natale A, *et al.* Ventricular fibrillation and polymorphic ventricular tachycardia with critical coronary artery stenosis: does bypass surgery suffice? *J Cardiovasc Electrophysiol.* 1994;**5**:988–94
90. Brugada J, *et al.* Coronary artery revascularization in patients with sustained ventricular arrhythmias in the chronic phase of a myocardial infarction: effects on the electrophysiologic substrate and outcome. *J Am Coll Cardiol.* 2001;**37**:529–33
91. Pouleur AC, *et al.* Pathogenesis of sudden unexpected death in a clinical trial of patients with myocardial infarction and left ventricular dysfunction, heart failure, or both. *Circulation.* 2010;**122**:597–602
92. Hohnloser SH, *et al.* Prophylactic use of an implantable cardioverter-defibrillator after acute myocardial infarction. *N Engl J Med.* 2004;**351**:2481–8
93. Steinbeck G, *et al.* Defibrillator implantation early after myocardial infarction. *N Engl J Med.* 2009;**361**:1427–36
94. Kumar S, *et al.* Electrophysiology-guided defibrillator implantation early after ST-elevation myocardial infarction. *Heart Rhythm.* 2010;**7**:1589–97
95. Gang UJ, *et al.* High-degree atrioventricular block complicating ST segment elevation myocardial infarction in the era of primary percutaneous coronary intervention. *Europace.* 2012;**14**:1639–45
96. Strauss DG *et al.* Right, but not left, bundle branch block is associated with large anteroseptal scar online first. *J Am Coll Cardiol.* 2013: doi:10.1016/j.jacc.2013.1004.1060.
97. Newby LK, *et al.* Cost effectiveness of early discharge after uncomplicated acute myocardial infarction. *N Engl J Med.* 2000;**342**:749–55
98. Scirica BM, *et al.* Vorapaxar for secondary prevention of thrombotic events for patients with previous myocardial infarction: a prespecified subgroup analysis of the TRA 2 degrees P-TIMI 50 trial. *Lancet.* 2012;**380**:1317–24
99. Dagenais GR, *et al.* Angiotensin-converting-enzyme inhibitors in stable vascular disease without left ventricular systolic dysfunction or heart failure: a combined analysis of three trials. *Lancet.* 2006;**368**:581–8
100. Pfeffer MA, *et al.* Valsartan, captopril, or both in myocardial infarction complicated by heart failure, left ventricular dysfunction, or both. *N Engl J Med.* 2003;**349**:1893–906
101. Pitt B, *et al.* Eplerenone reduces mortality 30 days after randomization following acute myocardial infarction in patients with left ventricular systolic dysfunction and heart failure. *J Am Coll Cardiol.* 2005;**46**:425–31
102. MRC/BHF heart protection study of cholesterol lowering with simvastatin in 20,536 high-risk individuals: a randomised placebo-controlled trial. *Lancet.* 2002;**360**:7–22
103. Ong HT. Beta blockers in hypertension and cardiovascular disease. *BMJ.* 2007;**334**:946–9
104. Bangalore S, *et al.* Beta blocker use and clinical outcomes in stable outpatients with and without coronary artery disease. *JAMA.* 2012;**308**:1340–9
105. Mega JL, *et al.* Rivaroxaban in patients with a recent acute coronary syndrome. *N Engl J Med.* 2012;**366**:9–19
106. Lamas GA, *et al.* Randomized comparison of high-dose oral vitamins versus placebo in the trial to assess chelation therapy (TACT). *ACC.* 2013.
107. Jeevanantham V, *et al.* Adult bone marrow cell therapy improves survival and induces long-term improvement in cardiac parameters: a systematic review and meta-analysis. *Circulation.* 2012;**126**:551–68

Chapter 29

Stable coronary artery disease

Definition

Stable coronary artery disease is a non-acute condition due to coronary artery atherosclerosis and is diagnosed following a diagnostic ischaemia test or an acute coronary syndrome.

Presentation

Patients with coronary artery disease (CAD) may be asymptomatic or present with angina pectoris or an acute coronary syndrome (unstable angina or MI), congestive heart failure, cardiac arrhythmias, or sudden death. **Angina pectoris** is characterized by substernal discomfort, heaviness, or a pressure-like feeling, which may radiate to the jaw, shoulder, back, or arm. It does not resemble localized, stabbing pain. These symptoms are usually brought on by exertion, emotional stress, cold, or a heavy meal and are relieved by rest or nitrates (Table 29.1). Angina equivalents are shortness of breath on exertion (SOBOE), epigastric discomfort, fatigue, or faintness, particularly in elderly patients. Pain that is stabbing, positional, or reproducible with palpation is usually non-cardiac.

Table 29.1 Grading of angina pectoris by the Canadian Cardiovascular Society classification system

Class I
Ordinary physical activity does not cause angina, such as walking, climbing stairs. Angina (occurs) with strenuous, rapid, or prolonged exertion at work or recreation.
Class II
Slight limitation of ordinary activity. Angina occurs on walking or climbing stairs rapidly, walking uphill, walking or stair climbing after meals or in cold, in wind, or under emotional stress, or only during the few hours after awakening. Angina occurs on walking more than two blocks on the level and climbing more than one flight of ordinary stairs at a normal pace and in normal condition.
Class III
Marked limitations of ordinary physical activity. Angina occurs on walking one to two blocks on the level and climbing one flight of stairs in normal conditions and at a normal pace.
Class IV
Inability to carry on any physical activity without discomfort—anginal symptoms may be present at rest.

Campeau L. The Canadian Cardiovascular Society grading of angina pectoris revisited 30 years later. *Can J Cardiol.* 2002;**18:**371–9.

Physical examination

May be unremarkable. Hypertension, xanthelasma, decreased peripheral pulses, carotid or renal artery bruits, and abdominal aortic aneurysm may be present. **History** may reveal smoking, diabetes, or family history of MI before age of 60 years.

Cardiac auscultation may reveal S_3 or S_4 or MR, particularly during an episode of chest pain (LV or papillary muscle dysfunction).

Crepitations over the lung bases in ischaemic heart failure.

Investigations

Basic biochemistry are essential (**FBC, lipids, glucose, creatinine, markers of myocardial damage** as well as **thyroid function tests** and **oral glucose tolerance test** if clinically indicated).

Diagnostic tests for the detection of myocardial ischaemia are most useful in patients with an intermediate pretest probability of CAD (Bayes theorem) and are recommended for all patients with an intermediate or high probability of CAD (Table 29.2, Figure 29.1). Sensitivity and specificity data of used tests are presented in Table 29.3. In patients in whom intervention is contemplated, stress echocardiography or perfusion imaging are indicated.

12-lead resting ECG is essential.[1,2] It is normal in approximately half of patients with stable angina, even with severe CAD. ST-T wave changes, Q waves, LV hypertrophy, LBBB, AV block, AF, and ventricular arrhythmias may be present and are associated with worse prognosis. During an episode of angina pectoris, 50% of patients with normal findings on resting electrocardiography develop ECG abnormalities, usually ST-T depression.

Chest X-ray is indicated in suspected heart failure, valvular heart disease, pericardial disease or aortic dissection/aneurysm, or clinical evidence of pulmonary disease.

Echocardiography LV function is the major predictor of long-term survival in patients with CAD, and LVESD is the best predictor of survival after MI. MR or other concomitant abnormalities may be seen (Table 29.4). Correspondence of LV segments with coronary arteries is presented in Figure 29.2.

Exercise treadmill test is indicated in all patients with angina or intermediate pretest probability of CAD (Tables 29.4

Table 29.2 ACCF/AHA 2012 GL on stable CAD. Pretest likelihood of coronary artery disease in symptomatic patients according to age and sex

	Non-anginal chest pain		Atypical angina		Typical angina	
Age (y)	Men	Women	Men	Women	Men	Women
30–39	4	2	34	12	76	26
40–49	13	3	51	22	87	55
50–59	20	7	65	31	93	73
60–69	27	14	72	51	94	86

2012 ACCF/AHA/ACP/AATS/PCNA/SCAI/STS Guideline for the diagnosis and management of patients with stable ischemic heart disease. *J Am Coll Cardiol.* 2012;**60**:e44–e164.

Risk factor	Score contribution	Individual's score
Comorbidity		
No	0	
Yes	86	
Diabetes		
No	0	
Yes	57	
Angina score		
Class I	0	
Class II	54	
Class III	91	
Duration of symptoms		
≥6 months	0	
<6 months	80	
Abnormal ventricular function		
No	0	
Yes	114	
ST depression or T wave inversion on resting electrocardiogram		
No	0	
Yes	34	
	Total =	

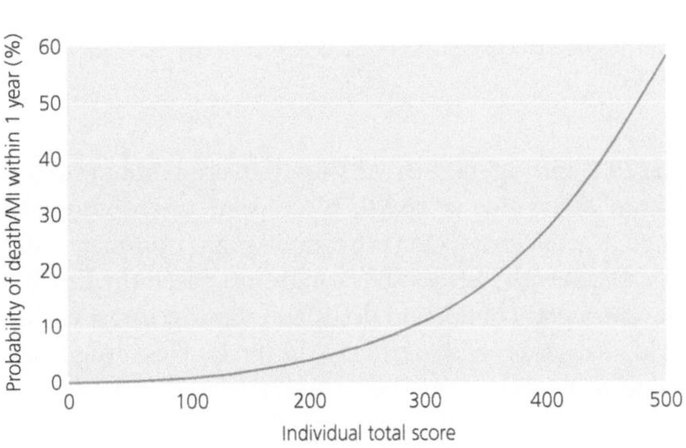

Figure 29.1 Left panel: Euro Heart score sheet to calculate risk score for patients presenting with stable angina (derived from 3779 patients with newly diagnosed SIHD).

* ≥1 of previous cerebrovascular event; hepatic disease defined as chronic hepatitis or cirrhosis or other hepatic disease causing elevation of transaminases ≥3 times upper limit of normal; PVD defined as claudication either at rest or on exertion, amputation for arterial vascular insufficiency, vascular surgery (reconstruction or bypass) or angioplasty to the extremities, documented aortic aneurysm, or non-invasive evidence of impaired arterial flow; chronic renal failure defined as chronic dialysis or renal transplantation or serum creatinine >200 mmol/L; chronic respiratory disease defined as a diagnosis previously made by physician or patient receiving bronchodilators or FEV_1 <75%, arterial pO_2 <60%, or arterial pCO_2 >50% predicted in previous studies; chronic inflammatory conditions defined as a diagnosis of rheumatoid arthritis, systemic lupus erythematosus or other connective tissue disease, polymyalgia rheumatica, and so on; malignancy defined as a diagnosis of malignancy within a year of active malignancy.

Right panel: risk of death or MI over 1 year after diagnosis of SIHD, according to Euro Heart score.

Plot to assign estimated probability of death or non-fatal MI within 1 year of presentation, according to a combination of clinical and investigative features in patients with stable angina.

MI indicates myocardial infacrtion; FEV_1, forced expiratory volume; pO_2, partial pressure of oxygen; pCO_2, partial pressure of carbon dioxide; and PVD, peripheral vascular disease.

Daly CA, *et al.* Predicting prognosis in stable angina—results from the Euro heart survey of stable angina:prospective observational study. *BMJ.* 2006;**332**:262–7.

Table 29.3 Sensitivity and specificity of non-invasive stress tests for the diagnosis of coronary artery disease

	Sensitivity (%)	Specificity (%)
Exercise electrocardiography	68	77
Exercise echocardiography	85	81
Dobutamine echocardiography	82	84
Exercise SPECT	87	73
Adenosine SPECT	89	75
Dobutamine magnetic resonance imaging	89	84
Adenosine magnetic resonance imaging	84	85
Adenosine PET	89	86

and 29.5, and Figure 29.3). All stress tests are contraindicated within 2 days after acute MI, in severe AS, and decompensated heart failure. Exercise treadmill test is non-diagnostic in patients with LBBB, WPW syndrome, paced rhythm, intraventricular conduction delay, and digoxin therapy. Due to low sensitivity and specificity, the test is of less prognostic value in low-risk populations, such as women. However, exercise testing is still the initial diagnostic strategy in symptomatic women with suspected CAD.[3] The use of myocardial perfusion imaging in this clinical setting should be reserved for those with abnormal, equivocal, or non-diagnostic studies.

The **Duke treadmill score** incorporates exercise capacity, ST segment deviation, and angina as major risk determinants. The score is calculated using the following formula:

Exercise time in minutes – (5 × the maximum ST segment deviation in millimetres) – (4 × the angina index [0, no pain; 1, angina; and 2, angina that caused discontinuation of the test]).

Low risk (≥5%) indicates a 97% 5-year survival, moderate risk (–10 to 4) 91%, and high risk (≤–11) 72% survival. Other risk factor determinants include extensive and prolonged ST segment depression, transient ST segment elevation, abnormal heart rate recovery, and delayed systolic blood pressure response to exercise. Stress test-induced ST elevation in lead aVR is highly suggestive of left main or ostial LAD disease.[4] The **exercise stress test is terminated** for one of the following reasons:[1]

Table 29.4 Echocardiography is stable CAD

ACCF/AHA 2013 GL on stable CAD. Resting imaging to assess cardiac structure and function	
Doppler echocardiography in patients with known or suspected IHD and a prior MI, pathological Q waves, symptoms or signs suggestive of heart failure, complex ventricular arrhythmias, or an undiagnosed heart murmur.	I-B
Echocardiography in hypertension or diabetes mellitus and abnormal ECG.	IIb-C
Measurement of LV function with radionuclide imaging in patients with a prior MI or pathological Q waves, provided there is no need to evaluate symptoms or signs suggestiveof heart failure, complex ventricular arrhythmias, or an undiagnosed heart murmur.	IIb-C
Echocardiography, radionuclide imaging, CMR, and cardiac computed tomography are not recommended for routine assessment of LV function in patients with a normal ECG, no history of MI, no symptoms or signs suggestive of heart failure, and no complex ventricular arrhythmias.	III-C
Routine reassessment (<1 year) of LV function with echocardiography, radionuclide imaging, CMR, or cardiac computed tomography in patients with no change in clinical status and for whom no change in therapy is contemplated.	III-C
ESC 2006 GL on stable CAD. recommendations for echocardiography for initial diagnostic assessment of angina	
Patients with abnormal auscultation, suggesting valvular heart disease or HCM.	I-B
Patients with suspected heart failure.	I-B
Patients with prior MI.	I-B
Patients with LBBB, Q waves, or other significant pathological changes on ECG, including ECG LVH (level of evidence C).	I-C

2012 ACCF/AHA/ACP/AATS/PCNA/SCAI/STS Guideline for the diagnosis and management of patients with stable ischemic heart disease. *J Am Coll Cardiol*. 2012;**60**:e44–e164.
Guidelines on the management of stable angina pectoris: executive summary: the Task Force on the management of stable angina pectoris of the European Society of Cardiology. *Eur Heart J*. 2006;**27**:1341–81.

- Symptom limitation, e.g. pain, fatigue, dyspnoea, and claudication
- Combination of symptoms, such as pain with significant ST changes
- Marked ST depression (>2 mm ST depression can be taken as a relative indication for termination and >4 mm as an absolute indication to stop the test)
- ST elevation ≥1 mm
- Significant arrhythmia
- Sustained fall in systolic blood pressure >10 mmHg
- Marked hypertension (>250 mmHg systolic or >115 mmHg diastolic)
- Achievement of maximum predicted heart rate.

Stress echocardiography The most popular test is dobutamine stress echocardiography (DSE) which is more

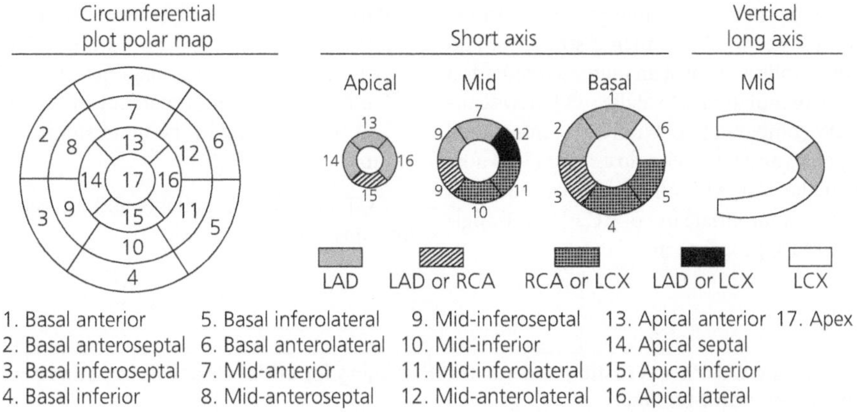

Figure 29.2 Correspondence of left ventricular 17 myocardial segments with each coronary artery.
Pereztol-Valdés O, *et al.* Correspondence between left ventricular 17 myocardial segments and coronary arteries. *Eur Heart J.* 2005;**26**:2637–43

specific but less sensitive, than perfusion imaging for detection of ischaemia. Both ischaemia and myocardial viability can be assessed. Life-threatening events, mainly ventricular arrhythmias, are rare (0.01%),[5] and the prognostic significance of induced VT remains uncertain. The diagnostic accuracy of DSE is reduced in patients with poor acoustic window (obese, COPD), severe LV dysfunction, prior cardiac surgery, and severe hypertension (Table 29.5).

Myocardial perfusion tests Exercise myocardial perfusion is assessed with single photon emission tomography (SPECT) (Table 29.5). Technetium or thallium (better for detection of myocardial viabilty) are used, and there is a relatively good correlation of standardized left ventricular segments with each coronary artery.[6] Adenosine or dipyridamole nuclear perfusion imaging is the preferred test for patients with LBBB or ventricular paced rhythm because of increased false positive findings with exercise or dobutamine echocardiography. In asthmatics, adenosine may cause bronchospasm and dipyridamole is preferred, unless the patient has significant hepatic impairment. Nuclear imaging exposes the patient to a moderate amount of ionizing radiation (approximately 15 mSv). Attenuation artefacts (obese patients and women with large breasts) decrease the specificity of nuclear testing. Global ischaemia (left main or severe multivessel disease) may also produce false negative results. Because higher myocyte fraction is needed to maintain contractile reserve than to achieve radiotracer uptake, nuclear imaging has higher sensitivity but lower specificity than dobutamine stress echocardiography in the detection of viability. However, the predictive accuracy of dobutamine stress echocardiography for functional recovery is higher than SPECT.[7] **Myocardial contrast echocardiography** is a new modality for assessment of myocardial perfusion.

Magnetic resonance imaging is a new stress imaging technique that may be used for both adenosine perfusion and dobutamine wall motion imaging.[8] It has high spatial and temporal resolution and, apart from ischaemia, identifies non-viable scar tissue, identifies myocarditis, and detects subendocardial ischaemia that may be missed by other tests. It can be performed in patients with stents and most orthopaedic implants. Patients with pacemakers and defibrillators may also undergo CMR under specific conditions and protocols. Following the intravenous administration of gadolinium, first-pass perfusion sequences can identify myocardial perfusion abnormalities. Low-dose dobutamine, or late gadolinium-enhancement protocols are used. Administration of gadolinium is contraindicated in patients with a creatinine clearance >30 mL/min due to the rare, but potentially life-threatening, complication of nephrogenic systemic fibrosis. MRI may show false positive defects related to transient dark rim artefacts in the subendocardium. If not properly recognized, such artefacts may limit the specificity of MRI perfusion imaging for detecting small subendocardial perfusion defects.[9]

Ambulatory ECG monitoring may also be useful in suspected arrhythmias (ESC 2006 I-B) or vasospastic angina (ESC 2006 IIa-C).

Coronary artery computed tomography (CCT) with multidetector scanners may visualize the coronary artery lumen and detect calcification (Table 29.5).[10] It is still limited by a high number of false positive results (up to 50% with severe calcification and coronary stents). Furthermore, its prognostic value as a substitute for conventional angiography has not been validated in clinical studies. In patients with acute chest pain, CT angiography in an experienced centre is faster to obtain than a stress test and improves diagnostic ability, albeit at an increased radiation exposure.[11,12] Doses of radiation get smaller with new scanners, i.e. 1.5–7 mSv compared to 6–7 mSv of conventional coronary angiography, and CCT with doses <1 mSv is now possible.[13] In 2010, the ACC and other American societies published criteria for appropriate use of CCT.[14] CCT angiography is considered appropriate in:

- Patients with low or intermediate risk or pretest probability for CAD and stable disease or acute syndromes or positive imaging tests
- For evaluation of graft patency in symptomatic patients and stenting only in the main stem and with stents >3 mm.

CCT in high-risk patients and for general screening is not considered appropriate.

Table 29.5 Investigations

ACCF/AHA 2012 on stable CAD. Stress testing and advanced imaging for initial diagnosis in patients with suspected SIHD who require non-invasive testing

Test	**Exercise status**		**ECG interpretable**		**Pretest probability of IHD**			**COR-LOE**
	Able	**Unable**	**Yes**	**No**	**Low**	**Intermediate**	**High**	
Patients able to exercise*								
Exercise ECG	X		X			X		I-A
Exercise with nuclear MPI or echo	X			X		X	X	I-B
Exercise ECG	X		X		X			IIa-C
Exercise with nuclear MPI or echo	X		X			X	X	IIa-B
Pharmacological stress CMR	X			X		X	X	IIa-B
CCTA	X		Any			X		IIb-B
Exercise echo	X		X			X		IIb-C
Pharmacological stress with nuclear MPI, echo, or CMR	X		X		Any			III-C (no benefit)
Exercise stress with nuclear MPI	X		X		X			III-C (no benefit)
Patients unable to exercise								
Pharmacological stress with nuclear MPI or echo		X	Any			X	X	I
Pharmacological stress echo		X	Any		X			IIa
CCTA		X	Any		X	X		IIa
Pharmacological stress CMR		X	Any			X	X	IIa
Exercise ECG		X		X	Any			III-C (no benefit)
Other								
CCTA	Any		Any			X		IIa-C
If patient has any of the following:								
a) Continued symptoms with prior normal test, or								
b) Inconclusive exercise or pharmacological stress, or								
c) Unable to undergo stress with MPI or echo								
CAC score	Any		Any		X			IIb-C

* Patients are candidates for exercise testing if they are capable of performing at least moderate physical functioning (i.e. moderate household, yard, or recreational work **and** most activities of daily living) and have no disabling co-morbidity. Patients should be able to achieve 85% of age-predicted maximum heart rate.

CAC indicates coronary artery calcium; CCTA, cardiac computed tomography angiography; CMR, cardiac magnetic resonance imaging; COR, class of recommendation; ECG, electrocardiogram; echo, echocardiography; IHD, ischaemic heart disease; LOE, level of evidence; MPI, myocardial perfusion imaging; N/A, not available; and SIHD, stable ischaemic heart disease.

2012 ACCF/AHA/ACP/AATS/PCNA/SCAI/STS Guideline for the diagnosis and management of patients with stable ischemic heart disease. *J Am Coll Cardiol.* 2012;**60**:e44–e164.

Table 29.5 (Continued)

ACCF/AHA 2012 GL on stable CAD. Stress testing and advanced imaging for initial diagnosis in patients with suspected SIHD who require non-invasive testing

Test	Exercise status		ECG interpretable		COR-LOE	Additional considerations
	Able	Unable	Yes	No		
Patients able to exercise*						
Exercise ECG	X		X		I-B	
Exercise with nuclear MPI or echo	X			X	I-B	Abnormalities other than LBBB or ventricular pacing
Exercise with nuclear MPI or echo	X		X		IIa-B	
Pharmacological stress CMR	X			X	IIa-B	
CCTA	X			X	IIb-B	
Pharmacological stress imaging (nuclear MPI, echo, CMR) or CCTA	X		X		III-C (no benefit)	
Patients unable to exercise						
Pharmacological stress with nuclear MPI or echo		X	Any		I-B	
Pharmacological stress CMR		X	Any		IIa-B	
CCTA		X	Any		IIa-C	Without prior stress test
Regardless of patient's ability to exercise						
Pharmacological stress with nuclear MPI or echo	Any			X	I-B	LBBB present
Exercise/pharmacological stress with nuclear MPI, echo, or CMR	Any		Any		I-B	Known coronary stenosis of unclear physiological significance being considered for revascularization
CCTA	Any		Any		IIa-C	Indeterminate result from functional testing
CCTA	Any		Any		IIb-C	Unable to undergo stress imaging or as alternative to coronary catheterization when functional testing indicates moderate to high risk and angiographic coronary anatomy is unknown
Requests to perform multiple cardiac imaging or stress studies at the same time	Any		Any		III-C (no benefit)	

* Patients are candidates for exercise testing if they are capable of performing at least moderate physical functioning (i.e. moderate household, yard, or recreational work **and** most activities of daily living) and have no disabling co-morbidity. Patients should be able to achieve 85% of age-predicted maximum heart rate.

CCTA indicates cardiac computed tomography angiography; CMR, cardiac magnetic resonance imaging; COR, class of recommendation; ECG, electrocardiogram; echo, echocardiography; LBBB, left bundle branch block; LOE, level of evidence; MPI, myocardial perfusion imaging; and N/A, not available.

2012 ACCF/AHA/ACP/AATS/PCNA/SCAI/STS Guideline for the diagnosis and management of patients with stable ischemic heart disease. *J Am Coll Cardiol.*2012;**60**:e44–e164.

ESC 2006 GL on stable CAD. Recommendations for exercise ECG for initial diagnostic assessment of angina

Patients with angina and intermediate pretest probability of coronary disease, based on age, gender, and symptoms, unless unable to exercise or displays ECG changes which make ECG non-evaluable.	I-B
Patients with ≥1 mm ST depression on resting ECG or taking digoxin.	IIb-B
Patients with low pretest probability (<10% probability) of coronary disease, based on age, gender, and symptoms.	IIb-B

ESC Guidelines on the management of stable angina pectoris: executive summary: The Task Force on the Management of Stable Angina Pectoris of the European Society of Cardiology. *Eur Heart J.* 2006;**27**:1341–81.

(Continued)

Table 29.5 (Continued)

ESC 2010 GL on revascularization. Indications of different imaging tests for the diagnosis of obstructive coronary artery disease and for the assessment of prognosis in subjects without known coronary artery disease[a]

	Asymptomatic (screening)	Symptomatic			Prognostic value of positive result[a]	Prognostic value of negative result[a]
		Pretest likelihood[b] of obstructive disease				
		Low	Intermediate	High		
Anatomical test						
Invasive angiography	III-A	III-A	IIb-A	I-A	I-A	I-A
MDCT angiography	III-B[c]	IIb-B	IIa-B	III-B	IIb-B	IIa-B
MRI angiography	III-B	III-B	III-B	III-B	III-C	III-C
Functional test						
Stress echo	III A	III A	I A	III A[d]	I A	I A
Nuclear imaging	III A	III A	I A	III A[d]	I A	I A
Stress MRI	III B	III C	IIa B	III B[d]	IIa B	IIa B
PET perfusion	III B	III C	IIa B	III B[d]	IIa B	IIa B

[a] For the prognostic assessment of known coronary stenosis, functional imaging is similarly indicated.
[b] The pretest likelihood of disease is calculated based on symptoms, sex, and risk factors.
[c] This refers to MDCT angiography, not calcium scoring.
[d] In patients with obstructive CAD documented by angiography, functional testing may be useful in guiding the revascularization strategy, based on the extent, severity, and localization of ischaemia.
CAD, coronary artery disease; MDCT, multidetector computed tomography; MRI, magnetic resonance imaging; PET, positron emission tomography.
ESC/EACTS Guidelines on myocardial revascularization The Task Force on Myocardial Revascularization of the European Society of Cardiology (ESC) and the European Association for Cardio-Thoracic Surgery (EACTS). *European Heart Journal* 2010;**31**:2501–2555.

The detection of **coronary artery calcium** has prognostic significance,[15] and a calcium scoring system has been devised, based on the X-ray attenuation coefficient or CT number measured in Hounsfield units and the area of calcium deposits.[16] An Agatston score <100 indicates low risk and a score >300 high risk, and, in the MESA (Multi-Ethnic Study of Atherosclerosis) trial, addition of calcium score to traditional risk factors, such as blood pressure, smoking, and hypercholesterolaemia, improves classification of risk as estimated by the Framingham risk calculation (http://www.mesa-nhlbi.org). [15] Coronary artery calcification is also an independent stroke predictor in subjects at low or intermediate vascular risk.[17] However, in the recent CONFIRM trial, a score of 0 did not rule out the presence of significant coronary disease, and, in intermediate-risk populations, calcium score did not add incremental prognostic information to that provided by clinical risk factors and the severity of CAD.[18] Its presence does not, by itself, justify coronary angiography.[19]

Positron emission tomography stress has high sensitivity for detection of ischaemia and myocardial viability and perhaps characterization of atherosclerotic plaques. Disadvantages are the high cost and lack of clinical verification studies for its prognostic ability.

Coronary angiography is indicated for diagnostic purposes (Table 29.6) in patients with:

- Significant angina
- High-risk clinical characteristics or non-invasive testing criteria
- LV dysfunction (LVEF <45%) or CCF
- Aborted sudden death or VT/VF
- Inconclusive non-invasive testing
- Previous CABG or PCI with recurrent symptoms or at high risk of restenosis of a prognostically important site.

Serious complications of coronary angiography, such as death, MI or stroke, and aortic dissection or aortic valve avulsion, had been previously reported in the order of 0.1%[1] but are probably even less in modern catheter labs.

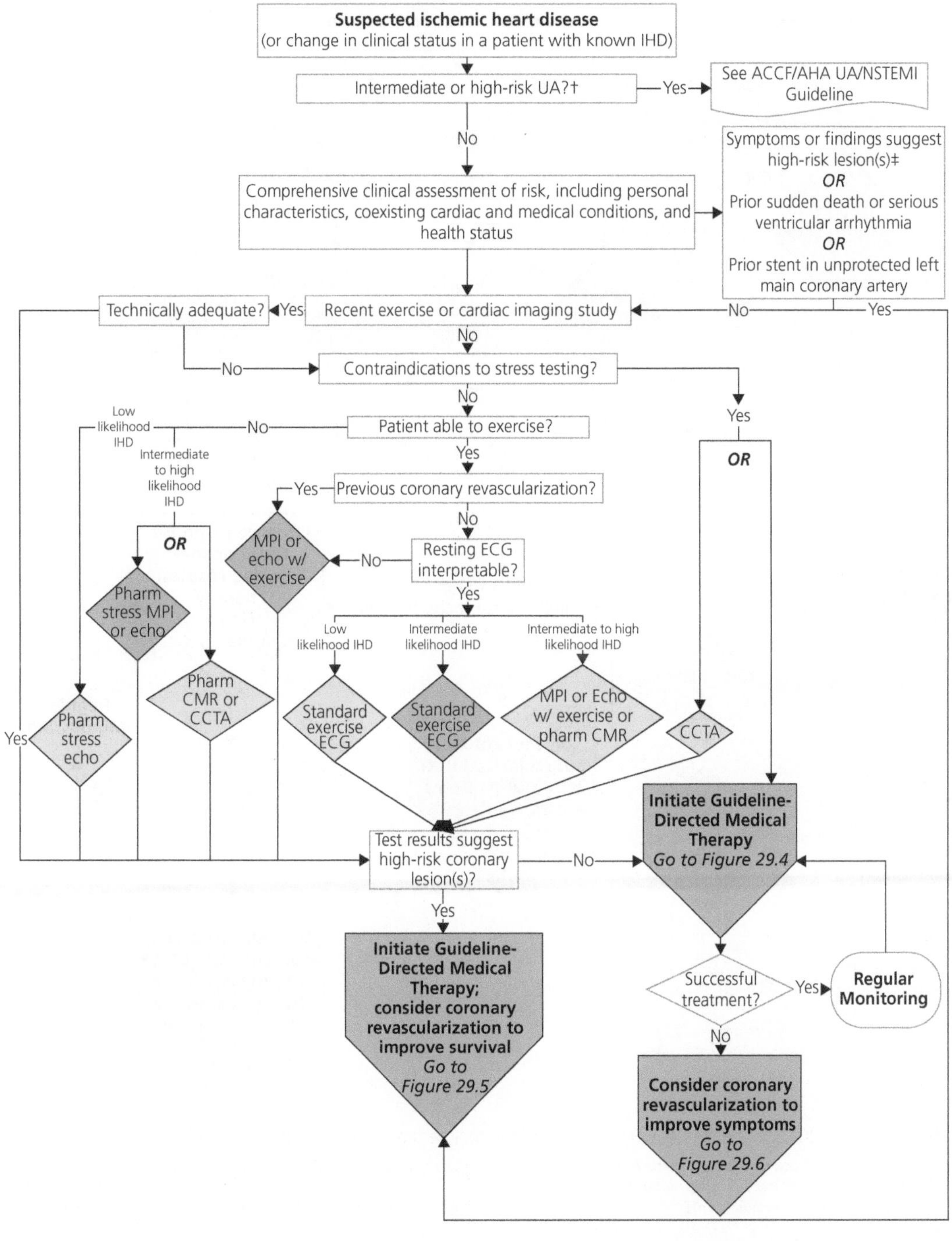

Figure 29.3a ACCF/AHA 2012 GL on Stable IHD. Diagnosis of Patients with Suspected IHD.

*: Colors correspond to the class of recommendations in the ACCF/AHA (ie green is for Class I, yellow for IIa). The algorithms do not represent a comprehensive list of recommendations (see full guideline text for all recommendations). †See Table 27.3 in UA/NSTEMI Chapter for short-term risk of death or nonfatal MI in patients with UA/NSTEMI.

‡CCTA is reasonable only for patients with intermediate probability of IHD. CCTA indicates computed coronary tomography angiography; CMR, cardiac magnetic resonance; ECG, electrocardiogram; Echo, echocardiography; IHD, ischaemic heart disease; MI, myocardial infarction; MPI, myocardial perfusion imaging; Pharm, pharmacological; UA, unstable angina; and UA/NSTEMI, unstable angina/non–ST elevation myocardial infarction.

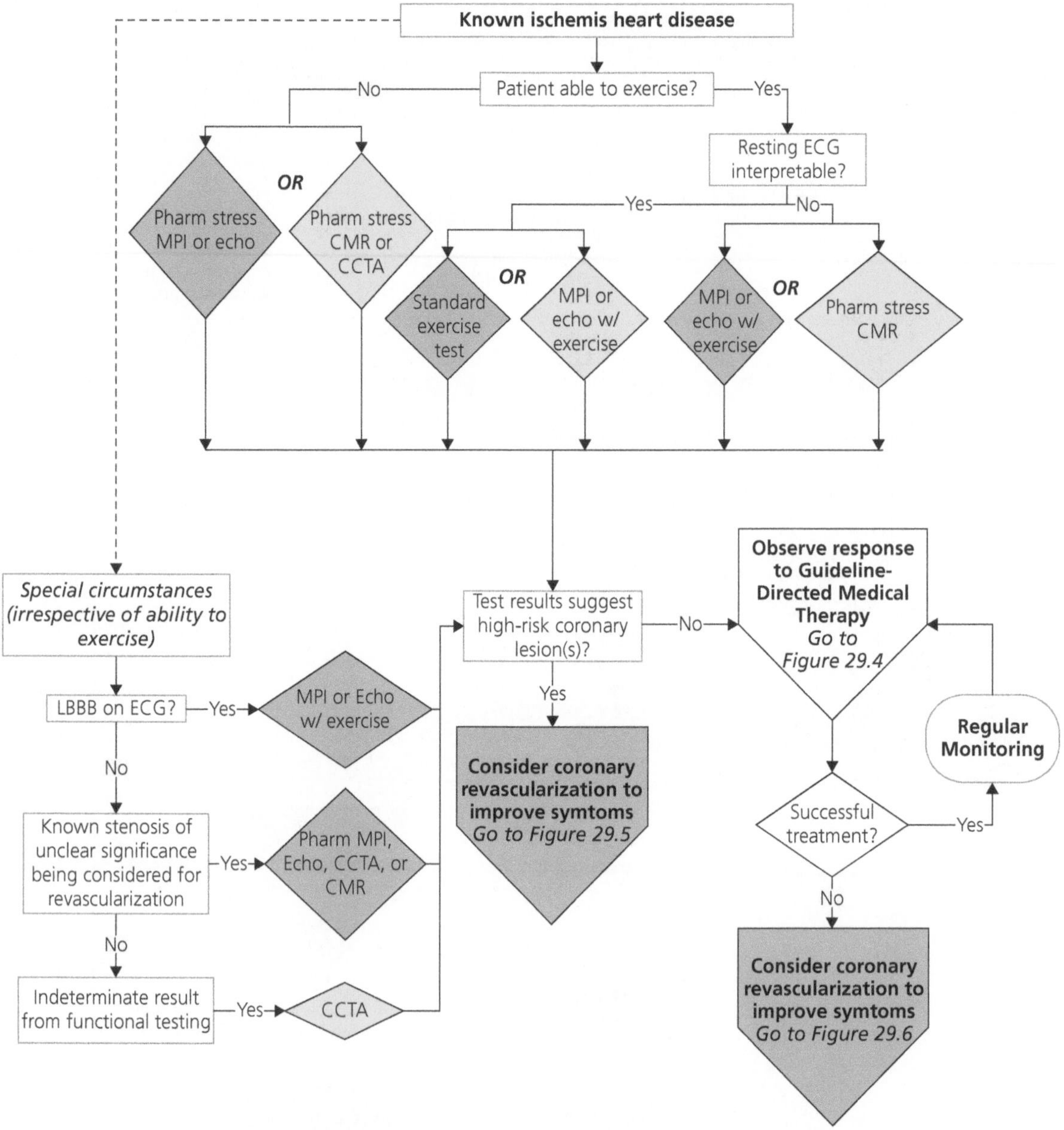

Figure 29.3b ACCF/AHA 2012 GL on stable IHD. Algorithm for risk assessment of patients with SIHD.*

* Colours correspond to the class of recommendations in the ACCF/AHA (ie green is for Class I, yellow for IIa). The algorithms do not represent a comprehensive list of recommendations (see full guideline text for all recommendations). CCTA indicates coronary computed tomography angiography; CMR, cardiac magnetic resonance; ECG, electrocardiogram; Echo, echocardiography; LBBB, left branch bundle block; MPI, myocardial perfusion imaging; and Pharm, pharmacological.

2012 ACCF/AHA/ACP/AATS/PCNA/SCAI/STS Guideline for the diagnosis and management of patients with stable ischemic heart disease. *J Am Coll Cardiol*. 2012;**60**:e44–e164.

Differential diagnosis

Cardiac causes of angina-like pain

Apart from epicardial coronary artery stenosis, other cardiac conditions that may cause myocardial ischaemia are:

- **Aortic stenosis, hypertension** and **LV hypertrophy** (reduced coronary blood flow)
- **Microvascular coronary dysfunction.** It has been attributed to endothelial dysfunction and carries adverse prognosis. More common in women (WISE study)[20]
- **Abnormal cardiac nociception.** Increased perception of pain centrally mediated or due to changed sensitivity of chemical and mechanical atrial and ventricular receptors
- **Coronary artery *spasm*** (smooth muscle dysregulation probably due to inflammation)
- **Congenital coronary abnormalities** Myocardial bridging involves a segment of a coronary artery, usually the LAD, embedded within the myocardium in a way that arterial compression occurs with systole.[21] With intense symptoms and documented ischaemia, CABG may be required. The value of stenting is debated. Fistulas, anomalous origins of coronary arteries, compression by the PA, as may happen with ASD, are other relevant anomalies (see Chapter 2).
- **Syndrome X** refers to exercise-induced angina-like symptoms in the context of ischaemic changes on treadmill stress testing and normal coronary arteries on angiography.[22] The exact cause is not known, but microvascular disease and endothelial dysfunction due to inflammation, hypercholesterolaemia, smoking, and obesity have been proposed. Insulin resistance, hormonal dysfunction, and psychological factors may also play a role. Microvascular coronary dysfunction is highly prevalent and associated with an adverse prognosis.[23] Coronary reactivity testing may be helpful in establishing the diagnosis of coronary spasm, microvascular dysfunction, or abnormal cardiac nociception. The test involves passing a Doppler flow wire into the coronary artery and assessing flow after injecting vasoactive agents that provoke spasm, such as acetylcholine (intracoronary incremental doses of 20–100 micrograms to the left and 20–50 micrograms to the right coronary artery over a period of 20 s) and ergonovine (20–60 micrograms to the left and 20–60 micrograms to RCA over a period of 2–5 min), or vasodilators, such as adenosine (150 micrograms/kg/min) and nitrates (Table 29.7). Provocations tests are considered safe, with an incidence of VT/VF or bradyarrhythmias of 3%.[24] Adenosine stress perfusion using MRI is also a promising modality for the detection of transmural coronary flow distribution (endocardial less than epicardial) due to microvascular coronary dysfunction.[23]
- **Prinzmetal's angina** refers to chest pain at rest, associated with ST elevation, and was thought to be due to coronary artery spasm (Table 29.7).

Table 29.6 Coronary angiography in patients with stable IHD

ACCF/AHA 2012 GL on stable CAD. Coronary angiography as an initial testing strategy to assess risk	
To assess cardiac risk in patients who have survived sudden cardiac death or potentially life-threatening ventricular arrhythmia.	I-B
Patients who develop symptoms and signs of heart failure should be evaluated to determine whether coronary angiography should be performed for risk assessment.	I-B
ACCF/AHA 2012 GL on stable CAD. Coronary angiography to assess risk after initial work-up with non-invasive testing	
Coronary arteriography is recommended for patients whose clinical characteristics and results of non-invasive testing indicate a high likelihood of severe IHD and when the benefits are deemed to exceed risk.	I-C
Patients with LVEF <50% and moderate risk criteria on non-invasive testing with demonstrable ischaemia.	IIa-C
Inconclusive prognostic information after non-invasive testing or non-invasive testing is contraindicated or inadequate.	IIa-C
Unsatisfactory quality of life due to angina, LVEF >50%, and intermediate-risk criteria on non-invasive testing.	IIa-C
Patients who elect not to undergo revascularization or who are not candidates for revascularization because of co-morbidities or individual preferences.	III-B
LVEF >50% and low-risk criteria on non-invasive testing.	III-B
Low risk according to clinical criteria and no non-invasive risk testing.	III-C
Asymptomatic patients with no evidence of ischaemia on non-invasive testing.	III-C
ESC 2006 GL on stable CAD. Recommendations for coronary arteriography for the purposes of establishing a diagnosis in stable angina	
Severe stable angina (≥Class 3 of CCS classification), with a high pretest probability of disease, particularly if the symptoms are inadequately responding to medical treatment.	I-B
Survivors of cardiac arrest.	I-B
Patients with serious ventricular arrhythmias.	I-C
Patients previously treated by myocardial revascularization (PCI, CABG) who develop early recurrence of moderate or severe angina pectoris.	I-C
Patients with an inconclusive diagnosis on non-invasive testing or conflicting results from different non-invasive modalities at intermediate to high risk of coronary disease.	IIa-C
Patients with a high risk of restenosis after PCI if PCI has been performed in a prognostically important site.	IIa-C

2012 ACCF/AHA/ACP/AATS/PCNA/SCAI/STS Guideline for the diagnosis and management of patients with stable ischemic heart disease. *J Am Coll Cardiol*. 2012;**60**:e44–e164.

Guidelines on the management of stable angina pectoris: executive summary: the Task Force on the management of stable angina pectoris of the European Society of Cardiology. *Eur Heart J*. 2006;**27**:1341–81.

Table 29.7 Syndrome X

ACCF/AHA 2012 GL on UA/NSTEMI. Cardiovascular 'syndrome X'	
Nitrates, beta blockers, and calcium channel blockers, alone or in combination.	I-B
Risk factor reduction.	I-B
Intracoronary ultrasound to assess the extent of atherosclerosis and rule out missed obstructive lesions.	IIb-B
Coronary angiography and provocative testing with acetylcholine, adenosine, or methacholine and 24 h ambulatory ECG.	IIb-C
Invasive physiological assessment (i.e. coronary flow reserve measurement) if coronary angiography does not reveal a cause of chest discomfort.	IIb-C
Imipramine or aminophylline for continued pain despite implementation of Class I measures.	IIb-C
Transcutaneous electrical nerve stimulation and spinal cord stimulation for continued pain, despite the implementation of Class I measures may be considered for patients with syndrome X.	IIb-B
Medical therapy with nitrates, beta blockers, and calcium channel blockers for patients with non-cardiac chest pain is not recommended.	III-C
ESC 2006 GL on stable CAD. Recommendations for investigation in patients with classical triad of syndrome X	
Resting echocardiogram to assess for ventricular hypertrophy and/or diastolic dysfunction.	I-C
Intracoronary acetylcholine during coronary arteriography to assess endothelium-dependent coronary flow reserve and exclude vasospasm.	IIb-C
Intracoronary ultrasound, coronary flow reserve, or FFR measurement to exclude suspected obstructive lesions (suspicious angiographic appearances or stress imaging).	IIb-C
ESC 2006 GL on stable CAD. Recommendations for diagnostic tests in suspected vasospastic angina	
ECG during angina if possible.	I-B
Coronary arteriography in patients with characteristic episodic chest pain and ST segment changes that resolve with nitrates and/or calcium antagonists to determine the extent of underlying coronary disease (level of evidence B).	I-B
Intracoronary provocative testing to identify coronary spasm in patients with clinical picture of coronary spasm.	IIa-B
Ambulatory ST segment monitoring to identify ST deviation.	IIa-C

2012 ACCF/AHA/ACP/AATS/PCNA/SCAI/STS Guideline for the diagnosis and management of patients with stable ischemic heart disease. *J Am Coll Cardiol*. 2012;**60**:e44–e164.
Guidelines on the management of stable angina pectoris: executive summary: the Task Force on the management of stable angina pectoris of the European Society of Cardiology. *Eur Heart J*. 2006;**27**:1341–81.

Non-cardiac causes of angina-like pain

- **Oesophageal reflux**, oesophagitis, and abnormal oesophageal motility have similar distribution with cardiac pain but are not related to exercise. These findings are common in patients, presenting with chest pain, but not necessarily the causative factor.
- **Duodenal ulcer** and **gall bladder pain.**
- **Pericardial pain.** Retrosternal or epigastric, precipitated by inspiration and relieved by sitting forward. May radiate to left shoulder.
- **Aortic dissection.** Tearing pain radiating to the back. Aortic aneurysms may also produce chronic pain.
- **Costochondritis.** Tenderness on palpation.
- **Pulmonary embolism** is usually associated with sudden onset of shortness of breath rather than pain.

A full list of conditions that may cause chest pain are presented in Table 29.8.

Risk stratification

The major clinical and angiographic predictors of survival of patients with CAD are:

- LV function
- Anatomical extent and severity of coronary atherosclerosis
- Severity of documented ischaemia
- Severity of angina.

LV function and viability

Echocardiographic LVEF <50% is considered abnormal. LVEF <35% denotes patients at high risk and is an independent predictor of mortality. Dobutamine stress echocardiography, myocardial perfusion tests, cardiac magnetic resonance, and positron emission tomography are used for assessment of viability of apparently scarred ventricular tissue.[25] The demonstration of viable myocardium in patients with coronary artery disease and LV dysfunction consistently identifies patients with poor prognosis that usually,[25–27] although not invariably,[28–31] improve with revascularization (see Therapy).

Coronary anatomy indices

The extent of significant lesions on the coronary arteries has been correlated with long-term mortality,[32] and risk stratification can be based on coronary anatomy (Table 29.9). Coronary stenoses are now considered haemodynamically significant when >50% diameter stenosis of the left main and >70% diameter stenosis of the other epicardial arteries.[33] However, intermediate angiographic stenosis (30–70%), either by quantitative coronary angiography or by subjective assessment at time of angiography, are not reliable criteria for risk stratification. The **SYNTAX score** is an angiographic grading tool, calculated as the sum of the points assigned to each lesion identified in the 16 segments of the coronary tree with greater than 50% diameter narrowing in vessels with a diameter greater than 1.5 mm (http://www.syntaxscore.com) (Table 29.10). The **clinical SYNTAX score** (SYNTAX score II) combines the angiographic SYNTAX Score with a clinical risk score incorporating age, ejection fraction, and creatinine clearance. It is calculated as:

Table 29.8 Causes of chest pain

Cardiovascular
Acute coronary syndrome
Aortic stenosis
Hypertension
Aortic dissection
Myocarditis
Pericarditis
Hypertrophic cardiomyopathy
Musculoskeletal
Cervical disc disease
Costochondritis
Fibrositis
Herpes zoster (before the rash)
Neuropathic pain
Rib fracture
Pulmonary
Pneumonia
Pulmonary embolism
Tension pneumothorax
Pleuritis
Gastrointestinal
Cholecystitis
Cholangitis
Peptic ulcer
Gastro-oesophageal reflux
Oesophageal spasm
Boerhaave syndrome (oesophageal rupture with mediastinitis)
Pancreatitis
Psychiatric
Hyperventilation
Affective disorders (depression)
Anxiety disorder/panic attack
Somatization and psychogenic pain disorder
Thought disorders (fixed delusions)

$$\text{Clinical SYNTAX score} = \text{SYNTAX score} \times [(\text{Age}/\text{LVEF}) + 1 \text{ point for each 10 mL creatinine clearance} <60 \text{ mL.min}/1.73 \text{ mm}^2)].$$

It predicts major cardiac and cerebrovascular events and mortality better than angiographic score and has been proposed for use in patients with anticipated PCI.[34] Incorporating functional assessment by considering coronary lesions with **FFR** measurements <0.80 improves its clinical usefulness.[35] The specificity of the **coronary calcium score**, as identified by CCT for obstructive coronary lesions, is low. However, it may be useful in asymptomatic subjects classified in intermediate Framingham risk range.[36,37]

Extent of ischaemia

In longitudinal studies, in patients with known or suspected coronary artery disease, detection of ischaemia predicts a significantly higher overall mortality, cardiac death, or MI, even in the absence of angina, whereas normal scintigraphy studies identify patients with a good prognosis at a low risk for future cardiac events.[38,39] Myocardial ischaemia is an established cause of polymorphic ventricular tachycardia or fibrillation and sudden cardiac death.[40] The majority of sudden deaths due to ischaemic heart disease are not associated with an acute MI, but transient acute ischaemia is an important trigger, preceding 35 to 80% of deaths due to a ventricular tachyarrhythmia.[41] However, imaging tests, such as exercise scintigraphy results, do not correlate well with angiographic findings, both in patients with and without angina, and they may not identify the culprit lesion(s) with certainty in the presence of multivessel disease.[42] Fractional flow reserve shows modest concordance with imaging tests, such as perfusion scintigraphy and dobutamine stress echocardiography, and quantitative coronary angiography and fractional flow reserve, particularly with 30% to 70% diameter stenoses.[43] Thus, no single test can serve as a gold standard, particularly when equivocal or borderline results are produced (Table 29.11 and Figure 29.3). Recently, an analysis of the STICH trial cohort revealed that in patients with LVEF ≤35% (but not with left main stem significant stenosis or class II or greater angina), inducible myocardial ischemia does not identify patients with worse prognosis or those with greater benefit from CABG over optimal medical therapy.[44]

Therapy

Therapy of patients with CAD is aimed at alleviating ischaemia and affecting the natural history of the disease by improving endothelial function, stabilizing atherosclerotic plaques, and modifying risk factors.

Medical therapy

Lifestyle modification is essential for risk reduction and symptomatic relief (Tables 29.12 and 29.13 and Figure 29.4). **Smoking** cessation, regular **physical activity** 30–60 min daily for at least 5 days a week, loss of **weight** (aimed at a BMI 18.5–24.9 kg/m^2) and a waist circumference of <89 cm in women and <102 in men are essential, although BMI, waist circumference, and waist-to-hip ratio do not provide significant additional information about cardiovascular risk beyond that already provided by systolic blood pressure, diabetes, and lipids.[45] Reduction of calorie

Table 29.9 Coronary artery disease prognostic index with medical therapy

Extent of CAD	Prognostic weight (0–100)	5-year survival rate (%)
1-vessel disease, 75%	23	93
>1-vessel disease, 50% to 74%	23	93
1-vessel disease, 95%	32	91
2-vessel disease	37	88
2-vessel disease, both 95%	42	86
1-vessel disease, 95% proximal LAD	48	83
2-vessel disease, 95% LAD	48	83
2-vessel disease, 95% proximal LAD	56	79
3-vessel disease	56	79
3-vessel disease, 95% in at least 1	63	73
3-vessel disease, 75% proximal LAD	67	67
3-vessel disease, 95% proximal LAD	74	59

Califf RM, *et al.* Task Force 5. Stratification of patients into high-, medium-, and low-risk subgroups for purposes of risk factor management. *J Am Coll Cardiol.* 1996;**27**:964–1047.

Table 29.10 The SYNTAX score algorithm

1. Dominance
2. Number of lesions
3. Segments involved per lesion
Lesion characteristics
4. Total occlusion
i. Number of segments involved
ii. Age of the total occlusion (>3 months)
iii. Blunt stump
iv. Bridging collaterals
v. First segment beyond the occlusion visible by antegrade or retrograde filling
vi. Side branch involvement
5. Trifurcation
i. Number of segments diseased
6. Bifurcation
i. Type
ii. Angulation between the distal main vessel and the side branch <70°
7. Aorto-ostial lesion
8. Severe tortuosity
9. Length >20 mm
10. Heavy calcification
11. Thrombus
12. Diffuse disease/small vessels
i. Number of segments with diffuse disease/small vessels

uptake and regular exercise are the best means to lose weight. Although several drugs are currently approved in the USA to treat obesity, only orlistat is FDA-approved for long-term use.[46] Some physical activity is better than none, and additional benefits occur with more physical activity.[47] Women who smoke may have a 25% greater risk ratio of coronary artery disease than do male smokers, independent of other cardiovascular risk factors.[48] Recommended **diet** is low-fat Mediterranean diet with high fibre, fruits and vegetables, olive oil, and omega-3 fatty acids content. This reduces total mortality, as well as mortality from cardiovascular disease and cancer, and the incidence of parkinsonism and Alzheimer's.[49–51] Dietary supplementation with omega-3 fatty acids has been shown to reduce mortality after MI in some trials, but recent data refute any established benefit.[52–54] Vitamins B (that lower homocysteine), however, do not reduce risk in patients with a previous cardiovascular event.[55] **Moderate alcohol intake** (1 to 2 drinks per day for women and up to 2 to 3 drinks per day for men) reduces cardiovascular risk.[56] Flavanols are theoretically beneficial, but their role is not clinically established.[57] **Sedentary behaviour**, such as prolonged TV watching, increases the risk of cardiovascular disease, diabetes, and all-cause mortality.[58]

Blood pressure should be <140/90 mmHg (<130/80 mmHg in the presence of diabetes or chronic renal disease). In diabetics, a **HbA_{1c}** <7% used to be recommended, but recent guidelines emphasize changes in lifestyle and dietary measures rather than strict adherence to HbA_{1c} reduction.[59] However, in young patients, efforts to lower glycosylated haemoglobin (HbA_{1c}) to <7.0% are justified to reduce the incidence of microvascular complications. Ideally, preprandial and postprandial glucose should be maintained at <130 mg/dL and <180 mg/dL, respectively.[60] Pioglitazone achieves greater increases in HDL and reductions in glycated haemoglobin, triglycerides, and C-reactive protein compared to glimepiride, with a resultant slower progression of atherosclerosis.[61] However, thiazolidinediones increase the risk of heart failure and should not be used in the presence of impaired LV function. Pioglitazone is safer than rosiglitazone in this respect,[62] but concerns about association with bladder cancer have appeared, and its use has been banned in France. Early addition of insulin confers no benefit in patients with prediabetes (for definition see Chapter 24) or patients whose type 2 diabetes is well controlled on diet or medication.[63]

Aspirin (75–162 mg/d) should be continued indefinitely, unless contraindicated. In high-risk patients, it

Table 29.11 ACCF/AHA GL 2012 on stable IHD

Non-invasive risk stratification
High risk (>3% annual death or MI)
1. Severe resting LV dysfunction (LVEF <35%) not readily explained by non-coronary causes
2. Resting perfusion abnormalities ≥10% of the myocardium in patients without prior history or evidence of MI
3. Stress ECG findings, including ≥2 mm of ST segment depression at low workload or persisting into recovery, exercise-induced ST segment elevation, or exercise-induced VT/VF
4. Severe stress-induced LV dysfunction (peak exercise LVEF <45% or drop in LVEF with stress ≥10%)
5. Stress-induced perfusion abnormalities encumbering ≥10% myocardium or stress segmental scores indicating multiple vascular territories with abnormalities
6. Stress-induced LV dilation
7. Inducible wall motion abnormality (involving >2 segments or two coronary beds)
8. Wall motion abnormality developing at low dose of dobutamine (≤10 mg/kg/min) or at a low heart rate (<120 beats/min)
9. CAC score >400 Agaston units
10. Multivessel obstructive CAD (≥70% stenosis) or left main stenosis (≥50% stenosis) on CCTA
Intermediate risk (1% to 3% annual death or MI)
1. Mild/moderate resting LV dysfunction (LVEF 35–49%) not readily explained by non-coronary causes
2. Resting perfusion abnormalities in 5–9.9% of the myocardium in patients without a history or prior evidence of MI
3. ≥1 mm of ST segment depression occurring with exertional symptoms
4. Stress-induced perfusion abnormalities encumbering 5% to 9.9% of the myocardium or stress segmental scores (in multiple segments) indicating one vascular territory with abnormalities but without LV dilation
5. Small wall motion abnormality, involving one to two segments and only one coronary bed
6. CAC score 100 to 399 Agaston units
7. One-vessel CAD with ≥70% stenosis or moderate CAD stenosis (50% to 69% stenosis) in ≥2 arteries on CCTA
Low risk (<1% annual death or MI)
1. Low-risk treadmill score (score ≥5) or no new ST segment changes or exercise-induced chest pain symptoms when achieving maximal levels of exercise
2. Normal or small myocardial perfusion defect at rest or with stress encumbering <5% of the myocardium*
3. Normal stress or no change of limited resting wall motion abnormalities during stress
4. CAC score <100 Agaston units
5. No coronary stenosis >50% on CCTA

* Although the published data are limited, patients with these findings will probably not be at low risk in the presence of either a high-risk treadmill score or severe resting LV dysfunction (LVEF ≤35%).

CAC indicates coronary artery calcium; CAD, coronary artery disease; CCTA, coronary computed tomography angiography; LV, left ventricular; LVEF, left ventricular ejection fraction; and MI, myocardial infarction.

2012 ACCF/AHA/ACP/AATS/PCNA/SCAI/STS Guideline for the diagnosis and management of patients with stable ischemic heart disease. *J Am Coll Cardiol.* 2012;**60**:e44–e164.

reduces arterial thrombosis by 25% by inhibiting platelet cyclo-oxygenase-1 and decreasing synthesis of thromboxane A.[2, 64] After CABG, aspirin (100–325 mg/d) should be continued indefinitely (ACCF/AHA 2011 GL on CABG, I-A). Higher doses of aspirin are no more recommended following stent implantation (81 mg/day considered by the ACCF/AHA 2011 GL on PCI).

Clopidogrel (75 mg/d) may replace aspirin if aspirin is absolutely contraindicated. In patients receiving DES for a non-ACS indication, clopidogrel 75 mg daily should be added to aspirin and given for at least 12 months if patients are not at high risk of bleeding (ACCF/AHA 2011 on PCI). In patients receiving BMS, clopidogrel should be given for a minimum of 1 month and ideally up to 12 months (unless the patient is at increased risk of bleeding; then, it should be given for a minimum of 2 weeks) (ACCF/AHA 2011 on PCI). With BMS or new generation DES, continuation of clopidogrel beyond 1 year does not appear beneficial.[65]

Statins are the first choice for lipid management, aiming at LDL <100 mg/dL (or ideally <70 mg/dL). **LDL levels** are calculated by the Friedwald equation (LDL-C = total cholesterol – HDL-C – triglycerides/5), that underestimates

Table 29.12 ACCF/AHA 2012 GL on stable IHD. Treatment of patients with stable IHD (similar recommendations have been provided by AHA/ACCF 2011 GL on secondary prevention and risk reduction)

Patient education	
Patients should have an individualized education plan to optimize care and promote wellness, including:	
a. Education on the importance of medication adherence for managing symptoms and retarding disease progression.	I-C
b. An explanation of medication management and cardiovascular risk reduction strategies in a manner that respects the patient's level of understanding, reading comprehension, and ethnicity.	I-B
c. A comprehensive review of all therapeutic options.	I-B
d. A description of appropriate levels of exercise, with encouragement to maintain recommended levels of daily physical activity.	I-C
e. Introduction to self-monitoring skills.	I-C
f. Information on how to recognize worsening cardiovascular symptoms and take appropriate action.	I-C
Patients should be educated about the following lifestyle elements that could influence prognosis: weight control; maintenance of a body mass index of 18.5–24.9 kg/m^2 and maintenance of a waist circumference <100 cm (40 inches) in men and <88 cm (35 inches) in women (less for certain racial groups); lipid management; blood pressure control; smoking cessation and avoidance of exposure to second-hand smoke; individualized medical, nutrition, and lifestyle changes for patients with diabetes mellitus to supplement diabetes treatment goals and education.	I-C
It is reasonable to educate patients about:	
a. Adherence to a diet that is low in saturated fat, cholesterol, and trans fat; high in fresh fruits, whole grains, and vegetables; and reduced in sodium intake, with cultural and ethnic preferences incorporated.	IIa-B
b. Common symptoms of stress and depression to minimize stress-related angina symptoms.	IIa-C
c. Comprehensive behavioural approaches for the management of stress and depression.	IIa-C
d. Evaluation and treatment of major depressive disorder when indicated.	IIa-B
Risk factor modification	
Lipid management	
Lifestyle modifications, including daily physical activity and weight management.	I-B
Reduced intake of saturated fats (to <7% of total calories), *trans* fatty acids (to <1% of total calories), and cholesterol (to <200 mg/d).	I-B
Moderate or high dose of a statin in the absence of contraindications or documented adverse effects.	I-A
In statin intolerance, low density lipoprotein cholesterol-lowering therapy with bile acid sequestrants,* niacin,† or both.	IIa-B
Blood pressure management	
Lifestyle modification: weight control; increased physical activity; alcohol moderation; sodium reduction; and emphasis on increased consumption of fresh fruits, vegetables, and low-fat dairy products.	I-B
In blood pressure ≥140/90 mmHg, antihypertensive drug therapy in addition to, or after a trial of, lifestyle modifications.	I-A
Medications used for treatment of high blood pressure should be based on specific patient characteristics and may include ACE inhibitors and/or beta blockers, with addition of other drugs, such as thiazide diuretics or calcium channel blockers, to achieve a goal blood pressure <140/90 mmHg.	I-B
Diabetes management	
A goal HbA_{1c} of ≤7% for patients with a short duration of diabetes mellitus and a long life expectancy.	IIa-B
A goal HbA_{1c} 7% to 9% for certain patients according to age, history of hypoglycaemia, presence of microvascular or macrovascular complications, or coexisting medical conditions.	IIa-C
Initiation of pharmacotherapy interventions to achieve target HbA_{1c}.	IIb-A
Therapy with rosiglitazone should not be initiated in patients with stable IHD.	III-C
Physical activity	
For all patients, 30 to 60 minutes of moderate-intensity aerobic activity, such as brisk walking, at least 5 days, and preferably 7 days, per week, supplemented by an increase in daily lifestyle activities (e.g. walking breaks at work, gardening, household work) to improve cardiorespiratory fitness and move patients out of the least-fit, least-active, high-risk cohort (bottom 20%).	I-B
Risk assessment with a physical activity history and/or an exercise test to guide prognosis and prescription.	I-B
Medically supervised programs (cardiac rehabilitation) and physician-directed, home-based programmes for at-risk patients at first diagnosis.	I-A

(Continued)

Table 29.12 (Continued)

Risk factor modification	
Complementary resistance training at least 2 days per week.	IIa-C
Weight management	
Body mass index and/or waist circumference should be assessed at every visit. Encourage weight maintenance or reduction through an appropriate balance of lifestyle physical activity, structured exercise, caloric intake, and formal behavioural programmes when indicated to maintain or achieve a body mass index between 18.5 and 24.9 kg/m^2 and a waist circumference <102 cm (40 inches) in men and <88 cm (35 inches) in women (less for certain racial groups).	I-B
Initial goal of weight loss therapy to reduce body weight by 5% to 10% from baseline. With success, further weight loss can be attempted if indicated.	I-C
Smoking cessation counselling	
Smoking cessation and avoidance of exposure to environmental tobacco smoke at work and home. Follow-up, referral to special programmes, and pharmacotherapy and a stepwise strategy for smoking cessation (Ask, Advise, Assess, Assist, Arrange, Avoid).	I-B
Management of psychological factors	
Screening SIHD patients for depression and refer or treat when indicated.	IIa-B
Treatment of depression has not been shown to improve cardiovascular disease outcomes but might be reasonable for its other clinical benefits.	IIb-C
Alcohol consumption	
Non-pregnant women may have 1 drink (4 ounces of wine, 12 ounces of beer, or 1 ounce of spirits) a day and men 1 or 2 drinks a day, unless alcohol is contraindicated (such as in patients with a history of alcohol abuse or dependence or with liver disease).	IIb-C
Avoiding exposure to air pollution	
Avoid exposure to increased air pollution to reduce the risk of cardiovascular events.	IIa-C
Additional medical therapy to prevent MI and death	
Antiplatelet therapy	
Aspirin 75–162 mg daily indefinitely in the absence of contraindications.	I-A
Clopidogrel when aspirin is contraindicated.	I-B
Aspirin 75–162 mg daily and clopidogrel 75 mg daily in certain high-risk patients.	IIb-B
Dipyridamole is not recommended as antiplatelet therapy in stable IHD.	III-B
Beta blocker therapy	
Beta blockers for 3 years in all patients with normal LV function after MI or ACS.	I-B
Beta blockers in all patients with LVEF ≤40% with heart failure or prior MI, unless contraindicated. (Use should be limited to carvedilol, metoprolol succinate, or bisoprolol, which have been shown to reduce risk of death.)	I-A
Beta blockers as chronic therapy for all other patients with coronary or other vascular disease.	IIb-C
Renin-angiotensin-aldosterone blocker therapy	
ACE inhibitors in all patients with hypertension, diabetes mellitus, LV ejection fraction ≤40%, or chronic kidney disease, unless contraindicated.	I-A
ARBs for patients with hypertension, diabetes mellitus, LV systolic dysfunction, or chronic kidney disease and have indications for, but are intolerant of, ACE inhibitors.	I-A
ACE inhibitor in patients with both SIHD and other vascular disease.	IIa-B
ARBs in other patients who are ACE inhibitor intolerant.	IIa-C
Influenza vaccination	
Annual influenza vaccine for patients with SIHD.	I-B
Additional therapy to reduce risk of MI and death	
Oestrogen therapy in post-menopausal women with SIHD.	III-A
Vitamin C, vitamin E, and beta carotene supplementation.	III-A
Treatment of elevated homocysteine with folate or vitamins B6 and B12.	III-A
Chelation therapy	III-C
Treatment with garlic, coenzyme Q10, selenium, or chromium.	III-C

(Continued)

Table 29.12 (Continued)

Medical therapy for relief of symptoms	
Use of anti-ischaemic medications	
Beta blockers as initial therapy for relief of symptoms.	I-B
Calcium channel blockers or long-acting nitrates when beta blockers are contraindicated or cause unacceptable side effects.	I-B
Calcium channel blockers or long-acting nitrates, in combination with beta blockers, when initial treatment with beta blockers is unsuccessful.	I-B
Sublingual nitroglycerin or nitroglycerin spray for immediate relief of angina.	I-B
Long-acting non-dihydropyridine calcium channel blocker (verapamil or diltiazem) instead of a beta blocker as initial therapy.	IIa-B
Ranolazine as a substitute for beta blockers if initial treatment with beta blockers leads to unacceptable side effects or is ineffective or if initial treatment with beta blockers is contraindicated	IIa-B
Ranolazine in combination with beta blockers when initial treatment with beta blockers is not successful in patients with SIHD.	IIa-A
Alternative therapies for relief of symptoms in patients with fefractory angina	
Enhanced external counterpulsation for relief of refractory angina.	IIb-B
Spinal cord stimulation for relief of refractory angina.	IIb-C
Transmyocardial revascularization for relief of refractory angina.	IIb-B
Acupuncture for the purpose of improving symptoms or reducing cardiovascular risk.	III-C

* The use of bile acid sequestrant is relatively contraindicated when triglycerides are ≥200 mg/dL and is contraindicated when triglycerides are ≥500 mg/dL.
† Dietary supplement niacin must not be used as a substitute for prescription niacin.
2012 ACCF/AHA/ACP/AATS/PCNA/SCAI/STS Guideline for the diagnosis and management of patients with stable ischemic heart disease. *J Am Coll Cardiol.* 2012;**60**:e44–e164.

LDL when triglycerides are ≥150mg/dl.[66] The reduction of major cardiac events is proportional to the reduction of LDL cholesterol (Tables 29.12 and 29.13).[67] If triglycerides are >200 mg/dL, elimination of sugar and trans fats intake, as well as weight reduction and regular exercise, may achieve reductions of up to 50%. Tests of apolipoprotein B and A-I, lipoprotein(a), or lipoprotein-associated phospholipase A2 do not add significant improvement in CVD prediction.[68] The vascular benefits of statins may be independent of baseline CRP concentrations.[69,70] Elevated liver enzymes (up to 3 times normal values) due to non-alcoholic fatty liver disease do not constitute a contraindication (Table 29.13).[71] All statins may result in elevated CKB levels, but simvastatin has been particularly associated with myopathy,[72] and the FDA has warned against its use in high doses (80 mg od; 9 June 2011). Statins may be **lipophilic** (lovastatin, simvastatin, atorvastatin) or **hydrophilic** (pravastatin, rosuvastatin). Hydrophilic statins may have fewer side effects due to less muscle cell penetration and lower dependence on the cytochrome P450 enzyme, but differences between the two groups by means of clinical outcomes are not established. CYP3A4 inhibitors **ketoconazole, posaconazole, erythromycin, clarithromycin, telithromycin, nefazodone**, and especially **itraconazole, HIV protease inhibitors** (such as lopinavir, ritonavir, atazanavir, darunavir, and fosampenavir), and **hepatitis C virus protease inhibitors** (such as boceprevir and telaprevir) may significantly increase statin (and especially lovastatin and simvastatin) exposures and result in rhabdomyolysis. Fibrates typically increase the risk of myopathy. According to a FDA Drug Safety Communication (1 March 2012), the concomitant administration of lovastatin and simvastatin with HIV protease inhibitors or HCV protease inhibitors is contraindicated. Atorvastatin should be restricted to 20 mg od, rosuvastatin to 10 mg, and pravastatin does not need dosage modification, whereas no data are available for fluvastatin, in patients taking HIV or HCV protease inhibitors. Ciclosporin and, rarely, calcium antagonists, digoxin, and sildenafil may also increase the risk of myopathy. Statin therapy (as well as niacin) is associated with a slightly increased risk of development of **diabetes**, especially in high doses and in predisposed patients, but the risk is low, both in absolute terms and when compared with the reduction in coronary events.[73–75] Although there is probably a small increased risk of new-onset type 2 diabetes and statin medications, statins should not be stopped in high risk primary and secondary prevention patients. Regular screening of individuals with evidence of metabolic syndrome is reasonable. In a Drug Safety Communication (28 February 2012), FDA eliminated the requirement for routine monitoring of liver enzymes from the drug labels and added information about the potential for generally non-serious and reversible **cognitive side effects**, such as memory loss and reports of increased blood sugar and HbA_{1c} levels. Recently, in a retrospective observational

Table 29.13 ESC recommendations for patients with stable CAD

ESC 2006 GL on stable IHD. Recommendations for pharmacological therapy to improve prognosis in patients with stable angina

Aspirin 75 mg od in all patients without contraindications (i.e. active GI bleeding, aspirin allergy, or previous aspirin intolerance).	I-A
Statin therapy for all patients with coronary disease.	I-A
ACE inhibitor therapy in patients with hypertension, heart failure, LV dysfunction, prior MI with LV dysfunction, or diabetes.	I-A
Oral beta blocker therapy in patients post-MI or with heart failure.	I-A
ACE inhibitor therapy in all patients with angina and proven coronary disease.	IIa-B
Clopidogrel in patients who cannot take aspirin (e.g. aspirin allergic).	IIa-B
High-dose statin therapy in high-risk (>2% annual CV mortality) patients with proven coronary disease.	IIa-B
Fibrate therapy in patients with low HDL and high triglycerides who have diabetes or the metabolic syndrome.	IIb-B
Fibrate or nicotinic acid as adjunctive therapy to statin in patients with low HDL and high triglycerides at high risk (>2% annual CV mortality).	IIb-C

ESC Guidelines on the management of stable angina pectoris: executive summary: The Task Force on the Management of Stable Angina Pectoris of the European Society of Cardiology. *Eur Heart J*. 2006;**27**:1341–81.

ESC 2011 GL on revasularization. Long-term medical therapy after myocardial revascularization

ACE inhibitors in all patients with LVEF <40% and for those with hypertension, diabetes, or CKD, unless contraindicated.	I-A
ACE inhibitors in all patients, unless contraindicated.	IIa-A
Angiotensin receptor blockers in patients who are intolerant of ACE inhibitors and have HF or MI with LVEF <40%.	I-A
Angiotensin receptor blockers in all ACE inhibitor-intolerant patients.	IIa-A
Beta blocker therapy in all patients after MI or ACS or LV dysfunction, unless contraindicated.	I-A
High-dose lipid lowering drugs in all patients, regardless of lipid levels, unless contraindicated.	I-A
Fibrates and omega-3 fatty acids (1 g/day) in combination with statins and in patients intolerant of statins.	IIa-B
Niacin to increase HDL cholesterol.	IIb-B

ESC/EACTS Guidelines on myocardial revascularization The Task Force on Myocardial Revascularization of the European Society of Cardiology (ESC) and the European Association for Cardio-Thoracic Surgery (EACTS). *European Heart Journal* 2010;**31**:2501–2555.

ESC 2012 GL on CVD prevention. Recommendations on diet

- ◆ A healthy diet has the following characteristics:
- ◆ Saturated fatty acids to account for <10% of total energy intake through replacement by polyunsaturated fatty acids.
- ◆ Trans-unsaturated fatty acids: as little as possible, preferably no intake from processed food and <1% of total energy intake from natural origin.
- ◆ <5 g of salt per day.
- ◆ 30–45 g of fibre per day, from wholegrain products, fruits, and vegetables.
- ◆ 200 g of fruit per day (2–3 servings).
- ◆ 200 g of vegetables per day (2–3 servings).
- ◆ Fish at least twice a week, one of which to be oily fish.
- ◆ Consumption of alcoholic beverages should be limited to two glasses per day (20 g/day of alcohol) for men and one glass per day (10 g/day of alcohol) for women.

Energy intake should be limited to the amount of energy needed to maintain (or obtain) a healthy weight, i.e. a BMI <25 kg/m^2.
In general, when following the rules for a healthy diet, no dietary supplements are needed.
European Guidelines on cardiovascular disease prevention in clinical practice (version 2012). *Eur Heart J*. 2012;**33**:1635–701.

ESC 2012 GL on CVD prevention. The 'Five As' for a smoking cessation strategy

A-SK	Systematicaly inquire about smoking status at every opportunity.
A-ADVISE	Unequivocally urge all smokers to quit.
A-ASSESS	Determine the person's degree of addiction and readiness to quit.
A-ASSIST	Agree on a smoking cessation strategy, including setting a quit date, behavioural counselling, and pharmacological support.
A-ARRANGE	Arrange a schedule of follow-up.

(Continued)

Table 29.13 (Continued)

ESC 2012 GL on CVD prevention. Recommendations regarding physical activity	
Healthy adults of all ages should spend 2.5–5 h a week on physical activity or aerobic exercise training of at least moderate intensity or 1–2.5 h a week on vigorous intense exercise. Sedentary subjects should start light-intensity exercise programmes.	I-A
Physical activity/aerobic exercise training should be performed in multiple bouts, each lasting ≥10 min and evenly spread throughout the week, i.e. on 4–5 days a week.	IIa-A
Patients with previous acute myocardial infarction, CABG, PCI, stable angina pectoris, or stable chronic heart failure should undergo moderate to vigorous intensity aerobic exercise training ≥3 times a week and 30 min per session. Sedentary patients should start light-intensity exercise programmes after adequate exercise-related risk stratification.	I-A

ESC 2012 GL on CVD prevention. Recommendations on blood pressure	
Lifestyle measures, such as weight control, increased physical activity, alcohol moderation, sodium restriction, and increased consumption of fruits, vegetables, and low-fat dairy products, in all patients with hypertension and in individuals with high normal BP.	I-B
All major antihypertensive drug classes (i.e. diuretics, ACE inhibitors, calcium antagonists, angiotensin receptor antagonists, and beta blockers) do not differ significantly in their BP-lowering efficacy.	I-A
Beta blockers and thiazide diuretics are not recommended in hypertensive patients with multiple metabolic risk factors increasing the risk of new-onset diabetes.	III-A
In patients with diabetes, an ACE inhibitor or a renin-angiotensin receptor blocker.	I-A
Risk stratification using the SCORE risk chart as a minimal requirement in each hypertensive patient.	I-B
Subclinical organ damage predicts cardiovascular death independently of SCORE, and a search for subclinical organ damage should be encouraged, particularly in individuals at low or moderate risk (SCORE 1–4%).	IIa-B
Drug treatment to be initiated promptly in patients with grade 3 hypertension as well as in patients with grade 1 or 2 hypertension who are at high or very high total cardiovascular risk.	I-C
In patients with grade 1 or 2 hypertension and at moderate total cardiovascular risk, drug treatment may be delayed for several weeks and, in grade 1 hypertensive patients without any other risk factor, for several months while trying lifestyle measures.	IIb-C
Systolic BP should be lowered to <140 mmHg (and diastolic BP <90 mmHg) in all hypertensive patients.	IIa-A
All hypertensive patients with established cardiovascular disease or with type 2 diabetes or with an estimated 10-year risk of cardiovascular death ≥5% (based on the SCORE chart) should be considered for statin therapy.	IIa-B
Antiplatelet therapy, in particular low-dose aspirin, for hypertensive patients with cardiovascular events.	I-A
Antiplatelet therapy in hypertensive patients without a history of cardiovascular disease but with reduced renal function or at high cardiovascular risk.	IIb-A

ESC 2012 GL on CVD prevention. Recommendations on diabetes mellitus	
A target HbA_{1c} for the prevention of CVD in diabetes of <7.0% (<53 mmol/mol).	I-A
Statins to reduce cardiovascular risk in diabetes.	I-A
Hypoglycaemia and excessive weight gain must be avoided, and individual approaches (both targets and drug choices) may be necessary in patients with complex disease.	I-B
Metformin as first-line therapy if tolerated and not contraindicated.	IIa-B
Further reductions in HbA_{1c} to a target of <6.5% (<48 mmol/mol) (the lowest possible safely reached HbA_{1c}) may be useful at diagnosis. For patients with a long duration of diabetes, this target may reduce risk of microvascular outcomes.	IIb-B
BP targets in diabetes are <140/80 mmHg.	I-A
Target LDL cholesterol is <2.5 mmol/L, for patients without atherosclerotic disease total cholesterol may be <4.5 mmol/L, with a lower LDL cholesterol target of <1.8 mmol/L (using higher doses of statins) for diabetic patients at very high CVD risk.	IIb-B
Antiplatelet therapy with aspirin is not recommended for people with diabetes who do not have clinical evidence of atherosclerotic disease.	III-A

ACS, acute coronary syndrome; BP, blood pressure; CKD, chronic kidney disease; CVD, cardiovascular disease; HbA_{1c}, glycated haemoglobin; LDL, low density lipoprotein.

(Continued)

Table 29.13 (Continued)

ESC 2012 GL on CVD prevention. Recommendations on antithrombotic therapy	
In the acute phase of coronary artery syndromes and for the following 12 months, dual antiplatelet therapy with a P2Y12 inhibitor (ticagrelor or prasugrel) added to aspirin is recommended, unless contraindicated due to excessive risk of bleeding.	I-B
Clopidogrel (600 mg loading dose, 75 mg daily dose) for patients who cannot receive ticagrelor or prasugrel.	I-A
In the chronic phase (>12 months) after myocardial infarction, aspirin for secondary prevention.	I-A
In patients with non-cardioembolic transient ischaemic attack or ischaemic stroke, secondary prevention with either dipyridamole plus aspirin or clopidogrel alone.	I-A
In the case of intolerance to dipyridamole (headache) or clopidogrel, aspirin alone is recommended.	I-A
In patients with non-cardioembolic cerebral ischaemic events, anticoagulation is not superior to aspirin and is not recommended.	III-B
Aspirin or clopidogrel cannot be recommended in individuals without cardiovascular or cerebrovascular disease due to the increased risk of major bleeding.	III-B

European Guidelines on cardiovascular disease prevention in clinical practice (version 2012). *Eur Heart J*. 2012;**33**:1635–701.

ESC 2012 GL on CVD prevention.	
Recommendations on management of hyperlipidaemia	
The recommended target levels are <5 mmol/L (less than ~190 mg/dL) for total plasma cholesterol and <3 mmol/L (less than ~115 mg/dL) for LDL cholesterol for subjects at low or moderate risk.	I-A
In patients at high CVD risk, an LDL cholesterol goal <2.5 mmol/L (less than ~100 mg/dL) is recommended.	I-A
In patients at very high CVD risk, the recommended LDL cholesterol target is <1.8 mmol/L (less than ~70 mg/dL) or a ≥50% LDL cholesterol reduction when the target level cannot be reached.	I-A
All patients with familial hypercholesterolaemia must be recognized as high-risk patients and be treated with lipid-lowering therapy.	I-A
In patients with an ACS, statin treatment in high doses has to be initiated while the patients are in hospital.	I-A
Prevention of non-haemorrhagic stroke: treatment with statins must be started in all patients with established atherosclerotic disease and in patients at high risk for developing CVD. Treatment with statins must be started in patients with a history of non-cardioembolic ischaemic stroke.	I-A
Occlusive arterial disease of the lower limbs and carotid artery disease are CHD risk-equivalent conditions, and lipid-lowering therapy is recommended.	I-A
Statins as the first-line drugs in transplant patients with dyslipidaemia.	IIa-B
Chronic kidney disease (stages 2–5, i.e. GFR <90 mL/min/1.73 m^2) is acknowledged as a CHD risk-equivalent, and the LDL cholesterol target in these patients should be adapted to the degree of renal failure.	IIa-C

Selected drugs that may increase risk of myopathy and rhabdomyolysis when used concomitantly with statin (CYP3A4 inhibitors/substrates or other mechanisms)
Ciclosporin, tacrolimus
Macrolides (azithromycin, clarithromycin, erythromycin)
Azole antifungals (itraconazole, ketoconazole, fluconazole)
Calcium antagonists (mibefradil, diltiazem, verapamil)
Nefazodone
HIV protease inhibitors (amprenavir, indinavir, nelfinavir, ritonavir, saquinavir)
Sildenafil
Others
Digoxin, niacin, fibrates (particularly gemfibrozil)

(Continued)

Table 29.13 (Continued)

ESC/EAS 2011 GL on dyslipidaemias. Lipid analyses as treatment target in the prevention of CVD	
LDL-C is recommended as target for treatment.	I-A
TC should be considered as treatment target if other analyses are not available.	IIa-A
TG should be analysed during the treatment of dyslipidaemias with high TG levels.	IIa-B
Non-HDL-C should be considered as a secondary target in combined hyperlipidaemias, diabetes, the MetS, or CKD.	IIa-B
Apo B should be considered as a secondary treatment target.	IIa-B
HDL-C is not recommended as a target for treatment.	III-C
The ratios apo B/apo AI and non-HDL-C/HDL-C are not recommended as targets for treatment.	III-C

Apo, apolipoprotein: CKD, chronic kidney disease; CVD, cardiovascular disease; HDL-C, high density lipoprotein cholesterol; LDL-C, low density lipoprotein cholesterol; MetS, metabolic syndrome; TC, total cholesterol; TG, triglyceride.
ESC/EAS Guidelines for the management of dyslipidaemias: the Task Force for the management of dyslipidaemias of the European Society of Cardiology (ESC) and the European Atherosclerosis Society (EAS). *Eur Heart J*. 2011;32:1769–818.

ESC/EAS 2011 GL on dyslipidaemias. Impact of lifestyle changes on lipid levels

	Magnitude of the effect	Level of evidence
Lifestyle interventions to reduce TC and LDL-C levels		
Reduce dietary saturated fat	+++	A
Reduce dietary trans fat	+++	A
Increase dietary fibre	++	A
Reduce dietary cholesterol	++	B
Utilize functional foods enriched with phytosterols	+++	A
Reduce excessive body weight	+	B
Utilize soy protein products	+	B
Increase habitual physical activity	+	A
Utilize red yeast rice supplements	+	B
Utilize polycosanol supplements	–	B
Lifestyle interventions to reduce TG levels		
Reduce excessive body weight	+++	A
Reduce alcohol intake	+++	A
Reduce intake of mono- and disaccharides	+++	A
Increase habitual physical activity	++	A
Reduce total amount of dietary carbohydrate	++	A
Utilize supplements of n-3 polyunsaturated fat	++	A
Replace saturated fat with mono- or polyunsaturated fat	+	B
Lifestyle interventions to increase HDL-C levels		
Reduce dietary trans fat	+++	A
Increase habitual physical activity	+++	A
Reduce excessive body weight	++	A
Reduce dietary carbohydrates and replace them with unsaturated fat	++	A
Use alcohol with moderation	++	B
Among carbohydrate-rich foods, prefer those with low glycaemic index and high fibre content	+	C
Quit smoking	+	B
Reduce intake of mono- and disaccharides	+	C

(Continued)

Table 29.13 (Continued)

ESC/EAS 2011 GL on dyslipidaemias. Monitoring lipids and enzymes in patients on lipid-lowering therapy
Testing lipids
How often should lipids be tested?
◆ Before starting lipid-lowering drug treatment, at least two measurements should be made, with an interval of 1–12 weeks, with the exception of conditions where immediate drug treatment is suggested, such as in ACS.
How often should patients' lipids be tested after starting lipid-lowering treatment?
◆ 8 (± 4) weeks after starting drug treatment.
◆ 8 (± 4) weeks after adjustments to treatment until within the target range.
How often should cholesterol or lipids be tested once a patient has reached target or optimal cholesterol?
◆ Annually (unless there are adherence problems or another specific reason for more frequent reviews).
Monitoring liver and muscle enzymes
How often should liver enzymes (ALT) be routinely measured in patients taking lipid-lowering drugs?
◆ Before treatment.
◆ 8 weeks after starting drug treatment or after any dose increase.
◆ Annually thereafter if liver enzymes are <3 × ULN.
What if liver enzymes become raised in a person taking lipid-lowering drugs?
If <3 × ULN:
◆ Continue therapy.
◆ Recheck liver enzymes in 4–6 weeks.
If values rise to ≥3 × ULN:
◆ Stop statin or reduce dose; recheck liver enzymes within 4–6 weeks.
◆ Cautious reintroduction of therapy may be considered after ALT has returned to normal.
How often should CK be measured in patients taking lipid-lowering drugs?
Pre-treatment
◆ Before starting treatment.
◆ If baseline CK level >5 × ULN, do not start drug therapy; recheck.
Monitoring
◆ Routine monitoring of CK is not necessary.
◆ Check CK if patient develops myalgia.
Increase alertness regarding myopathy and CK elevation in patients at risk, such as elderly patients, concomitant interfering therapy, multiple medications, liver or renal disease.
Monitoring liver and muscle enzymes
What if CK becomes raised in a person taking lipid-lowering drugs?
If >5 × ULN:
◆ Stop treatment; check renal function, and monitor CK every 2 weeks.
◆ Consider the possibility of transient CK elevation for other reasons, such as muscle exertion.
◆ Consider secondary causes of myopathy if CK remains elevated.
If ≤5 × ULN:
◆ If no muscle symptoms, continue statin (patients should be alerted to report symptoms; consider further checks of CK).
◆ If muscle symptoms, monitor symptoms and CK regularly.

ACS, acute coronary syndrome; ALT, alanine aminotransferase; CK, creatine phospholdnase; ULN, upper limit of normal.
ESC/EAS Guidelines for the management of dyslipidaemias: the Task Force for the management of dyslipidaemias of the European Society of Cardiology (ESC) and the European Atherosclerosis Society (EAS). *Eur Heart J*. 2011;**32**:1769–818.

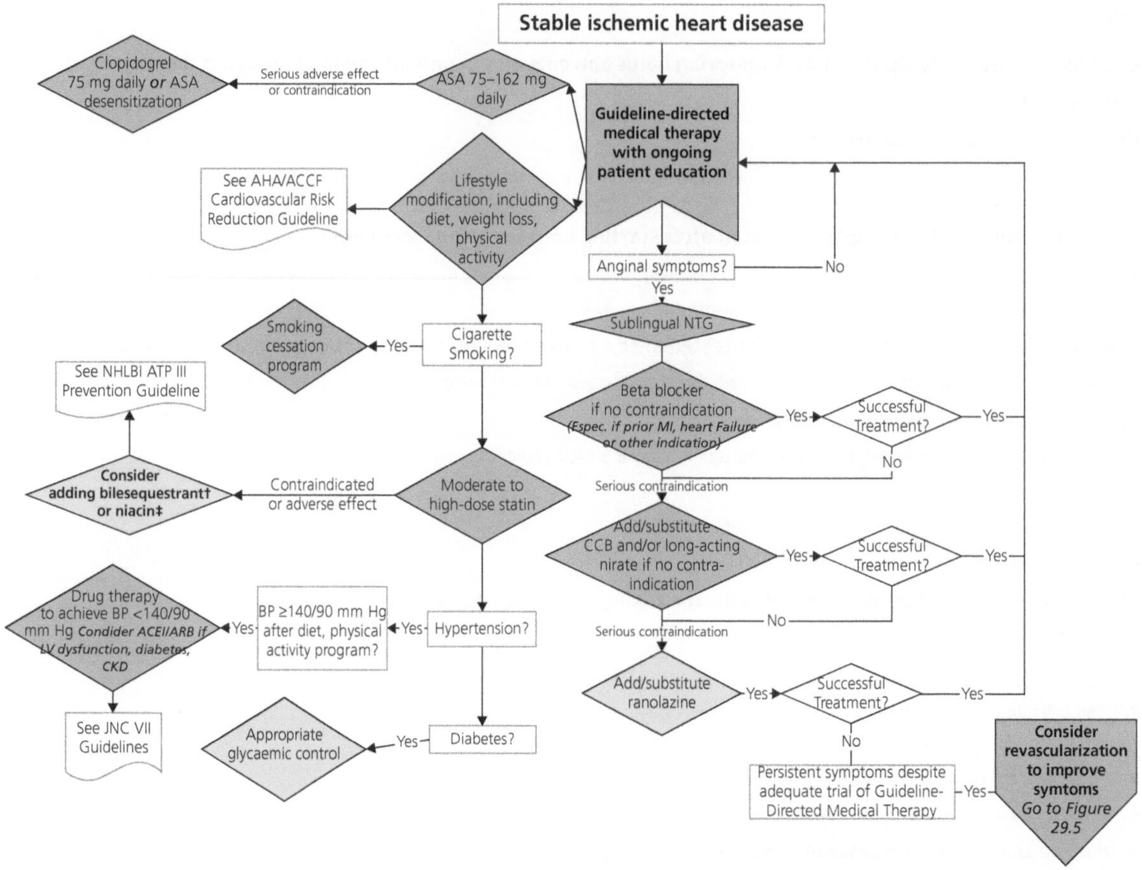

Figure 29.4 ACC/AHA 2012 GL on stable IHD. Algorithm for guideline-directed medical therapy for patients with SIHD.*

* Colours correspond to the class of recommendations in the ACCF/AHA. The algorithms do not represent a comprehensive list of recommendations (see full guideline text for all recommendations).

† The use of bile acid sequestrant is relatively contraindicated when triglycerides are ≥200 mg/dL and is contraindicated when triglycerides are ≥500 mg/dL.

‡ Dietary supplement niacin must not be used as a substitute for prescription niacin.

ACCF indicates American College of Cardiology Foundation; ACEI, angiotensin-converting enzyme inhibitor; AHA, American Heart Association; ARB, angiotensin receptor blocker; ASA, aspirin, ATP III, Adult Treatment Panel 3; BP, blood pressure; CCB, calcium channel blocker; CKD, chronic kidney disease; HDL-C, high density lipoprotein cholesterol; JNC VII, Seventh Report of the Joint National Committee on Prevention, Detection, Evaluation, and Treatment of High Blood Pressure; LDL-C, low density lipoprotein cholesterol; LV, left ventricular; MI, myocardial infarction; NHLBI, National Heart, Lung, and Blood Institute; and NTG, nitroglycerin.

2012 ACCF/AHA/ACP/AATS/PCNA/SCAI/STS Guideline for the diagnosis and management of patients with stable ischemic heart disease. *J Am Coll Cardiol.* 2012;**60**:e44–e164.

analysis of databases, an increased risk of **acute kidney injury** was found with high potency statins, defined as ≥10 mg rosuvastatin, ≥20 mg atorvastatin, and ≥40 mg simvastatin. This effect, was strongest in the first 120 days after initiation of treatment.[76] There is no increased risk of developing cognitive defects[77] or cancer with statins,[78] and these agents may actually reduce the risk of cancer in heart transplant recipients.[79] Statin exposure following ischaemic stroke was not associated with intracranial haemorrhage,[80] but avoiding statins should be considered for patients with a history of intracranial haemorrhage, particularly those cases with a lobar location.[81] Some worsening in energy and exertional fatigue, especially in women, may be seen.[82] **Fibrates** added to statin have not been found to reduce cardiovascular events (ACCORD trial),[83] and, according to new guidelines by the AHA, treatment with fibrates is indicated only for values >500 mg/dL.[84] Combinations of a statin with a fibrate might be considered in high-risk individuals, such as diabetics, with a high triglyceride/low HDL cholesterol pattern.[85,86] The combination (especially with gemfibrosil) increases the risk of myopathy, and fibrates increase homocysteine levels that may be prothrombotic; in addition, the ability of fibrates to increase HDL may be attenuated in patients with type 2 diabetes. [75] The addition of **ezetimibe** or **niacin** to statins is not beneficial (ENHANCE and

AIM-HIGH trials), despite significant improvements in HDL cholesterol and triglyceride levels,[87,88] and niacin has been recently shown to be associated with significant adverse events such as new-onset diabetes, infections, and GI and intracranial bleeding.[89] Addition of **n-3 fatty acids** to statins may also have beneficial effects, regardless of possible triglyceride reduction, but their clinical value is not proven.[90] **Plant sterol (phytosterols)** supplements reduce cholesterol absorption by competitive inhibition and transcriptional induction of genes implicated in cholesterol metabolism, but concerns have been raised that they may be atherogenic, although no association between cardiovascular disease and serum sterol concentration was detected in a recent meta-analysis.[91] Recently, a fully human **proprotein convertase subtilisin/kexin 9 (PCSK9) monoclonal antibody** was found to increase the recycling of low density lipoprotein receptors and reduce LDL cholesterol levels to a higher degree than atorvastatin.[92]

Beta blockers should be given in patients with a past MI, acute coronary syndrome, or LV dysfunction in the context of coronary artery disease, unless contraindicated (severe asthma, sick sinus syndrome, AV block). Metoprolol and bisoprolol have been shown to reduce adverse effects in stable patients.[93] However, they confer no survival benefit in patients with CAD without prior MI or in patients with a remote MI (>1 year).[94]

ACE inhibitors should be given indefinitely in patients with LVEF <40% or hypertension, diabetes, chronic kidney, and possibly to all patients with CAD disease, unless contraindicated. **Angiotensin II receptor blockers** may be used in patients intolerant of ACE inhibitors. Aldosterone blockers are recommended in all patients with LVEF <40% and diabetes or heart failure but without renal dysfunction or hyperkalaemia.

Calcium channel blockers If beta blocker treatment is unsuccessful or contraindicated. Long-acting non-dihydropyridines can be used instead of beta blockers. When dihydropyridines are used, they should be combined preferably with a beta blocker.

Nitrates are useful for immediate angina relief. Short-acting nitrates are preferred. They may be also considered for long-acting therapy if beta blocker treatment is unsuccessful or contraindicated but with adequate nitrate-free interval to decrease nitrate tolerance. However, prolonged exposure to nitrates induces endothelial dysfunction, and long-term therapy may worsen the prognosis of patients with CAD.[95,96]

Ranolazine For chronic angina relief, usually in addition to, or instead of, beta blockers. Ranolazine is a sodium ion channel inhibitor that does not affect heart rate or blood pressure. It does not affect the incidence of cardiac mortality or MI (MERLIN-TIMI 36). Initial evidence suggesting that it may suppress reentrant and EAD-induced multifocal VF needs to be verified.[97]

Nicorandil and **ivabradine** are new anti-ischaemic drugs, but clinical experience is rather limited.

Vorapaxar, an inhibition of the protease-activated receptor PAR-1 through which thrombin activates platelets, reduced the risk of cardiovascular death or ischaemic events in patients with stable atherosclerosis who were receiving standard therapy but also increased the risk of moderate or severe bleeding, including intracranial haemorrhage.[98]

Proton pump inhibitors are given in patients on dual antiplatelet therapy and at high risk of GI bleed (advanced age, warfarin, steroids, NSAIDs, peptic ulcer). Routine use is not recommended (ACC/AHA 2011 on PCI, III-C).

NSAIDs (both non-selective and selective COX-2 inhibitors) are associated with an increased thrombotic risk, with diclofenac conferring the highest risk, and naproxen being the safest agent.[99] Since the withdrawal of COX-2 inhibitor rofecoxib due to increased incidence of MIs, concerns have also been raised about celecoxib that inhibits neointimal formation, and thus theoretically stent restenosis, but has been associated with a higher thrombotic risk.[100] In a recent meta-analysis, naproxen was the safest agent whereas diclofenac and, probably, ibuprofen conferred the same risk as coxibs.[101]

Influenza vaccine Annually for all patients with CAD. Hormone therapy with oestrogen plus progestin, or oestrogen alone, should not be given, and the value of antioxidant vitamin supplements (vitamins E, C, or beta carotene) or folic acid, with or without B6 and B12, is not proven. Chelation therapy (ethylenediamine tetraacetic acid or EDTA) is not indicated and may be harmful because of its potential to cause hypocalcaemia. Specific guidelines on CAD prevention have been published by ACC/AHA and ESC.[59,102] All patients should be screened for depression, particularly following an ACS.

In **syndrome X**, nitrates, beta blockers, and calcium channel blockers nay be used but with variable success (ESC 2006 GL on stable CAD, I-B). Nicorandil (ESC 2006 GL on stable CAD, IIa-C), aminophylline (ESC 2006 GL on stable CAD, IIb-C), and imipramine (ESC 2006 GL on stable CAD, IIa-C) may also be tried. Recommendations of ACCF/AHA are similar (Table 29.7).

Revascularization

Studies considering both CABG and PCI for revascularization usually,[103–106] although not invariably,[107] show a greater survival benefit than medical therapy in patients with significant inducible ischaemia (>10% of LV myocardium). As a general rule, the greater the risk, the greater the benefit by revascularization (Tables 29.14 to 29.18 and Figures 29.4 to 29.6). The use of **myocardial viability testing** in guiding revascularization has been questioned,[28–31] although concerns about the limitations of these trials have been raised.[7]

The issue of **complete revascularization** is not settled in patients with stable coronary artery disease, as opposed to those with acute coronary syndromes. Although there has been some evidence of improved survivalwith complete revascularization in some studies, this is not established either for CABG,[108–110] or PCI.[111–113] In a recent study on asymptomatic patients (33% of them diabetic) who had been subjected to previous revascularization with CABG or PCI the detection of inducible ischemia on myocardial perfusion scintifraphy did not indicate a survival benefit from repeat revascularization.[114]

Surgical revascularization

The earliest trials of coronary artery bypass grafting (CABG) vs medical therapy in patients with chronic stable angina were conducted in the 1970s and 1980s.[115–117] Despite major advances in medical therapy (especially antiplatelet and lipid-lowering therapy) and surgical techniques (including the use of the internal mammary artery), the overall conclusions from these trials and associated registry studies remain valid today. Symptomatic relief was better with CABG; however, no overall difference was observed in survival or freedom from MI with CABG vs medical therapy, except in patients with:

- **Left main disease (VA trial),**
- **Multivessel disease plus LV dysfunction but not overt heart failure (35% < LVEF <50%) (VA and CASS trials), and**
- **Probably proximal LAD disease in conjunction with multivessel disease (European trial).**

Revascularization may also offer a survival benefit to patients with severe or post-infarction angina. It is now accepted that in high- and medium-risk patients, CABG (particularly left main or three-vessel disease or one or two-vessel disease with proximal LAD involvement) decreases mortality compared to medical therapy. In low-risk patients, it is detrimental.[118,119] In the STICH trial on patients with LVEF ≤35%, the value of CABG over medical therapy was not proven by means of reducing total mortality (although cardiac mortality is reduced), even if performed in patients with proven myocardial viability.[28,29] However, CABG may offer improved survival/MI/stroke rates in diabetics with extensive coronary disease or impaired LV function (BARI 2D trial).[120] The beneficial effects of CABG do not last beyond 10 years after surgery, presumably due to the limited longevity of used grafts (Table 29.16). Furthermore, grafting a coronary artery increases the risk of disease progression 3 to 6 times, especially in the right coronary artery.[121] Saphenous vein graft intimal hyperplasia is not reduced by the addition of clopidogrel to aspirin (CASCADE).[122] CABG procedures carry a **3% perioperative mortality**, 0–10% risk of myocardial infarction, 5% risk of need for prolonged intubation, 2–6% of re-operation for bleeding, 1–4% of wound infection, 0.5–1% renal failure, 1.6% of stroke, and a 6% risk of residual cognitive defects that may not be less, even with beating heart procedures.[123] One year after coronary surgery, 10–20% of saphenous vein grafts fail while, at 10 years, only about half of saphenous vein grafts are patent, and, of those, only half are free of angiographic arteriosclerosis.[124,125] Vein graft failure is associated with repeat revascularization but not

Table 29.14 Revascularization in CAD

ACC/AHA 2012 GL on stable IHD. Revascularization to improve survival compared with medical therapy		
Anatomical setting		
UPLM or complex CAD		
CABG and PCI	Heart Team approach recommended	I-C
CABG and PCI	Calculation of the STS and SYNTAX scores	IIa-B
UPLM* (>50% diameter stenosis)		
CABG		I-B
PCI	for SIHD when **both** of the following are present: ◆ Anatomical conditions associated with a low risk of PCI procedural complications and a high likelihood of good long-term outcome (e.g. a low SYNTAX score of ≤22, ostial or trunk left main CAD) ◆ Clinical characteristics that predict a significantly increased risk of adverse surgical outcomes (e.g. STS-predicted risk of operative mortality ≥5%)	IIa-B
	for UA/NSTEMI if not a CABG candidate	IIa-B
	for STEMI when distal coronary flow is TIMI flow grade 3 and PCI can be performed more rapidly and safely than CABG	IIa-C

(Continued)

Table 29.14 (Continued)

Anatomical setting		
UPLM* (>50% diameter stenosis)		
PCI	for SIHD when **both** of the following are present: ◆ Anatomical conditions associated with a low to intermediate risk of PCI procedural complications and intermediate to high likelihood of good long-term outcome (e.g. low-intermediate SYNTAX score of <33, bifurcation left main CAD) ◆ Clinical characteristics that predict an increased risk of adverse surgical outcomes (e.g. moderate-severe COPD, disability from prior stroke, or prior cardiac surgery; STS-predicted risk of operative mortality >2%)	IIb-B
	for SIHD in patients (versus performing CABG) with unfavourable anatomy for PCI and who are good candidates for CABG	III-B (harm)
3-vessel disease (>70% diameter stenoses) with or without proximal LAD artery disease*		
CABG		I-B
	choose CABG over PCI in patients with complex 3-vessel CAD (e.g. SYNTAX >22) who are good candidates for CABG	IIa-b
PCI	of uncertain benefit	IIb-B
2-vessel disease (>70% diameter stenoses) with proximal LAD artery disease*		
CABG		I-B
PCI	of uncertain benefit	IIb-B
2-vessel disease (>70% diameter stenoses) without proximal LAD artery disease*		
CABG	with extensive ischaemia (e.g., high-risk criteria on stress testing, abnormal intracoronary hemodynamic evaluation, or 20% perfusion defect by myocardial perfusion stress imaging) or target vessels supplying a large area of viable myocardium	IIa-B
	of uncertain benefit without extensive ischaemia	IIb-C
PCI	of uncertain benefit	IIb-B
1-vessel proximal LAD artery disease (>70% diameter stenosis)		
CABG	with LIMA for long-term benefit in the presence of extensive ischemia	IIa-B
PCI	of uncertain benefit	IIb-B
1-vessel disease (>70% diameter stenosis) without proximal LAD artery involvement		
CABG		III-B (harm)
PCI		III-B (harm)
LV dysfunction		
CABG	EF 35% to 50% and multivessel CAD or proximal LAD coronary artery stenosis, when viable myocardium is present in the region of intended revascularization	IIa-B
CABG	EF <35% without significant left main CAD whether or not viable myocardium is present.	IIb-B
PCI	Insufficient data	
Survivors of sudden cardiac death with presumed ischaemia-mediated VT		
CABG		I-B
PCI		I-C
No anatomical or physiological criteria for revascularization		
	(e.g. <70% diameter non-left main coronary artery stenosis, fractional flow reserve >0.80, no or only mild ischaemia on non-invasive testing)	
CABG		III-B (harm)
PCI		III-B (harm)
Previous CABG and extensive anterior wall ischemia		
CABG		IIb-B
PCI		IIb-B

* In patients with multivessel disease who also have diabetes, it is reasonable to choose CABG (with LIMA) over PCI (Class IIa/LOE: B).

CABG indicates coronary artery bypass graft; CAD, coronary artery disease; COPD, chronic obstructive pulmonary disease; EF, ejection fraction; LAD, left anterior descending; LIMA, left internal mammary artery; LV, left ventricular; N/A, not applicable; PCI, percutaneous coronary intervention; SIHD, stable ischaemic heart disease; STEMI, ST elevation myocardial infarction; STS, Society of Thoracic Surgeons; SYNTAX, Synergy between percutaneous coronary intervention with TAXUS and cardiac surgery; TIMI, Thrombolysis In Myocardial Infarction; UA/NSTEMI, unstable angina/non-ST elevation myocardial infarction; UPLM, unprotected left main; and VT, ventricular tachycardia.

Table 29.14 (Continued)

ACC/AHA 2012 GL on stable IHD. Revascularization to improve symptoms with significant anatomical (>50% left main or >70% non-left main CAD) or physiological (FFR <0.80) coronary artery stenoses	
Clinical setting	
≥1 significant stenoses amenable to revascularization and unacceptable angina despite GDMT	I-A (CABG) I-A (PCI)
≥1 significant stenoses and unacceptable angina in whom GDMT cannot be implemented because of medication contraindications, adverse effects, or patient preferences	IIa-C (CABG) IIa-C (PCI)
Previous CABG with ≥1 significant stenoses associated with ischaemia and unacceptable angina despite GDMT	IIa-C (PCI) IIb-C (CABG)
Complex 3-vessel CAD (e.g. SYNTAX score >22) with or without involvement of the proximal LAD artery and a good candidate for CABG	IIa-B (CABG preferred over PCI)
Viable ischaemic myocardium that is perfused by coronary arteries that are not amenable to grafting	IIb-B (TMR as an adjunct to CABG)
No anatomical or physiological criteria for revascularization	III-C (harm-CABG) III-C (harm-PCI)

CABG indicates coronary artery bypass graft; CAD, coronary artery disease; COR, class of recommendation; FFR, fractional flow reserve; GDMT, guideline-directed medical therapy; LOE, level of evidence; N/A, not applicable; PCI, percutaneous coronary intervention; SYNTAX, Synergy between Percutaneous Coronary Intervention with TAXUS and Cardiac Surgery; and TMR, transmyocardial laser revascularization.
2012 ACCF/AHA/ACP/AATS/PCNA/SCAI/STS Guideline for the diagnosis and management of patients with stable ischemic heart disease. J Am Coll Cardiol. 2012; **60** :e44–e164.

ESC 2010 GL on revascularization. Indications for revascularization in stable angina or silent ischaemia		
	Subset of CAD by anatomy	
For prognosis	Left main >50%[a]	I-A
	Any proximal LAD >50%[a]	I-A
	2VD or 3VD with impaired LV function[a]	I-B
	Proven large area of ischaemia (>10% LV)	I-B
	Single remaining patent vessel >50% stenosis[a]	I-C
	IVD without proximal LAD and without >10% ischaemia	III-A
For symptoms	Any stenosis >50% with limiting angina or angina equivalent, unresponsive to OMT	I-A
	Dyspnoea/CHF and >10% LV ischaemia/viability supplied by >50% stenotic artery	IIa-B
	No limiting symptoms with OMT	III-C

[a] With documented ischaemia or FFR 0.80 for angiographic diameter stenoses 50–90%.
CAD, coronary artery disease; CHF, chronic heart failure; FFR, fractional flow reserve; LAD, left anterior descending; LV, left ventricle; OMT, optimal medical therapy; VD, vessel disease.

ESC 2010 GL on revascularization. Indications for coronary artery bypass grafting vs percutaneous coronary intervention in stable patients with lesions suitable for both procedures and low predicted surgical mortality

Subset of CAD by anatomy	**Favours CABG**	**Favours PCI**
IVD or 2VD—non-proximal LAD	IIb-C	I-C
IVD or 2VD—proximal LAD	I-A	IIa-B
3VD simple lesions, full functional revascularization achievable with PCI, SYNTAX score ≥22	I-A	IIa-B
3VD complex lesions, incomplete revascularization achievable with PCI, SYNTAX score >22	I-A	III-A

(Continued)

Table 29.14 (Continued)

Subset of CAD by anatomy	Favours CABG	Favours PCI
Left main (isolated or IVD, ostium/shaft)	I-A	IIa-B
Left main (isolated or IVD, distal bifurcation)	I-A	
Left main + 2VD or 3VD, SYNTAX score ≤32	I-A	IIa-B
Left main + 2VD or 3VD, SYNTAX score ≥33	I-A	

CABG, coronary artery bypass graft; CAD, coronary artery disease; LAD, left anterior descending; PCI, percutaneous coronary intervention; VD, vessel disease.

ESC 2010 GL on revascularization. Crossed revascularization procedures	
Following CABG	
In early graft failure	
Coronary angiography is indicated for highly symptomatic patients or in the event of post-operative instability or with abnormal biomarkers/ECG suggestive of perioperative MI.	I-C
Decision of redo CABG or PCI should be made by the Heart Team.	I-C
PCI is a superior alternative to reoperation in patients with early ischaemia after CABG.	I-B
The preferred target for PCI is the native vessel or ITA graft, not the freshly occluded SVG.	I-C
For freshly occluded SVG, redo CABG is recommended, rather than PCI, if the native artery appears unsuitable for PCI or several important grafts are occluded.	I-C
In late graft failure following CABG	
PCI or redo CABG is indicated in patients with severe symptoms or extensive ischaemia despite OMT.	I-B
PCI is recommended as a first choice, rather than redo CABG.	I-B
PCI of the bypassed native artery is the preferred approach when stenosed grafts >3 years old.	I-B
ITA is the conduit of choice for redo CABG.	I-B
Redo CABG should be considered for patients with several diseased grafts, reduced LV function, several CTO, or absence of a patent ITA.	IIa-C
PCI should be considered in patients with patent left ITA and amenable anatomy.	IIa-C
Following PCI	
In early failure following PCI	
Repeat PCI is recommended for early symptomatic restenosis after PCI.	I-B
Immediate CABG is indicated if failed PCI is likely to cause a large MI.	I-C
In late failure following PCI	
Patients with intolerable angina or ischaemia will eventually require CABG if:	
(a) Lesions are unsuitable for PCI.	I-C
(b) There is additional non-discrete disease progression in other vessels.	I-C
(c) Restenoses are repetitive, and interventional options are not favourable.	I-C

CABG, coronary artery bypass grafting; CTO, chronic total occlusion; ECG, electrocardiogram; ITA, internal thoracic artery; LV, left ventricle; MI, myocardial infarction; OMT, optimal medical therapy; PCI, percutaneous coronary intervention; SVG, saphenous vein graft.
ESC/EACTS Guidelines on myocardial revascularization The Task Force on Myocardial Revascularization of the European Society of Cardiology (ESC) and the European Association for Cardio-Thoracic Surgery (EACTS). *European Heart Journal*. 2010;**31**:2501–2555.

Table 29.15 Revascularization in special patient subsets

ESC 2010 GL on revascularization. Specific recommendations for diabetic patients	
Revascularization in stable patients with extensive CAD to improve MACCE-free survival.	I-A
Use of DES to reduce restenosis and repeat TVR.	I-A
In patients on metformin, renal function should be carefully monitored after coronary angiography/PCI.	I-C
CABG, rather than PCI, when the extent of the CAD justifies a surgical approach (especially MVD) and the patient's risk profile is acceptable.	IIa-B
In patients with known renal failure undergoing PCI, metformin may be stopped 48 h before the procedure.	IIb-C

(Continued)

Table 29.15 (Continued)

ESC 2010 GL on revascularization. Specific recommendations for diabetic patients	
Systematic use of GIK in diabetic patients undergoing revascularization.	III-B

DES, drug-eluting stent; GIK, glucose-insulin potassium; MACCE, major adverse cardiac and cerebral event; MVD, multivessel disease; MI, myocardial infarction; TVR, target vessel revascularization.

ESC 2010 GL on Revascularization. Specific recommendations for patients with mild to moderate chronic kidney disease	
CABG, rather than PCI, when the extent of the CAD justifies a surgical approach, the patient's risk profile is acceptable, and life expectancy is reasonable.	IIa-B
Off-pump CABG rather than on-pump CABG.	IIb-B
For PCI, DES rather than BMS.	IIb-C
ACCF/AHA 2011 GL on CABG. Renal dysfunction	
Off-pump CABG in patients with preoperative renal dysfunction (creatinine clearance <60 mL/min).	IIb-B
Maintenance of a perioperative haematocrit >19% and mean arterial pressure >60 mmHg in patients undergoing on-pump CABG.	IIb-C
Delay of surgery after coronary angiography until the effect of radiographic contrast material on renal function is assessed.	IIb-B
The effectiveness of pharmacological agents to provide renal protection during cardiac surgery is uncertain	IIb-B
ACCF/AHA 2011 GL on CABG. Patients with end-stage renal disease on dialysis	
CABG to improve survival rate in patients with end-stage renal disease undergoing CABG for left main coronary artery stenosis ≥50%.	IIb-C
CABG to improve survival rate or to relieve angina despite GDMT for patients with end-stage renal disease with significant stenoses (>70%) in three major vessels or in the proximal LAD artery plus one other major vessel, regardless of LV systolic function.	IIb-B
CABG in patients with end-stage renal disease whose life expectancy is limited by non-cardiac issues.	III-C

2011 ACCF/AHA Guideline for Coronary Artery Bypass Graft Surgery. *J Am Coll Cardiol*. 2011;**58**:e123–210.
ESC/EACTS Guidelines on myocardial revascularization The Task Force on Myocardial Revascularization of the European Society of Cardiology (ESC) and the European Association for Cardio-Thoracic Surgery (EACTS). *European Heart Journal*. 2010;**31**:2501–2555.

Table 29.16 Graft patency after CABG

Graft	Patency	Patency	Patency
	At 1 year	At 4–5 years	At 10–15 years
SVG	>90	65–80	25–50
Radial artery	86–96	89	ND
Left ITA	>91	88	88
Right ITA	ND	96	65

ITA, internal thoracic artery; ND, no data.
ESC/EACTS Guidelines on myocardial revascularization The Task Force on Myocardial Revascularization of the European Society of Cardiology (ESC) and the European Association for Cardio-Thoracic Surgery (EACTS). *European Heart Journal* 2010;**31**:2501–2555.

Table 29.17 Combined CABG and valve surgery

ACCF/AHA 2011 GL on CABG. Patients with concomitant valvular disease	
Cconcomitant aortic valve replacement in patients undergoing CABG who have at least moderate aortic stenosis.	I-B
Concomitant mitral valve repair or replacement at the time of CABG, in patients undergoing CABG who have severe ischaemic mitral valve regurgitation not likely to resolve with revascularization.	I-B
Concomitant mitral valve repair or replacement at the time of CABG, in patients undergoing CABG who have moderate ischaemic mitral valve regurgitation not likely to resolve with revascularization.	IIa-B
Concomitant aortic valve replacement when evidence (e.g. moderate-severe leaflet calcification) suggests that progression of the aortic stenosis may be rapid and the risk of the combined procedure is acceptable in patients undergoing CABG who have mild aortic stenosis.	IIb-C

2011 ACCF/AHA Guideline on CABG. *Circulation*. 2011;**124**:2610–42.

(Continued)

Table 29.17 (Continued)

ESC 2010 GL on revascularization. Recommendations for combined valve surgery and coronary artery bypass grafting	
Combined valve surgery and:	
CABG in patients with a primary indication for aortic/mitral valve surgery and coronary artery diameter stenosis >70%.	I-C
CABG in patients with a primary indication for aortic/mitral valve surgery and coronary artery diameter stenosis 50–70%.	IIa-C
Combined CABG and:	
Mitral valve surgery in patients with a primary indication for CABG and severe ischaemic mitral regurgitation and EF >30%.	I-C
Mitral valve surgery in patients with a primary indication for CABG and moderate ischaemic mitral regurgitation, provided valve repair is feasible and performed by experienced operators.	IIa-C
Aortic valve surgery in patients with a primary indication for CABG and moderate aortic stenosis (mean gradient 30–50 mmHg or Doppler velocity 3–4 m/s or heavily calcified aortic valve, even when Doppler velocity 2.5–3 m/s).	IIa-C

ESC Guidelines on myocardial revascularization. *Eur Heart J*.2010;**31**:2501–55.

Table 29.18 Technical aspects of CABG

ACCF/AHA 2011 GL on CABG	
The role of preoperative carotid artery non-invasive screening in CABG patients	
A multidisciplinary team approach (consisting of a cardiologist, cardiac surgeon, vascular surgeon, and neurologist) for patients with clinically significant carotid artery disease for whom CABG is planned.	I-C
Carotid artery duplex scanning in selected patients with high-risk features, i.e. age >65 years, left main coronary stenosis, peripheral artery disease, history of cerebrovascular disease (transient ischaemic attack, stroke, etc.), hypertension, smoking, and diabetes mellitus).	IIa-C
In previous transient ischaemic attack or stroke and a significant (50% to 99%) carotid artery stenosis, consider carotid revascularization in conjunction with CABG. The sequence and timing (simultaneous or staged) of carotid intervention and CABG should be determined by the patient's relative magnitudes of cerebral and myocardial dysfunction.	IIa-C
If there is no history of transient ischaemic attack or stroke, carotid revascularization may be considered in the presence of bilateral severe (70% to 99%) carotid stenoses or a unilateral severe carotid stenosis with a contralateral occlusion.	IIb-C
Patients with chronic obstructive pulmonary disease/respiratory insufficiency	
Preoperative intensive inspiratory muscle training is reasonable to reduce the incidence of pulmonary complications in patients at high risk for respiratory complications after CABG.	IIa-B
After CABG, non-invasive positive pressure ventilation may be reasonable to improve pulmonary mechanics and to reduce the need for reintubation.	IIb-B
High thoracic epidural analgesia may be considered to improve lung function after CABG.	IIb-B
Bypass graft conduit	
The left internal mammary artery (LIMA) should be used to bypass the LAD.	I-B
The right internal mammary artery to bypass the LAD when the LIMA is unavailable or unsuitable.	IIa-C
Use of a second internal mammary artery to graft the left circumflex or right coronary artery is reasonable.	IIa-B
Complete arterial revascularization in patients ≤60 years of age with few or no co-morbidities.	IIb-C
Arterial grafting of the right coronary artery may be reasonable when a critical (≥90%) stenosis is present.	IIb-B
Contraindicated in <90% RCA stenosis.	III-C
Use of a radial artery graft may be reasonable when grafting left-sided coronary arteries with severe stenoses (>70%) and right-sided arteries with critical stenoses (≥90%).	IIb-B
Preoperative antiplatelet therapy	
Aspirin (100 mg to 325 mg daily) to CABG patients preoperatively.	I-B
In patients referred for elective CABG, clopidogrel and ticagrelor should be discontinued for at least 5 days before surgery.	I-B
Prasugrel should be discontinued for at least 7 days	I-C
In patients referred for urgent CABG, clopidogrel and ticagrelor should be discontinued for at least 24 hours.	I-B

(Continued)

Table 29.18 (Continued)

In patients referred for CABG, short-acting intravenous glycoprotein IIb/IIIa inhibitors (eptifibatide or tirofiban) should be discontinued for at least 2 to 4 hours before surgery and abciximab for at least 12 hours beforehand.	I-B
In patients referred for urgent CABG, it may be reasonable to perform surgery less than 5 days after clopidogrel or ticagrelor has been discontinued and less than 7 days after prasugrel has been discontinued.	IIb-C
Perioperative beta blockers and antiarrhythmic drugs	
Beta blockers should be administered for at least 24 hours before CABG and should be reinstituted as soon as possible after CABG to all patients without contraindications to reduce the incidence or clinical sequelae of post-operative AF.	I-B
Beta blockers should be prescribed to all CABG patients without contraindications at the time of hospital discharge.	I-C
Beta blockers in patients without contraindications, particularly in those with LVEF >30% for reducing the risk of in-hospital mortality and perioperative myocardial ischaemia.	IIa-B
Intravenous administration of beta blockers in clinically stable patients unable to take oral medications is reasonable in the early post-operative period.	IIa-B
The effectiveness of preoperative beta blockers in reducing in-hospital mortality rate in patients with LVEF less than 30% is uncertain.	IIb-B
Preoperative administration of amiodarone to reduce the incidence of post-operative AF is reasonable for patients at high risk for post-operative AF who have contraindications to beta blockers.	IIa-B
Digoxin and non-dihydropyridine calcium channel blockers can be useful to control the ventricular rate in the setting of AF but are not indicated for prophylaxis.	IIa-B

2011 ACCF/AHA Guideline on CABG. *Circulation*. 2011;**124**:2610–42.

ESC 2010 GL on revascularization. Technical considerations for CABG	
Procedures should be performed in a hospital structure and by a team specialized in cardiac surgery, using written protocols.	I-B
Arterial grafting to the LAD system.	I-A
Complete revascularization with arterial grafting to non-LAD coronary systems in patients with reasonable life expectancy.	I-A
Minimization of aortic manipulation is recommended.	I-C
Graft evaluation before leaving the operating theatre.	I-C
ESC 2010 GL on revascularization. Prevention of AF after CABG	
Beta blockers to decrease the incidence of AF after CABG.	I-A
Sotalol to decrease the incidence of AF after CABG.	IIa-A
Amiodarone to decrease the incidence of AF after CABG.	IIa-A
Statins to decrease the incidence of AF after CABG.	IIa-B
Corticosteroids to decrease the incidence of AF after CABG.	IIb-B
Restoring sinus rhythm in patients having CABG in order to increase survival.	IIb-B
AF ablation during CABG may be considered an effective strategy.	IIb-C

ESC Guidelines on myocardial revascularization. *Eur Heart J*.2010;**31**:2501–55.

with death and/or MI.[126] The use of the **left internal thoracic artery** to the LAD is superior to venous grafts, and the right internal thoracic artery is preferable to the radial to the best recipient vessel after the LAD.[125,127] The use of bilateral internal thoracic arteries is safe, even in diabetics, despite a trend for more deep wound infections,[128–130] and multiple arterial grafts improve survival compared to vein grafts.[131] Bilateral internal thoracic artery grafting should also be considered even in patients >65 years of age.[132] A reduced risk of stroke with off-pump beating heart bypass surgery (**OPCAB**), that was suggested by a recent meta-analysis,[133] has not been verified in the largest randomized trials so far. Similar (CORONARY and GOPCABE trials)[134,135] or even worse outcomes (ROOBY trial)[136] with OPCAB have been reported, and the issue of less effective revascularization with this approach has been raised. However, off-pump surgery may be protective against new-onset ventricular arrhythmias,[137] and may be preferable in high-risk patients. In patients with a patent LIMA to the LAD artery and ischaemia in the distribution of the right or left circumflex coronary arteries, it is reasonable to recommend reoperative CABG to treat angina if medical therapy has failed and the coronary stenoses are not amenable to PCI (ACCF/AHA 2011 on CABG, IIa-B).

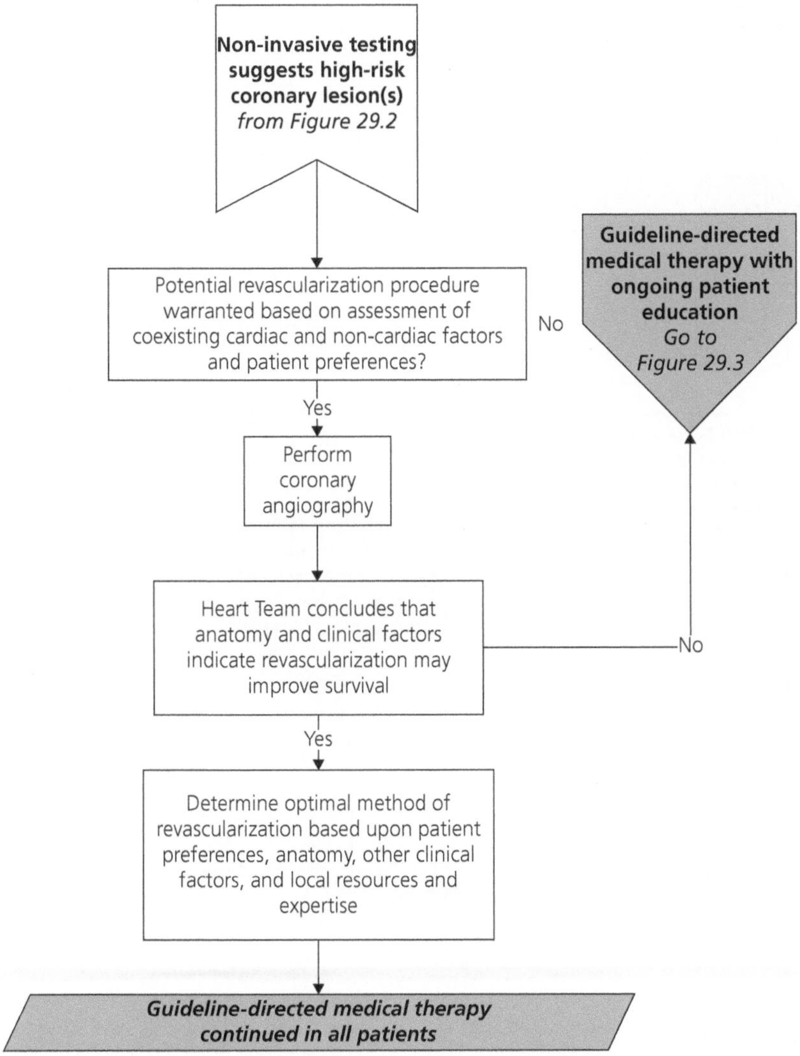

Figure 29.5 ACC/AHA GL 2012 on stable IHD. Algorithm for revascularization to improve survival of patients with SIHD.*

* Colours correspond to the class of recommendations in the ACCF/AHA (ie green is for Class I, yellow for IIa). The algorithms do not represent a comprehensive list of recommendations (see full guideline text for all recommendations).

2012 ACCF/AHA/ACP/AATS/PCNA/SCAI/STS Guideline for the diagnosis and management of patients with stable ischemic heart disease. *J Am Coll Cardiol.* 2012;**60**:e44–e164.

The European System for Cardiac Operative Risk Evaluation, **logistic EuroSCORE and EuroSCORE II** (http://www.euroscore.org) and the Society of Thoracic Surgeons **STS score** (http://riskcalc.sts.org) that is probably more accurate in high risk patients are useful guides for calculation of the intraoperative risk. If the patient has already received a stent, cangrelor, a selective P2Y12 inhibitor, may be more effective as bridging therapy than heparin.[138] Aortocoronary **saphenous vein graft aneurysms** occur, with an approximate incidence of 0.07%, as a late complication of CABG. They are associated with significant morbidity and mortality since they grow with time, and percutaneous or surgical management is recommended.[100] After CABG, patients should receive beta blockers (that should be started at least 24 h pre-op to reduce post-op AF, ACCF/AHA on CABG 2011 I-B), statins (ACCF/AHA 2011 I-A), and IV insulin to maintain a blood glucose <180 mg/dL while avoiding hypoglycaemia (ACCF/AHA 2011 I-B). Indications for concomitant valve surgery are presented in Table 29.17.

Choice of the graft conduit and perioperative medication are presented in Table 29.18.

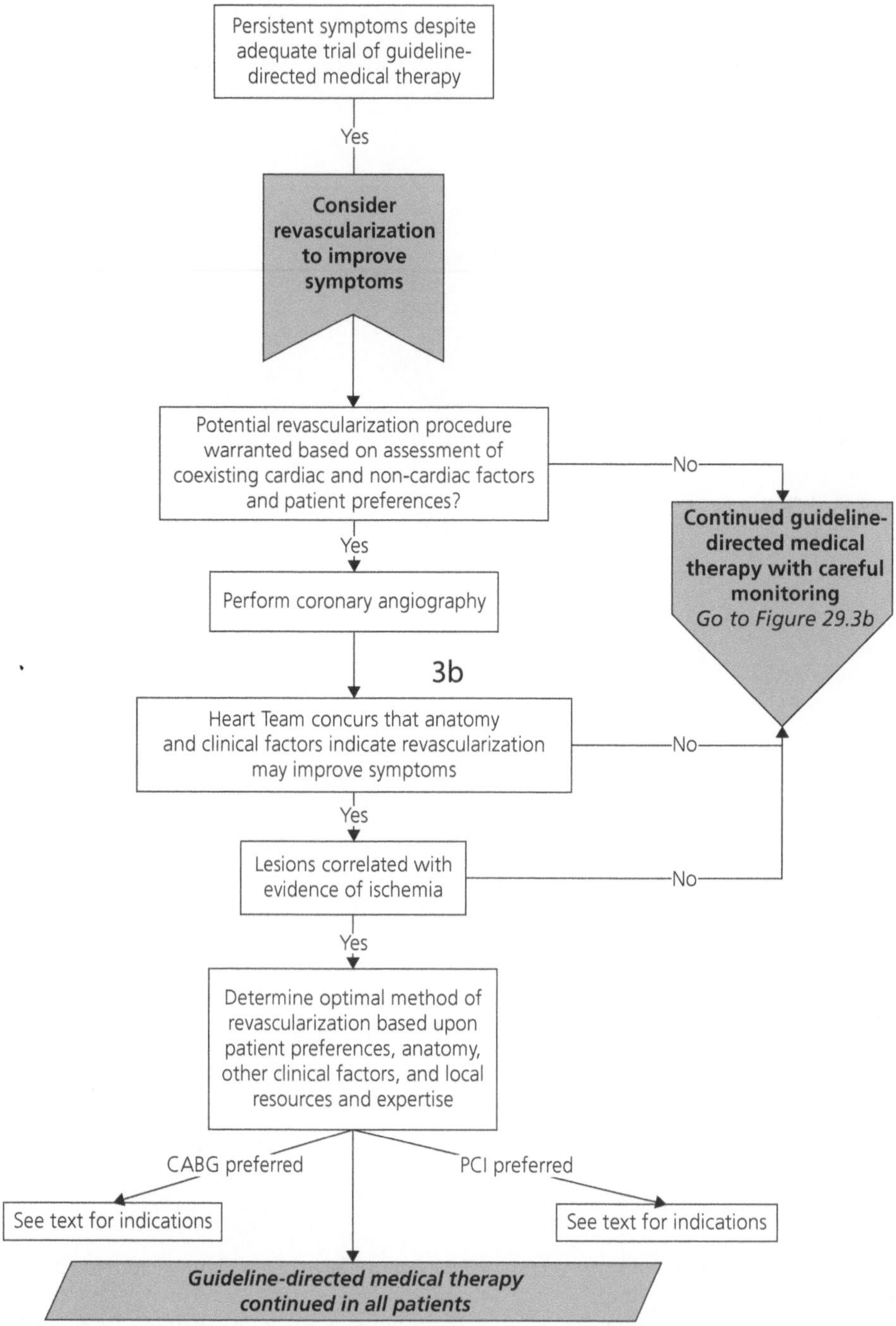

Figure 29.6 ACC/AHA 2012 GL on stable IHD. Algorithm for revascularization to improve symptoms of patients with SIHD.*

* Colours correspond to the class of recommendations in the ACCF/AHA. The algorithms do not represent a comprehensive list of recommendations (see full guideline text for all recommendations).

2012 ACCF/AHA/ACP/AATS/PCNA/SCAI/STS Guideline for the diagnosis and management of patients with stable ischemic heart disease. *J Am Coll Cardiol*. 2012;**60**:e44–e164.

Percutanous coronary intervention (PCI)

General recommendations on PCI are presented in Table 29.19. In the absence of acute coronary syndrome or recent myocardial infarction, elective percutaneous coronary intervention with balloon, bare meta stents (BMS), or drug-eluting stents (DES) has not been shown to improve survival or decrease the risk of MI compared to medical therapy alone, regardless of the use of stents.[139–142] PCI is associated with greater freedom from angina compared with medical therapy, although this benefit is attenuated with the use of modern, evidence-based medications.[143] BMS is superior to balloon, and DES is superior to BMS by decreasing target lesion revascularization but without any effect on mortality or the risk of MI.[144] The COURAGE trial enrolled 2287 patients with greater than 70% coronary stenosis in at least one proximal epicardial coronary artery and evidence of myocardial ischaemia or angina. For the composite of death and non-fatal MI, no statistical difference was found between the two groups after a mean follow-up of 4.6 years. Rates of angina were consistently lower in the PCI group than in the medical therapy group during follow-up but were no longer statistically significant at 5 years. Rates of subsequent revascularization were also lower in the PCI group.[145] There was a trend for better survival in a subgroup of patients with substantial ischaemia (>10% myocardium).[146] PCI may be beneficial in stable patients who had an MI within the previous 3 months,[139] particularly in the presence of residual ischaemia.[147] However, opening of an occluded artery beyond 24 hours after the MI in patients without residual ischaemia does not decrease the risk of death, re-infarction rate, or development of LV failure (Occluded Artery Trial).[148,149] Coronary lesions with fractional flow reserve (FFR) >0.8 can be safely left on medical therapy without intervention (DEFER, FAME, and FAME II trials).[150] Lesions with FFR<0.80 should be treated with PCI.[151] Approximately 12–38% of PCI performed on stable patients in the USA may not fulfill the appropriateness criteria of ACC.[152]

Although MIs frequently occur at sites of mild to moderate stenoses,[153,154] post-mortem examinations have demonstrated that ruptured plaques that lead to thrombosis more likely occur within the segment of significant stenoses.[155,156] The majority of ruptured plaques and half of thin cap fibroatheromas (i.e. vulnerable plaques) exhibit a >50% diameter stenosis.[157] Thus, subtotal occlusions of a vessel supplying non-infarcted myocardium, stenoses greater than 90% that, by definition, represent vulnerable plaques,[158] significant, complex lesions that are prone to develop total occlusions,[159] and stenoses with unequivocally reduced fractional flow reserve (<0.75%)[160] may represent optimal targets for PCI. However, randomized studies of PCI vs medical therapy to support this view are missing, although observational studies on registries argue in favour of PCI.[161] Possible explanations for the failure of PCI to improve prognosis might be the limited number of patients with proven ischaemia enrolled in these trials and the adoption of complex, elaborate techniques that have not proved their usefulness, but expose the patient to additional risk of iatrogenic MI (approximately 7% measured my CK-MB elevation)[162] that has prognostic significance, regardless of its extent.[163–166] PCI may reduce spontaneous MI compared to medical therapy, but at the expence of procedural MI that results in no difference in MI in total.[166] Additionally, PCI is directed at the lesions that cause ischaemic symptoms and does not change the natural history of coronary atherosclerosis in which non-obstructive lesions might progress suddenly to high-grade stenoses or vessel occlusion. These sites might have been bypassed by a coronary graft. The **in-hospital mortality of PCI is estimated 0.4–1.9% whereas periprocedural infarction is 0.4–4.9%**, and emergency CABG is required in 0.3% of patients.[27,167] In the National Cardiovascular Data Registry report, PCI in-hospital mortality was 1.27%, ranging from 0.65% in elective PCI to 4.81% in ST-segment elevation myocardial infarction patients.[168] Stent thrombosis with DES is 0.3–0.6% per year but with a potentially continuous steady rate up to 5 years.[169] Independent risk factors are acute coronary syndrome and target of proximal left anterior descending coronary artery for early and side branch stenting, diabetes mellitus, and end-stage renal disease, with or without haemodialysis, for late stent thrombosis, smoking, and total stent length >28 mm for late stent thrombosis.[153] Following stenting, clinical events occur in 25% of patients within the next 5 years, with a 10% incidence of death and 8.4% of myocardial infarction. New ischaemic perfusion defects (usually silent) are expected in 23% of patients, and 40% of them are due to disease progression not related to stents.[170] **DES** have been traditionally associated with a higher stent thrombosis rate than BMS (Figure 29.3), but this may not be true with second generation DES, such as cobalt-chromium everolimus-eluting stents, and dual antiplatelet therapy for at least 1 year after stent implantation.[171] IV cangrelor added to clopidogrel for PCI may reduce periprocedural ischemic events; the potential value of this strategy is not known when prasugrel or ticagrelor are used.[172]

PCI should be performed by operators with a workload of at least 75 cases per year in an institution performing more than 400, and certainly not less than 200, cases per year. On-site surgical backup is no more mandatory for elective PCI, provided there have been plans for rapid transport to a cardiac surgery operating room in a nearby hospital (Table 29.19). Rates of in-hospital mortality and emergency CABG for primary and non-primary PCI appear similar at centres with and without on-site surgery (CPORT and MASS COMM trials).[173–176]

Table 29.19 Technical aspects of PCI

ACCF/AHA/SCAI 2011 GL for PCI. Summary of recommendations for preprocedural considerations and interventions in patients undergoing PCI	
Contrast-induced AKI	
Patients should be assessed for risk of contrast-induced AKI before PCI.	I-C
Patients undergoing cardiac catheterization with contrast media should receive adequate preparatory hydration.	I-B
In patients with CKD (creatinine clearance <60 mL/min), the volume of contrast media should be minimized.	I-B
Administration of N-acetyl-L-cysteine is not useful for the prevention of contrast-induced AKI.	III-A (no benefit)
Anaphylactoid reactions	
Patients with prior evidence of an anaphylactoid reaction to contrast media should receive appropriate prophylaxis before repeat contrast administration.	I-B
In patients with a prior history of allergic reactions to shellfish or seafood, anaphylactoid prophylaxis for contrast reaction is not beneficial.	III-A (no benefit)
Statins	
Administration of a high-dose statin before PCI to reduce the risk of periprocedural MI.	IIa-A (statin-naive patient) IIa-B (chronic statin therapy)
Bleeding risk	
All patients should be evaluated for risk of bleeding before PCI.	I-C
CKD	
In patients undergoing PCI, the glomerular filtration rate should be estimated and the dosage of renally cleared medications should be adjusted.	I-B

AKI indicates acute kidney injury; CKD, chronic kidney disease; COR, class of recommendation; LOE, level of evidence; MI, myocardial infarction; N/A, not applicable; and PCI, percutaneous coronary intervention.

ACCF/AHA/SCAI 2011 GL on PCI. Antiplatelet and Antithrombin Pharmacotherapy at the time of PCI	
Oral antiplatelet agents	
Patients already on daily aspirin therapy, 81 mg to 325 mg before PCI.	I-B
Patients not on aspirin therapy, non-enteric aspirin 325 mg before PCI.	I-B
Loading dose of a P2Y 12 inhibitor with stenting.	I-A
Clopidogrel—600 mg loading dose.	I-B
Prasugrel—contraindicated in patients with prior TIA/CVA (III-B) Not recommended in patients >75 years of age. Lower maintenance dose in persons weighing <60 kg	I-B
Ticagrelor—issuess of patient compliance may be especially important.	I-B
GP IIb/IIIa inhibitors (abciximab, double-bolus eptifi batide, high-bolus dose tirofiban)	
No clopidogrel pre-treatment	IIa-B
Clopidogrel pretreatment	IIb-B
Antithrombin agents	
UFH Dosing based on whether or not GPI was administered	I- C
Bivalirudin—lower bleeding rates associated with bivalirudin are mitigated when used concomitantly with a GPI.	I -B
Enoxaparin—an additional dose of 0.3 mg/kg IV enoxaparin should be administered at the time of PCI to patients who have received <2 therapeutic SC doses (e.g. 1 mg/kg) or received the last SC enoxaparin dose 8 to 12 h before PCI (I-B) Patients treated with SC enoxaparin within 12 h of PCI should not receive additional treatment 'with UFH during PCI ('stacking') (III-B)	IIb-B
Anti-Xa inhibitors	
Fondaparinux—PCI should not be performed with fondaparinux as the sole antithrombin agent in patients treated with upstream fondaparinux. An additional anticoagulant with anti-IIa activity should beadministered.	III-C (harm)

ACT indicates activated clotting time; COR, class of recommendation; CVA, cerebrovascular accident; FDA, U.S. Food and Drug Administration; GP, glycoprotein; GPI, glycoprotein IIb/IIIa inhibitor; IC, intracoronary; IV, intravenous; LOE, level of evidence; MI, myocardial infarction; N/A, not applicable; PCI, percutaneous coronary intervention; SC, subcutaneous; SIHD, stable ischemic heart disease; STEMI, ST-elevation myocardial infarction; TIA, transient ischemic attack; UA/NSTEMI, unstable angina/non–ST-elevation myocardial infarction; and UFH, unfractionated heparin.

(Continued)

Table 29.19 (Continued)

Vascular access	
Use of radial artery access to decrease access site complications.	IIa-A
Adjunctive diagnostic/therapeutic devices	
Fractional flow reserve to assess angiographic intermediate coronary lesions (50% to 70% diameter stenosis) and can be useful for guiding revascularization decisions in patients with SIHD.	IIa-A
IVUS for the assessment of angiographically indeterminant left main CAD.	IIa-B
IVUS and coronary angiography 4 to 6 weeks and 1 year after cardiac transplantation to exclude donor CAD, detect rapidly progressive cardiac allograft vasculopathy, and provide prognostic information.	IIa-B
IVUS to determine the mechanism of stent restenosis.	IIa-C
IVUS for the assessment of non-left main coronary arteries with angiographically intermediate coronary stenosis (50% to 70% diameter stenosis).	IIb-B
IVUS for guidance of coronary stent implantation, particularly in cases of left main coronary artery stenting.	IIb-B
IVUS to determine the mechanism of stent thrombosis.	IIb-C
Not recommended when PCI or CABG is not being contemplated	III-C
Rotational atherectomy for fibrotic or heavily calcified lesions that might not be crossed by a balloon catheter or adequately dilated before stent implantation.	IIa-C
Rotational atherectomy should not be performed routinely for *de novo* lesions or in-stent restenosis.	III-A
Laser angioplasty for fibrotic or moderately calcified lesions that cannot be crossed or dilated with conventional balloon angioplasty.	IIb-C
Laser angioplasty should not be used routinely during PCI.	III-A
Cutting balloon angioplasty to avoid slippage-induced coronary artery trauma during PCI for in-stent restenosis or ostial lesions in side branches.	IIb-C
Cutting balloon angioplasty should not be used routinely during PCI.	III-A
Percutaneous haemodynamic support devices	
Elective insertion of an appropriate haemodynamic support device as an adjunct to PCI in carefully selected high-risk patients.	IIb-C
No-reflow pharmacological therapies	
Administration of an intracoronary vasodilator (adenosine, calcium channel blocker, or nitroprusside) to treat PCI-related no-reflow that occurs during primary or elective PCI.	IIa-B
Chronic total occlusions	
PCI of a chronic total occlusion in patients with appropriate clinical indications and suitable anatomy when performed by operators with appropriate expertise.	IIa-B
Saphenous vein grafts	
Embolic protection devices should be used during saphenous vein graft PCI when technically feasible.	I-B
Platelet GP IIb/IIIa inhibitors are not beneficial as adjunctive therapy during saphenous vein graft PCI.	III-B
PCI is not recommended for chronic saphenous vein graft occlusions.	III-C
Bifurcation lesions	
Provisional side branch stenting should be the initial approach inpatients with bifurcation lesions when the side branch is not large and has only mild or moderate focal disease at the ostium.	I-A
Vascular Bifurcation lesions	
Use elective double stenting in patients with complex bifurcation morphology involving a large side branch where the risk of side branch occlusion is high and the likelihood of successful side branch reaccess is low.	IIa-B
Aorto-ostial stenoses	
IVUS for the assessment of angiographically indeterminant IIa-B left main CAD.	IIa-B
Use of DES when PCI is indicated in patients with an aorto-ostial stenosis.	IIa-B
Coronary stents	
DES in high risk of restenosis and the patient is likely to be able to tolerate and comply with prolonged DAPT.	

(Continued)

Table 29.19 (Continued)

Elective PCI and STEMI.	I-A
UA/NSTEMI.	I-C
Balloon angioplasty or BMS in patients with high bleeding risk, inability to comply with 12 months of DAPT, or anticipated invasive or surgical procedures within the next 12 months.	I-B
PCI with coronary stenting should not be performed if the patient is not likely to be able to tolerate and comply with DAPT.	III-B
DES should not be implanted if the patient is not likely to be able to tolerate and comply with prolonged DAPT or this cannot be determined before stent implantation.	III-B
Restenosis	
Patients who develop clinical restenosis after balloon angioplasty should be treated with BMS or DES if anatomical factors are appropriate and if the patient is able to comply with and tolerate DAPT.	I-B
Patients who develop clinical restenosis after BMS should be treated with DES if anatomical factors are appropriate and the patient is able to comply with and tolerate DAPT.	I-A
Patients who develop clinical restenosis after DES may be considered for repeat PCI with balloon angioplasty, BMS, or DES containing the same drug or an alternative antiproliferative drug if anatomical factors are appropriate and the patient is able to comply with and tolerate DAPT.	IIb-C
Vascular closure devices	
Patients considered for vascular closure devices should undergo a femoral angiogram to ensure their anatomical suitability for deployment.	I-C
Use of vascular closure devices for the purposes of achieving faster haemostasis and earlier ambulation compared with the use of manual compression.	IIa-B
The routine use of vascular closure devices is not recommended for the purpose of decreasing vascular complications, including bleeding.	III-B
Clopidogrel genetic testing	
Genetic testing to identify whether a patient at high risk for poor clinical outcomes is predisposed to inadequate platelet inhibition with clopidogrel.	IIb-C
When a patient predisposed to inadequate platelet inhibition with clopidogrel is identified by genetic testing, treatment with an alternate P2Y12 inhibitor (e.g. prasugrel or ticagrelor).	IIb-C
Platelet function testing	
Platelet function testing may be considered in patients at high risk for poor clinical outcomes.	IIb-C
In patients treated with clopidogrel with high platelet reactivity, alternative agents, such as prasugrel or ticagrelor, might be considered.	IIb-C
Operator and institutional competency and volume	
Elective/urgent PCI should be performed by operators with an acceptable annual volume (≥75 procedures) at high-volume centres (>400 procedures) with on-site cardiac surgery.	I-C
Elective/urgent PCI should be performed by operators and institutions whose current risk-adjusted outcomes statistics are comparable to those reported in contemporary national data registries.	I-C
Primary PCI for STEMI should be performed by experienced operators who perform more than 75 elective PCI procedures per year and, ideally, at least 11 PCI procedures for STEMI per year. Ideally, these procedures should be performed in institutions that perform more than 400 elective PCIs per year and more than 36 primary PCI procedures for STEMI per year.	I-C
It is reasonable that operators with acceptable volume (≥75 PCI procedures/year) perform elective/urgent PCI at low-volume centres (200 to 400 PCI procedures/year) with on-site cardiac surgery.	IIa-C
Low-volume operators (≥75 PCI procedures per year) perform elective/urgent PCI at high-volume centres (>400 PCI procedures per year) with on-site cardiac surgery. Ideally, operators with an annual procedure volume of fewer than 75 procedures per year should only work at institutions with an activity level of more than 600 procedures per year. Operators who perform fewer than 75 procedures per year should develop a defined mentoring relationship with a highly experienced operator who has an annual procedural volume of at least 150 procedures.	IIa-C
The benefit of primary PCI for STEMI patients eligible for fibrinolysis when performed by an operator who performs fewer than 75 procedures per year (<11 PCIs for STEMI per year) is not well established.	IIb-C
It is not recommended that elective/urgent PCI be performed by low-volume operators (<75 procedures per year) at low-volume centres (200 to 400 procedures per year) with or without on-site cardiac surgery. An institution with a volume of fewer than 200 procedures per year, unless in a region that is underserved because of geography, should carefully consider whether it should continue to offer this service.	III-C

(Continued)

Table 29.19 (Continued)

PCI in hospitals without on-site surgical backup	
Primary PCI is reasonable in hospitals without on-site cardiac surgery, provided that appropriate planning for programme development has been accomplished.	IIa-B
Elective PCI might be considered in hospitals without on-site cardiac surgery, provided that appropriate planning for programme development has been accomplished and rigorous clinical and angiographic criteria are used for proper patient selection.	IIb-B
Primary or elective PCI should not be performed in hospitals without on-site cardiac surgery capabilities without a proven plan for rapid transport to a cardiac surgery operating room in a nearby hospital or without appropriate haemodynamic support capability for transfer.	III-C

2011 ACCF/AHA/SCAI Guideline for Percutaneous Coronary Intervention. A Report of the American College of Cardiology Foundation/American Heart Association Task Force on Practice Guidelines and the Society for Cardiovascular Angiography and Interventions. *J Am Coll Cardiol* 2011;**58**:e44–122.

ESC 2010 GL on revascularization. Specific PCI devices and pharmacotherapy

FFR-guided PCI is recommended for detection of ischaemia-related lesion(s) when objective evidence of vessel-related ischaemia is not available.	I-A
DES[d] are recommended for reduction of restenosis/reocclusion if no contraindication to extended DAPT.	I-A
Distal embolic protection is recommended during PCI of SVG disease to avoid distal embolization of debris and prevent MI.	I-B
Rotablation is recommended for preparation of heavily calcified or severely fibrotic lesions that cannot be crossed by a balloon or adequately dilated before planned stenting.	I-C
Manual catheter thrombus aspiration should be considered during PCI of the culprit lesion in STEMI.	IIa-A
For PCI of unstable lesions, IV abciximab should be considered for pharmacological treatment of no-reflow.	IIa-B
Drug-eluting balloons[d] should be considered for the treatment of in-stent restenosis after prior BMS.	IIa-B
Proximal embolic protection may be considered for preparation before PCI of SVG disease.	IIb-B
For PCI of unstable lesions, intracoronary or IV adenosine may be considered for pharmacological treatment of no-reflow.	IIb-B
Tornus catheter may be used for preparation of heavily calcified or severely fibrotic lesions that cannot be crossed by a balloon or adequately dilated before planned stenting.	IIb-C
Cutting or scoring balloons may be considered for dilatation of in-stent restenosis, to avoid slipping-induced vessel trauma of adjacent segments.	IIb-C
IVUS-guided stent implantation may be considered for unprotected left main PCI.	IIb-C
Mesh-based protection may be considered for PCI of highly thrombotic or SVG lesions.	IIb-C
For PCI of unstable lesions, intracoronary nitroprusside or other vasodilators may be considered for pharmacological treatment of no-reflow.	IIb-C

ESC/EACTS Guidelines on myocardial revascularization The Task Force on Myocardial Revascularization of the European Society of Cardiology (ESC) and the European Association for Cardio-Thoracic Surgery (EACTS). *European Heart Journal* 2010;**31**: 2501–2555.

a: Recommendation is only valid for specific devices with proven efficacy/safety profile, according to the respective lesion characteristics of the studies.

DAPT, dual antiplatelet therapy; DES, drug-eluting stent; FFR, fractional flow reserve; IVUS, intravascular ultrasound; MI, myocardial infarction; PCI, percutaneous coronary intervention; STEMI, ST-segment elevation myocardial infarction; SVG, saphenous vein graft.

ESC 2010 GL on revascularization. Recommendations for prevention of contrast-induced nephropathy

All patients with CKD		
OMT (including statins, beta blockers, and ACE inhibitors or sartans) is recommended.	Dose according to clinical indications.	I-A
Hydration with isotonic saline is recommended.	1 mL/kg/h 12 h before and continued for 24 h after the procedure (0.5 mL/kg/h if EF <35% or NYHA >2).	I-A
N-acetylcysteine administration may be considered.	600–1200 mg 24 h before and continued for 24 h after the procedure.	IIb-A
Infusion of sodium bicarbonate 0.84% may be considered.	1 h before: bolus = body weight in kg × 0.462 mEq IV infusion for 6 h after the procedure = body weight in kg × 0.154 mEq per hour.	IIb-A

(Continued)

Table 29.19 (Continued)

Patients with mild, moderate, or severe CKD		
Use of LOCM or IOCM is recommended.	<350 mL or <4 mL/kg	I^d-A^d
Patients with severe CKD		
Prophylactic haemofiltration 6 h before complex PCI should be considered.	Fluid replacement rate 1000 mL/h without weight loss and saline hydration, continued for 24 h after the procedure.	IIa-B
Elective haemodialysis is not recommended as a preventive measure.		III-B

ESC/EACTS Guidelines on myocardial revascularization The Task Force on Myocardial Revascularization of the European Society of Cardiology (ESC) and the European Association for Cardio-Thoracic Surgery (EACTS). *European Heart Journal* 2010: **31**: 2501–2555.

There has been some evidence that concomitant balloon counterpulsation may improve long-term outcomes in high-risk patients undergoing PCI.[177,178] In patients with chronic kidney disease, either an isosmolar or a low molecular weight, other than ioxaglate or iohexol, contrast medium has been previously recommended, but subsequent studies on this issue have been contradictory to allow certain recommendations. N-acetylcysteine does not appear to be beneficial.[179] A recently verified policy is to administer 250 mL of normal saline solution over 30 min and IV furosemide (0.5 mg/kg up to a maximum of 50 mg), approximately 90 min before the coronary procedure, and perform the procedure when a urine output >300 mL/h is achieved. Additional doses of furosemide (up to a maximal cumulative dose of 2.0 mg/kg) are given in cases where the urine output is <300 mL/h during treatment, and matched hydration is continued for 4 h after the last contrast dose.[180] High-dose statin such as atorvastatin 80 mg within 24 hour preprocedure, may also reduce contrast-induced renal injury.[181] Although the use of closure devices is not recommended on a routine basis by the ACC/AHA/SCAI 2011 guideline on PCI, their use may decrease complications, even after elective intervention.[182]

PCI vs CABG

Studies comparing CABG to PCI with balloon or BMS, in general, have shown similar 5-year mortality rates in patients with single or multivessel disease.[183–186] Repeat revascularization is consistently lowered with CABG but at a probable risk of higher stroke rate compared to PCI.[182–185] The large New York state registry of 60 000 patients has reported an advantage of CABG in the presence of two-vessel disease with proximal LAD stenosis.[187] No difference in outcome after CABG or PCI has been shown in patients with isolated proximal LAD disease.[189] CABG is superior in patients with severe, multivessel disease, and especially diabetics.[189-193] The BARI 2D trial in diabetics detected similar rates of death and major adverse cardiac events between PCI or CABG and optimum pharmacological therapy. Repeat revascularizations were more frequent in the drug treatment group, and patients with more complex coronary artery disease, as treated by CABG, had a greater benefit of early revascularization.[189] In the FREEDOM trial, 1900 patients with diabetes were randomLy assigned to undergo either CABG or PCI with DES.[190] After 5 years of follow-up, the 947 patients assigned to undergo CABG had significantly lower mortality (10.9% vs 16.3%) and fewer myocardial infarctions (6.0% vs 13.9%) than the 953 patients assigned to undergo PCI. However, patients in the CABG group had significantly more strokes (5.2% vs 2.4%), mostly because of strokes that occurred within 30 days after revascularization. In the SYNTAX trial, 1800 patients with previously untreated left main stem or three-vessel disease were randomly assigned to undergo CABG or PCI with DES.[194] Five-year all-cause mortality and stroke were not significantly diferent between CABG (11.4% and 3.7%, respectively) and PCI (13.9% and 2.4%, respectively. Major adverse cerebrovascular and cardiac rates were significantly increased with PCI in patients with intermediate SYNTAX Score, ie23–32, (36.0% vs 25.8%, p=0.008) or high ie >33 SYNTAX Score (44.0% vs 26.8%, <0.0001). Adverse rates were not significantly different for patients with a low (0–22) baseline SYNTAX score. A higher rate of stroke in the CABG group was detected at the first year of follow-up. These results suggest that CABG remains the standard of care for patients with complex disease (intermediate or high SYNTAX scores); however, PCI may be an acceptable alternative revascularization method to CABG when treating patients with less complex disease, but its superiority over medical therapy alone is not proven. The SYNTAX II Score may be a more useful guide for decision making between CABG and PCU in this respect.[195] The ASCERT study recently reported results from the ACC PCI and STS CABG registries: among patients older than 65 years and with two- or three-vessel CAD that did not require emergency therapy, CABG offered a better survival compared to PCI (mortality rates 16.4% vs 20.7%, RR: 0.79, 95% CI: 0.76–0.82).[196] In a recent extensive analysis of Medicare beneficiaries, aged >=66 years, multivessel CABG was associated with lower long-term mortality than multivessel PCI. Patients with diabetes, heart failure, peripheral arterial disease, or tobacco use had the largest predicted differences in survival after CABG, whereas those with none of these factors had slightly better survival after PCI.[194] Thus, PCI is considered inappropriate for left main stenosis and additional CAD with intermediate to high CAD burden (multiple diffuse lesions, presence of chronic total occlusion, or high SYNTAX score), or triple-vessel CAD and high CAD burden.[33] PCI may also be used for unprotected left main stem lesions[198] (see Table 29.14), and double kissing crush stenting is preferred for unprotected distal left main bifurcation lesions.[199] In conclusion, according to available evidence:

- No revascularization is indicated in asymptomatic or mildly symptomatic patients, no **moderate or significant ischaemia on non-invasive testing or only a small area of viable myocardium or one- or two-vessel CAD without proximal LAD involvement, or an occluded vessel after MI and no significant residual ischaemia.**
- **In left main disease (>50% and demonstration of ischaemia) or triple-vessel disease with LVEF < 50% or proximal LAD involvement, or triple-vessel CAD with high CAD burden, or triple-vessel CAD in diabetics,** CABG is indicated.
- **For patients with one- or two-vessel disease,** data are not definitive and the superiority of revascularization over medical therapy is not proven. CABG is probably indicated in patients with symptoms and documented extensive ischaemia and with two-vessel disease with LVEF <50%, particularly in the presence of proximal LAD disease, and probably diabetes. PCI may be indicated in one- or two-vessel disease with FFR <0.80, or in the presence of significant ischaemia, or if angina persists despite optimum medical therapy.

Hybrid coronary revascularization

Hybrid coronary revascularization (defined as the planned combination of LIMA-to-LAD artery grafting and PCI of ≥1 non-LAD coronary arteries) is reasonable in patients with heavily calcified proximal aorta or poor target vessels for CABG (but amenable to PCI) or unfavourable LAD artery for PCI (i.e. excessive vessel tortuosity or chronic total occlusion (ACCF/AHA 2011 on CABG, IIa-B). It can also be considered as an alternative to multivessel PCI or CABG in an attempt to improve the overall risk-benefit ratio of the procedures (ACCF/AHA 2011 on CABG, IIb-C, ESC 2010 on revascularization IIb-B).

Long-term therapy

Measures for secondary prevention are implemented, as described in Tables 29.12 and 29.13. Detailed recommendations on prevention have been released by the ACC/AHA[59] and the ESC.[200] Echocardiography and tests for ischaemia are indicated when new symptoms appear (Table 29.20). Annual treadmill exercise testing in patients who have no change in clinical status may also be performed in moderate- or high-risk patients. In patients entering a formal cardiac rehabilitation programme after PCI, treadmill exercise testing is reasonable (ACCF/AHA 2011 PCI, IIa-C), but routine periodic stress testing of asymptomatic patients after PCI without specific clinical indications are not recommended (ACCF/AHA 2011 PCI, III-C). Sexual activity is allowed in patients who can exercise >3 to 5 METS without angina, excessive dyspnoea, ischaemic ST segment changes, cyanosis, hypotension, or arrhythmia (AHA 2012 on sexual activity and CVD, IIa-C), 1 or more weeks after uncomplicated MI (IIa-C), several days after PCI if the vascular access site is without complications (IIa-C), and 6–8 weeks after CABG, provided the sternotomy is well healed (IIa-B).

Evaluation and risk assessment before non-cardiac surgery

Although current perioperative risk prediction models place greater emphasis on CAD, patients with HF or AF have a significantly higher risk of post-operative mortality than patients with CAD, and even minor procedures carry a risk higher than previously appreciated.[201] Recommendations by the ACC/AHA 2009 guidelines on perioperative cardiovascular evaluation are presented in Tables 29.21 to 29.23 and Figure 29.7.[202] The role of preoperative beta blockers has been questioned,[203] and the ESC guidelines are being reconsidered in this respect.[204] There has also been recent evidence that the earliest optimal time for elective surgery is 46 to 180 days after bare metal stent implantation or >180 days after drug-eluting stent implantation (Figure 29.8).[202] Recommendations on cardiac disease evaluation and management in kidney and liver transplantation candidates have been recently published by AHA/ACCF.[205] Transplantation is generally not recommended 4 weeks after balloon angioplasty, 3 months after BMS, and 12 months after DES. In case of urgent surgery, however, clopidogrel must be stopped for 5 days, or even continued in case of low bleeding risk.

Table 29.20 Follow-up of CAD patients

ACCF/AHA 2012 GL on stable CAD. Follow-up non-invasive testing in patients with known SIHD: new, recurrent, or worsening symptoms not consistent with UA

Test	Exercise status		ECG interpretable			Additional considerations
	Able	Unable	Yes	No		
Patients able to exercise*						
Exercise ECG	X		X		I-B	
Exercise with nuclear MPI or echo	X			X	I-B	
Exercise with nuclear MPI or echo	X		Any		IIa-B	◆ Prior requirement for imaging with exercise ◆ Known or at high risk for multivessel disease
Pharmacological stress nuclear MPI/echo/CMR	X		X		III-C (no benefit)	
Patients unable to exercise						
Pharmacological stress nuclear MPI or echo		X	Any		I-B	
Pharmacological stress CMR		X	Any		IIa-B	
Exercise ECG		X		X	III-C (no benefit)	
Irrespective of ability to exercise						
CCTA	Any		Any		IIb-B	Patency of CABG or coronary stent ≥3 mm diameter
CCTA	Any		Any		IIb-B	In the absence of known moderate or severe calcification and intent to assess coronary stent <3 mm in diameter
CCTA	Any		Any		III-C (no benefit)	Known moderate or severe native coronary calcification or assessment of coronary stent <3 mm in diameter in patients who have new or worsening symptoms not consistent with UA

* Patients are candidates for exercise testing if they are capable of performing at least moderate physical functioning (i.e. moderate household, yard, or recreational work **and** most activities of daily living) and have no disabling co-morbidity. Patients should be able to achieve 85% of age-predicted maximum heart rate.
CABG indicates coronary artery bypass graft surgery; CCTA, cardiac computed tomography angiography; CMR, cardiac magnetic resonance; ECG, electrocardiogram; echo, echocardiography; MPI, myocardial perfusion imaging; N/A, not available; SIHD, stable ischaemic heart disease; and UA, unstable angina.
2012 ACCF/AHA/ACP/AATS/PCNA/SCAI/STS Guideline for the diagnosis and management of patients with stable ischemic heart disease. *J Am Coll Cardiol.* 2012;**60**:e44–e164.

Non-invasive testing in known SIHD: asymptomatic (or stable symptoms)

Test	Exercise status		ECG interpretable		Pretest probability of ischaemia		Additional considerations
	Able*	Unable	Yes	No			
Exercise or pharmacological stress with nuclear MPI, echo, or CMR at ≥2-year intervals		X		X	Prior evidence of silent ischaemia or high risk for recurrent cardiac event. Meets criteria listed in additional considerations.	IIa-C	a) Unable to exercise to adequate workload, or b) Uninterpretable ECG, or c) History of incomplete coronary revascularization
Exercise ECG at ≥1-year intervals	X		X		Any	IIb-C	a) Prior evidence of silent ischaemia, OR b) At high risk for recurrent cardiac event

(Continued)

Table 29.20 (Continued)

Test	Exercise status		ECG interpretable		Pretest probability of ischaemia		Additional considerations
	Able*	**Unable**	**Yes**	**No**			
Exercise ECG	X		X		No prior evidence of silent ischaemia and not at high risk of recurrent cardiac event.	IIb-C	For annual surveillance
Exercise or pharmacological stress with nuclear MPI, echo, or CMR or CCTA	Any		Any		Any	III-C (no benefit)	a) <5-year intervals after CABG, or b) <2-year intervals after PCI

* Patients are candidates for exercise testing if they are capable of performing at least moderate physical functioning (i.e. moderate household, yard, or recreational work **and** most activities of daily living) and have no disabling co-morbidity. Patients should be able to achieve 85% of age-predicted maximum heart rate.

CABG indicates coronary artery bypass graft surgery; CCTA, cardiac computed tomography angiography; CMR, coronary magnetic resonance; CCTA, computed tomography angiography; CMR, cardiac magnetic resonance; ECG, electrocardiogram; echo, echocardiography; MPI, myocardial perfusion imaging; N/A, not available; PCI, percutaneous coronary intervention; and SIHD, stable ischaemic heart disease.

ESC 2010 GL on revasularization

Strategies for follow-up and management in asymptomatic patients after myocardial revascularization	
Stress imaging (stress echo or MPS) should be used rather than stress ECG.	I-A
With low-risk findings (+) at stress testing, it is recommended to reinforce optimal medical therapy and lifestyle changes.	IIa-C
With high- to intermediate-risk findings (++) at stress testing, coronary angiography is recommended.	IIa-C
Early imaging testing should be considered in specific patient subsets.*	IIa-C
Routine stress testing may be considered >2 years after PCI and >5 years after CABG.	IIb-C
Strategies for follow-up and management in symptomatic patients after myocardial revascularization	
Stress imaging (stress echo or myocardial perfusion stress) rather than stress ECG.	I-A
It is recommended to reinforce optimal medical therapy and lifestyle changes in patients with low-risk findings (+) at stress testing.	I-B
With intermediate- to high-risk findings (++) at stress testing, coronary angiography is recommended.	I-C
Emergent coronary angiography is recommended in patients with STEMI.	I-A
Early invasive strategy is indicated in high-risk NSTE-ACS patients.	I-A
Elective coronary angiography is indicated in low-risk NSTE-ACS patients.	I-C

* Specific patient subsets indicated for early stress testing with imaging:
- Predischarge or early post-discharge imaging stress test in STEMI patients treated with primary PCI or emergency CABG;
- Patients with safety critical professions (e.g. pilots, drivers, divers) and competitive athletes;
- Users of 5-phosphodiesterase inhibitors;
- Patients who would like to be engaged in recreational activities for which high oxygen consumption is required;
- Patients resuscitated from sudden death;
- Patients with incomplete or suboptimal revascularization, even if asymptomatic;
- Patients with a complicated course during revascularization (perioperative MI, extensive dissection during PCI, endarterectomy during CABG, etc.);
- Patients with diabetes (especially those requiring insulin);
- Patients with MVD and residual intermediate lesions or with silent ischaemia.

(+) Low-risk findings at stress imaging are ischaemia at high workload, late-onset ischaemia, single zone of low-grade wall motion abnormality or small reversible perfusion defect, or no evidence of ischaemia.

(++) Intermediate- and high-risk findings at stress imaging are ischaemia at low workload, early-onset ischaemia, multiple zones of high-grade wall motion abnormality, or reversible perfusion defect.

ESC/EACTS Guidelines on myocardial revascularization The Task Force on Myocardial Revascularization of the European Society of Cardiology (ESC) and the European Association for Cardio-Thoracic Surgery (EACTS). *European Heart Journal* 2010; **31**: 2501–2555.

Table 29.21 ACCF/AHA 2009 GL on perioperative cardiovascular evaluation. Cardiac risk (combined incidence of cardiac death and nonfatal MI) stratification for non-cardiac surgical procedures

Risk stratification	Procedure examples
Vascular (reported cardiac risk often more than 5%)	Aortic and other major vascular surgery Peripheral vascular surgery
Intermediate (reported cardiac risk generally 1% to 5%)	Intraperitoneal and intrathoracic surgery Carotid endarterectomy Head and neck surgery Orthopaedic surgery Prostate surgery
Low† (reported cardiac risk generally less than 1%)	Endoscopic procedures Superficial procedure Cataract surgery Breast surgery Ambulatory surgery

† These procedures do not generally require further preoperative cardiac testing.
2009 ACCF/AHA focused update on perioperative beta blockade incorporated into the ACC/AHA 2007 guidelines on perioperative cardiovascular evaluation and care for noncardiac surgery. *J Am Coll Cardiol*. 2009; **54**: e13-e118.

Table 29.22 ACCF/AHA 2009. Perioperative cardiovascular evaluation

Patients who have a need for emergency non-cardiac surgery should proceed to the operating room and continue perioperative surveillance and post-operative risk stratification and risk factor management.	I-C
Patients undergoing low-risk surgery are recommended to proceed to planned surgery.	I-B
Patients with poor (<4 METs) or unknown functional capacity and no clinical risk factors* should proceed with planned surgery.	I-B
Patients with functional capacity ≥4 METs without symptoms proceed to planned surgery.	I-B
Preoperative resting 12-lead ECG is recommended for patients with at least one clinical risk factor.*	I-B
Patients with poor (<4 METs) or unknown functional capacity and no clinical risk factors should proceed with planned surgery.	I-B
LV function assessment is indicated in patients with dyspnoea of unknown origin to undergo preoperative evaluation of LV function.	I-C
Patients with poor (<4 METs) or unknown functional capacity and three, or more, clinical risk factors who are scheduled for intermediate-risk surgery proceed with planned surgery with heart rate control.	IIa-B
Stress testing may be considered for patients with at least one to two clinical risk factors and poor functional capacity (less than 4 METs) who require intermediate-risk or vascular surgery.	IIb-B

* Clinical risk factors include history of ischaemic heart disease, history of compensated or prior heart failure, history of cerebrovascular disease, diabetes mellitus, and renal insufficiency (defined in the Revised Cardiac Risk Index as a preoperative serum creatinine of greater than 2 mg/dL).
2009 ACCF/AHA focused update on perioperative beta blockade incorporated into the ACC/AHA 2007 guidelines on perioperative cardiovascular evaluation and care for noncardiac surgery. *J Am Coll Cardiol*. 2009; **54**: e13-e118.

Table 29.23 Revascularization before non-cardiac surgery

ACCF/AHA 2011 GL on PCI. Revascularization before non-cardiac surgery	
For patients who require PCI and are scheduled for elective non-cardiac surgery in the subsequent 12 months, a strategy of balloon angioplasty, or BMS implantation followed by 4 to 6 weeks of DAPT, is reasonable.	IIa-B
For patients with DES who must undergo urgent surgical procedures that mandate the discontinuation of DAPT, it is reasonable to continue aspirin if possible and restart the P2Y12 inhibitor as soon as possible in the immediate post-operative period.	IIa-C
Routine prophylactic coronary revascularization should not be performed in patients with stable CAD before non-cardiac surgery.	III-B
Elective non-cardiac surgery should not be performed in the 4 to 6 weeks after balloon angioplasty or BMS implantation or the 12 months after DES implantation in patients in whom the P2Y12 inhibitor will need to be discontinued perioperatively.	III-B
ACCF/AHA 2009 GL on perioperative evaluation. Recommendations for perioperative beta blocker therapy	
Beta blockers should be continued in patients undergoing surgery who are receiving beta blockers for treatment of conditions with AACF/AHA Class I indications.	I-C
Beta blockers titrated to heart rate and blood pressure are probably recommended for patients undergoing vascular** or intermediate-risk surgery who are at high cardiac risk due to coronary artery disease, positive cardiac ischaemia tests, or >1 clinical factor.*	IIa-B
The usefulness of beta blockers is uncertain in the presence of a single clinical risk factor but absence of coronary artery disease.	IIb-C

* Clinical risk factors include history of ischaemic heart disease, history of compensated or prior heart failure, history of cerebrovascular disease, diabetes mellitus, and renal insufficiency (defined in the Revised Cardiac Risk Index as a preoperative serum creatinine of greater than 2 mg/dL).
** Vascular surgery is defined by emergency aortic and other major vascular surgery and peripheral vascular surgery.
2011 ACCF/AHA/SCAI Guideline on percutaneous coronary intervention. *J Am Coll Cardiol*. 2011; **58**:e44–122.
2009 ACCF/AHA focused update on perioperative beta blockade incorporated into the ACC/AHA 2007 guidelines on perioperative cardiovascular evaluation and care for noncardiac surgery. *J Am Coll Cardiol*. 2009; **54**:e13–e118.

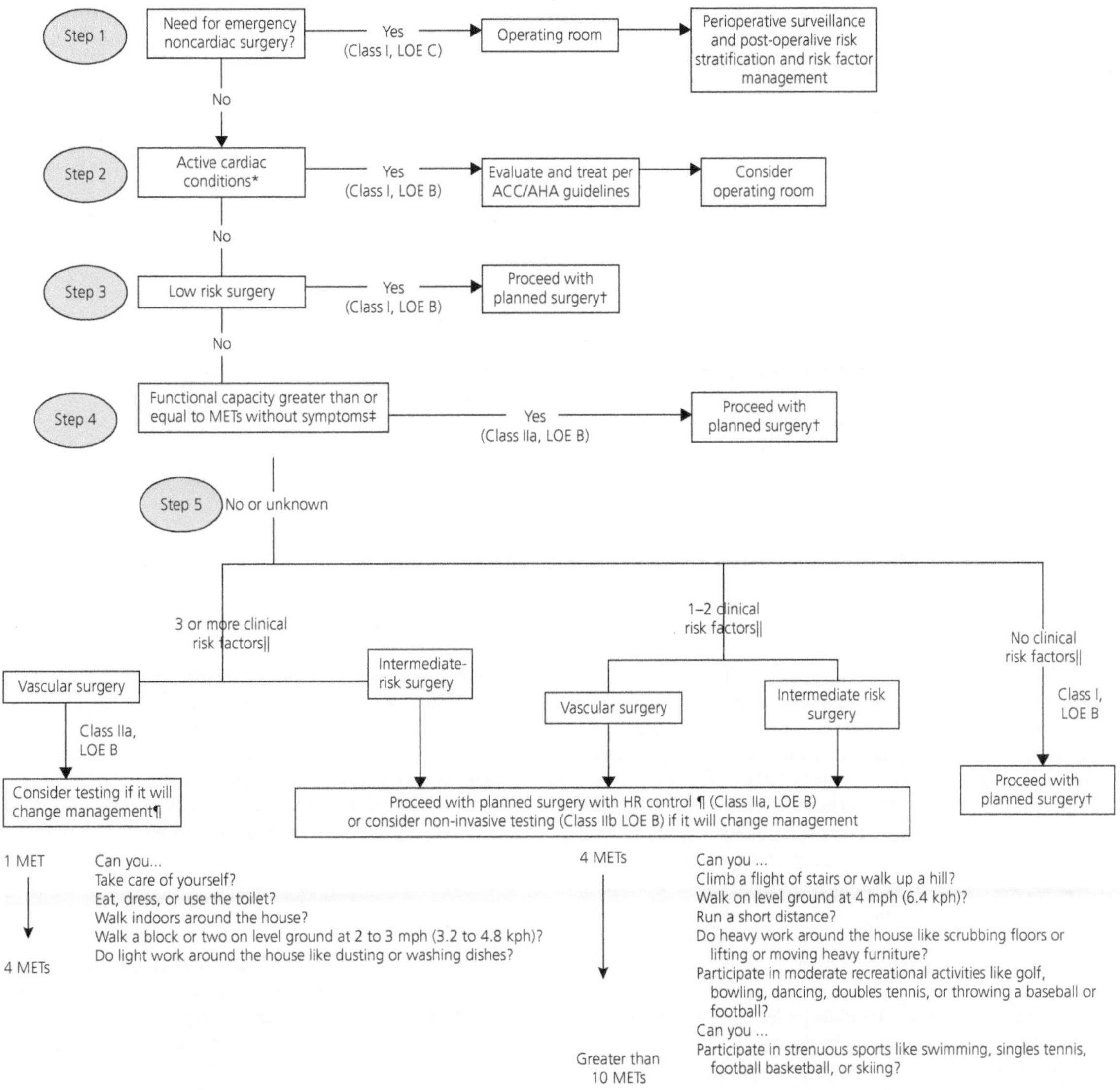

Figure 29.7 ACC/AHA 2009 on perioperative cardiovascular evaluation. Cardiac evaluation and care algorithm for non-cardiac surgery based on active clinical conditions, known cardiovascular disease, or cardiac risk for patients 50 years of age or greater.

‡ MET level equivalent are indicated.

§ Non-invasive testing may be considered before surgery in specific patients with risk factors if it will change management.

//Clinical risk factors include ischaemic heart disease, compensated or prior heart failure, diabetes mellitus, renal insufficiency, and cerebrovascular disease.

¶ Consider perioperative beta blockade for populations in which this has been shown to reduce cardiac morbidity/mortality.

HR, heart rate; LOE, level of evidence; and MET, metabolic equivalent.
2009 ACCF/AHA focused update on perioperative beta blockade incorporated into the ACC/AHA 2007 guidelines on perioperative cardiovascular evaluation and care for noncardiac surgery. *J Am Coll Cardiol*. 2009; 24;**54**:e13–e118.

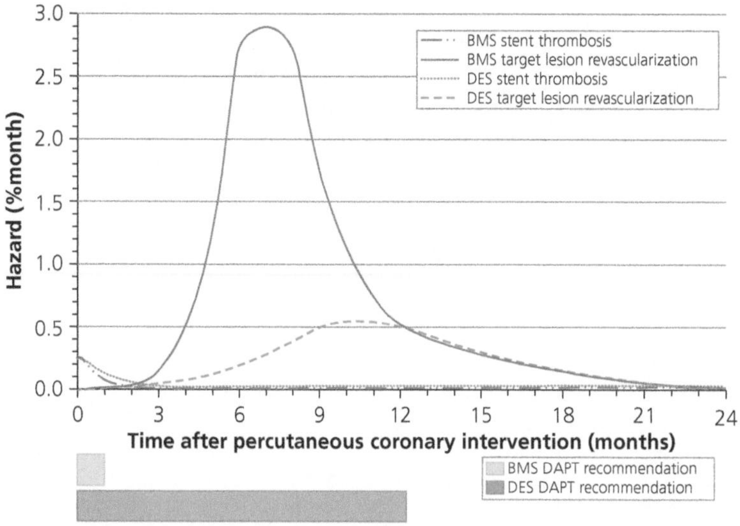

Figure 29.8 Hazard of stent thrombosis and target lesion revascularization over time according to type of stent.
Matteau A, Mauri L. Optimal timing of noncardiac surgery after stents, *Circulation*. 2012;**126**:1322–4.

References

1. Fox K, *et al.* Guidelines on the management of stable angina pectoris: executive summary: the Task Force on the management of stable angina pectoris of the European Society of Cardiology. *Eur Heart J.* 2006;**27**:1341–81
2. Fihn SD GJ, *et al.* ACCF/AHA/ACP/AATS/PCNA/SCAI/STS guideline for the diagnosis and management of patients with stable ischaemic heart disease: a report of the American College of Cardiology Foundation/American Heart Association Task Force on Practice Guidelines, and the American College of Physicians, American Association for Thoracic Surgery, Preventive Cardiovascular Nurses Association, Society for Cardiovascular Angiography and Interventions, and Society of Thoracic Surgeons. *J Am Coll Cardiol.* 2012;**60**:e44–164.
3. Shaw LJ, *et al.* Comparative effectiveness of exercise electrocardiography with or without myocardial perfusion single photon emission computed tomography in women with suspected coronary artery disease: results from the What Is the Optimal Method for Ischemia Evaluation in Women (WOMEN) trial. *Circulation.* 2011;**124**:1239–49
4. Uthamalingam S, *et al.* Exercise-induced ST-segment elevation in ECG lead aVR is a useful indicator of significant left main or ostial LAD coronary artery stenosis. *JACC Cardiovasc Imaging.* 2011;**4**:176–86
5. Sicari R, *et al.* Stress echocardiography expert consensus statement: European Association of Echocardiography (EAE) (a registered branch of the ESC). *Eur J Echocardiogr.* 2008;**9**:415–37
6. Pereztol-Valdes O, *et al.* Correspondence between left ventricular 17 myocardial segments and coronary arteries. *Eur Heart J.* 2005;**26**:2637–43
7. Shah BN, *et al.* The hibernating myocardium: Current concepts, diagnostic dilemmas, and clinical challenges in the post-STICH era. *Eur Heart J.* 2005;**26**:2637–43
8. Hundley WG, *et al.* ACCF/ACR/AHA/NASCI/SCMR 2010 expert consensus document on cardiovascular magnetic resonance: a report of the American College of Cardiology Foundation Task Force on Expert Consensus Documents. *Circulation.* 2010;**121**:2462–508
9. Blankstein R, *et al.* Selecting a non-invasive imaging study after an inconclusive exercise test. *Circulation.* 2010;**122**:1514–18
10. Mark DB, *et al.* ACCF/ACR/AHA/NASCI/SAIP/SCAI/SCCT 2010 expert consensus document on coronary computed tomographic angiography: a report of the American College of Cardiology Foundation Task Force on Expert Consensus Documents. *Circulation.* 2010;**121**:2509–43
11. Hoffmann U, *et al.* Coronary CT angiography versus standard evaluation in acute chest pain. *N Engl J Med.* 2012;**367**:299–308
12. Litt HI, *et al.* CT angiography for safe discharge of patients with possible acute coronary syndromes. *N Engl J Med.* 2012;**366**:1393–403
13. Achenbach S, *et al.* Coronary computed tomography angiography with a consistent dose below 1 msv using prospectively electrocardiogram-triggered high-pitch spiral acquisition. *Eur Heart J.* 2010;**31**:340–6
14. Taylor AJ, *et al.* ACCF/SCCT/ACR/AHA/ASE/ASNC/NASCI/SCAI/SCMR 2010 appropriate use criteria for cardiac computed tomography. A report of the American College of Cardiology Foundation Appropriate Use Criteria Task Force, the Society of Cardiovascular Computed Tom-

ography, the American College of Radiology, the American Heart Association, the American Society of Echocardiography, the American Society of Nuclear Cardiology, the North American Society for Cardiovascular Imaging, the Society for Cardiovascular Angiography and Interventions, and the Society for Cardiovascular Magnetic Resonance. *J Am Coll Cardiol.* 2010;**56**:1864–94
15. Polonsky TS, *et al.* Coronary artery calcium score and risk classification for coronary heart disease prediction. *JAMA.* 2010;**303**:1610–16
16. Agatston AS, *et al.* Quantification of coronary artery calcium using ultrafast computed tomography. *J Am Coll Cardiol.* 1990;**15**:827–32
17. Hermann DM, *et al.* Coronary artery calcification is an independent stroke predictor in the general population. *Stroke.* 2013; **44**: 1008–13
18. Villines TC, *et al.* Prevalence and severity of coronary artery disease and adverse events among symptomatic patients with coronary artery calcification scores of zero undergoing coronary computed tomography angiography: results from the CONFIRM (Coronary CT Angiography Evaluation for Clinical Outcomes: An International Multicenter) registry. *J Am Coll Cardiol.* 2011;**58**:2533–40
19. Patel MR, *et al.* ACCF/SCAI/AATS/AHA/ASE/ASNC/HFSA/HRS/SCCM/SCCT/SCMR/STS 2012 appropriate use criteria for diagnostic catheterization: a report of the American College of Cardiology Foundation Appropriate Use Criteria Task Force, Society for Cardiovascular Angiography and Interventions, American Association for Thoracic Surgery, American Heart Association, American Society of Echocardiography, American Society of Nuclear Cardiology, Heart Failure Society of America, Heart Rhythm Society, Society of Critical Care Medicine, Society of Cardiovascular Computed Tomography, Society for Cardiovascular Magnetic Resonance, and Society of Thoracic Surgeons. *J Am Coll Cardiol.* 2012;**59**:1995–2027
20. Gulati M, *et al.* Adverse cardiovascular outcomes in women with nonobstructive coronary artery disease: a report from the Women's Ischemia Syndrome Evaluation Study and the St James Women Take Heart Project. *Arch Intern Med.* 2009;**169**:843–50
21. Alegria JR, *et al.* Myocardial bridging. *Eur Heart J.* 2005;**26**:1159–68
22. Kaski JC. Pathophysiology and management of patients with chest pain and normal coronary arteriograms (cardiac syndrome X). *Circulation.* 2004;**109**:568–72
23. Bairey Merz CN, *et al.* Syndrome X and microvascular coronary dysfunction. *Circulation.* 2011;**124**:1477–80
24. Takagi Y, *et al.* Clinical implications of provocation tests for coronary artery spasm: safety, arrhythmic complications, and prognostic impact: multicentre registry study of the Japanese Coronary Spasm Association. *Eur Heart J.* 2013;**34**:258–67.
25. Allman KC, *et al.* Myocardial viability testing and impact of revascularization on prognosis in patients with coronary artery disease and left ventricular dysfunction: a meta-analysis. *J Am Coll Cardiol.* 2002;**39**:1151–8
26. Hillis LD, *et al.* 2011 ACCF/AHA Guideline for Coronary Artery Bypass Graft Surgery: a report of the American College of Cardiology Foundation/American Heart Association Task Force on Practice Guidelines. *Circulation.* 2011;**124**:e652–35
27. Wijns W, *et al.* Guidelines on myocardial revascularization. *Eur Heart J.* 2010;**31**:2501–55
28. Bonow RO, *et al.* Myocardial viability and survival in ischaemic left ventricular dysfunction. *N Engl J Med.* 2011;**364**:1617–25
29. Velazquez EJ, *et al.* Coronary-artery bypass surgery in patients with left ventricular dysfunction. *N Engl J Med.* 2011;**364**:1607–16
30. Cleland JG CM, *et al.* The heart failure revascularisation trial (HEART). *Eur J Heart Fail.* 2011;**13**:227–33
31. Beanlands RS NG, et al. F-18-fluorodeoxyglucose positron emission tomography imaging-assisted management of patients with severe left ventricular dysfunction and suspected coronary disease: A randomized, controlled trial (PARR-2). *J Am Coll Cardiol Cardiovasc Interv.* 2007;**50**:2002–12
32. Min JK, *et al.* Prognostic value of multidetector coronary computed tomographic angiography for prediction of all-cause mortality. *J Am Coll Cardiol.* 2007;**50**:1161–70
33. Patel MR, *et al.* ACCF/SCAI/STS/AATS/AHA/ASNC/HFSA/SCCT 2012 Appropriate use criteria for coronary revascularization focused update: a report of the American College of Cardiology Foundation Appropriate Use Criteria Task Force, Society for Cardiovascular Angiography and Interventions, Society of Thoracic Surgeons, American Association for Thoracic Surgery, American Heart Association, American Society of Nuclear Cardiology, and the Society of Cardiovascular Computed Tomography. *J Am Coll Cardiol.* 2012;**59**:857–81
34. Garg S, *et al.* A new tool for the risk stratification of patients with complex coronary artery disease: the Clinical SYNTAX Score. *Circ Cardiovasc Interv.* 2010;**3**:317–26
35. Nam CW, *et al.* Functional SYNTAX Score for risk assessment in multivessel coronary artery disease. *J Am Coll Cardiol.* 2011;**58**:1211–18
36. Elias-Smale SE, *et al.* Coronary calcium score improves classification of coronary heart disease risk in the elderly: the Rotterdam study. *J Am Coll Cardiol.* 2010;**56**:1407–14
37. Erbel R, *et al.* Coronary risk stratification, discrimination, and reclassification improvement based on quantification of subclinical coronary atherosclerosis: the Heinz Nixdorf Recall study. *J Am Coll Cardiol.* 2010;**56**:1397–406
38. Jahnke C, *et al.* Prognostic value of cardiac magnetic resonance stress tests: adenosine stress perfusion and dobutamine stress wall motion imaging. *Circulation.* 2007;**115**:1769–76
39. Sajadieh A, *et al.* Prevalence and prognostic significance of daily-life silent myocardial ischaemia in middle-aged and elderly subjects with no apparent heart disease. *Eur Heart J.* 2005;**26**:1402–09
40. Camm A, *et al.* Risk stratification of patients with ventricular arrhythmias. In: Zipes DP, Jalife J. Clinical electrophysiology. From cell to bedside. 3rd edition. pp. 808–27, Saunders, Philadelphia, 2000
41. Spaulding CM, *et al.* Immediate coronary angiography in survivors of out-of-hospital cardiac arrest. *N Engl J Med.* 1997;**336**:1629–33

42. Blumenthal RS, *et al.* Detecting occult coronary disease in a high-risk asymptomatic population. *Circulation.* 2003;**107**:702–07
43. Christou MA, *et al.* Meta-analysis of fractional flow reserve versus quantitative coronary angiography and non-invasive imaging for evaluation of myocardial ischaemia. *Am J Cardiol.* 2007;**99**:450–56
44. Panza JA, *et al.* Inducible myocardial ischemia and outcomes in patients with coronary artery disease and left ventricular dysfunction. *J Am Coll Cardiol.* 2013;**61**:1860–70
45. Wormser D, *et al.* Separate and combined associations of body-mass index and abdominal adiposity with cardiovascular disease: collaborative analysis of 58 prospective studies. *Lancet.* 2011;**377**:1085–95
46. Bray GA, *et al.* Medical therapy for the patient with obesity. *Circulation.* 2012;**125**:1695–703
47. Sattelmair J, *et al.* Dose response between physical activity and risk of coronary heart disease: a meta-analysis. *Circulation.* 2011;**124**:789–95
48. Huxley RR, *et al.* Cigarette smoking as a risk factor for coronary heart disease in women compared with men: a systematic review and meta-analysis of prospective cohort studies. *Lancet.* 2011;**378**:1297–305
49. Crowe FL, *et al.* Fruit and vegetable intake and mortality from ischaemic heart disease: results from the European Prospective Investigation into Cancer and Nutrition (EPIC)-Heart study. *Eur Heart J.* 2011;**32**:1235–43
50. Sofi F, *et al.* Adherence to Mediterranean diet and health status: meta-analysis. *BMJ.* 2008;**337**:a1344
51. Estruch RRE, *et al.* Primary prevention of cardiovascular disease with a Mediterranean diet. *N Engl J Med.* 2013 Feb 25;[Epub ahead of print]
52. Bosch J, *et al.* N-3 fatty acids and cardiovascular outcomes in patients with dysglycemia. *N Engl J Med.* 2012;**367**:309–18
53. Rizos EC, *et al.* Association between omega-3 fatty acid supplementation and risk of major cardiovascular disease events: a systematic review and meta-analysis. *JAMA.* 2012;**308**:1024–33
54. Group TRaPSC. N-3 fatty acids in patients with multiple cardiovascular risk factors. *N Engl J Med.* 2013;**368**:1800–8
55. Galan P, *et al.* Effects of b vitamins and omega 3 fatty acids on cardiovascular diseases: a randomised placebo controlled trial. *BMJ.* 2010;**341**:c6273
56. Costanzo S, *et al.* Cardiovascular and overall mortality risk in relation to alcohol consumption in patients with cardiovascular disease. *Circulation.* 2010;**121**:1951–59
57. Heiss C, *et al.* Flavanols and cardiovascular disease prevention. *Eur Heart J.* 2010;**31**:2583–92
58. Grontved A, *et al.* Television viewing and risk of type 2 diabetes, cardiovascular disease, and all-cause mortality: a meta-analysis. *JAMA.* 2011;**305**:2448–55
59. Smith SC, Jr., *et al.* AHA/ACCF Secondary Prevention and Risk Reduction Therapy for Patients with Coronary and other Atherosclerotic Vascular Disease: 2011 update: a guideline from the American Heart Association and American College of Cardiology Foundation. *Circulation.* 2011;**124**:2458–73
60. Inzucchi SE, *et al.* Management of hyperglycaemia in type 2 diabetes: a patient-centered approach. Position statement of the American Diabetes Association (ADA) and the European Association for the Study of Diabetes (EASD). *Diabetologia.* 2012;**55**:1577–96
61. Nicholls SJ, *et al.* Lowering the triglyceride/high-density lipoprotein cholesterol ratio is associated with the beneficial impact of pioglitazone on progression of coronary atherosclerosis in diabetic patients: insights from the PERISCOPE (Pioglitazone Effect on Regression of Intravascular Sonographic Coronary Obstruction Prospective Evaluation) study. *J Am Coll Cardiol.* 2011;**57**:153–9
62. Loke YK, *et al.* Comparative cardiovascular effects of thiazolidinediones: systematic review and meta-analysis of observational studies. *BMJ.* 2011;**342**:d1309
63. Gerstein HC, *et al.* Basal insulin and cardiovascular and other outcomes in dysglycemia. *N Engl J Med.* 2012;**367**: 319–28
64. Collaborative meta-analysis of randomised trials of antiplatelet therapy for prevention of death, myocardial infarction, and stroke in high risk patients. *BMJ.* 2002;**324**:71–86
65. Valgimigli M, *et al.* Short- versus long-term duration of dual-antiplatelet therapy after coronary stenting: a randomized multicentre trial. *Circulation.* 2012;**125**:2015–26
66. Martin SS, *et al.* Friedewald estimated versus directly measured low-density lipoprotein cholesterol and treatment implications. *J Am Coll Cardiol.* 2013; doi:10.1016/j.jacc.2013.1001.1079
67. Baigent C, *et al.* Efficacy and safety of more intensive lowering of LDL cholesterol: a meta-analysis of data from 170,000 participants in 26 randomised trials. *Lancet.* 2010;**376**:1670–81
68. Emerging Risk Factors Collaboration. Lipid-related markers and cardiovascular disease prediction. *JAMA.* 2012;**307**:2499–506
69. Heart Protection Study Collaborative G, *et al.* C-reactive protein concentration and the vascular benefits of statin therapy: an analysis of 20,536 patients in the Heart Protection Study. *Lancet.* 2011;**377**:469–76
70. Sever PS, *et al.* Evaluation of C-reactive protein prior to and on-treatment as a predictor of benefit from atorvastatin: observations from the Anglo-Scandinavian Cardiac Outcomes Trial. *Eur Heart J.* 2012;**33**:486–94
71. Calderon RM, *et al.* Statins in the treatment of dyslipidemia in the presence of elevated liver aminotransferase levels: a therapeutic dilemma. *Mayo Clin Proc.* 2010;**85**:349–56
72. Armitage J BL, Wallendszus K,, *et al.* Intensive lowering of LDL cholesterol with 80 mg versus 20 mg simvastatin daily in 12,064 survivors of myocardial infarction: a double-blind randomised trial. *Lancet.* 2010; **376**:1658–69
73. Preiss D, *et al.* Risk of incident diabetes with intensive-dose compared with moderate-dose statin therapy: a meta-analysis. *JAMA.* 2011;**305**:2556–64
74. Sattar N, *et al.* Statins and risk of incident diabetes: a collaborative meta-analysis of randomised statin trials. *Lancet.* 2010;**375**:735–42
75. Waters DD, *et al.* Predictors of new-onset diabetes in patients treated with atorvastatin: results from 3 large randomized clinical trials. *J Am Coll Cardiol.* 2011;**57**:1535–45
76. Hemmelgarn BR, *et al.* Use of high potency statins and rates of admission for acute kidney injury: Multicenter, retro-

spective observational analysis of administrative database. *BMJ*. 2013;**346**:f880. doi: 810.1136/bmj.f1880
77. Jukema JW, *et al.* The controversies of statin therapy: weighing the evidence. *J Am Coll Cardiol*. 2012;**60**:875–81
78. Marelli C, *et al.* Statins and risk of cancer: a retrospective cohort analysis of 45,857 matched pairs from an electronic medical records database of 11 million adult Americans. *J Am Coll Cardiol*. 2011;**58**:530–37
79. Frohlich GM, *et al.* Statins and the risk of cancer after heart transplantation. *Circulation*. 2012;**126**:440–7
80. Hackam DG, *et al.* Statins and intracerebral haemorrhage: a retrospective cohort study. *Arch Neurol*. 2012;**69**: 39–45
81. Westover MB, *et al.* Statin use following intracerebral haemorrhage: a decision analysis. *Arch Neurol*. 2011;**68**:573–9
82. Golomb BA, *et al.* Effects of statins on energy and fatigue with exertion: results from a randomized controlled trial. *Arch Intern Med*. 2012;**172**:1180–2
83. Ginsberg HN, *et al.* Effects of combination lipid therapy in type 2 diabetes mellitus. *N Engl J Med*. 2010;**362**:1563–74
84. Miller M, *et al.* Triglycerides and cardiovascular disease: a scientific statement from the American Heart Association. *Circulation*. 2011;**123**:2292–33
85. Jun M, *et al.* Effects of fibrates on cardiovascular outcomes: a systematic review and meta-analysis. *Lancet*. 2010;**375**:1875–84
86. Reiner Z, *et al.* ESC/EAS Guidelines for the management of dyslipidaemias: the Task Force for the management of dyslipidaemias of the European Society of Cardiology (ESC) and the European Atherosclerosis Society (EAS). *Eur Heart J*. 2011;**32**:1769–818
87. Boden WE, *et al.* Niacin in patients with low HDL cholesterol levels receiving intensive statin therapy. *N Engl J Med*. 2011;**365**:2255–67
88. Kastelein JJ, *et al.* Simvastatin with or without ezetimibe in familial hypercholesterolaemia. *N Engl J Med*. 2008;**358**:1431–43
89. Armitage J, *et al.* Hps2-thrive: Randomized placebo-controlled trial of ER niacin and laropriprant in 25,673 patients with pre-existing cardiovascular disease. *ACC*. 2013
90. Saravanan P, *et al.* Cardiovascular effects of marine omega-3 fatty acids. *Lancet*. 2010;**376**:540–50
91. Genser B, *et al.* Plant sterols and cardiovascular disease: a systematic review and meta-analysis. *Eur Heart J*. 2012;**33**:444–51
92. Roth EM, *et al.* Atorvastatin with or without an antibody to PCSK9 in primary hypercholesterolemia. *N Engl J Med*. 2012;**367**:1891–900
93. Ong HT. Beta blockers in hypertension and cardiovascular disease. *BMJ*. 2007;**334**:946–9
94. Bangalore S, *et al.* Beta blocker use and clinical outcomes in stable outpatients with and without coronary artery disease. *JAMA*. 2012;**308**:1340–9
95. Munzel T, *et al.* Nitrate therapy: new aspects concerning molecular action and tolerance. *Circulation*. 2011;**123**:2132–44
96. Nakamura Y, *et al.* Long-term nitrate use may be deleterious in ischemic heart disease: A study using the databases from two large-scale postinfarction studies. Multicenter Myocardial Ischemia Research Group. *Am Heart J*. 1999;**138**:577–85
97. Morita N, *et al.* Suppression of re-entrant and multifocal ventricular fibrillation by the late sodium current blocker ranolazine. *J Am Coll Cardiol*. 2011;**57**:366–75
98. Morrow DA, *et al.* Vorapaxar in the secondary prevention of atherothrombotic events. *N Engl J Med*. 2012;**366**:1404–13
99. Schjerning Olsen AM, *et al.* Duration of treatment with nonsteroidal anti-inflammatory drugs and impact on risk of death and recurrent myocardial infarction in patients with prior myocardial infarction: a nationwide cohort study. *Circulation*. 2011;**123**:2226–35
100. Ramirez FD, *et al.* Natural history and management of aortocoronary saphenous vein graft aneurysms: a systematic review of published cases. *Circulation*. 2012;**126**:2248–56
101. Coxib and traditional NSAID Trialists' (CNT) Collaboration. Vascular and upper gastrointestinal effects of non-steroidal anti-inflammatory drugs: meta-analyses of individual participant data from randomised trials. *Lancet*. 2013 May 29. doi:pii: S0140-6736(13)60900-9.
102. Graham I, *et al.* European guidelines on cardiovascular disease prevention in clinical practice: executive summary: Fourth Joint Task Force of the European Society of Cardiology and Other Societies on Cardiovascular Disease Prevention in Clinical Practice (Constituted by representatives of nine societies and by invited experts). *Eur Heart J*. 2007;**28**:2375–414
103. Davies RF, *et al.* Asymptomatic Cardiac Ischemia Pilot (ACIP) study two-year follow-up: outcomes of patients randomized to initial strategies of medical therapy versus revascularization. *Circulation*. 1997;**95**:2037–43
104. Hachamovitch R, *et al.* Comparison of the short-term survival benefit associated with revascularization compared with medical therapy in patients with no prior coronary artery disease undergoing stress myocardial perfusion single photon emission computed tomography. *Circulation*. 2003;**107**:2900–7
105. Hueb W, *et al.* Ten-year follow-up survival of the Medicine, Angioplasty, or Surgery Study (MASS II): a randomized controlled clinical trial of 3 therapeutic strategies for multivessel coronary artery disease. *Circulation*. 2010;**122**:949–57
106. Jeremias A, *et al.* The impact of revascularization on mortality in patients with nonacute coronary artery disease. *Am J Med*. 2009;**122**:152–61
107. Mahmarian JJ, *et al.* An initial strategy of intensive medical therapy is comparable to that of coronary revascularization for suppression of scintigraphic ischaemia in high-risk but stable survivors of acute myocardial infarction. *J Am Coll Cardiol*. 2006;**48**:2458–67
108. Bell MR, *et al.* Effect of completeness of revascularization on long-term outcome of patients with three-vessel disease undergoing coronary artery bypass surgery. A report from the Coronary Artery Surgery Study (CASS) Registry. *Circulation*. 1992;**86**:446–57
109. Kleisli T CW, *et al.* In the current era, complete revascularization improves survival after coronary artery bypass surgery. *J Thorac Cardiovasc Surg* 2005;**129**:1283–91
110. Vander Salm TJ, *et al.* What constitutes optimal surgical revascularization? Answers from the Bypass Angioplasty

Revascularization Investigation (BARI). *J Am Coll Cardiol.* 2002;**39**:565–72

111. Hannan EL, *et al.* Incomplete revascularization in the era of drug-eluting stents: impact on adverse outcomes. *JACC Cardiovasc Interv.* 2009;**2**:17–25
112. Kim YH, *et al.* Impact of angiographic complete revascularization after drug-eluting stent implantation or coronary artery bypass graft surgery for multivessel coronary artery disease. *Circulation.* 2011;**123**:2373–81
113. van den Brand MJ, *et al.* The effect of completeness of revascularization on event-free survival at one year in the ARTS trial. *J Am Coll Cardiol.* 2002;**39**:559–64
114. Aldweib N, *et al.* Impact of repeat myocardial revascularization on outcome in patients with silent ischemia after previous revascularization. *J Am Coll Cardiol.* 2013;**61**:1616–23
115. Eighteen-year follow-up in the Veterans Affairs Cooperative Study of Coronary Artery Bypass Surgery for stable angina. The VA Coronary Artery Bypass Surgery Cooperative Study Group. *Circulation.* 1992;**86**:121–30
116. Alderman EL, *et al.* Ten-year follow-up of survival and myocardial infarction in the randomized Coronary Artery Surgery Study. *Circulation.* 1990;**82**:1629–46
117. Varnauskas E. Twelve-year follow-up of survival in the randomized European Coronary Surgery Study. *N Engl J Med.* 1988;**319**:332–7
118. Hillis LD, *et al.* 2011 ACCF/AHA guideline for coronary artery bypass graft surgery: executive summary: a report of the American College of Cardiology Foundation/American Heart Association Task Force on Practice Guidelines. *J Thorac Cardiovasc Surgery.* 2012;**143**:4–34
119. Yusuf S, *et al.* Effect of coronary artery bypass graft surgery on survival: overview of 10-year results from randomised trials by the Coronary Artery Bypass Graft Surgery Trialists Collaboration. *Lancet.* 1994;**344**:563–70
120. Brooks MM, *et al.* Clinical and angiographic risk stratification and differential impact on treatment outcomes in the Bypass Angioplasty Revascularization Investigation 2 Diabetes (BARI 2D) trial. *Circulation.* 2012;**126**:2115–24
121. Kroncke GM, *et al.* Five-year changes in coronary arteries of medical and surgical patients of the Veterans Administration Randomized Study of Bypass Surgery. *Circulation.* 1988;**78**:I144–50
122. Kulik A, *et al.* Aspirin plus clopidogrel versus aspirin alone after coronary artery bypass grafting: the clopidogrel after surgery for coronary artery disease (CASCADE) trial. *Circulation.* 2010;**122**:2680–87
123. Roach GW, *et al.* Adverse cerebral outcomes after coronary bypass surgery. Multicenter Study of Perioperative Ischemia Research Group and the Ischemia Research and Education Foundation Investigators. *N Engl J Med.* 1996;**335**:1857–63.
124. Mehta RH, *et al.* Saphenous vein grafts with multiple versus single distal targets in patients undergoing coronary artery bypass surgery: one-year graft failure and five-year outcomes from the Project of Ex-Vivo Vein Graft Engineering via Transfection (PREVENT) IV trial. *Circulation.* 2011;**124**:280–8
125. Sabik JF, 3rd, *et al.* Comparison of saphenous vein and internal thoracic artery graft patency by coronary system. *Ann Thorac Surg.* 2005;**79**:544–51; discussion 544–51
126. Lopes RD, *et al.* Relationship between vein graft failure and subsequent clinical outcomes after coronary artery bypass surgery. *Circulation.* 2012;**125**:749–56
127. Ruttmann E, *et al.* Second internal thoracic artery versus radial artery in coronary artery bypass grafting: a long-term, propensity score-matched follow-up study. *Circulation.* 2011;**124**:1321–29
128. Dorman MJ, *et al.* Bilateral internal mammary artery grafting enhances survival in diabetic patients: a 30-year follow-up of propensity score-matched cohorts. *Circulation.* 2012;**126**:2935–42
129. Ioannidis JP, *et al.* Early mortality and morbidity of bilateral versus single internal thoracic artery revascularization: propensity and risk modeling. *J Am Coll Cardiol.* 2001;**37**:521–8
130. Taggart DP, *et al.* Randomized trial to compare bilateral vs. single internal mammary coronary artery bypass grafting: 1-year results of the Arterial Revascularisation Trial (ART). *Eur Heart J.* 2010;**31**:2470–81
131. Locker C, *et al.* Multiple arterial grafts improve late survival of patients undergoing coronary artery bypass graft surgery: analysis of 8622 patients with multivessel disease. *Circulation.* 2012;**126**:1023–30
132. Medalion B, *et al.* Should bilateral internal thoracic artery grafting be used in elderly patients undergoing coronary artery bypass grafting? *Circulation.* 2013;**127**:2186–93
133. Afilalo J, *et al.* Off-pump vs On-pump coronary artery bypass surgery: an updated meta-analysis and meta-regression of randomized trials. *Eur Heart J.* 2012; **33**:1257–67
134. Diegeler A, *et al.* for the GOPCABE Study Group. Off-pump versus on-pump coronary-artery bypass grafting in elderly patients. *New Engl J Med.* 2013; doi: 10.1056/NEJMoa1211666
135. Lamy A, *et al.* for the CORONARY Investigators. Effects of off-pump and on-pump coronary-artery bypass grafting at 1 year. *New Engl J Med.* 2013; doi: 10.1056/NEJMoa1301228
136. Hattler B, *et al.* Off-Pump coronary artery bypass surgery is associated with worse arterial and saphenous vein graft patency and less effective revascularization: Results from the Veterans Affairs Randomized On/Off Bypass (ROOBY) trial. *Circulation.* 2012;**125**:2827–35
137. El-Chami MF, *et al.* Ventricular arrhythmia after cardiac surgery: incidence, predictors, and outcomes. *J Am Coll Cardiol.* 2012;**60**:2664–71
138. Angiolillo DJ, *et al.* Bridging antiplatelet therapy with cangrelor in patients undergoing cardiac surgery: a randomized controlled trial. *JAMA.* 2012;**307**:265–74
139. Katritsis DG, *et al.* Percutaneous coronary intervention versus conservative therapy in nonacute coronary artery disease: a meta-analysis. *Circulation.* 2005;**111**:2906–12
140. Katritsis DG, *et al.* PCI for stable coronary disease. *N Engl J Med.* 2007;**357**:414–15; author reply 417–18

141. Stergiopoulos K, *et al.* Initial coronary stent implantation with medical therapy vs medical therapy alone for stable coronary artery disease: meta-analysis of randomized controlled trials. *Arch Intern Med.* 2012;**172**:312–19
142. Trikalinos TA, *et al.* Percutaneous coronary interventions for non-acute coronary artery disease: a quantitative 20-year synopsis and a network meta-analysis. *Lancet.* 2009;**373**:911–18
143. Wijeysundera HC, *et al.* Meta-analysis: Effects of percutaneous coronary intervention versus medical therapy on angina relief. *Ann Intern Med.* 2010;**152**:370–9
144. Kirtane AJ, *et al.* Safety and efficacy of drug-eluting and bare metal stents: comprehensive meta-analysis of randomized trials and observational studies. *Circulation.* 2009;**119**:3198–206
145. Boden WE, *et al.* Optimal medical therapy with or without PCI for stable coronary disease. *N Engl J Med.* 2007;**356**:1503–16
146. Shaw LJ, *et al.* Optimal medical therapy with or without percutaneous coronary intervention to reduce ischemic burden: results from the Clinical Outcomes Utilizing Revascularization and Aggressive Drug Evaluation (COURAGE) trial nuclear substudy. *Circulation.* 2008;**117**:1283–91
147. Erne P, *et al.* Effects of percutaneous coronary interventions in silent ischemia after myocardial infarction: the SWISSI II randomized controlled trial. *JAMA.* 2007;**297**:1985–91
148. Ioannidis JP, *et al.* Percutaneous coronary intervention for late reperfusion after myocardial infarction in stable patients. *Am Heart J.* 2007;**154**:1065–71
149. Menon V, *et al.* Lack of benefit from percutaneous intervention of persistently occluded infarct arteries after the acute phase of myocardial infarction is time independent: insights from Occluded Artery Trial. *Eur Heart J.* 2009;**30**:183–91
150. De Bruyne B, *et al.* Fractional flow reserve-guided PCI versus medical therapy in stable coronary disease. *N Engl J Med.* 2012;**367**:991–1001
151. Li J EM, *et al.* Long-term outcomes of fractional flow reserve-guided vs. Angiography-guided percutaneous coronary intervention in contemporary practice. *Eur Heart J.* 2013;**34**:1375–83
152. Chan PS, *et al.* Appropriateness of percutaneous coronary intervention. *JAMA.* 2011;**306**:53–61
153. Ambrose JA, *et al.* Angiographic progression of coronary artery disease and the development of myocardial infarction. *J Am Coll Cardiol.* 1988;**12**:56–62
154. Little WC, *et al.* Can coronary angiography predict the site of a subsequent myocardial infarction in patients with mild-to-moderate coronary artery disease? *Circulation.* 1988;**78**:1157–66
155. Falk E. Plaque rupture with severe pre-existing stenosis precipitating coronary thrombosis. Characteristics of coronary atherosclerotic plaques underlying fatal occlusive thrombi. *Br Heart J.* 1983;**50**:127–34
156. Qiao JH, *et al.* The severity of coronary atherosclerosis at sites of plaque rupture with occlusive thrombosis. *J Am Coll Cardiol.* 1991;**17**:1138–42
157. Finn AV, *et al.* Concept of vulnerable/unstable plaque. *Arterioscler Thromb Vasc Biol.* 2010;**30**:1282–92
158. Naghavi M, *et al.* From vulnerable plaque to vulnerable patient: a call for new definitions and risk assessment strategies: part I. *Circulation.* 2003;**108**:1664–72
159. Kaski JC, *et al.* Rapid angiographic progression of coronary artery disease in patients with angina pectoris. The role of complex stenosis morphology. *Circulation.* 1995;**92**:2058–65
160. Tonino PA, *et al.* Fractional flow reserve versus angiography for guiding percutaneous coronary intervention. *N Engl J Med.* 2009;**360**:213–24
161. Hannan EL, *et al.* Comparative outcomes for patients who do and do not undergo percutaneous coronary intervention for stable coronary artery disease in New York. *Circulation.* 2012;**125**:1870–9
162. Park DW, *et al.* Frequency, causes, predictors, and clinical significance of peri-procedural myocardial infarction following percutaneous coronary intervention. Eur Heart J. 2013;34:1662–9.
163. Ioannidis JP, *et al.* Mortality risk conferred by small elevations of creatine kinase-MB isoenzyme after percutaneous coronary intervention. *J Am Coll Cardiol.* 2003;**42**:1406–11
164. Katritsis DG, *et al.* Percutaneous coronary intervention for stable coronary artery disease. *J Am Coll Cardiol.* 2008;**52**:889–3
165. Katritsis DG, *et al.* Double versus single stenting for coronary bifurcation lesions: a meta-analysis. *Circ Cardiovasc Interv.* 2009;**2**:409–15
166. Bangalore S, *et al.* Percutaneous coronary intervention versus optimal medical therapy for prevention of spontaneous myocardial infarction in subjects with stable ischemic heart disease. *Circulation.* 2013;**127**:769–81
167. Levine GN, *et al.* 2011 ACCF/AHA/SCAI Guideline for Percutaneous Coronary Intervention: a report of the American College of Cardiology Foundation/American Heart Association Task Force on Practice Guidelines and the Society for Cardiovascular Angiography and Interventions. *Circulation.* 2011;**124**:e574–651
168. Peterson ED, *et al.* NCDR registry participants. Contemporary mortality risk prediction for percutaneous coronary intervention: Results from 588,398 procedures in the national cardiovascular data registry. *J Am Coll Cardiol.* 2010;**18**:1923–32
169. Kimura T, *et al.* Very late stent thrombosis and late target lesion revascularization after sirolimus-eluting stent implantation: five-year outcome of the j-Cypher Registry. *Circulation.* 2012;**125**:584–91
170. Zellweger MJ, *et al.* Coronary artery disease progression late after successful stent implantation. *J Am Coll Cardiol.* 2012;**59**:793–99
171. Palmerini T, *et al.* Stent thrombosis with drug-eluting and bare-metal stents: evidence from a comprehensive network meta-analysis. *Lancet.* 2012;**379**:1393–402
172. Bhatt DL, *et al.*, for the CHAMPION PHOENIX Investigators. Effect of platelet inhibition with cangrelor during pci on ischemic events. *N Engl J Med.* 2013; doi: 10.1056/NEJMoa1300815

173. Aversano T, *et al.* Outcomes of PCI at hospitals with or without on-site cardiac surgery. *N Engl J Med.* 2012;**366**:1792–802
174. Singh M, *et al.* Percutaneous coronary intervention at centres with and without on-site surgery: a meta-analysis. *JAMA.* 2011;**306**:2487–94
175. Jacobs AK *et al.* Nonemergency PCI at hospitals with or without on-site cardiac surgery. *N Engl J Med.* 2013; doi: 10.1056/NEJMoa1300610
176. Shahian DM, *et al.* Percutaneous coronary interventions without on-site cardiac surgical backup. N Engl J Med. 2012;**366**:1814–23
177. O'Neill WW, *et al.* A prospective, randomized clinical trial of hemodynamic support with Impella 2.5 versus intra-aortic balloon pump in patients undergoing high-risk percutaneous coronary intervention: the PROTECT II study. *Circulation.* 2012;**126**:1717–27.
178. Perera D, *et al.* Long-term mortality data from the balloon pump-assisted coronary intervention study (BCIS-1): a randomized, controlled trial of elective balloon counterpulsation during high-risk percutaneous coronary intervention. *Circulation.* 2013;**127**:207–12.
179. Acetylcysteine for prevention of renal outcomes in patients undergoing coronary and peripheral vascular angiography: main results from the randomized Acetylcysteine for Contrast-induced nephropathy Trial (ACT). *Circulation.* 2011;**124**:1250–9
180. Marenzi G, *et al.* Prevention of contrast nephropathy by furosemide with matched hydration: the MYTHOS (Induced Diuresis With Matched Hydration Compared to Standard Hydration for Contrast Induced Nephropathy Prevention) trial. *JACC Cardiovasc Interv.* 2012;**5**:90–7
181. Quintavalle C FD, *et al.* Impact of a high loading dose of atorvastatin on contrast-induced acute kidney injury. *Circulation.* 2012;**126**:3008–16
182. Smilowitz NR, *et al.* Practices and complications of vascular closure devices and manual compression in patients undergoing elective transfemoral coronary procedures. *Am J Cardiol.* 2012;**110**:177–82
183. Bravata DM, *et al.* Systematic review: the comparative effectiveness of percutaneous coronary interventions and coronary artery bypass graft surgery. *Ann Intern Med.* 2007;**147**:703–16
184. Hlatky MA, *et al.* Coronary artery bypass surgery compared with percutaneous coronary interventions for multivessel disease: a collaborative analysis of individual patient data from ten randomised trials. *Lancet.* 2009;**373**:1190–7
185. Palmerini T, *et al.* Risk of stroke with coronary artery bypass graft surgery compared with percutaneous coronary intervention. *J Am Coll Cardiol.* 2012;**60**:798–805
186. Park SJ, *et al.* Randomized trial of stents versus bypass surgery for left main coronary artery disease. *N Engl J Med.* 2011;**364**:1718–27
187. Hannan EL, *et al.* Long-term outcomes of coronary-artery bypass grafting versus stent implantation. *N Engl J Med.* 2005;**352**:2174–83
188. Kapoor JR, *et al.* Isolated disease of the proximal left anterior descending artery comparing the effectiveness of percutaneous coronary interventions and coronary artery bypass surgery. *JACC Cardiovasc Interv.* 2008;**1**:483–91
189. Chaitman BR, *et al.* The Bypass Angioplasty Revascularization Investigation 2 Diabetes randomized trial of different treatment strategies in type 2 diabetes mellitus with stable ischemic heart disease: impact of treatment strategy on cardiac mortality and myocardial infarction. *Circulation.* 2009;**120**:2529–40
190. Farkouh ME, *et al.* Strategies for multivessel revascularization in patients with diabetes. *N Engl J Med.* 2012;**367**:2375–84
191. Kappetein AP, *et al.* Comparison of coronary bypass surgery with drug-eluting stenting for the treatment of left main and/or three-vessel disease: 3-year follow-up of the SYNTAX trial. *Eur Heart J.* 2011;**32**:2125–34
192. Kapur A, *et al.* Randomized comparison of percutaneous coronary intervention with coronary artery bypass grafting in diabetic patients. 1-year results of the CARDia (Coronary Artery Revascularization in Diabetes) trial. *J Am Coll Cardiol.* 2010;**55**:432–40
193. Lee MS, *et al.* Meta-analysis of studies comparing coronary artery bypass grafting with drug-eluting stenting in patients with diabetes mellitus and multivessel coronary artery disease. *Am J Cardiol.* 2010;**105**:1540–44
194. Mohr FW MM, *et al.* Coronary artery bypass graft surgery versus percutaneous coronary intervention in patients with three-vessel disease and left main coronary disease: 5-year follow-up of the randomised, clinical syntax trial. *Lancet.* 2013;**381**:629–38
195. Farooq V, *et al.* Anatomical and clinical characteristics to guide decision making between coronary artery bypass surgery and percutaneous coronary intervention for individual patients: Development and validation of SYNTAX SCORE II. *Lancet.* 2013;**381**:639–50
196. Weintraub WS, *et al.* Comparative effectiveness of revascularization strategies. *N Engl J Med.* 2012;**366**:1467–76
197. Hlatky MA, *et al.* Comparative effectiveness of multivessel coronary bypass surgery and multivessel percutaneous coronary intervention: A cohort study. *Ann Intern Med.* 2013 April 23;[Epub ahead of print]
198. Bittl JA, et al.; American College of Cardiology Foundation/American Heart Association Task Force on Practice Guidelines. Bayesian methods affirm the use of percutaneous coronary intervention to improve survival in patients with unprotected left main coronary artery disease. Circulation. 2013;127:2177–85.
199. Chen S-L, *et al.* Comparison of double kissing crush versus culotte stenting for unprotected distal left main bifurcation lesions: Results from a multicenter, randomized, prospective DKCRUSH-III study. *J Am Coll Cardiol.* 2013; doi: 10.1016/j.jacc.2013.1001.1023
200. Perk J, *et al.* European Guidelines on cardiovascular disease prevention in clinical practice (version 2012). The Fifth Joint Task Force of the European Society of Cardiology and Other Societies on Cardiovascular Disease

Prevention in Clinical Practice (constituted by representatives of nine societies and by invited experts). *Eur Heart J*. 2012;**33**:1635–701

201. van Diepen S, *et al.* Mortality and readmission of patients with heart failure, atrial fibrillation, or coronary artery disease undergoing noncardiac surgery: an analysis of 38 047 patients. *Circulation*. 2011;**124**:289–96
202. Fleisher LA, *et al.* 2009 ACCF/AHA focused update on perioperative beta blockade incorporated into the ACC/AHA 2007 guidelines on perioperative cardiovascular evaluation and care for noncardiac surgery. *J Am Coll Cardiol*. 2009;**54**:e13–118
203. Bouri S, *et al.* Meta-analysis of secure randomised controlled trials of β-blockade to prevent perioperative death in non-cardiac surgery. *Heart* 2013;:doi:10.1136/heartjnl-2013-304262
204. The Task Force for Preoperative Cardiac Risk Assessment and Perioperative Cardiac Management in Non-cardiac Surgery of the European Society of Cardiology (ESC) and endorsed by the European Society of Anaesthesiology (ESA). Guidelines for pre-operative cardiac risk assessment and perioperative cardiac management in non-cardiac surgery. *Eur Heart J*. 2013;**30**:2769–812
205. Lentine KL, *et al.* Cardiac disease evaluation and management among kidney and liver transplantation candidates: a scientific statement from the American Heart Association and the American College of Cardiology Foundation: endorsed by the American Society of Transplant Surgeons, American Society of Transplantation, and National Kidney Foundation. *Circulation*. 2012;**126**:617–63

Part V

Heart failure

Relevant guidelines

ACCF/AHA 2013 guideline on heart failure

2013 ACCF/AHA Guideline for the Management of Heart Failure. *JACC* 2013; doi: 10.1016/j.jacc.2013.05.019

ESC 2012 guidelines on heart failure

ESC Guidelines for the diagnosis and treatment of acute and chronic heart failure 2012. *Eur Heart J*. 2012;**33**:1787–847.

ACCF/AHA/HRS 2012 guidelines for device-based therapy of cardiac rhythm abnormalities

2012 ACCF/AHA/HRS focused update incorporated into the ACCF/AHA/HRS 2008 guidelines for device-based therapy of cardiac rhythm abnormalities. *J Am Coll Cardiol*. 2013;**61**:e6–75

ESC 2013 guidelines on pacing and cardiac resynchronization

2013 ESC Guidelines on cardiac pacing and cardiac resynchronization therapy. *Eur Heart J* 2013. doi:10.1093/eurheartj/eht150

AHA 2012 scientific statement on sexual activity and cardiovascular disease

Sexual activity and cardiovascular disease: a scientific statement from the American Heart Association. *Circulation*. 2012;**125**:1058–72.

ESC 2011 guidelines on pregnancy

ESC Guidelines on the management of cardiovascular diseases during pregnancy. *Eur Heart J*. 2011;**32**:3147–97.

2012 EHRA/HRS expert consensus statement on cardiac resynchronization therapy in heart failure

2012 EHRA/HRS expert consensus statement on cardiac resynchronization therapy in heart failure: implant and follow-up recommendations and management. *Europace*. 2012;**14**:1236–86.

Chapter 30

Classification, epidemiology, and pathophysiology of heart failure

Definitions and classification

Heart failure is a complex clinical syndrome that results from any structural or functional impairment of ventricular filling or ejection of blood. There is a consequent failure to deliver oxygen according to metabolic requirements, despite normal filling pressures (or only at the expense of increased filling pressures).[1, 2] Patients have the following features:

- **Typical symptoms** (breathlessness at rest or on exercise, fatigue, tiredness, ankle oedema), and
- **Typical signs** (tachycardia, tachypnoea, pulmonary rales, pleural effusion, raised jugular venous pressure, peripheral oedema, hepatomegaly, and
- **Objective evidence of a structural or functional abnormality of the heart at rest** (cardiomegaly, third heart sound, cardiac murmurs, abnormality on the echocardiogram, such as reduced LVEF or valve disease or other structural disorder, raised natriuretic peptide concentration).

Heart failure with reduced ejection fraction (<40%) (HFrEF)

Also referred to as **systolic HF**. Randomized clinical trials have mainly enrolled patients with HF*r*EF, and it is only in these patients that efficacious therapies have been demonstrated to date.[1]

Heart failure with preserved ejection fraction (>40%) (HFpEF)

Also referred to as **diastolic HF** (Figure 30.1). To date, efficacious therapies have not been identified. The ACCF/AHA[1] have further subdivided this category into:

- **HFpEF, borderline 41–49%.** Borderline or intermediate group with characteristics, treatment patterns, and outcomes similar to those of patients with HF*p*EF.
- **HFpEF, improved >40%.** A subset of patients with HF*p*EF who previously had HF*r*EF. These patients with improvement or recovery in EF may be clinically distinct from those with persistently preserved or reduced EF.

Left heart failure refers to predominant congestion of the pulmonary veins with fluid retention and pulmonary oedema. **Right heart failure** refers to predominant congestion of the systemic veins with fluid retention and peripheral oedema.[4] These conditions may coexist, and the most common cause of right ventricular failure is raised pulmonary artery pressure due to left ventricular failure. **High-output heart failure** refers to the syndrome caused by circulatory high-output conditions, such as anaemia, thyrotoxicosis, septicaemia, arteriovenous shunts, liver failure, Paget's disease, and beriberi.

Preload refers to left and/or right atrial pressures (volume overload) and **afterload** to the work of the myocardium (pressure overload or high impedance).

Epidemiology

The prevalence of heart failure is 1–2% of the adult population in developed countries and rises to ≥10% in persons of 70 years or older.[5] The lifetime risk of developing heart failure is estimated to be 20% for all persons older than 40 years.[6] In the USA, approximately 5.1 million have heart failure that leads to 271 000 deaths per year.[7] With an ageing population, there is a shift towards heart failure with preserved LVEF that predominates in patients over 70 years old.[3] Although there is a trend for reduction of hospitalization for HF both in Europe and the US, it is still the most common cause of hospitalization after normal delivery.[8] The incidence of heart failure has not declined in the past 20 years, and, despite recent advances in its management, the 5-year mortality after hospitalization exceeds 40%.[2]

Pathophysiology

The previously normal heart is subject to either an acute (e.g. myocardial infarction) or a chronic insult (e.g. hypertension) that results in altered loading conditions. These activate compensatory mechanisms, such as increased ventricular preload, or the Frank–Starling mechanism, by ventricular dilatation and volume expansion, peripheral vasoconstriction, renal sodium and water retention to enhance ventricular preload, and initiation of the adrenergic nervous system which raises heart rate and contractile function. These processes are controlled mainly by activation of various neurohormonal vasoconstrictor systems, including RAAS, the adrenergic nervous system, and non-osmotic release of arginine-vasopressin. Initially, these mechanisms are beneficial and adaptive,

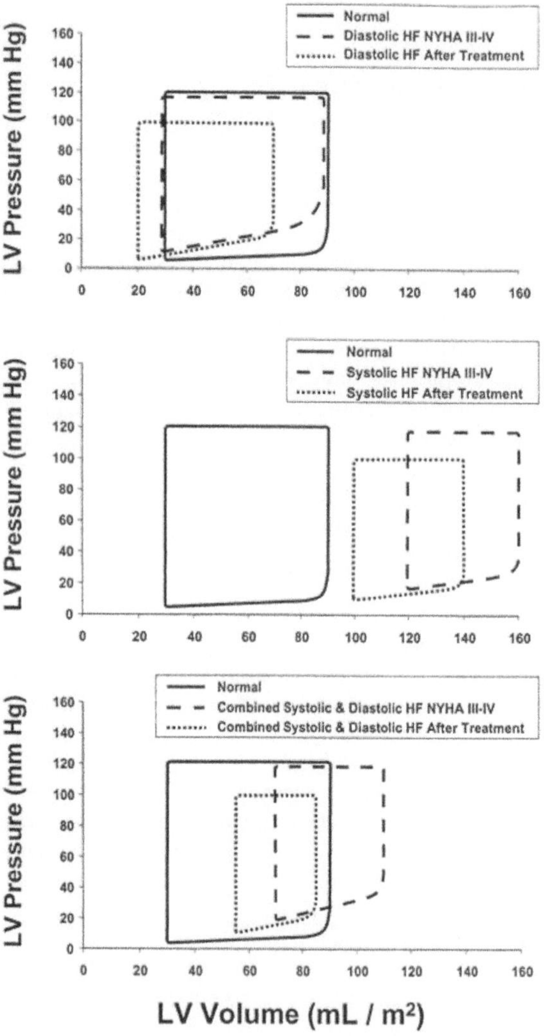

Figure 30.1 Pressure-volume loops contrasting isolated diastolic heart failure (A) with systolic heart failure (B) and combined systolic and diastolic heart failure (C).

Zile MR, Brutsaert DL. New concepts in diastolic dysfunction and diastolic heart failure: Part I: diagnosis, prognosis, and measurements of diastolic function. *Circulation*. 2002;**105**:1387–93.

sustaining heart rate, blood pressure, and cardiac output, and thus maintaining organ perfusion. In the long term, they result in disruptions of β-adrenergic signalling and impaired mobilization of intracellular calcium, with consequent myocyte hypertrophy to preserve wall stress as the heart dilates, apoptosis, fibroblast proliferation, and interstitial collagen accumulation. Changes in size, shape, and pump function of the heart define cardiac remodelling, a determinant of the clinical course of heart failure.[9] The consequences of these structural changes are a reduction in stroke volume, an increase in systemic vascular resistance, and the development of signs and symptoms of congestion and tissue hypoperfusion. Eventually, in untreated cases, cardiac cachexia develops due to activation of proinflammatory cytokines, such as tumour necrosis factor alpha and interleukin 2, with consequent cardiac cell death.[8] Misfolded proteins that are central in the pathophysiology of neurodegenerative disorders such as Parkinson's and Alzheimer disease, have also been found to play a role in pathologic cardiac hypertrophy and dilated and ischemic cardiomyopathies, thus leading to the suggestion that proteotoxicity is a key contributor to the progression of heart failure.[10] Apart from causing further myocardial injury, activation of neurohormonal vasoconstrictor systems has detrimental effects on other organs such as the kidneys, liver, muscles, intestines, and lungs, and create a 'vicious cycle', that accounts for many of the clinical features of heart failure, including cardiac electrical instability. Heart failure may cause renal failure (cardiorenal syndrome) and the opposite may occur (renocardiac syndrome), and abnormal liver function tests (albumin, bilirubin, aminotransferases, and alkaline phosphatase) are frequently seen in patients with chronic and, especially, acute heart failure, and are associated with adverse prognosis.[11]

Both systolic and diastolic heart failure may occur, and a decrease in LVEF to <55%, as well as any worsening of diastolic LV function are independently associated with increased mortality.[12] In addition to being a marker of increased risk due to its association with hypertension, diabetes mellitus, ischemia, and reduced systolic function, diastolic dysfunction may also be a direct contributor to adverse outcomes by limiting cardiac output reserve, accelerating neuroendocrine activation, and promoting physical inactivity. RV hypertrophy predicts an increased risk of heart failure which is usually attributable to LV dysfunction.[13]

Aetiology

Hypertension and **coronary artery disease** are the commonest causes of heart failure in industrialized countries whereas, in underdeveloped countries, other causes, such as **infectious diseases**, are more important.[14–16] Extensive myocardial necrosis can result in pump failure. Small infarctions may also cause regional contractile dysfunction and adverse remodelling with myocyte hypertrophy, apoptosis, and deposition of extracellular matrix. Long-standing untreated hypertension is associated with both systolic and diastolic heart failure, and 75% of patients presenting with heart failure have hypertension.[15] Even modest decreases in systolic blood pressure reduce mortality and risk for heart failure.[17,18] **Valvular heart disease**, **cardiomyopathies**, and **congenital heart disease** are also important causes. Patients with **diabetes mellitus** have a four times higher risk for heart failure and higher mortality compared to non-diabetics.[19] An association of **thiazolidinediones** with heart failure is well established. **Alcohol** is a direct myocardial toxin and a reversible cause of heart failure.[20, 21] **Tobacco** and **cocaine** increase the risk for CAD, which can lead to heart failure. Long-term use of cocaine results in activation of the sympathetic nervous system, causing left ventricular dysfunction both directly and through promotion of coronary thrombosis, coronary spasm, and atherosclerosis.[20] Chemotherapeutic agents, such as **anthracyclines (doxorubicin, daunorubicin)** and **trastuzumab** may also increase the risk of heart failure.[22–24] Anthracyclines impair left ventricular function due to the generation of reactive oxygen species, disruption of mitochondria, and uncoupling of the electron transport chain. Anthracycline cardiotoxicity is dose-dependent, with intermittent high doses and higher cumulative doses increasing the risk of cardiomyopathy and lethal arrhythmias.[25, 26] Risk factors include younger age, female gender, and use of trastuzumab.[26] This form of cardiomyopathy can occur acutely soon after treatment, within a few months of treatment, or many years later, and may be prevented by carvedilol (a beta blocker with antioxidant properties) with an ACE inhibitor.[27] **Antiangiogenic** and **anti-vascular endothelial growth factor (VEGF)** chemotherapy agents (such as bevacizumab and sunitinib) may also cause secondary hypertension and LV failure.[24, 28] Both **hyperthyroidism** and **hypothyroidism** can be reversible causes of heart failure.[29] **Increased resting heart rate** is associated with cardiovascular morbidity and mortality in the general population and in patients with cardiovascular disease.[30] **Persistent tachycardias**, both supraventricular and ventricular, are established causes of heart failure (tachycardiopathies), and atrial fibrillation is independently associated withy an adverse outcome in patients hospitalized for heart failure.[11] **Pulmonary arterial hypertension** may lead to RV failure. **Male sex, less education, physical inactivity**, and **overweight** have also been identified as independent risk factors for CHF.[14] **Long-chain monosaturated fatty acids (LCMUFAs)** such as erucic acid that is a component of rapeseed oil (also found in low quantities in Canola oil) are cardiotoxic and have been associated with heart failure.[31] LCMUFAs are present in mustard oils and related products, some fish species, and processed meat and poultry products. Obstructive **sleep apnoea** is associated with hypertension and a higher incidence of heart failure.[32] Patients with **metabolic syndrome** (abdominal adiposity, hypertriglyceridaemia, low HDL, hypertension, and fasting hyperglycaemia) are at higher risk of cardiovascular disease and heart failure. **HIV infection** is also an important cause of left or biventricular dysfunction.[33]

References

1. Yancy CW, *et al.* 2013 ACCF/AHA guideline for the management of heart failure. *JACC.* 2013; doi: 10.1016/j.jacc.2013.1005.1019
2. McMurray JJ, *et al.* ESC guidelines for the diagnosis and treatment of acute and chronic heart failure 2012: the Task Force for the diagnosis and treatment of acute and chronic heart failure 2012 of the European Society of Cardiology. Developed in collaboration with the Heart Failure Association (HFA) of the ESC. *Eur J Heart Fail.* 2012;**14**:803–69
3. Zile MR, *et al.* New concepts in diastolic dysfunction and diastolic heart failure: part I: diagnosis, prognosis, and measurements of diastolic function. *Circulation.* 2002;**105**:1387–93
4. Voelkel NF, *et al.* Right ventricular function and failure: report of a National Heart, Lung, and Blood Institute Working Group on cellular and molecular mechanisms of right heart failure. *Circulation.* 2006;**114**:1883–91
5. Mosterd A, *et al.* Clinical epidemiology of heart failure. *Heart.* 2007;**93**:1137–46
6. Lloyd-Jones DM, *et al.* Lifetime risk for developing congestive heart failure: the Framingham Heart Study. *Circulation.* 2002;**106**:3068–72
7. Go AS, *et al.* Heart disease and stroke statistics—2013 update: a report from the American Heart Association. *Circulation.* 2013;**127**:e6–e245
8. Braunwald E. Research advances in heart failure: a compendium. *Circ Res.* 2013; Jul 25. [Epub ahead of print]
9. Cohn JN, *et al.* Cardiac remodeling—concepts and clinical implications: a consensus paper from an international forum on cardiac remodeling. Behalf of an International Forum on Cardiac Remodeling. *J Am Coll Cardiol.* 2000;**35**:569–82
10. Willis MS, Patterson C. Proteotoxicity and cardiac dysfunction — alzheimer's disease of the heart? *N Engl J Med.* 2013;**368**:455–64
11. Mountanonakis SE, *et al.* Presence of atrial fibrillation is independently associated with adverse outcomes in patients hospitalized with heart failure. *Circ Heart Failure.* 2012;**5**:191–201
12. Aljaroudi W, *et al.* Impact of progression of diastolic dysfunction on mortality in patients with normal ejection fraction. *Circulation.* 2012;**125**:782–8
13. Kawut SM, *et al.* Right ventricular structure is associated with the risk of heart failure and cardiovascular death: the Multi-Ethnic Study of Atherosclerosis (MESA)—right ventricle study. *Circulation.* 2012;**126**:1681–8
14. He J, *et al.* Risk factors for congestive heart failure in us men and women: NHANES I epidemiologic follow-up study. *Arch Intern Med.* 2001;**161**:996–1002
15. Krum H, *et al.* Heart failure. *Lancet.* 2009;**373**:941–55
16. Ramani GV, *et al.* Chronic heart failure: contemporary diagnosis and management. *Mayo Clin Proc.* 2010;**85**:180–95
17. Chobanian AV, *et al.* The seventh report of the Joint National Committee on prevention, detection, evaluation, and treatment of high blood pressure: The JNC 7 report. *JAMA.* 2003;**289**:2560–72
18. Dagenais GR, *et al.* Effects of ramipril on coronary events in high-risk persons: results of the Heart Outcomes Prevention Evaluation Study. *Circulation.* 2001;**104**:522–6

19. Thrainsdottir IS, *et al.* The association between glucose abnormalities and heart failure in the population-based Reykjavik study. *Diabetes Care.* 2005;**28**:612–16
20. Awtry EH, *et al.* Alcoholic and cocaine-associated cardiomyopathies. *Prog Cardiovasc Dis.* 2010;**52**:289–99
21. Walsh CR, *et al.* Alcohol consumption and risk for congestive heart failure in the Framingham Heart Study. *Ann Intern Med.* 2002;**136**:181–91
22. Choueiri TK, *et al.* Congestive heart failure risk in patients with breast cancer treated with bevacizumab. *J Clin Oncol.* 2011;**29**:632–8
23. Hunt SA, *et al.* 2009 focused update incorporated into the ACC/AHA 2005 guidelines for the diagnosis and management of heart failure in adults: A report of the American College Of Cardiology Foundation/American Heart Association task force on practice guidelines: Developed in collaboration with the International Society for Heart and Lung Transplantation. *Circulation.* 2009;**119**:e391–479
24. Suter TM, Ewer MS. Cancer drugs and the heart: importance and management. *Eur Heart J.* 2013;**34**:1102–11
25. Khouri MG, *et al.* Cancer therapy-induced cardiac toxicity in early breast cancer: addressing the unresolved issues. *Circulation.* 2012;**126**:2749–63
26. Lipshultz SE, *et al.* Female sex and drug dose as risk factors for late cardiotoxic effects of doxorubicin therapy for childhood cancer. *N Engl J Med.* 1995;**332**:1738–43
27. Bosch X, *et al.* Enalapril and carvedilol for preventing chemotherapy-induced left ventricular systolic dysfunction in patients with malignant hemopathies. The overcome trial. *J Am Coll Cardiol.* 2013; doi:pii: S0735–1097 (0713)01398–01393
28. Nazer B, *et al.* Effects of novel angiogenesis inhibitors for the treatment of cancer on the cardiovascular system: focus on hypertension. *Circulation.* 2011;**124**:1687–91
29. Klein I, *et al.* Thyroid hormone and the cardiovascular system. *N Engl J Med.* 2001;**344**:501–9
30. Custodis F, *et al.* Vascular pathophysiology in response to increased heart rate. *J Am Coll Cardiol.* 2010;**56**: 1973–83
31. Imamura F, *et al.* Long-chain monounsaturated fatty acids and incidence of congestive heart failure in 2 prospective cohorts / clinical perspective. *Circulation.* 2013;**127**: 1512–21
32. Bradley TD, *et al.* Obstructive sleep apnoea and its cardiovascular consequences. *Lancet.* 2009;**373**:82–93
33. Sliwa K, *et al.* Contribution of the human immunodeficiency virus/acquired immunodeficiency syndrome epidemic to de novo presentations of heart disease in the Heart of Soweto Study cohort. *Eur Heart J.* 2012;**33**: 866–74

Chapter 31

Chronic heart failure

Presentation

Presenting symptoms of heart failure, such as **dyspnoea**, **exercise intolerance**, and **fatigue**, are non-specific and mimicked by many other conditions, especially in the elderly. Several classification schemes (the most popular being by the New York Heart Association (NYHA), Canadian Cardiovascular Society (CCS), and Killip) have been presented for a semi-quantitative assessment of symptom severity (Table 31.1).

Orthopnoea, dyspnoea that occurs in the recumbent position, is a later manifestation. It may also be seen in patients with COPD and abdominal obesity or ascites. **Paroxysmal nocturnal dyspnoea** refers to acute episodes of dyspnoea and coughing that occur at night and awaken the patient. It is relatively specific for heart failure. **Pulmonary oedema** may develop in acute exacerbations of heart failure. Minor episodes of haemoptysis may represent transient, exercise-induced pulmonary oedema. **Cardiac asthma** refers to wheezing due to bronchospasm or increased pressure in the bronchial arteries. **Cheyne-Stokes respiration** is periodic respiration with apnoeic phases during which the arterial PO_2 and the PCO_2 rises. It is due to diminished sensitivity of the respiratory centre to arterial PCO_2 and occurs with advanced failure. **Altered mental status** may reflect hypoperfusion. **Anorexia** or **nausea** and **right upper quadrant pain** and **ascites** reflect bowel and liver congestion. **Cardiac cachexia** may be seen with advanced failure. A careful history is mandatory.

Physical examination

Physical signs are also non-specific:

- Sinus tachycardia or AF in 30% of patients with advanced disease
- Raised jugular venous pulse
- Third heart sound (S_3)
- Basal pulmonary rales
- Peripheral oedema with ankle swelling and hepatomegaly.

Table 31.1 Classifications of heart failure

NYHA functional classification	
Class I Patients with cardiac disease but no resulting limitation of physical activity. Ordinary physical activity does not cause undue fatigue, palpitation, dyspnoea, or anginal pain.	
Class II Patients with cardiac disease resulting in slight limitation of physical activity. Comfortable at rest, but ordinary physical activity results in fatigue, palpitation, dyspnoea, or anginal pain. **By limiting activity, patients still able to lead a normal social life.**	
Class III Patients with cardiac disease resulting in marked limitation of physical activity. Comfortable at rest, but less-than-ordinary physical activity results in fatigue, palpitation, dyspnoea, or anginal pain. **Patients unable to do any housework.**	
Class IV Patients with cardiac disease resulting in inability to carry out any physical activity without symptoms. Dyspnoea or angina may be present, even at rest. Comfortable at rest, but less-than-ordinary physical activity results in fatigue, palpitation, dyspnoea, or anginal pain. **Patients incapacitated and virtually confined to bed or a chair.**	
ACC/AHA stages of heart failure	
Stage A At high risk for developing heart failure. No identified structural or functional abnormality; no signs or symptoms.	
Stage B Developed structural heart disease that is strongly associated with the development of heart failure but without signs or symptoms.	
Stage C Symptomatic heart failure associated with underlying structural heart disease.	
Stage D Advanced structural heart disease and marked symptoms of heart failure at rest despite maximal medical therapy.	
Killip classification of the severity of heart failure in the context of myocardial infarction	
Stage I	No heart failure.
	No clinical signs of cardiac decompensation.
Stage II	Heart failure.
	Diagnostic criteria include rales, S_3 gallop, and pulmonary venous hypertension.
	Pulmonary congestion with wet rales in the lower half of the lung fields.
Stage III	Severe heart failure.
	Frank pulmonary oedema with rales throughout the lung fields.
Stage IV	Cardiogenic shock.
	Signs include hypotension (SBP <90 mmHg) and evidence of peripheral vasoconstriction, such as oliguria, cyanosis, and sweating.

Pulmonary rales may be absent despite elevated left-sided filling pressures due to chronic lymphatic hypertrophy, which prevents alveolar oedema despite elevated interstitial pressures.[1] **Ankle oedema** may be caused by heart or renal failure and pericardial constriction, particularly with elevated JVP, chronic venous insufficiency, calcium channel blockers, IVC obstruction, prolonged air travel, idiopathic, liver congestion and hypoalbuminaemia, secondary hyperaldosteronism. Anasarca is rare in cardiac failure, unless untreated, and there is concomitant hypoalbuminaemia. **Unilateral ankle oedema** may be due to venous thrombosis, lymphatic obstruction, and saphenous vein harvesting for CABG. Young patients may be not edematous despite intravascular volume overload. In obese patients and elderly patients, edema may reflect peripheral rather than cardiac causes.

The Framingham criteria emphasized the importance of jugular venous pressure elevation, an S_3 gallop, and a positive hepatojugular reflex in establishing a diagnosis while minimizing the importance of lower extremity oedema. The **jugular venous pressure** is measured as the vertical distance between the venous pulsation and the sternal angle of Louis (where the manubrium meets the sternum), with the patient semi-recumbent at an angle of about 45°. A distance >3 cm (cm of blood or water) is considered abnormal (1.36 cmH_2O = 1 mmHg). Alternatively, the ability to see venous pulsations above the clavicle in the seated position denotes raised JVP since the clavicle is at least 10 cm above the right atrium.

- **a wave:** atrial contraction, coincident with the P wave of the ECG. Large a wave indicates increased right ventricular end-diastolic pressure (RVEDP) as in pulmonary hypertension and pulmonary valve stenosis, or TS. Cannon a waves are seen in AV dissociation. Absent in AF.
- **c wave:** not visible (TV closure).
- **x descent:** atrial diastolic suction due to ventricular contraction that pools the TV and RA floor downward.
- **v wave:** atrial filling. Smaller than the a wave; equal in ASD. Accentuated in TR (merges with a wave to produce the s wave).
- **y descent:** reflects fall in right atrial pressure after TV opening. Blunted in TS or tamponade, steep in early

diastolic filling as in pericardial constriction (pericardial knock).

The normal JVP should fall by at least 3 mmHg with inspiration. A rise or failure to decrease with inspiration is a sign of constrictive pericarditis (**Kussmaul sign**), but it can also be seen in restrictive cardiomyopathy, massive pulmonary embolus, and RV failure. The **abdomino-jugular reflex** refers to sustained rise of >3 cm of JVP for at least 15 s after release of consistent pressure over the upper abdomen for at least 10 s.

Physical examination is not helpful in discriminating between systolic and diastolic heart failure.

Investigations

Haematocrit and leukocyte count, blood urea nitrogen and creatinine, glucose and HbA_{1c} serum electrolytes, liver function tests, lipid profile, and thyroid function tests are taken routinely (Tables 31.2, 31.3, and 31.4). Natriuretic peptide (**BNP**) and its precursor N terminal **pro-BNP** are sensitive and specific indices for discriminating between causes of dyspnoea (Figure 31.1).[4] Low BNP (<100 pg/mL or NT-pro-BNP <400 pg/mL) has a very high negative predictive value, making it a useful rule-out test. This peptide is raised with advanced age, female sex, and renal insufficiency and lowered with obesity. A normal BNP

Table 31.2 ACC/AHA 2013 GL on HF. Initial and serial evaluation of the heart failure patient

Clinical evaluation	
History and physical examination	
Thorough history and physical examination to identify cardiac and non-cardiac disorders or behaviours that might cause or accelerate the development or progression of HF.	I-C
In patients with idiopathic dilated cardiomyopathy (DCM), a 3-generational family history should be obtained for familial DCM.	I-C
Volume status and vital signs should be assessed at each patient encounter. This include serial assessment of weight, jugular venous pressure and peripheral edema or orthopnea	I-B
Risk scoring	
Validated multivariable risk scores to estimate subsequent risk of mortality in abulatory or hospitalized patients with HF.	IIa-B
Diagnostic tests	
Complete blood count, urinalysis, serum electrolytes (including calcium and magnesium), blood urea nitrogen, serum creatinine, glucose, fasting lipid profile, liver function tests, and thyroid-stimulating hormone as initial laboratory evaluation.	I-C
Serial monitoring should include serum electrolytes and renal function.	I-C
A 12-lead ECG initially on all patients presenting with HF.	I-C
Screening for hemochromatosis or HIV.	IIa-C
Diagnostic tests for rheumatologic diseases, amyloidosis, or pheochromocytoma in clinical suspicion of these diseases.	IIa-C

Biomarkers

Biomarker, application	Setting	
Natriuretic peptides		
Diagnosis or exclusion of HF	Ambluatory, acute	I-A
Prognosis of HF	Ambluatory, acute	I-A
Achieve GDMT	Ambulatory	IIa-B
Guidance for acute decompensated HF therapy	Acute	IIb-C
Biomarkers of myocardial injury		
Additive risk stratification	Acute, ambulatory	I-A
Biomarkers of myocardial fibrosis		
Additive risk stratification	Ambulatory	IIb-B
	Acute	IIb-A

GDMT, guideline-directed medical therapy; HF, heart failure.

(Continued)

Table 31.2 (Continued)

Selected causes of elevated natriuretic peptide concentrations	
Cardiac	**Non-cardiac**
Heart failure, including RV syndromes	Advancing age
Acute coronary syndrome	Anemia
Heart muscle disease, including LVH	Renal failure
Valvular heart disease	Pulmonary: obstructive sleep apnea, severe pneumonia, pulmonary hypertension
Pericardial disease	Critical illness
Atrial fibrillation	Bacterial sepsis
Myocarditis	Severe burns
Cardiac surgery	Toxic-metabolic insults, including cancer chemotherapy and envenomation
Cardioversion	

LVH: left ventricular hypertrophy; RV: right ventricular
2013 ACCF/AHA Guideline for the Management of Heart Failure. *JACC* 2013; doi: 10.1016/j.jacc.2013.05.019.

Table 31.3 ESC 2012 GL on HF

Common laboratory test abnormalities in heart failure		
Abnormality	**Causes**	**Clinical implications**
Renal/kidney impairment (creatinine >150 μmol/L/1.7 mg/dL, eGFR <60 mL/min/1.73 m^2)	Renal disease Renal congestion ACE inhibitor/ARB, MRA Dehydration NSAIDs and other nephrotoxic drugs	Calculate eGFR Consider reducing ACE inhibitor/ARB or MRA dose (or postpone dose uptitration) Check potassium and BUN Consider reduding diuretic dose if dehydrated, but, if renal congestion, more diuresis may help Review drug therapy
Anaemia (<13 g/dL or 8.0 mmol/L in men; <12 g/dL or 7.4 mmol/L in women)	Chronic HF, haemodilution, iron loss or poor utilization, renal failure, chronic disease, malignancy	Diagnostic work-up Consider treatment
Hyponatraemia (<135 mmol/L)	Chronic HF, haemodilution, AVP release, diuretics (especially thiazides) and other drugs	Consider water restriction, adjusting diuretic dosage Ultrafiltration, vasopressin antagonist Review drug therapy
Hypernatraemia (>150 mmol/L)	Water loss/inadequate water intake	Assess water intake Diagnostic work-up
Hypokalaemia (<3.5 mmol/L)	Diuretics, secondary hyperaldosteronism	Risk of arrhythmia Consider ACE inhibitor/ARB, MRA, potassium supplements
Hyperkalaemia (>5.5 mmol/L)	Renal failure, potassium supplement, renin-angiotensin-aldosterone system blockers	Stop potassium supplements/potassium-sparing diuretic Reduce dose of/stop ACE inhibitor/ARB, MRA Assess renal function and urine pH Risk of bradycardia and serious arrhythmias
Hyperglycaemia (>6.5 mmol/L/117 mg/dL)	Diabetes, insulin resistance	Evaluate hydration, treat glucose intolerance
Hyperuricaemia (>500 μmol/L/8.4 mg/dL)	Diuretic treatment, gout, malignancy	Allopurinol Reduce diuretic dose
Albumin high (>45 g/L)	Dehydration, myeloma	Rehydrate Diagnostic work-up
Albumin low (<30 g/L)	Poor nutrition, renal loss	Diagnostic work-up
Transaminase increase	Liver dysfunction Liver congestion Drug toxicity	Diagnostic work-up Liver congestion Review drug therapy

(Continued)

Table 31.3 (Continued)

Common laboratory test abnormalities in heart failure		
Abnormality	**Causes**	**Clinical implications**
Elevated troponins	Myocyte necrosis Prolonged ischaemia, severe HF, myocarditis, sepsis, renal failure	Evaluate pattern of increase (mild increases common in severe HF) Perfusion/viability studies Coronary angiography Evaluation for revascularization
Elevated creatine kinase	Inherited and acquired myopathies (including myositis)	Consider genetic cardiomyopathy (laminopathy, desminopathy, dystrophinopathy), muscular dystrophies Statin use
Abnormal thyroid tests	Hyper-/hypothyroidism Amiodarone	Treat thyroid abnormality Reconsider amiodarone use
Urine analysis	Proteinuria, glycosuria, bacteria	Diagnostic work-up Rule out infection, diabetes
International normalized ratio >3.5	Anticoagulant overdose Liver congestion/disease Drug interactions	Review anticoagulant dose Assess liver function Review drug therapy
CRP >10 mg/L, neutrophilic leukocytosis	Infection, inflammation	Diagnostic work-up

AV, atrioventricular; CMR, cardiac magnetic resonance; CRT-P, cardiac resynchronization therapy pacemaker; CRT-D, cardiac resynchronization therapy defibrillator; ECG, electrocardiogram; HF, heart failure; ICD, implantable cardioverter-defibrillator; LBBB, left bundle branch block; LV, left ventricular.
ESC guidelines for the diagnosis and treatment of acute and chronic heart failure 2012. *Eur Heart J.* 2012;33:1787–847.

Table 31.4 ESC 2012 GL on HF

Recommendations for the diagnostic investigations in ambulatory patients suspected of having heart failure[a]	
Investigations to consider in all patients	
Transthoracic echocardiography to evaluate cardiac structure and function, including diastolic function, and to measure LVEF to make the diagnosis of HF, assist in planning and monitoring of treatment, and to obtain prognostic information.	I-C
A 12-lead ECG to determine heart rhythm, heart rate, QRS morphology, and QRS duration, and to detect other relevant abnormalities. This information also assists in planning treatment and is of prognostic importance. A completely normal ECG makes systolic HF unlikely.	I-C
Measurement of blood chemistry (including sodium, potassium, calcium, urea/blood urea nitrogen, creatinine/estimated glomerular filtration rate, liver enzymes and bilirubin, ferritin/TIBC) and thyroid function to:	I-C
(i) Evaluate patient suitability for diuretic, renin-angiotensin-aldosterone antagonist, and anticoagulant therapy (and monitor treatment).	
(ii) Detect reversible/treatable causes of HF (e.g. hypocalcaemia, thyroid dysfunction) and co-morbidities (e.g. iron deficiency).	
(iii) Obtain prognostic information.	
A complete blood count to:	I-C
(i) Detect anaemia, which may be an alternative cause of the patient's symptoms and signs and may cause worsening of HF.	
(ii) Obtain prognostic information.	
Measurement of natriuretic peptide (BNP, NT-pro-BNP, or MR-pro-ANP) should be considered to:	IIa-C
(i) Exclude alternative causes of dyspnoea (if the level is below the exclusion cut-point, HF is very unlikely).	
(ii) Obtain prognostic information.	
A chest radiograph (X-ray) to detect/exclude certain types of lung disease, e.g. cancer (does not exclude asthma/COPD). It may also identify pulmonary congestion/oedema and is more useful in patients with suspected HF in the acute setting.	IIa-C

(Continued)

Table 31.4 (Continued)

Recommendations for the diagnostic investigations in ambulatory patients suspected of having heart failure[a]	
Investigations to consider in selected patients	
CMR imaging to evaluate cardiac structure and function, to measure LVEF, and to characterize cardiac tissue, especially in subjects with inadequate echocardiographic images or where the echocardiographic findings are inconclusive or incomplete (but taking account of cautions/contraindications to CMR).	I-C
Coronary angiography in patients with angina pectoris, who are considered suitable for coronary revascularization, to evaluate the coronary anatomy.	I-C
Myocardial perfusion/ischaemia imaging (echocardiography, CMR, SPECT, or PET) in patients thought to have CAD and who are considered suitable for coronary revascularization to determine whether there is reversible myocardial ischaemia and viable myocardium.	IIa-C
Left and right heart catheterization in patients being evaluated for heart transplantation or mechanical circulatory support to evaluate right and left heart function and pulmonary arterial resistance.	I-C
Exercise testing:	IIa-C
(i) To detect reversible myocardial ischaemia.	
(ii) As part of the evaluation of patients for heart transplantation and mechanical circulatory support.	
(iii) To aid in the prescription of exercise training.	
(iv) To obtain prognostic information.	

BNP, B-type natriuretic peptide: CAD, coronary artery disease; CMR, cardiac magnetic resonance: COPD, chronic obstructive pulmonary disease: BCG, electrocardiogram; HF, heart failure; LV, left vertricular; LVEF, left ventricular ejection fraction: MR-pro-ANP, mid-regional pro-atrial natriuretic peptide; NT-pro-BNP, N-terminal pro-B-type natriuretic peptide; PET, position emission tomography: SPECT, single photon emission computed tomography: TIBC, total iron-binding capacity.

[a] This list is not exclusive, and other investigations are discussed in the text. Additional investigations may be indicated in patients with suspected acute HF in the emergency department/hospital, including troponins and D-dimer measurement and right heart catheterization.

ESC guidelines for the diagnosis and treatment of acute and chronic heart failure 2012. *Eur Heart J*. 2012;**33**:1787–847.

Table 31.5 ACCF/AHA 2013 GL on heart failure

Recommendations for noninvasive cardiac imaging	
Patients with suspected, acute, or new-onset HF should undergo a chest X-ray	I-C
A 2-D echocardiogram with Doppler for initial evaluation of HF	I-C
Repeat measurement of EF in patients with who have had a significant change in clinical status or received treatment that might affect cardiac function or for consideration of device therapy	I-C
Noninvasive imaging to detect myocardial ischemia and viability in HF and CAD	IIa-C
Viability assessment before revascularization in HF patients with CAD	IIa-B
Radionuclide ventriculography or MRI to assess LVEF and volume	IIa-C
MRI when assessing myocardial infiltration or scar	IIa-B
Routine repeat measurement of LV function assessment should not be performed	III-B (no benefit)

Recommendations for invasive evaluation	
Monitoring with a pulmonary artery catheter in patients with respiratory distress or impaired systemic perfusion when clinical assessment is inadequate	I-C
Invasive hemodynamic monitoring for carefully selected patients with acute HF with persistent symptoms and/or when hemodynamics are uncertain	IIa-C
When ischemia may be contributing to HF, coronary arteriography	IIa-C
Endomyocardial biopsy in patients with HF when a specific diagnosis is suspected that would influence therapy	IIa-C
Routine use of invasive hemodynamic monitoring is not recommended in normotensive patients with acute HF	III-B (no benefit)
Endomyocardial biopsy should not be performed in the routine evaluation of HF	III-C (harm)

CAD indicates coronary artery disease; EF, ejection fraction; HF, heart failure; LV, left ventricular; LVEF, left ventricular ejection fraction; and MRI, magnetic resonance imaging.

2013 ACCF/AHA Guideline for the Management of Heart Failure. *JACC 2013*; doi: 10.1016/j.jacc.2013.05.019

in an untreated patient virtually excludes cardiac disease. High values (BNP >400 pg/mL or NT-pro-BNP >2000 pg/mL) suggest that heart failure is likely, whereas the diagnosis is uncertain with intermediate values. For patients presenting with acute onset or worsening of symptoms, the optimal exclusion cut-off point is 300 pg/mL for NT-pro-BNP and 100 pg/mL for BNP. For patients presenting in a non-acute way, the optimum exclusion cut-off point is 125 pg/mL for NT-pro-BNP and 35 pg/mL for BNP.[2] The sensitivity and specificity of BNP and NT-pro-BNP for the diagnosis of HF are lower in non-acute patients, and their value to guide therapy is not well established. **Cardiac troponins** are detected in most heart failure patients and their values have prognostic significance.[5] Other biomarkers In

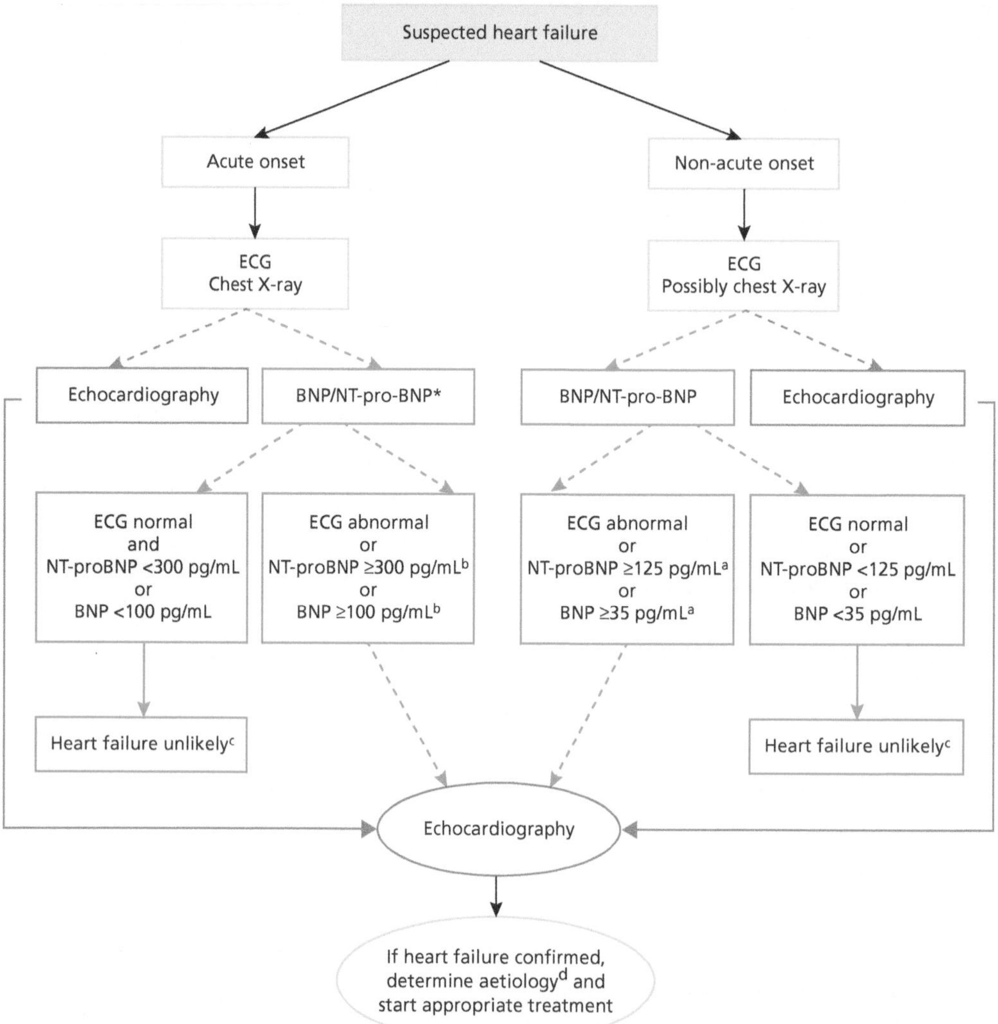

*In the acute setting, MR-proANP may also be used (cut-off point 120 pmol/L. i.e. <120 pmol/L = heart failure unlikely),
BNP = B-type natriuretic peptide; ECG = electrocardiogram; HF = heart failure; MR-proANP= mid-regional pro atrial natriuretic peptide;
NT-proBNP = N-terminal pro B-type natriuretic peptide.
[a]Exclusion cut-off points for natriuretic peptides are chosen to minimize the false-negative rate while reducing unnecessary referrals for echocardiography.
[b]Other causes of elevated natriuretic peptide levels in the acute setting are an acute coronary syndrome, atrial or ventricular arrhythmias, pulmonary embolism and severe chronic obstructive pulmonary disease with elevated right heart pressures, renal failure, and sepsis. Other causes of an elevated natriuetic level in the non-acute setting are: old age (>75 years), atrial arrhythmias, left ventricular hypertrophy, chronic obstrutive pulmonary disease, and chronic kindney disease.
[c]Treatment may reduce natriuretic peptide concentration, and natriuretic peptide concentrations may not be markedly elevated in patients with HF-PEF.
[d]See Section 3.5 and Web Table 3.

Figure 31.1 ESC 2012 GL on HF. Diagnostic flowchart for patients with suspected heart failure—showing alternative 'echocardiography first' (blue) or 'natriuretic peptide first' (red) approaches.

ESC guidelines for the diagnosis and treatment of acute and chronic heart failure 2012. *Eur Heart J*. 2012;**33**:1787–847.

Table 31.6 ESC 2012 GL on HF. Common echocardiographic measures of LV diastolic dysfunction

Measurement	**Abnormality**	**Clinical implications**
e′	Decreased (<8 cm/s septal, <10 cm/s lateral, or <9 cm/s average)	Delayed LV relaxation
E/e′ ratio[a]	High (>15)	High LV filling pressure
	Low (<8)	Normal LV filling pressure
	Intermediate (8–15)	Grey zone (additional parameters necessary)
Mitral inflow E/A ratio[b]	'Restrictive' (>2)	High LV filling pressure
		Volume overload
	'Impaired relaxation' (<1)	Delayed LV relaxation
		Normal LV filling pressure
	Normal (1–2)	Inconclusive (may be 'pseudonormal')
Mitral inflow during Valsalva manoeuvre	Change of the 'pseudonormal' to the 'impaired relaxation' pattern (with a decrease in E/A ratio ≥0.5)	High LV filling pressure (unmasked through Valsalva)
(A pulm–A mitral) duration	>30 ms	High LV filling pressure

A pulm–A mitral, time difference between pulmonary vein flow A-wave duration and mitral flow A-wave duration; E/A, ratio of early to late diastolic mitral inflow waves; e′, early diastolic velocity of mitral annulus; E/e′, ratio of the mitral inflow E wave to the tissue Doppler e′ wave; HF, heart failure; LV, left ventricular.

[a] Different cut-off points exist in different consensus documents; for the cut-off points mentioned in this table, both septal and average e′ may be used.

[b] Highly variable and unsuitable for diagnosis on its own; largely depending on its own; largely depending on loading conditions; age-corrected normal values exist.

ESC guidelines for the diagnosis and treatment of acute and chronic heart failure 2012: *Eur Heart J*. 2012;**33**:1787–847.

ambulatory chronic heart failure patients, a score derived from multiple biomarkers such as high-sensitivity C-reactive protein, myeloperoxidase, B-type natriuretic peptide, soluble fms-like tyrosine kinase receptor-1, troponin I, soluble toll-like receptor-2, creatinine, and uric acid, may also improve prediction of adverse events.[6] Screening for *haemochromatosis, sleep-disturbed breathing, HIV, rheumatological diseases, amyloidosis, or phaeochromocytoma* is also undertaken when there is a clinical suspicion of these diseases.

ECG Left ventricular hypertrophy, atrial enlargement, previous myocardial infarction, active ischaemia, conduction abnormalities, and arrhythmias may be present. An entirely normal ECG makes the diagnosis of systolic dysfunction unlikely (<10%).

Chest radiography may reveal cardiomegaly and/or pulmonary congestion (Kerley B lines and interstitial oedema with upper lobe blood diversion). Pleural effusions may be present, with biventricular failure.

Echocardiography, especially three-dimensional echo,[5] may provide important information about ventricular dimensions, extent of systolic dysfunction, whether dysfunction is global or segmental, the status of valves, and estimates of pulmonary artery pressure (Table 31.4). It is most specific for diagnosis of LV systolic dysfunction. Radionuclide ventriculography can also be performed to assess LVEF and volumes. Assessment of diastolic dysfunction still remains rather elusive, even with tissue Doppler imaging that provides information on patterns of diastolic relaxation and filling and ventricular dyssynchrony (Figure 31.2 and Table 31.6) (see also Chapter 32).

MRI provides the most accurate estimate of ventricular structure and function. The use of gadolinium contrast allows detection of inflammation and scarring. It cannot be used in the presence of implanted devices, although now this can be overcome with special techniques. MRI-assessed 4D flow is a novel method for assessment of diastolic dysfunction.[6]

Maximal exercise testing, ideally with respiratory gas exchange, is useful to document the contribution of HF to exercise limitation and identify high-risk patients. Metabolic stress testing with respiratory gas analysis is useful to differentiate between cardiac or pulmonary limitation to exercise and to determine functional class in patients who are candidates for cardiac transplantation or in whom the cause of exercise intolerance is unclear. Peak oxygen uptake (peak VO_2), anaerobic threshold, and VE/VCO_2 slope (ventilatory response to exercise) are useful indicators of the functional capacity of the patient with prognostic significance.

Holter monitoring may be considered in patients who are being investigated for ventricular arrhythmias.

Selected ion-flow tube mass-spectrometry (SIFT-MS) of exhaled breath samples (collected within 24 h of hospital admission and following an 8-h fast and before the administration of morning pharmacotherapy) has been recently proposed as simple test that allows detection of patients with impending decompensation and development of acute HF.[7]

Coronary angiography is indicated when the patient has angina or coronary artery disease is suspected (Table 31.4).

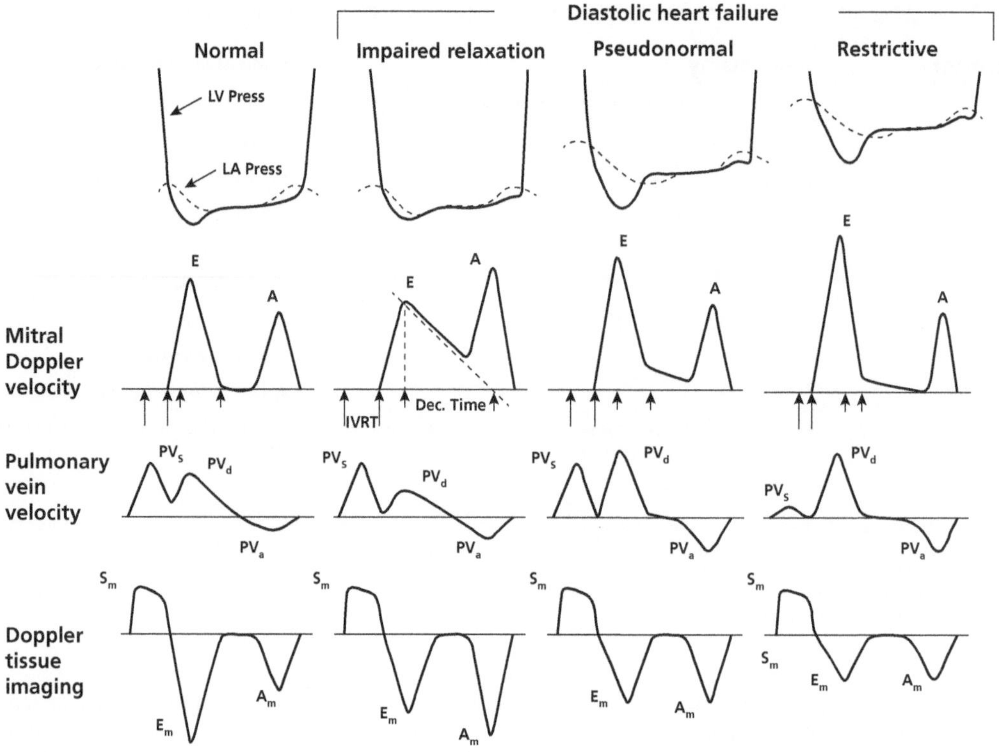

Figure 31.2 LV and left atrial (LA) pressures during diastole, transmitral Doppler LV inflow velocity, pulmonary vein Doppler velocity, and Doppler tissue velocity. IVRT indicates isovolumic relaxation time; Dec. Time, e-wave deceleration time; E, early LV filling velocity; A, velocity of LV filling contributed by atrial contraction; PVs, systolic pulmonary vein velocity; PVd, diastolic pulmonary vein velocity; PVa, pulmonary vein velocity resulting from atrial contraction; Sm, myocardial velocity during systole; Em, myocardial velocity during early filling; and Am, myocardial velocity during filling produced by atrial contraction.

Zile MR, Brutsaert DL. New concepts in diastolic dysfunction and diastolic heart failure: Part I: diagnosis, prognosis, and measurements of diastolic function. *Circulation*. 2002;**105**:1387–93.

Cardiac catheterization may also be needed when echocardiography is insufficient to define the severity of valve disease and/or pulmonary pressures.

Myocardial ischaemia and viability studies are required in ischaemic patients in whom intervention is planned. Imaging modalities with comparable diagnostic accuracy are dobutamine echocardiography, nuclear imaging by SPECT and/or by PET, MRI with dobutamine and/or with contrast agents, CT with contrast agents (Table 31.4).

Cardiac biopsy on a routine basis is not recommended in CCF. It is only needed when specific cause is considered, mainly giant cell myocarditis.

Prognosis

Conditions associated with a poor prognosis in heart failure are as age, aetiology, NYHA class, LVEF, key co-morbidities (renal dysfunction, diabetes, anaemia, hyperuricaemia), and plasma natriuretic peptide concentration. Common comorbidities are presented in Table 31.7. Several risk scores for predicting survival in heart failure have been developed,[8] one of the most useful ones being that of MAGGIC (www.heartfailure.org).[9]

Therapy

General measures

Patients with heart failure should be enrolled in a multidisciplinary care management programme to reduce the risk of heart failure hospitalization GL (ESC 2012 GL on HF, I-A).[8,10,11] Regular **aerobic exercise** is beneficial for patients with stable, non-decompensated heart failure (ESC 2012 on HF I-A),[12] through various mechanisms such as maintaining protein folding in the heart and preventing premature cell death.[13] Sexual activity is not

Table 31.7 ACCF/AHA 2013 GL on HF. Ten most common co-occurring chronic conditions among medicare beneficiaries with heart failure (N=4,947,918), 2011

Beneficiaries Age ≥65 y (N=4,376,150)*			**Beneficiaries Age <65 y (N=571,768)†**		
	N	**%**		**N**	**%**
Hypertension	3,685,373	84.2	Hypertension	461,235	80.7
Ischemic heart disease	3,145,718	71.9	Ischemic heart disease	365,889	64.0
Hyperlipidemia	2,623,601	60.0	Diabetes	338,687	59.2
Anemia	2,200,674	50.3	Hyperlipidemia	325,498	56.9
Diabetes	2,027,875	46.3	Anemia	284,102	49.7
Arthritis	1,901,447	43.5	Chronic kidney disease	257,015	45.0
Chronic kidney disease	1,851,812	42.3	Depression	207,082	36.2
COPD	1,311,118	30.0	Arthritis	201,964	35.3
Atrial fibrillation	1,247,748	28.5	COPD	191,016	33.4
Alzheimer's disease/dementia	1,207,704	27.6	Asthma	88,816	15.5

*Mean No. of conditions is 6.1; median is 6.
†Mean No. of conditions is 5.5; median is 5.
Data source: CMS administrative claims data, January 2011-December 2011, from the Chronic Condition Warehouse (CCW), ccwdata.org. CMS indicates Centers for Medicare and Medicaid Services; and COPD, chronic obstructive pulmonary disease.
2013 ACCF/AHA Guideline for the Management of Heart Failure. *JACC* 2013; doi: 10.1016/j.jacc.2013.05.019

advised for patients with decompensated or advanced (NYHA class III or IV) heart failure (AHA 2012 on Sexual Activity and CDV, III-C). **Salt restriction** is usually advisable, especially in patients with stages C and D, although more data are needed to support a specific sodium intake level.[14] **Fluid restriction** to 1.5–2 L/day may be considered only in patients with severe symptoms and hyponatraemia. **Weight loss** is initially advisable in patients with coronary artery disease, but, in established heart failure, wasting is an independent risk factor.[15] **Alcohol** has a direct toxicity on myocardium and, at high doses, may cause hypertension and arrhythmias. It should be restricted to 2 units a day and avoided in alcohol-related dilated cardiomyopathy. **Smoking cessation, avoidance of high altitude** (>1500 m), and **vaccination against influenza and pneumococcus** are recommended. **Pregnancy** carries a high risk in patients with heart failure, and any decision should be discussed on an individual basis. **Contraception** with combined hormonal contraceptives is contraindicated due to fluid retention and increased thrombotic risk. Progesterone-only forms are probably safer but still carry a risk of thrombotic risk and osteopaenia.[16] Copper intrauterine devices or transcervical tubal occlusion are relatively safer.[16] Patients with **diabetes** should be treated appropriately for blood pressure, lipid and glycemic control, but avoiding hypoglycaemia potentially associated with drug therapy, targeting a HbA_{1c} <6.5.[17] An association of thiazolidinediones with heart failure is well established. Recent evidence indicates that rosiglitazone, in addition, increases the risk of stroke and total mortality.[18] Pioglitazone appears to be a safer alternative with favourable effects on atheroma progression,[19] but, recently, its use was suspended in France due to concerns about increased risk of bladder cancer. In established heart failure, all thiazolidinediones should be avoided. Metformin can be used as long as LV dysfunction is not severe and renal function adequate (creatinine <1.5 mg/dL in men and <1.4 mg/dL in women).[20] **Non-steroidal anti-inflammatory drugs (including COX-2 inhibitors)** as well as **corticosteroids** and **herbal preparations** (licorice, ginseng, ma huang) cause salt and water retention and should be used with much caution. In gout attacks, **colchicine** is preferred to NSAIDs in symptomatic heart failure patients. Although there has been some evidence that **aspirin** may interfere with prostaglandin synthesis, leading to a reduced effectiveness of ACE inhibition, the clinical significance of this observation is probably negligible.[21, 22] Ischaemic patients are treated with antiplatelet agents. **Tricyclic antidepressants** are contraindicated due to proarrhythmic potential. Use of **dexrazoxane** might be cardioprotective against anthracycline-induced cardiomyopathy by attenuation of the formation of free radicals.[23] The value of enhancement of **erythropoiesis** in anemia is controversial. Erythropoiesis stimulation with darbepoetin alfa corrects hemoglobin deficiency in systolic heart failure but fails to improve mortality or hospitalization rates and may increase thromboembolic risk.[24]

Drug therapy

Beta blockers and angiotensin-converting enzyme inhibitors (ACEI) or angiotensin receptor blockers (ARB) are the cornerstones of heart failure therapy (Figures 31.3, 31.4, 31.5, Tables 31.8–12).[8, 14, 15, 25]

Angiotensin-converting enzyme inhibitors (ACEI) have multiple pleiotropic actions, including improved endothelial function, antiproliferative effects on smooth muscle cells, and antithrombotic effects. They decrease mortality in established heart failure (up to 23%) as well as in post-MI patients with reduced LVEF.[26] Enalapril, captopril, and lisinopril have been mostly studied in CCF trials and ramipril and trandolapril in post-MI trials, but their benefits appear to be a class effect without differences between tissue or non-tissue ACEI. Patients with heart failure may have increased plasma angiotensin II and, consequently, poor prognosis despite chronic ACE inhibitor therapy.[27]

Angiotensin receptor blockers (ARB) bind competitively to the AT1 receptor and should avoid this escape phenomenon. ARBs also reduce mortality in heart failure, are equally effective with ACEI in randomized trials,[28] and are very suitable for patients unable to tolerate ACEI due to cough (occurs in 10% in whites, up to 50% in Chinese).[8] Mainly studied agents in CCF are valsartan and candesartan. Irbesartan has been mainly studied in hypertension and diabetic nephropathy trials. Losartan has produced controversial results on mortality at low doses. Studies on the combination of ACEI and ARB have been controversial, and this combination should be probably avoided in patients already taking beta blockers (triple neurohormonal blockade).[29,30] In patients with LVEF ≤40% who remain symptomatic on ACEI and beta blockers, addition of eplerenone is preferred to an ARB. The addition of an ARB (or renin inhibitor) to the combination of an ACEI and a mineralocorticoid antagonist is also not recommended because of the risk of renal dysfunction and hyperkalaemia. However, a combination of ACEI, ARB, beta blockade, and spironolactone has been successfully tried, together with continuous flow LV assist device for reversal of end-stage heart failure.[31] In haemodialysis patients with heart failure and LVEF ≤40%, the

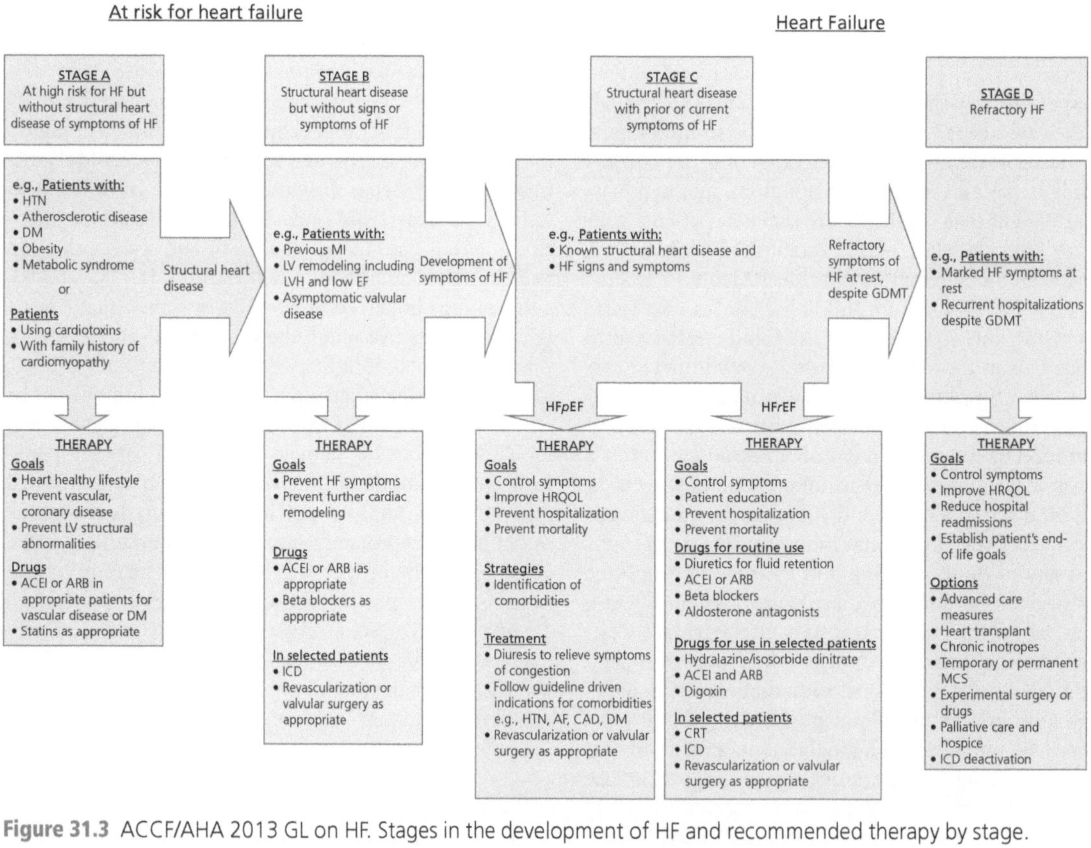

Figure 31.3 ACCF/AHA 2013 GL on HF. Stages in the development of HF and recommended therapy by stage.

ACEI indicates angiotensin-converting enzyme inhibitor; AF, atrial fibrillation; ARB, angiotensin-receptor blocker; CAD, coronary artery disease; CRT, cardiac resynchronization therapy; DM, diabetes mellitus; EF, ejection fraction; GDMT, guideline-directed medical therapy; HF, heart failure; HF**p** EF, heart failure with preserved ejection fraction; HF**r** EF, heart failure with reduced ejection fraction; HRQOL, health-related quality of life; HTN, hypertension; ICD, implantable cardioverter-defibrillator; LV, left ventricular; LVH, left ventricular hypertrophy; MCS, mechanical circulatory support; and MI, myocardial infarction.

2013 ACCF/AHA Guideline for the Management of Heart Failure. *JACC* 2013; doi: 10.1016/j.jacc.2013.05.019

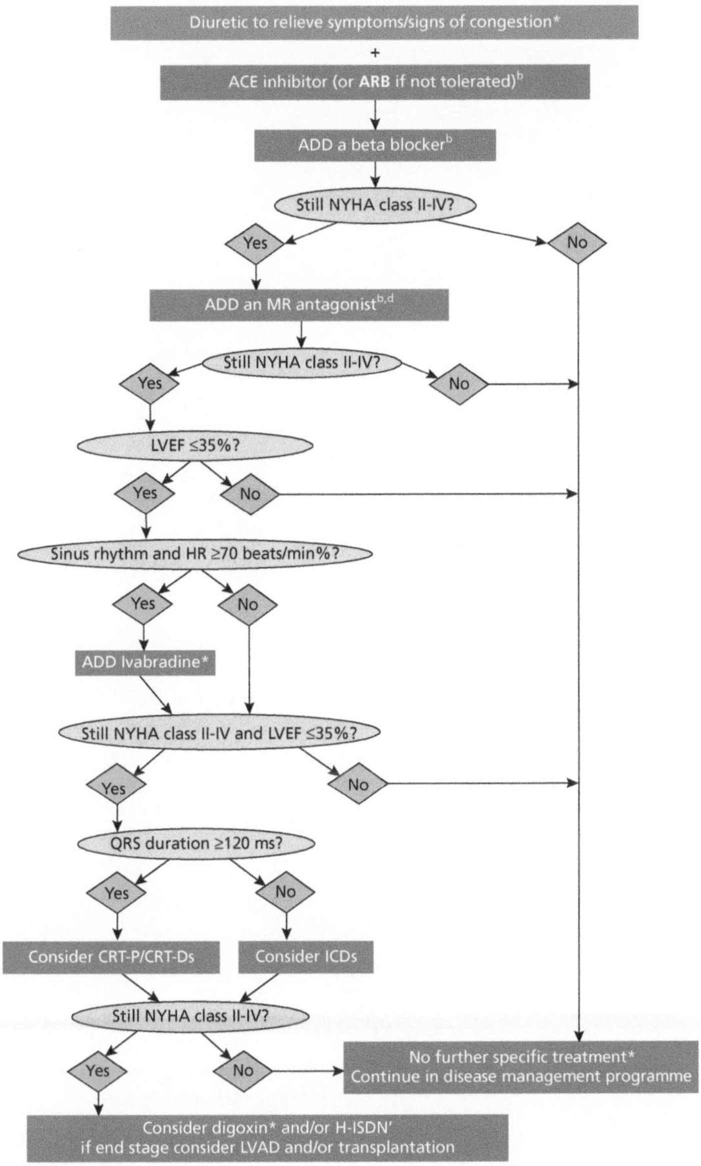

Figure 31.4 ESC 2012 guidelines on HF. Treatment options for patients with chronic symptomatic systolic heart failure (NYHA functional class II–IV).

ACE, angiotensin-converting enzyme; ARB, angiotensin receptor blocker; CRT-D, cardiac resynchronization therapy defibrillator; CRT-P, cardiac resynchronization therapy pacemaker; H-ISDN, hydralazine and isosorbide dinitrate; HR, heart rate; ICD, implantable cardioverter-defibrillator; LBBB, left bundle branch block; LVAD, left ventricular assist device; LVEF, left ventricular ejection fraction; MR antagonist, mineralocorticoid receptor antagonist; NYHA, New York Heart Association. (a) Diuretics may be used, as needed, to relieve the signs and symptoms of congestion, but they have not been shown to reduce hospitalization or death. (b) Should be titrated to evidence-based dose or maximum tolerated dose below the evidence-based dose. (c) Asymptomatic patients with an LVEF ≤35% and a history of myocardial infarction should be considered for an ICD. (d) If mineralocorticoid receptor antagonist is not tolerated, an ARB may be added to an ACE inhibitor as an alternative. (e) European Medicines Agency has approved ivabradine for use in patients with a heart rate ≥75 bpm. May also be considered in patients with a contraindication to a beta blocker or beta blocker intolerance. (f) Indication differs according to heart rhythm, NYHA class, QRS duration, QRS morphology, and LVEF. (g) Not indicated in NYHA class IV. (h) Digoxin may be used earlier to control the ventricular rate in patients with atrial fibrillation—usually in conjunction with a beta blocker. (i) The combination of hydralazine and isosorbide dinitrate may also be considered earlier in patients unable to tolerate an ACEI or an ARB.

ESC guidelines for the diagnosis and treatment of acute and chronic heart failure 2012. *Eur Heart J*. 2012;**33**:1787–847.

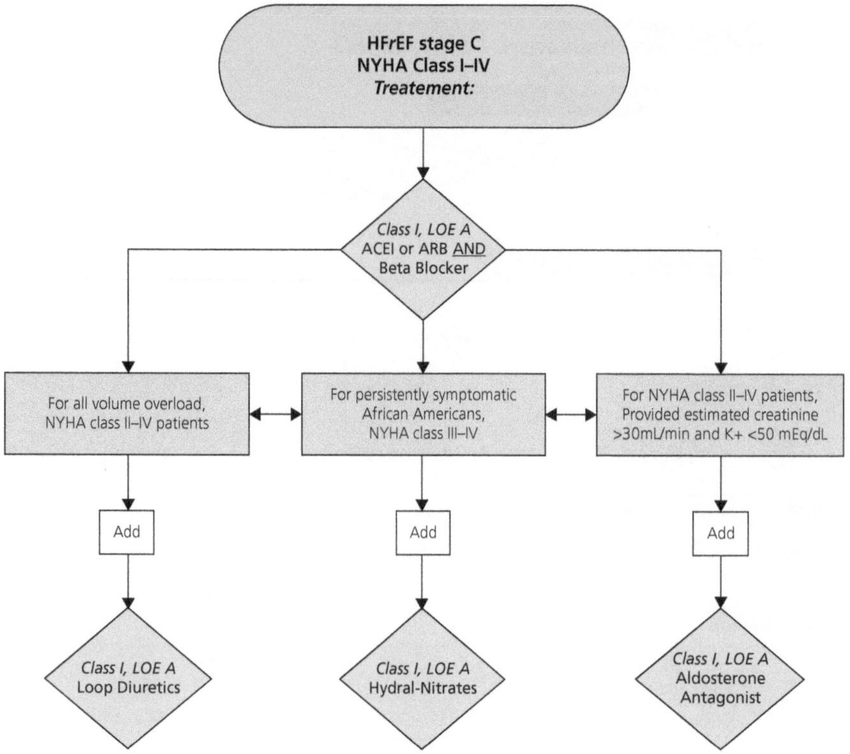

Figure 31.5 ACCF/AHA 2013 GL on HF. Stage C HF with reduced EF: evidence-based, guideline-directed medical therapy.

ACEI indicates angiotensin-converting enzyme inhibitor; ARB, angiotensin-receptor blocker; HFr EF, heart failure with reduced ejection fraction; Hydral-Nitrates, hydralazine and isosorbide dinitrate; LOE, Level of Evidence; and NYHA, New York Heart Association.
2013 ACCF/AHA Guideline for the Management of Heart Failure. *JACC* 2013; doi: 10.1016/j.jacc.2013.05.019

Table 31.8 ACC/AHA 2013 on HF

Medical therapy for Stage C HFrEF: magnitude of benefit demonstrated in RCTs

GDMT	RR reduction in mortality (%)	NNT for mortality reduction (standardized to 36 mo)	RR reduction in HF hospitalizations
ACE inhibitor or ARB	17	26	31
Beta blocker	34	9	41
Aldosterone antagonist	30	6	35
Hydralazine/nitrate	43	7	33

ACE indicates angiotensin-converting enzyme; ARB, angiotensin-receptor blocker; GDMT, guideline directed medical therapy; HF, heart failure; HFrEF, heart failure with reduced ejection fraction; NNT, number needed to treat; RCTs, randomized controlled trials; and RR, relative risk

Drugs commonly used for Stage C HFrEF

Drug	Initial daily dose(s)	Maximum dose(s)	Mean doses achieved in clinical trials
ACE inhibitors			
Captopril	6.25 mg 3 times	50 mg 3 times	122.7 mg/d
Enalapril	2.5 mg twice	10–20 mg twice	16.6 mg/d
Fosinopril	5–10 mg once	40 mg once	N/A

(Continued)

Table 31.8 (Continued)

Drug	Initial daily dose(s)	Maximum dose(s)	Mean doses achieved in clinical trials
Lisinopril	2.5–5 mg once	20–40 mg once	32.5–35.0 mg/d
Perindopril	2 mg once	8–16 mg once	N/A
Quinapril	5 mg once	20 mg twice	N/A
Ramipril	1.25–2.5 mg once	10 mg once	N/A
Trandolapril	1 mg once	4 mg once	N/A
ARBs			
Candesartan	4–8mg once	32 mg once	24 mg/d
Losartan	25–50 mg once	50–150 mg once	129 mg/d
Valsartan	20–40 mg twice	160 mg twice	254 mg/d
Aldosterone antagonists			
Spironolactone	12.5–25.0 mg once	25 mg once or twice	26 mg/d
Eplerenone	25 mg once	50 mg once	42.6 mg/d
Beta blockers			
Bisoprolol	1.25 mg once	10 mg once	8.6 mg/d
Carvedilol	3.125 mg twice	50 mg twice	37 mg/d
Carvedilol CR	10 mg once	80 mg once	N/A
Metoprolol succinate extended release (metoprolol CR/XL)	12.5–25 mg once	200 mg once	159 mg/d
Hydralazine and isosorbide dinitrate			
Fixed-dose combination	37.5 mg hydralazine/20 mg isosorbide dinitrate 3 times daily	75 mg hydralazine/40 mg isosorbide dinitrate 3 times daily	~175 mg hydralazine/90 mg isosorbide dinitrate daily
Hydralazine and isosorbide dinitrate	Hydralazine: 25–50 mg, 3 or 4 times daily and isosorbide dinitrate: 20–30 mg 3 or 4 times daily	Hydralazine: 300 mg daily in divided doses and isosorbide dinitrate 120 mg daily in divided doses	N/A

ACE indicates angiotensin-converting enzyme; ARB, angiotensin-receptor blocker; CR, controlled release; CR/XL, controlled release/extended release; HFr EF, heart failure with reduced ejection fraction; and N/A, not applicable.

Recommendations for treatment of Stage A HF

Hypertension and lipid disorders should be controlled in accordance with contemporary guidelines to lower the risk of HF	I-A
Other conditions that may lead to or contribute to HF, such as obesity, diabetes mellitus, tobacco use, and known cardiotoxic agents, should be controlled or avoided	I-C

Recommendations for treatment of Stage B HF

In patients with a history of MI and reduced EF, ACE inhibitors or ARBs to prevent HF	I-A
In patients with MI and reduced EF, evidence-based beta blockers to prevent HF	I-B
In patients with MI, statins to prevent HF	I-A
Blood pressure control to prevent symptomatic HF	I-A
ACE inhibitors in all patients with a reduced EF to prevent HF	I-A

(Continued)

Table 31.8 (Continued)

Beta blockers in all patients with a reduced EF to prevent HF	I-C
ICD in patients with asymptomatic ischemic cardiomyopathy, at least 40 d post-MI, LVEF ≤30%, and on GDMT	IIa-B
Nondihydropyridine calcium channel blockers in patients with low LVEF	III-C (harm)

ACE indicates angiotensin-converting enzyme; ARB, angiotensin-receptor blocker; COR, Class of Recommendation; EF, ejection fraction; GDMT, guideline-directed medical therapy; HF, heart failure; ICD, implantable cardioverter-defibrillator; LOE, Level of Evidence; LVEF, left ventricular ejection fraction; MI, myocardial infarction.

Recommendations for treatment of Stage C HF

Nonpharmacological interventions	
Patients with HF should receive specific education to facilitate HF self-care	I-B
Exercise training (or regular physical activity) is safe and effective for patients who are able to participate to improve functional status	I-A
Sodium restriction in symptomatic HF to reduce congestive symptoms	IIa-C
Continuous positive airway pressure (CPAP) to increase LVEF and improve functional status in patients with HF and sleep apnea	IIa-B
Cardiac rehabilitation in clinically stable patients to improve functional capacity, exercise duration, health-related quality of life, and mortality	IIa-B
Pharmacological treatment for stage C HFrEF	
Measures listed as Class I recommendations for patients in stages A and B are recommended where appropriate for patients in stage C	I-A/B/C
Guideline-directed medical therapy	I-A

Recommendations for Pharmacological Therapy for Management of Stage C HFrEF

Diuretics	
Diuretics in patients with HFrEF with fluid retention	I-C
ACE inhibitors	
ACE inhibitors for all patients with HFrEF	I-A
ARBs	
ARBs in patients with HFrEF who are ACE inhibitor intolerant	I-A
ARBS as alternatives to ACE inhibitors as first-line therapy in HFrEF	IIa-A
Addition of an ARB in persistently symptomatic patients with HFrEF on GDMT	IIb-A
Routine combined use of an ACE inhibitor, ARB, and aldosterone antagonist for all stable patients	III-C (harm)
Beta blockers	
Use of 1 of the 3 beta blockers proven to reduce mortality for all stable patients	I-A
Aldosterone receptor antagonists	
Aldosterone receptor antagonists in patients with NYHA class II–IV who have LVEF ≤35%	I-A
Aldosterone receptor antagonists following an acute MI who have LVEF ≤40% with symptoms of HF or DM	I-B
Inappropriate use of aldosterone receptor antagonists may be harmful	III-B (harm)
Hydralazine and isosorbide dinitrate	
The combination of hydralazine and isosorbide dinitrate for African Americans with NYHA class III–IV HFrEF on GDMT	I-A
A combination of hydralazine and isosorbide dinitrate in patients with HFrEF who cannot be given ACE inhibitors or ARBs	IIa-B
Digoxin	
Digoxin in patients with HFrEF	IIa-B

(Continued)

Table 31.8 (Continued)

Anticoagulation	
Patients with chronic HF with permanent/persistent/paroxysmal AF and an additional risk factor for cardioembolic stroke should receive chronic anticoagulant therapy*	I-A
The selection of an anticoagulant agent should be individualized	I-C
Chronic anticoagulation for patients with chronic HF who have permanent/persistent/paroxysmal AF but are without an additional risk factor for cardioembolic stroke*	IIa-B
Anticoagulation is not recommended in patients with chronic HFrEF without AF, a prior thromboembolic event, or a cardioembolic source	III-B (no benefit)
Statins	
Statins are not beneficial as adjunctive therapy when prescribed solely for HF	III-A (no benefit)
Omega-3 fatty acids	
Omega-3 PUFA supplementation as adjunctive therapy in HFrEF or HFpEF patients	IIa-B
Other drugs	
Nutritional supplements as treatment for HF are not recommended in HFrEF	III-B (no benefit)
Hormonal therapies other than to correct deficiencies are not recommended in HFrEF	III-C (no benefit)
Drugs known to adversely affect the clinical status of patients with HFrEF are potentially harmful and should be avoided or withdrawn	III-B (harm)
Long-term use of an infusion of a positive inotropic drug is not recommended and may be harmful except as palliation	III-C (harm)
Calcium channel blockers	
Calcium channel blocking drugs are not recommended as routine treatment in HFrEF	III-A (no benefit)

*In the absence of contraindications to anticoagulation.
ACE indicates angiotensin-converting enzyme; AF, atrial fibrillation; ARB, angiotensin-receptor blocker; COR, Class of Recommendation; DM, diabetes mellitus; GDMT, guideline-directed medical therapy; HF, heart failure; HFpEF, heartfailure with preserved ejection fraction; HFr EF, heart failure with reduced ejection fraction; LOE, Level of Evidence; LVEF, left ventricular ejection fraction; MI, myocardial infarction; N/A, not available; NYHA, New York Heart Association; and PUFA, polyunsaturated fatty acids.

Strategies for achieving optimal guideline-directed medical therapy (GDMT)

1. Uptitrate in small increments to the recommended target dose or the highest tolerated dose for those medications listed in Table 15 with an appreciation that some patients cannot tolerate the full recommended doses of all medications, particularly patients with low baseline heart rate or blood pressure or with a tendency to postural symptoms.
2. Certain patients (e.g., the elderly, patients with chronic kidney disease) may require more frequent visits and laboratory monitoring during dose titration and more gradual dose changes. However, such vulnerable patients may accrue considerable benefits from GDMT. Inability to tolerate optimal doses of GDMT may change after diseasemodifying interventions such as CRT.
3. Monitor vital signs closely before and during uptitration, including postural changes in blood pressure or heart rate, particularly in patients with orthostatic symptoms, bradycardia, and/or "low" systolic blood pressure (e.g., 80 to 100 mm Hg).
4. Alternate adjustments of different medication classes (especially ACE inhibitors/ARBs and beta blockers) listed in Table 15. Patients with elevated or normal blood pressure and heart rate may tolerate faster incremental increases in dosages.
5. Monitor renal function and electrolytes for rising creatinine and hyperkalemia, recognizing that an initial rise in creatinine may be expected and does not necessarily require discontinuation of therapy; discuss tolerable levels of creatinine above baseline with a nephrologist if necessary.
6. Patients may complain of symptoms of fatigue and weakness with dosage increases; in the absence of instability in vital signs, reassure them that these symptoms are often transient and usually resolve within a few days of these changes in therapy.
7. Discourage sudden spontaneous discontinuation of GDMT medications by the patient and/or other clinicians without discussion with managing clinicians.
8. Carefully review doses of other medications for HF symptom control (e.g., diuretics, nitrates) during uptitration.
9. Consider temporary adjustments in dosages of GDMT during acute episodes of noncardiac illnesses (e.g., respiratory infections, risk of dehydration, etc.).
10. Educate patients, family members, and other clinicians about the expected benefits of achieving GDMT, including an understanding of the potential benefits of myocardial reverse remodeling, increased survival, and improved functional status and HRQOL.

ACE indicates angiotensin-converting enzyme; ARB, angiotensin-receptor blocker; CRT, cardiac resynchronization therapy; and HRQOL, health-related quality of life.
2013 ACCF/AHA Guideline for the Management of Heart Failure. *JACC* 2013; doi: 10.1016/j.jacc.2013.05.019

Table 31.9 ESC recommendations on therapy

ESC 2012 GL on HF. Drug therapy of heart failure	
ACEIs in LVEF ≤40%, given with a beta blocker	I-A
Beta blockers in LVEF ≤40%, given with ACEI (or ARB)	I-A
MRA in NYHA II–IV and LVEF ≤35% despite treatment with ACEI (or ARB) and beta blocker	I-A
ARBs in LVEF ≤40% and ACEI intolerance, given with a beta blocker and MRA	I-A
ARBs in NYHA II–IV and LVEF ≤40% despite treatment with ACEI and beta blocker and MRA intolerance	I-A
Ivabradine in SR and LVEF ≤35% and HR ≥70 bpm, NYHA II–IV despite beta blocker (max dose) and ACEI (or ARB) and MRA (or ARB)*	IIa-B
Ivabradine in SR and LVEF ≤35% and HR ≥70 bpm and beta blocker intolerance, given with ACEI (or ARB) and MRA*	IIb-C
Digoxin in SR and LVEF ≤45% and beta blocker intolerance, given with ACE (or ARB) and MRA (or ARB)*	IIb-B
Digoxin in LVEF ≤45% and NYHA II–IV despite beta blocker and ACEI (or ARB) and MRA (or ARB)*	IIb-B
Hydralazine-ISDN as an alternative to an ACE or ARB, if neither is tolerated, in EF ≤45% and dilated LV (or EF ≤35%), given with a beta blocker and an MRA	IIb-B
Hydralazine-ISDN in EF ≤45% and dilated LV (or EF ≤35%) and NYHA II-IV despite beta blocker and ACEI (or ARB) and MRA (or ARB)	IIb-B
n-3 PUFA (with ACEI or ARB and beta blocker and MRA (or ARB))	IIb-B
ESC 2012 GL on HF. Harmful treatments in heart failure	
Thiazolidinediones (glitazones)	III-A
Most CCBs (with the exception of amlodipine and felodipine)	III-B
NSAIDs and COX-2 inhibitors (fluid retention and renal dysfunction)	III-B
Addition of an ARB (or renin inhibitor) to the combination of an ACE inhibitor AND a mineralocorticoid antagonist (renal dysfunction and hyperkalaemia)	III-C

* For reduction of hospitalization only.
MRA, mineralocorticoid receptor blocker; HR, heart rate; SR, sinus rhythm.

Table 31.10 ESC 2012 GL on HF

Recommendations for the treatment of hypertension in patients with symptomatic HF (NYHA functional class II–IV) and LV systolic dysfunction	
Step 1	
One or more of an ACE inhibitor (or ARB), beta blocker, and MRA as first-, second-, and third-line therapy (reducing the risk of HF hospitalization and reducing the risk of premature death).	I-A
Step 2	
A thiazide diuretic (or if the patient is treated with a thiazide diuretic, switching to a loop diuretic) is when hypertension persists despite treatment with a combination of as many as possible of an ACE inhibitor (or ARB), beta blocker, and MRA.	I-C
Step 3	
When hypertension persists despite treatment with a combination of as many as possible of an ACE inhibitor (or ARB), beta blocker, MRA, and diuretic.	
Amlodipine	I-A
Hydralazine	I-A
Felodipine	IIa-B
Moxonidine is not recommended (increased mortality)	III-B
Alpha-adrenoceptor antagonists are not recommended (neurohumoral activation, fluid retention, worsening HF)	III-A

ACE, angiotensin-converting enzyme; ARB, angiotensin receptor blocker; HF, heart failure; LV, left ventricular; LVEF, left ventricular ejection fraction; MRA, mineralocorticoid receptor antagonist.
ESC guidelines for the diagnosis and treatment of acute and chronic heart failure 2012, *Eur Heart J*. 2012;**33**:1787–847.

Table 31.11 Dosages of ACEI/ARB and beta blockers in heart failure

	Starting dose (mg)	Target dose (mg)
ACEI		
Captopril	6.25 tds	50 tds
Enalapril	2.5 bd	10–20 bd
Lisinopril	2.5–5.0 od	20–40 od
Ramipril	2.5 od	10 od or 5 bd
Trandolapril	0.5 od	4 od
Perindopril	2 od	16 od
Quinapril	5 bd	20 bd
Fosinopril	5–10 od	40 od
ARB		
Candesartan	4–8 od	32 od
Valsartan	20–40 bd	160 bd
Irbesartan	75 od	300 od
Losartan	50 od	150 od
Beta blocker		
Bisoprolol	1.25 od	10 od
Carvedilol	3.125 bd	25–50 bd
Metoprolol succinate (SR)	12.5–25 od	200 od
Nebivolol	1.25 od	10 od

Doses of diuretics in heart failure

Oral doses	Starting dose (mg)	Maximum dose (mg)
Aldosterone antagonists		
Eplerenone	25 od*	50
Spironolactone	12.5–25 od*	50
Other potassium-sparing diuretics		
Amiloride	2.5 od	20
Triamterene	25 bd	200
Loop diuretics		
Furosemide	20–40 od or bd	600
Bumetanide	0.5–1.0 od or bd	10
Torsemide	10–20 od	200
Thiazide diuretics		
Chlorothiazide	250–500 od or bd	1000
Hydrochlorothiazide	25 mg od or bd	200
Bendrofluazide	2.5 od	10
Thiazide-like		
Metolazone	2.5 mg od	20 mg
Indapamide	2.5 mg od	5 mg
Chlorthalidone	12.5–25 od	100
IV doses		
Furosemide	Max single dose 160–200 mg, or 40 mg load followed by 10–40 mg/h infusion	
Bumetanide	Max single dose 4–8 mg, or 1 mg load followed by 0.5–2 mg/h infusion	
Torsemide	Max single dose of 100–200, or 20 mg load followed by 5–20 mg/h infusion	
Chlorothiazide	500–1000 mg od	

*: If eGFR >=50 mL/min/1.73 m2. If eGFR=30–49 mL/min/1.73 m2, eplerenone 25 mg od every other day or spironolactone 12.5 mg od or every other day.

After dose initiation for K+, increase ≤ 6.0 mEq/L or worsening renal function, hold until K+ <5.0 mEq/L. Consider restarting reduced dose after confirming resolution of hyperkalemia/renal insufficiency for at least 72 h.

Table 31.12 ACC/AHA 2013 GL on HF

Strategies for minimizing the risk of hyperkalaemia in patients treated with aldosterone antagonists
1. Impaired renal function is a risk factor for hyperkalemia during treatment with aldosterone antagonists. The risk of hyperkalemia increases progressively when serum creatinine is >1.6 mg/dL.* In elderly patients or others with low muscle mass in whom serum creatinine does not accurately reflect glomerular filtration rate, determination that glomerular filtration rate or creatinine clearance is >30 mL/min/1.73 m^2 is recommended.
2. Aldosterone antagonists would not ordinarily be initiated in patients with baseline serum potassium >5.0 mEq/L.
3. An initial dose of spironolactone of 12.5 mg or eplerenone 25 mg is typical, after which the dose may be increased to spironolactone 25 mg or eplerenone 50 mg if appropriate.
4. The risk of hyperkalemia is increased with concomitant use of higher doses of ACE inhibitors (captopril ≥75 mg daily; enalapril or lisinopril ≥10 mg daily).
5. In most circumstances, potassium supplements are discontinued or reduced when initiating aldosterone antagonists.
6. Close monitoring of serum potassium is required; potassium levels and renal function are most typically checked in 3 d and at 1 wk after initiating therapy and at least monthly for the first 3 mo.

*Although the entry criteria for the trials of aldosterone antagonists included creatinine <2.5 mg/dL, the majority of patients had much lower creatinine; in 1 trial (425), 95% of patients had creatinine ≤1.7 mg/dL.

ACE indicates angiotensin-converting enzyme.

2013 ACCF/AHA Guideline for the Management of Heart Failure. *JACC* 2013; doi: 10.1016/j.jacc.2013.05.019

addition of telmisartan to ACE significantly reduced all-cause and cardiac mortality and hospital stays.[32] ARBs are not removed by dialysis. Intravenous ferric carboxymaltose improves quality of life in iron-deficient patients with heart failure.[33]

Contraindications to the use of ACEI/ARB are bilateral renal stenosis, serum potassium >5 mmol/L, and serum creatinine >2.5 mg/dL (relative contraindication). A history of angioedema or the development of severe cough are contraindications for an ACEI. Angioedema is extremely rare with ARB. If creatinine rises above 3 mg/dL or K >5.5 mmol/L, the dose of ACE should be halved. With values >3.5 mg/dL creatinine or >6 mmol/L K, ACEI should be stopped.[15] However, there is evidence that the use of low-dose (15 to 25% of maximal dose) ACEI or ARB in patients with advanced renal disease (creatinine up to 5 mg/mL) may be beneficial.[34] In this case, once-daily morning dosing is considered (reduced ACE inhibition in the evening permits increased renal excretion of renal potassium), and concomitant use of a loop diuretic and restriction of dietary potassium intake (24-hour urine collection <40 mEq/day) are recommended.[34]

For ACEIs/ARBs, as well other drugs for CCF, see also Chapter 24 on hypertension.

Beta blockers upregulate β-1 receptor density, blunt norepinephrine and renin production, and mitigate the production of deleterious cytokines, including tumour necrosis factor alpha. They reduce mortality (up to 35%) in heart failure, in addition to that offered by ACEI. Carvedilol, bisoprolol, and long-acting metoprolol unequivocally reduce mortality.[35–37] In patients with LVEF ≤30%, QRS ≥130 ms, and LBBB, carvedilol has been found more effective than metoprolol in reducing hospitalization and ventricular arrhythmias.[38] In addition, co-administration of carvedilol with enalapril has been reported to prevent the cardiotoxicity of anthracycline chemotherapy.[24] Nebivolol have also been found efficacious in the elderly.[39] Xamoterol, a beta blocker with intrinsic sympathomimetic activity, and bucindolol, a non-selective beta blocker, have not been found beneficial. Beta blockers are started on low doses (i.e. carvedilol 3.125 mg bd) and titrated upwards every 2 weeks. In patients with newly diagnosed heart failure, it is safe to use either an ACE inhibitor or a beta blocker as first-line therapy.[37]

Contraindications to the use of beta blockers are asthma (but not COPD), second- or third-degree AV block, sick sinus syndrome (bradycardia <50 bpm) without permanent pacing, phaechromocytoma, and cocaine use (unopposed alpha receptors causing vasoconstriction).

Mineralocorticoid receptor antagonists (MRA) The secondary hyperaldosteronism seen in patients with heart failure promote sodium retention and endothelial dysfunction and may contribute to myocardial fibrosis. Both the selective agent **eplerenone** and the non-selective antagonist **spironolactone** reduce mortality in post-MI patients with LVEF <40% and severe or mild symptoms or in patients with advanced heart failure (Table 31.8).[40–42] Spironolactone may cause painful gynaecomastia in men (antagonist of aldosterone and androgen and progesterone receptors). Renal function and serum potassium levels must be closely monitored due to the risk of hyperkalaemia, especially when these agents are used together with an ACE or ARB.

Contraindications to aldosterone antagonists:
Hyperkalaemia (K >5 mmol/L), creatinine >2.5 mg/dL, and concomitant use of a combination of ACE and ARB.

Loop diuretics, such as furosemide, are the only therapy that can acutely produce symptomatic improvement. However, no clinical trial has assessed their effect on mortality in heart failure. They should not be used alone in heart failure since they do not prevent the progression of disease or maintain clinical stability over time. Torsemide has better absorption than furosemide, and bumetanide is a more powerful diuretic. They should be used in patients not responsive to furosemide. Renal function and electrolytes should be regularly measured with the use of diuretics due to the risk of hyperkalaemia, elevation of BUN, and dilutional hyponatraemia.

In patients resistant to loop diuretics, a thiazide may be added in combination. Several effects, such as the braking phenomenon (acute reduction in diuretic efficacy with repeated loop diuretic dosing), post-diuretic effect (increased sodium retention after the loop diuretic has worn off), rebound sodium retention (increased distal nephron sodium reabsorption due to factors, such as distal tubule hypertrophy), increased angiotensin II levels due to persistent volume reduction, and renal adaptation (hypertrophy and hyperfunction of distal tubule cells, causing increased local sodium uptake and aldosterone secretion) lead to diuretic resistance.[43] By blocking distal tubule sodium reabsorption, thiazides or thiazide-like drugs such as metolazone (up to 10 mg daily for 3–5 days), can antagonize the renal adaptation to chronic loop diuretic therapy and potentially improve diuretic resistance due to rebound sodium retention, even in patients with renal failure (Figure 31.6).[43] There is increased risk of hypokalaemia, worsening of renal function, fluid depletion that may require fluid resuscitation, and hyponatraemia. Addition of an aldosterone antagonist may reduce hypokalaemia and improve natriuresis. Diuretic combinations may improve symptoms but do not decrease mortality in heart failure.

Digoxin may still have a role in patients with systolic heart failure and concomitant atrial fibrillation. In patients with sinus rhythm, digoxin (concentrations of 0.5–0.8 micrograms/L) has been shown to offer a reduction of hospital admissions, without any impact on mortality.[44] Digoxin blocks the sodium-potassium (Na-K) ATPase, raising intracellular sodium, and reduces Ca

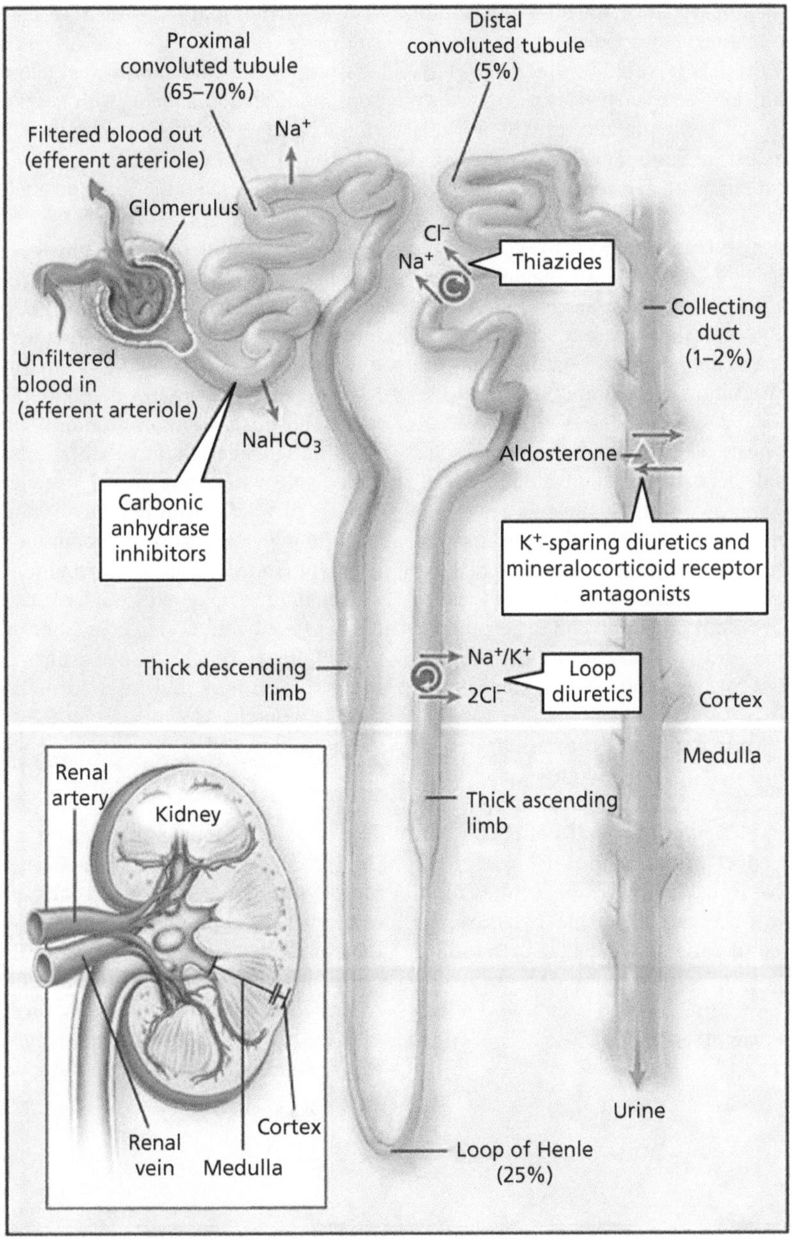

Figure 31.6 Sites of diuretic action in the nephron. The percentage of sodium reabsorbed in a given region is indicated in parentheses. 'K^+-sparing agents' collectively refers to the epithelial sodium channel inhibitors (e.g. amiloride and triamterene) and mineralocorticoid receptor antagonists (e.g. spironolactone and eplerenone). Sodium is reabsorbed in the distal tubule and collecting ducts through an aldosterone-sensitive sodium channel and by activation of an ATP-dependent sodium-potassium pump. Through both mechanisms, potassium is secreted into the lumen to preserve electroneutrality. Sodium channel inhibitors preserve potassium by interfering with the sodium-potassium pump whereas mineralocorticoid receptor antagonists spare potassium through their inhibitory effect on aldosterone. $NaHCO_3$ denotes sodium bicarbonate.

Ernst ME, Moser M. Use of diuretics in patients with hypertension. *N Engl J Med*. 2009;**361**:2153–64.

efflux by sodium-calcium exchange. Calcium overload of the sarcoplasmic reticulum may trigger arrhythmias. In a recent analysis of the AFFIRM study, digoxin was associated with a significant increase in all-cause mortality in patients with AF, even in the presence of HF,[45] but this finding was not verified in another analysis of the same study.[46] If used in patients with HF and AF, serum levels should be <1 ng/mL.

Hydralazine and nitrates are inferior to ACE inhibitors. However, in African-American heart failure patients (who generally have low plasma renin concentrations and, thus, are theoretically less responsive to RAAS blockade), hydralazine and nitrates are helpful.[47] Complications are arthralgia and increased antinuclear antibodies (lupus-like syndrome is rare).

Ivabradine High heart rate, that has been identified as a risk factor in chronic heart failure, and ivabradine, a selective inhibitor of hyperpolarization-activated cyclic-nucleotide-gated funny current (I*f*) involved in pacemaking generation and responsiveness of the sinoatrial node have been found to improve outcome (composite of cardiac death or hospital admission)[48] or admission to hospital for myocardial infarction and coronary revascularization.[49] More data are needed for its adoption in routine clinical practice.

Other **antiarrhythmic drugs** are contraindicated in heart failure due to proarrhythmic potential and negative inotropic effects. **Amiodarone** decreased mortality in the GESICA trial (60% non-ischaemic patients) [50] but had no significant effect in the SCD-HeFT trial (70% ischaemic patients).[51] It may increase non-cardiac mortality in patients with NYHA class III heart failure.[52] It is still recommended in patients with an ICD to reduce shocks or in patients with VT in whom ICD is not an option (Table 31.13). Dofetilide has also been found not to affect mortalitry in patients with HF and AF,[53] but clinical experience is limited.

Allopurinol that increases ATP conservation is under study.[54]

Verapamil and **diltiazem** are negative inotropes and are contraindicated in patients with heart failure. Dihydropyridine calcium channel blockers, such as **amlodipine** and **felodipine**, may be used safely (e.g. for systemic hypertension and angina), but they have no effect on mortality (Table 31.14).

The use of **inotropes** and **phosphodiesterase inhibitors** in chronic heart failure is not indicated since it is associated with increased mortality.[55] The PROMISE study found that oral milrinone increases mortality[56] whereas oral enoximone does not offer any improvement.[54] Oral levosimendan may improve symptoms but without any effect on hospitalizations or mortality (PERSIST).[57]

Although heart failure is accompanied by a hypercoagulable state, there are no sufficient data to support the use of **warfarin** in patients in normal sinus rhythm without a history of thromboembolic events or echocardiographic evidence of LV thrombus.[21, 22] A reduced risk of ischaemic stroke with warfarin used instead of aspirin is offset by an increased risk of major haemorrhage (WARCEF trial).[21] The use of aspirin is safe in heart failure, [21, 22] and it should be used definitely in ischaemic cardiomyopathy.

Atrial fibrillation and ventricular arrhythmias

The prevalence of atrial fibrillation in heart failure is 5% (NYHA I) to 25–50% (NYHA III/IV). New-onset AF is most probably associated with increased subsequent risk of mortality and morbidity.[58] It is very important to detect those patients with fast AF who have developed heart failure due to tachycardia-induced cardiomyopathy. Atrial kick contributes up to 30% of stroke volume, and an analysis of the CHF-STAT trial indicated that patients with heart failure who maintained sinus rhythm on amiodarone had improved

Table 31.13 ESC 2012 GL on HF

Ventricular arrhythmias	
Correction of potential aggravating/precipitating factors (e.g. electrolyte disorders, use of proarrhythmic drugs, myocardial ischaemia)	I-C
Optimization of therapy with ACEI (or ARB), beta-blocker, and MRA	I-A
Coronary revascularization in patients with coronary artery disease	I-C
ICD in symptomatic or sustained VT or VF	I-A
Amiodarone in patients with an ICD, who continue to have symptomatic ventricular arrhythmias or recurrent shocks despite optimal treatment and device re-programming	I-C
Catheter ablation in patients with an ICD who continue to have ventricular arrhythmias causing recurrent shocks not preventable by optimal treatment device re-programming and amiodarone	I-C
Amiodarone in optimally treated patients in whom an ICD is not appropriate	IIb-C
Routine use of amiodarone in patients with non-sustained ventricular arrhythmias (lack of benefit and potential drug toxicity)	III-A
Other antiarrhythmic drugs (particularly class IC agents and dronedarone) in systolic HF (worsening HF, proarrhythmia, and death)	III-A

Table 31.14 ESC 2012 GL on HF

Recommendations for the pharmacological treatment of stable angina pectoris in patients with symptomatic HF (NYHA functional class II–IV) and LV systolic dysfunction	
Step 1: a beta blocker*	
Preferred first-line treatment to relieve angina (reduces the risk of HF hospitalization and premature death).	I-A
Alternatives to a beta blocker	
(i) Ivabradine in patients in SR who cannot tolerate a beta blocker (effective antianginal treatment and safe in HF).	IIa-A
(ii) Oral or transcutaneous nitrate in patients unable to tolerate a beta blocker (effective antianginal treatment and safe in HF).	IIa-A
(iii) Amlodipine in patients unable to tolerate a beta blocker (effective antianginal treatment and safe in HF).	IIa-A
(iv) Nicorandil in patients unable to tolerate a beta blocker (effective antianginal treatment but safety in HF uncertain).	IIb-C
(v) Ranolazine in patients unable to tolerate a beta blocker (effective antianginal treatment but safety in HF uncertain).	IIb-C
Step 2: add a second antianginal drug when angina persists, despite treatment with a beta blocker or alternative (taking account of the combinations not recommended below)	
Ivabradine	I-A
Oral or transcutaneous nitrate	I-A
Amlodipine	I-A
Nicorandil	IIb-C
Ranolazine	IIb-C
Step 3: coronary revascularization	
Coronary revascularization is recommended when angina persists, despite treatment with two antianginal drugs.	I-A
Alternatives to coronary revascularization	
A third antianginal drug from those listed above may be considered when angina persists, despite treatment with two antianginal drugs (excluding the combinations not recommended below).	IIb-C
The following are NOT recommended	
Combination of any of ivabradine, ranolazine, and nicorandil (unknown safety),	III-C
Combination of nicorandil and a nitrate (lack of additional efficacy),	III-C
Diltiazem or verapamil (negative inotropic action and risk of worsening HF),	III-B

* Nitrates and beta blockers are also recommended for angina by ACC/AHA 2009 (I-B).

ESC guidelines for the diagnosis and treatment of acute and chronic heart failure 2012. *Eur Heart J*. 2012;**33**:1787–847.

survival.[59] Maintenance of sinus rhythm with dofetilide in patients with LVEF <35% was also associated with reduced mortality in the DIAMOND trial.[60] However, rhythm control has not been found superior to rate control in the randomized AF-CHF trial.[61] In patients with AF and heart failure, **dronedarone** increased mortality,[62] whereas **dofetilide** prevented AF recurrences without any effect on mortality.[53] **Amiodarone** is the only agent that is recommended for prevention of atrial arrhythmia recurrence in patients with heart failure and/or reduced LVEF. The recommendations of ESC 2012 GL on heart failure for patients with AF are presented in Table 31.15. The ACCF/AHA recommendations are presented in Chapter 52 on AF. If restoration of SR is required, **electrical cardioversion** in urgent cases (TOE is required if >48 h duration) or IV amiodarone are used.

A combination of beta blocker and digoxin is used for rate control. A non-dihydropyridine calcium channel blocker with digoxin may be considered in patients with heart failure and preserved LVEF. Catheter modification of the AV node and pacing may be considered in drug-refractory cases; however, pulmonary vein isolation with catheter ablation is preferable to AV nodal modification and biventricular pacing.[63] In patients with AF and heart failure in the presence of normal LVEF, restoration and maintenance of sinus rhythm may be useful for symptomatic relief.

Anticoagulation with warfarin is recommended in the presence of heart failure and an additional risk factor, such as age ≥75 years, hypertension, LVEF <35%, diabetes mellitus, by the ACC/AHA/HRS 2011[64] and the ESC 2010[65] guidelines on AF. Heart failure guidelines (ACC/AHA 2009 and EC 2012) recommend routine anticoagulation in all patients with heart failure and AF,[8, 15] and this is probably the safest approach.

Recommendations for patients with heart failure and ventricular arrhythmias are presented in Table 31.13. Recommendations for cardiac resynchronization therapy are discussed in the relevant section.

Surgical therapy

Revascularization is thought to improve survival in patients with ischaemic cardiomyopathy and proven myocardial viability by perfusion tests, stress echocardiography, or MRI.[66, 67] However, the STICH trial failed to detect any impact of CABG on total mortality in patients with LVEF ≤35% (although cardiac mortality was reduced), even if performed in patients with proven myocardial viability.[68, 69] In patients with LVEF ≥35%, indications for CABG are as in IHD (Table 31.16).

Functional MR is characterized by annular dilatation and leaflet non-coaptation in the setting of anatomically normal papillary muscles and valve leaflets. In patients who are not candidates for surgical coronary revascularization, mitral valve repair remains controversial.

Ischaemic MR (or infarct-related MR) is typically associated with leaflet tethering and displacement related to abnormal LV wall motion and geometry or papillary muscle dysfunction. MV repair can be added to CABG in this group of high-risk patients without increasing mortality, but its impact on late survival and functional class may be limited.[70] In heart failure due to valve disease (e.g. AS

Table 31.15 ESC 2012 GL on HF

Pharmacological rate control during atrial fibrillation	
Step 1	
Beta blocker	I-A
Alternative step 1	
Digoxin in beta blocker intolerance.	I-B
Amiodarone in beta blocker and digoxin intolerance.	IIb-C
AV node ablation (possibly CRT) in beta blocker, digoxin, and amiodarone intolerance.	IIb-C
Step 2	
Digoxin, in addition to beta blocker, in beta blocker inadequacy.	I-B
Alternative step 2	
Amiodarone, in addition to either beta blocker or digoxin (but not both). In beta blocker and digoxin inadequacy.	IIb-C
AV node ablation (possibly CRT) in inadequate response to two of beta blocker, digoxin, and amiodarone.	IIb-C
No more than two of beta blocker, digoxin, and amiodarone (or any other drug-suppressing cardiac conduction) should be combined due to risk of bradycardia, AV block, and asystole.	IIa-C
Rhythm control	
Electrical cardioversion or pharmacological cardioversion with amiodarone in persisting symptoms and/or signs of HF, despite optimum pharmacological treatment and adequate rate control.	IIb-C
Amiodarone prior to (and following) successful electrical cardioversion to maintain SR.	IIb-C
Dronedarone is not recommended (increased risk of hospital admissions and premature death).	III-A
Class I antiarrhythmic agents (increased risk of premature death).	III-A
Prevention of thromboembolism	
The CHA2DS2-VASc and HAS-BLED scores are recommended to determine the likely risk-benefit of oral anticoagulation.	I-B
An oral anticoagulant for all patients with paroxysmal or persistent/permanent AF and a CHA2DS2-VASc score ≥1, without contraindications and irrespective of whether a rate or rhythm management strategy is used (including after successful cardioversion).	I-A
In patients with AF of ≥48 h duration or when the known duration of AF is unknown, an oral anticoagulant at a therapeutic dose for ≥3 weeks prior to electrical or pharmacological cardioversion.	I-C
Intravenous heparin or LMWH for patients who have not been treated with an anticoagulant and require urgent electrical or pharmacological cardioversion.	I-C
Alternative to IV heparin or LMWH	
A TOE-guided strategy may be considered for patients who have not been treated with an anticoagulant and require urgent electrical or pharmacological cardioversion.	IIb-C
Combination of an oral anticoagulant and an antiplatelet agent in patients with chronic (>12 months after an acute event) coronary or other arterial disease (high risk of bleeding).	III-A

Table 31.16 Revascularization in heart failure

ACCF/AHA 2013 GL on HF. Recommendations for surgical/percutaneous/transcather interventional treatments of HF	
CABG or percutaneous intervention for HF patients on GDMT with angina and suitable coronary anatomy, especially significant left main stenosis or left main equivalent	I-C
CABG to improve survival in patients with mild to moderate LV systolic dysfunction and significant multivessel CAD or proximal LAD stenosis when viable myocardium is present	IIa-B
CABG or medical therapy to improve morbidity and mortality for patients with severe LV dysfunction (EF <35%), HF, and significant CAD	IIa-B
Surgical aortic valve replacement for patients with critical aortic stenosis and a predicted surgical mortality of no greater than 10%	IIa-B
Transcatheter aortic valve replacement for patients with critical aortic stenosis who are deemed inoperable	IIa-B
CABG in patients with ischemic heart disease, severe LV systolic dysfunction, and operable coronary anatomy whether or not viable myocardium is present	IIb-B
Transcatheter mitral valve repair or mitral valve surgery for functional mitral insufficiency is of uncertain benefit	IIb-B
Surgical reverse remodelling or LV aneurysmectomy in HFrEF for specific indications, including intractable HF and ventricular arrhythmias	IIb-B

CABG indicates coronary artery bypass graft; CAD, coronary artery disease; COR, Class of Recommendation; EF, ejection fraction; GDMT, guideline-directed medical therapy; HF, heart failure; HFr EF, heart failure with reduced ejection fraction; LAD, left anterior descending; LOE, Level of Evidence; and LV, left ventricular.

ESC 2012 GL on heart failure. Myocardial revascularization in chronic HF and systolic LV dysfunction	
CABG for patients with angina and significant left main stenosis, who are suitable for surgery and expected to survive >1 year with good functional status.	I-C
CABG for patients with angina and two- or three-vessel coronary disease, including a LAD stenosis, who are suitable for surgery and expected to survive >1 year with good functional status.	I-B
PCI as an alternative to CABG in the above categories of patients unsuitable for surgery.	IIb-C
CABG and PCI are NOT recommended in patients without angina AND without viable myocardium.	III-C

ESC guidelines for the diagnosis and treatment of acute and chronic heart failure 2012. *Eur Heart J*. 2012;**33**:1787–847.

or MS), surgical or interventional correction may restore almost normal heart function. In patients with ischaemic cardiomyopathy subjected to CABG, surgical LV reconstruction reduces LV volumes and LV wall stress but offers no benefit in mortality or hospitalizations (STICH).[71] Thus, routine LV reconstruction is not recommended. LV volume reduction may still play a role when non-viability of the akinetic segment can be established and when the procedure is likely to provide a volume reduction of a magnitude approaching 30%.[14] Ventricular reshaping techniques with new devices are under study.[72]

Device therapy

Cardiac resynchronization therapy (CRT)

Mechanical dyssynchrony refers to non-synchronous contraction of the wall segments of the left ventricle (intraventricular) or between the left and right ventricles (interventricular). Dyssynchrony impairs systolic function and ventricular filling, increases wall stress, and worsens mitral regurgitation. It is most readily defined by the presence of QRS widening (>120 ms) and LBBB configuration on the electrocardiogram and can be visualized on two-dimensional echocardiography. Biventricular pacing by atrial synchronized pacing of the RV and the LV via the coronary sinus to the basal or mid-ventricular but not apical LV region[73] accomplishes reverse remodelling of the LV. This remodelling effect, as well as survival benefit, is greater in non-ischaemic patients,[74] although clinical improvement with CRT has been shown in both ischaemic and non-ischaemic heart failure. The use of the posterior or lateral LV regions is also associated with decreased risk of arrhythmic events in comparison with anterior lead location and ICD-only patients.[75] In patients with NYHA III or IV heart failure and LVEF <35%, and QRS > 120 ms, CRT reduces morbidity and mortality (up to 36%), even without a defibrillator (CARE-HF trial, and others) (Table 31.17 and Figure 31.7).[76–80]

Approximately 20–30% of patients are 'non-responders', in whom CRT fails to result in benefit despite appropriate indications for therapy. The presence of RBBB, initial r wave in lead V_1, advanced heart failure (NYHA IV), advanced age, male gender, and ischaemic cardiomyopathy are predictors of poor outcome with CRT whereas LBBB and QRS >150 s are predictors of response.[10,81–83] In patients with LVEF ≤35%, symptoms of heart failure, but a QRS duration <120 milliseconds, cardiac resynchronization therapy may be detrimental (LESSER-EARTH trial).[6] **Echocardiography indices** commonly used to detect dyssynchrony are a septal to later LV wall delay in peak systolic velocity of 65 ms by tissue Doppler imaging and maximal delay in peak systolic velocity of 12 LV segments of 100 ms. Echocardiography techniques for measurements of intra- and interventricular delay do not reliably identify responders to CRT, and the mortality benefit of CRT may occur in the absence of prospective echocardiographic predictors (PROSPECT and SMART-AV).[84, 85] In addition to the ability to accurately detect mechanical delay, successful CRT also is affected by myocardial scar burden and lead position relative to dyssynchronous segments. Thus, decisions to use CRT should not be based on currently available echocardiographic/Doppler variables. However, echo-derived LV dyssynchrony (maximum delay between peak systolic velocities of the septal and the lateral walls >60 ms) may still be clinically important, especially in patients in whom it is detected following CRT.[86] Technological advances, such as *speckle tracking strain and real-time three-dimensional imaging*, are under study,[87] and there has been evidence that the use of speckle-tracking echocardiography to the target LV lead placement may yield improved clinical outcome (TARGET trial).[88] Recommendations for CRT optimization are presented in Table 31.18.

In summary, biventricular pacing is indicated in SR, QRS >150 ms, LBBB, LVEF ≤35%, and NYHA II–IV.

It is also reasonable in QRS ≥120 ms and LBBB, LVEF ≤35% or non-LBBB but QRS ≥150 ms and LVEF ≤30% (Table 31.17). There has also been evidence that patients with QRS >130 ms may also respond to CRT even if LVEF >30%.[89] Randomized studies on CRT have been almost exclusively restricted to patients with SR. CRT may be beneficial in patients with atrial fibrillation and QRS >120 ms and LVEF ≤35%, although no data on the effect on mortality exist.[90,91] The benefits of CRT appear to be attenuated in patients with AF. The presence of AF is associated with an increased risk of clinical non-response and death than in patients without AF. AV nodal ablation in CRT patients may be associated with reductions in mortality (Figure 31.8).[92] Also, no data exist to guide therapy by means of rate or rhythm control in patients with QRS >130 ms.

Recommendations on lead placement and follow-up of CRT devices have been published.[93]

CRT with ICD

The incremental benefits of combined CRT plus implantable cardioverter-defibrillator (ICD) devices vs CRT-alone devices in patients with LV systolic dysfunction remain uncertain.[79, 80]

However, in certain patients with heart failure, an ICD is indicated for either **secondary (after VT/VF) or primary prevention** (patients without heart failure, but with LVEF <30% at least 40 days post-MI, or with heart failure NYHA II or III and LVEF <35% at least 40 days post-MI). In these patients, an ICD is indicated; when CRT is also indicated, a combined device with ICD capabilities (CRT-D) should be implanted (Table 31.17). CRT-C should also be considered, if indicated, when an ICD is planned (ESC 2013 GL on pacing and CRT, I-B)

In trials of **primary prevention** in patients with heart failure, ICD reduced mortality in post-MI patients with LVEF <30% (MADIT II)[94] and ischaemic or non-ischaemic cardiomyopathy with LVEF <35% (SCD-HeFT).[51] There was also a trend for reduced mortality with ICD in non-ischaemic heart failure and LVEF <35% and non-sustained VT (DEFINITE).[91] In patients with LVEF <35%, advanced heart failure (NYHA class III or IV) due to ischaemic or non-ischaemic cardiomyopathies, and a QRS interval >120 ms, the presence of ICD capabilities also reduced mortality (COMPANION).[96] Thus, in patients with an indication for ICD, the addition of CRT is beneficial in the presence of QRS >120 ms (and especially 150 ms) or paced QRS >200 ms and LVEF <35%.

In patients with **mild to moderate heart failure (NYHA II or III)**, CRT-D improves survival, albeit at a cost of increased implantation-related complications (RAFT).[97]

In **mildly symptomatic patients (NYHA I or II)** who fulfill the above criteria, CRT improves LV structure and function but without affecting mortality (MADIT-CRT, REVERSE, MIRACLE-ICD).[98–100]

Patients who meet criteria for both CRT and ICD should receive CRT-D.

Indications for CRT-D:

- Spontaneous or inducible VF or sustained VT, and/or
- QRS >150 ms, LBBB, LVEF ≤35%, and NYHA II–IV, and/or
- LVEF ≤30% and NYHA I.

In ischaemic patients, ICD should be considered if indications exist at least 40 days after MI. A possible exemption to this rule are post-MI (>48h) patients who develop sustained VT/VF, provided the arrhythmia is not due to transient or reversible ischemia, reinfarction, or metabolic abnormalities (ACCF/AHA 2013 GL on STEMI, I-B).

In patients with end-stage heart failure (NYHA IV), the risks of multiple shocks and quality of life deterioration must be carefully weighed against the survival benefits. ICD may aggravate heart failure either by right ventricular apical pacing that produces dyssynchrony or multiple shocks. Thus, in patients with advanced heart failure, especially non-ischaemic, and major comorbidities such as need for renal dialysis, frailty and cachexia, CRT-D is not indicated.[10]

Advanced heart failure

Definition and identification of patients with advanced HF are presented in Table 31.19. The INTERMACS classification is presented in Table 31.20. Principles of therapy are indicated in Tables 31.21 and 31.22. Acute heart failure and cardiogenic shock are discussed in Chapter 33.

Table 31.17 Device therapy in HF patients receiving optimal, guideline-directed medical therapy

ACCF/AHA 2103 GL on HF and ACCF/AHA 2012 GL on Device Therapy. Recommendations for Device Therapy for Management of Stage C HF

Indications for ICD*	
HFrEF at least 40 d post-MI, LVEF ≤35%, NYHA II/III	I-A
HFrEF at least 40 d post-MI, LVEF ≤30%, NYHA I	I-B
Asymptomatic ischemic cardiomyopathy, at least 40 d post-MI, and with LVEF ≤30%	IIa-B
Patients with a high risk of nonsudden death such as frequent hospitalizations, frailty, or severe comorbidities**	IIb-B

* In patients expected to live >1 y. **Counseling should be specific to each individual patient and should include documentation of a discussion about the potential for sudden death and nonsudden death from HF or noncardiac conditions. Information should be provided about the efficacy, safety, and potential complications of an ICD and the potential for defibrillation to be inactivated if desired in the future, notably when a patient is approaching end of life. This will facilitate shared decision making between patients, families, and the medical care team about ICDs.

Indications for CRT	
SR, LVEF ≤35%, LBBB, QRS ≥150 ms, NYHA III/IV	I-A
SR, LVEF ≤35%, LBBB, QRS ≥150 ms, NYHA II	I-B
SR, LVEF ≤35%, LBBB, QRS 120–149 ms, NYHA II/III/IV	IIa-B
SR, LVEF ≤30%, LBBB, QRS ≥150 ms, ischaemic HF, NYHA I	IIb-C
SR, LVEF ≤35%, non-LBBB, QRS ≥150 ms, NYHA III/IV	IIa-A
SR, LVEF ≤35%, non-LBBB, QRS 120–149 ms, NYHA III/IV	IIb-B
SR, LVEF ≤35%, non-LBBB, QRS ≥150 ms, NYHA II	IIb-B
LVEF ≤35%, undergoing new or replacement device with anticipated ventricular pacing >40%	IIa-C
AF, LVEF ≤35%, if the patients requires ventricular pacing or otherwise meets CRT criteria and AV nodal ablation or rate control allows near 100% ventricular pacing	IIa-B
Non-LBBB, QRS<150 ms, NYHA I/II	III-B (no benefit)
Patients whose comorbidities and/or frailty limit survival to <1 y	III-C (no benefit)

2013 ACCF/AHA Guideline for the Management of Heart Failure. *JACC* 2013; doi: 10.1016/j.jacc.2013.05.019
2012 ACCF/AHA/HRS focused update incorporated into the ACCF/AHA/HRS 2008 guidelines for device-based therapyof cardiac rhythm abnormalities. *J Am Coll Cardiol*. 2013;**61**:e6–75

ESC 2012 GL on HF. Device therapy in heart failure

Indications for ICD*	
Ventricular arrhythmia causing haemodynamic instability	I-A
Symptomatic ischemic HF (NYHA class II–III) >40 days after acute MI, and an EF ≤35% despite ≥3 months of treatment with optimal pharmacological therapy	I-A
Symptomatic non-ischemic HF (NYHA class II–III), and an EF ≤35% despite ≥3 months of treatment with optimal pharmacological therapy	I-B

*in patients with expectation of survival >1 year with good functional status

ESC Guidelines for the diagnosis and treatment of acute and chronic heart failure 2012. *Eur Heart J*. 2012; **33**:1787–847.

ESC 2013 GL on Cardiac Pacing and CRT . Indications and optimization of CRT (almost similar recommendations have been provided by the ESC 2012 GL on HF).

Indications for CRT in patients in sinus rhythm*	
QRS > 150 ms, LBBB, NYHA II–IV, EF <35%	I-A
QRS 120–150 ms, LBBB, NYHA II–IV, EF <35%	I-B
QRS > 150 ms, non-LBBB, NYHA II–IV, EF <35%	IIa-B
QRS 120–150 ms, LBBB, NYHA II–IV, EF <35%	IIb-B
QRS < 120 ms	III-B

(Continued)

Table 31.17 (Continued)

Indications for CRT in patients in permanent AF*	
QRS ≥120, LVEF≤35%, NYHA III/IV provided that a BiV pacing as close to 100% as possible can be achieved	IIa-B
AV junction ablation should be added in case of incomplete BiV pacing	IIa-B
Uncontrolled heart rate and reduced LVEF who are candidates for AV junction ablation for rate control	IIa-B
Indication for upgraded or de novo CRT in patients with conventional pacemaker indications and heart failure*	
Upgrade from conventional PM or ICD LVEF <35%, NYHA III/IV and high percentage of ventricular pacing	I-B
De novo CRT Reduced EF and expected high percentage of ventricular pacing in order to decrease the risk of worsening HF	IIa-B
Choice of pacing mode (and cardiac resynchronization therapy optimization)	
Achieve BiV pacing as close to 100% as possible (survival benefit and reduction in hospitalization are strongly associated with an increasing percentage of BiV pacing)	IIa-B
Apical position of the LV lead should be avoided	IIa-B
LV lead placement targeted at the latest activated LV segment	IIb-B

*Patients should generally not be implanted during admission for acute decompensated HF. In such patients, guideline-indicated medical treatment should be optimized and the patient reviewed as an out-patient after stabilization. It is recognized that this may not always be possible.
2013 ESC Guidelines on cardiac pacing and cardiac resynchronization therapy. *Eur Heart J*. 2013. doi:10.1093/eurheartj/eht150

Table 31.18 ESC 2013 GL on cardiac pacing and CRT

Summary of current evidence for CRT optimization

Parameter	Standard (current practice)	CRT optimization	Additional clinical benefit (compared to standard)
LV lead position	Posterolateral	• Avoid apical • Target latest activated area	Benefit likely (less hospitalization for HF) Benefit likely (one RCT more responders, less hospitalization for HF)
AV delay	Fixed empirical AV interval 120 ms (range 100–120 ms)	• Echo-Doppler: shortest AV delay without truncation of the A-wave (Ritter's method) or change in LV systolic function	• Uncertain or mild (one small RCT and several observational positive)
		• Device-based algorithms (SmartDelay, QuickOpt)	• Uncertain (two RCTs negative)
VV delay	Simultaneous BiV	• Echo: residual LV dyssynchrony	• Uncertain or mild (one RCT showed mild benefit)
		• Echo-Doppler: largest stroke volume	• Uncertain (one RCT negative, one controlled positive)
		• ECG: narrowest LV-paced QRS; difference between BiV and preimplantation QRS	• Unknown (no comparative study)
		• Device-based algorithms (Expert-Ease, Quick-Opt, Peak endocardial acceleration)	• Uncertain (three RCTs negative)
LV pacing alone	Simultaneous BiV	n.a.	Non-inferior

AV, atrioventricular; BiV, biventricular; CRT, cardiac resynchronization therapy; DTI, tissue Doppler imaging; HF, heart failure; LV, left ventricular; n.a., not available; RCT, randomized controlled trial; VV, interventricular delay.

2013 ESC Guidelines on cardiac pacing and cardiac resynchronization therapy. *Eur Heart J*. 2013. doi:10.1093/eurheartj/eht150

Inotrope-dependent patients (i.e. levels 1 to 3 according to the Interagency Registry for Mechanical Assist Devices—INTERMACS classification, Table 31.20) who can be maintained on a single inotropic agent can be discharged home either on long-term IV inotropic support or on oral levosimendan but with detrimental or no effect on mortality. Left ventricular assist devices are portable blood pumps that can be used in patients with end-stage heart failure:[101,102]

- As bridge to recovery in people with potentially reversible forms of heart failure, such as myocarditis or post-partum cardiomyopathy
- As bridge to transplantation within the next weeks
- As destination therapy for patients unsuitable for transplantation.

The randomized REMATCH trial in patients with end-stage heart failure unsuitable for transplantation detected a

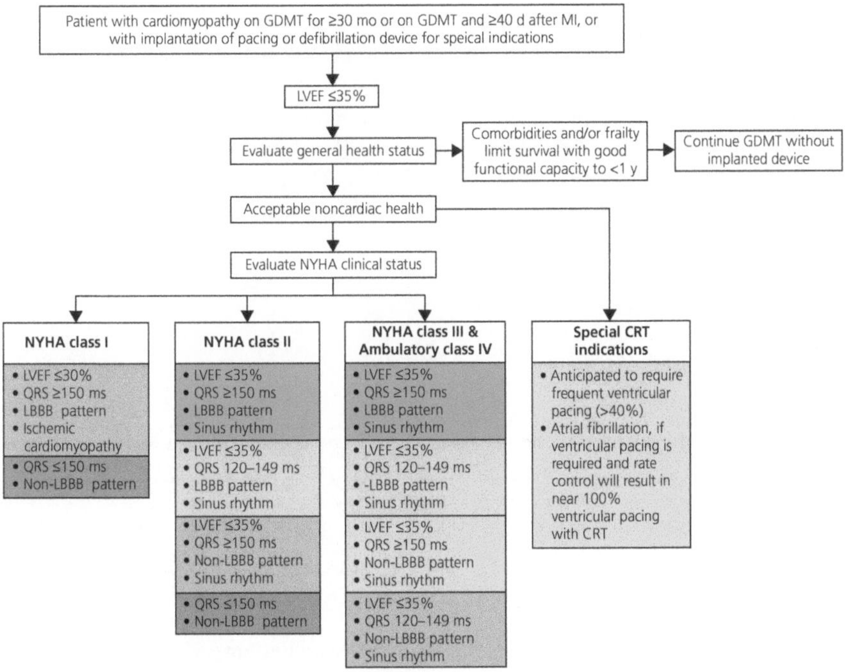

Colors correspond to the class of recommendations in the ACCF/AHA table 1.

Benefit for NYHA class I and II patients has only been shown in CRT-D trials, and while patients may not experience immediate symptomatic benefit, late remodeling may be avoided along with long-term HF consequences. There are no trials that support CRT-pacing (without ICD) in NYHA class I and II patients. Thus, it is anticipated these patients would receive CRT-D unless clinical reasons or personal wishes make CRT-pacing more appropriate. In patients who are NYHA class III and ambulatory class IV, CRT-D may be chosen but clinical reasons and personal wishes may make CRT-paci]ng appropriate to improve symptoms and quality of life when an ICD is not expected to produce meaningful benefit in survival.

Figure 31.7 ACCF/AHA 2013 on HF. Indications for CRT therapy algorithm.

CRT indicates cardiac resynchronization therapy; CRT-D, cardiac resynchronization therapy-defibrillator; GDMT, guideline-directed medical therapy; HF, heart failure; ICD, implantable cardioverter-defibrillator; LBBB, left bundle-branch block; LV, left ventricular; LVEF, left ventricular ejection fraction; MI, myocardial infarction; and NYHA, New York Heart Association.

2013 ACCF/AHA Guideline for the Management of Heart Failure. *JACC* 2013; doi: 10.1016/j.jacc.2013.05.019

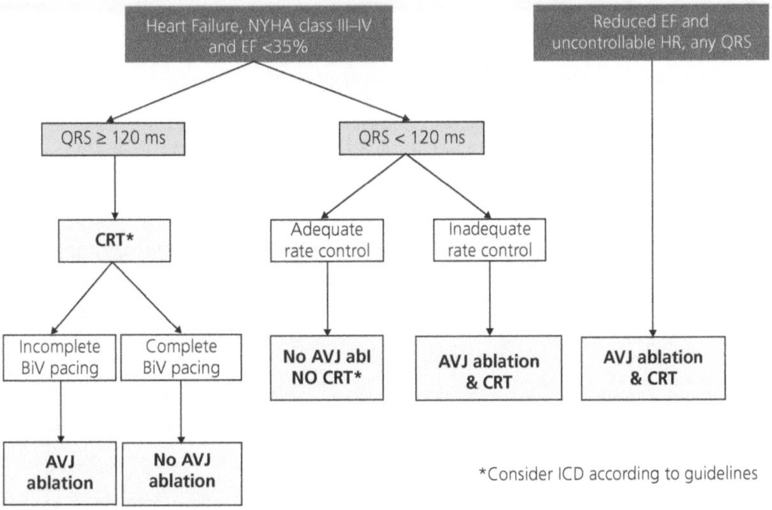

Figure 31.8 ESC 2013 GL on cardiac pacing and CRT.

Indication for atrioventricular junction (AVJ) ablation in patients with symptomatic permanent atrial fibrillation (AF) and optimal pharmacological therapy.

BiV, biventricular; CRT, cardiac resynchronization therapy; EF, ejection fraction; HR, heart rate; ICD, implantable cardioverter defibrillator; NYHA, New York Heart Association.

Table 31.19 Advanced HF

Definition of Advanced HF proposed by the Heart Failure Association of the ESC and adopted by the ACCF/AHA 2013 GL on HF
1. Severe symptoms of HF with dyspnea and/or fatigue at rest or with minimal exertion (NYHA class III or IV)
2. Episodes of fluid retention (pulmonary and/or systemic congestion, peripheral edema) and/or reduced cardiac output at rest (peripheral hypoperfusion)
3. Objective evidence of severe cardiac dysfunction shown by at least 1 of the following: a. LVEF <30% b. Pseudonormal or restrictive mitral inflow pattern c. Mean PCWP >16 mm Hg and/or RAP >12 mm Hg by PA catheterization d. High BNP or NT-proBNP plasma levels in the absence of noncardiac causes
4. Severe impairment of functional capacity shown by 1 of the following: a. Inability to exercise b. 6-Minute walk distance ≤ 300 m c. Peak VO2 <12 to 14 mL/kg/min
5. History of ≥ 1 HF hospitalization in past 6 mo
6. Presence of all the previous features despite "attempts to optimize" therapy, including diuretics and GDMT, unless these are poorly tolerated or contraindicated, and CRT when indicated

BNP indicates B-type natriuretic peptide; CRT, cardiac resynchronization therapy; GDMT, guideline-directed medical therapy; HF, heart failure; LVEF, left ventricular ejection fraction; NT-proBNP, N3 terminal pro-B-type natriuretic peptide; NYHA, New York Heart Association; PA, pulmonary artery; PWCP, pulmonary capillary wedge pressure; and RAP, right atrial pressure.
Metra M, *et al.* Advanced chronic heart failure: A position statement from the Study Group on Advanced Heart Failure of the Heart Failure Association of the European Society of Cardiology. *Eur J Heart Fail.* 2007;**9**:684–94.

ACCF/AHA 2013 FL on HF. Clinical events and findings useful for identifying patients with advanced HF
Repeated (≥2) hospitalizations or ED visits for HF in the past year
Progressive deterioration in renal function (e.g., rise in BUN and creatinine)
Weight loss without other cause (e.g., cardiac cachexia)
Intolerance to ACE inhibitors due to hypotension and/or worsening renal function
Intolerance to beta blockers due to worsening HF or hypotension
Frequent systolic blood pressure <90 mm Hg
Persistent dyspnea with dressing or bathing requiring rest
Inability to walk 1 block on the level ground due to dyspnea or fatigue
Recent need to escalate diuretics to maintain volume status, often reaching daily furosemide equivalent dose >160 mg/d and/or use of supplemental metolazone therapy
Progressive decline in serum sodium, usually to <133 mEq/L
Frequent ICD shocks

ACE indicates angiotensin-converting enzyme; BUN, blood urea nitrogen; ED, emergency department; HF, heart failure; and ICD, implantable cardioverter-defibrillator
2013 ACCF/AHA Guideline for the Management of Heart Failure. *JACC* 2013; doi: 10.1016/j.jacc.2013.05.019
ESC Guidelines for the diagnosis and treatment of acute and chronic heart failure 2012. *Eur Heart J.* 2012; **33**:1787–847.

Table 31.20 Interagency Registry for Mechanical assist Devices (INTERMACS)

Levels of limitation and time frame of need for consideration of mechanical circulatory support		
INTERMACS profile level	**Status**	**Time frame**
1	Critical cardiogenic shock	Hours
2	Progressive decline	Days to week
3	Stable but inotrope-dependent	Weeks
4	Recurrent advanced heart failure	Weeks to few months if baseline restored
5	Exertion intolerant	Weeks to months
6	Exertion limited	Months if nutrition and activity maintained
7	Advanced NYHA class III	

Alba AC, *et al.* Usefulness of the INTERMACS scale to predict outcomes after mechanical assist device implantation. *J Heart Lung Transplant.* 2009;**28**:827–33.

(*Continued*)

Table 31.20 (Continued)

INTERMACS profiles		
Profile*	**Profile description**	**Features**
1	Critical cardiogenic shock ("Crash and burn")	Life-threatening hypotension and rapidly escalating inotropic/pressor support, with critical organ hypoperfusion often confirmed by worsening acidosis and lactate levels
2	Progressive decline ("Sliding fast" on inotropes)	"Dependent" on inotropic support but nonetheless shows signs of continuing deterioration in nutrition, renal function, fluid retention, or other major stress indicator. Can also apply to a patient with refractory volume overload, perhaps with evidence of impaired perfusion, in whom inotropic infusions cannot be maintained due to tachyarrhythmias, clinical ischemia, or other intolerance
3	Stable but inotrope dependent	Clinicall stable on mild-moderate doses of intravenous inotropes (or has a temporary circulatory support device) after repeated documentation of failure to wean without symptomatic hypotension, worsening symptoms, or progressive organ dysfunction (usually renal)
4	Resting symptoms onoral therapy at home	Patient who is at home on oral therapy but frequently has symptoms of congestion at rest or with activities of daily living (dressing or bathing). He or she may have orthopnea, shortness of breath during dressing or bathing, gastrointestinal symptoms (abdominal disconfirm, nausea, poor appetite), disabling ascites, or severe lower-extremity edema
5	Exertion intolerant ("housebound")	Patient who is comfortable at rest but unable to engage in any activity, living predominantly within the house or housebound
6	Exertion limited ("walking wounded")	Patient who is comfortable at rest without evidence of fluid overload but who is able to do some mild activity. Activities of daily living are comfortable and minor activities outside the home such as visiting friends or going to a restaurant can be performed, but fatigure results within a few minutes or with any meaningful physical exertion
7	Advanced NYHA class III	Patient who is clinically stable with a reasonable level of comfortable activity, despite a history of previous decompensation that is not recent. This patient is usually able to walk more than a block. Any decompensation requiring intravenous diuretics or hospitalization within the previous month should make this person a Patient Profile 6 or lower.

*Modifier options: Profiles 3–6 can be modified with the designation FF (frequent flyer) for 1 patients with recurrent decompensations leading to frequent (generally at least 2 in last 3 mo or 3 in last 6 mo) emergency department visits or hospitalizations for intravenous diuretics, ultrafiltration, or brief inotropic therapy. Profile 3 can be modified in this fashion if the patient is usually at home. If a Profile 7 patient meets the definition of FF, the patient should be moved to Profile 6 or worse. Other modifier options include A (arrhythmia), which should be used in the presence of recurrent ventricular tachyarrhythmias contributing to the overall clinical course (e.g., frequent ICD shocks or requirement of external defibrillation, usually more than twice weekly); or TCS (temporary circulatory support) for hospitalized patients profiles 1–3.

ICD indicates implantable cardioverter-defibrillator; INTERMACS, Interagency Registry for Mechanically Assisted Circulatory Support; and NYHA, New York Heart Association.

Table 31.21 ACCF/AHA 2013

Therapy of advanced heart failure	
Fluid restriction	
Fluid restriction (1.5 to 2 L/d) in stage D, especially in patients with hyponatremia, to reduce congestive symptoms	IIa-C
Inotropic support	
Cardiogenic shock pending definitive therapy or resolution	I-C
BTT or MCS in stage D refractory to GDMT	IIa-B
Short-term support for threatened end-organ dysfunction in hospitalized patients with stage D and severe HFrEF	IIb-B
Long-term support with continuous infusion palliative therapy in select stage D HF	IIb-B
Routine intravenous use, either continuous or intermittent, is potentially harmful in stage D HF	III-B (harm)
Short-term intravenous use in hospitalized patients without evidence of shock or threatened end-organ performance is potentially harmful	III-B (harm)
MCS	
MCS is beneficial in carefully selected* patients with stage D HF in whom definitive management (e.g., cardiac transplantation) is anticipated or planned	IIa-B
Nondurable MCS is reasonable as a "bridge to recovery" or "bridge to decision" for carefully selected* patients with HF and acute profound disease	IIa-B
Durable MCS is reasonable to prolong survival for carefully selected* patients with stage D HFrEF	IIa-B

(Continued)

Table 31.21 (Continued)

Cardiac transplantation	
Evaluation for cardiac transplantation is indicated for carefully selected patients with stage D HF despite GDMT, device, and surgical management	I-C

*Although optimal patient selection for MCS remains an active area of investigation, general indications 1 for referral for MCS therapy include patients with LVEF <25% and NYHA class III-IV functional status despite GDMT, including, when indicated, CRT, with either high predicted 1- to 2-y mortality (as suggested by markedly reduced peak oxygen consumption, clinical prognostic scores, etc.) or dependence on continuous parenteral inotropic support. Patient selection requires a multidisciplinary team of experienced advanced HF and transplantation cardiologists, cardiothoracic surgeons, nurses, and, ideally, social workers and palliative care clinicians.

MCS indicates mechanical circulatory support; BTT, bridge to transplant; COR, Class of Recommendation; CRT, cardiac resynchronization therapy; EF, ejection fraction; GDMT, guideline-directed medical therapy; HF, heart failure; HFrEF, heart failure with reduced ejection fraction; LOE, Level of Evidence; MCS, mechanical circulatory support; and NYHA, New York Heart Association.

Intravenous inotropic agents used in management of HF

	Dose			Effects					
Inotropic agent	**Bolus**	**Infusion (/min)**	**Drug kinetics and metabolism**	**CO**	**HR**	**SVR**	**PVR**	**Adverse effects**	**Special considerations**
Adrenergic agonists									
Dopamine	N/A	5 to 10	$t_{1/2}$: 2 to 20 min R, H, P	↑	↑	↔	↔	T, HA, N, tissue necrosis	Caution: MAO-I
	N/A	10 to 15		↑	↑	↑	↔		
Dobutamine	N/A	2.5 to 5.0	$t_{1/2}$: 2 to 3 min H	↑	↑	↓	↔	↑/↓BP, HA, T, N, F, hypersenstivity	Caution: MAO-I; CI: sulfite allergy
	N/A	5 to 20		↑	↑	↔	↔		
PDE inhibitor									
Milrinone	N/R	0.125 to 0.75	$t_{1/2}$: 2.5 h H	↑	↑	↓	↓	T, ↓BP	Renal dosing, monitor LFTs

$t_{1/2}$ indicates elimination half-life; BP, blood pressure; CI, contraindication; CO, cardiac output; F, fever; H, hepatic; HA, headache; HF, heart failure; HR, heart rate; :LFT, liver function test; MAO-I, monoamine oxidase inhibitor; N, nausea; N/A, not applicable; N/R, not recommended; P, plasma; PDE, phosphodiesterase; PVR, pulmonary vascular resistance; R, renal; SVR, systemic vascular resistance; and T, tachyarrhythmias

2013 ACCF/AHA Guideline for the Management of Heart Failure. *JACC*. 2013; doi: 10.1016/j.jacc.2013.05.019

Table 31.22 ESC 2012 GL on HF

Ventricular assist devices

Ventricular assist device indications

LVAD or BiVAD in selected patients with end-stage HF, despite optimal pharmacological and device treatment and who are otherwise suitable for heart transplantation.	I-B
LVAD in highly selected patients who have end-stage HF, despite optimal pharmacological and device therapy, and who are not suitable for heart transplantation but are expected to survive >1 year with good functional status.	IIa-B

Patients potentially eligible for implantation of a ventricular assist device

Patients with >2 months of severe symptoms, despite optimal medical and device therapy, and more than one of the following:
LVEF <25% and, if measured, peak VO_2 <12 mL/kg/min
≥3 HF hospitalizations in previous 12 months without an obvious precipitating cause
Dependence on IV inotropic therapy
Progressive end-organ dysfunction (worsening renal and/or hepatic function) due to reduced perfusion and not to inadequate ventricular filling pressure (PCWP ≥20 mmHg and SBP ≤80–90 mmHg or CI ≤2 L/min/m^2)
Deteriorating right ventricular function

ESC guidelines for the diagnosis and treatment of acute and chronic heart failure 2012. *Eur Heart J*. 2012;**33** :1787–847.

Table 31.23 Short-term and long-term mechanical support devices

Device	Location and implantation	Flow type and maximal cardiac output	Configuration	Duration	Uses
Impella (Abiomed Inc, Danvers, MA)	Intracorporeal, percutaneous, or surgical placement	Axial flow LVAD 3- to 5-d BTR, 2.5 or 5 L/min	LVAD	Short	BTR/BTD/BIT
TandemHeart (Cardiac Assist, Inc, Pittsburgh, PA)	Extracorporeal, percutaneous, or surgical placement	Centrifugal flow LVAD, 3- to 5-d BTR, 4 L/min	LVAD	Short	BTR/BTD/BIT
Centrimag (Levitronix LLC, Waltham, MA)	Extracorporeal, surgical placement	Centrifugal flow, 10 L/min	LVAD ± RVAD	Short	BTR/BTD/BIT
Thoratec PVAD (Thoratec Corp, Pleasanton, CA)	Extracorporeal, surgical placement	Pulsatile flow, 6–7 L/min	LVAD ± RVAD	Internediate to long	BTT
Abiomed BVS 5000 (Abiomed Inc, Danvers, MA)	Extracorporeal, surgical placement	Pulsatile flow, 6–7 L/min	LVAD ± RVAD	Intermediate to long	BTT
Heartmate II (Thoratec Corp, Pleasanton, CA)	Intracorporeal, surgical placement	Axial flow, 10 L/min	LVAD	Long	BTT, DT
Heartmate XVE (Thoratec Corp, Pleasanton, CA)	Intracorporeal, surgical placement	Pulsatile 10 L/min	LVAD	Long	BTT, DT
Heartware HVAD (Heartware Inc, Miami Lakes, PL)	Intracorporeal, surgical placement	Centrifugal flow, 10 L/min	LVAD	Long	BTT (D)
Jarvik 2000 Flowmaker (Jarvik Heart Inc, New York, NY)	Intracorporeal, surgical placement	Axial flow, 7 L/min	LVAD	Long	BTT (D)
Duraheart LVAS (Terumo Heart Inc, Ann Arbor, MI)	Intracorporeal, surgical placement	Centrifugal flow, 10 L/min	LVAD	Long	BTT (D)
CardioWest (Syncardia Systems, Tucson, AZ)	Intracorporeal, surgical placement	Pulsatile, >9 L/min	TAH	Long	BTT

LVAD indicates left ventricular assist device; BTR, bridge to recovery; BTD, bridge to decision; BTT, bridge to transplantation; RVAD, right ventricular assist device; DT, destination therapy; ID, investigational device; and TAH, total artificial heart.
Ahmad T, *et al.* When the heart runs out of heartbeats: treatment options for refractory end-stage heart failure. *Circulation*. 2012;**125**:2948–55.

Table 31.24 ESC 2012 GL on HF

Heart transplantation: indications and contraindications
Patients to consider
End-stage heart failure with severe symptoms, a poor prognosis, and no remaining alternative treatment options
Motivated, well informed, and emotional stable
Capable of complying with the intensive treatment required post-operatively
Contraindications
Active infection
Severe peripheral arterial or cerebrovascular disease
Current alcohol or drug abuse
Treated cancer in previous 5 years
Unhealed peptic ulcer
Recent thromboembolism
Significant renal failure (e.g. creatinine clearance <50 mL/min)
Significant liver disease
Systemic disease with multiorgan involvement
Other serious co-morbidity with poor prognosis
Emotional instability or untreated mental illness
High, fixed pulmonary vascular resistance (>4–5 Wood Units and mean transpulmonary gradient >15 mmHg)

ESC Guidelines for the diagnosis and treatment of acute and chronic heart failure 2012. *Eur Heart J*. 2012;**33**:1787–847.

Table 31.25 ESC 2011 GL on pregnancy

Recommendations for the management of cardiomyopathies and heart failure	
Anticoagulation in patients with intracardiac thrombus detected by imaging or with evidence of systemic embolism.	I-A
Women with HF during pregnancy should be treated according to current guidelines for non-pregnant patients, respecting contraindications for some drugs in pregnancy.	I-B
Women with DCM should be informed about the risk of deterioration of the condition during gestation and peripartum.	I-C
In patients with a past history or family history of sudden death, close surveillance with prompt investigation is recommended if symptoms of palpitations or presyncope are reported.	I-C
LMWH or vitamin K antagonists, according to stage of pregnancy, for patients with AF.	I-C
Delivery with β-blocker protection in women with HCM.	IIa-C
β-blockers in all patients with HCM and more than mild LVOTO or maximal wall thickness >15 mm to prevent sudden pulmonary congestion.	IIa-C
In HCM, cardioversion should be considered for persistent atrial fibrillation.	IIa-C
Due to high metabolic demands of lactation and breastfeeding, preventing lactation may be considered in post-partum cardiomyopathy (PPCM).	IIb-C
Subsequent pregnancy is not recommended if LVEF does not normalize in women with PPCM.	III-C

ESC Guidelines on the management of cardiovascular diseases during pregnancy: the Task Force on the Management of Cardiovascular Diseases during Pregnancy of the European Society of Cardiology (ESC), *Eur Heart J*. 2011;**32**:3147–97.

significantly better survival at 1 and 2 years in the device group than in the medical therapy group (52% vs 25% at 1 year and 23% vs 8% at 2 years, respectively.[103] New, intrapericardial systems or non-pulsatile devices may yield better clinical outcomes.[31, 104–107] Potential complications are haemorrhage due to acquired von Willebrand's disease, platelet damage, and development of mucosal AV malformations.[108, 109] Device infection occurs in 22% of patients per year despite the use of newer, smaller devices, and affects mortality.[110] Thrombosis, device failure, and RV failure may also occur. Although the long-term efficacy and safety of LVADs as an alternative to heart transplantation or medical therapy remains uncertain, the limited availability of organs and their use as bridge to recovery, especially before terminal stages of the disease, suggest expansion of their use.[111, 112] However, their cost-effectiveness is still not established.[113]

Heart transplantation

Approximately 5% and 10% of all patients with heart failure have advanced disease, which is associated with a very high mortality and very poor quality of life. Heart transplantation has been the only means of improving the quality of life and survival in these patients. With the advances in immunosuppression therapy, 1-year survival after cardiac transplantation approaches 90%, with 50% of patients surviving >11 years.[114, 115] The listing criteria and evaluation and management of patients undergoing cardiac transplantation have been described in detail by the International Society for Heart and Lung Transplantation.[116] Indications and contraindications for transplantation by the ESC are also presented in Table 31.24. Heart transplantation is indicated in hospitalized patients with status I classification (United Network of Organ Sharing), who need intravenous inotropes or a circulatory support device. In ambulatory (status II) patients, transplantation does not improve survival; these patients might benefit from long-term LVAD unloading that may allow recovery of myocardial contractility in patients with dilated cardiomyopathy.

Stem cell therapy

Preliminary data suggested that autologous stem cell intracoronary transplantation may improve survival in patients with ischaemic heart failure,[117] but recent results have been disappointing.[118]

Pregnancy

Recommendations for pregnant women with heart failure are presented in Table 31.25.[119]

References

1. Stevenson LW, *et al.* The limited reliability of physical signs for estimating haemodynamics in chronic heart failure. *JAMA*. 1989;**261**:884–8
2. Kim HN, *et al.* Natriuretic peptide testing in heart failure. *Circulation*. 2011;**123**:2015–19
3. Kociol RD, *et al.* Troponin elevation in heart failure prevalence, mechanisms, and clinical implications. *J Am Coll Cardiol*. 2010;**56**:1071–8
4. Ky B, *et al.* Multiple biomarkers for risk prediction in chronic heart failure. *Circ Heart Fail*. 2012;**5**:183–90
5. Dorosz JL, *et al.* Performance of 3-dimensional echocardiography in measuring left ventricular volumes and ejection fraction: a systematic review and meta-analysis. *J Am Coll Cardiol*. 2012;**59**:1799–808
6. Kumar R, *et al.* Assessment of left ventricular diastolic function using 4-dimensional phase-contrast cardiac magnetic resonance. *J Comput Assist Tomogr*. 2011;**35**: 108–12

7. Larsen TB, *et al.* Efficacy and safety of dabigatran etexilate and warfarin in 'real world' patients with atrial fibrillation: A prospective nationwide cohort study. *J Am Coll Cardiol.* 2013;doi: 10.1016/j.jacc.2013.1003.1020
8. Yancy CW, *et al.* 2013 ACCF/AHA guideline for the management of heart failure. JACC. 2013; doi: 10.1016/j.jacc.2013.1005.1019
9. Pocock SJ, *et al.* Predicting survival in heart failure: A risk score based on 39 372 patients from 30 studies. *Eur Heart J.* 2013;1404–13
10. 2013 ESC guidelines on cardiac pacing and cardiac resynchronization therapy. *Eur Heart J* 2013:doi:10.1093/eurheartj/eht1150
11. McMurray, *et al.* ESC guidelines for the diagnosis and treatment of acute and chronic heart failure 2012: the Task Force for the diagnosis and treatment of acute and chronic heart failure 2012 of the European Society of Cardiology. Developed in collaboration with the Heart Failure Association (HFA) of the ESC. *Eur J Heart Fail.* 2012;**14**:803–69
12. O'Connor CM, *et al.* Efficacy and safety of exercise training in patients with chronic heart failure: HF-ACTION randomized controlled trial. *JAMA.* 2009;**301**:1439–50
13. Willis MS, Patterson C. Proteotoxicity and cardiac dysfunction—alzheimer's disease of the heart? *N Engl J Med.* 2013;**368**:455–64
14. Gupta D, *et al.* Dietary sodium intake in heart failure. *Circulation.* 2012;**126**:479–85
15. Krum H, *et al.* Heart failure. *Lancet.* 2009;**373**:941–55
16. Sedlak T, *et al.* Contraception in patients with heart failure. *Circulation.* 2012;**126**:1396–400
17. Zoungas S, *et al.* Severe hypoglycemia and risks of vascular events and death. *N Engl J Med.* 2010;**363**:1410–18
18. Nissen SE, *et al.* Rosiglitazone revisited: an updated meta-analysis of risk for myocardial infarction and cardiovascular mortality. *Arch Intern Med.* 2010;**170**:1191–201
19. Loke YK, *et al.* Comparative cardiovascular effects of thiazolidinediones: systematic review and meta-analysis of observational studies. *BMJ.* 2011;**342**:d1309
20. Inzucchi SE, *et al.* Management of hyperglycaemia in type 2 diabetes: a patient-centred approach. Position statement of the American Diabetes Association (ADA) and the European Association for the Study of Diabetes (EASD). *Diabetologia.* 2012;**55**:1577–96
21. Homma S, *et al.* Warfarin and aspirin in patients with heart failure and sinus rhythm. *N Engl J Med.* 2012;**366**:1859–69
22. Massie BM, *et al.* Randomized trial of warfarin, aspirin, and clopidogrel in patients with chronic heart failure: the Warfarin and Antiplatelet Therapy in Chronic Heart Failure (WATCH) trial. *Circulation.* 2009;**119**:1616–24
23. Gianni L, *et al.* Anthracycline cardiotoxicity: from bench to bedside. *J Clin Oncol.* 2008;**26**:3777–84
24. Swedberg K, *et al.*, for the RED-HF Committees and Investigators. Treatment of anemia with darbepoetin alfa in systolic heart failure. *N Engl J Med.* 2013;**doi:** 10.1056/NEJMoa1214865
25. Ramani GV, *et al.* Chronic heart failure: contemporary diagnosis and management. *Mayo Clin Proc.* 2010;**85**:180–95
26. Garg R, *et al.* Overview of randomized trials of angiotensin-converting enzyme inhibitors on mortality and morbidity in patients with heart failure. Collaborative group on ACE inhibitor trials. *JAMA.* 1995;**273**:1450–6
27. Roig E, *et al.* Clinical implications of increased plasma angiotensin II despite ACE inhibitor therapy in patients with congestive heart failure. *Eur Heart J.* 2000;**21**:53–7
28. Lee VC, *et al.* Meta-analysis: angiotensin-receptor blockers in chronic heart failure and high-risk acute myocardial infarction. *Ann Intern Med.* 2004;**141**:693–704
29. Cohn JN, *et al.* A randomized trial of the angiotensin-receptor blocker valsartan in chronic heart failure. *N Engl J Med.* 2001;**345**:1667–75
30. McMurray JJ, *et al.* Effects of candesartan in patients with chronic heart failure and reduced left-ventricular systolic function taking angiotensin-converting-enzyme inhibitors: the CHARM-ADDED trial. *Lancet.* 2003;**362**:767–71
31. Birks EJ, *et al.* Reversal of severe heart failure with a continuous-flow left ventricular assist device and pharmacological therapy: a prospective study. *Circulation.* 2011;**123**:381–90
32. Cice G, *et al.* Effects of telmisartan added to angiotensin-converting enzyme inhibitors on mortality and morbidity in haemodialysis patients with chronic heart failure a double-blind, placebo-controlled trial. *J Am Coll Cardiol.* 2010;**56**:1701–8
33. Comin-Colet J, *et al.* The effect of intravenous ferric carboxymaltose on health-related quality of life in patients with chronic heart failure and iron deficiency: a subanalysis of the FAIR-HR study. *Eur Heart J.* 2013;**34**:30–8
34. Hebert LA. Optimizing ACE-inhibitor therapy for chronic kidney disease. *N Engl J Med.* 2006;**354**:189–91
35. Hjalmarson A, *et al.* Effects of controlled-release metoprolol on total mortality, hospitalizations, and well-being in patients with heart failure: the Metoprolol CR/XL Randomized Intervention Trial in congestive heart failure (MERIT-HF). MERIT-HF Study Group. *JAMA.* 2000;**283**:1295–302
36. Packer M, *et al.* Effect of carvedilol on survival in severe chronic heart failure. *N Engl J Med.* 2001;**344**:1651–8
37. Willenheimer R, *et al.* Effect on survival and hospitalization of initiating treatment for chronic heart failure with bisoprolol followed by enalapril, as compared with the opposite sequence: results of the randomized Cardiac Insufficiency Bisoprolol Study (CIBIS) III. *Circulation.* 2005;**112**:2426–35
38. Ruwald MH, *et al.* Effect of metoprolol versus carvedilol on outcomes in madit-crt (multicenter automatic defibrillator implantation trial with cardiac resynchronization therapy). *J Am Coll Cardiol.* 2013;**61**:doi: doi:10.1016/j.jacc.2013.1001.1020
39. Flather MD, *et al.* Randomized trial to determine the effect of nebivolol on mortality and cardiovascular hospital admission in elderly patients with heart failure (seniors). *Eur Heart J.* 2005;**26**:215–25
40. Pitt B, *et al.* Eplerenone, a selective aldosterone blocker, in patients with left ventricular dysfunction after myocardial infarction. *N Engl J Med.* 2003;**348**:1309–21
41. Pitt B, *et al.* The effect of spironolactone on morbidity and mortality in patients with severe heart failure. Randomized aldactone evaluation study investigators. *N Engl J Med.* 1999;**341**:709–17
42. Zannad F, *et al.* Eplerenone in patients with systolic heart failure and mild symptoms. *N Engl J Med.* 2011; **364**:11–21
43. Jentzer JC, *et al.* Combination of loop diuretics with thiazide-type diuretics in heart failure. *J Am Coll Cardiol.* 2010;**56**:1527–34

44. The effect of digoxin on mortality and morbidity in patients with heart failure. The Digitalis Investigation Group. *N Engl J Med.* 1997;**336**:525–33
45. Whitbeck MG, *et al.* Increased mortality among patients taking digoxin—analysis from the AFFIRM study. *Eur Heart J.* 2013;34:1481–8
46. Gheorghiade M, *et al.* Lack of evidence of increased mortality among patients with atrial fibrillation taking digoxin: Findings from post hoc propensity-matched analysis of the AFFIRM trial. *Eur Heart J.* 2013;34:1489–97
47. Taylor AL, *et al.* Combination of isosorbide dinitrate and hydralazine in blacks with heart failure. *N Engl J Med.* 2004;**351**:2049–57
48. Bohm M, *et al.* Heart rate as a risk factor in chronic heart failure (SHIFT): the association between heart rate and outcomes in a randomised placebo-controlled trial. *Lancet.* 2010;**376**:886–94
49. Fox K, *et al.* Ivabradine for patients with stable coronary artery disease and left-ventricular systolic dysfunction (BEAUTIFUL): a randomised, double-blind, placebo-controlled trial. *Lancet.* 2008;**372**:807–16
50. Doval HC, *et al.* Randomised trial of low-dose amiodarone in severe congestive heart failure. Grupo de Estudio de la Sobrevida en la Insuficiencia Cardiaca en Argentina (GESICA). *Lancet.* 1994;**344**:493–8
51. Bardy GH, *et al.* Amiodarone or an implantable cardioverter-defibrillator for congestive heart failure. *N Engl J Med.* 2005;**352**:225–37
52. Packer DL, *et al.* Impact of implantable cardioverter-defibrillator, amiodarone, and placebo on the mode of death in stable patients with heart failure: analysis from the sudden cardiac death in heart failure trial. *Circulation.* 2009;**120**:2170–6
53. Torp-Pedersen C, *et al.* Dofetilide in patients with congestive heart failure and left ventricular dysfunction. Danish Investigations of Arrhythmia and Mortality on Dofetilide Study Group. *N Engl J Med.* 1999;341:857–65
54. Hirsch GA, *et al.* Allopurinol acutely increases adenosine triphospate energy delivery in failing human hearts. *J Am Coll Cardiol.* 2012;**59**:802–8
55. Toma M, *et al.* Inotropic therapy for end-stage heart failure patients. *Curr Treat Options Cardiovasc Med.* 2010;**12**:409–19
56. Packer M, *et al.* Effect of oral milrinone on mortality in severe chronic heart failure. The PROMISE Study Research Group. *N Engl J Med.* 1991;**325**:1468–75
57. Nieminen MS, *et al.* Oral levosimendan in patients with severe chronic heart failure—the PERSIST study. *Eur J Heart Fail.* 2008;**10**:1246–54
58. Swedberg K, *et al.* Prognostic relevance of atrial fibrillation in patients with chronic heart failure on long-term treatment with beta-blockers: results from COMET. *Eur Heart J.* 2005;**26**:1303–8
59. Deedwania PC, *et al.* Spontaneous conversion and maintenance of sinus rhythm by amiodarone in patients with heart failure and atrial fibrillation: observations from the veterans affairs congestive heart failure survival trial of antiarrhythmic therapy (CHF-STAT). The Department of Veterans Affairs CHF-STAT Investigators. *Circulation.* 1998;**98**:2574–9
60. Pedersen OD, *et al.* Does conversion and prevention of atrial fibrillation enhance survival in patients with left ventricular dysfunction? Evidence from the Danish Investigations of Arrhythmia and Mortality ON Dofetilide/(DIAMOND) study. *Card Electrophysiol Rev.* 2003;**7**:220–4
61. Roy D, *et al.* Rhythm control versus rate control for atrial fibrillation and heart failure. *N Engl J Med.* 2008;**358**:2667–77
62. Kober L, *et al.* Increased mortality after dronedarone therapy for severe heart failure. *N Engl J Med.* 2008;**358**:2678–87
63. Khan MN, *et al.* Pulmonary-vein isolation for atrial fibrillation in patients with heart failure. *N Engl J Med.* 2008;**359**:1778–85
64. Fuster V, *et al.* 2011 ACCF/AHA/HRS focused updates incorporated into the ACC/AHA/ESC 2006 guidelines for the management of patients with atrial fibrillation: a report of the American College of Cardiology Foundation/American Heart Association Task Force on practice guidelines. *Circulation.* 2011;**123**:e269–367
65. Camm AJ, *et al.* Guidelines for the management of atrial fibrillation: the Task Force for the management of atrial fibrillation of the European Society of Cardiology (ESC). *Eur Heart J.* 2010;**31**:2369–429
66. Allman KC, *et al.* Myocardial viability testing and impact of revascularization on prognosis in patients with coronary artery disease and left ventricular dysfunction: a meta-analysis. *J Am Coll Cardiol.* 2002;**39**:1151–8
67. Buckley O, *et al.* Predicting benefit from revascularization in patients with ischaemic heart failure: imaging of myocardial ischaemia and viability. *Circulation.* 2011;**123**:444–50
68. Bonow RO, *et al.* Myocardial viability and survival in ischaemic left ventricular dysfunction. *N Engl J Med.* 2011;**364**:1617–25
69. Velazquez EJ, *et al.* Coronary-artery bypass surgery in patients with left ventricular dysfunction. *N Engl J Med.* 2011;**364**:1607–16
70. Diodato MD, *et al.* Repair of ischaemic mitral regurgitation does not increase mortality or improve long-term survival in patients undergoing coronary artery revascularization: a propensity analysis. *Ann Thorac Surg.* 2004;**78**:794–99; discussion 794–9
71. Jones RH, *et al.* Coronary bypass surgery with or without surgical ventricular reconstruction. *N Engl J Med.* 2009; **360**:1705–17
72. Grossi EA, *et al.* Outcomes of the RESTOR-MV trial (Randomized Evaluation of a Surgical Treatment for Off-Pump Repair of the Mitral Valve). *J Am Coll Cardiol.* 2010;**56**:1984–93
73. Singh JP, *et al.* Left ventricular lead position and clinical outcome in the multicentre automatic defibrillator implantation trial-cardiac resynchronization therapy (MADIT-CRT) trial. *Circulation.* 2011;**123**:1159–66
74. McLeod CJ, *et al.* Differential outcome of cardiac resynchronization therapy in iischaemic cardiomyopathy and idiopathic dilated cardiomyopathy. *Heart Rhythm.* 2011;**8**: 377–82
75. Kutyifa V, *et al.* Left ventricular lead location and the risk of ventricular arrhythmias in the MADIT-CRT trial. *Eur Heart J.* 2013;**34**:184–90
76. 2012 ACCF/AHA/HRS focused update incorporated into the ACCF/AHA/HRS 2008 guidelines for device-based therapy of cardiac rhythm abnormalities. *J Am Coll Cardiol.* 2013;**61**:e6–75
77. Cleland JG, *et al.* Clinical trials update from the American Heart Association meeting 2010: EMPHASIS-HF, RAFT, TIM-HF, tele-HF, ASCEND-HF, ROCKET-AF, and PROTECT. *Eur J Heart Fail.* 2011;**13**:460–65

78. Epstein AE, *et al.* ACC/AHA/HRS 2008 guidelines for device-based therapy of cardiac rhythm abnormalities: executive summary. *Heart Rhythm.* 2008;**5**:934–55
79. Lam SK, *et al.* Combined resynchronisation and implantable defibrillator therapy in left ventricular dysfunction: Bayesian network meta-analysis of randomised controlled trials. *BMJ.* **2007;335**:925
80. McAlister FA, *et al.* Cardiac resynchronization therapy for patients with left ventricular systolic dysfunction: a systematic review. *JAMA.* 2007;**297**:2502–14
81. Bilchick KC, *et al.* Bundle-branch block morphology and other predictors of outcome after cardiac resynchronization therapy in Medicare patients. *Circulation.* 2010;**122**:2022–30
82. Perrin MJ, *et al.* Greater response to cardiac resynchronization therapy in patients with true complete left bundle branch block: a PREDICT substudy. *Europace.* 2012;**14**:690–5
83. Sipahi I, *et al.* Impact of QRS duration on clinical event reduction with cardiac resynchronization therapy: meta-analysis of randomized controlled trials. *Arch Intern Med.* 2011;**171**:1454–62
84. Chung ES, *et al.* Results of the predictors of response to CRT (PROSPECT) trial. *Circulation.* 2008;**117**:2608–16
85. Ellenbogen KA, *et al.* Primary results from the SmartDelay determined AV optimization: a comparison to other AV delay methods used in cardiac resynchronization therapy (SMART-AV) trial: a randomized trial comparing empirical, echocardiography-guided, and algorithmic atrioventricular delay programming in cardiac resynchronization therapy. *Circulation.* 2010;**122**:2660–8
86. Auger D, *et al.* Effect of cardiac resynchronization therapy in patients without left intraventricular dyssynchrony. *Eur Heart J.* 2012;**33**:913–20
87. Delgado V, *et al.* Relative merits of left ventricular dyssynchrony, left ventricular lead position, and myocardial scar to predict long-term survival of ischaemic heart failure patients undergoing cardiac resynchronization therapy. *Circulation.* 2011;**123**:70–8
88. Khan FZ, *et al.* Targeted left ventricular lead placement to guide cardiac resynchronization therapy: the TARGET study: a randomized, controlled trial. *J Am Coll Cardiol.* 2012;**59**:1509–18
89. Kutyifa V, *et al.* The influence of left ventricular ejection fraction on the effectiveness of cardiac resynchronization therapy MADIT-CRT (Multicenter Automatic Defibrillator Implantation Trial with Cardiac Resynchronization Therapy). *J Am Coll Cardiol.* 2013;**61**:936–44
90. Dickstein K, *et al.* 2010 focused update of ESC guidelines on device therapy in heart failure: an update of the 2008 ESC guidelines for the diagnosis and treatment of acute and chronic heart failure and the 2007 ESC guidelines for cardiac and resynchronization therapy. Developed with the special contribution of the Heart Failure Association and the European Heart Rhythm Association. *Eur Heart J.* 2010;**31**:2677–87
91. Tracy CM, *et al.* 2012 ACCF/AHA/HRS focused update incorporated into the ACCF/AHA/HRS 2008 guidelines for device-based therapy of cardiac rhythm abnormalities: A Report Of The American College of Cardiology Foundation/American Heart Association Task Force on practice guidelines and the Heart Rhythm Society. *J Am Coll Cardiol.* 2012
92. Ganesan AN, *et al.* Role of AV nodal ablation in cardiac resynchronization in patients with coexistent atrial fibrillation and heart failure a systematic review. *J Am Coll Cardiol.* 2012;**59**:719–26
93. Daubert JC, *et al.* 2012 EHRA/HRS expert consensus statement on cardiac resynchronization therapy in heart failure: implant and follow-up recommendations and management. *Europace.* 2012;**14**:1236–86
94 Moss AJ, *et al.* Prophylactic implantation of a defibrillator in patients with myocardial infarction and reduced ejection fraction. *N Engl J Med.* 2002;**346**:877–83
95. Kadish A, *et al.* Prophylactic defibrillator implantation in patients with nonischaemic dilated cardiomyopathy. *N Engl J Med.* 2004;**350**:2151–8
96. Bristow MR, *et al.* Cardiac-resynchronization therapy with or without an implantable defibrillator in advanced chronic heart failure. *N Engl J Med.* 2004;**350**:2140–50
97. Tang AS, *et al.* Cardiac-resynchronization therapy for mild-to-moderate heart failure. *N Engl J Med.* 2010;**363**: 2385–95
98. Abraham WT, *et al.* Effects of cardiac resynchronization on disease progression in patients with left ventricular systolic dysfunction, an indication for an implantable cardioverter-defibrillator, and mildly symptomatic chronic heart failure. *Circulation.* 2004;**110**:2864–8
99. Linde C, *et al.* Randomized trial of cardiac resynchronization in mildly symptomatic heart failure patients and in asymptomatic patients with left ventricular dysfunction and previous heart failure symptoms. *J Am Coll Cardiol.* 2008;**52**:1834–43
100. Moss AJ, *et al.* Cardiac-resynchronization therapy for the prevention of heart-failure events. *N Engl J Med.* 2009;**361**:1329–38
101. Birks EJ. Left ventricular assist devices. *Heart.* 2010;**96**:63–71
102. Estep JD, *et al.* Imaging for ventricular function and myocardial recovery on nonpulsatile ventricular assist devices. *Circulation.* 2012;**125**:2265–77
103. Rose EA, *et al.* Long-term use of a left ventricular assist device for end-stage heart failure. *N Engl J Med.* 2001;**345**:1435–43
104. Miller LW. Left ventricular assist devices are underutilized. *Circulation.* 2011;**123**:1552–58; discussion 1558
105. Naidu SS. Novel percutaneous cardiac assist devices: the science of and indications for haemodynamic support. *Circulation.* 2011;**123**:533–43
106. Stewart GC, *et al.* Mechanical circulatory support for advanced heart failure: patients and technology in evolution. *Circulation.* 2012;**125**:1304–15
107. Stewart GC, *et al.* Keeping left ventricular assist device acceleration on track. *Circulation.* 2011;**123**:1559–68; discussion 1568
108. Ahmad T, *et al.* When the heart runs out of heartbeats: treatment options for refractory end-stage heart failure. *Circulation.* 2012;**125**:2948–55
109. Eckman PM, *et al.* Bleeding and thrombosis in patients with continuous-flow ventricular assist devices. *Circulation.* 2012;**125**:3038–47
110. Gordon RI, *et al,* the Ventricular Assist Device Infection Study Group. Prospective, multicenter study of ventricular assist device infections. *Circulation.* 2013;**127**:691–702

111. Owens AT, *et al.* Should left ventricular assist device be standard of care for patients with refractory heart failure who are not transplantation candidates?: left ventricular assist devices should not be standard of care for transplantation-ineligible patients. *Circulation.* 2012;**126**: 3088–94
112. Mehra MR, *et al.* Should left ventricular assist device should be standard of care for patients with refractory heart failure who are not transplantation candidates?: left ventricular assist devices should be considered standard of care for patients with refractory eart failure who are not transplantation candidates. *Circulation.* 2012;**126**:3081–7
113. Miller LW, *et al.* Cost of ventricular assist devices: Can we afford the progress?. *Circulation.* 2013;**127**:743–8
114. Mancini D, *et al.* Selection of cardiac transplantation candidates in 2010. *Circulation.* 2010;**122**:173–83
115. Strueber M, *et al.* Multicentre evaluation of an intrapericardial left ventricular assist system. *J Am Coll Cardiol.* 2011;**57**:1375–82
116. Mehra MR, *et al.* Listing criteria for heart transplantation: International Society for Heart and Lung Transplantation guidelines for the care of cardiac transplant candidates—2006. *J Heart Lung Transplant.* 2006;**25**:1024–42
117. Strauer BE, *et al.* The acute and long-term effects of intracoronary stem cell transplantation in 191 patients with chronic heart failure: the STAR-HEART study. *Eur J Heart Fail.* 2010;**12**:721–9
118. Perin EC, *et al.* Effect of transendocardial delivery of autologous bone marrow mononuclear cells on functional capacity, left ventricular function, and perfusion in chronic heart failure: the FOCUS-CCTRN trial. *JAMA.* 2012;**307**:1717–26
119. Regitz-Zagrosek V, *et al.* Esc guidelines on the management of cardiovascular diseases during pregnancy: the Task Force on the management of cardiovascular diseases during pregnancy of the European Society of Cardiology (ESC). *Eur Heart J.* 2011;**32**:3147–97

Chapter 32

Heart failure with preserved LVEF

Definition

Heart failure with preserved ejection fraction (>50% although definitions vary), (HFpEF), or diastolic HF is seen in approximately 50% of patients with HF.[1] The diagnosis of HFpEF is challenging because it is largely one of excluding other potential noncardiac causes of symptoms suggestive of HF. To date, efficacious therapies have not been identified. The ACCF/AHA have further subdivided this category into HFpEF, borderline 41–49%, and HFpEF, improved >40% (see Chapter 30 on classification of HF).

Aetiology and pathophysiology

Heart failure with preserved LVEF may be seen in various conditions, such as diastolic dysfunction, pressure overload hypertrophy from valvular disease (especially AS), pericardial disease, and RV dysfunction. **Diastolic dysfunction** is caused by a decrease in ventricular relaxation and/or an increase in ventricular stiffness probably due to fibrosis and myocardial hypertrophy. Common causes are long-standing arterial hypertension, ischemic heart disease, diabetes, severe sepsis, and increased age (Table 32.1). **Diastolic heart failure** occurs when the ventricular chamber is unable to accept an adequate volume of blood during diastole at normal diastolic pressures and at volumes sufficient to maintain an appropriate stroke volume (see Figure 30.1 in Chapter 30).[2–4] Systolic dysfunction may coexist: LVEF is an imperfect measure of systolic function, and stroke volume and cardiac output may be reduced despite a normal LVEF.

Epidemiology

The prevalence of heart failure with preserved LVEF is estimated to be 50% among heart failure populations, and its pathophysiology is incompletely understood.[5] It is dominant in the elderly who have multiple non-cardiac co-morbidities that mainly affect their prognosis.[6] The mortality rate for patients with diastolic heart failure is slightly better than those with systolic heart failure (approaching 30% in 1 year compared with 1% for age-matched controls).[7, 8] However, progression from normal to abnormal diastolic function is an independent predictor of mortality in patients with normal LVEF.[9]

Clinical presentation

May be identical to that of systolic heart failure.

Table 32.1 ACC/AHA 2009 Guideline on HF. Differential diagnosis in a patient with heart failure and normal left ventricular ejection fraction

Incorrect diagnosis of HF
Inaccurate measurement of LVEF
Primary valvular disease
Restrictive (infiltrative) cardiomyopathies
Amyloidosis, sarcoidosis, haemochromatosis
Pericardial constriction
Episodic or reversible LV systolic dysfunction
Severe hypertension, myocardial ischaemia
HF associated with high metabolic demand (high-output states)
Anaemia, thyrotoxicosis, arteriovenous fistulae
Chronic pulmonary disease with right HF
Pulmonary hypertension associated with pulmonary vascular disorders
Atrial myxoma
Diastolic dysfunction of uncertain origin
Obesity

2009 Focused update incorporated into the ACC/AHA 2005 Guidelines for the Diagnosis and Management of Heart Failure in Adults, *J Am Coll Cardiol.* 2009:**53**:e1–e90.

Table 32.2 ACC/AHA 2013 Guideline on HF

Recommendations for treatment of HFpEF	
Systolic and diastolic blood pressure should be controlled according to published clinical practice guidelines	I-B
Diuretic for relief of symptoms due to volume overload	I-C
Coronary revascularization for patients with CAD in whom angina or demonstrable myocardial ischemia is present despite GDMT	IIa-C
Management of AF according to published clinical practice guidelines for HFpEF to improve symptomatic HF	IIa-C
Use of beta-blocking agenets, ACE inhibitors, and ARBs for hypertension in HFpEF	IIa-C
ARBs to decrease hospitalizations in HFpEF	IIb-B
Nutrutional supplementation is not recommended in HFpEF	III-C (no benefit)

ACE indicates angiotensin-converting enzyme; AF, atrial fibrillation; ARBs, angiotensin-receptor blockers; CAD, coronary artery disease; COR, Class of Recommendation; GDMT, guideline-directed medical therapy; HF, heart failure; HFpEF, heart failure with preserved ejection fraction; and LOE, Level of Evidence.

Diagnosis

The ESC has proposed the following criteria:[10]

- Symptoms and signs of heart failure, LVEF >45%, and the presence of abnormal LV relaxation or diastolic stiffness
- Others have adopted an LVEF >50%.[3]

Proposed criteria vary and are mostly empiric.

Echocardiographic indices indicative of diastolic dysfunction include transmitral and pulmonary venous Doppler filling profiles and tissue Doppler imaging that provides information on patterns of diastolic relaxation and filling and ventricular dyssynchrony (see Fig. 32.2, and Table 31.6). However, assessment of diastolic dysfunction remains still rather elusive.

Plasma BNP amounts are raised in patients with heart failure with preserved LVEF but, in general, to a lesser extent than in systolic heart failure.

Therapy

Therapy of heart failure with preserved systolic function is not satisfactory (Table 32.2). Blood pressure control, rate/rhythm control in underlying AF, control of pulmonary congestion with diuretic agents, and revascularization, when indicated, are recommended.[10, 11] Blood pressure control improves diastolic function, irrespective of the type of antihypertensive agent used.[12] ARBs, beta-blockers to control tachycardia and increase the duration of diastole, diuretics in smaller doses than in systolic heart failure (aldosterone antagonists are promising), and calcium channel blockers (diltiazem or verapamil) are used for symptomatic relief. Despite a lower rate of hospitalizations, no reduction in mortality has been shown with ACEI or ARBs or beta-blockers.[13–15]

References

1. Yancy CW, *et al.* 2013 ACCF/AHA guideline for the management of heart failure. *JACC.* 2013; doi: 10.1016/j.jacc.2013.1005.10192. Borlaug BA, *et al.* Diastolic and systolic heart failure are distinct phenotypes within the heart failure spectrum. *Circulation.* 2011;**123**:2006–13; discussion 2014
3. Vasan RS, *et al.* Defining diastolic heart failure: a call for standardized diagnostic criteria. *Circulation.* 2000;**101**:2118–21
4. Zile MR, *et al.* New concepts in diastolic dysfunction and diastolic heart failure: part I: diagnosis, prognosis, and measurements of diastolic function. *Circulation.* 2002;**105**:1387–93
5. Owan TE, *et al.* Epidemiology of diastolic heart failure. *Prog Cardiovasc Dis.* 2005;**47**:320–32
6. Ather S, *et al.* Impact of non-cardiac co-morbidities on morbidity and mortality in a predominantly male population with heart failure and preserved versus reduced ejection fraction. *J Am Coll Cardiol.* 2012;**59**:998–1005
7. Bhatia RS, *et al.* Outcome of heart failure with preserved ejection fraction in a population-based study. *N Engl J Med.* 2006;**355**:260–9
8. Owan TE, *et al.* Trends in prevalence and outcome of heart failure with preserved ejection fraction. *N Engl J Med.* 2006;**355**:251–9
9. Aljaroudi W, *et al.* Impact of progression of diastolic dysfunction on mortality in patients with normal ejection fraction. *Circulation.* 2012;**125**:782–8

10. McMurray JJV, *et al.* ESC guidelines for the diagnosis and treatment of acute and chronic heart failure 2012: the Task Force for the diagnosis and treatment of acute and chronic heart failure 2012 of the European Society of Cardiology. Developed in collaboration with the Heart Failure Association (HFA) of the ESC. *Eur J Heart Fail.* 2012;**14**:803–69
11. Hunt SA, *et al.* 2009 focused update incorporated into the ACC/AHA 2005 guidelines for the diagnosis and management of heart failure in adults: a report of the American College of Cardiology Foundation/American Heart Association Task Force on practice guidelines: developed in collaboration with the International Society for Heart and Lung Transplantation. *Circulation.* 2009;**119**:e391–479
12. Solomon SD, *et al.* Effect of angiotensin receptor blockade and antihypertensive drugs on diastolic function in patients with hypertension and diastolic dysfunction: a randomised trial. *Lancet.* 2007;**369**:2079–87
13. Hernandez AF, *et al.* Clinical effectiveness of beta-blockers in heart failure: findings from the OPTIMIZE-HF (organized program to initiate lifesaving treatment in hospitalized patients with heart failure) registry. *J Am Coll Cardiol.* 2009;**53**:184–92
14. Massie BM, *et al.* Irbesartan in patients with heart failure and preserved ejection fraction. *N Engl J Med.* 2008;**359**: 2456–67
15. Yusuf S, *et al.* Effects of candesartan in patients with chronic heart failure and preserved left ventricular ejection fraction: the CHARM–PRESERVED trial. *Lancet.* 2003;**362**:777–81

Chapter 33

Acute heart failure and cardiogenic shock

Acute heart failure

Definition

Acute decompensated heart failure is a clinical syndrome resulting from decreased cardiac performance, renal dysfunction, and alterations in vascular compliance (Table 33.1 and Figure 33.1). In-hospital mortality is 4%, and 1-year mortality approaches 50%.[1] The **cardiorenal syndrome** is recognized as a complication of acute heart failure, although not all patients have a low cardiac output.[2] It is exacerbated by continuing use of diuretics that reduce glomerular filtration rate.

Aetiology and prognosis

The most common co-morbid conditions are hypertension (73%), coronary artery disease (57%), and diabetes (44%). Preserved systolic function is found in up to 50% of patients and carries a better prognosis.[3] Renal dysfunction, systolic blood pressure <115 mmHg, and an elevated troponin level are associated with worse outcome.[1,3]

Low perfusion at rest? (e.g. narrow pulse pressure, cool extremities, hypotension)	Congestion at rest? (e.g. orthopnea, elevated jugular venous pressure, pulmonary rales, S3 gallop, edema): No	Congestion at rest?: Yes
No	Warm and dry	Warm and wet
Yes	Cold and dry	Cold and wet

Figure 33.1 ACCF/AHA 2013 GL on HF. Classification of patients presenting with acutely decompensated HF

2013 ACCF/AHA Guideline for the Management of Heart Failure. *JACC* 2013; doi: 10.1016/j.jacc.2013.05.019

Table 33.1 ESC 2012 GL on HF

Precipitants and causes of acute heart failure
Events usually leading to rapid deterioration
◆ Rapid arrhythmia or severe bradycardia/conduction disturbance
◆ Acute coronary syndrome
◆ Mechanical complication of acute coronary syndrome (e.g. rupture of interventricular septum, mitral valve chordal rupture, right ventricular infarction)
◆ Acute pulmonary embolism
◆ Hypertensive crisis
◆ Cardiac tamponade
◆ Aortic dissection
◆ Surgery and perioperative problems
◆ Peripartum cardiomyopathy
Events usually leading to less rapid deterioration
◆ Infection (including infective endocarditis)
◆ Exacerbation of COPD/asthma
◆ Anaemia
◆ Kidney dysfunction
◆ Non-adherence to diet/drug therapy
◆ Iatrogenic causes (e.g. prescription of an NSAID or corticosteroid; drug interactions)
◆ Arrhythmias, bradycardia, and conduction disturbances not leading to sudden, severe change in heart rate
◆ Uncontrolled hypertension
◆ Hypothyroidism or hyperthyroidism
◆ Alcohol and drug abuse

AHF, acute heart failure; COPD, chronic obstructive pulmonary disease; NSAID, non-steroidal anti-inflammatory drug.
ESC guidelines for the diagnosis and treatment of acute and chronic heart failure 2012. *Eur Heart J.* 2012;**33**:1787–847.

Therapy

General principles are presented in Tables 33.2 and 33.3 and Figures 33.2 and 33.3. See also advanced HF in Chapter 31. For post-MI cardiogenic shock see also chapter on MI. Routine use of pulmonary artery catheter is not recommended and should be restricted to cases that do not respond to IV diuretics.[4] Pulmonary capillary wedge pressure is not an accurate reflection of LV end-diastolic pressure in patients with mitral stenosis, aortic regurgitation, pulmonary venous occlusive disease, ventricular interdependence, high airway pressure, respiratory treatment, or a poorly compliant LV.

Oxygen is administered via a nasal cannula (4 L/min). Non-invasive ventilation is more effective in improving symptoms but has no effect on outcome (a PEEP of 5–10 cmH_2O; FiO_2 delivery ≥0.40, usually for 30 min/h). Potential complications are worsening of right ventricular failure and pneumothorax. Care should be taken in serious obstructive airways disease to avoid hypercapnia.

Non-invasive ventilation (NIV) refers to all modalities that assist ventilation without the use of an endotracheal tube but rather with a sealed face mask. NIV is more effective in improving symptoms but has no effect on outcome (a PEEP of 5–10 cmH_2O; FiO_2 delivery ≥0.40, usually for 30 min/h). With PEEP, it improves LV function by reducing LV afterload. NIV with positive end-expiratory pressure (PEEP) should be considered as early as possible in every patient with acute cardiogenic pulmonary oedema and hypertensive AHF, as it improves clinical parameters, including respiratory distress. It should be used with caution in cardiogenic shock and right ventricular failure.

Morphine may be required for alleviation of acute symptoms but has been associated with worse outcome.[5]

Intravenous **loop diuretics** are essential. When large doses are required, a continuous infusion has greater efficacy and is less ototoxicity than IV boluses. High doses of IV loop diuretics do not substantially worsen renal failure.[6] Additional use of a thiazide, such as **metolazone**, provides a synergistic effect. Diuresis is continued until physical findings (JVP) and biomarker trends suggest euvolaemia. Weight loss is desirable but cannot be used as a surrogate marker for clinical outcomes. A urinary catheter is helpful.

Vasodilators, such as **nitroglycerin**, starting with 10–20 mcg/min IV and targeting a systolic BP not lower than 95 mmHg. Tolerance is being developed on continuous use after 24–48 h, and the efficacy and safety of IV nitrates is uncertain.[7] Alternatively, **nitroprusside** (starting dose 0.1–0.3 micrograms/kg/min with BP monitoring through an arterial line) can be given. It is light-sensitive, and the administration line should be covered. **Nesiritide** is a recombinant BNP (bolus, followed by 0.01 micrograms/kg/min) that was approved for normotensive patients who do not respond to adequate doses of diuretics, but no benefit was seen in the ASCEND-HF trial.[8]

Ultrafiltration is an invasive fluid removal technique implemented through two large-bore, peripherally inserted venous lines. It may supplement or obviate the need for diuretic therapy, particularly in non-responders,[9] but its efficacy and safety are virtually unknown.[7]

Beta-blockers are discontinued only in haemodynamically unstable patient. Withdrawal of beta-blocker in patients with decompensated heart failure is associated with increased mortality.[10]

Inotropes are **synthetic cathecholamines**, **phosphodiesterase inhibitors**, and **calcium sensitizers**. They are indicated in the development of cardiogenic shock, e.g. low cardiac output with hypotension and/or pulmonary congestion despite appropriate afterload reduction, and development of cardiorenal syndrome. They should be used with caution, even in the short term, since they increase both in-hospital

Table 33.2 ESC 2012 GL on HF. Acute heart failure

Patients with pulmonary congestion/oedema without shock	
IV loop diuretic. Symptoms, urine output, renal function, and electrolytes should be monitored regularly.	I-B
High-flow oxygen in oxygen saturation <90% or PaO_2 <60 mmHg (8.0 kPa).	I-C
Thromboembolism prophylaxis (e.g. LMWH) in patients not already anticoagulated and with no contraindication to anticoagulation.	I-A
Non-invasive ventilation (e.g. CPAP) in dyspnoeic patients with pulmonary oedema and a respiratory rate >20 breaths/min. Should not be used in systolic BP <85 mmHg (and BP should be monitored regularly).	IIa-B
IV opiate (with an antiemetic) in particularly anxious, restless, or distressed patients. Alertness and ventilatory effort should be monitored frequently.	IIa-C
IV infusion of a nitrate in pulmonary congestion/oedema and systolic BP >110 mmHg, in the absence severe mitral or aortic stenosis. Symptoms and BP should be monitored frequently.	IIa-B
IV infusion of sodium nitroprusside in pulmonary congestion/oedema and systolic BP >110 mmHg, in the absence severe mitral or aortic stenosis. Caution in acute MI. Symptoms and BP should be monitored frequently.	IIa-B
Inotropic agents not recommended, unless the patient is hypotensive (systolic BP <85 mmHg), hypoperfused, or shocked (risk of atrial and ventricular arrhythmias, myocardial ischaemia, and death).	III-C
Patients with hypotension, hypoperfusion or shock	
Electrical cardioversion if an atrial or ventricular arrhythmia is contributing to haemodynamic compromise.	I-C
IV infusion of an inotrope (e.g. dobutamine) in hypotension (systolic BP <85 mmHg) and/or hypoperfusion. The ECG should be monitored continuously (risk of arrhythmias and myocardial ischaemia).	IIa–C
Short-term mechanical circulatory support (as a 'bridge to recovery') in patients severely hypoperfused despite inotropic therapy and with a potentially reversible cause (e.g. viral myocarditis) or a potentially surgically correctable cause.	IIa-C
IV infusion of levosimendan (or a phosphodiesterase inhibitor) to reverse the effect of beta-blockade if beta-blockade is contributing to hypoperfusion. ECG (risk of arrhythmias and myocardial ischaemia) and BP (vasodilation and hypotension) should be monitored continuously.	IIb-C
A vasopressor (e.g. dopamine or norepinephrine) in cardiogenic shock despite treatment with an inotrope. ECG should be monitored (risk of arrhythmias and myocardial ischaemia), and intra-arterial blood pressure measurement should be considered.	IIb-C
Short-term mechanical circulatory support (as a 'bridge to decision') in patients deteriorating rapidly before a full diagnostic and clinical evaluation can be made.	IIb-C
Patients with an ACS	
Immediate primary PCI (or CABG in selected cases) is recommended if there is an ST elevation or a new LBBB ACS.	I-A
Alternative to PCI or CABG: Intravenous thrombolytic therapy (if PCI/CABG cannot be performed), if there is ST segment elevation or new LBBB.	I-A
Early PCI (or CABG in selected patients) if there is non-ST elevation ACS. Urgent revascularization if the patient is haemodynamically unstable.	I-A
Eplerenone in EF ≤40%.	I-B
ACE inhibitor (or ARB) in EF ≤40%, after stabilization.	I-A
Beta-blocker in EF ≤40%, after stabilization.	I–B
IV opiate (along with an antiemetic) in patients with ischaemic chest pain. Alertness and ventilatory effort should be monitored frequently.	IIa-C
Patients with AF and a rapid ventricular rate	
Full anticoagulation (e.g. with IV heparin), if not already anticoagulated and with no contraindication to anticoagulation.	I-A
Electrical cardioversion in patients haemodynamically compromised by AF.	I-C
Electrical cardioversion or pharmacological cardioversion with amiodarone to restore sinus rhythm non-urgently ('rhythm control' strategy). Only with a first episode of AF of <48 h duration (or no evidence of left atrial appendage thrombus on TOE).	I-C
IV administration of a cardiac glycoside for rapid control of the ventricular rate.	I-C
Dronedarone is not recommended (increased risk of hospital admission and premature death), particularly in patients with an EF ≤40%.	III-A
Class I antiarrhythmic agents are not recommended (increased risk of premature death), particularly in patients with LV systolic dysfunction.	III-A
Patients with severe bradycardia or heart block	
Pacing in haemodynamical compromised by severe bradycardia or heart block.	I-C

ESC guidelines for the diagnosis and treatment of acute and chronic heart failure 2012, *Eur Heart J*. 2012;**33**:1787–847.

Table 33.3 ACCF/AHA 2013 GL on HF

Recommendation for therapies in the hospitalized patient	
HF patients hospitalized with fluid overload should be treated with intravenous diuretics	I-B
HF patients receiving loop diuretic therapy should receive an initial parenteral dose greater than or equal to their chronic oral daily dose; then should be serially adjusted	I-B
HFrEF patients requiring HF hospitalization on GDMT should continue GDMT unless hemodynamic instability or contraindicated	I-B
Initiation of beta-blocker therapy at a low dose is recommended after optimization of volume status and discontinuation of intravenous agents	I-B
Thrombosis/thromboembolism prophylaxis is recommended for patients hospitalized with HF	I-B
Serum electrolytes, urea nitrogen, and creatinine should be measured during titration of HF medications, including diuretics	I-C
When diuresis is inadequate, it is reasonable to a) Give higher doses of intravenous loop diuretics; or b) Add a second diuretic (e.g., thiazide)	IIa-B
Low-dose dopamine infusion may be considered with loop diuretics to improve diuresis	IIb-B
Ultrafiltration may be considered for patients with obvious volume overload	IIb-B
Ultrafiltration may be considered for patients with refractory congestion	IIB-C
Intravenous nitroglycerin, nitroprusside, or nesiritide may be considered an adjuvant to diuretic therapy for stable patients with HF	IIB-A
In patients hospitalized with volume overload and severe hyponatremia, vasopressin antagonists may be considered	IIb-B

COR indicates Class of Recommendation; GDMT, guideline-directed medical therapy; HF, heart failure; HFrEF, heart failure with reduced ejection fraction; LOE, Level of Evidence; and N/A, not available.

Recommendation for hospital discharge	
Performance improvement systems in the hospital and early postdischarge outpatient setting to identify HF for GDMT	I-B
Before hospital discharge, at the first postdischarge visit, and in subsequent follow-up visits, the following should be addressed: a. Initiation of GDMT if not done or contraindicated; b. Causes of HF, barriers to care, and limitations in support; c. Assessment of volume status and blood pressure with adjustment of HF therapy; d. Optimization of chronic oral HF therapy; e. Renal function and electrolytes; f. Management of comorbid conditions; g. HF education, self-care, emergency plans, and adherence; and h. Palliative or hospice care	I-B
Multidisciplinary HF disease-management programs for patients at high risk for hospital readmission are recommended	I-B
A follow-up visit within 7 to 14 d and/or a telephone follow-up within 3d of hospital discharge is reasonable	IIa-B
Use of clinical risk-prediction tools and/or biomarkers to identify higher-risk patients is reasonable	IIa-B

COR indicates Class of Recommendation; GDMT, guideline-directed medical therapy; HF, heart failure; and LOE, level of evidence
2013 ACCF/AHA Guideline for the Management of Heart Failure. *JACC* 2013; doi: 10.1016/j.jacc.2013.05.019

and post-discharge mortality, particularly with long-term therapy.[11,12] Beta-blockers should not be used concomitantly with inotropes to avoid competitive binding of beta receptors.[13]

Catecholamines mediate their cardiovascular actions through alpha1-, beta 1-, and beta 2-adrenergic, and dopaminergic receptors.[14] Beta 1-adrenergic receptor stimulation results in enhanced myocardial contractility through Ca-mediated facilitation of the actin-myosin complex binding with troponin C and enhanced chronotropy through Ca channel activation. Beta 2-adrenergic receptor stimulation on vascular smooth muscle cell results in increased Ca uptake by the sarcoplasmic reticulum and vasodilation. Activation of alpha1-adrenergic receptors on arterial vascular smooth muscle cells results in smooth muscle contraction and an increase in systemic vascular resistance. Stimulation of D1 and D2 dopaminergic receptors in the kidney and splanchnic vasculature probably

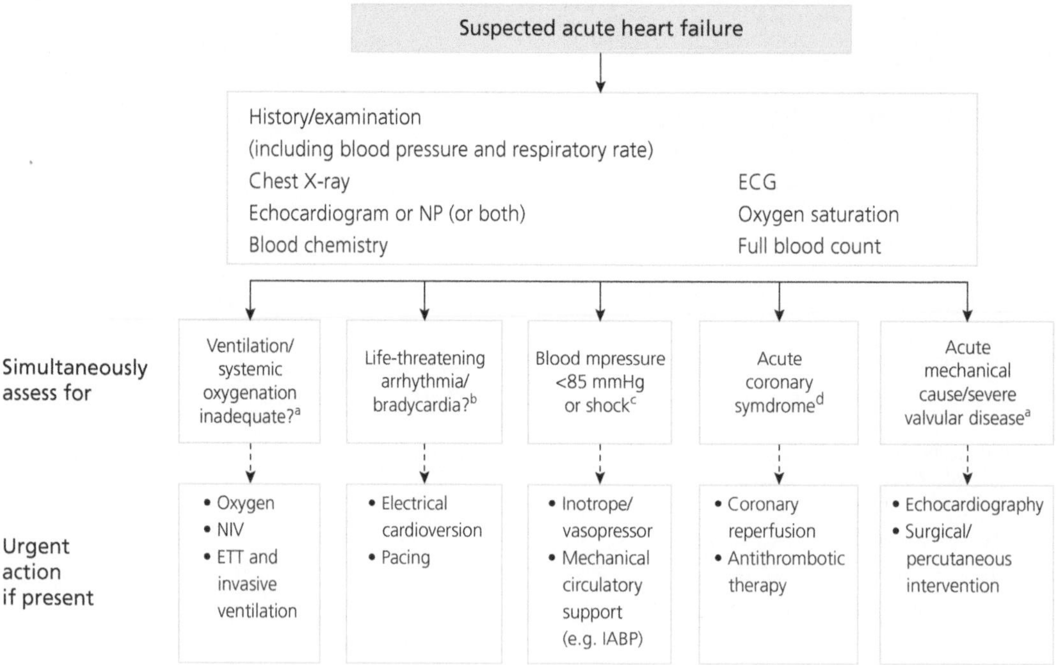

Figure 33.2 ESC 2012 guidelines on HF. Initial assessment of patient with suspected acute heart failure. (a) For example, respiratory distress, confusion, SpO_2 <90%, or PaO_2 <60 mmHg (8.0 kPa). (b) For example, ventricular tachycardia, third-degree atrioventricular block. (c) Reduced peripheral and vital organ perfusion—patients often have cold skin and urine output ≤15 mL/h and/or disturbance of consciousness. (d) Percutaneous coronary revascularization (or thrombolysis) indicated if ST segment elevation or new left bundle branch block. (e) Vasodilators should be used with great caution, and surgery should be considered for certain acute mechanical complications (e.g. interventricular septal rupture, mitral valve papillary muscle rupture). ECG, electrocardiogram; ETT, endotracheal tube; IABP, intra-aortic balloon pump; NIV, non-invasive ventilation; NP, natriuretic peptide.

ESC guidelines for the diagnosis and treatment of acute and chronic heart failure, *Eur Heart J.* 2012;**33:**1787–847.

Figure 33.3 ESC 2012 guidelines on HF. Algorithm for management of acute pulmonary oedema/congestion. (1) In patients already taking diuretic, 2.5 times existing oral dose recommended. Repeat as needed. (2) Pulse oximeter oxygen saturation <90% or PaO_2 <60 mmHg (<8.0 kPa). (3) Usually start with 40–60% oxygen, titrating to SpO_2 >90%; caution required in patients at risk of CO_2 retention. (4) For example, 4–8 mg of morphine plus 10 mg of metoclopramide; observe for respiratory depression. Repeat as needed. (5) Cold skin, low pulse volume, poor urine output, confusion, myocardial ischaemia. (6) For example, start an IV infusion of dobutamine 2.5 micrograms/kg/min, doubling dose every 15 min according to response or tolerability (dose titration usually limited by excessive tachycardia, arrhythmias, or ischaemia). A dose >20 micrograms/kg/min is rarely needed. Even dobutamine may have mild vasodilator activity as a result of beta2 adrenoceptor stimulation.
(7) Patient should be kept under regular observation (symptoms, heart rate/rhythm, SpO_2, SBP, urine output) until stabilized and recovered. (8) For example, start IV infusion at 10 micrograms/min and doubled every 10 min according to response and tolerability (usually dose uptitration is limited by hypotension). A dose of >100 micrograms/min is rarely needed.
(9) An adequate response includes reduction in dyspnoea and adequate diuresis (>100 mL/h urine production in first 2 h), accompanied by an increase in oxygen saturation (if hypoxaemic) and usually a reduction in heart and respiratory rate (which should occur in 1–2 h). Peripheral blood flow may also increase, as indicated by a reduction in skin vasoconstriction, an increase in skin temperature, and improvement in skin colour. There may also be a decrease in lung crackles. (10) Once the patient is comfortable and a stable diuresis has been established, withdrawal of IV therapy can be considered (with substitution of oral diuretic treatment). (11) Assess for symptoms relevant to HF (dyspnoea, orthopnoea, paroxysmal nocturnal dyspnoea), associated co-morbidity (e.g. chest pain due to myocardial ischaemia), and treatment-related adverse effects (e.g. symptomatic hypotension). Assess for signs of peripheral and pulmonary congestion/oedema, heart rate and rhythm, blood pressure, peripheral perfusion, respiratory rate, and respiratory effort. An ECG (rhythm/ischaemia and infarction) and blood

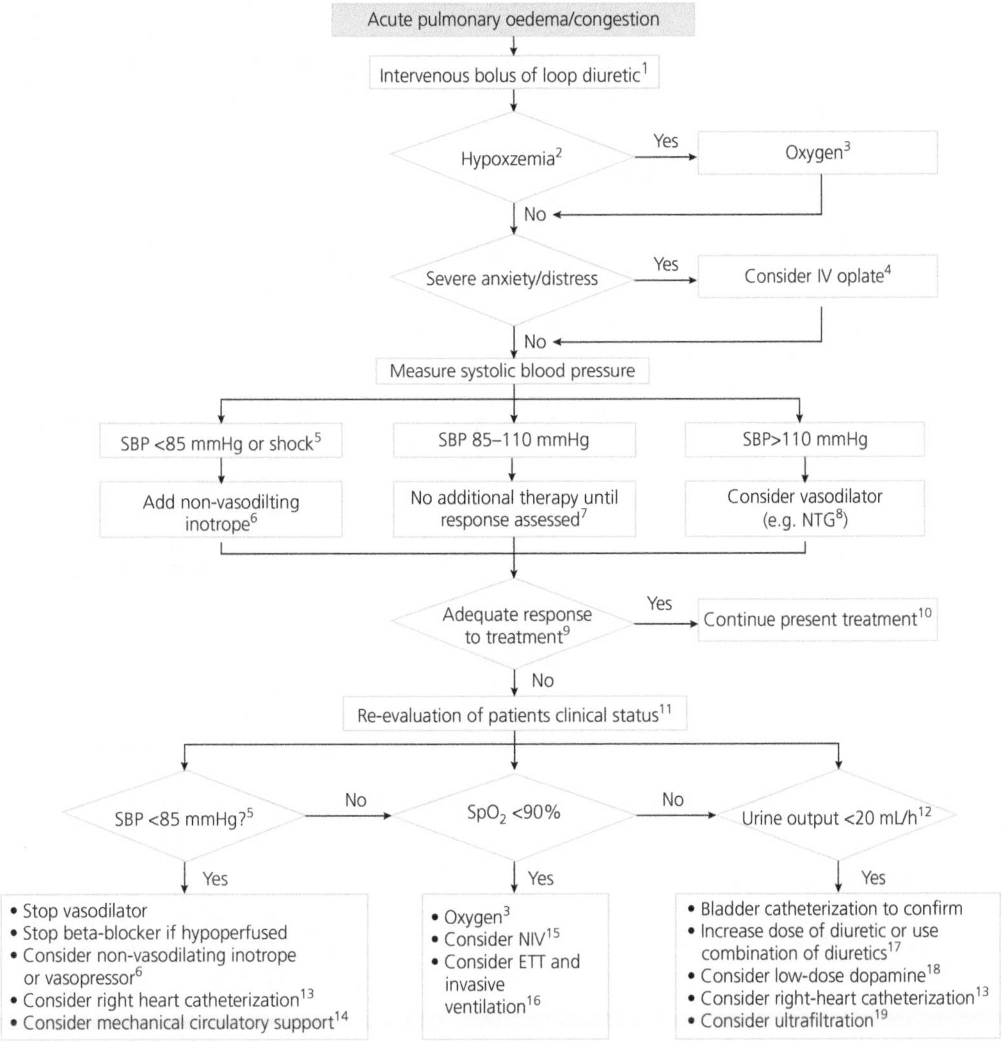

Figure 33.3 (Continued)

chemistry/haematology (anaemia, electrolyte disturbances, kidney failure) should also be examined. Pulse oximetry (or arterial blood gas measurements) should be checked and echocardiography performed (if not already carried out). (12) Less than 100 mL/h over 1–2 h is an inadequate initial response to IV diuretic (confirm if inadequate by catheterizing bladder). (13) In patients with persistently low blood pressure/shock, consider alternative diagnoses (e.g. pulmonary embolism), acute mechanical problems, and severe valve disease (particularly aortic stenosis). Pulmonary artery catheterization may identify patients with an inadequate left ventricular filling pressure (and characterize the patient's haemodynamic pattern, enabling more precise tailoring of vasoactive therapy). (14) An intra-aortic balloon pump or other mechanical circulatory support should be considered in patients without contraindications. (15) CPAP or NIPPV should be considered in patients without contraindications. (16) Consider endotracheal intubation and invasive ventilation if worsening hypoxaemia, failing respiratory effort, increasing confusion, etc. (17) Double dose of loop diuretic up to equivalent of furosemide 500 mg (doses of 250 mg and above should be given by infusion over 4 h). (18) If no response to doubling of dose of diuretic despite adequate left ventricular filling pressure (either inferred or measured directly), start IV infusion of dopamine 2.5 micrograms/kg/min. Higher doses are not recommended to enhance diuresis. (19) If steps 17 and 18 do not result in an adequate diuresis and the patient remains in pulmonary oedema, venovenous isolated ultrafiltration should be considered.

CPAP, continuous positive airway pressure; ETT, endotracheal tube; IV, intravenous; NIPPV, non-invasive positive pressure ventilation; NIV, non-invasive ventilation; NTG, nitroglycerine; PaO_2, partial pressure of oxygen; SBP, systolic blood pressure; SpO_2, saturation of peripheral oxygen.

ESC guidelines for the diagnosis and treatment of acute and chronic heart failure *Eur Heart J.* 2012;**33:**1787–847.

results in renal and mesenteric vasodilation through activation of complex second messenger systems, although the mode of action of dopamine is debated. cAMP stimulation by these agents, and consequent Ca overload of the sarcoplasmic reticulum and release of Ca into the cytoplasm, may trigger arrhythmias and increase mortality.

Dobutamine binds beta 1 and beta 2 receptors at a 3:1 ratio. It has minor effect on alpha1 receptors, and, at doses <5 micrograms/kg/min, the net effect is mild vasodilation. At doses <15 micrograms/kg/min, it increases cardiac contractility without affecting peripheral resistance. It can be given by a peripheral IV line. Tolerance may develop after a few days, and arrhythmias may occur at any dose as with any other inotrope.[14]

Dopamine binds beta 1, beta 2, alpha 1, and dopaminergic receptors. It is indicated in severe hypotension and worsening of renal function (cardiorenal syndrome). In 'renal' doses (0.5–3 micrograms/kg/min), dopamine promotes vasodilation and increased blood flow to renal tissue and has natriuretic effects on renal tubules. However, it does not increase glomerular filtration rate, and a renal protective effect has not been demonstrated.[15] At doses of 3–10 micrograms/kg/min, there is increased cardiac contractility and systemic vascular resistance. Dopamine should be given through a central line to avoid tissue extravasation. Combination of dobutamine (7.5 micrograms/kg/min) and dopamine (7.5 micrograms/kg/min) is better than one only agent at higher doses in cardiogenic shock. If, despite this, the blood pressure remains <70 mmHg, **norepinephrine** (0.01–3 micrograms/kg/min) is preferred to epinephrine that may promote coronary thrombosis.[16]

Milrinone inhibits phosphodiesterase 3, an enzyme in the sarcoplasmic reticulum that breaks down cAMP into AMP. It has inotropic, vasodilator (especially pulmonary), and lusitropic (improvement of diastolic relaxation) effects. It causes more significant RV afterload reduction and less myocardial oxygen consumption than the cathetholamines, and no tolerance is developed with prolonged use. However, outcomes are similar to those with dobutamine in acute decompensated failure.[17] It may be deleterious in ischaemic cardiomyopathy.[18]

Levosimendan is a calcium sensitizer that improves contractility by enhancing binding of calcium to troponin C. Its superiority over dobutamine is controversial,[19,20] and its efficacy and safety uncertain.[7]

Vasopressin (antidiuretic hormone) causes vascular smooth muscle constriction (V1 receptors) and water reabsorption (V2 receptors). It causes less coronary and cerebral vasoconstriction than cathecholamines. It is mainly used in cardiopulmonary arrest (40 U bolus).

Serelaxin, a recombinant human relaxin-2 and vasoactive peptide hormone, was recently associated with a reduction of 180 day mortality in patients admitted with acute heart failure (RELAX-HF trial).[21]

Intra-aortic balloon counterpulsation may be required in non-responsive cases. It can be used up to 3–4 weeks. Contraindicated in AR or aortic dissection.

Cardiogenic shock

Definition

Cardiogenic shock is a state of systemic hypoperfusion due to cardiac failure.

Aetiology and pathophysiology

Cardiogenic shock occurs in 5–8% of patients with ST elevation myocardial infarction and 2.5% of non-STEMI. Predominant RV shock represents 5% of all cardiogenic shock cases.[22] Risk factors for development of shock in the context of MI include delayed reperfusion, old age, anterior MI, hypertension, diabetes mellitus, multivessel coronary artery disease, history of prior MI or heart failure, and left bundle branch block. Mechanical complications of MI, including rupture of the ventricular septum (mortality >80%), free wall, or papillary muscles and chordae cause 12% of cardiogenic shock cases. Abnormalities of ventricular relaxation and compliance, neurohormonal changes, excessive nitric oxide production, and inappropriate vasodilation as part of the systemic inflammatory response syndrome caused by MI, and excessive use of medications, such as beta-blockers, ACE inhibitors, morphine, and diuretics, have been postulated as additional responsive factors. Although LVEF may be moderately depressed (in the SHOCK trial, mean LVEF was 30%), it is still a prognostic indicator.[23]

Presentation

The patient typically presents with cool extremities, decreased urine output, and altered mental status. Haemodynamic status:

- Systolic blood pressure <80 mmHg or mean arterial pressure 30 mmHg lower than baseline
- Cardiac index <1.8 L/min/m^2 without support or <2.0 to 2.2 L/min/m^2 with support)
- Adequate or elevated filling pressure (e.g. LVEDP >18 mmHg or right ventricular end-diastolic pressure >10 to 15 mmHg).

Cinical examination and chest radiograph are not reliable predictors of pulmonary capillary wedge pressure. Pulmonary artery and pulmonary wedge pressures can be measured with a pulmonary catheter or with Doppler echocardiography. A short mitral deceleration time (≤140 ms) is highly predictive of pulmonary capillary wedge pressure ≥20 mmHg in cardiogenic shock.

Therapy

Mortality is approximately 50%.

Use of **intra-aortic balloon** pumping improves coronary and peripheral perfusion via diastolic balloon inflation and augments LV performance via systolic balloon deflation with an acute decrease in afterload. Its use is recommended by both the ACC/AHA and ESC guidelines; however, in the IABP-SHOCK II randomized trial, intra-aortic balloon counterpulsation did not significantly reduce 30 day mortality in patients with cardiogenic shock complicating acute myocardial infarction for whom an early revascularization strategy was planned.[24]

In post–MI shock, **early revascularization** with PCI or CABG (even in suitable patients >75 years of age) remains the cornerstone of therapy, offering >10% increases in survival.[23] The survival benefit may be seen as long as 48 hours after MI and 18 hours after shock onset. In cases of septal rupture, percutaneous VSD closure is also an evolving therapeutic modality.

Arterial oxygenation and near-normal pH should be maintained, if necessary, with **mechanical ventilation via mask or intubation**. Positive end-expiratory pressure decreases preload and afterload. **Fluid administration**, in order to ensure adequate right-sided filling pressure and LV preload, is necessary; however, when the RVEDP is >20 mmHg, ventricular septum shift towards the LV may impair systolic function. **Intensive insulin therapy** improves survival in hyperglycaemic, critically ill patients and is recommended for use in complicated MI.

Inotropic, and especially **vasopressor**, agents should be used in the lowest possible doses. Preferred agents are dopamine, with or without dobutamine, and noradrenaline for more severe hypotension.

Percutaneous ventricular assist devices may also be used,[25] although the role of LVAD in cardiogenic shock is not clear.[26]

References

1. Adams KF, Jr., *et al.* Characteristics and outcomes of patients hospitalized for heart failure in the United States: rationale, design, and preliminary observations from the first 100 000 cases in the Acute Decompensated Heart Failure National Registry (ADHERE). *Am Heart J.* 2005;**149**:209–16
2. Ramani GV, *et al.* Chronic heart failure: contemporary diagnosis and management. *Mayo Clin Proc.* 2010;**85**:180–95
3. Yancy CW, *et al.* Clinical presentation, management, and in-hospital outcomes of patients admitted with acute decompensated heart failure with preserved systolic function: a report from the Acute Decompensated Heart Failure National Registry (ADHERE) database. *J Am Coll Cardiol.* 2006;**47**:76–84
4. Binanay C, *et al.* Evaluation study of congestive heart failure and pulmonary artery catheterization effectiveness: the ESCAPE trial. *JAMA.* 2005;**294**:1625–33
5. Peacock WF, *et al.* Morphine and outcomes in acute decompensated heart failure: an ADHERE analysis. *Emerg Med J.* 2008;**25**:205–9
6. Felker GM, *et al.* Diuretic strategies in patients with acute decompensated heart failure. *N Engl J Med.* 2011;**364**:797–805
7. McMurray JJ, *et al.* ESC guidelines for the diagnosis and treatment of acute and chronic heart failure 2012: the Task Force for the diagnosis and treatment of acute and chronic heart failure 2012 of the European Society of Cardiology. Developed in collaboration with the Heart Failure Association (HFA) of the ESC. *Eur J Heart Fail.* 2012;**14**:803–69
8. Cleland JG, *et al.* Clinical trials update from the American Heart Association meeting 2010: emphasis-HF, RAFT, TIM-HF, TELE-HF, ASCEND-HF, ROCKET-AF, and PROTECT. *Eur J Heart Fail.* 2011;**13**:460–5
9. Costanzo MR, *et al.* Ultrafiltration versus intravenous diuretics for patients hospitalized for acute decompensated heart failure. *J Am Coll Cardiol.* 2007;**49**:675–83
10. Fonarow GC, *et al.* Influence of beta-blocker continuation or withdrawal on outcomes in patients hospitalized with heart failure: findings from the OPTIMIZE-HF program. *J Am Coll Cardiol.* 2008;**52**:190–9
11. Abraham WT, *et al.* In-hospital mortality in patients with acute decompensated heart failure requiring intravenous vasoactive medications: an analysis from the Acute Decompensated Heart Failure National Registry (ADHERE). *J Am Coll Cardiol.* 2005;**46**:57–64
12. Cuffe MS, *et al.* Short-term intravenous milrinone for acute exacerbation of chronic heart failure: a randomized controlled trial. *JAMA.* 2002;**287**:1541–7
13. Ahmad T, *et al.* When the heart runs out of heartbeats: treatment options for refractory end-stage heart failure. *Circulation.* 2012;**125**:2948–55
14. Overgaard CB, *et al.* Inotropes and vasopressors: review of physiology and clinical use in cardiovascular disease. *Circulation.* 2008;**118**:1047–56
15. Bellomo R, *et al.* Low-dose dopamine in patients with early renal dysfunction: a placebo-controlled randomised trial. Australian and New Zealand Intensive Care Society (ANZICS) Clinical Trials Group. *Lancet.* 2000;**356**:2139–43
16. Lin H, *et al.* Opposing effects of plasma epinephrine and norepinephrine on coronary thrombosis *in vivo. Circulation.* 1995;**91**:1135–42
17. Yamani MH, *et al.* Comparison of dobutamine-based and milrinone-based therapy for advanced decompensated congestive heart failure: haemodynamic efficacy, clinical outcome, and economic impact. *Am Heart J.* 2001;**142**:998–1002
18. Felker GM, *et al.* Heart failure etiology and response to milrinone in decompensated heart failure: results from the OPTIME-CHF study. *J Am Coll Cardiol.* 2003;**41**:997–1003
19. Follath F, *et al.* Efficacy and safety of intravenous levosimendan compared with dobutamine in severe low-output heart failure (the LIDO study): a randomised double-blind trial. *Lancet.* 2002;**360**:196–202
20. Mebazaa A, *et al.* Levosimendan vs dobutamine for patients with acute decompensated heart failure: the SURVIVE randomized trial. *JAMA.* 2007;**297**:1883–91

21. Metra M, *et al.* Effect of serelaxin on cardiac, renal, and hepatic biomarkers in the relaxin in acute heart failure (RELAX-AHF) development program: correlation with outcomes. *J Am Coll Cardiol.* 2013;**61**:196–206.
22. Reynolds HR, *et al.* Cardiogenic shock: current concepts and improving outcomes. *Circulation.* 2008;**117**:686–97
23. Hochman JS, *et al.* Early revascularization in acute myocardial infarction complicated by cardiogenic shock. SHOCK Investigators. Should we emergently revascularize occluded coronaries for cardiogenic shock. *N Engl J Med.* 1999;**341**:625–34
24. Thiele H, *et al.* Intra-aortic balloon support for myocardial infarction with cardiogenic shock. *N Engl J Med.* 2012;**367**:1287–96
25. Kar B, *et al.* Percutaneous circulatory support in cardiogenic shock: interventional bridge to recovery. *Circulation.* 2012;**125**:1809–17
26. Thiele H, *et al.* Randomized comparison of intra-aortic balloon support with a percutaneous left ventricular assist device in patients with revascularized acute myocardial infarction complicated by cardiogenic shock. *Eur Heart J.* 2005;**26**:1276–83

Part VI

Cardiomyopathies

Relevant guidelines

ACCF/AHA 2011 guidelines on HCM

2011 ACCF/AHA guideline for the diagnosis and treatment of hypertrophic cardiomyopathy. *J Am Coll Cardiol.* 2011;**58**:e212–60.

ESC 2013 guidelines on pacing and cardiac resynchronization

2013 ESC Guidelines on cardiac pacing and cardiac resynchronization therapy. *Eur Heart J 2013.* doi:10.1093/eurheartj/eht150

ACC/AHA/HRS 2012 for device-based therapy of cardiac rhythm abnormalities

2012 ACCF/AHA/HRS focused update incorporated into the ACCF/AHA/HRS 2008 guidelines for device-based therapy of cardiac rhythm abnormalities. *J Am Coll Cardiol.* 2013;**61**:e6–75.

HRS/EHRA 2011 expert consensus statement on the state of genetic testing for the channelopathies.

HRS/EHRA expert consensus statement on the state of genetic testing for the channelopathies and cardiomyopathies *Heart Rhythm.* 2011;**8**:1308–39.

ESC 2011 guidelines on the management of cardiovascular diseases during pregnancy

ESC guidelines on the management of cardiovascular diseases during pregnancy. *Eur Heart J.* 2011;**32**:3147–97.

ACC/AHA ESC 2006 guidelines for management of patients with ventricular arrhythmias

ACC/AHA/ESC 2006 guidelines for management of patients with ventricular arrhythmias and the prevention of sudden cardiac death. *Circulation.* 2006;**114**:e385–484.

ACCF/AHA 2013 guideline on heart failure

2013 ACCF/AHA Guideline for the Management of Heart Failure. *JACC* 2013. DOI: 10.1016/j.jacc.2013.05.019.

Chapter 34

Classification of cardiomyopathies

Introduction

Proposals by the AHA and ESC have replaced the 1995 WHO definition and classification scheme.

American Heart Association (2006)

Definition

A heterogeneous group of diseases of the myocardium associated with mechanical and/or electrical dysfunction that usually (but not invariably) exhibit inappropriate ventricular hypertrophy or dilatation and are due to a variety of causes that frequently are genetic. Cardiomyopathies either are confined to the heart or are part of generalized systemic disorders, often leading to cardiovascular death or progressive heart failure-related disability.[1]

Classification

- **Primary cardiomyopathies** are those solely, or predominantly, confined to heart muscle.
- **Secondary cardiomyopathies** show pathological myocardial involvement as part of a large number and variety of generalized systemic (multiorgan) disorders.

Ion channelopathies are considered forms of primary genetic cardiomyopathy.[2]

European Society of Cardiology (2008)

Definition

Myocardial disorders, in which the heart muscle is structurally and functionally abnormal, in the absence of coronary artery disease, hypertension, valvular disease, and congenital heart disease sufficient to cause the observed myocardial abnormality.[3]

Classification

Cardiomyopathies are classified into the conventional phenotypes of **hypertrophic cardiomyopathy**, **dilated cardiomyopathy**, **arrhythmogenic right ventricular dysplasia**, and **unclassified forms** (such as non-compaction) (Figure 34.1). Each phenotype is then subclassified into familial and non-familial forms.

Familial refers to the occurrence, in more than one family member, of either the same disorder or a phenotype that is (or could be) caused by the same genetic mutation and not to acquired cardiac or systemic diseases in which the

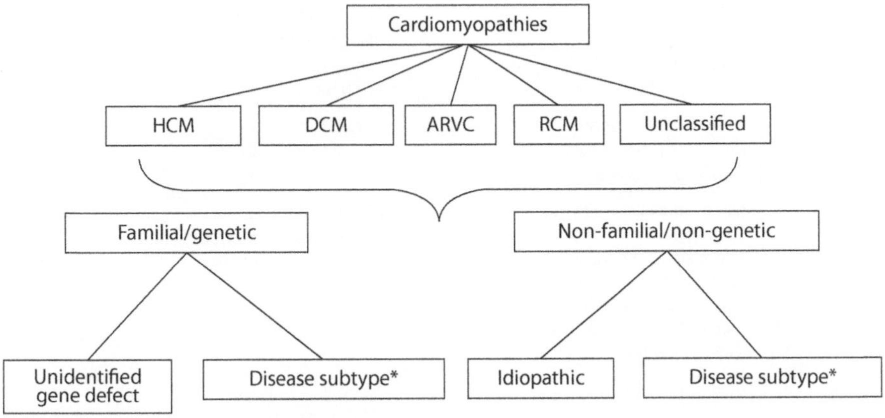

Figure 34.1 Summary of proposed classification system.

ARVC, arrhythmogenic right ventricular cardiomyopathy; DCM, dilated cardiomyopathy; HCM, hypertrophic cardiomyopathy; RCM, restrictive cardiomyopathy.
* Refers to subtypes of each phenotype, e.g. cardiomyopathy in the context of glycogen storage disease in HOCM, peripartum cardiomyopathy in DCM, etc.
Elliott P, *et al*. Classification of the cardiomyopathies: a position statement from the European Society Of Cardiology Working Group on Myocardial and Pericardial Diseases. *Eur Heart J*. 2008;**29**:270–6.

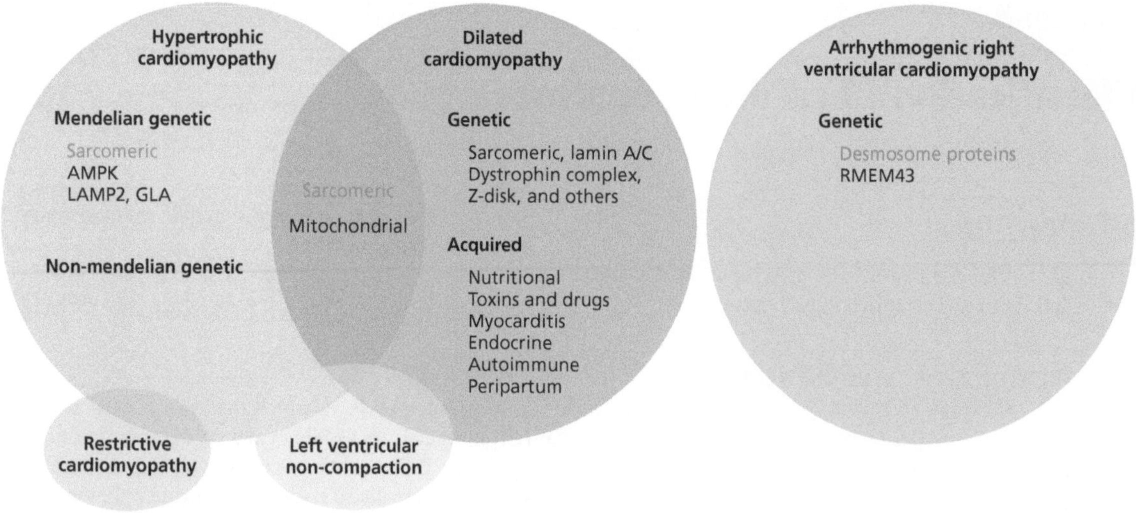

Figure 34.2 Clinical categories of inherited cardiomyopathies and their genetic basis. The clinical entities hypertrophic cardiomyopathy and dilated cardiomyopathy share some disease genes with each other, as well as with restrictive cardiomyopathy and left ventricular non-compaction, which are less common. Arrhythmogenic right ventricular cardiomyopathy appears to be a genetically distinct category, although its clinical phenotype cannot always be easily distinguished from that of dilated cardiomyopathy.

AMPK denotes AMP-activated protein kinase; GLA α-galactosidase A; LAMP2, lysosomal-associated membrane protein 2; TMEM43, transmembrane protein 43. Classes of genes shown in red are the overwhelmingly predominant cause of disease within the respective categories.

Watkins H, *et al*. Inherited cardiomyopathies. *N Engl J Med.*;**364**:1643–56

Table 34.1. Examples of signs and symptoms that should raise the suspicion of specific diagnoses grouped according to the main echocardiographic phenotype

	Main echocardiographic phenotype			
Finding	**HCM**	**DCM**	**ARVC**	**RCM**
Learning difficulties, mental retardation	Mitochondrial diseases Noonan syndrome Danon disease	Dystrophinopathies Mitochondrial diseases Myotonic dystrophy ACTN mutation		Noonan syndrome
Sensorineural deafness	Mitochondrial diseases Anderson–Fabry disease LEOPARD syndrome	Epicardin mutation Mitochondrial diseases		
Visual impairment	Mitochondrial diseases (retinal disease, optic nerve) TTR-related amyloidosis (vitreous opacities, cotton wool type) Danon disease (retinitis pigmentosa) Anderson — Fabry disease (cataracts, corneal opacities)	CRYAB (polar cataract) Type 2 *myotonic dystrophy* (subcapsular cataract)		
Gait disturbance	Friedreich's ataxia	Dystrophinopathies Sarcoglycanopathies Myofibrillar myopathies		
Myotonia (involuntary muscle contraction with delayed relaxation)		Myotonic dystrophy (type 1 and type 2)		

(Continued)

Table 34.1 (Continued)

Finding	Main echocardiographic phenotype HCM	DCM	ARVC	RCM
Paraesthesiae/sensory abnormalities/neuropathic pain	Amyloidosis Anderson — Fabry disease			Amyloidosis
Carpal tunnel syndrome (bilateral)	TTR-related amyloidosis			Amyloidosis
Muscle weakness	Mitochondrial diseases Glycogenosis *FHL*1 mutation	Dystophinopathies Sarcoglycanopathies Laminopathies Myotonic dystrophy Desminopathy		Desminopathies (generally distal progressing to proximal)
Palpebral ptosis	Mitochondrial diseases Myotonic dystrophy			
Lentigines/café au lait spots	LEOPARD syndrome			
Angiokeratomata	Anderson – Fabry disease			
Hypohidrosis				
Pigmentation of skin and scars		Haemochromatosis		
Palmoplantar keratoderma and woolly hair		Carvajal syndrome	Naxos and Carvajal Syndromes	

ARVC, arrhythmogenic right ventricular cardiomyopathy; DCM, dilated cardiomyopathy; HCM, hypertrophic cardiomyopathy; RCM, restrictive cardiomyopathy; TTR, transthyretin.

Rapezzi C, *et al.* Diagnostic work-up in cardiomyopathies: bridging the gap between clinical phenotypes and final diagnosis. A position statement from the ESC Working Group on Myocardial and Pericardial Diseases. *Eur Heart J* 2013; 34: 1448–1458.

Table 34.2. Electrocardiographic abnormalities that suggest specific diagnoses, grouped according to the main cardiac phenotype

Main phenotype	Finding	Specific diseases to be considered
HCM	Short P-R /preexcitation	Glycogenosis; Danon disease; PRKAG2; Anderson–Fabry disease Mitochondrial disease
	AV block	Amyloidosis Late-stage Anderson–Fabry disease Danon disease Acute myocarditis
	Extreme LVH (Sokolow >100)	Danon disease; Pompe
	Low QRS voltage (or normal voltages despite increased LV wall thickness)	Amyloidosis
	Extreme superior ('North-West') QRS axis deviation	Noonan syndrome
DCM	AV block	Laminopathy Emery Dreifuss 1 Myocarditis, particularly Trypanosoma cruzi, Diphtheria and Lyme disease Sarcoidosis Desminopathy Myotonic dystrophy
	Low P wave amplitude	Emery Dreifuss 1 and 2

(Continued)

Table 34.2 (Continued)

Main phenotype	Finding	Specific diseases to be considered
	Atrial standstill	Emery Dreifuss 1 and 2
	'Posterolateral infarction'	Dystrophin-related cardiomyopathy Limb-girdle muscular dystrophy Sarcoidosis
	Low QRS voltage + 'atypical RBBB'	ARVC with biventricular involvement
	Extremely low QRS amplitude	PLN mutation (very rare)
ARVC	Inverted T waves in inferolateral leads	ARVC with biventricular involvement
	Epsilon waves in inferolateral leads	ARVC with biventricular involvement
RCM	AV block	Desmin-related cardiomyopathy Amyloidosis

ARVC, arrhythmogenic right ventricular cardiomyopathy; AV, atrioventricular; DCM, dilated cardiomyopathy; HCM, hypertrophic cardiomyopathy; PLN, phospholamban; RBBB, right bundle branch block; RCM, restrictive cardiomyopathy.
Rapezzi C, *et al.* Diagnostic work-up in cardiomyopathies: bridging the gap between clinical phenotypes and final diagnosis. A position statement from the ESC Working Group on Myocardial and Pericardial Diseases. *Eur Heart J* 2013; 34: 1448–1458.

Table 34.3 First-level (to be performed in each patient) and second-level examinations (to be performed in selected patients that show features suggesting specific diagnoses)

	HCM	DCM	RCM
First level	CK Rental function Proteinuria Liver function tests	CK Rental function Proteinuria Liver function tests Haemoglobin and white blood cell count Serum iron, ferritin Calcium, phosphates, thyroid stimulating hormone	CK Rental function; Proteinuria Liver function tests Haemoglobin and white blood cell count Serum iron, ferritin Urine and plasma protein immunofixation,[a] free light chains[a]
Second level	alpha-Galactosidase A levels (or DNA for AFD suspected in women) Latic acid[b]; myoglobinuria[b] Urine and plasma protein immunofiaxation,[a] free light chains[a]	Organ and non-organ specific serum autoantibodies; titres for suspected infection; coxsadcievirus, echovirus, influenza virus; HIV; Borrelia bugdorferi (suspected Lyme disease), Changas disease (geographic exposure). Thiamine (alcohol abuse, nutritional deficiency). Uninary/plasma catecholamines (suspected phaeochromocytoma) Serum angiotensin converting enzyme (sarcoidosis)	Serum angiotensin converting enzyme (sarcoidosis) Organ and non-organ specific serum autoantibodies

AFD, Anderson-Fabry disease; CK, creatine kinase; DCM, dilated cardiomyopathy; HCM, hypertrophic cardiomyopathy; RCM, restrictive cardiomyopathy; TTR, transthyretin.
[a] AL amyloidosis.
[b] Mitochondrial diseases.
Rapezzi C, *et al.* Diagnostic work-up in cardiomyopathies: bridging the gap between clinical phenotypes and final diagnosis. A position statement from the ESC Working Group on Myocardial and Pericardial Diseases. *Eur Heart J* 2013; 34: 1448–1458.

clinical phenotype is influenced by genetic polymorphism. Traditionally, most familial cardiomyopathies are considered **monogenic** disorders (the gene defect is sufficient by itself to cause the trait). A monogenic cardiomyopathy can be sporadic when the causative mutation is *de novo*, i.e. has occurred in an individual for the first time within the family (or at the germinal level in one of the parents). Patients with identified *de novo* mutations are assigned to the familial category, as their disorder can be subsequently transmitted to their offspring. There has been evidence, however, that inherited cardiomyopathies are genetically heterogeneous; within each category, there are multiple disease genes and many different mutations, each of which is uncommon. The degree of genetic heterogeneity varies among the cardiomyopathies and determines the extent to which a final common pathway of pathogenesis can be identified for each condition (Figure 34.2).[5] A glossary of genetic terms used is provided in Chapter 56 on genetic channelopathies.

Table 34.4 Abnormalities in routine laboratory tests that should raise suspicion of specific cardiomyopathies, grouped according to the main cardiac phenotype

	Main cardiac phenotype		
Finding	**HCM**	**DCM**	**RCM**
↑ Creatine kinase	Mitochondrial diseases Glycogenosis Danon disease	Dystrophinopathies Sarcoglycanopathies Zaspopathies (*LDB3* gene) Laminopathies Myotonic dystrophy *FKTN* mutations Desminopathies Myofibrillar myopathies	Desminopathies
Proteinuria with/without ↓ glomerular filtration rate ↑ Transaminase	Anderson–Fabry disease Amyloidosis Mitochondrial diseases Glycogenosis Danon disease		Amyloidosis
High transferring saturation/ hyperferritinaemia		Haemochromatosis	Haemochromatosis
Lactic acidosis	Mitochondrial diseases	Mitochondrial diseases	
Myoglobinuria	Mitochondrial diseases	Mitochondrial diseases	
Leucocytopenia	Mitochondrial diseases (*TAZ* gene/Barth Syndrome)	Mitochondrial diseases (*TAZ* gene/Barth Syndrome)	

DCM, dilated cardiomyopathy; HCM, hypertrophic cardiomyopathy; RCM, restrictive cardiomyopathy.
Rapezzi C, *et al.* Diagnostic work-up in cardiomyopathies: bridging the gap between clinical phenotypes and final diagnosis. A position statement from the ESC Working Group on Myocardial and Pericardial Diseases. *Eur Heart J* 2013; **34**: 1448–1458

Table 34.5 Echocardiographic clues to diagnosis grouped according to main morphological phenotype

Main cardiac phenotype	Finding	Specific diseases to be considered
HCM	Increased interatrial septum thickness	Amyloidosis
	Increased atrioventricular valve thickness	Amyloidosis; Anderson–Fabry disease
	Increased RV free wall thickness	Amyloidosis; myocarditis, Anderson–Fabry disease
	Mild – moderate pericardial effusion	Amyloidosis; myocarditis
	Ground-glass appearance of ventricular myocardium	Amyloidosis
	Concentric LVH	Glycogenosis, Anderson–Fabry disease
	Extreme concentric LVH	Danon disease, Pompe disease
	Global hypokinesia (with/without LV dilatation)	Anderson– Fabry; mitochondrial disease; TTR-related amyloidosis; PRKAG2 mutations; Danon disease; myocarditis; end-stage sarcomeric HCM
DCM	LV non-compaction	Genetic DCM (more frequently sarcomeric mutations)
	Postero-lateral akinesia/dyskinesia	Dystrophin-related cardiomyopathy
	Mild (absent) dilatation + akinetic/dyskinetic segments with non-coronary distribution	Myocarditis Sarcoidosis
ARVC	Coexistent LV segment dysfunction	Biventricular ARVC
RCM	Partial LV or RV apical obliteration	Endomyocardial fibrosis/hyperosinophilia

ARVC, arrhythmogenic right ventricular cardiomyopathy; DCM, dilated cardiomyopathy; HCM, hypertrophic cardiomyopathy; LV, left ventricular; LVH, left ventricular hypertrophy; RCM, restrictive cardiomyopathy; RV, right ventricular; TTR, transthyretin.
Rapezzi C, *et al.* Diagnostic work-up in cardiomyopathies: bridging the gap between clinical phenotypes and final diagnosis. A position statement from the ESC Working Group on Myocardial and Pericardial Diseases. *Eur Heart J* 2013; 34: 1448–1458

Non-familial cardiomyopathies are clinically defined by the presence of cardiomyopathy and absence of disease in other family members (based on pedigree analysis and clinical evaluation). They are subdivided into **idiopathic** (no identifiable cause) and **acquired** cardiomyopathies in which ventricular dysfunction is a complication, rather than an intrinsic feature, of the disease. A diagnostic work up for specific cardiomyopathy diagnoses has been proposed by the ESC Working Group on Myocardial and Pericardial Diseases (Tables 34.1–4).[4]

References

1. Maron BJ, *et al.* Contemporary definitions and classification of the cardiomyopathies: an American Heart Association scientific statement from the Council on Clinical Cardiology, Heart Failure and Transplantation Committee; Quality of Care and Outcomes Research and Functional Genomics and Translational Biology Interdisciplinary Working Groups; and Council on Epidemiology and Prevention. *Circulation.* 2006;**113**:1807–16
2. Lehnart SE, *et al.* Inherited arrhythmias: a National Heart, Lung, and Blood Institute and Office of Rare Diseases Workshop consensus report about the diagnosis, phenotyping, molecular mechanisms, and therapeutic approaches for primary cardiomyopathies of gene mutations affecting ion channel function. *Circulation.* 2007;**116**: 2325–45
3. Elliott P, *et al.* Classification of the cardiomyopathies: a position statement from the European Society of Cardiology Working Group on myocardial and pericardial diseases. *Eur Heart J.* 2008;**29**:270–6
4. Rapezzi C, *et al.* Diagnostic work-up in cardiomyopathies: Bridging the gap between clinical phenotypes and final diagnosis. A position statement from the esc working group on myocardial and pericardial diseases. *Eur Heart J.* 2013;**34**:1448–58
5. Watkins H, *et al.* Inherited cardiomyopathies. *N Engl J Med.* 2011;**364**:1643–56

Chapter 35

Dilated cardiomyopathy

Definition

Dilated cardiomyopathy (DCM) is characterized by left ventricular dilatation and systolic dysfunction in the absence of hypertension, coronary artery disease, valve disease, congenital heart disease, and other overloading conditions. Left ventricular diastolic dysfunction may coexist, and atrial dilation as well as right ventricular dilation and dysfunction can also develop.

Epidemiology

Dilated cardiomyopathy is the most common cardiomyopathy worldwide and accounts for 25% of heart failure cases in the USA. Prevalence in adults is 1:2500, with an incidence of 7:100 000 per year.[1] This disorder develops at any age and in either sex but more commonly in men than in women. In children, two-thirds of cases are idiopathic.

Aetiology and pathophysiology

Familial and genetic

Inherited dilated cardiomyopathy accounts for 20–35% of all cases, with mutations identified in more than 30 genes.[2–4] Most mutations are private missense, nonsense, or short insertion/deletions. Autosomal dominant inheritance is the predominant pattern of transmission. X-linked, autosomal recessive, and mitochondrial inheritance are less common. At presentation, a family history and screening of first-degree relatives (for ventricular dilation, conduction disturbances, and skeletal myopathy) should be considered.[5]

Causative genes in dilated cardiomyopathy seem to predominantly encode cytoskeletal and sarcomeric proteins, with subsequent defects of force generation and transmission (Table 35.1), but it seems that none of the known disease-associated genes has been shown to account for ≥5% of this disease.[6] Recently, however, TTN truncating mutations were detected in approximately 25% of familial cases of idiopathic dilated cardiomyopathy and in 18% of sporadic cases.[7] Metabolic abnormalities and disturbed calcium homeostasis are additional mechanisms for cardiomyopathy. In the case of sarcomere-encoding genes, the same genes identified for hypertrophic cardiomyopathy seem to be responsible and support the concept of a 'final common pathway' of genetically determined cardiomyopathies: dilated cardiomyopathy is mainly a cytoskeletal disease, hypertrophic cardiomyopathy a sarcomeric disease, and arrhythmogenic right ventricular

Table 35.1 Genetic causes of dilated cardiomyopathy. Autosomal inheritance is usually dominant

Gene	Protein	Location and function
Autosomal		
LMNA*	Lamin A and C	Nuclear
TMPO	Thymopoietin	Nuclear
MYPN	Myopalladin	Z disc
DES	Desmin	Cytoskeleton, dystrophin-associated
SGCD	δ-sarcoglycan	Cytoskeleton, dystrophin-associated
LAMA4	Laminin alpha 4	Cytoskeleton
ILK	Integrin-linked kinase	Cytoskeleton
CRP3	Muscle-LIM protein	Z disc
VCL	Metavinculin	Z disc
ZASP/Cypher (LDB3)	LIM domain-binding protein 3	Z disc
ACTN2	a-actinin 2	Z disc
TCAP	Titin cap	Z disc
ACTC	Cardiac actin	Z disc
ANKRD1	Cardiac ancyring repeat protein	Z disc
TTN	Titin	Sarcomere (giant filament)
MYBPC3	Myosin-binding protein C	Sarcomere (thick filament)
MYH6	α-myosin heavy chain	Sarcomere (thick filament)
TNNT2	Cardiac troponin T	Sarcomere (thin filament)
MYH7	β-myosin heavy chain	Sarcomere (thick filament)
TPM1	α-tropomyosin	Sarcomere (thin filament)
TNNC1	Cardiac troponin C	Sarcomere (thin filament)
TNNI3	Cardiac troponin I	Sarcomere (thin filament)
PLN	Phospholamban	Sarcoplasmic reticulum Ca^{++} regulator
SCN5A*	$Na_v1.5$	Inward sodium current (I_{Na})
ABCC9	Sulfonylurea receptor 2A	Inward potassium-rectifying current (I_{KATP})
PSEN1/2	Presenillin 1/2	Transmembrane protein
RBM20	RNA-binding protein	Nuclear protein
X-linked		
TAZ G4.5	Tafazzin	Mitochondrial (Barth syndrome)
DMD	Dystrophin	Cytoskeleton

* These mutations account for 10–20% of cases of dilated cardiomyopathy associated with cardiac conduction defect.

cardiomyopathy/dysplasia a desmosomal disease, although several exceptions exist (Figure 35.1).

When the disease is associated with atrioventricular block, with or without limb girdle muscular dystrophy, the most frequently identified gene is the **LMNA** encoding for lamin proteins A and C.[8] These mutations also cause Emery–Dreifuss muscular dystrophy and limb girdle muscular dystrophy. Patients with the LMNA gene are also prone to AF and subsequently thromboembolism and ventricular arrhythmias and sudden death. Mutations in the **tafazzin (TAZ) gene** are responsible for the Barth syndrome that presents in male infants as heart failure associated with cyclic neutropenia and cardiolipin abnormalities and mitochondrial dysfunction. The **dystrophin gene** is responsible for Duchenne and Becker muscular dystrophy and X-linked dilated cardiomyopathy that develops in young men, with rapid progression from heart failure to death due to ventricular tachycardia or ventricular failure. These patients are identified by raised amounts of the muscle isoform of serum creatine kinase. Other mutations with pleiotropic cardiac manifestations, such as those of the SCN5A gene that has been implicated in various arrhythmia syndromes (long QT, Brugada, idiopathic VF, conduction system disease, sick sinus syndrome, and AF),[9] are presented in Table 35.1.

Infectious causes

Myocarditis is characterized by pathological inflammation of the myocardium, leading to chronic heart failure in a substantial number of patients younger than 40 years. Bacterial, fungal, parasitic, rickettsial, and spirochetal infections may be implicated, but the more common cause in the western world is **viral** infection (see Chapter 44). Although the causative relationship between viral infection and myocarditis is not unequivocally established, identification of the causative virus with polymerase chain reaction (PCR) indicates that some cases of dilated cardiomyopathy are the result of chronic myocarditis and subsequent cardiac injury either due to autoimmune reactions or direct viral tissue injury. Viral persistence in the myocardium has been associated with progressive cardiac dysfunction.[10] The most common viruses are parvovirus B19, adenovirus, coxsackie B, and other enteroviruses.[10, 11] Presentation of disease can vary, ranging from minor symptoms of malaise to acute heart failure. **Chagas' cardiomyopathy**, caused by the protozoan *Trypanosoma cruzi*, remains the leading cause of chronic systolic heart failure in endemic areas. The annual incidence of Chagas cardiomyopathy is 1.85% and is driven prinmarily by mild cardiomyopathy.[12] Approximately 25% of asymptomatic, *T cruzi*-seropositive persons will develop cardiomyopathy within the next 10 years.[12]

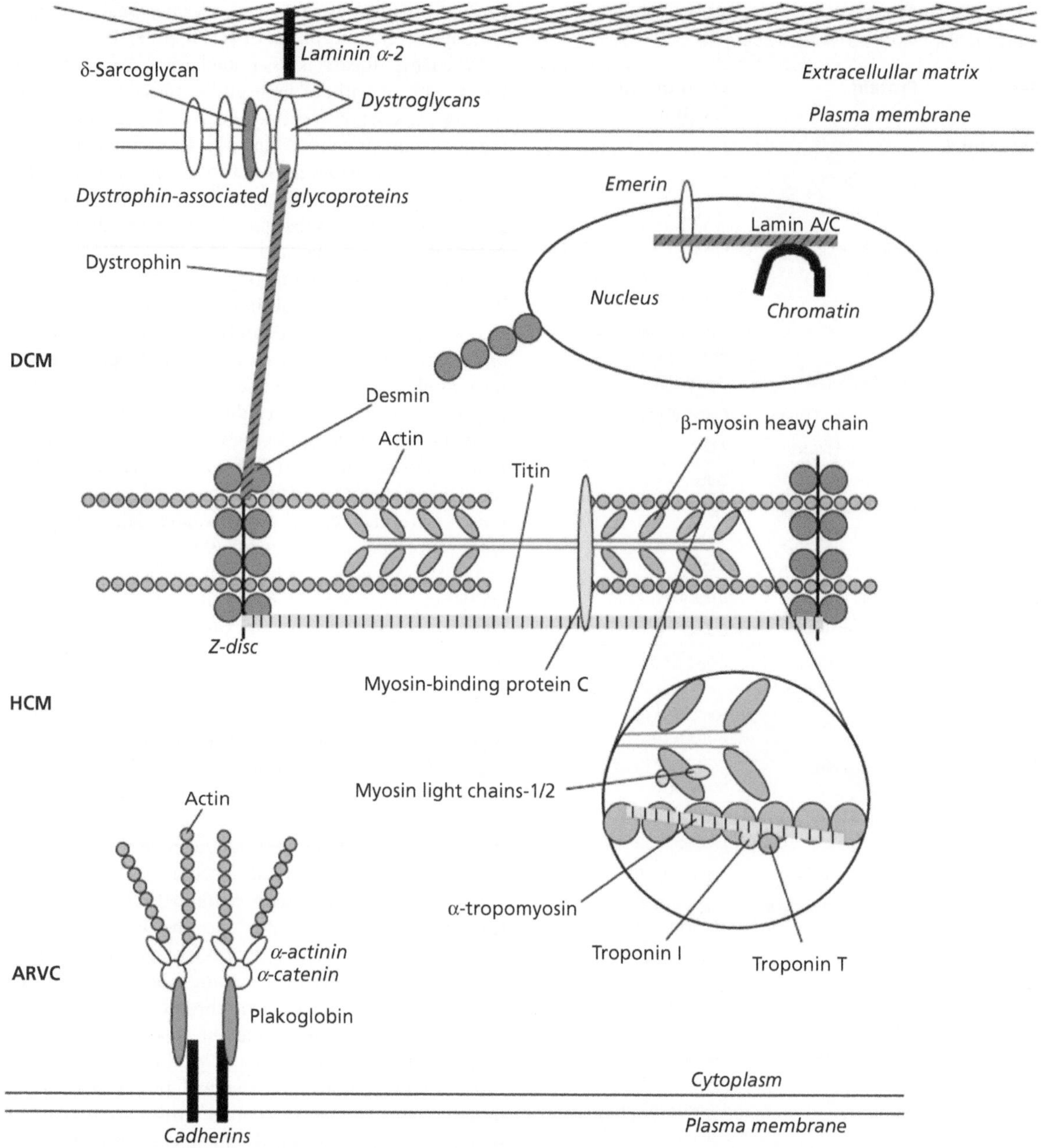

Figure 35.1 The final common pathway involved in cardiomyopathies. Cardiac myocytes are surrounded by the sarcolemma and contain myofibrils that are formed by repeating sarcomeres, the basic contractile units consisting of thin (actin, a–tropomyosin, and troponins) and thick (myosin and myosin-binding proteins) filaments. Titin is the supporting protein that extends from the Z disc (at the borders of the sarcomere in the thin filament) to the M disc (in the thick filament). Cardiac myocytes join each other at the intercalated disks that contain gap junctions (connexins), mechanical junctions (N-cadherin, catenins, vinculin), and desmosomes (desmin, desmoplakin, desmocolin, and desmoglein). As the dystrophin-associated protein complex links the basal lamina, sarcolemma, and sarcomere, mutant proteins (sarcomeric, cytosolic, or nuclear) cause dilated, hypertrophic, or a combined cardiomyopathy. Defective proteins in red cause DCM; those in yellow cause mainly HOCM but may also cause DCM; those in blue cause either HOCM or DCM, and those in green cause ARVD.
Franz *et al*. Cardiomyopathies: from genetics to the prospect of treatment. *Lancet* 2001; **358**:1627–1637.

Autoimmunity

Diagnosis for both viral and non-viral causes is based on histological, immunological, and immunohistochemical criteria for endomyocardial biopsy samples. Autoimmune-mediated chronic myocarditis is characterized by autoantibodies to cardiac myosin and other heart antigens.[1] Whether patients develop heart disease because they possess harmful antibodies against this receptor or whether they develop these antibodies as a result of cardiac tissue injury remains unclear. However, circulating cardiac autoantibodies are identified in dilated cardiomyopathy and myocarditis patients at a higher frequency than in patients with non-inflammatory heart disease. Furthermore, in healthy relatives of dilated cardiomyopathy patients, serum antiheart autoantibodies are an independent predictor for development of this disease.[13]

Cytotoxicity

Chronic alcohol abuse (more than 3 units a day) is one of the most important causes of dilated cardiomyopathy in developed countries.[14, 15] The exact mechanism is not known: direct toxicity and increased cellular apoptosis, acetaldehyde-mediated cardiac calcium regulation disruption, and neurohormonal activation have been proposed. A genetic background may also coexist. Recent data indicate that the outcome is worse than in idiopathic dilated cardiomyopathy, and the estimated 4-year mortality rate approaches 50% in patients without complete abstinence after diagnosis.[14, 16] The cardiac toxicity of drugs, such as **cocaine**, **anthracyclines (doxorubicin and daunorubicin)**, **trastazumab**, and **anti-vascular endothelial growth factor (VEGF)** chemotherapy agents (bevacizumab, sorafenib, sunitinib, pazopanib), is discussed in Chapter 31 on CCF.

HIV infection, hyper- and hypothyroidism, infiltrative disease, such as **haemochromatosis, rheumatological disease, mitochondrial dysfunction,** and **metabolic storage diseases,** are more rare causes.

Despite complete evaluation, including history, physical examination, echocardiography, coronary angiography, and endomyocardial biopsy, approximately 50% of patients with dilated cardiomyopathy have no aetiology identified.[17]

Peripartum cardiomyopathy and **tachycardiomyopathies** and **stress-induced cardiomyopathy** are discussed in relevant chapters.

Presentation

Patients present with **SOBOE** and **fatigue** or signs of **overt heart failure.**

Physical examination

It may be unremarkable or reveal the signs of heart failure (see Chapter 31 on CCF). Additional signs that may be present are described in Table 34.1.

Investigations

Electrocardiography No ECG abnormalities are specific for DCM. First- or second-degree AV block, intraventricular block, ST-T wave changes, Q waves, atrial fibrillation, or ventricular arrhythmias may be seen (Table 34.2). New ventricular arrhythmias or second-degree or third-degree heart block in patients with apparently chronic dilated cardiomyopathy suggests sarcoidosis. AF is seen in patients with the LMNA gene. Monomorphic sustained VT is due to bundle branch reentry but is rare and also suggests sarcoidosis, Chagas' disease, or LV-dominant ARVC.

Echocardiography The left ventricle is dilated and more spherical than usual, with raised wall stress and depressed systolic function with or without mitral regurgitation (Table 34.5). Usually, contractility is globally reduced without segmental abnormalities. Additionally, pericardial effusion (especially in myocarditis) and signs of right heart failure may be present.

MRI provides the most accurate estimate of ventricular structure and function and allows detection of inflammation and scarring (see Chapter 31 on CCF).

Endomyocardial biopsy is controversial. It can be used to distinguish between disease processes that need alternative treatment strategies, such as storage diseases, sarcoidosis, and haemochromatosis (see Chapter 31 on CCF). It is reasonable in patients with new-onset cardiomyopathy and fulminant heart failure who may benefit from an early diagnosis. Usually, however, microscopic examination reveals areas of interstitial and perivascular fibrosis and sometimes areas of necrosis and cellular infiltrate. Myocardial fibrosis is the presumed substrate of VF in DCM.

Electrophysiology study is indicated in patients with sustained palpitations, wide-QRS-complex tachycardia, presyncope, or syncope (ACC/AHA/ESC 2006 GL on ventricular arrhythmias, I-C). It may be also needed to diagnose bundle-branch reentrant tachycardia and to guide ablation.

Additionally, testing for secondary or specific causes that mimic dilated cardiomyopathy may be warranted (Tables 34.3 and 34.4).

Risk stratification

Risk stratification of patients with DCM is discussed in Chapter 31 on CCF. The main risk stratifier is LVEF. As in other primary myocardial disorders, programmed ventricular stimulation has no role in predicting SCD, and the independent predictive ability of NSVT is not established.[18] Cardiac magnetic resonance may be a predictor of SCD by means of detecting myocardial fibrosis.[19]

Genetic counselling

Familial dilated cardiomyopathy demonstrates incomplete penetrance (i.e. not all mutations carriers are affected by the disease), with variable phenotypic expression, and significant locus and allelic heterogeneity, making genetic diagnosis complex. For pure dilated cardiomyopathy the diagnostic yield of **genetic testing** is 20%.

Relatives of patients with DCM should undergo clinical examination, ECG, and echocardiographic screening, and, when a highly positive family history is present, referral to a cardiovascular genetics centre for genetic testing is indicated. Recent developments on TTN truncating mutations are exciting in this respect.[7] In the presence of premature conduction disturbances and ventricular arrhythmias, screening for mutations in the SCN5A or LMNA genes may be useful. The HRS/EHRA recommendations are presented in Table 35.2.

Therapy

Treatment of heart failure has been described in the section on Heart failure. Treatment of myocarditis is described in Chapter 44. Immunosuppresion with steroids and azathioprine may be useful only in dilated cardiomyopathy patients with evidence of HLA upregulation on biopsy samples or virus-negative myocarditis and chronic inflammatory cardiomyopathy.[20, 21] Intravenous immunoglobulin is not effective in recent-onset dilated cardiomyopathy.[22] In chronic dilated cardiomyopathy and persistent viral genomes, treatment with interferon resulted in the elimination of the viral genomes and improved left ventricular function.[23] Immunoadsorption with subsequent immunoglobulin G substitution is another possibility for patients with cardiodepressant autoantibodies detected in myocardial biopsy specimens.[24] Patients with the LMNA gene (and, in particular, mutation c.908–909delCT) and perhaps other X-linked familial forms should be considered for ICD at diagnosis.[25] Independent risk factors for malignant arrhythmias in lamin A/C mutation carriers are NSVT, LVEF <45% at the first clinical contact, male sex, and non-missense mutations (ins-del/truncating or mutations affecting splicing).[26] Patients with muscular dystrophies should be closely followed for consideration of the need of pacing or ICD. Beta-blockers are avoided in cocaine-related cardiomyopathy (unopposed alpha receptors), and benzodiazepines are used to blunt adrenergic excess in cocaine-associated heart failure.[14] Left ventricular volume procedures (such as the Batista or Dor) have not offered improved survival whereas percutaneous mitral annuloplasty with new devices for functional MR is being studied.[27] Gene and stem cell

Table 35.2 Genetic testing for DCM

HRS/EHRA 2011 statement on genetic testing. State of genetic testing for dilated cardiomyopathy	
Comprehensive or targeted (LMNA and SCN5A) DCM genetic testing for patients with DCM and significant cardiac conduction disease (i.e. first-, second-, or third-degree heart block) and/or a family history of premature unexpected sudden death.	I
Mutation-specific genetic testing for family members and appropriate relatives following the identification of a DCM causative mutation in the index case.	I
Genetic testing for patients with familial DCM to confirm the diagnosis, to recognize those who are at highest risk of arrhythmia and syndromic features, to facilitate cascade screening within the family, and to help with family planning.	IIa

HRS/EHRA 2011 expert consensus statement on the state of genetic testing for the channelopathies and cardiomyopathies. *Heart Rhythm*. 2011;**8**:1308–39.
2013 ACCF/AHA Guideline for the Management of Heart Failure. *JACC* 2013. DOI: 10.1016/j.jacc.2013.05.019.

ACCF/AHA 2013 GL on HF. Screening of Family Members and Genetic Testing in Patients With Idiopathic or Familial DCM

	Screening for family members	**Genetic testing**
Familial DCM	First-degree relatives not known to be affected should undergo periodic, serial echocardiographic screening with assessment of LV function and size.	Genetic testing may be considered inconjunction with genetic counseling
	Frequency of screening is uncertain, but every 3–5 y is reasonable	
Idiopathic DCM	Patients should inform first-degree relatives of their diagnosis.	The utility of genetic testing in this setting remains uncertain
	Relatives should update their clinicians and discuss whether they should undergo screening by echocardiography.	Yield of genetic testing may be higher in patients with significant cardiac conduction disease and/or a family history of premature sudden cardiac death.

2013 ESC Guidelines on cardiac pacing and cardiac resynchronization therapy. **Eur Heart J** 2013. doi:10.1093/eurheartj/eht150

Table 35.3 ESC 2011 GL on cardiovascular disease during pregnancy

Recommendations for the management of cardiomyopathies and heart failure	
Anticoagulation in patients with intracardiac thrombus detected by imaging or with evidence of systemic embolism.	I-A
Women with HF during pregnancy should be treated according to current guidelines for non-pregnant patients, respecting contraindications for some drugs in pregnancy.	I-B
Women with DCM should be informed about the risk of deterioration of the condition during gestation and peripartum.	I-C
In patients with a past history or family history of sudden death, close surveillance with prompt investigation is recommended if symptoms of palpitations or presyncope are reported.	I-C
LMWH or vitamin K antagonists according to stage of pregnancy for patients with AF.	I-C
Delivery with beta-blocker protection in women with HCM.	IIa-C
Beta-blockers in all patients with HCM and more than mild LVOTO or maximal wall thickness >15mm to prevent sudden pulmonary congestion.	IIa-C
In HCM, cardioversion should be considered for persistent atrial fibrillation.	IIa-C
Due to high metabolic demands of lactation and breastfeeding, preventing lactation may be considered in post-partum cardiomyopathy (PPCM).	IIb-C
Subsequent pregnancy is not recommended if LVEF does not normalize in women with PPCM.	III-C

ESC guidelines on the management of cardiovascular diseases during pregnancy: *Eur Heart J.* 2011;**32**:3147–97.

therapy are also under investigation. Indications for ICD and cardiac resynchronization pacing (CRT) are presented in Chapter 31 on heart failure. Although meta-analyses have indicated potential benefit, no single trial has documented improved survival with primary ICD implantation in dilated, as opposed to ischaemic, cardiomyopathy (see Chapter 68). ICD is clearly indicated in patients with sustained VT/VF (ACCF/AHA 2012 GL on Devices, I-C). It may also be indicated in patients with unexplained syncope and significant LV dysfunction (AACF/AHA 2012 GL on Devices, IIa-B).

Prognosis

Prognosis is variable, depending on the cause of DCM, with an average annual mortality of 10–30%, which, however, becomes consistently lower with time (5-year mortality at 20%).[28,29] SCD accounts for, at least, 30% of the overall mortality in DCM.[30] Approximately 30% of new-onset DCM cases may have substantial recovery. Patients with cardiomyopathy due to infiltrative myocardial diseases, HIV infection, or doxorubicin therapy have an especially poor prognosis.[17] Framingham data suggest that survival is worse in non-ischaemic than ischaemic cardiomyopathy,[16] although this is debatable.[17]

Pregnancy

It is not absolutely contraindicated any more, depending on the type of cardiomyopathy and underlying risk factors (Table 35.3).[31,32] Careful considerations to maintain normovolaemia and lumbar epidural anaesthesia are preferred. Caesarian delivery may be needed to avoid the undesirable circulatory effects of the Valsalva manoeuvre.

References

1. Jefferies JL, *et al.* Dilated cardiomyopathy. *Lancet.* 2010;**375**:752–62
2. Hershberger RE, *et al.* Clinical and genetic issues in dilated cardiomyopathy: a review for genetics professionals. *Genet Med.* 2010;**12**:655–67
3. Hershberger RE, *et al.* Update 2011: clinical and genetic issues in familial dilated cardiomyopathy. *J Am Coll Cardiol.* 2011;**57**:1641–9
4. Kamisago M, *et al.* Mutations in sarcomere protein genes as a cause of dilated cardiomyopathy. *N Engl J Med.* 2000;**343**:1688–96
5. Burkett EL, *et al.* Clinical and genetic issues in familial dilated cardiomyopathy. *J Am Coll Cardiol.* 2005;**45**:969–81
6. Ackerman MJ, *et al.* HRS/EHRA expert consensus statement on the state of genetic testing for the channelopathies and cardiomyopathies; this document was developed as a

partnership between the Heart Rhythm Society (HRS) and the European Heart Rhythm Association (EHRA). *Heart Rhythm*. 2011;**8**:1308–39

7. Herman DS, *et al.* Truncations of titin causing dilated cardiomyopathy. *N Engl J Med*. 2012;**366**:619–28
8. Taylor MR, *et al.* Natural history of dilated cardiomyopathy due to lamin a/c gene mutations. *J Am Coll Cardiol*. 2003;**41**:771–80
9. Olson TM, *et al.* Sodium channel mutations and susceptibility to heart failure and atrial fibrillation. *JAMA*. 2005;**293**:447–54
10. Kuhl U, *et al.* Viral persistence in the myocardium is associated with progressive cardiac dysfunction. *Circulation*. 2005;**112**:1965–70
11. Mahrholdt H, *et al.* Presentation, patterns of myocardial damage, and clinical course of viral myocarditis. *Circulation*. 2006;**114**:1581–90
12. Sabino EC, *et al.* Ten-year incidence of chagas cardiomyopathy among asymptomatic trypanosoma cruzi-seropositive blood donors. *Circulation*. 2013;**127**:1105–1115.
13. Caforio AL, *et al.* Prospective familial assessment in dilated cardiomyopathy: cardiac autoantibodies predict disease development in asymptomatic relatives. *Circulation*. 2007;**115**:76–83
14. Awtry EH, *et al.* Alcoholic and cocaine-associated cardiomyopathies. *Prog Cardiovasc Dis*. 2010;**52**:289–99
15. Laonigro I, *et al.* Alcohol abuse and heart failure. *Eur J Heart Fail*. 2009;**11**:453–62
16. Ho KK, *et al.* Survival after the onset of congestive heart failure in Framingham Heart Htudy subjects. *Circulation*. 1993;**88**:107–15
17. Felker GM, *et al.* Underlying causes and long-term survival in patients with initially unexplained cardiomyopathy. *N Engl J Med*. 2000;**342**:1077–84
18. Katritsis D, *et al.* Non-sustained ventricular tachycardia. *J Am Coll Cardiol*. 2012;**60**:1993–2004
19. Assomull RG, *et al.* Cardiovascular magnetic resonance, fibrosis, and prognosis in dilated cardiomyopathy. *J Am Coll Cardiol*. 2006;**48**:1977–85
20. Frustaci A, *et al.* Randomized study on the efficacy of immunosuppressive therapy in patients with virus-negative inflammatory cardiomyopathy: the TIMIC study. *Eur Heart J*. 2009;**30**:1995–2002
21. Wojnicz R, *et al.* Randomized, placebo-controlled study for immunosuppressive treatment of inflammatory dilated cardiomyopathy: two-year follow-up results. *Circulation*. 2001;**104**:39–45
22. McNamara DM, *et al.* Controlled trial of intravenous immune globulin in recent-onset dilated cardiomyopathy. *Circulation*. 2001;**103**:2254–9
23. Kuhl U, *et al.* Interferon-beta treatment eliminates cardiotropic viruses and improves left ventricular function in patients with myocardial persistence of viral genomes and left ventricular dysfunction. *Circulation*. 2003;**107**:2793–8
24. Ameling S *et al.* Myocardial gene expression profiles and cardiodepressant autoantibodies predict response of patients with dilated cardiomyopathy to immunoadsorption therapy. *European Heart Journal* 2013;**34**:666–675
25. Antoniades L, *et al.* Malignant mutation in the lamin a/c gene causing progressive conduction system disease and early sudden death in a family with mild form of limb girdle muscular dystrophy. *J Interv Card Electrophysiol*. 2007;**19**:1–7
26. van Rijsingen IA, *et al.* Risk factors for malignant ventricular arrhythmias in lamin a/c mutation carriers a European cohort study. *J Am Coll Cardiol*. 2012;**59**:493–500
27. Schofer J, *et al.* Percutaneous mitral annuloplasty for functional mitral regurgitation: results of the Carillon Mitral Annuloplasty Device European Union Study. *Circulation*. 2009;**120**:326–33
28. Dec GW, *et al.* Idiopathic dilated cardiomyopathy. *N Engl J Med*. 1994;**331**:1564–75
29. Di Lenarda A, *et al.* Changing mortality in dilated cardiomyopathy. The Heart Muscle Disease Study Group. *Br Heart J*. 1994;**72**:S46–51
30. Sen-Chowdhry S, *et al.* Sudden death from genetic and acquired cardiomyopathies. *Circulation*. 2012;**125**:1563–76
31. Regitz-Zagrosek V, *et al.* ESC guidelines on the management of cardiovascular diseases during pregnancy: the Task Force on the management of cardiovascular diseases during pregnancy of the European Society of Cardiology (ESC). *Eur Heart J*. 2011;**32**:3147–97
32. Stergiopoulos K, *et al.* Pregnancy in patients with pre-existing cardiomyopathies. *J Am Coll Cardiol*. 2011;**58**: 337–50

Chapter 36

Hypertrophic cardiomyopathy

Definition

Hypertrophic cardiomyopathy (HOCM) is a disease characterized by idiopathic hypertrophy of the left (≥15 mm), and occasionally right, ventricle in the absence of haemodynamic stress that is sufficient to account for the degree of hypertrophy.[1,2]

Other typical findings such as LV wall thickness ≥15 mm, usually due to basal septal hypertrophy with myocyte disarray, LVOT obstruction with gradient ≥30 mm Hg at rest or exercise (labile obstruction), and mitral valve systolic anterior motion, are common but not obligatory for a diagnosis of HOCM.

There are several patterns of hypertrophy, such as asymmetrical septal hypertrophy with or without LVOT obstruction, mid-ventricular hypertrophy, apical hypertrophy, LV free wall hypertrophy, posterobasal left ventricular free wall hypertrophy, segmental hypertrophy with normal LV mass on MRI, and, rarely, concentric hypertrophy similar to that found in systemic hypertension.[3,4]

Epidemiology

HOCM is the most common genetic cardiomyopathy. The prevalence of the disorder is estimated to be 0.2%, but this figure may be an underestimate. [4] The prevalence of HOCM in phenotype-negative children relatives at risk of developing HOCM is 6% at 12 years follow-up.[5]

Aetiology

It most commonly affects the cardiac sarcomere, with considerable heterogeneity in phenotypic expression and clinical course. It is often inherited in an **autosomal dominant** pattern with variable expressivity, but patients with new mutations (i.e. without any relatives with the disease) do exist. Every offspring has a 50% chance of developing the disease later in life (age-dependent penetrance). Familial disease is less frequent in children than in adults, with various modes of inheritance. In adults, 50–60% of cases are due to more than 1400 mutations in over 11 genes that encode for sarcomeric or other myocyte proteins (Table 36.1).[6,7] Inheritance is autosomal dominant. Several hundred mutations in MYH7 and MYBPC3 that encode for the β-myosin heavy chain and the myosin binding protein C are responsible for half the cases of HOCM (Figure 35.1 of Chapter 35 on DCM). Most of mutations are missence (substitution of one amino acid by another), but insertion/deletion mutations may also occur. Heterogenous expression of these mutations, as well as modifier genes and environmental factors, contribute to the characteristic diversity of HOCM phenotype. The reasons for the development of hypertrophy due to sarcomeric mutations are not clear, and the same genes may be responsible for dilated, or other forms of, cardiomyopathies. Reduced contractile function and activation of various signalling pathways are speculated.[8] Inherited non-sarcomeric disease, such as mutations of genes encoding for other cytosolic proteins, **Fabry's disease** (deficiency of alpha-galactosidase), and mitochondrial disease, may also result in similar cardiac hypertrophy (Table 36.2). **Friedreich's ataxia** is an autosomal recessive neurodegenerative disease caused by a defect in the gene encoding for the mitochondrial protein frataxin (MICONOS study group). Myocardial involvement is well documented, with concentric left ventricular hypertrophy as the dominating cardiac finding. Average life expectancy in patients with cardiac involvement is considerably reduced to 29–38 years.[9] **Mitochondrial disease** includes clinical disorders that occur as a result of dysfunctional cellular oxidative phosphorylation due to defects in mitochondrial (or rarely nuclear) DNA. Hypertrophic remodelling is the dominant pattern of cardiomyopathy in all forms of mitochondrial disease.[10] Most cases of left ventricular hypertrophy in children are associated with congenital malformations, inherited metabolic disorders, and neuromuscular diseases (Table 36.3).

Pathophysiology

Left ventricular hypertrophy is typically characterized by **myocyte disarray**, with cardiomyocytes varying in size

Table 36.1 Genetic causes of hypertrophic cardiomyopathy

Gene	Protein	Location and function
MYH7 (20–45% of patients)	β-myosin heavy chain	Sarcomere (thick filament)
MYBPC3 (15–20% of patients)	Myosin binding protein C	Sarcomere (thick filament)
TNNT2 (1–7% of patients)	Cardiac troponin T type 2	Sarcomere (thin filament)
TNNI3 (1–7% of patients)	Cardiac troponin I type 3	Sarcomere (thin filament)
MYL2	Regulatory myosin light chain	Sarcomere (thick filament)
MYL3	Essential myosin light chain	Sarcomere (thick filament)
TPM1	α-tropomyosin	Sarcomere (thin filament)
ACTC	Cardiac actin	Sarcomere (thin filament)
MYH6	α-myosin heavy chain	Sarcomere (thick filament)
TNNC1	Cardiac troponin C	Sarcomere (thin filament)
TTN	Titin	Sarcomere (giant filament)
ACTN2	a-actinin 2	Z disk
MYOZ2	Myozenin 2	Z disk
TCAP	Telethonin	Z disk
CRP3	Muscle-LIM protein	Z disk
ANKRD1	Cardiac ankyrin repeat protein	Z disk
VCL	Metavinculin	Z disk
PLN	Phospholamban	Ca^{++} handling/ regulatory proteins
CALR3	Calreticulin 3	Ca^{++} handling/ regulatory proteins
CASQ2	Calreticulin 3	Ca^{++} handling/ regulatory proteins
JPH2	Junctophilin 2	Ca^{++} handling/ regulatory proteins
RYR 2	Ryanodine receptor 2	Ca^{++} handling/ regulatory proteins

In bold are genes with strongest evidence of pathogenicity.
Maron BJ, *et al*. Genetics of hypertrophic cardiomyopathy after 20 years: clinical perspectives. *J Am Coll Cardiol*. 2012 Aug 21;**60**:705–15.

Table 36.2 HOCM phenocopy genes (diseases that can masquerade as HOCM)

Gene	Syndrome
LAMP2 (lysosome-associated membrane protein)	Danon disease
DTNA (a-dystrobrevin)	Barth syndrome/LV non-compaction
TAZ (tafazzin)	Barth syndrome
GLA (alpha-galactosidase A)	Fabry's disease
AGL (amylo-1,6-glucosidase)	Forbes' disease
FXN (frataxin)	Friedreich's ataxia
KRAS/SOS1	Noonan's
PTPN11/RAF1	Noonan's, LEOPARD
GAA	Pompe's disease
PRKAG2	Wolff–Parkinson–White

Landstrom AP, Ackerman MJ. Mutation type is not clinically useful in predicting prognosis in hypertrophic cardiomyopathy. *Circulation*. 2010;**122**:2441–9.

Table 36.3 Causes of left ventricular hypertrophy in children and adults

Familial sarcomeric disease
Metabolic disease
Infant of diabetic mother
Glycogen storage disease II (Pompe's disease) and III (Forbes' disease)
Anderson–Fabry disease
Carnitine deficiency
Phosphorylase B kinase deficiency
AMP kinase (WPW and conduction disease)
Debrancher enzyme deficiency
Hurler's syndrome
Hurler–Scheie disease
Hunter's syndrome
Mannosidosis
Fucosidosis
Total lipodystrophy
Mitochondrial cytopathy
MELAS (mitochondrial encephalomyopathy, lactic acidosis, and stroke-like episodes)
MERRF (myoclonic epilepsy and ragged red fibres)
LHON (Leber's hereditary optic neuropathy)
Syndromic HCM
Noonan's syndrome
LEOPARD syndrome
Friedreich's ataxia

(Continued)

Table 36.3 (Continued)

Beckwith–Wiedermann syndrome
Swyer's syndrome (pure gonadal dysgenesis)
Miscellaneous
Amyloidosis
Phaeochromocytoma
Obesity
Athletic training

Maron MS, *et al.* Mitral valve abnormalities identified by cardiovascular magnetic resonance represent a primary phenotypic expression of hypertrophic cardiomyopathy. *Circulation*. 2011;**124**:40–7.

and shape and forming abnormal intercellular connections, usually with expansion of the interstitial compartment and areas of replacement fibrosis (Figure 36.1).[11] There is also small vessel disease, in which intramural coronary vessels are apparently narrowed by medial hypertrophy.[11] Myocyte disarray is characteristic of, but not confined to, HOCM. It can be seen in patients with other diseases, such Noonan's syndrome, Friedreich's ataxia, and congenital disorders.

Systolic septal bulging into the LVOT and hyperdynamic LV contraction (causing the Venturi effect) contribute to the creation of a variable **LVOT gradient** that increases with decreased afterload. Approximately 25% of patients have dynamic LVOT obstruction caused by contact between the anterior or, less commonly, the posterior mitral valve leaflet and the interventricular septum during systole **(systolic anterior motion—SAM)**. Severe LV hypertrophy results in increased chamber stiffness and diastolic dysfunction. Intrinsic abnormalities of the mitral apparatus, including fibrous leaflet thickening, prolapse, and malposition of the anterior papillary muscle, occur in an estimated 20% of patients with HCM and contribute to the obstruction. MRI may also detect mitral leaflet elongation that is independent of other disease variables.[12] Dyspnoea occurs with exertion and may result from limitation of cardiac output due to the low end-diastolic volume of a non-compliant LV, high pulmonary venous pressure due to diastolic dysfunction, and mitral regurgitation. Angina may result from an inability of the narrowed coronary microcirculation to supply the hypertrophied myocardium in the context of high myocardial oxygen demand associated with elevated LV systolic pressure. Atrial fibrillation or flutter is associated with a worsening of symptoms because these patients are depended on atrial transport due to the concomitant diastolic dysfunction, an important pathophysiological feature of HOCM. Presyncopal episodes and syncope are due to LVOT obstruction, myocardial ischaemia, inappropriate systemic vasodilation, and ventricular arrhythmias. Myocardial fibrosis and, especially, disarray are most probably the arrhythmogenic substrates. Abnormal blood pressure response during exercise, defined as fall or failure to rise >20 mmHg, may be seen in up to 25% of patients with HCM and is attributed to autonomic dysfunction. Approximately 10% of patients with HOCM will develop end-stage morphology, with LV dilation and wall thinning, that is associated with worse outcome.[13]

Presentation and natural history

Patients may be asymptomatic or present with dyspnoea and angina, with a characteristic day-to-day variation in the activity needed to cause symptoms. Presyncope or syncope may also be the presenting symptom and is a marker for risk of sudden death.

There are three relatively discrete, but not mutually exclusive, pathways of clinical progression:[2]

1. **Sudden cardiac death (SCD)** due to unpredictable ventricular tachyarrhythmias, most commonly in young asymptomatic patients <35 years of age (including competitive athletes). The estimated rate of SCD is 1% per year in the overall HCM population but probably higher in those at greatest risk. Sex is not a major determinant of the risk of SCD. Most events, even in athletes, are not related to strenuous exercise.
2. **Heart failure** characterized by exertional dyspnoea (with or without chest pain) that may be progressive, despite preserved systolic function and sinus rhythm, or, in a small proportion of patients, heart failure may progress to the end stage, with LV remodelling and systolic dysfunction caused by extensive myocardial scarring.
3. **AF**, either paroxysmal or chronic, is also associated with various degrees of heart failure and an increased risk of systemic thromboembolism and both fatal and non-fatal stroke.
4. Patients surviving into the seventh decade with this genetic disease are at low risk for HCM-related mortality and morbidity, including sudden death (even when conventional risk factors are present).[14]

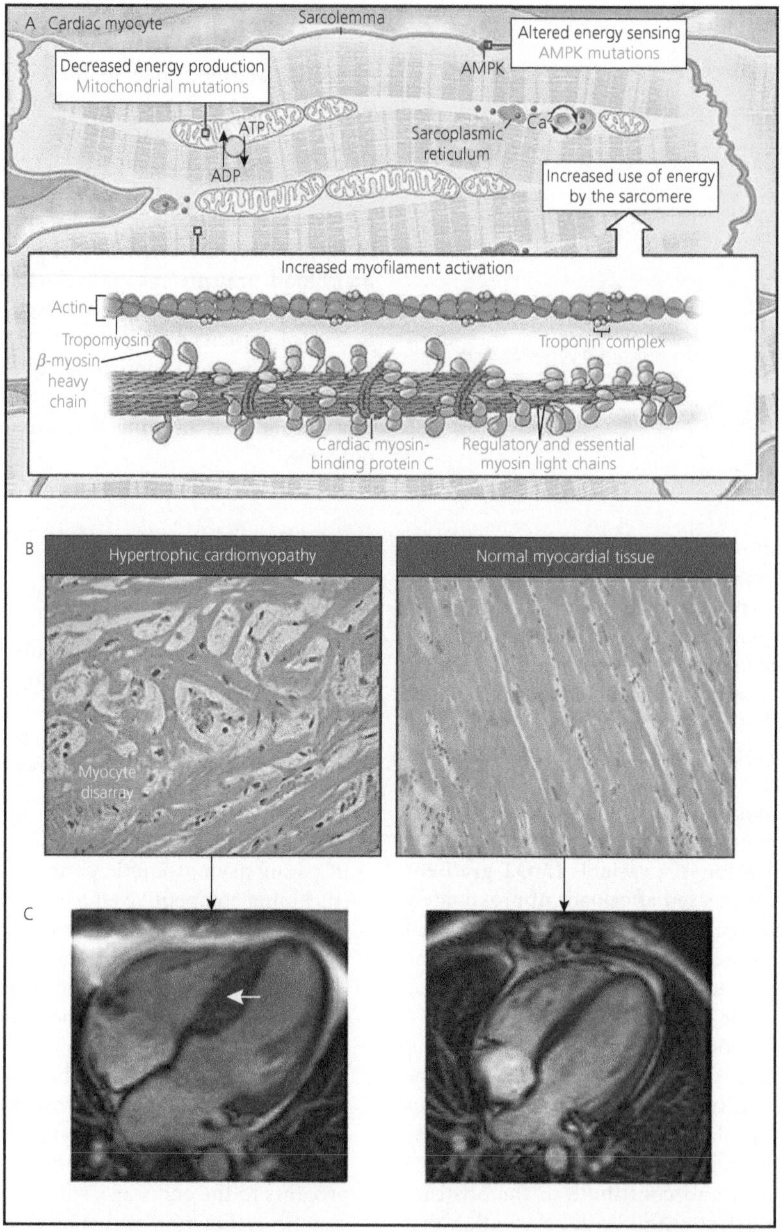

Figure 36.1 Pathogenesis of hypertrophic cardiomyopathy. In hypertrophic cardiomyopathy, mutations in sarcomeric proteins generally increase myofilament activation and result in myocyte hypercontractility and excessive energy use (panel A). Alterations in myocardial energy status can also result from primary mutations affecting myocardial energy generation (e.g. mitochondrial transfer RNA mutations). These mitochondrial defects and mutations in the cardiac energy-sensing apparatus (e.g. AMP-activated protein kinase [AMPK]) recapitulate a hypertrophic cardiomyopathy-like phenotype. Alterations in myocardial energetics and in calcium handling, combined with stimulation of signalling pathways (e.g. the Janus-associated kinase signal transducers and activators of transcription [JAK-STAT] signalling pathway) diminish myocyte relaxation and promote myocyte growth, with aberrant tissue architecture (i.e. myofibrillar disarray and myocardial fibrosis) (panel B, haematoxylin and eosin). In patients with hypertrophic cardiomyopathy, these changes often result in gross hypertrophy, with especially prominent septal hypertrophy (arrow) as compared with the normal heart, as shown on the cardiac magnetic resonance images (panel C).

Watkins H, *et al*. Inherited cardiomyopathies. *N Engl J Med*.;**364**:1643–56.

Physical examination

Examination may be unremarkable or reveal:

- **Bisferiens pulse** with dynamic obstruction
- Prominent **a wave** in JVP
- **Systolic murmur** at left sternal edge. It is distinguished from all other systolic murmurs (apart from this of mitral valve prolapse) by an increase in intensity with the Valsalva manoeuvre and during squatting-to-standing and by a decrease in intensity during standing-to-squatting action, passive leg elevation, and handgrip.
- **Pansystolic murmur** of MR.

Investigations

A **12-lead ECG** is abnormal in 75–95% of patients, and may show left atrial enlargement, repolarization abnormalities, and inferolateral Q waves. The PR may be short, and giant T waves may be present (distal hypertrophy—Japanese variant). QT prolongation (>480 ms) may be seen in 25% of patients.[15] ECG is essential (ACCF/AHA 2011 I-C) and should be repeated every year once the diagnosis has been established to evaluate for asymptomatic changes in conduction or rhythm (ACCF/AHA 2001, IIa-C).

Holter monitoring (ACCF/AHA 2011, I-B), to detect paroxysmal AF or non-sustained VT, should be repeated every 1–2 years (ACCF/AHA 2011, IIa-C). Frequent and prolonged (>10 beats) episodes of NSVT are a marker of sudden death.

Echocardiography LV wall thickness >15 mm in any segment is diagnostic. Patients with LVOT obstruction ≥30 mmHg at rest are at greater risk for heart failure or stroke death in comparion with patients without obstruction.[16] LVOT obstruction is usually associated with variable degrees of mitral regurgitation, which, when due to SAM, is usually directed posteriorly. Thickening of the mitral leaflets and anomalous papillary muscle origin may coexist and contribute to obstruction. When due to SAM, the jet is directed posteriorly, unless structural abnormalities of the mitral valve are present. LVOT flow gradient without SAM suggests other valvular or subvalvular causes of obstruction.[3] Transthoracic echo is recommended in the initial evaluation of all patients with suspected HCM (ACCF/AHA 2011, I-B) and should be repeated every 1–2 years (ACCF/AHA 2011, IIa-C). If the resting instantaneous peak LVOT gradient is ≤50 mmHg, it is reasonable to perform **exercise echocardiography** for detection of exercise-induced dynamic LVOT obstruction (ACCF/AHA 2011, I-B). Diastolic dysfunction is frequent and can dominate the clinical picture to resemble restrictive cardiomyopathy.[2] **Tissue Doppler imaging** may identify mutation carriers prior to development of hypertrophy by detecting reduced long axis systolic and early diastolic velocities and velocity gradients.[17]

Transoesophageal echocardiography is useful if transthoracic echo is inconclusive for clinical decision-making about medical therapy and in situations, such as planning for myectomy, exclusion of subaortic membrane, mitral regurgitation secondary to structural abnormalities of the mitral valve apparatus, or in assessment for the feasibility of alcohol septal ablation (Class IIa-C, ACC/AHA 2011). It is essential for intraoperative guidance of septal myectomy (Class I-B, ACC/AHA 2011) and for the intraprocedural guidance of alcohol septal ablation with intracoronary contrast injection of the septal perforator(s) (Class I-B, ACC/AHA 2011).

Exercise testing with simultaneous respiratory gas analysis is useful for demonstration of exercise-induced obstruction, assessment of functional capacity and risk stratification (Class IIa-B, ACC/AHA 2011), and for the differential diagnosis of unexplained hypertrophy. Up to 25% of patients with HOCM have an abnormal blood pressure response during upright exercise (systolic blood pressure fails to rise >20–25 mmHg from baseline or falls), either due to abnormal vasodilatation in non-exercising muscles or impaired cardiac output, and a reduction in peak oxygen consumption compared with healthy controls. However, respiratory gas profiles indicative of severe and premature lactic acidaemia can be the only clue to a diagnosis of mitochondrial myopathy.[8, 10] ***BNP***, an independent predictor of survival in HOCM, can identify patients who have poor cardiopulmonary exercise tolerance.[18]

Cardiac magnetic resonance can identify focal hypertrophy as well as hypertrophy particularly in the anterolateral free wall and apex, which is not well appreciated by two-dimensional echocardiography. It is essential in controversial cases (Class I-B, ACC/AHA 2011). CMR can also provide detailed characterization of other myocardial structures, such as the papillary muscles, and enables an accurate assessment of total LV mass. Delayed gadolinium enhancement sequences can characterize areas of myocardial fibrosis/scarring and have been associated with ventricular tachyarrhythmias and the risk of sudden death.[19]

Coronary angiography is indicated in the presence of chest pain in patients with a high likelihood of coronary artery disease (Class I-C, ACC/AHA 2011). Angina may also be caused by myocardial bridging that is common in HCM HCM,[20] or supply/demand mismatch due to the hypetrophy.

Myocardial perfusion studies are indicated only in the presence of chest pain or high likelihood of coronary artery disease (Class IIa-C, ACC/AHA 2011), not as a routine test for the detection of silent coronary disease.

Programmed ventricular stimulation has no role in risk stratification (see also ICD therapy).[2]

Differential diagnosis

Diseases resulting in LV hypertrophy are presented in Table 36.3. The likelihood of HCM can be determined by the identification of a diagnostic sarcomere mutation or inferred by marked LV thickness >25 mm and/or LVOT obstruction with systolic anterior motion and mitral-septal contact. However, in clinical practice, the most commonly encountered conditions that may resemble HCM are essential hypertension and the athletic heart. The **elderly** may also present with sigmoid or hypertrophied septum and make diagnosis difficult.[21] Symmetric LV hypertrophy, thickened valves, and moderately depressed LV function in males >65 years old suggest senile or transthyretin-related amyloidosis rather than HCM.[22] Long-standing **arterial hypertension** produces concentric hypertrophy of the LV, but wall thickness >15 mm is rare. However, HCM can present with wall thickness <15 mm, and, particularly in black patients, diagnosis can be made by discovery of a non-hypertensive first-degree relative or by genetic testing.

The **athletic heart** results from intense training. Wall thickness resembling cardiomyopathy may occur in sporting disciplines that combine isometric and isotonic activity, such as cycling and rowing. Sudden cardiac death in young competitive athletes is an important, although rare, public health problem. The single most common cardiovascular cause of these unexpected catastrophes is HCM, accounting for about one-third of cases.[23, 24] Since the phenotypic expression of HOCM is variable, and not uncommonly includes patients with mild and localized left ventricular hypertrophy, the differential diagnosis with athlete's heart may be difficult. By contrast with most patients with HCM, athletes have increased left and right ventricular cavity dimensions and normal diastolic function and rarely have ECG changes suggestive of myocardial disease.[23–25] Physiological left ventricular hypertrophy can also be differentiated from hypertrophic cardiomyopathy by tissue Doppler imaging velocity measurements.[17] In some cases, protracted deconditioning may be the only way to establish a diagnosis. Unexplained, symmetrical LV hypertrophy not fulfilling standard criteria for HOCM and organ involvement, such as diabetes and deafness, should also alert the cardiologist to the possibility of **mitochondrial DNA disease.**[10] Left ventricular hypertrophy in the context of childhood neuropathy, corneal opacities, proteinuria, hearing loss, and small vascular lesions on the buttocks suggest Fabry disease.[26]

Therapy

The management of patients with HOCM is aimed at activity restriction, with avoidance of volume depletion, symptomatic relief, prevention of sudden death, and screening of relatives. With the exception of ICD, no pharmacological, or other, strategies offer protection from sudden death.[24] In asymptomatic HCM patients, benefit from beta blockers or L-type calcium channel blockers has not been established (Table 36.4), but beta blockers are first-line agents for the management of symptomatic (angina or dyspnoea) patients with HCM. Vasodilators, including dihydropyridine calcium channel blockers and angiotensin-converting enzyme inhibitors, are potentially harmful in those with evidence of LVOT obstruction (Table 36.4, Figure 36.2).

Beta blockers, particularly without intrinsic sympathomimetic activity and aimed at heart rate <60–65 bpm, improve ventricular relaxation, increase diastolic filling time, and should theoretically reduce susceptibility to ventricular arrhythmias. They are the mainstay of treatment for symptomatic improvement (Table 36.4).

L-type calcium channel blockers, such as **verapamil** (starting in low doses and titrating up to 480 mg/day) and **diltiazem**, are beneficial due to negative inotropic and chronotropic effects and improved diastolic function and are used instead of, or with, beta blockers. They may, however, exacerbate LVOT gradient due to vasodilation. They are particularly useful in the non-obstructive form.

Disopyramide, in combination with beta blockers, reduces LVOT gradient and improves symptoms by its negative inotropic action. Although it has not been considered proarrhythmic in HOCM,[27] concerns about the inherent proarrhythmia of Class IA agents cannot be ignored. Significant vagolytic side effects, such as dry mouth and prostatism, occur in 5% of patients.

Septal myectomy is considered for patients with significant LVOT gradients (≥50 mmHg, Table 36.5) or ≥30 mmHg at rest or ≥50 mmHg during exercise, and symptoms refractory to medical therapy (Table 36.5).[28] Operative mortality in experienced centres is <1.5%, and the risk of VSD is 1% and of complete heart block 6%.[28, 29] Mitral valve replacement has been used to manage HOCM in the unusual patient whose septal thickness is 16–18 mm, if a significant mid-cavity gradient is present, or if a significant gradient or substantial mitral regurgitation persists after adequate myectomy.[28]

Transcatheter septal ablation with alcohol infusion can be considered in symptomatic patients with accessible septal branch and septal thickness ≥15 mm, significant LVOT gradient (≥30 mmHg at rest or ≥50 mmHg on provocation), and in the absence of intrinsic abnormality of the mitral valve and of proximal left anterior descending coronary artery stenosis.[30–32] It has uncertain effectiveness with marked septal hypertrophy (>30 mm). Mortality is <3% and the risk of permanent pacemaker 10–30%, but it is reduced with contrast

Table 36.4 ACCF/AHA 2011 GL on HCM

Management of HCM	
Asymptomatic patients	
Co-morbidities (hypertension, diabetes, hyperlipidaemia, obesity) should be appropriately treated	I-C
Low-intensity aerobic exercise	IIa-C
Usefulness of beta blockade and calcium channel blockers not well established	IIb-C
Septal reduction therapy should not be performed for asymptomatic adult and paediatric patients with HCM with normal effort tolerance	III-C
In patients with resting or provocable outflow tract obstruction, pure vasodilators and high-dose diuretics are potentially harmful	III-C
Symptomatic patients	
Beta blockers in adults for symptoms, with caution in sinus bradycardia or severe conduction disease	I-B
If low doses ineffective, titrate to a resting heart rate <60–65 bpm	I-B
Verapamil (starting in low doses and titrating up to 480 mg/day) for symptoms. If no response or contraindication to beta blockers, with caution in high gradients, advanced heart failure, or sinus bradycardia	I-B
IV phenylephrine (or another pure vasoconstricting agent) for the treatment of acute hypotension in patients who do not respond to fluid administration	I-B
Disopyramide with a beta blocker or verapamil in patients who do not respond to beta blockers or verapamil alone	IIa-B
Diuretics in non-obstructive HCM when dyspnoea persists despite the use of beta blockers or verapamil or their combination	IIa-C
Beta blockers in children or adolescents monitored for depression, fatigue, or impaired scholastic performance	IIb-C
Diuretics in non-obstructive HCM when dyspnoea persists despite the use of beta blockers or verapamil or their combination	IIb-C
ACEI or ARB with resting or provocable LVOT obstruction	IIb-C
Diltiazem if verapamil is not tolerated	IIb-C
Nifedipine or other dihydropyridine calcium channel blockers	III-C
Verapamil in the setting of systemic hypotension or severe dyspnoea at rest	III-C
Digitalis in the absence of AF	III-B
Disopyramide alone without beta blockers or verapamil in AF	III-B
Dopamine, dobutamine, norepinephrine, and other IV inotropes for acute hypotension in patients with obstructive HCM	III-B

ACCF/AHA 2011 Guideline for the Diagnosis and Treatment of Hypertrophic Cardiomyopathy. *J Am Coll Cardiol*. 2011 13;**58**:e212–60.

echocardiography and slow ethanol injection.[32] There is always the theoretical risk of ventricular arrhythmias arising at the borders of the iatrogenic scar, although this has not been seen in clinical studies so far. Thus, this option is not recommended in young patients. However, in a recent non-randomized comparison at Mayo Clinic, long-term survival offered by septal ablation was favourable and similar to that of an age- and sex-matched general population and to patients undergoing surgical myectomy as well, without an increased risk of sudden cardiac death.[33] In patients with pre-existing risk factors for sudden death, an ICD should be implanted before septal ablation. Radiofrequency septal ablation is also under study.[34]

DDD pacing with a short AV delay has been shown to decrease LVOT gradient and symptoms in most, but not all, randomized comparisons.[35, 36] It may be useful in the elderly without short PR intervals (Table 36.6). It is recommended in medically refractory symptomatic patients with LVOT obstruction who are suboptimal candidates for septal reduction therapy.[2, 37]

Atrial fibrillation occurs in 20% of patients with HOCM (4-fold increase than in the general population).[16] AF can cause sudden, and sometimes severe, deterioration in symptoms and exercise capacity and is associated with a high risk of thromboembolism. Restoration of sinus rhythm usually results in a substantial improvement in symptoms, and amiodarone is effective in preventing recurrences.[38] Control of the ventricular rate with beta blockers, calcium antagonists, or both is almost as effective. Because of the potentially adverse effects of digoxin in patients with hypertrophic cardiomyopathy and normal

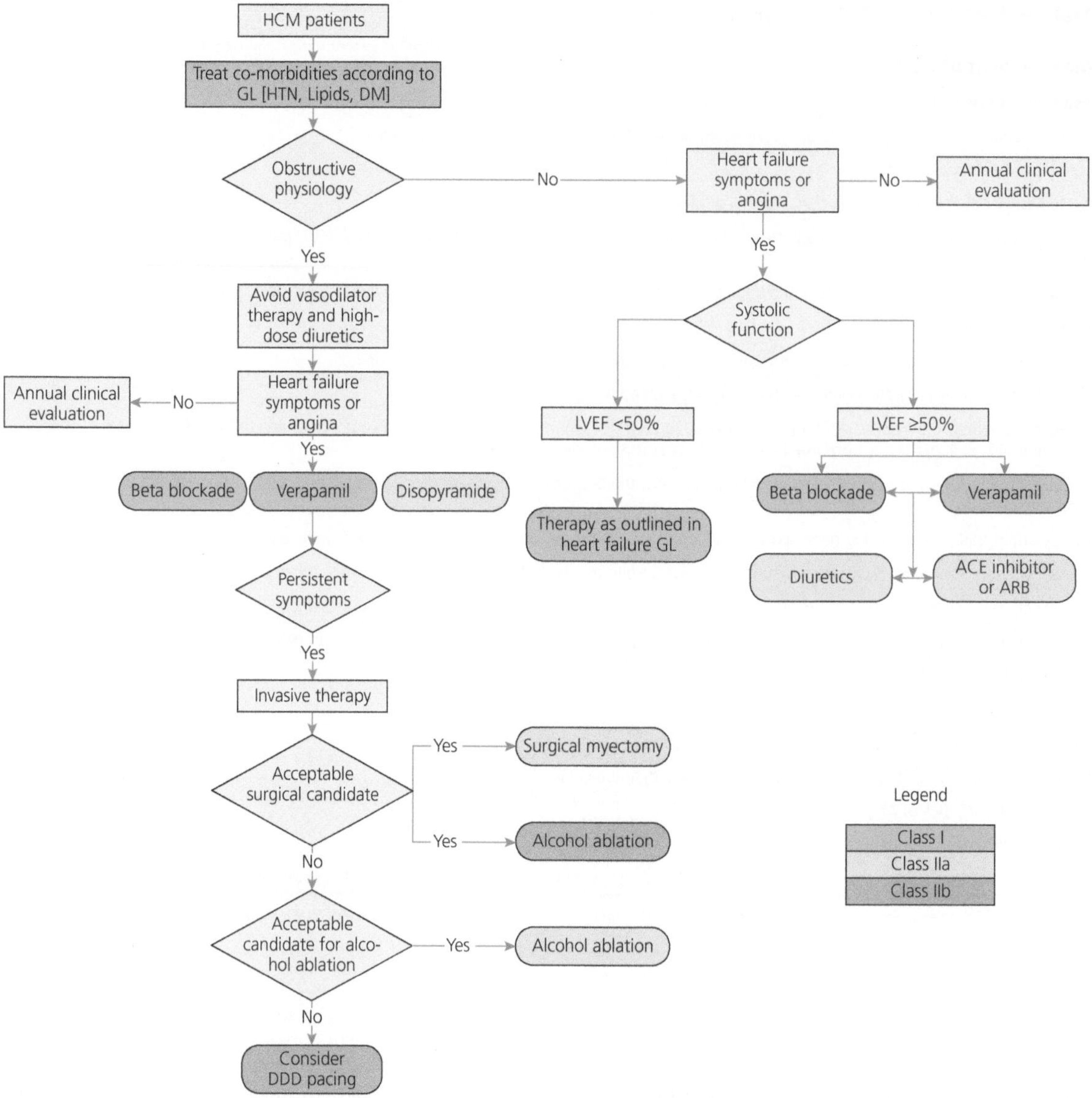

Figure 36.2 Treatment algorithm.
ACE indicates angiotensin-converting enzyme; ARB, angiotensin receptor blocker; DM, diabetes mellitus; EF, ejection fraction; GL, guidelines; HCM, hypertrophic cardiomyopathy; HTN, hypertension; LV, left ventricular.
ACCF/AHA 2011 Guideline for the Diagnosis and Treatment of Hypertrophic Cardiomyopathy. *J Am Coll Cardiol.* 2011;**58**:e212–60

systolic function, this drug is not routinely recommended for rate control. All patients with permanent or paroxysmal AF, in the context of an enlarged atrium, should be anticoagulated (Table 36.7, Figure 36.3). Catheter ablation may offer restoration of sinus rhythm and improvement of symptomatic status in up to 50% of patients.[39]

ICD HOCM is the most common cause of sudden death in young people (≤1% annually and predominantly in patients <25 years), including competitive athletes. Sudden death is paradoxically low in patients >60 years of age.[16] It is caused by fast VT or VF that are caused by reentry in the electrophysiological substrate of scarring and disarray. There is no evidence that bradyarrhythmias play a role.[24]

High risk factors are:

- Previous cardiac arrest (although most are lethal)
- Unexplained syncope
- Massive LV hypertrophy (≥30 mm)

Table 36.5 ACC/AHA 2011 GL on HCM

Invasive therapies	
Septal reduction therapy should be performed only by experienced operators* in the context of a comprehensive HCM clinical programme and only for the treatment of eligible patients with severe drug-refractory symptoms and LVOT obstruction.†	I-C
Consultation with centres experienced in performing both surgical septal myectomy and alcohol septal ablation.	IIa-C
Surgical septal myectomy at experienced centres is the first consideration for the majority of eligible patients with severe drug-refractory symptoms and LVOT obstruction.	IIa-B
Surgical septal myectomy at experienced centres in symptomatic children with severe resting obstruction (>50 mmHg)	IIa-C
Alcohol septal ablation at experienced centres when surgery is contraindicated or high-risk and NYHA III/IV.	IIa-B
Patient's preference for septal ablation with severe drug-refractory symptoms and LVOT obstruction.	IIb-B
Alcohol septal ablation in patients with HCM with marked (i.e. >30 mm) septal hypertrophy is discouraged.	IIb-C
Septal reduction for patients minimally or asymptomatic or controlled on optimal medical therapy.	III-C
Septal reduction therapy in inexperienced centres.	III-C
Mitral valve replacement for relief of LVOT obstruction in patients in whom septal reduction therapy is an option.	III-C
Alcohol septal ablation in patients in need of cardiac surgery (mitral or CABG).	III-C
Alcohol septal ablation in patients <21 years of age and in adults <40 years of age if myectomy is a viable option.	III-C

* Experienced operators are defined as an individual operator with a cumulative case volume of at least 20 procedures or an individual operator who is working in a dedicated HCM programme with a cumulative total of at least 50 procedures.

† Eligible patients are defined by all of the following: a. Clinical: severe dyspnoea or chest pain (usually NYHA functional classes III or IV) or occasionally other exertional symptoms (such as syncope or near syncope) that interfere with everyday activity or quality of life despite optimal medical therapy; b. Haemodynamic: dynamic LVOT gradient at rest or with physiological provocation 50 mmHg associated with septal hypertrophy and SAM of the mitral valve; c. Anatomical: targeted anterior septal thickness sufficient to perform the procedure safely and effectively in the judgement of the individual operator.

ACCF/AHA 2011 Guideline for the Diagnosis and Treatment of Hypertrophic Cardiomyopathy. *J Am Coll Cardiol*. 2011 13;**58**:e212–60.

Table 36.6 Pacing

ACCF/AHA 2011 GL on HCM	
In patients with a dual-chamber device implanted for non-HCM indications, consider a trial of dual-chamber atrial-ventricular pacing (from the right ventricular apex) for the relief of symptoms attributable to LVOT obstruction.	IIa-B
Permanent pacing in medically refractory symptomatic patients with obstructive HCM who are suboptimal candidates for septal reduction therapy.	IIb-B
Permanent pacemaker implantation for the purpose of reducing gradient in asymptomatic or medically controlled patients.	III-C
Permanent pacemaker implantation as a first-line therapy to relieve symptoms in medically refractory symptomatic patients with HCM and LVOT obstruction who are candidates for septal reduction.	III-B
ESC 2013 GL on Cardiac Pacing and CRT	
AV pacing with short AV interval in patients with resting or provocable LVOT obstruction and drug-refractory symptoms who:	
a) have contraindications for septal alcohol ablation or septal myectomy	IIb-B
b) or are at high risk of developing heart block following septal alcohol ablation or septal myectomy	IIb-C
In ICD indication, a dual-chamber ICD should be considered	IIa-C

ACCF/AHA 2011 Guideline for the Diagnosis and Treatment of Hypertrophic Cardiomyopathy. *J Am Coll Cardiol*. 2011 13; **58**:e212–60.
2013 ESC Guidelines on cardiac pacing and cardiac resynchronization therapy. *Eur Heart* J 2013. doi:10.1093/eurheartj/eht150

- Family history of HOCM-related sudden cardiac death
- Frequent and prolonged (>10 beats) episodes of non-sustained VT on Holter
- Hypotensive or attenuated blood pressure response to upright exercise.

Although no randomized studies exist in populations (as in **ischaemic** cardiomyopathy), there is a consensus that, in high-risk patients defined as those with a history of cardiac arrest or with ≥2 risk factors, ICD are lifesaving (Table 36.8, Figure 36.4). An exemption may be LAMP2 cardiomyopathy that is largely refractory to ICD therapy and has a poor prognosis.[40, 41] The presence of LV apical aneurysm, end-stage disease with widespread LV scarring, and delayed gadolinium enhancement in MRI are probably additional important risk factors. Sustained VT has a similar prognostic impact to SCD, although it is relatively uncommon in HCM and raises suspicion of a left ventricular apical aneurysm.[42] Three of the five principal risk predictors (NSVT, abnormal blood pressure response to exercise, and marked LV hypertrophy) have significantly

Table 36.7 ACCF/AHA 2011 GL on HCM

Management of AF	
Vitamin K antagonists (i.e. warfarin, to INR 2.0–3.0) in patients with paroxysmal, persistent, or chronic AF. Direct thrombin inhibitors (i.e dabigatran§) may represent another option, but data for patients with HCM are not available.	I-C
Ventricular rate control in patients with AF is for rapid ventricular rates. High doses of beta antagonists and non-dihydropyridine calcium channel blockers.	I-C
Disopyramide (with ventricular rate-controlling agents) and amiodarone for AF.	IIa-B
Radiofrequency ablation for AF in patients with refractory symptoms or inability to take antiarrhythmic drugs.	IIa-B
Maze procedure with closure of LA appendage in patients with a history of AF, either during septal myectomy or as an isolated procedure in selected patients.	IIa-C
Sotalol, dofetilide, and dronedarone as alternative antiarrhythmic agents in patients with HCM, especially in those with an ICD, but clinical experience is limited.	IIb-C

§ Dabigatran should not be used in patients with prosthetic valves, haemodynamically significant valve disease, advanced liver failure, or severe renal failure (creatinine clearance <15 mL/min).
ACCF/AHA 2011 Guideline for the Diagnosis and Treatment of Hypertrophic Cardiomyopathy. *J Am Coll Cardiol*. 2011;**58**:e212–60.

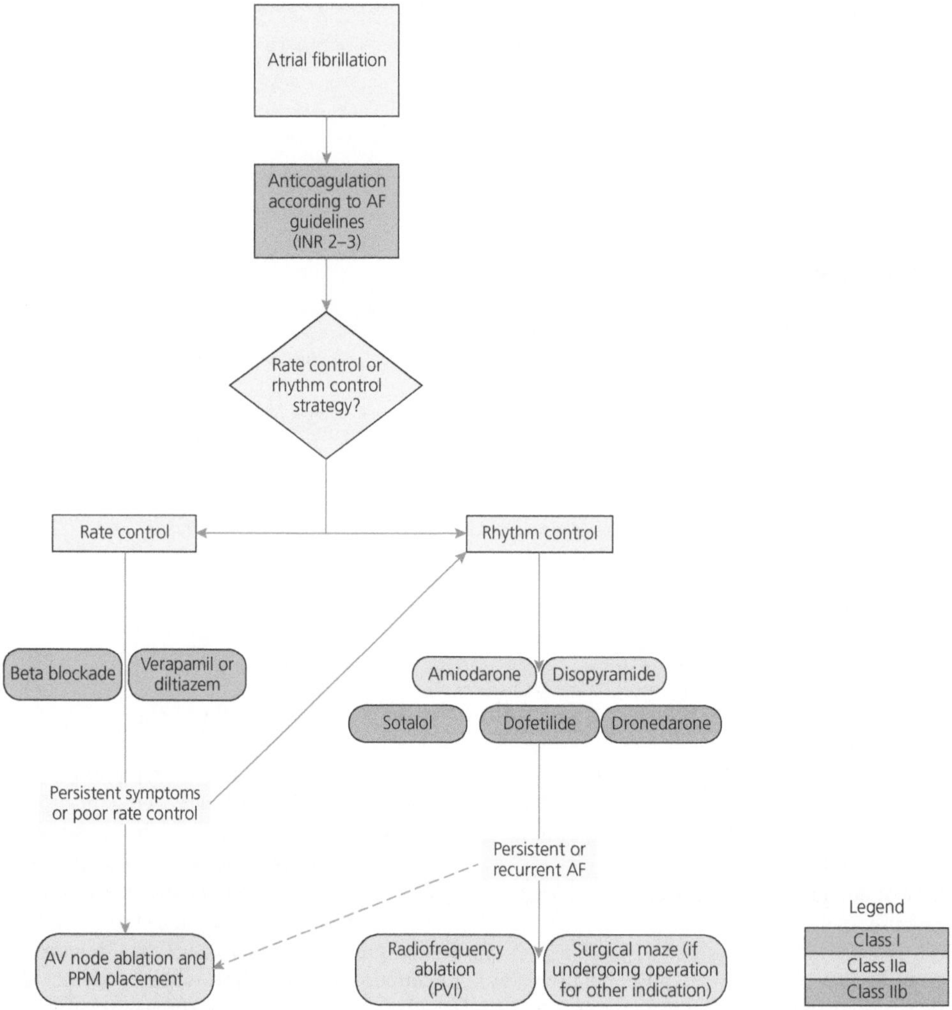

Figure 36.3 Management of AF in HCM.

AF indicates atrial fibrillation; AV, atrioventricular; INR, international normalized ratio; PPM, permanent pacemaker; and PVI, pulmonary vein isolation.
ACCF/AHA 2011 Guideline for the Diagnosis and Treatment of Hypertrophic Cardiomyopathy. *J Am Coll Cardiol*. 2011;**58**:e212–60

Table 36.8 ACC/AHA 2011 GL on HCM

Prevention of SCD	
SCD risk stratification	
Comprehensive SCD risk stratification at initial evaluation to determine the presence of the following:	I-B
a. A personal history for ventricular fibrillation, sustained VT, or SCD events, including appropriate ICD therapy for ventricular tachyarrhythmias.†	
b. A family history for SCD events, including appropriate ICD therapy for ventricular tachyarrhythmias.†	
c. Unexplained syncope.	
d. Documented NSVT (3 or more beats at ≥ 120 bpm on ambulatory (Holter) ECG.	
e. Maximal LV wall thickness ≥ 30 mm.	
Assessment of blood pressure response during exercise as part of SCD risk stratification.	IIa-B
SCD risk stratification on a periodic basis (every 12 to 24 months) for patients who have not undergone ICD implantation but would otherwise be eligible in the event that risk factors are identified (12 to 24 months).	IIa-C
Potential SCD risk in selected patients for whom risk remains borderline after documentation of conventional risk factors:	
a. CMR imaging with LGE.	IIb-C
b. Double and compound mutations (i.e. >1).	IIb-C
c. Marked LVOT obstruction.	IIb-B
Invasive electrophysiologic testing as routine SCD risk stratification.	III-C
Selection of patients for ICD*	
Application of individual clinical judgement and discussion of the strength of evidence, benefits, and risks to allow informed patient's active participation in decision-making.	I-C
ICD placement is recommended for patients with HCM with prior documented cardiac arrest, VF, or haemodynamically significant VT.	I-C
ICD for patients with:	IIa-C
a. Sudden death, presumably caused by HCM in one, or more, first-degree relatives.	
b. A maximum LV wall thickness ≥30 mm.	
c. One, or more, recent and unexplained syncopal episodes.	
Select patients with NSVT (particularly those <30 years of age) in the presence of other SCD risk factors or modifiers.	IIa-C
ICD in select patients with an abnormal blood pressure response with exercise in the presence of other SCD risk factors or modifiers.	IIa-C
ICD for high-risk children with HCM, based on unexplained syncope, massive LV hypertrophy, or family history of SCD, after taking into account the relatively high complication rate of long-term ICD implantation.	IIa-C
ICD in patients with isolated bursts of NSVT in the absence of any other SCD risk factors or modifiers.	IIb-C
ICD in patients with an abnormal blood pressure response with exercise in the absence of any other SCD risk factors or modifiers, particularly in the presence of significant outflow obstruction.	IIb-C
ICD as a routine strategy in patients with HCM without an indication of increased risk is potentially harmful.	III-C
ICD as a strategy to permit patients with HCM to participate in competitive athletics.	III-C
ICD in patients who have an identified HCM genotype in the absence of clinical manifestations of HCM.	III-C
Selection of ICD device type	
Single-chamber devices in younger patients without a need for atrial or ventricular pacing.	IIa-B
Dual-chamber ICDs for patients with sinus bradycardia and/or paroxysmal AF.	IIa-C
Dual-chamber ICDs for patients with elevated resting outflow gradients >50 mmHg and significant heart failure symptoms who may benefit from RV pacing (most commonly, but not limited to, patients >65 years of age).	IIa-B

* The ACCF/AHA/HRS 2012 GL on Device Therapy recommend ICD in patients with spontaneous VT/VF (I-A/B) and in patients with one or more risk factors (IIa-C).

† Appropriate ICD discharge is defined as ICD therapy triggered by VT or ventricular fibrillation, documented by stored intracardiac electrogram or cycle length data, in conjunction with the patient's symptoms immediately before and after device discharge.

ACCF/AHA 2011 Guideline for the Diagnosis and Treatment of Hypertrophic Cardiomyopathy. *J Am Coll Cardiol*. 2011;**58**:e212–60.

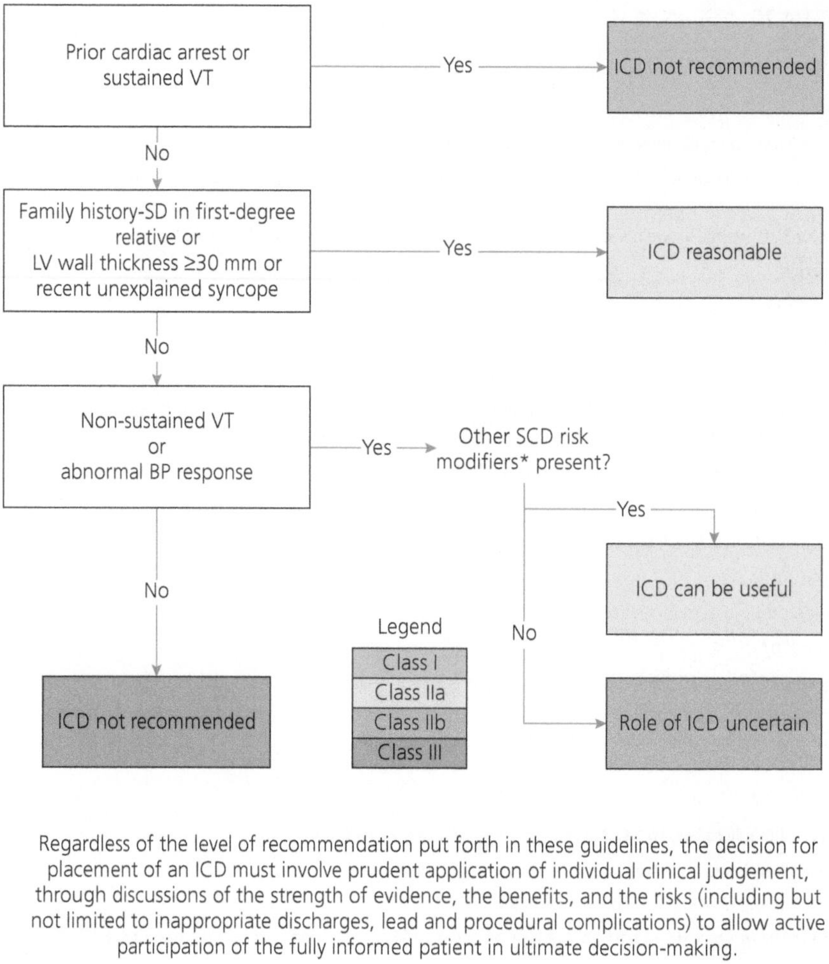

Figure 36.4 Indications for ICDs in HCM. *SCD risk modifiers include established risk factors and emerging risk modifiers. BP indicates blood pressure; ICD, implantable cardioverter-defibrillator; LV, left ventricular; SCD, sudden cardiac death; SD, sudden death; and VT, ventricular tachycardia.
ACCF/AHA 2011 Guideline for the Diagnosis and Treatment of Hypertrophic Cardiomyopathy. *J Am Coll Cardiol*. 2011;**58**:e212–60

higher predictive potential in young adult HCM patients than the >50 age group, and a family history of SCD is also considered less relevant with advancing years.[36] In patients >60 years of age, the risk of HOCM-related sudden death is very low.[14] Asymptomatic patients with none of these factors are at low risk (<0.5%/year), although risk factors are not identified in 3% of SCD victims.[24, 42] Results from a recent multicentre registry indicated that an important proportion of ICD discharges occurred in primary prevention patients who had undergone implantation for a single risk factor, except abnormal blood pressure response.[43] Potential complications of ICD therapy are pneumothorax, haematoma, lead revisions, and infection. The main concern, however, is inappropriate shocks that may occur in up to 36% of patients, with a rate of 5% per year.[44] Extreme LV hypertrophy is the most common risk factor in children and an ICD when indicated can be lifesaving. However, the complication rate (inappropriate shocks and lead malfunction) may be up to 3-fold higher that interventions for VT/VF.[45] **Amiodarone** is not considered a therapeutic option for prevention of sudden death in HOCM anymore.[2]

LV dysfunction and heart failure Recommendations are provided in Table 36.9. Heart transplantation is the last option for patients with irreversible heart failure due to systolic dysfunction.

Table 36.9 ACC/AHA 2011 on HCM

Patients with LV systolic dysfunction	
Patients with systolic dysfunction with EF ≤50% are treated as for adults with other forms of heart failure with reduced EF, including angiotensin-converting enzyme inhibitors, angiotensin receptor blockers, beta blockers, and other indicated drugs.	I-B
Other concomitant causes of systolic dysfunction (such as CAD) are considered as potential contributors to systolic dysfunction in patients with HCM.	I-C
ICD in adult patients with advanced (as defined by NYHA III or IV heart failure) non-obstructive HCM on maximal medical therapy and EF ≤50%, who do not otherwise have an indication for an ICD.	IIb-C
Reassess the use of negative inotropic agents (i.e. verapamil, diltiazem, or disopyramide), and consider discontinuing in patients who develop systolic dysfunction.	IIb-C
Selection of patients for heart transplantation	
Consideration for heart transplantation of patients with advanced heart failure (end-stage*) and non-obstructive HCM not otherwise amenable to other treatment/interventions, with EF ≤50% (or occasionally with preserved EF).	I-B
Consideration for heart transplantation of symptomatic children with HCM with restrictive physiology who are not responsive to, or appropriate candidates for, other therapeutic interventions.	I-C
Heart transplantation in mildly symptomatic patients of any age.	III-C

* Characterized by systolic dysfunction (EF ≤50%), often associated with LV remodelling, including cavity enlargement and wall thinning, and because of diffuse myocardial scarring.

ACCF/AHA 2011 Guideline for the Diagnosis and Treatment of Hypertrophic Cardiomyopathy. *J Am Coll Cardiol*. 2011;**58** (2):e212–60.

Experimental therapies ARBs, aldosterone antagonists, statin, and especially N-acetylcysteine have been shown in animal models to achieve reversal or prevention of hypertrophy and fibrosis in HOCM.[46] Pilot studies are being conducted.

Physical activity and sports

Patients are allowed to participate in low-intensity competitive sports (Class IIa-C, ACC/AHA 2011). Intensive competitive sports should be avoided, regardless of age, LVOT obstruction severity, or prior septal reduction intervention (Table 36.10). For sports classification, see also Chapter 81 on athlete's heart in Miscellaneous Topics.

Family counselling and genetic testing

Family counselling is essential when the diagnosis of HOCM is established (Table 36.11). Clinical assessment of all first-degree relatives (particularly those <25 years) is necessary. It is recommended that clinical screening should start between 10–12 years, and then repeated every 2 years until the age of 20 and every 5 years until the age of 60.[47] However, the majority of child carriers of sarcomere gene mutations and child relatives with unknown genetic status do not develop HOCM, at least within the next 12 years of follow-up.[5] Advances in DNA sequencing techniques (deep or massive parallel sequencing) have made genetic screening practical, with a diagnostic yield of 50–60% with familial HOCM but lower (30%) when sporadic disease is considered (see http://www.genetests.org). In familial HOCM, genetic screening of the clinically normal family members could lead to early identification of those with the causal mutation. Although genetic testing is a powerful tool for both diagnosis and future treatment options, it has several limitations. Application of genetic testing is relevant whenever one of the known causal genes is responsible for HOCM in the family. Pathognomonic mutations are not be identified in up to 50% of clinically affected probands.[4] In addition, not all genetic variants, including non-synonymous variants in sarcomeric genes, cause HOCM, and many could be benign variants. Therefore, identification of a non-synonymous variant in a known gene for HOCM in an individual alone is not sufficient to establish the causal role, and a specific mutation in isolation has no prognostic utility.[48] Recent data suggest that the penetrance of the disease is much less than previously thought, and the SCD event rate in predictively tested mutation-carrying relatives is lower than in probands.[49] Whether gene-positive, phenotype-negative individuals carry a higher risk of sudden death in is not known. Finally, the absence of a known mutation present in the family does not offer 100% security since there is possible presence of a second mutation and/or technical errors. Thus, the value of genetic screening is debatable.[50] Recommendations of HRS/EHRA are presented (Table 36.12). Genetic testing may also be useful when metabolic storage disorders with either a very bad prognosis (LAMP2 cardiomyopathy) or the possibility of therapy (Fabry's disease) are suspected.

Table 36.10 Physical activity and sports

ACC/AHA 2011 GL on HCM

Participation in competitive or recreational sports and physical activity

Low-intensity competitive sports (e.g. golf and bowling).	IIa-C
Recreational sporting activities.	IIa-C
Intense competitive sports, regardless of age, sex, race, presence or absence of LVOT obstruction, prior septal reduction therapy, or implantation of a cardioverter-defibrillator for high-risk status.	III-C

ACCF/AHA 2011 GL on HCM

Recommendations for the acceptability of recreational (non-competitive) sports activities and exercise in patients with HCM*

Intensity level	Eligibility scale for HCM†	Intensity level	Eligibility scale for HCM†
High		Modest hiking	4
Basketball (full court)	0	Motorcycling‡	3
Basketball (half court)	0	Jogging	3
Body building‡	1	Sailing§	3
Gymnastics	2	Surfing§	2
Ice hockey‡	0	Swimming (laps)§	5
Racquetball/squash	0	Tennis (doubles)	4
Rock climbing‡	1	Treadmill/stationary bicycle	5
Running (sprinting)	0	Weightlifting (free weights)‡$	1
Skiing (downhill)‡	2	Low	
Skiing (cross-country)	2	Bowling	5
Soccer	0	Brisk walking	5
Tennis (singles)	0	Golf	5
Touch (flag) football	1	Horseback riding‡	3
Windsurfing§	1	Scuba diving§	0
Moderate		Skating¶	5
Baseball/softball	2	Snorkelling§	5
Biking	4	Weights (non-free weights)	4
Hiking	3		

* Recreational sports are categorized according to high, moderate, and low levels of exercise and graded on a relative scale (from 0 to 5) for eligibility, with 0 to 1 indicating generally not advised or strongly discouraged; 4 to 5, probably permitted; and 2 to 3, intermediate and to be assessed clinically on an individual basis. The designations of high, moderate, and low levels of exercise are equivalent to an estimated >6, 4 to 6, and <4 metabolic equivalents, respectively.

† Assumes absence of laboratory DNA genotyping data, therefore, limited to clinical diagnosis.

‡ These sports involve the potential for traumatic injury, which should be taken into consideration for individuals with a risk for impaired consciousness.

§ The possibility of impaired consciousness occurring during water-related activities should be taken into account with respect to the individual patient's clinical profile.

$ Recommendations generally differ from those for weight-training machines (non-free weights), based largely on the potential risks of traumatic injury associated with episodes of impaired consciousness during bench-press manoeuvres; otherwise, the physiological effects of all weight-training activities are regarded as similar with respect to the present recommendations.

¶ Individual sporting activity not associated with the team sport of ice hockey.

ACCF/AHA 2011 Guideline for the Diagnosis and Treatment of Hypertrophic Cardiomyopathy. *J Am Coll Cardiol*. 2011;**58**:e212–60.

Table 36.11 ACCF/AHA 2011 GL on HCM. Proposed clinical screening strategies with echocardiography (and 12-lead ECG) for detection of hypertrophic cardiomyopathy with left ventricular hypertrophy in families*

Age <12 y
Optional unless:
Malignant family history of premature death from HCM or other adverse complications
Patient is a competitive athlete in an intense training programme
Onset of symptoms
Other clinical suspicion of early LV hypertrophy
Age 12 to 18–21 years†
Every 12–18 mo
Age >18–21 years
At onset of symptoms or at least every 5 years. More frequent intervals are appropriate in families with a malignant clinical course or late-onset HCM.

* When pathologic mutations are not identified or genetic testing is either ambiguous or not performed.
† Age range takes into consideration individual variability in achieving physical maturity and, in some patients, may justify screening at an earlier age.
Initial evaluation should occur no later than early pubescence.
ECG indicates electrocardiogram; HCM, hypertrophic cardiomyopathy; and LV, left ventricular.
ACCF/AHA 2011 Guideline for the Diagnosis and Treatment of Hypertrophic Cardiomyopathy. *J Am Coll Cardiol*. 2011;**58**:e212–60.

Table 36.12 Genetic screening

ACCF/AHA 20011 GL on HCM **Genetic testing strategies/family screening**	
Evaluation of familial inheritance and genetic counselling.	I-B
Patients who undergo genetic testing should also undergo counselling by someone knowledgeable in the genetics of cardiovascular disease so that results and their clinical significance can be appropriately reviewed with the patient.	I-B
Screening (clinical, with or without genetic testing) in first-degree relatives of patients with HCM.	I-B
Genetic testing for HCM and other genetic causes of unexplained cardiac hypertrophy is recommended in patients with an atypical clinical presentation of HCM or when another genetic condition is suspected to be the cause.	I-B
Genetic testing in the index patient to facilitate the identification of first-degree family members at risk for developing HCM.	IIa-B
The usefulness of genetic testing in the assessment of risk of SCD in HCM is uncertain.	IIb-B
Genetic testing in relatives when the index patient does not have a definitive pathogenic mutation.	III-B
Ongoing clinical screening in genotype-negative relatives in families with HCM.	III-B
Genotype-positive/phenotype-negative patients	
Serial ECG, TTE, and clinical assessment at periodic intervals (12 to 18 months in children and adolescents and about every 5 years in adults), based on the patient's age and change in clinical status, in individuals with pathogenic mutations who do not express the HCM phenotype.	I-B
HRS/EHRA 2011 statement on genetic testing for the channelopathies **State of genetic testing for hypertrophic cardiomyopathy**	
Comprehensive or targeted (MYBPC3, MYH7, TNNI3, TNNT2, TPM1)	I

HCM genetic testing for any patient in whom a cardiologist has established a clinical diagnosis of HCM based on examination of the patient's clinical history, family history, and electrocardiographic/echocardiographic phenotype.
Mutation-specific genetic testing for family members and appropriate relatives following the identification of the HCM-causative mutation in an index case.
ACCF/AHA 2011 Guideline for the Diagnosis and Treatment of Hypertrophic Cardiomyopathy. *J Am Coll Cardiol*. 2011;**58**:e212–60.
HRS/EHRA expert consensus statement on the state of genetic testing for the channelopathies and cardiomyopathies. *Heart Rhythm*. 2011;**8**:1308–39.

Table 36.13 ACC/AHA 2011 GL on HCM

Pregnancy/delivery	
In women who are asymptomatic or whose symptoms are controlled with beta-blocking drugs, the drugs should be continued during pregnancy, but increased surveillance for fetal bradycardia or other complications is warranted.	I-C
Genetic counselling before planned conception (for mother or father with HCM).	I-C
In women with HCM and resting or provocable LVOT obstruction ≥50 mmHg and/or cardiac symptoms not controlled by medical therapy alone, pregnancy is associated with increased risk, and these patients should be referred to a high-risk obstetrician.	I-C
The diagnosis of HCM among asymptomatic women is not considered a contraindication for pregnancy, but patients should be carefully evaluated in regard to the risk of pregnancy.	I-C
For women whose symptoms are controlled (mild to moderate), pregnancy is reasonable, but expert maternal/fetal medical specialist care, including cardiovascular and prenatal monitoring, is advised.	IIa-C
For women with advanced heart failure symptoms and HCM, pregnancy is associated with excess morbidity/mortality.	III-C

ACCF/AHA 2011 Guideline for the Diagnosis and Treatment of Hypertrophic Cardiomyopathy. *J Am Coll Cardiol.* 2011;**58**:e212–60.

The potential association of double, triple or compound sarcomere mutations (5% of patients with HOCM) with a higher risk is under study.[4]

Pregnancy

It is not contraindicated. Serious complications are rare (1–2%); caution is needed in patients with significant gradient when administering epidural anaesthesia that induces peripheral vasodilation (Table 36.13).[51, 52] See also Table 35.3.

References

1. Maron BJ, *et al.* American College of Cardiology/European Society of Cardiology Clinical Expert Consensus Document on hypertrophic cardiomyopathy. A report of the American College of Cardiology Foundation Task Force on Clinical Expert Consensus Documents and the European Society of Cardiology Committee for Practice Guidelines. *J Am Coll Cardiol.* 2003;**42**:1687–713
2. Gersh BJ, *et al.* 2011 ACCF/AHA guideline for the diagnosis and treatment of hypertrophic cardiomyopathy: a report of the American College of Cardiology Foundation/American Heart Association Task Force on Practice Guidelines. Developed in collaboration with the American Association for Thoracic Surgery, American Society of Echocardiography, American Society of Nuclear Cardiology, Heart Failure Society of America, Heart Rhythm Society, Society for Cardiovascular Angiography and Interventions, and Society of Thoracic Surgeons. *J Am Coll Cardiol.* 2011;**58**:e212–60
3. Maron BJ, *et al.* Novel hypertrophic cardiomyopathy phenotype: segmental hypertrophy isolated to the posterobasal left ventricular free wall. *Am J Cardiol.* 2010;**106**:750–2
4. Maron BJ, Maron MS. Hypertrophic cardiomyopathy. *Lancet.* 2013;**381**:242–55
5. Jensen MK, *et al.* Penetrance of hypertrophic cardiomyopathy in children and adolescents: a 12-year follow-up study of clinical screening and predictive genetic testing. *Circulation.* 2013;**127**:48–54
6. Ackerman MJ, *et al.* HRS/EHRA expert consensus statement on the state of genetic testing for the channelopathies and cardiomyopathies this document was developed as a partnership between the Heart Rhythm Society (HRS) and the European Heart Rhythm Association (EHRA). *Heart Rhythm.* 2011;**8**:1308–39
7. Marian AJ. Hypertrophic cardiomyopathy: from genetics to treatment. *Eur J Clin Invest.* 2010;**40**:360–9
8. Elliott P, *et al.* Hypertrophic cardiomyopathy. *Lancet.* 2004;**363**:1881–91
9. Weidemann F, *et al.* The heart in Friedreich ataxia: definition of cardiomyopathy, disease severity, and correlation with neurological symptoms. *Circulation.* 2012;**125**:1626–34
10. Bates MG, *et al.* Cardiac involvement in mitochondrial DNA disease: clinical spectrum, diagnosis, and management. *Eur Heart J.* 2012;**33**:3023–33
11. Varnava AM, *et al.* Hypertrophic cardiomyopathy: the interrelation of disarray, fibrosis, and small vessel disease. *Heart.* 2000;**84**:476–82
12. Maron MS, *et al.* Mitral valve abnormalities identified by cardiovascular magnetic resonance represent a primary phenotypic expression of hypertrophic cardiomyopathy. *Circulation.* 2011;**124**:40–7
13. Harris KM, *et al.* Prevalence, clinical profile, and significance of left ventricular remodeling in the end-stage phase of hypertrophic cardiomyopathy. *Circulation.* 2006;**114**:216–25
14. Maron BJ, *et al.* Risk stratification and outcome of patients with hypertrophic cardiomyopathy ≥60 years of age. *Circulation.* 2013;**127**:585–93
15. Johnson JN, *et al.* Prevalence and clinical correlates of QT prolongation in patients with hypertrophic cardiomyopathy. *Eur Heart J.* 2011;**32**:1114–20
16. Maron BJ, *et al.* Evolution of hypertrophic cardiomyopathy to a contemporary treatable disease. *Circulation.* 2012;**126**:1640–4
17. Nagueh SF, *et al.* Tissue Doppler imaging predicts the development of hypertrophic cardiomyopathy in subjects with subclinical disease. *Circulation.* 2003;**108**:395–8

18. Gekke JB, *et al.* B-type natriuretic peptide and survival in hypertrophic cardiomyopathy. *J Am Coll Cardiol.* 2013 April 16; [Epub ahead of print]
19. O'Hanlon R, *et al.* Prognostic significance of myocardial fibrosis in hypertrophic cardiomyopathy. *J Am Coll Cardiol.* 2010;**56**:867–74
20. Basso C, *et al.* Myocardial bridging, a frequent component of the hypertrophic cardiomyopathy phenotype, lacks systematic association with sudden cardiac death. *Eur Heart J.* 2009;**30**:1627–34
21. Gupta RM, *et al.* Still a kid at heart: hypertrophic cardiomyopathy in the elderly. *Circulation.* 2011;**124**:857–63
22. Rapezzi C, *et al.* Disease profile and differential diagnosis of hereditary transthyretin-related amyloidosis with exclusively cardiac phenotype: An Italian perspective. *Eur Heart J.* 2013;**34**:520–8
23. Maron BJ. Distinguishing hypertrophic cardiomyopathy from athlete's heart physiological remodelling: clinical significance, diagnostic strategies and implications for preparticipation screening. *Br J Sports Med.* 2009;**43**:649–56
24. Maron BJ. Contemporary insights and strategies for risk stratification and prevention of sudden death in hypertrophic cardiomyopathy. *Circulation.* 2010;**121**:445–56
25. Pelliccia A, *et al.* The upper limit of physiologic cardiac hypertrophy in highly trained elite athletes. *N Engl J Med.* 1991;**324**:295–301
26. Yousef Z, *et al.* Left ventricular hypertrophy in fabry disease: A practical approach to diagnosis. *Eur Heart J.* 2013;**34**:802–8
27. Sherrid MV, *et al.* Multicenter study of the efficacy and safety of disopyramide in obstructive hypertrophic cardiomyopathy. *J Am Coll Cardiol.* 2005;**45**:1251–8
28. Fifer MA, *et al.* Management of symptoms in hypertrophic cardiomyopathy. *Circulation.* 2008;**117**:429–39
29. Woo A, *et al.* Clinical and echocardiographic determinants of long-term survival after surgical myectomy in obstructive hypertrophic cardiomyopathy. *Circulation.* 2005;**111**:2033–41
30. Ball W, *et al.* Long-term survival in patients with resting obstructive hypertrophic cardiomyopathy comparison of conservative versus invasive treatment. *J Am Coll Cardiol.* 2011;**58**:2313–21
31. Nagueh SF, *et al.* Alcohol septal ablation for the treatment of hypertrophic obstructive cardiomyopathy. a multicenter North American registry. *J Am Coll Cardiol.* 2011;**58**:2322–28
32. Nagueh SF, *et al.* Comparison of ethanol septal reduction therapy with surgical myectomy for the treatment of hypertrophic obstructive cardiomyopathy. *J Am Coll Cardiol.* 2001;**38**:1701–06
33. Sorajja P, *et al.* Survival after alcohol septal ablation for obstructive hypertrophic cardiomyopathy. *Circulation.* 2012;**126**:2374–80
34. Lawrenz T, *et al.* Endocardial radiofrequency ablation for hypertrophic obstructive cardiomyopathy: acute results and 6 months' follow-up in 19 patients. *J Am Coll Cardiol.* 2011;**57**:572–6
35. Gadler F, *et al.* Significant improvement of quality of life following atrioventricular synchronous pacing in patients with hypertrophic obstructive cardiomyopathy. Data from 1 year of follow-up. PIC Study Group. Pacing in cardiomyopathy. *Eur Heart J.* 1999;**20**:1044–50
36. Maron BJ, *et al.* Assessment of permanent dual-chamber pacing as a treatment for drug-refractory symptomatic patients with obstructive hypertrophic cardiomyopathy. A randomized, double-blind, crossover study (M-PATHY). *Circulation.* 1999;**99**:2927–33
37. Brignole M, *et al.* 2013 ESC Guidelines on cardiac pacing and cardiac resynchronization therapy. *Eur Heart J* 2013. doi:10.1093/eurheartj/eht150
38. Robinson K, *et al.* Atrial fibrillation in hypertrophic cardiomyopathy: a longitudinal study. *J Am Coll Cardiol.* 1990;**15**:1279–85
39. Di Donna P, *et al.* Efficacy of catheter ablation for atrial fibrillation in hypertrophic cardiomyopathy: impact of age, atrial remodelling, and disease progression. *Europace.* 2010;**12**:347–55
40. Ho CY. Hypertrophic cardiomyopathy in 2012. *Circulation.* 2012;**125**:1432–8
41. Maron BJ, *et al.* Clinical outcome and phenotypic expression in LAMP2 cardiomyopathy. *JAMA.* 2009;**301**:1253–59
42. Sen-Chowdhry S, *et al.* Sudden death from genetic and acquired cardiomyopathies. *Circulation.* 2012;**125**:1563–76
43. Maron BJ, *et al.* Implantable cardioverter-defibrillators and prevention of sudden cardiac death in hypertrophic cardiomyopathy. *JAMA.* 2007;**298**:405–12
44. Lin G, *et al.* Device complications and inappropriate implantable cardioverter defibrillator shocks in patients with hypertrophic cardiomyopathy. *Heart.* 2009;**95**:709–14
45. Maron BJ, *et al.* Prevention of sudden cardiac death with implantable cardioverter-defibrillators in children and adolescents with hypertrophic cardiomyopathy. *J Am Coll Cardiol.* 2013;**61**: doi: 10.1016/j.jacc.2013.1001.1037
46. Marian AJ. Experimental therapies in hypertrophic cardiomyopathy. *J Cardiovasc Transl Res.* 2009;**2**:483–92
47. Charron P, *et al.* Genetic counselling and testing in cardiomyopathies: a position statement of the European Society of Cardiology Working Group on myocardial and pericardial diseases. *Eur Heart J.* 2010;**31**:2715–26
48. Landstrom AP, *et al.* Mutation type is not clinically useful in predicting prognosis in hypertrophic cardiomyopathy. *Circulation.* 2010;**122**:2441–9; discussion 2450
49. Christiaans I, *et al.* Manifest disease, risk factors for sudden cardiac death, and cardiac events in a large nationwide cohort of predictively tested hypertrophic cardiomyopathy mutation carriers: determining the best cardiological screening strategy. *Eur Heart J.* 2011;**32**:1161–70
50. Jacoby D, *et al.* Genetics of inherited cardiomyopathy. *Eur Heart J.* 2012;**33**:296–304
51. Regitz-Zagrosek V, *et al.* ESC guidelines on the management of cardiovascular diseases during pregnancy: the Task Force on the management of cardiovascular diseases during pregnancy of the European Society of Cardiology (ESC). *Eur Heart J.* 2011;**32**:3147–97
52. Stergiopoulos K, *et al.* Pregnancy in patients with pre-existing cardiomyopathies. *J Am Coll Cardiol.* 2011;**58**:337–50

Chapter 37

Restrictive cardiomyopathy

Definition

Restrictive cardiomyopathy (RCM) is defined as heart muscle disease that results in impaired ventricular filling, with normal or decreased diastolic volume of either or both ventricles. Systolic function usually remains normal, at least early in the disease, and wall thickness may be normal or increased, depending on the underlying cause.[1, 2] Restrictive cardiomyopathies are the least common of the cardiomyopathic disorders.

Pathophysiology

In typical RCM, systolic function is less affected than diastolic function, and usually there is an abnormality of filling rather than of relaxation. Thus, in most cases, there is rapid completion of filling of a poorly compliant ventricle in early diastole (E wave), with little or no further filling in late diastole (A wave). Though there is poor compliance of the ventricles, the peak filling rate is higher than normal, possibly as a result of augmented ventricular diastolic suction. The situation is thus analogous to pericardial disease causing constriction or tamponade. Usually, patients with restrictive cardiomyopathy have normal ventricular volumes but raised filling pressures. In both constriction and restriction, there is characteristically rapid completion of ventricular filling in early diastole so that the ventricular diastolic waveform has a dip and plateau (square root sign) configuration, but this is not always present.[2] Since the condition affects either or both ventricles, it may cause symptoms and signs of right or left ventricular failure. Infiltrative cardiac diseases may also produce hypertrophic or dilated cardiomyopathy patterns. Some of them increase ventricular wall thickness without actual myocyte hypertrophy and, occasionally, even produce dynamic left ventricular outflow obstruction (as may happen in amyloidosis) while others cause chamber enlargement with secondary wall thinning and global or regional wall motion abnormalities (as may happen in sarcoidosis).[3]

Aetiology

Conditions associated with restrictive cardiomyopathy are presented in Table 37.1. Infiltrative cardiomyopathies are characterized by the deposition of abnormal substances that cause the ventricular walls to become progressively rigid, thereby impeding ventricular filling.

Amyloidosis is the most common cause in the western world and, apart from diastolic, may also cause systolic ventricular abnormalities. Cardiac involvement is more common in **primary amyloidosis**, which is caused by the production of immunoglobulin light chains (AL) by plasma cells, often in the context of multiple myeloma.[1] Restrictive cardiomyopathy results from replacement of normal myocardial contractile elements by infiltrative interstitial deposits that begins in the subendocardium and extends in the myocardium. Survival is poor in the presence of cardiac involvement and heart failure symptoms <1 year after diagnosis. **Secondary amyloidosis** is caused by the deposition of a non-immunoglobulin protein (AA) and can be **hereditary**, **senile**, or due to a **chronic inflammatory process.**[4, 5] **Hereditary** transtyretin-related amyloidosis (ATTR) is due to amyloid derived from a mutation (usually V30M) in the gene encoding for the hepatically produced protein transthyretin. It can occur with or without peripheral neuropathy. It is autosomal dominant but sporadic mutations may also occur thus making a negative family history not a useful screening method. **Senile systemic amyloidosis** (SSA) is probably due to age-related thransthyretin misaggregation. Development of cardiomyopathy is less common with secondary amyloidosis and prognosis much better. Symmetric LV hypertrophy, thickened valves, and moderately depressed LV function in males >65 years old suggest ATTR or SSA rather than HCM.[6] Amyloid infiltration of the heart is common in the elderly.

Sarcoidosis affects the basal septum, atrioventricular node and His bundle, focal regions in the ventricular free walls, and the papillary muscles. Two-dimensional echocardiographic characteristics of cardiac sarcoid vary according to disease activity, and include wall thickening (>13 mm) due to granulomatous expansion and wall thinning (<7 mm) due to fibrosis. With scar retraction, aneurysms may develop, especially if the patient has been treated with corticosteroids. Cardiac involvement is clinically apparent in only 5% of patients with systemic sarcoidosis, but, on autopsy, the prevalence of cardiac disease of approximately 25%.[7]

Fabry's disease is an X-linked autosomal recessive disease that results from the progressive accumulation of glycosphingolipids due to lysosomal alpha-galactosidase A deficiency. Affected patients have microvascular disease of the kidneys, heart, and brain. Cardiac involvement is not manifested until the third or fourth decade of life and may mimic hypertrophic cardiomyopathy.

Primary (idiopathic) restrictive cardiomyopathy is expressed morphologically as myocyte hypertrophy and

Table 37.1 Types of restrictive cardiomyopathy

Myocardial
Noninfiltrative
Idiopathic cardiomyopathy
Familial cardiomyopathy (sarcomeric or other mutations)
Scleroderma
Pseudoxanthoma elasticum
Diabetic cardiomyopathy
Infiltrative
Amyloidosis
Sarcoidosis
Gaucher's disease
Mucopolysacharidoses (Hurler–Scheie syndrome)
Fatty infiltration
Storage diseases
Iron overload cardiomyopathy (primary haemochromatosis, beta thalassaemia, and other anaemias)
Fabry's disease
Glycogen storage disease
Myocardial oxalosis (primary hyperoxaluria)
Endomyocardial
Endomyocardial fibrosis
Radiation
Cardiotoxicity of anthracyclines
Hypereosinophilic syndrome
Carcinoid heart disease
Metastatic cancers
Drugs causing fibrous endocarditis (serotonin, methysergide, ergotamine, mercurial agents, busulfan)

Underlined are the most common conditions.
Kushwaha et al. Restrictive cardiomyopathy. *NEJM* 1997; **336**:267–276.

interstitial fibrosis.[8] It can be familial, with dominant inheritance and incomplete penetrance, and associated with skeletal myopathy and complete heart block.

Sarcomeric mutations There is now clinical and genetic evidence demonstrating that restrictive cardiomyopathy is part of the spectrum of sarcomeric disease and frequently coexists with hypertrophic cardiomyopathy in affected families.[9] To date, mutations have been identified in the cardiac genes for the sarcomeric proteins a-actin, troponin I and troponin T as well as for desmin (a cytosolic protein) (Figure 35.1 of Chapter 35 on DCM, Table 37.2).

Endomyocardial fibrosis and **Löffler's endocarditis** (eosinophilic cardiomyopathy) are the main causes of

Table 37.2 Genetic causes of restrictive cardiomyopathy

Gene	Protein	Location and function
Autosomal		
MYH7 (5% of patients)	Beta-myosin heavy chain	Sarcomere
TNNI3 (5% of patients)	Cardiac troponin I	Sarcomere
DES	Desmin	Cytoskeleton, dystrophin-associated
TNNT2	Cardiac troponin T	Sarcomere
ACTC	Cardiac actin	Sarcomere

obliterative cardiomyopathy. They are both associated with eosinophilia (>1.5 x 10^9/L for, at least, 6 months) that is either primary (Loffler's) or secondary due to parasitic infections, lymphomas, or vasculitis. [1,2] The intracytoplasmic granular content of activated eosinophils is responsible for the toxic damage to the heart, with initial myocarditis and arteritis that are followed by a thrombotic stage and eventually formation of extensive fibrosis that promotes further thrombotic material formation. Endomyocardial fibrosis is endemic in equatorial Africa, South America, and Asia.

Anthracyclines can cause dilated cardiomyopathy or endomyocardial fibrosis. Diastolic dysfunction may persist, even years, after therapy with anthracyclines. The risk is greatly increased when there is a history of **irradiation** that causes myocardial and endocardial fibrosis, particularly in the right ventricle.[1]

Carcinoid heart disease occurs as a late complication of the carcinoid syndrome in up to half of cases, with tricuspid regurgitation as the predominant lesion.[1] The development of cardiac lesions is correlated with circulating levels of serotonin and its principal metabolite 5-hydroxyindoleacetic acid. The pathological lesion consists of fibrous plaques involving the tricuspid and pulmonary valves and the right ventricular endocardium.

Chloroquine and **hydroxychloroquine** in large cumulative doses (kg) may cause skeletal myopathy and restrictive cardiomyopathy.[10]

Presentation

The diagnosis of restrictive cardiomyopathy should be considered in a patient presenting with **heart failure but no evidence of cardiomegaly or systolic dysfunction**. Usually, patients present with **fatigue** and **dyspnoea**. Angina does not occur, except in amyloidosis in which it may be the presenting symptom.[2] Patients may also present with thromboembolic complications. Cardiac conduction disturbances and AF are particularly common in idiopathic restrictive cardiomyopathy and amyloidosis. Heart block and ventricular arrhythmias are also common in cardiac sarcoidosis.

Physical examination

- **JVP** is elevated. A rapid 'x' descent and especially a prominent 'y' descent may be present in sinus rhythm.
- **Kussmaul's sign**, i.e. a rise or failure of JVP to decrease with inspiration, may be present but typically occurs in constrictive pericarditis.
- S_3 of LV or RV origin may be present.
- **Peripheral oedema** or **ascites** and **enlarged and pulsatile liver** may be seen in progressed disease.

In advanced cases, all typical signs of heart failure are present, except cardiomegaly, although dilated ventricles may develop at later stages, particularly in patients with amyloidosis or sarcoidosis.

Investigations

Chest X-ray reveals a normal cardiac size with possible atrial enlargement. Pulmonary congestion and pleural effusions may be present.

ECG shows non-specific ST-T changes with or without conduction abnormalities. The absence of increased voltage on ECG, despite the appearance of echocardiographic hypertrophy, can be the first clue to certain infiltrative diseases, such as cardiac amyloid or Friedreich's ataxia. Low voltage and prolonged PR interval and a pseudoinfarction pattern in the inferoseptal wall are typical signs of advanced amyloidosis. A decrease in QRS complex amplitude occurs because of myocyte atrophy, along with decreased conduction velocity and dyssynchronous activation resulting from amyloid deposition. However, infiltrative cardiomyopathies associated with increased size of cardiac myocytes may have increased voltage (e.g. Fabry's disease).[3]

Two-dimensional echocardiography Ventricles are small, with normal or increased wall thickness, and the atria are usually dilated. Valvular regurgitation and atrial enlargement are more common in RCM than in constrictive pericarditis.

In **amyloidosis**, the ventricular walls are thickened, and pericardial effusion may coexist. In advanced cardiac amyloidosis, the typical ground glass (granular or sparkling) appearance of the myocardium as well as pericardial effusion may be seen.[11]

Two-dimensional echocardiography is diagnostic in the **hypereosinophilic syndrome**, revealing the typical packing of both ventricular apices due to thrombus and usually significant MR.

Akinetic segments interspersed with normokinetic segments, resulting in an uneven wall motion abnormality, may be seen in **sarcoidosis.**

Doppler echocardiography The pattern of mitral inflow velocity reveals increased early diastolic filling velocity (E wave ≥1 m/s), decreased late filling velocity (A wave ≤0.5 m/s), increased E/A ratio (≥2), decreased deceleration time (≤150 ms), and decreased isovolumic relaxation time (≤70 ms). Pulmonary or hepatic vein patterns show that systolic forward flow is less than diastolic forward flow, with increased reversal of diastolic flow after atrial contraction during inspiration.

In patients with amyloidosis, Doppler variables of shortened deceleration time and increased early diastolic filling velocity to atrial filling velocity ratio are stronger predictors of cardiac death than were the two-dimensional echocardiographic variables of mean left ventricular wall thickness and fractional shortening.[12] New modalities, such as **strain rate** and **speckle tracking**, may be useful in diagnosing early amyloid infiltration.[11]

Cardiac catheterization The characteristic haemodynamic feature is a deep and rapid early decline in ventricular pressure at the onset of diastole, with a rapid rise to a plateau in early diastole. This is manifested as a prominent y descent, followed by a rapid rise to a plateau, i.e. the dip and plateau or square root sign. However, filling and the ventricular diastolic waveform are affected by heart rate, degree of hydration, and stage in the disease process so that, in some individuals, filling is more gradual. The right atrial pressure is elevated, and the wave form is M- or W-shaped, as in constrictive pericarditis. Usually, respiratory variation of venous pressure is absent, but the y descent may become deeper during inspiration.

Cardiac magnetic resonance has a higher resolution than echocardiography and detects the presence of myocardial fibrosis.[13] It is particularly useful in the diagnosis of infiltrative diseases, such as sarcoidosis, radiation-induced fibrosis, iron-loaded cardiomyopathy, amyloidosis, and constrictive pericarditis. **PET imaging** is also useful in this respect.[5]

Cardiac biopsy may be required for distinguishing restrictive cardiomyopathy types from constrictive pericarditis. A specific condition, such as amyloidosis, iron storage disease, Fabry's disease, sarcoidosis, or glycogen storage disease, may be diagnosed. However, non-specific histological features, such as interstitial fibrosis and myocyte hypertrophy, are common, and patchy infiltration, as typically occurs in sarcoidosis, may obscure the diagnosis. Amyloidosis cannot be excluded purely on the basis of light microscopy. Electron microscopy of myocardial tissue can confirm the diagnosis when light microscopy is negative, though care should be taken to distinguish between recently formed perimyocyte collagen and amyloid. The presence or absence of amyloid deposits in other organs is not absolutely predictive of cardiac involvement.

Recommendations for genetic testing are presented in Table 37.3.[14]

Differential diagnosis

Restrictive haemodynamic characteristics may also be seen in cases of dilated or hypertrophic cardiomyopathy. However, the main problem is the distinction of RCM from constrictive pericarditis. Differences are summarized in Table 37.4, but no test is absolutely diagnostic. The two conditions may also coexist, as happens in the cases of radiation fibrosis.[2]

In the elderly, restrictive cardiomyopathy should be differentiated from age-related changes in diastolic

Table 37.3 HRS/EHRA 2011 statement on genetic testing for the channelopathies

State of genetic testing for restrictive cardiomyopathy	
Mutation-specific genetic testing for family members and appropriate relatives following the identification of an RCM causative mutation in the index case.	I
Patients in whom a cardiologist has established a clinical index of suspicion for RCM based on examination of the patient's clinical history, family history, and electrocardiographic/echocardiographic phenotype.	IIb

HRS/EHRA 2011 expert consensus statement on the state of genetic testing for the channelopathies and cardiomyopathies. *Heart Rhythm*. 2011;**8**:1308–39.

Table 37.4 Differential diagnosis of restrictive cardiomyopathy and constrictive pericarditis

	Restrictive cardiomyopathy	Constrictive pericarditis
Physical examination	Kussmaul's sign may be present	Kussmaul's sign usually present
	Apical impulse may be prominent	Apical impulse usually not palpable
	S_3 may be present, rarely S_4	Pericardial knock may be present
	Regurgitant murmurs more common	Regurgitant murmurs uncommon
Electrocardiography	Low voltage (especially in amyloidosis), pseudoinfarction, left axis deviation, atrial fibrillation, and conduction disturbances common. Low voltage (<50%)	
Echocardiography	Increased wall thickness	Normal wall thickness (especially thickened interatrial septum in amyloidosis)
Pericardial thickening may be seen	Thickened cardiac valves (amyloidosis)	Prominent early diastolic filling with abrupt displacement of interventricular septum Granular sparkling texture (amyloid)
Atrial dilation and MR/TR common	Atrial dilation, MR/TR uncommon Decreased systolic RV and LV velocities with inspiration	Increased RV velocity and decreased LV velocity with inspiration
	Inspiratory augmentation of hepatic vein diastolic flow	Expiratory augmentation of hepatic vein diastolic flow reversal Reversal
E is diminished with expiration (cut-off value of 7 cm/s)	Preserved or increased early diastolic filling (E)	
Velocity of propagation of early ventricular inflow	Velocity of propagation of early ventricular inflow and early mitral annular velocity reduced and early mitral annular velocity normal	
Cardiac catheterization	LVEDP often <5 mmHg greater than RVEDP, but RVEDP >1/3 of RV systolic pressure Concordant pressure change between LV and RV	RVEDP and LVEDP usually equal, maybe identical RV systolic pressure <50 mm Hg
		Discordant pressure change between LV and RV during inspiration and expiration
Endomyocardial biopsy	May reveal specific cause of restrictive cardiomyopathy	May be normal or show non-specific myocyte hypertrophy or myocardial fibrosis
CT/MRI	Pericardium usually normal	Pericardium may be thickened May reveal significant myocardial fibrosis

Modified from Kushwaha *et al*. *NEJM* 1997; **336**:267–276, and Talreja *et al*. *JACC* 2008;**51**:315–9

Table 37.5 Differential diagnosis of cardiac amyloidosis, HOCM, and hypertensive heart disease

	Amyloidosis	Hypertensive heart disease	Hypertrophic cardiomyopathy
Distribution of LV thickening	Global	Global	Usually regional
LV cavity size	Normal to small	Normal; may dilate in end stage	Normal; may dilate in end stage
Ejection fraction	Low normal or mildly ↓	Ranges from hyperdynamic to low	Often hyperdynamic
RV thickness	Often ↑	Normal	Rarely ↑
Myocardial echogenicity	Often ↑	Normal	Normal
Longitudinal strain/tissue Doppler velocity	Severely ↓	Mildly to moderately ↓	Regionally ↓
Valve abnormalities	May be uniformly thickened	No specific abnormality	Mitral regurgitation if systolic anterior motion
	Mitral regurgitation rarely more than mild		
Diastolic function	Often restrictive (grade 3 or 4)	Grade 1 or 2 most common	No specific common pattern
ECG voltage	Frequently low in limb leads	LVH	LVH
Blood pressure	Normal to low; rarely elevated	High	Normal
Cardiac MRI	Frequent, widespread delayed gadolinium enhancement, including RV and atria	Mild or no late enhancement	Varying, often mild, late enhancement, usually localized to LV

LV indicates left ventricular; RV, right ventricular; MRI, magnetic resonance imaging; and LVH, left ventricular hypertrophy.
Falk RH. Cardiac amyloidosis: a treatable disease, often overlooked. *Circulation*. 2011;**124**:1079–85.

compliance. Cardiac amyloidosis may mimic hypertrophic cardiomyopathy or hypertensive heart disease (Table 37.5).

Therapy

Diuretics are used with caution to avoid inadvertent reduction of ventricular filling pressures. There may be also extreme sensitivity to **beta blockers. ACEI/ARBs** may also be used with caution.

In AL amyloidosis, possibly because of an associated autonomic neuropathy, ACEIs and ARBs are rarely tolerated and may provoke profound hypotension, even when prescribed in small doses. Beta-blockade is of no proven use and may aggravate hypotension whereas calcium channel blockers generally worsen congestive heart failure.[4]

Digoxin is potentially arrhythmogenic, particularly in amyloidosis.

Anticoagulation is recommended because of the propensity for thrombus formation in all types of RCM and particularly in endomyocardial fibrosis.

AF reduces cardiac output, and rhythm control is recommended. Cardioversion in amyloidosis should be performed under cover of ventricular or transthoracic pacing with patches.

Permanent pacing and/or **ICD** may be required in conduction disturbances (mainly in amyloidosis, idiopathic RCM, and sarcoidosis), sick sinus syndrome (mainly amyloidosis), and arrhythmias (mainly in sarcoidosis, see Table 49.17).

Transplantation may increase survival, but, in systemic disorders, such as amyloidosis or sarcoidosis, recurrences may be seen in the transplanted heart. **Autologous stem cell transplantation** may also be helpful in amyloidosis.

Amyloidosis has a poor prognosis, particularly in the presence of a monoclonal light chain in serum or urine, multiple myeloma, and hepatic involvement. Untreated patients have a median survival of less than 6 months after the onset of heart failure.[15] Median survival is less than 50% in 2 years despite therapy with melphalan, steroids, immunomodulating agents (lenalidomide and/or bortezomib), and stem cell transplantation.[15, 16]

Prognosis of idiopathic cardiomyopathy is better than in amyloidosis but relatively poor in children.[17] Transplantation is the only therapeutic option in advanced cases.

Loffler's endocarditis may respond to steroids at early stages. Surgical decortication may be required in advanced cases of endomyocardial fibrosis, but operative mortality is high (15–25%).[2] Most patients with this condition are dead within 2 years.[2]

Replacement of alpha-galactosidase A reduces wall thickness in Fabry's disease.[12]

References

1. Kushwaha SS, *et al.* Restrictive cardiomyopathy. *N Engl J Med.* 1997;**336**:267–76
2. Wilmshurst PT, *et al.* Restrictive cardiomyopathy. *Br Heart J.* 1990;**63**:323–4
3. Seward JB, *et al.* Infiltrative cardiovascular diseases: cardiomyopathies that look alike. *J Am Coll Cardiol.* 2010;**55**:1769–79
4. Falk RH. Cardiac amyloidosis: a treatable disease, often overlooked. *Circulation.* 2011;**124**:1079–85
5. Ruberg FL, *et al.* Transthyretin (TTR) cardiac amyloidosis. *Circulation.* 2012;**126**:1286–300
6. Rapezzi C, *et al.* Disease profile and differential diagnosis of hereditary transthyretin-related amyloidosis with exclusively cardiac phenotype: An Italian perspective. *Eur Heart J.* 2013;**34**:520–8
7. Britton KA, *et al.* Clinical problem-solving. The beat goes on. *N Engl J Med.* 2010;**362**:1721–6
8. Katritsis D, *et al.* Primary restrictive cardiomyopathy: clinical and pathologic characteristics. *J Am Coll Cardiol.* 1991;**18**:1230–5
9. Sen-Chowdhry S, *et al.* Genetics of restrictive cardiomyopathy. *Heart Fail Clin.* 2010;**6**:179–86
10. Newton-Cheh C, *et al.* Case records of the Massachusetts General Hospital. Case 11-2011. A 47 year old man with systemic lupus erythematosus and heart failure. *N Engl J Med.* 2011;**364**:1450–60
11. Nihoyannopoulos P, *et al.* Restrictive cardiomyopathies. *Eur J Echocardiogr.* 2009;**10**:III23–33
12. Klein AL, *et al.* Prognostic significance of Doppler measures of diastolic function in cardiac amyloidosis. A Doppler echocardiography study. *Circulation.* 1991;**83**:808–16
13. Moreo A, *et al.* Influence of myocardial fibrosis on left ventricular diastolic function: non-invasive assessment by cardiac magnetic resonance and echo. *Circ Cardiovasc Imaging.* 2009;**2**:437–43
14. Ackerman MJ, *et al.* HRS/EHRA expert consensus statement on the state of genetic testing for the channelopathies and cardiomyopathies; this document was developed as a partnership between the Heart Rhythm Society (HRS) and the European Heart Rhythm Association (EHRA). *Heart Rhythm.* 2011;**8**:1308–39
15. Skinner M, *et al.* Treatment of 100 patients with primary amyloidosis: a randomized trial of melphalan, prednisone, and colchicine versus colchicine only. *Am J Med.* 1996;**100**:290–8
16. Palladini G, *et al.* Treatment with oral melphalan plus dexamethasone produces long-term remissions in AL amyloidosis. *Blood.* 2007;**110**:787–8
17. Cetta F, *et al.* Idiopathic restrictive cardiomyopathy in childhood: diagnostic features and clinical course. *Mayo Clin Proc.* 1995;**70**:634–40

Chapter 38

Arrhythmogenic right ventricular cardiomyopathy/dysplasia

Definition

Arrhythmogenic right ventricular cardiomyopathy or dysplasia (ARVC/D) is predominantly a genetically determined heart muscle disorder that is characterized mainly by fibrofatty replacement of the right ventricular myocardium. This results in abnormalities ranging from regional wall motion abnormalities and aneurysms to global dilation and dysfunction, with or without left ventricular involvement.[1, 2]

Epidemiology

The estimated prevalence of ARVC/D in the general population ranges from 0.1 to 0.02%.[3] ARVC is one of the most arrhythmogenic forms of human heart disease and a major cause of sudden death in the young.[4] The annual incidence of SCD is not known, with reported rates ranging from 0.08 to 1.5%, although, in ICD recipients, the annual rate of intervention is up to 5%.[5, 6]

Aetiology

Several causative **desmosomal genes** (encoding for proteins of the cell adhesion complex) have been identified Since only 30–50% of patients have one of these gene abnormalities, it is assumed that there are also other genes not yet identified. Frequently patients with ARVC/D have more than one genetic defect in the same gene (compound heterozygosity) or in a second complementary gene (digenic heterozygosity).[7] In addition, a family member may have an ARVC gene defect and develop the disease or have no or minimal manifestations of the disease.[7] ARVC is inherited as an **autosomal dominant** trait with variable, age-dependent penetrance, meaning that the risk of a family member inheriting an abnormal gene is 50% for all offspring of the genetically affected proband. There are also recessive forms such as **Naxos disease** (palmoplantar keratosis, wooly hair and ARVC/D) and **Carvajal syndrome** that are associated with a cutaneous phenotype.[8]

Extradesmosomal gene mutations have also been described (Table 38.1). In a recent extensive study in Dutch families, mutations mainly affected placophilin-2 (truncating PKP2 mutations). [9] Radical mutations in apparently healthy subjects are high-probability ARVC-associated mutations, whereas rare missense mutations should be interpreted in the context of race and ethnicity, mutation location, and sequence conservation.[10] Recently, LMNA mutations were also found in severe forms of ARVC, also indicating that it is not just a disease of desmosomal proteins.[11] In addition, DES-encoding desmin, TTN-encoding titin, and PLN-encoding phospholamban have been suggested as novel ARVC genes.[1] However, they all account for overlap syndromes characterized mostly by a dilated cardiomyopathy phenotype and a high prevalence of conduction disease. The exact role of inflammatory (viral myocarditis) or immune mechanisms that may be present is not known.

Table 38.1 Genetic causes of ARVC/D

Autosomal dominant		
ARVD 1	TGFβ3	Transforming growth factor β3*
ARVD 2	RyR2	Cardiac ryanodine receptor*
ARVD 3	Unnamed; maps to 14q12–q22	
ARVD 4	Unnamed; maps to 2q32.1–q32.3	
ARVD 5	TNEM 43	Transmembrane 43*
ARVD 6	Unnamed; maps to 10p14–p12	
ARVD 7	Unnamed; maps to 10q22.3	
ARVD 8 (2–12% of patients)	DSP	Desmoplakin
ARVD 9 (25–40% of patients)	PKP-2	Plakophilin
ARVD 10 (5–10% of patients)	DSG-2	Desmoglein 2
ARVD 11 (2–7% of patients)	DSC-2	Desmocolin 2
ARVD 12	JUP	Plakoglobin
Autosomal recessive		
Naxos disease	JUP	Plakoglobin
Carvajal syndrome	DSP	Desmoplakin

* Extradesmosomal genes.
Modified from Sen-Chowdhry S, McKenna WJ. Sudden death from genetic and acquired cardiomyopathies. *Circulation*. 2012;**125**:1563–76.

Compared with other familial cardiomyopathies and ion channelopathies associated with sudden death, arrhythmogenic cardiomyopathy has low penetrance and unusually variable disease expression, even within members of the same family who carry the same disease-associated mutation, presumably due to genetic and/or epigenetic modifiers that interact with environmental factors.[4] Thus, ARVC does not appear to be a monogenic disease, but rather a complex genetic disease, characterized by marked intrafamilial and interfamilial phenotype diversity.

Pathophysiology

Desmosomal proteins are the primary cause of ARVC derangement. Desmosomes are cellular complexes that primarily serve to link intermediate filaments to the plasma membrane and create strong intercellular linkages (intercellular cardiac glue) that allow transmission of force through the cardiac syncytium.[12] Intercellular junctions are composed of a core region, which mediates cell to cell adhesion, and a plaque region which provides attachment to the intermediate filament cytoskeleton (Figure 38.1). Three separate groups of proteins assemble to form the desmosome: transmembrane proteins, i.e. desmosomal cadherins, such as desmoglein and desmocollin; desmoplakin, a plakin family protein that binds directly to intermediate filaments; and linker proteins, i.e. armadillo proteins, such as plakoglobin and plakophilin, which mediate interactions between the desmosomal cadherin tails and desmoplakin.[8, 10]

The mechanism whereby mutations affecting components of the cardiac desmosome result in ARVC/D is not known. It is believed that the lack of the protein or the incorporation of defective proteins into cardiac desmosomes may provoke detachment of myocytes at the intercalated discs, particularly under mechanical stress conditions. Histologically, there is presence of replacement type fibrosis and myocyte degenerative changes, together with substantial fat replacement. The replacement of the right ventricular myocardium by fibrofatty tissue is progressive, starting from the epicardium or mid-myocardium and then extending to become transmural. It eventually leads to wall thinning and aneurysms, typically located at the inferior, apical, and infundibular walls (so-called triangle of dysplasia), the hallmark of ARVC/D.[8] The fibrofatty replacement interferes with electrical impulse conduction and is the key cause of epsilon waves, right bundle branch block, late potentials, and reentrant ventricular arrhythmias, also possibly due to gap junction remodelling. Left ventricular involvement, usually confined to the posterolateral subepicardium, is present

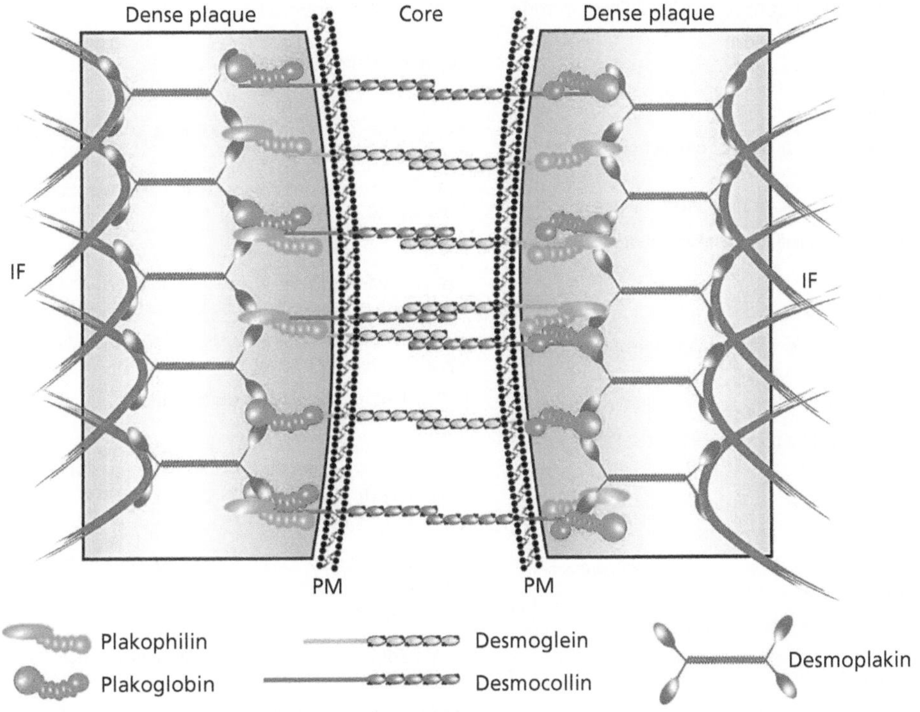

Figure 38.1 Schematic representation of the intracellular and intercellular components of the desmosomal plaque.

IF, intermediate filaments; PM, cytoplasmic membrane.

Basso C, *et al.* Arrhythmogenic right ventricular cardiomyopathy. *Lancet*. 2009;**373**:1289–300.

in more than half of cases. Predominant LV disease is also recognized. Thus, the term ARVC refers to RV, biventricular, and LV dominant subtypes. Mechanical stress may impact cellular junctions, and exercise may exacerbate the progression of the disease.[12]

Presentation

Patients usually present between the second and fourth decades of life due to **palpitations with ventricular ectopic beats or runs of ventricular tachycardia.** Arrhythmias occur early in the natural history of arrhythmogenic cardiomyopathy, often preceding structural remodelling of the myocardium, and **sudden death** by VF may also be seen in the asymptomatic young people and athletes. There is a predilection for the male sex in the second to the fourth decades of life.[1] Patients with ARVC may present with asymptomatic NSVT, despite only subtle RV abnormalities, and have a trend for an increased arrhythmic risk and a rate of appropriate ICD intervention of 3.7%/year.[5] Disease progression may occur during exacerbations that are usually clinically silent or characterized by the appearance of life-threatening arrhythmias and chest pain. Environmental factors, such as exercise or inflammation, might facilitate disease progression. **Progressive heart failure** may occur in <10% of patients.[13]

Investigations

Investigations and diagnostic criteria for ARVC/D are presented in Table 38.2 and Figure 38.2. Clinical diagnosis of ARVC/D may be difficult due to the broad spectrum of phenotypic manifestations, ranging from severe to concealed forms.

ECG depolarization abnormalities result from delayed right ventricular activation and include RBBB, prolongation of right precordial QRS duration (110 ms or more), and epsilon waves, defined as small amplitude potentials occurring after the QRS complex and before the onset of the T waves. Usually, these patients have inverted T waves over V_1–V_3. S wave duration >55 ms in V_1–V_3 is also a marker of the disease.

Holter monitoring may reveal ventricular ectopic beats or runs of VT with LBBB morphology and inferior or superior axis.

On **echocardiography**, the more common structural changes in the right ventricle consist of wall motion abnormalities, trabecular derangement, and diastolic dilatation

Table 38.2 Revised (2010) International Task Force criteria for diagnosis of ARVC/D

Definitive diagnosis: 2 major, or 1 major and 2 minor criteria, or 4 minor from different categories
Borderline: 1 major and 1 minor or 3 minor criteria from different categories
Possible: 1 major or 2 minor criteria from different categories
I. Global or regional dysfunction and structural alterations*
Major
By 2D echo:
Regional RV akinesia, dyskinesia, or aneurysm and one of the following (end diastole):
PLAX RVOT ≥32 mm (corrected for body size [PLAX/BSA] ≥19 mm/m^2)
PSAX RVOT ≥36 mm (corrected for body size [PSAX/BSA] ≥21 mm/m^2), or
Fractional area change ≤33%
By MRI:
Regional RV akinesia or dyskinesia or dyssynchronous RV contraction and one of the following:
Ratio of RV end–diastolic volume to BSA ≥110 mL/m^2 (male) or ≥100 mL/m^2 (female), or
RV ejection fraction ≤40%
By RV angiography:
Regional RV akinesia, dyskinesia, or aneurysm.
Minor
By 2D echo:
Regional RV akinesia or dyskinesia and one of the following (end diastole):
PLAX RVOT ≥29 to <32 mm (corrected for body size [PLAX/BSA] ≥16 to <19 mm/m^2)
PSAX RVOT ≥32 to <36 mm (corrected for body size [PSAX/BSA] ≥18 to <21 mm/m^2), or
Fractional area change >33% to ≤40%
By MRI:
Regional RV akinesia or dyskinesia or dyssynchronous RV contraction and one of the following:
Ratio of RV end–diastolic volume to BSA ≥100 to <110 mL/m^2 (male) or ≥90 to <100 mL/m^2 (female), or
RV ejection fraction >40% to ≤45%
II. Tissue characterization of wall
Major
Residual myocytes <60% by morphometric analysis (or <50% if estimated), with fibrous replacement of the RV free wall myocardium in ≥1 sample, with or without fatty replacement of tissue on endomyocardial biopsy.
Minor
Residual myocytes 60–75% by morphometric analysis (or 50–65% if estimated), with fibrous replacement of the RV free wall myocardium in ≥1 sample, with or without fatty replacement of tissue on endomyocardial biopsy.
III. Repolarization abnormalities
Major
Inverted T waves in right precordial leads (V_1, V_2, and V_3) or beyond in individuals
>14 years of age (in the absence of complete right bundle branch block QRS ≥120 ms)
Minor
Inverted T waves in leads V_1 and V_2 in individuals >14 years of age (in the absence of complete right bundle branch block) or in V_4, V_5, or V_6.
Inverted T waves in leads V_1, V_2, V_3, and V_4 in individuals >14 years of age in the presence of complete right bundlebranch block.
IV. Depolarization/conduction abnormalities
Major
Epsilon wave (reproducible low-amplitude signals between end of QRS complex to onset of the T wave) in the right precordial leads (V_1 to V_3).
Minor
Late potentials by SAECG in ≥1 of 3 parameters in the absence of QRS duration of ≥110 ms on the standard ECG.
Filtered QRS duration (fQRS) ≥114 ms.
Duration of terminal QRS, 40 mV (low-amplitude signal duration) ≥38 ms.
Root mean square voltage of terminal 40 ms ≤20 mV.
Terminal activation duration of QRS ≥55 ms, measured from the nadir of the S wave to the end of the QRS, including R_0, in V_1, V_2, or V_3, in the absence of complete right bundle branch block.
V. Arrhythmias
Major
Non-sustained or sustained ventricular tachycardia of left bundle branch morphology with superior axis (negative or indeterminate QRS in leads II, III, and aVF and positive in lead aVL).
Minor
Non-sustained or sustained ventricular tachycardia of RV outflow configuration, LBBB morphology with inferior axis (positive QRS in leads II, III, and aVF and negative in lead aVL) or of unknown axis.
>500 ventricular extrasystoles per 24 hours (Holter).
VI. Family history
Major
ARVC/D confirmed in a first-degree relative who meets current Task Force criteria
ARVC/D confirmed pathologically at autopsy or surgery in a first-degree relative
Identification of a pathogenic mutation† categorized as associated or probably associated with ARVC/D in the patient under evaluation
Minor
History of ARVC/D in a first-degree relative in whom it is not possible or practical to determine whether the family member meets current Task Force criteria
Premature sudden death (<35 years of age) due to suspected ARVC/D in a first-degree relative

(*Continued*)

Table 38.2 (Continued)

ARVC/D confirmed pathologically or by current Task Force criteria in second-degree relative

PLAX indicates parasternal long-axis view; RVOT, RV outflow tract; BSA, body surface area; PSAX, parasternal short-axis view; aVF, augmented voltage unipolar left foot lead; and aVL, augmented voltage unipolar left arm lead.

* Hypokinesis is not included in this or subsequent definitions of RV regional wall motion abnormalities for the proposed modified criteria.
† A pathogenic mutation is a DNA alteration associated with ARVC/D that alters or is expected to alter the encoded protein, is unobserved or rare in a large non-ARVC/D control population, and either alters or is predicted to alter the structure or function of the protein, or has demonstrated linkage to the disease phenotype in a conclusive pedigree.
Marcus FI, *et al*. Diagnosis of arrhythmogenic right ventricular cardiomyopathy/dysplasia: proposed modification of the Task Force criteria. *Eur Heart J*. 2010;**31**: 806–14.

of the RVOT, but the ventricle may be normal in mild forms of ARVC/D. Typically, the inferior subtricuspid, antero-apical, and mid-outflow tract regions are affected **(triangle of dysplasia)**. In the early stages of ARVC/D, overall right ventricular function may be normal, with local or regional wall motion abnormalities, and these are difficult to quantify.[14] As the disease progresses, RV dilatation and failure may occur. Although ARVC was originally described as a right ventricular disease, it is now recognized to include a spectrum of biventricular and left dominant forms that may be misdiagnosed as dilated cardiomyopathy.

Cardiac magnetic resonance is very useful by means of detecting fatty tissue and, with gadolinium, intramyocardial fibrosis. This is very important since intramyocardial fat without fibrosis is present in the right ventricular anterolateral and apical region, even in a normal heart, and increases with age and body weight.[15] Thus, caution is needed in patients with misdiagnoses of ARVC mostly based on cardiac imaging/CMR features.[16]

Electroanatomical mapping can reveal low-voltage areas, either endocardially or epicardially, that correspond to fibrofatty myocardial replacement and could assist in the differential diagnosis with idiopathic right ventricular outflow tract tachycardia.[17]

Endomyocardial biopsy has not been consistently useful because the structural changes in ARVC tend to spare the subendocardium and do not typically involve the interventricular septum.

Immunohistochemical analysis of endomyocardial biopsy samples has been recently found to be a sensitive and specific diagnostic test for ARVC/D by means of detecting defective desmosomal proteins at intercalated discs.[18]

Differential diagnosis

It is aimed at exclusion of idiopathic right ventricular outflow tract tachycardia that is benign and displays LBBB morphology with inferior axis. The absence of ECG repolarization and depolarization abnormalities and of right ventricular structural changes, recording of a single VT morphology and non-inducibility at programmed ventricular stimulation, and a normal voltage map provide evidence for the idiopathic nature of the VT.[4] Table 38.3 and Figure 38.3 present proposed criteria for distinguishing idiopathic VT from VT in ARVC.[19] A score ≥5 suggests ARVC (see also Chapter 55 on VT). Other conditions to be excluded are **Ebstein's anomaly, atrial septal defect, Uhl's disease** (isolated right ventricular enlargement and failure, with partial or total absence of right ventricular myocardium due to apoptotic anomalies), **pulmonary hypertension, right ventricular infarction, dilated cardiomyopathy, myocarditis, sarcoidosis, Chagas' disease,** and **Brugada syndrome**. In black athletes without concomitant symptoms or family history, T-wave inversion and RV enlargement may be a bening finding.[20]

Risk stratification

Cardiac arrest due to VF can occur at any time during the disease course. The prognostic value of proposed risk factors (Table 38.4), such as previous cardiac arrest, syncope, participation in competitive sports, young age, VT, severe right ventricular dysfunction, left ventricular involvement, and QRS dispersion of 40 ms or more, has not been prospectively assessed.[8] The value of programmed ventricular stimulation is debatable, with both negative[11] and positive[17] results reported. Family history is of rather limited value in predicting SCD.[5] Although LV involvement has been considered for a long time as an expression of the advanced disease phase, it is now accepted that ARVC can start with isolated or predominant LV involvement since the early stages.[1]

Therapy

Asymptomatic patients or healthy gene carriers do not require prophylactic treatment. They should undergo cardiac follow-up, including medical history, 12-lead ECG, 24-hour Holter monitoring, exercise testing, and echocardiography, on a regular basis. Data on antiarrhythmic drug therapy are limited. The prophylactic value of beta-blockers remains unknown, and only amiodarone has been shown to prevent ventricular arrhythmias in ARVC/D patients treated with ICD.[21] Sotalol at high doses (320–480 mg daily) has also been found partially effective.[22] Treatment with ICD is indicated in patients with cardiac arrest, syncope, or haemodynamically poorly tolerated VT, or severe right or biventricular dysfunction (Table 38.5).[23, 24]

A potential problem with ICD in ARVC is that the disease is often progressive, leading to loss of myocardium and reduced ventricular R wave sensing over time. Catheter

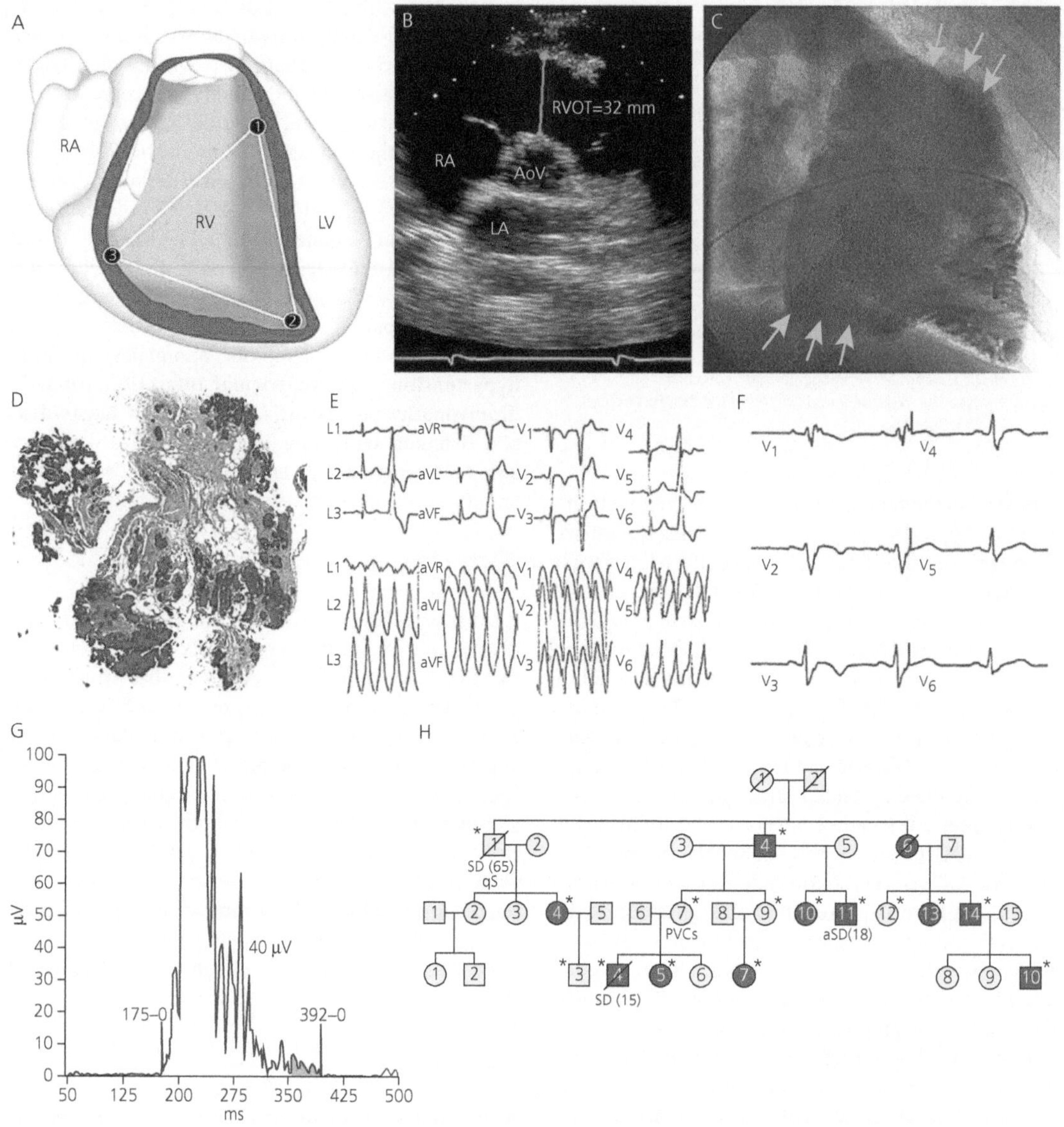

Figure 38.2 Features of arrhythmogenic right ventrical cardiomyopathy. Diagnostic morphofunctional, electrocardiographic, and tissue characteristic features of arrhythmogenic right ventricular cardiomyopathy. (A) Triangle of dysplasia, which shows the characteristic areas for structural and functional abnormalities of the right ventricle. RA, right atrium; RV, right ventricle; LV, left ventricle. (B) Two-dimensional echocardiography showing right ventricular outflow tract enlargement from the parasternal short axis view. AoV, aortic valve; LA, left atrium; RVOT, right ventricular outflow tract. (C) Right ventricular contrast angiography (30° right anterior oblique view) showing a localized right ventricular outflow tract aneurysm (arrows) and inferobasal akinesia (arrows) with mild tricuspid regurgitation. (D) Endomyocardial biopsy sample with extensive myocardial atrophy and fibrofatty replacement (trichrome; ×6). (E) 12-lead ECG with inverted T waves (V_1, V_2, V_3), with left bundle branch block morphology, premature ventricular complexes, and VT. (F) ECG tracing showing post-excitation epsilon wave in precordial leads V_1, V_2, V_3 (arrows). (G) Signal-averaged ECG with late potentials (40 Hz high-pass filtering); filtered QRS duration (QRSD) = 217 ms; low amplitude signal (LAS) = 107 ms; and root mean square voltage of terminal 40 ms (RMS) = 4 μV. (H) Family pedigree of arrhythmogenic right ventricular cardiomyopathy: note the autosomal dominant inheritance of the disease.

SD, sudden death; aSD, aborted sudden death; PVC, premature ventricular complexes; qS, qS in inferior leads. * Gene mutation carrier.

Basso C, *et al.* Arrhythmogenic right ventricular cardiomyopathy. *Lancet*. 2009;**373**:1289–300.

ablation of VT, when feasible, is successful in reducing further episodes but cannot offer absolute protection without ICD backup since the progressive course of the disease precludes any curative role. When ICD therapy is not feasible, amiodarone or soatalol may be used (IIa-C by the ACC/AHA/ESC GL on ventricular arrhythmias). Heart failure is treated according to standard recommendations (see Chapter 31). Cardiac transplantation may be needed in patients with intractable arrhythmias or heart failure. **Physical activity** is restricted to mild cardiovascular sports for weight management with a low static component (see Chapter 81 on athlete's heart for sports classification).[12] The relative risk of SCD from ARVC is 5-fold higher in athletes than in non-athletes,[25] and competitive sports are prohibited.

Table 38.3 Electrocardiographic scoring system for distinguishing RVOT arrhythmias in patients with ARVC from idiopathic VT

ECG characteristic	Points
Anterior T wave inversions (V_1–V_3) in sinus rhythm	3
VT/PVC:	
Lead I QRS duration ≥120 ms	2
QRS notching (multiple leads)	2
V_5 transition or later	1

Anterior T wave inversion is defined as T wave negativity in, at least, leads V_1, V_2, and V_3.
Lead I QRS duration ≥120 ms is defined as the duration from the initial deflection of the QRS complex to the end of the QRS complex in lead I.
QRS notching in multiple leads is defined as a QRS complex deflection on the upstroke or downstroke of >0.5 mV that did not cross baseline occurring in, at least, two leads (Figure 38.3).
The precordial transition point is designated as the earliest precordial lead where the R wave amplitude exceeded the S wave amplitude.
Hoffmayer KS, *et al*. An electrocardiographic scoring system for distinguishing right ventricular outflow tract arrhythmias in patients with arrhythmogenic right ventricular cardiomyopathy from idiopathic ventricular tachycardia. *Heart Rhythm*. 2013;**10**:477–82.

Genetic testing

Molecular genotyping is currently applied to relatives of a proband with a known mutation probably associated with ARVC/D for risk assessment (presymptomatic test) while it is not routinely used in isolated cases with a borderline phenotype for confirming the diagnosis. However, a negative genetic test does not exclude the possibility that the phenotype is due to a mutation of unknown, and thus untested, disease-causing genes. Approximately 50% of ARVC/D probands do not carry any known causative gene mutations.[24] The certainty of detecting causative mutation carriers is further limited by the difficulty in distinguishing causative mutations (mostly missense gene variants) from polymorphisms as well as by the potential presence of an undetected second pathogenetic mutation in the same or another gene. There is a low signal to noise ratio, with mutations in a recent series identified in 43% of ARVC cases and in 16% of controls.[10] There is no evidence that the genotype may help with management strategies. Recommendations by HRS/EHRA are presented in Table 38.6.[26]

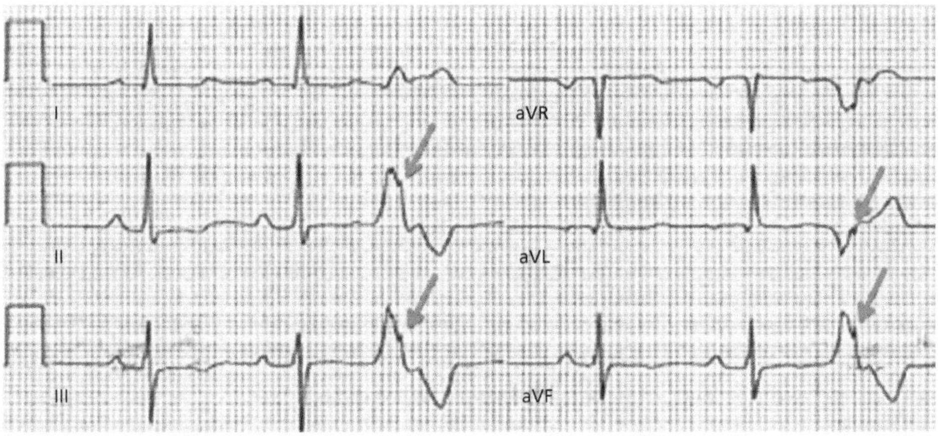

Figure 38.3 Example of QRS notching. Arrows show QRS notching in lead II, III, aVF, and aVL.

Hoffmayer KS, *et al*. An electrocardiographic scoring system for distinguishing right ventricular outflow tract arrhythmias in patients with arrhythmogenic right ventricular cardiomyopathy from idiopathic ventricular tachycardia. *Heart Rhythm*. 2013;**10**:477–82.

Table 38.4 Risk stratification and ICD indications in ARVC/D

Arrhythmic risk	Characteristics	ICD implantation
High (8–10%/year)	Aborted sudden death	Mandatory
	Haemodynamically unstable sustained VT	
	Syncope	
Intermediate (<2%/year)	Haemodynamically stable sustained VT	Individualized
	Non-sustained VT	
	Severe dilation and/or dysfunction of RV, LV, or bothEarly onset (<35 years) severe disease	
Low (<1%/year)	Probands or relatives fulfilling Task Force criteria for ARVC/D Regardless of family history of sudden death or inducibility at EPS (in the absence of syncope, VT, or severe ventricular dysfunction)	Unjustified

Corrado D, *et al.* Molecular biology and the clinical management of arrhythmogenic right ventricular cardiomyopathy/dysplasia. *Heart.* 2011;**97**:530–9.

Table 38.5 ACC/AHA 2012 GL on devices

Indications for ICD	
Survivors of cardiac arrest due to VF or unstable VT without reversible cause	I-A
Spontanous sustained VT stable or unstable	I-B
One or more risk factors for SCD	IIa-C

2012 ACCF/AHA/HRS focused update incorporated into the ACCF/AHA/HRS 2008 guidelines for device-based therapy of cardiac rhythm abnormalities. *J Am Coll Cardiol.* 2013;**61**:e6–75.

Table 38.6 HRS/EHRA 2011 statement on genetic testing

State of genetic testing for arrhythmogenic cardiomyopathy (ACM)/arrhythmogenic right ventricular cardiomyopathy	
Family members and appropriate relatives following the identification of the ACM/ARVC causative mutation in an index case.	I
Comprehensive or targeted (DSC2, DSG2, DSP, JUP, PKP2, and TMEM43) ACM/ARVC genetic testing for patients satisfying Task Force diagnostic criteria for ACM/ARVC.	IIa
Patients with possible ACM/ARVC (1 major or 2 minor criteria) according to the 2010 Task Force criteria.	IIb
Patients with only a single minor criterion according to the 2010 Task Force criteria.	III

HRS/EHRA 2011 expert consensus statement on the state of genetic testing for the channelopathies and cardiomyopathies. *Heart Rhythm.* 2011;**8**: 1308–39.

Pregnancy

It is well tolerated, but clinical follow-up is recommended in the last trimester and puerperium because of a reported increased risk of ventricular arrhythmias. See Table 35.3.

References

1. Basso C, *et al.* Arrhythmogenic right ventricular cardiomyopathy. *Circ Arrhythm Electrophysiol.* 2012;**5**:1233–46
2. Marcus FI, *et al.* Diagnosis of arrhythmogenic right ventricular cardiomyopathy/dysplasia: proposed modification of the Task Force criteria. *Eur Heart J.* 2010;**31**:806–14
3. Corrado D, *et al.* Trends in sudden cardiovascular death in young competitive athletes after implementation of a preparticipation screening program. *JAMA.* 2006;**296**:1593–601
4. Saffitz JE. Arrhythmogenic cardiomyopathy: advances in diagnosis and disease pathogenesis. *Circulation.* 2011;**124**:e390–2
5. Corrado D, *et al.* Prophylactic implantable defibrillator in patients with arrhythmogenic right ventricular cardiomyopathy/dysplasia and no prior ventricular fibrillation or sustained ventricular tachycardia. *Circulation.* 2010;**122**:1144–52
6. Sen-Chowdhry S, *et al.* Sudden death from genetic and acquired cardiomyopathies. *Circulation.* 2012;**125**:1563–76
7. Marcus FI, *et al.* Genetics of arrhythmogenic right ventricular cardiomyopathy: A practical guide for physicians. *JACC.* 2013; doi: 10.1016/j.jacc.2013.1001.1073
8. Basso C, *et al.* Arrhythmogenic right ventricular cardiomyopathy. *Lancet.* 2009;**373**:1289–300
9. Cox MG, *et al.* Arrhythmogenic right ventricular dysplasia/cardiomyopathy: pathogenic desmosome mutations in index-patients predict outcome of family screening: Dutch arrhythmogenic right ventricular dysplasia/cardiomyopathy genotype-phenotype follow-up study. *Circulation.* 2011;**123**:2690–700
10. Kapplinger JD, *et al.* Distinguishing arrhythmogenic right ventricular cardiomyopathy/dysplasia-associated mutations from background genetic noise. *J Am Coll Cardiol.* 2011;**57**:2317–27
11. Quarta G, *et al.* Mutations in the lamin A/C gene mimic arrhythmogenic right ventricular cardiomyopathy. *Eur Heart J.* 2012;**33**:1128–36
12. Webster G, *et al.* An update on channelopathies: from mechanisms to management. *Circulation.* 2013;**127**:126–40

13. Hulot JS, *et al.* Natural history and risk stratification of arrhythmogenic right ventricular dysplasia/cardiomyopathy. *Circulation*. 2004;**110**:1879–84
14. Marcus FI, *et al.* Arrhythmogenic right ventricular cardiomyopathy/dysplasia clinical presentation and diagnostic evaluation: results from the North American Multidisciplinary Study. *Heart Rhythm*. 2009;**6**:984–92
15. Sen-Chowdhry S, *et al.* Cardiovascular magnetic resonance in arrhythmogenic right ventricular cardiomyopathy revisited: comparison with Task Force criteria and genotype. *J Am Coll Cardiol*. 2006;**48**:2132–40
16. Marcus F, *et al.* Pitfalls in the diagnosis of arrhythmogenic right ventricular cardiomyopathy/dysplasia. *Am J Cardiol*. 2010;**105**:1036–9
17. Corrado D, *et al.* Three-dimensional electroanatomical voltage mapping and histologic evaluation of myocardial substrate in right ventricular outflow tract tachycardia. *J Am Coll Cardiol*. 2008;**51**:731–9
18. Asimaki A, *et al.* A new diagnostic test for arrhythmogenic right ventricular cardiomyopathy. *N Engl J Med*. 2009;**360**:1075–84
19. Hoffmayer KS, *et al.* An electrocardiographic scoring system for distinguishing right ventricular outflow tract arrhythmias in patients with arrhythmogenic right ventricular cardiomyopathy from idiopathic ventricular tachycardia. *Heart Rhythm*. 2013;**10**:477–82
20. Zaidi A, *et al.* Physiological right ventricular adaptation in elite athletes of African and Afro-Caribbean origin/clinical perspective. *Circulation*. 2013;**127**:1783–92
21. Marcus GM, *et al.* Efficacy of antiarrhythmic drugs in arrhythmogenic right ventricular cardiomyopathy: a report from the North American ARVC Registry. *J Am Coll Cardiol*. 2009;**54**:609–15
22. Wichter T, *et al.* Efficacy of antiarrhythmic drugs in patients with arrhythmogenic right ventricular disease. Results in patients with inducible and noninducible ventricular tachycardia. *Circulation*. 1992;**86**:29–37
23. Bhonsale A, *et al.* Incidence and predictors of implantable cardioverter-defibrillator therapy in patients with arrhythmogenic right ventricular dysplasia/cardiomyopathy undergoing implantable cardioverter-defibrillator implantation for primary prevention. *J Am Coll Cardiol*. 2011;**58**:1485–96
24. Corrado D, *et al.* Does sports activity enhance the risk of sudden death in adolescents and young adults? *J Am Coll Cardiol*. 2003;**42**:1959–63
25. Corrado D, *et al.* Molecular biology and clinical management of arrhythmogenic right ventricular cardiomyopathy/dysplasia. *Heart*. 2011;**97**:530–9
26. Ackerman MJ, *et al.* HRS/EHRA expert consensus statement on the state of genetic testing for the channelopathies and cardiomyopathies; this document was developed as a partnership between the Heart Rhythm Society (HRS) and the European Heart Rhythm Association (EHRA). *Heart Rhythm*. 2011;**8**:1308–39

Chapter 39

Peripartum cardiomyopathy

Definition

Peripartum cardiomyopathy is a distinct cardiomyopathy, the cardiac phenotype of which resembles dilated cardiomyopathy.[1]

National Heart, Lung, and Blood Institute and the Office of Rare Diseases (2000)

- Development of heart failure in the last month of pregnancy or within 5 months post-partum
- Absence of an identifiable cause of heart failure
- Absence of recognizable heart disease prior to the last month of pregnancy
- LVEF <45%, fractional shortening <30%, or both, with or without an LVEDD >2.7 cm/m^2 body surface area.[1]

Heart Failure Association of the European Society of Cardiology (2010)

Peripartum cardiomyopathy is an idiopathic cardiomyopathy, presenting with heart failure secondary to left ventricular systolic dysfunction towards the end of pregnancy or in the months following delivery, where no other cause of heart failure is found. It is a diagnosis of exclusion. The left ventricle may not be dilated, but the ejection fraction is nearly always reduced below 45%.[2,3]

Epidemiology

The incidence of peripartum cardiomyopathy varies from 1 in 2500–4000 in the USA to 1 in 1000 in South Africa, and 1 in 300 in Haiti.[3,4]

Aetiology

Peripartum cardiomyopathy continues to be a cardiomyopathy of unknown cause. Various pathophysiologic mechanisms have been proposed, such as excessive prolactin (reduced myocardial STAT3 protein levels and activated oxidative stress-cathepsin D-16 kDA prolactin cascade), cytokine-mediated inflammation, viral myocarditis, and autoimmune mechanisms. A genetic background has been suggested.

Prolonged tocolysis, advanced maternal age, high gravidity/parity, multipregnancy, race, socio-economic status, gestational hypertension, and cocaine abuse are risk factors associated with the development of peripartum cardiomyopathy.[4]

Presentation

Clinical presentation is extremely variable, from mild symptoms that can be attributed to pregnancy to acute heart failure. Elevated JVP, S_3, and basal rales can be normal in pregnancy. Most often, patients present with NYHA III or IV symptoms. Patients may also present with ventricular arrhythmias, systemic embolism due to LV thrombus, or pulmonary embolism. Most cases occur in the puerperium.[4]

Investigations

Diagnosis is being put by exclusion (Table 39.1).

- **ECG** is seldom normal, usually displaying ST-T abnormalities or LV hypertrophy voltage criteria.
- **Echocardiography** is essential for LV assessment.
- **MRI** allows more accurate measurements, but gadolinium crosses the placenta and is not recommended during pregnancy.[2]
- **BNP** and **NT-pro-BNP** levels are raised.

Therapy

After delivery, peripartum cardiomyopathy is treated conventionally (see Chapter 31 on CCF).

During pregnancy precautions are needed:

Furosemide in congestion—caution is needed in pre-eclampsia due to concern for decreased placental perfusion. **Thiazides** carry a possible risk of birth defects or fetal thrombocytopenia. **Spironolactone** may cause feminization of male fetus. No data for **eplerenone.**

Hydralazine and **nitrates** to maintain a systolic blood pressure <110 mmHg. **Amlodipine** can also be used. **ACEI** and **ARB** are teratogenic.

Beta 1-selective beta-blockers, such as **metoprolol**, that are compatible with breastfeeding are used. Neonates should be monitored for bradycardia, hypoglycaemia, and growth retardation. Beta 2 receptor blockade has anti-tocolytic action, and carvedilol may be teratogenic at high doses.[4]

Digoxin may be used.

Bromocriptine (2.5 mg twice daily for 2 weeks, followed by 2.5 daily for 4 weeks), a dopamine D2 receptor agonist, has prevented the onset of disease in experimental models of peripartum cardiomyopathy and appears successful and safe in initial trials with patients.[5]

The addition of **pentoxyfylline** to conventional therapy has also been shown to improve outcome in patients with peripartum cardiomyopathy.[6]

Table 39.1 Differential diagnosis of peripartum cardiomyopathy (PPCM)

Distinguishing features	
Pre-existing idiopathic dilated cardiomyopathy (IDC) unmasked by pregnancy presents by the 2nd trimester	PPCM most commonly presents post-partum whereas IDC (unmasked by pregnancy) usually presents during pregnancy with larger cardiac dimensions than PPCM
Pre–existing familial dilated cardiomyopathy (FDC) unmasked by pregnancy. FDC usually presents during pregnancy with larger cardiac dimensions than PPCM	PPCM most commonly presents post-partum whereas FDC usually presents by 2nd trimester
HIV/AIDS cardiomyopathy ventricles	HIV cardiomyopathy presents often with non-dilated ventricles
Pre-existing valvular heart disease unmasked by pregnancy	Rheumatic mitral valve disease is often unmasked by pregnancy; PPCM most commonly presents post-partum whereas valvular heart disease usually presents by 2nd trimester
Hypertensive heart disease	Exclude pre-existing severe hypertension in those presenting before delivery
Pre-existing unrecognized congenital heart disease	Previously unrecognized congenital heart disease often has associated pulmonary hypertension; PPCM most commonly presents post-partum whereas congenital heart disease usually presents by 2nd trimester
Pregnancy-associated myocardial infarction	
Pulmonary embolus	

Subcutaneous **LMWH** are used in LVEF <30% or AF.

In acute heart failure, **dobutamine** and **dopamine** may be used. **Norepinephrine** decreases placental blood flow. **CRT with or without ICD** is considered in patients who fulfill criteria 6 months following presentation.

Therapy with standard heart failure medications should be continued probably for a minimum of 12 months.[7] If cardiac function does not normalize within 6–12 months, heart failure medications should likely be continued indefinitely.

Delivery

Unless there is deterioration in the maternal or fetal condition, there is no need for early delivery. Urgent delivery, irrespective of gestation, may need to be considered in women presenting or remaining in advanced HF with haemodynamic instability. In general, spontaneous vaginal birth is preferable in stable women, but assisted second stage is recommended to reduce maternal efforts and shorten labour. Caesarean section is preferred for patients who are critically ill and in need of inotropic therapy or mechanical support.[2]

Prognosis

The prognosis is better than with other causes of dilated cardiomyopathy, with normalization of LV function in >50% of patients, mostly occurring within 2 to 6 months after diagnosis, although later recovery is also possible.[8] With contemporary therapy, reported mortality is 4–6% at 4 to 5 years.[9, 10] Approximately 10% of the patients may require transplanantion.[9] Most patients experience partial recovery, and 30% complete recovery; half of patients may not recover normal function within 6 months. Outcomes for **subsequent pregnancies** after peripartum cardiomyopathy are better for women who have fully recovered heart function after their initial presentation. In general, a subsequent pregnancy carries a recurrence risk for post-partum cardiomyopathy of 30–50%.[3] Factors associated with lack of recovery at initial assessment are LVEDD >5.6 cm, the presence of LV thrombus, and African-American race. Pregnancy is discouraged in women with LVEF <25% at diagnosis that has not been normalized at 2 months.[2, 8] However, even if the LVEF is normalized, there is still a need for counselling because of the risk of recurrence with a new pregnancy.[3] Patients who decide to become pregnant again should undergo baseline echocardiography and determination of serum BNP level before or early in pregnancy. Patients should be followed with repeat echocardiography during the early second and third trimesters, during the last gestational month, early after delivery, and at any time if new symptoms of heart failure develop. Early termination of an unintentional pregnancy should be considered to prevent worsening of LV function and potential maternal mortality, especially in patients with persistent LV dysfunction.

References

1. Pearson GD, *et al.* Peripartum cardiomyopathy: National Heart, Lung, and Blood Institute and Office of Rare Diseases (National Institutes of Health) Workshop recommendations and review. *JAMA*. 2000;**283**:1183–8
2. Sliwa K, *et al.* Current state of knowledge on aetiology, diagnosis, management, and therapy of peripartum cardiomyopathy: a position statement from the Heart Failure Association of the European Society of Cardiology Working Group on peripartum cardiomyopathy. *Eur J Heart Fail.* 2010;**12**:767–78
3. Regitz-Zagrosek V, *et al.* ESC guidelines on the management of cardiovascular diseases during pregnancy: the Task Force on the management of cardiovascular diseases during pregnancy of the European Society of Cardiology (ESC). *Eur Heart J*. 2011;**32**:3147–97
4. Cruz MO, *et al.* Update on peripartum cardiomyopathy. *Obstet Gynecol Clin North Am*. 2010;**37**:283–303
5. Sliwa K, *et al.* Evaluation of bromocriptine in the treatment of acute severe peripartum cardiomyopathy: a proof-of-concept pilot study. *Circulation*. 2010;**121**:1465–73
6. Sliwa K, *et al.* The addition of pentoxifylline to conventional therapy improves outcome in patients with peripartum cardiomyopathy. *Eur J Heart Fail.* 2002;**4**:305–9
7. Blauwet LA, *et al.* Diagnosis and management of peripartum cardiomyopathy. *Heart*. 2011;**97**:1970–81
8. Elkayam U. Clinical characteristics of peripartum cardiomyopathy in the United States: diagnosis, prognosis, and management. *J Am Coll Cardiol.* 2011;**58**:659–70
9. Amos AM, *et al.* Improved outcomes in peripartum cardiomyopathy with contemporary. *Am Heart J*. 2006;**152**:509–13
10. Felker GM, *et al.* Underlying causes and long-term survival in patients with initially unexplained cardiomyopathy. *N Engl J Med*. 2000;**342**:1077–84

Chapter 40

Tachycardiomyopathy

Definition

The term denotes tachycardia-induced cardiomyopathy. Tachycardia is a reversible cause of impaired left ventricular function that can lead to heart failure and death. Very frequent premature ventricular conductions may also be a cause of cardiomyopathy.

Epidemiology

The incidence of tachycardiomyopathy is unknown, but it has been reported in any age group, from the fetus to the elderly.

Aetiology

The syndrome has been initially described with the so-called persistent reciprocating junctional tachycardia, a term that denoted both atrioventricular reentry due to a septal decremental pathway and fast-slow atrioventricular nodal reentry. We know now that any chronic cardiac arrhythmia may cause tachycardia-induced cardiomyopathy: **incessant atrioventricular reentrant tachycardia due to septal accessory pathways, rapid atrial fibrillation, idiopathic ventricular tachycardia, inappropriate sinus nodal tachycardia, atrial flutter**, and **persistent ectopic beats** are the most described causes.[1–3]

Pathophysiology

Rapid pacing in animal models have documented cytoskeletal changes and remodelling of the extracellular matrix attributed to abnormal calcium cycling, increased catecholamines and decreased beta 1-adrenergic receptor density, oxidative stress, depletion of myocardial energy stores, and myocardial ischaemia due to increased heart rate.[3, 4] However, it is not known why the majority of patients with frequent PVCs have a benign course whereas up to 30% of them may develop cardiomyopathy.[5]

Presentation

Patients present with possibly unexplained left ventricular dilatation and systolic dysfunction and a history of paroxysmal tachycardias or permanent AF. Heart failure develops slowly, but sudden death is possible.[2]

Diagnosis

No strict criteria exist. Diagnosis is established by excluding other causes of cardiomyopathy and demonstrating recovery of LV function after eradication of the arrhythmia or control of the ventricular rate. The ventricular rate that causes cardiomyopathy is not known, although rates >100 bpm for prolonged periods are considered to be responsible.[3] PVCs should be >20 000 beats/day to be accounted for the cardiomyopathy (or alternatively a 24-hour burden of >24% on Holter),[6] although ectopy-induced cardiomyopathy has been reported in a patient with only 5502 beats/day.[7] Worsening of the LV function has been reported with >1000 beats/day,[8] but the clear-cut point that marks the critical frequency for cardiomyopathy is not known. Usually, LVEDD is <65 and LVESD <50 mm in patients with LVEF <30% due to TIC.[1] Larger values suggest dilated cardiomyopathy, although overlapping exists.

Therapy

There is considerable evidence that LV function improves approximately 3 months following restoration of normal heart rate. In inappropriate sinus nodal tachycardia, beta-blockers are indicated. Sinus nodal modification with catheter ablation carries a 10% risk of sinus nodal damage and need of a PPM. Catheter ablation is indicated in cases of accessory pathways, idiopathic VT, and monomorphic VPBs. In AF, both pulmonary vein isolation[9] and AV nodal modification [10] improve LV function, but PV isolation has been found superior to AV nodal ablation and biventricular pacing in this respect.[11]

Long-term medical therapy with beta-blockers and ACE inhibitors or ARBs is indicated before and after successful ablation attempts for LV remodelling purposes.

References

1. Lishmanov A, *et al.* Tachycardia-induced cardiomyopathy: evaluation and therapeutic options. *Congest Heart Fail.* 2010;**16**:122–6
2. Nerheim P, *et al.* Heart failure and sudden death in patients with tachycardia-induced cardiomyopathy and recurrent tachycardia. *Circulation.* 2004;**110**:247–52
3. Shinbane JS, *et al.* Tachycardia-induced cardiomyopathy: a review of animal models and clinical studies. *J Am Coll Cardiol.* 1997;**29**:709–15

4. Gopinathannair R, *et al.* Tachycardia-mediated cardiomyopathy: recognition and management. *Curr Heart Fail Rep.* 2009;**6**:257–64
5. Lee GK, *et al.* Premature ventricular contraction-induced cardiomyopathy: a treatable condition. *Circ Arrhythm Electrophysiol.* 2012;**5**:229–36
6. Baman TS, *et al.* Relationship between burden of premature ventricular complexes and left ventricular function. *Heart Rhythm.* 2010;**7**:865–9
7. Yarlagadda RK, *et al.* Reversal of cardiomyopathy in patients with repetitive monomorphic ventricular ectopy originating from the right ventricular outflow tract. *Circulation.* 2005;**112**:1092–7
8. Niwano S, *et al.* Prognostic significance of frequent premature ventricular contractions originating from the ventricular outflow tract in patients with normal left ventricular function. *Heart.* 2009;**95**:1230–7
9. Hsu LF, *et al.* Catheter ablation for atrial fibrillation in congestive heart failure. *N Engl J Med.* 2004;**351**:2373–83
10. Wood MA, *et al.* Clinical outcomes after ablation and pacing therapy for atrial fibrillation : a meta-analysis. *Circulation.* 2000;**101**:1138–44
11. Khan MN, *et al.* Pulmonary vein isolation for atrial fibrillation in patients with heart failure. *N Engl J Med.* 2008;**359**:1778–85

Chapter 41

Stress cardiomyopathy

Definition

Stress cardiomyopathy, also referred to as Takotsubo cardiomyopathy, transient apical ballooning, or broken heart syndrome, is a disorder associated with transient left ventricular dysfunction. It occurs more often in old women after emotional or physical stress, but it also happens in men <50 year old and in the absence of stress.[1] LV ballooning may be apical, mid-ventricular, or basal.

Pathophysiology

The mechanisms of disease remain unclear, and the cause has not been established. An excessive release of catecholamines (stress, exogenous cathecholamines administered during diagnostic test, and beta-receptor agonists)[2] seems to have a pivotal role in the development of stress cardiomyopathy. In-hospital mortality is 2%, and 2-year mortality is approximately 10%.[1,3]

Diagnosis

Usually, patients present with chest pain or exertional dyspnoea, but the condition can be asymptomatic.

The **ECG** shows signs of acute or anterior myocardial infarction or ST-T changes.

Troponin elevation (0.01–5.3 ng/mL) is the rule.[1]

Cardiac MRI and **echocardiography** display characteristic figures (Figure 41.1). Average LVEF is 32–36%.[1,3] Approximately 4% have right or left ventricular thrombus.

Therapy

Beta-blockers are essential, but they do not offer absolute protection.[1]

Anticoagulation should be considered in the presence of ventricular thrombus or embolic events. Standard heart failure therapy is administered when needed. Early restoration of normal ventricular function is the rule, but, in 5% of the patients, it can be delayed (>2 months). Approximately 5% of patients have a recurrence 3 weeks to 4 years after the first event.[1]

References

1. Sharkey SW, *et al.* Natural history and expansive clinical profile of stress (takotsubo) cardiomyopathy. *J Am Coll Cardiol.* 2010;**55**:333–41
2. Abraham J, *et al.* Stress cardiomyopathy after intravenous administration of catecholamines and beta-receptor agonists. *J Am Coll Cardiol.* 2009;**53**:1320–5
3. Parodi G, *et al.* Natural history of takotsubo cardiomyopathy. *Chest.* 2011;**139**:887–92

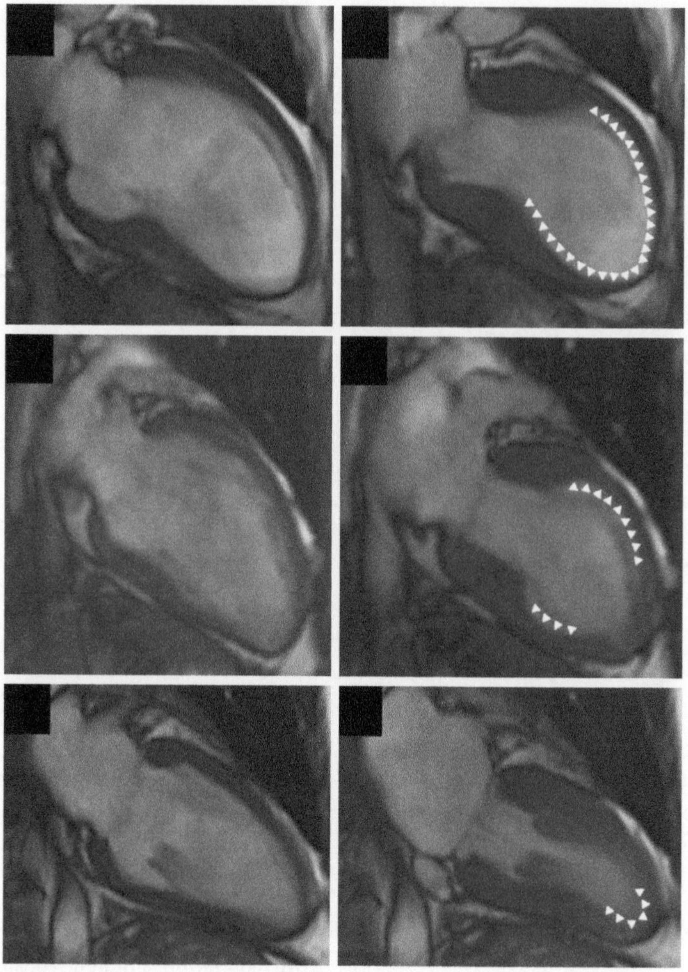

Figure 41.1 Diversity of LV contraction patterns in stress cardiomyopathy, as demonstrated by cardiac magnetic resonance in vertical long-axis view (A, C, and E) diastole; (B, D, and F) systole. Three types are depicted: (A, B) most common pattern of mid- and apical left ventricular (LV) akinesia (arrowheads); (C, D) mid-LV akinesia (arrowheads) with sparing of apical region; and (E, F) apical LV contraction abnormality only (arrowheads).
Sharkey SW, *et al*. Natural history and expansive clinical profile of stress (tako-tsubo) cardiomyopathy. *J Am Coll Cardiol*. 2010;**55**:333–41

Chapter 42

Iron overload cardiomyopathies

Definition

Iron overload cardiomyopathies are due to increased gastrointestinal (GI) iron absorption (haemochromatosis) or excess administration of exogenous iron by dietary sources or red blood cell (RBC) transfusions (haemosiderosis). They have either a restrictive or dilated phenotype that usually develops at later stages of the disease.[1]

Aetiology

The incidence of iron overload cardiomyopathy is increasing worldwide. Chronic blood transfusion is the main treatment for hereditary anaemias, such as thalassaemia and sickle cell disease, that, although prevalent in the Mediterranean basin, are also seen in other parts of the western world due to immigration. Causes of iron overload cardiomyopathy are presented in Table 42.1. Hereditary haemochromatosis is an autosomal disorder in which mutations, usually of the HFE gene of specific cause increased GI absorption of iron. Chronic transfusion is mandatory for the anaemias listed. A unit of packed RBCs consists of 200 to 250 mg of elemental iron that accumulates in the body because there is no active excretion of iron.

Pathophysiology

Cardiac iron is regulated through transferrin-mediated uptake mechanisms. During iron overload, transferrin is saturated, and non-transferrin-bound iron is released into the circulation and enters cardiac myocytes in the ferrous form through L-type calcium channels. Iron is then bound to ferritin and transported to lysosomes for degradation and long-term storage in the cardiac myocyte. When the antioxidant capacity of the cell is exceeded, iron is catalyzed by the rapid Fenton reaction producing hydroxyl ions, which is an extremely reactive free radical species that causes cell damage and death. Pathologic iron deposition begins initially within the epicardium and extends to the myocardium and then the endocardium, which helps explain the preservation of systolic function until very late in the disease. Thus, iron deposition is a problem of probably reversible storage than infiltration.[1,2]

A restrictive pattern with LV diastolic dysfunction is usually seen, and the condition may later progress to dilated cardiomyopathy, although both forms may be independently seen. Iron accumulation occurs initially the ventricular myocardium and then the conduction system and the atrial myocardium, thus creating both conduction disorders and tachyarrhythmias due to inhomegeneity of conduction and refractoriness. Right heart failure can also be present early in the course of disease and be independent of left heart failure.

Presentation

Patients may be asymptomatic or present with **exertional shortness of breath**. Severely overloaded patients develop **advanced heart failure** if left untreated, and average survival is less than a year. Paroxysmal **atrial fibrillation** is the most common form of arrhythmia seen and is invariably associated with myocardial damage.

Diagnosis

Iron overload is considered when plasma **transferrin saturation is >55%** and **serum ferritin >200 ng/mL in women or 300 ng/mL in men.**[3,4] Myocardial overload cannot be detected based upon these measurements.

Liver biopsy is the gold standard for diagnosing haemochromatosis, but cardiac biopsy may be negative due to the patchy nature of the disease.

Echocardiography may reveal restrictive or dilated pattern.

Cardiac magnetic resonance is the only non-invasive method, with the potential to assess quantitatively myocardial iron load by using techniques, such as special small magnetic fields called gradients (gradient echo-GE) at specific time intervals (echo time-TE). The time constant of decay for GE-induced relaxation time is known as T2*. The following stratification scheme has been proposed:[5]

- T2* >20 ms indicates low risk for the imminent development of congestive heart failure
- T2* = 10–20 ms indicates intermediate risk of cardiac failure
- T2* <10 ms indicates high risk that needs intensification of chelation therapy.

Therapy

Dietary interventions to minimize or eliminate iron ingestion are not feasible or useful.

Table 42.1 Aetiology of iron overload disorders

Disease	Mechanism	Molecular correlate	Iron deposition
Primary			
Hereditary haemochromatosis	Increased GI absorption with normal diet	Missense mutation	Liver, heart, endocrine glands
Type 1 (*HFE*-related) (AR)		◆ C282Y homozygosity	
		◆ H63D homozygosity	
		◆ C282Y/H63D heterozygosity	
		◆ Other mutations of *HFE*	
Type 2 (juvenile haemochromatosis) (AR)	Increased GI absorption with normal diet	Mutation on *HJV* gene, which encodes for haemojuvelin	Liver, heart, endocrine glands
		Rare form where hepcidin is inactivated	
Type 3 (AR)	Increased GI absorption with normal diet	Mutation of transferrin receptor-2	Liver, heart, endocrine glands
Type 4 (AD)	Increased GI absorption with normal diet	Mutation of *SLC40A1*, which encodes for ferroportin	Macrophages, liver, heart, endocrine glands
Secondary			
a. Iron-loading anaemias (transfusion-related)	Transfusion-related	Mutation causing defect in synthesis of alpha- and beta-globin chains of haemoglobin	Heart, pancreas, pituitary, liver
Thalassaemia	In severe thalassaemia, can have increased GI absorption		
Sickle cell anaemia	Transfusion-related	Substitution of a valine for glutamic acid as the 6th amino acid on the beta-globin chain (HbS)	Liver, heart
Sideroblastic anaemia	Transfusion-related	Hereditary or acquired	Neurons, heart, mitochondria
	Increased GI absorption with normal diet	Ineffective erythropoiesis	
Diamond-Blackfan anaemia	Transfusion-related	Congenital hypoplastic anaemia with decreased erythroid precursors	Heart, liver
Congenital dyserythropoiesis anaemia	Transfusion-related	Ineffective erythropoiesis	Liver, heart, endocrine
Post-stem cell transplant patients	Transfusion-related		Liver, heart
Chronic kidney disease/end-stage renal failure/dialysis	Oral and IV iron supplementation	Decreased erythropoietin	Heart, liver
	Transfusion-related		
b. Dietary overload	Increased dietary intake	Increased diet with predisposing genetic factors (proposed mechanism)	Heart, liver, endocrine
African iron overload			
c. Miscellaneous			
Aceruloplasminaemia (AR)	Inhibition of iron oxidation	Mutations of ceruloplasmin gene	Liver, heart, pancreas
Congenital atransferrinaemia (AR)	Inhibition of iron transportation	Mutations of transferrin gene	Liver, heart, pancreas
Chronic liver diseases			
Hepatitis C and B	In part, increased GI absorption	Not applicable	Liver
Alcohol-induced liver disease	In part, increased GI absorption	Not applicable	Liver
Porphyria cutanea tarda	In part, increased GI absorption	Not established, some are part AD	Liver
Fatty liver disease	In part, increased GI absorption	Not applicable	Liver

AD, autosomal dominant; AR, autosomal recessive; GI, gastrointestinal; IV, intravenous.
Gujja P, *et al*. Iron overload cardiomyopathy: better understanding of an increasing disorder. *J Am Coll Cardiol*. 2010;**56**:1001–12

Phlebotomy removes 400–500 mL of blood (200–250 mg of iron) at each session, thus mobilizing iron from the organs where it is stored for the production of haemoglobin. Early in the disease, this procedure is done up to 1–2 times a week to obtain a target ferritin below 20 ng/mL, and then maintenance phlebotomy is performed 2–4 times a year.[6] Routine monitoring of haemoglobin, ferritin, and haematocrit is essential during maintenance phlebotomy.

Chelation therapy is used in patients not suitable for required phlebotomy, such as those with significant anaemia or malignancy. It removes iron by binding to it and then excreting the compound in urine and bile. Presently available chelators include deferoxamine (subcutaneous or IV) and oral deferiprone.[1]

New therapeutic modalities being studied are: Erythrocytapheresis, novel chelating agents, calcium cannel blockers, hepcidin induction (a gene regulating iron homeostasis in the body), gene therapy in beta thalassaemia or sickle cell disease (genetically modulating autologous stem cells implanted by a vector into the target cell), and donor-matched healthy stem cell transplantation.

References

1. Gujja P, *et al.* Iron overload cardiomyopathy: better understanding of an increasing disorder. *J Am Coll Cardiol.* 2010;**56**:1001–12
2. Wood JC, *et al.* Physiology and pathophysiology of iron cardiomyopathy in thalassemia. *Ann N Y Acad Sci.* 2005;**1054**:386–95
3. Qaseem A, *et al.* Screening for hereditary haemochromatosis: a clinical practice guideline from the American College of Physicians. *Ann Intern Med.* 2005;**143**:517–21
4. Schmitt B, *et al.* Screening primary care patients for hereditary haemochromatosis with transferrin saturation and serum ferritin level: systematic review for the American College of Physicians. *Ann Intern Med.* 2005;**143**:522–36
5. Wood JC. Magnetic resonance imaging measurement of iron overload. *Curr Opin Hematol.* 2007;**14**:183–90
6. Porter JB. Practical management of iron overload. *Br J Haematol.* 2001;**115**:239–52

Chapter 43

Left ventricular non-compaction

Definition

Left ventricular non-compaction (LVNC) (spongy myocardium or fetal myocardium) represents an arrest in the normal process of myocardial compaction, the final stage of myocardial morphogenesis, resulting in persistence of many prominent ventricular trabeculations and deep intertrabecular recesses.[1, 2] There is a bilayered LV wall, consisting of a thick endocardial layer with prominent intertrabecular recesses, with a thin, compact epicardial layer. Trabeculations are typically most evident in the apical portion of the LV (Figure 43.1). Histology is not specific.

Epidemiology

Its prevalence is estimated to be 0.05% in adults,[3] although it is now thought to be higher. However, uncertainty about the assessment of trabeculations that can occur in normal subjects makes true diagnosis difficult to be established.[4]

Aetiology

Left ventricular non-compaction is predominantly a genetic cardiomyopathy with variable presentation, ranging from asymptomatic to severe, and mostly an autosomal dominant mode of inheritance. It has been associated with mutations in sarcomere genes.[5]

Presentation

LVNC presents in several subtypes, such as isolated LVNC with or without arrhythmias, dilated LVNC, hypertophic LVNC, restrictive LVNC, and in association with congenital defects, such as ASD, VSD, AS, and coarctation.

Clinical features include **heart failure, arrhythmias,** and **thromboembolic events**. In infancy, LVNC presents with heart failure.

Diagnosis

The **ECG** is typically abnormal and may show giant voltages.

Echocardiographic diagnosis is based on the presence of:[4,6]

- At least three trabeculations, with a ratio of the distance from the epicardial surface to the trough of the trabecular areas divided by the distance from

the epicardial surface to the trough of the trabecular areas ≤5
- A two-layer structure and a maximal end-systolic ratio of non-compacted to compacted layers of >2
- Colour Doppler evidence of deep perfused intertrabecular recesses.

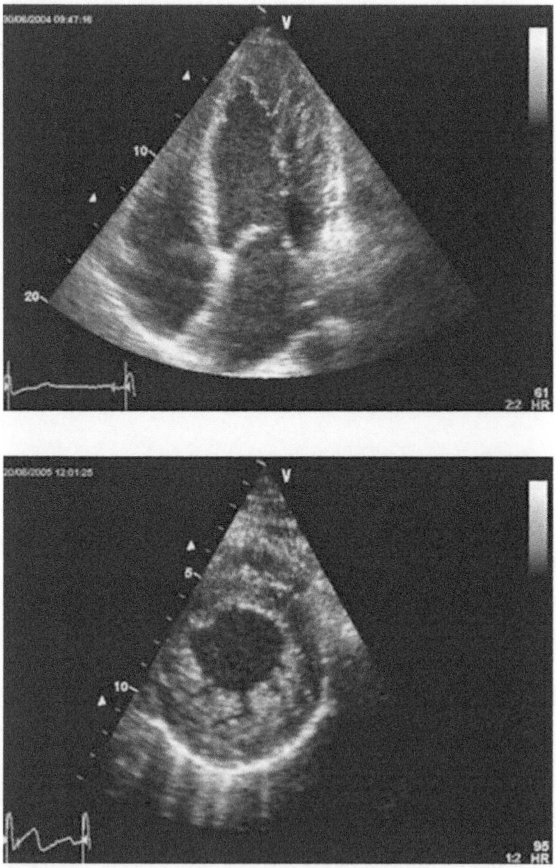

Figure 43.1 Apical echocardiographic view of a non-compacted left ventricle with extended and prominent trabeculations in the apical region and in the lateral wall. Two-layered appearance of the myocardium in a short-axis view of the left ventricle.

Pantazis AA, Elliott PM. Left ventricular noncompaction. *Curr Opin Cardiol.* 2009;**24**:209–13

Such findings, however, can also be found in up to 8% of normal subjects.[4]

Cardiac MRI offers better spatial resolution than echocardiograpy.

Recommendations for **genetic testing** are provided in Table 43.1.[7]

Therapy

Aspirin is administered in all patients while anticoagulation is indicated in patients with dilated LV and LVEF <40% or history of thromboembolism. If LV dysfunction is present, the management is that of heart failure. Arrhythmias are managed as in other cardiomyopathies, and ICD may be considered (ACC/AHA 2008 IIb-C).

The diagnosis of LVNC requires genetic counselling, DNA diagnostics, and cardiological family screening. Prognosis depends on the degree of ventricular dysfunction; reported mortality within 6 years is up to 47%.[2]

References

1. Pantazis AA, *et al.* Left ventricular noncompaction. *Curr Opin Cardiol.* 2009;**24**:209–13
2. Towbin JA. Left ventricular non-compaction: a new form of heart failure. *Heart Fail Clin.* 2010;**6**:453–69, viii
3. Ritter M, *et al.* Isolated non-compaction of the myocardium in adults. *Mayo Clin Proc.* 1997;**72**:26–31
4. Kohli SK, *et al.* Diagnosis of left ventricular non-compaction in patients with left ventricular systolic dysfunction: time for a reappraisal of diagnostic criteria? *Eur Heart J.* 2008;**29**:89–95
5. Hoedemaekers YM, *et al.* The importance of genetic counseling, DNA diagnostics, and cardiologic family screening in left ventricular non-compaction cardiomyopathy. *Circ Cardiovasc Genet.* 2010;**3**:232–9
6. Jenni R, *et al.* Echocardiographic and pathoanatomical characteristics of isolated left ventricular non-compaction: a step towards classification as a distinct cardiomyopathy. *Heart.* 2001;**86**:666–71
7. Ackerman MJ, *et al.* HRS/EHRA expert consensus statement on the state of genetic testing for the channelopathies and cardiomyopathies; this document was developed as a partnership between the Heart Rhythm Society (HRS) and the European Heart Rhythm Association (EHRA). *Heart Rhythm.* 2011;**8**:1308–39

Table 43.1 HRS/EHRA 2011 statement on genetic testing

State of genetic testing for left ventricular non-compaction (LVNC)	
Family members and appropriate relatives following the identification of a LVNC causative mutation in the index case.	I
Patients in whom a cardiologist has established a clinical diagnosis of LVNC, based on examination of the patient's clinical history, family history, and electrocardiographic/echocardiographic phenotype.	IIa

HRS/EHRA 2011 expert consensus statement on the state of genetic testing for the channelopathies and cardiomyopathies. *Heart Rhythm.* 2011;**8**:1308–39.

Part VII

Myocarditis

Relevant guidelines

AHA/ACC/ESC 2007 scientific statement

The role of endomyocardial biopsy in the management of cardiovascular disease: a scientific statement from the American Heart Association, the American College of Cardiology, and the European Society of Cardiology. Endorsed by the Heart Failure Society of America and the Heart Failure Association of the European Society of Cardiology. *Eur Heart J.* 2007;**28**:3076–93.

ACC/AHA/HRS 2008 guidelines for device-based therapy

ACC/AHA/HRS 2008 guidelines for device-based therapy of cardiac rhythm abnormalities: executive summary. *Heart Rhythm.* 2008;**5**:934–55.

Chapter 44

Acute myocarditis

Definition and classification

Myocarditis refers to inflammation of the heart muscle due to exposure to external or self-antigens. Diagnosis is currently based on clinical presentation and non-invasive imaging findings, such as cardiac magnetic resonance.[1,2] Endomyocardial biopsy is subject to sampling error, and the conventional Dallas criteria have been abandoned.[3] Immunohistochemical staining for characterization of inflammation and polymerase chain reaction (PCR) for viral genome detection are more sensitive criteria with prognostic significance.[4]

Clinicopathological classifications were based on early studies that used myocardial biopsies and conventional histology. Lymphocytic infiltration was the more common finding, usually in myocarditis due to viral, immune, or systemic disorders. Eosinophilic (hypereosinophilic syndrome or allergic reactions) and giant cell myocarditis (autoimmune) were also seen. **Fulminant lymphocytic myocarditis** is characterized by fever, rapid onset of syndromes (within 2 weeks), and severe heart failure with haemodynamic compromise. It is thought to be due to high cytokine production, and aggressive treatment with haemodynamic support leads to recovery and good prognosis in most patients.[5] **Acute (non-fulminant) lymphocytic myocarditis** does not have a distinct onset and haemodynamic compromise. The mild form has good prognosis but often results in death or the need for cardiac transplantation when presented with symptoms and LVEF <45%.[6] **Giant cell myocarditis** leads to severe heart failure, ventricular tachycardia or block and has an ominous prognosis, with a mean survival less than 6 months without a transplant.[7] Atrial giant cell myocarditis represents a more benign form.[8] **Acute necrotizing eosinophilic myocarditis** is an aggressive form of eosinophilic myocarditis with acute onset and ominous prognosis.[9] We know now that these well-defined conditions are rare, and patients without distinct clinical pathological manifestations encompass a much broader category.[3,9]

Epidemiology

The true incidence of myocarditis is difficult to determine and is basically unknown, with estimates ranging from 0.12 to 12%.[1] It can be the cause of sudden death in approximately 10% of adults.[1,10]

In patients with human immunodeficiency virus infection, myocarditis was observed in >50% of performed autopsies.[11]

Aetiology

Several infectious and non-infectious diseases can cause myocarditis. Table 44.1 presents the most common ones. In the western world, the most common cause is viral infections. The predominant viral cause of this disease seems to change every decade (coxsackie in the 1980s, adenovirus in the 1990s, and parvovirus B19 since 2000).[12,13] PCR analysis of viral genomes in myocardial tissue from endomyocardial biopsy samples has now replaced viral culture and serial serological testing. The most common viruses identified by this method are parvovirus B19, adenovirus, coxsackie B and other enteroviruses, and human herpes virus 6, cytomegalovirus, hepatitis C, influenza A virus, and HIV. The question of whether these viruses are innocent bystanders or pathological agents still remains.

Pathophysiology

It is not completely understood. Acute infection results in myocyte death and activation of the innate immune response, including interferon gamma, and mobilization of natural killer cells with phagocytosis of released viral particles and cardiac proteins. Most patients recover, but a subset has progression to a second phase, consisting of an adaptive immune response. In this response, antibodies to viral proteins and to some cardiac proteins (including cardiac myosin and β1 or muscarinic receptors) are produced, and effector T cells proliferate. Eventually, the immune response is downregulated, and fibrosis replaces a cellular infiltrate in the myocardium. Under neurohumoral stimulation and haemodynamic stress, the ventricles dilate and may lead to chronic cardiomyopathy.

Presentation

Presentation of disease can vary, ranging from minor symptoms of malaise to acute heart failure. In adults, symptoms of viraemia, such as fever, myalgias, arthralgias, fatigue, and respiratory or gastrointestinal symptoms, frequently, but not always, precede the onset of myocarditis by several days to a few weeks. Children, particularly infants, have a more fulminant presentation than adults. Patients may

Table 44.1 Aetiology of myocarditis

Viral infections
Parvovirus B19
Adenoviruses
Enteroviruses (coxsackie B)
Human herpesvirus 6
Hepatitis C
CMV
Influenza A
EBV
HIV
Bacterial infections
Corynobacterium diphtheria
Mycobacterium
Streptococcus A
Streptococcus pneumoniae
Spirochetal infections
Borrelia burgdorferi (Lyme disease)
Rickettsial infections
Coxiella burnetii (Q fever)
Protozoal Infections
Trypanosoma cruzi (Chagas' disease)
Toxoplasma gondii
Drugs
Anthracyclines
Clozapine
Mesalamine
Ethanol
Hypersensitivity reactions
Smallpox vaccination
Autoimmune diseases
Giant cell myocarditis
Systemic lupus erythematosus
Churg–Strauss syndrome
Systemic diseases
Coeliac disease
Hypereosinophilic syndrome with eosinophilic endomyocardial disease
Sarcoidosis (idiopathic granulomatous myocarditis)

present with dyspnoea, chest pain, palpitations, and decreased exercise tolerance. Fulminant cases are relatively rare. Ocasionally, the condition resembles myocardial infarction. Patients who present with apparently chronic dilated cardiomyopathy, yet with new ventricular arrhythmias or second-degree or third-degree heart block or who do not have a response to optimal care, are more likely to have cardiac sarcoidosis, a granulomatous myocarditis, or, rarely, Chagas' or Lyme disease.[9] Myocarditis may also occur concomitantly with other cardiomyopathies, such as arrhythmogenic right ventricular dysplasia, hypertrophic cardiomyopathy and amyloidosis, or myocardial infarction.[9]

Physical examination

Physical examination may be unremarkable. Fever, tachycardia, S_3 or S_4 gallop, and pulmonary congestion may be present.

Investigations

ECG findings are usually non-specific ST-T changes. Occasionally, ECG changes may mimic myocardial infarction or display arrhythmias or LBBB. Q waves or new LBBB are ominous prognostic signs.[14]

Echocardiography may show global or segmental hypokinesia with or without pericardial effusion. Patients with fulminant myocarditis usually have small cardiac chambers and thickened walls, whereas in acute myocarditis there is marked left ventricular dilation and normal wall thickness.[15] Diastolic filling patterns are abnormal in most patients, and the presence of right ventricular dysfunction is an ominous prognostic sign. Atrial dilatation with atrial wall thickening may suggest atrial giant cell myocarditis.[8]

Cardiac biomarkers of myocardial injury are elevated in up to 35% patients with myocarditis. Increased serum concentrations of troponin T (TnT), and especially troponin I (TnI), are more common than increased levels of CK-MB in both adults and children with acute myocarditis.[16] Serum levels of interleukin-10 on admission are a prognostic predictor of human fulminant myocarditis.[1]

Cardiac MRI provides information about tissue necrosis and fibrosis, hyperaemia, and interstitial oedema, and is a useful prognostic tool.[17] The T2-weighted oedema imaging is used as a tool for evaluating the presence of acute myocardial inflammation. Proposed criteria are presented in Table 44.2.

Endomyocardial biopsy The usefulness of biopsy is limited by sampling error but is necessary in certain conditions, such as suspicion of giant cell or fulminant myocarditis (Table 44.3). There is a reported mortality risk of 0.3% with cardiac biopsy.[18]

Therapy

Because of the high incidence of LV dysfunction, standard therapy for heart failure is administered. Beta-blocker treatment should be avoided in the acute phase of

Table 44.2 Lake Louis CMR diagnostic criteria for myocarditis

In the setting of clinically suspected myocarditis, cardiac MRI findings are consistent with myocardial inflammation if, at least, two of the following criteria are present:
1. Regional or global myocardial signal intensity increase in T2-weighted images
2. Increased global myocardial early enhancement ratio between myocardium and skeletal muscle in gadolinium-enhanced T1-weighted images
3. There is at least one focal lesion with non-ischaemic regional distribution in inversion recovery-prepared gadolinium-enhanced T1-weighted images (late gadolinium enhancement)
Cardiac MRI study is consistent with myocyte injury and/or scar caused by myocardial inflammation if criterion 3 is present
A repeat cardiac MRI study between 1 to 2 weeks after the initial cardiac MRI study is recommended if one if the criteria is present or none of the criteria is present, but onset of symptoms is very recent, and there is strong clinical evidence for myocardial inflammation
The presence of left ventricular dysfunction or pericardial effusion provides additional, supportive evidence for myocarditis

Friedrich MG, *et al*; International Consensus Group on Cardiovascular Magnetic Resonance in Myocarditis. Cardiovascular magnetic resonance in myocarditis: A JACC White Paper. *J Am Coll Cardiol*. 2009;**53**:1475–87.

Table 44.3 AHA/ACC/ESC 2007

Indications for endomyocardial biopsy	
New-onset heart failure of <2 weeks duration associated with a normal-sized or dilated LV and haemodynamic compromise	I-B
New-onset heart failure of 2 weeks to 3 months' duration, associated with a dilated LV left ventricle and new ventricular arrhythmias, second- or third-degree heart block, or failure to respond to usual care within 1–2 weeks	I-B
Heart failure of <3 months duration, associated with a dilated LV and new ventricular arrhythmias, second- or third-degree heart block, or failure to respond to usual care within 1 to 2 weeks	IIa-C
Heart failure associated with a DCM of any duration, associated with suspected allergic reaction and/or eosinophilia	IIa-C
Heart failure associated with suspected anthracycline cardiomyopathy	IIa-C
Heart failure associated with unexplained restrictive cardiomyopathy	IIa-C
Suspected cardiac tumours	IIa-C
Unexplained cardiomyopathy in children	IIa-C
New-onset heart failure of 2 weeks to 3 months' duration, associated with a dilated LV, without new ventricular arrhythmias or second- or third-degree heart block, that responds to usual care within 1 to 2 weeks	IIb-B
Heart failure of <3 months duration, associated with a dilated LV, without new ventricular arrhythmias or second- or third-degree heart block, that responds to usual care within 1 to 2 weeks	IIb-C
Heart failure associated with unexplained HCM, suspected ARVC/D, unexplained ventricular arrhythmias	IIb-C
Unexplained atrial fibrillation	III-C

AHA/ACC/ESC 2007 scientific statement. The role of endomyocardial biopsy in the management of cardiovascular disease. *Eur Heart J*. 2007;**28**:3076–93.

decompensated heart failure and in the very early treatment of fulminant myocarditis.[19] In patients with suspected myocarditis, however, the lack of beta-blocker treatment is associated with poor outcome.[4] Digitalis is contraindicated whereas dihydropyridines may be beneficial but not in acute heart failure.[1] In animal studies, NSAIDs have increased inflammation and mortality and should be given at the lowest required dose in patients with perimyocarditis in whom LV function is clearly normal and who have prominent chest pain from pericarditis.[19]

Physical activity is avoided in the acute phase.

Antiviral therapy (ribavirin) has not proven effective. Interferon has resulted in the elimination of the viral genomes and improved left ventricular function in patients with chronic dilated cardiomyopathy and persistent viral genomes.[20]

Immunosuppressive therapy has not proved useful in patients with acute myocarditis and reduced LV function.[6] However, immunosuppresion with steroids and azathioprine has been found effective in patients with biopsy-proven virus-negative myocarditis and chronic dilated cardiomyopathy.[21,22] It may also be useful in giant-cell myocarditis and sarcoidosis.[19]

In recent-onset dilated cardiomyopathy or myocarditis, **intravenous immune globulin** did not improve LV function.[23] However, in children with acute myocarditis, high-dose gamma-globulin (2 g/kg over 24 hours) resulted in improvement of LV function and a tendency to better survival in the first year after treatment.[24] ICD implantation is indicated in patients with giant cell myocarditis, regardless of LVEF.[25]

Prognosis

It is excellent for adult patients with mild acute lymphocytic myocarditis with preserved LV function. Presentation with heart failure and LVEF >45% carries a bad prognosis, with mortality 50% at 4 years. NYHA class, immunohistological signs of inflammation, and lack of beta-blocker therapy, but not histology (positive Dallas criteria) or viral genome detection, have been related to poor outcome within the next 5 years.[4] Recently, the presence of late gadolinium enhancement on cardiac MRI was found to be the best independent predictor of mortality in biopsy-proven viral myocarditis.[17] Viral persistence in the myocardium has been associated with progressive cardiac dysfunction,[12] and biopsy-proven myocarditis is associated with a 19% mortality over the next 4.7 years.[17] Patients with fulminant viral myocarditis with severe haemodynamic compromise have an excellent long-term prognosis and are more likely to experience complete recovery than patients with acute (non-fulminant) myocarditis;[5] aggressive haemodynamic support is warranted for patients with this condition. In patients with cardiac sarcoidosis or giant cell myocarditis, prognosis depends probably on an early initiated treatment (immunosuppressive therapy or heart transplantation).

References

1. Blauwet LA, *et al.* Myocarditis. *Prog Cardiovasc Dis.* 2010;**52**:274–88
2. Friedrich MG, *et al.* Cardiovascular magnetic resonance in myocarditis: a JACC White Paper. *J Am Coll Cardiol.* 2009;**53**:1475–87
3. Baughman KL. Diagnosis of myocarditis: death of Dallas criteria. *Circulation.* 2006;**113**:593–5
4. Kindermann I, *et al.* Predictors of outcome in patients with suspected myocarditis. *Circulation.* 2008;**118**:639–48
5. McCarthy RE, 3rd, *et al.* Long-term outcome of fulminant myocarditis as compared with acute (non-fulminant) myocarditis. *N Engl J Med.* 2000;**342**:690–5
6. Mason JW, *et al.* A clinical trial of immunosuppressive therapy for myocarditis. The Myocarditis Treatment Trial Investigators. *N Engl J Med.* 1995;**333**:269–75
7. Cooper LT, Jr., *et al.* Idiopathic giant cell myocarditis—natural history and treatment. Multicenter Giant Cell Myocarditis Study Group Investigators. *N Engl J Med.* 1997;**336**:1860–6
8. Larsen BT, *et al.* Atrial giant cell myocarditis: a distinctive clinicopathologic entity. *Circulation.* 2013;**127**:39–47
9. Cooper LT, Jr. Myocarditis. *N Engl J Med.* 2009;**360** :1526–38
10. Fabre A, *et al.* Sudden adult death syndrome and other non-ischaemic causes of sudden cardiac death. *Heart.* 2006;**92**:316–20
11. Anderson DW, *et al.* Prevalent myocarditis at necropsy in the acquired immunodeficiency syndrome. *J Am Coll Cardiol.* 1988;**11**:792–9
12. Kuhl U, *et al.* Viral persistence in the myocardium is associated with progressive cardiac dysfunction. *Circulation.* 2005;**112**:1965–70
13. Mahrholdt H, *et al.* Presentation, patterns of myocardial damage, and clinical course of viral myocarditis. *Circulation.* 2006;**114**:1581–90
14. Nakashima H, *et al.* Q wave and non-Q wave myocarditis with special reference to clinical significance. *Jpn Heart J.* 1998;**39**:763–74
15. Felker GM, *et al.* Echocardiographic findings in fulminant and acute myocarditis. *J Am Coll Cardiol.* 2000; **36**:227–32
16. Smith SC, *et al.* Elevations of cardiac troponin I associated with myocarditis. Experimental and clinical correlates. *Circulation.* 1997;**95**:163–8
17. Grun S, *et al.* Long-term follow-up of biopsy-proven viral myocarditis: predictors of mortality and incomplete recovery. *J Am Coll Cardiol.* 2012;**59**:1604–15
18. Cooper LT, *et al.* The role of endomyocardial biopsy in the management of cardiovascular disease: a scientific statement from the American Heart Association, the American College of Cardiology, and the European Society of Cardiology endorsed by the Heart Failure Society of America and the Heart Failure Association of the European Society of Cardiology. *Eur Heart J.* 2007;**28**:3076–93
19. Kindermann I, *et al.* Update on myocarditis. *J Am Coll Cardiol.* 2012;**59**:779–92
20. Kuhl U, *et al.* Interferon-beta treatment eliminates cardiotropic viruses and improves left ventricular function in patients with myocardial persistence of viral genomes and left ventricular dysfunction. *Circulation.* 2003;**107**:2793–8
21. Frustaci A, *et al.* Randomized study on the efficacy of immunosuppressive therapy in patients with virus-negative inflammatory cardiomyopathy: the TIMIC Study. *Eur Heart J.* 2009;**30**:1995–2002
22. Schultheiss HP, *et al.* The management of myocarditis. *Eur Heart J.* 2011;**32**:2616–25
23. McNamara DM, *et al.* Controlled trial of intravenous immune globulin in recent-onset dilated cardiomyopathy. *Circulation.* 2001;**103**:2254–9
24. Drucker NA, *et al.* Gamma-globulin treatment of acute myocarditis in the pediatric population. *Circulation.* 1994;**89**:252–7
25. ACCF/HRS/AHA/ASE/HFSA/SCAI/SCCT/SCMR. 2013 appropriate use criteria for implantable cardioverter-defibrillators and cardiac resynchronization therapy. *J Am Coll Cardiol.* 2013; doi:10.1016/j.jacc.2012.1012.1017

Part VIII

Pericardial disease

Relevant guidelines

ESC 2004 guidelines on pericardial disease

Guidelines on the diagnosis and management of pericardial diseases executive summary; the Task Force on the diagnosis and management of pericardial diseases of the European Society of Cardiology. *Eur Heart J.* 2004;**25**:587–610.

Chapter 45

Pericardial anatomy and congenital pericardial defects

Pericardial anatomy

The pericardium consists of two layers: the **visceral pericardium** or epicardium, a serous layer that is adjacent to the heart and proximal great vessels, and the **parietal pericardium** which is formed by the outer fibrous sac and the continuation of the visceral pericardium as it reflects back near the origin of the great vessels to form the inner layer of the parietal pericardium. The visceral and parietal layers are separated by the pericardial cavity, which, in healthy people, contains 15 to 50 mL of a plasma ultrafiltrate.[1,2] Intrapericardial pressure is normally similar to pleural pressure, varying from -6 mmHg at end inspiration to -3mm Hg at end expiration. Apart from restraining the heart, the normal pericardium is an important determinant of cardiac filling by limiting chamber dilation and equalizing compliance between the right and left ventricle.

Congenital pericardial defects

They comprise partial left (70%) or right (17%) pericardial absence and have a prevalence of 0.001%. **Total pericardial absence** is rare but predisposes the patient to traumatic aortic dissection.[3] **Partial left side defects** can be complicated by herniation and strangulation of the heart and the coronaries and may require surgical pericardioplasty. On echocardiography, there are prominent right cardiac chambers that may lead to the erroneous diagnosis of RV volume overload or ASD. A **pericardial cyst** is a benign abnormality that is detected as an incidental mass lesion on chest radiography, usually at the right costophrenic angle. The differential diagnosis includes tumours, cardiac chamber enlargement, and diaphragmatic hernia, as well as inflammatory (tuberculosis, cardiac surgery) and echinococcal cysts.

References

1. Khandaker MH, *et al.* Pericardial disease: diagnosis and management. *Mayo Clin Proc.* 2010;**85**:572–93
2. Troughton RW, *et al.* Pericarditis. *Lancet.* 2004;**363**:717–27
3. Maisch B, *et al.* Guidelines on the diagnosis and management of pericardial diseases executive summary; the Task Force on the diagnosis and management of pericardial diseases of the European Society of Cardiology. *Eur Heart J.* 2004;**25**:587–610

Chapter 46

Acute and relapsing pericarditis

Acute pericarditis

Definition

Pericarditis indicates inflammation of the pericardium due to various causes.

Epidemiology

Pericarditis is diagnosed in 0.1% of hospitalized patients and in 5% of patients seen in the emergency room with chest pain but without myocardial infarction.[1]

Aetiology

Causes and estimated incidence of acute pericarditis are presented in Table 46.1. In 80– 90% of patients, the cause is either viral or unknown (idiopathic). Idiopathic pericarditis is thought to be very common because the yield of diagnostic tests to confirm aetiology is relatively low. The major specific causes to be ruled out are tuberculous pericarditis, metastatic neoplasia, and connective tissue disorders.[2]

Presentation

Fever, myalgia, and malaise may occur as a prodromal phase. Body temperature >38°C is uncommon and may indicate purulent pericarditis.

Chest pain is usually sudden in onset, retrosternal, typically accentuated by inspiration and attenuated by leaning forward. Radiation of the pain to trapezius muscle ridges is

Table 46.1 Aetiology and estimated incidence of acute pericarditis

Condition	Estimated incidence (%)
Idiopathic	Most common (>75)[a]
Infectious	
Viral Echovirus and Coxsackievirus, influenza, EBV, CMV, adenovirus, varicella, rubella, mumps, HBV, HCV, HIV, parvovirus B19, and human herpes virus 6	Very common[1]
Bacterial	5–10
Tuberculous,[b] Coxiella burnetii, and rarely: pneumococcus, meningococcus, gonococcus, Haemophilus, staphylococci, Chlamydia, mycoplasma, Legionella, Leptospira, Listeria	5
Fungal Histoplasma and in immunosuppressed patients: aspergillosis, blastomycosis, candida	Rare
Parasites Echinococcus, toxoplasma	Very rare
Autoimmune Mainly systemic sclerosis, SLE, RA	3–5
Myocarditis	30
Myocardial infarction	5–10
Post-cardiotomy	1–1.5
Neoplastic disease	5–7
Metastatic Lung, breast, lymphoma	
Primary Pericardial mesothelioma	Rare
Metabolic	
Uraemia	
Before dialysis	5
After initiation of dialysis	13
Myxoedema	30
Chest wall trauma	Rare
Aortic dissection	Rare
Irradiation	Rare
Drug-related Procainamide, hydralazine, isoniazid, phenytoin (lupus-like syndrome), penicillins (hypersensitivity pericarditis with eosinophilia), doxorubicin, and daunorubicin	Rare

Estimated incidence is derived from studies excluding patients with renal failure, neoplasia, trauma, or radiation.

1: Most idiopathic cases are thought to be viral.

2: In developing countries, the prevalence of tuberculous pericarditis is high: 70–80% of pericarditis in sub-Saharan Africa and ≥90% when associated with HIV infection.

3: Incidence of pericarditis in patients with the specific condition, i.e. myocarditis, myocardial infarction, or myxoedema.

HBV, hepatitis B; HCV, hepatitis C; CMV, cytomegalovirus; HIV, human immunodeficiency virus, SLE, systemic lupus erythematosus; RA, rheumatoid arthritis.

Adapted from: Khandaker MH, *et al.* Pericardial disease: diagnosis and management. *Mayo Clin Proc.* 2010;**85**:572–93,

Guidelines on the diagnosis and management of pericardial diseases executive summary; the Task Force on the diagnosis and management of pericardial diseases of the European Society of Cardiology. *Eur Heart J.* 2004;**25**:587–610,

Imazio M, *et al.* Controversial issues in the management of pericardial diseases. *Circulation.* 2010;**121**:916–28.

probably due to pericarditis because the phrenic nerve that innervates these muscles traverses the pericardium.[3] Dull pain, imitating myocardial ischaemia, may also occur.

Pericardial friction rub is a high-pitched, scratchy sound heard at the left sternal border. It is present in up to 85% of patients but may be transient (repeat examinations are required) and mono-, bi-, or triphasic (corresponding to atrial systole, ventricular systole, and rapid ventricular filling). It is audible throughout the respiratory cycle whereas a pleural rub is absent when respirations are suspended.

Investigations

Diagnostic criteria for pericarditis are:

- Typical chest pain
- Pericardial friction rub
- Suggestive ECG changes (typically widespread ST segment elevation, PR depression)
- New or worsening pericardial effusion (not necessary)
- Elevated CRP (not specific).

ECG Four stages have been described:

- **Stage 1:** diffuse ST segment elevation (epicardial inflammation) and PR segment depression, with reciprocal ST segment depression in the aVR and V_1 leads, within the first hours to days (present in 80% of patients with pericarditis). There can also be PR segment elevation in the aVR (atrial injury)
- **Stage 2:** the ST and PR segments normalize
- **Stage 3:** T wave inversions
- **Stage 4:** ECG normal or T wave inversions persist indefinitely.

Differential diagnosis from myocardial infarction

In MI:

- ST segment elevations are often convex, rather than concave, and regional, rather than widespread
- Q wave formation and loss of R wave voltage often occur
- T wave inversions appear before the ST segments return to baseline
- PR segment depression is uncommon
- Atrioventricular block or ventricular arrhythmias may be seen.

A ratio of the height of the ST segment junction to the height of the apex of the T wave of more than 0.25 in lead V_6 is suggestive of pericarditis (Figure 46.1).[1,4]

Chest X-ray shows cardiomegaly only with effusions >250 mL.

Echocardiography may be normal or show a small effusion. A paediatric transoesophageal echo probe inserted into a chest drain in the pericardial space allows rapid assessment of post-operative effusions.[4]

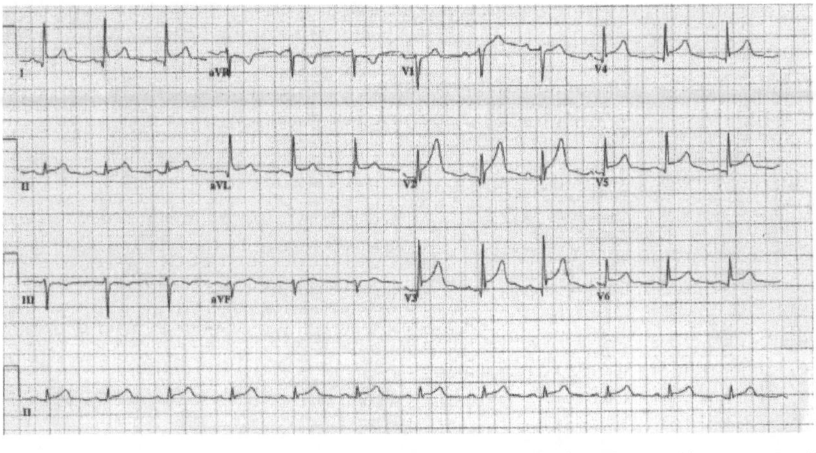

Figure 46.1 Apparently idiopathic acute pericarditis: nearly ubiquitous J (ST) elevations, with corresponding J (ST) depression in aVR. As is common in III and aVF when the QRS axis is horizontal (or these leads are of small voltage), the J (ST) is not elevated. The height of J (ST) is >25% of the height of the T wave peak in V5 and V6. Most PR segments are slightly depressed with respect to the T-P baseline (corresponding PR elevation in aVR). In the clinical setting, a spectrum of myopericardial inflammatory syndromes can be encountered, ranging from pure pericarditis to forms with increasing myocardial involvement (sometimes mimicking an acute coronary syndrome).

Imazio M, *et al*. Controversial issues in the management of pericardial diseases. *Circulation*. 2010;**121**:916–28.

Cardiac CT and MR provide excellent visualization of the pericardium and pericardial space. Normal pericardial thickness is usually 1–2 mm (<4 mm). Delayed gadolinium enhancement on CMR is the most sensitive method for diagnosis of acute pericarditis.[3]

Troponin concentrations are elevated in 30–50% of cases (CK-MB less often) due to epicardial inflammation. Persistence for more than 2 weeks suggests myocarditis. Unlike acute coronary syndromes, troponin elevation is not a negative prognostic marker in myopericardial inflammatory syndromes. Myopericardial inflammatory syndromes (myopericarditis/perimyocarditis) are rather benign clinical syndromes that can be frequently encountered in patients with an initial suspicion of pericarditis.[5]

Viral cultures and **antibody** testing are not useful clinically.

WBC, ESR, and CRP are usually elevated. Marked WBC elevation may suggest purulent pericarditis.

Antinuclear antibody and **rheumatoid factor**, **tuberculin skin test** or **QuantiFERON-TB assay**, and **HIV** testing should be ordered only if the clinical presentation is suggestive of these diseases.

Pericardiocentesis is indicated in tamponade or if purulent, tuberculous, or neoplastic pericarditis is suspected.[3] Pericardial fluid is analysed for cell count, microscopy (including Gram and Ziehl–Nielsen stain), bacterial culture, and cytological examination. PCR techniques can identify causative viruses and *M. tuberculosis* (see also Chapter 47). Immunohistochemistry techniques can identify antibodies to myolemma and sarcolemma in immune-mediated pericarditis.[4] Concentrations of adenosine deaminase activity >30 U/L in pericardial fluid are specific for *M. tuberculosis* and can predict constriction. Carcinoembryonic antigen concentrations are higher (5 ng/mL) in neoplastic than in benign effusions.

Measurements of pH, glucose, protein, and lactic dehydrogenase are also routinely done, but no accepted criteria link such measures to specific causes of pericarditis.[1]

Pericardial biopsy should be considered for patients who have recurrent tamponade despite treatment. In subjects with tamponade of unknown cause, pericardiocentesis and pericardial biopsy provided a diagnosis in 29% and 54% of cases, respectively.[1]

Therapy

When the aetiology is identified, therapy is directed towards treating the underlying cause. Patients with idiopathic or viral myocarditis can be managed as outpatients. **Aspirin** (800 mg every 8 h for 7 days, followed by gradual tapering for 1 additional week) or an NSAID such as **ibuprofen** (400–800 mg tds) for 1–2 weeks, with gastroprotection, usually with proton pump inhibitors, are preferred. Indomethacin should be avoided in patients with coronary artery disease because it decreases coronary blood flow.[2]

In patients who do not respond to aspirin or NSAID therapy for 1 week, **colchicine** (0.5 or 0.6 mg mg bd) is added for up to 3 months. It reduces recurrences and the risk of tamponade or constriction.[6] Its efficacy is greatest in familial Mediterranean fever, but it is also recommended as initial management of acute idiopathic pericarditis in combination with an NSAID.[7] Most common side effect is diarrhoea (8%). It is avoided in patients with severe renal insufficiency, hepatobiliary dysfunction, blood dyscrasias, and gastrointestinal motility disorders.[3] Reduced dosage is recommended for patients < 70 kg (0.5 mg od), or with advanced renal dysfunction or concurrent therapy with moderate to strong inhibitors of CYP3A4 (eg, protease inhibitors, ketoconazole, fluconazole, erythromycin, diltiazem, verapamil) or P-glycoprotein inhibitors (eg, cyclosporine).[7] **Corticosteroids** increase the risk of relapsing pericarditis and should be used only in severely symptomatic cases not responsive to aspirin or NSAIDs. Prednisolone (0.25–0.5 mg/kg/day) with slow tapering (5–10 mg every week) is given for 4 weeks. As initial treatment, steroids should be used only when the underlying cause is an immune-mediated disease, a connective tissue disorder, or uraemic pericarditis.[8] They have also been reported to reduce the incidence of constriction in tuberculous pericarditis.[4]

Relapsing pericarditis

Definition

Relapsing pericarditis is diagnosed when there is a documented first attack of acute pericarditis and evidence of either recurrence or continued activity of pericarditis by means of recurrent pain and one, or more, of the following signs: fever, pericardial friction rub, electrocardiographic changes, echocardiographic evidence of pericardial effusion, and elevations in WBC or ESR or CRP.

Presentation

Recurrences occur in up to 25% of patients with acute pericarditis and usually occur less than 6 weeks after discontinuation or reduction of treatment but may also appear as late as 20 months after the initial attack.[3] They are often seen at discontinuation of, or attempts to wean patients from, anti-inflammatory treatment. Prognosis is good in idiopathic cases, and there is no risk of constriction.

Therapy

Aspirin or a NSAID are given for 2–4 weeks and colchicine is added for up to 6 months.[9] Long-term colchicine is ususally well tolerated with rare discontinuation required for diarroea. Hepatotoxicity and myelosuppression may occur in patients with chronic renal failure. If aspirin or a NSAID is contraindicated, prednisone may be added to colchicine for 2–6 weeks. All doses are as described for acute pericarditis. In truly refractory cases (patients who require prednisolone >25 mg daily), triple therapy with aspirin or NSAID, colchicines, and prednisolone should be administered. Alternatively, azathioprine or methotrexate or cyclophosphamide may be empirically tried.[2]

Rarely, a pericardial window, or even pericardiectomy, may be needed.[8]

References

1. Lange RA, *et al.* Clinical practice. Acute pericarditis. *N Engl J Med.* 2004;**351**:2195–202
2. Imazio M, *et al.* Controversial issues in the management of pericardial diseases. *Circulation.* 2010;**121**:916–28
3. Khandaker MH, *et al.* Pericardial disease: diagnosis and management. *Mayo Clin Proc.* 2010;**85**:572–93
4. Troughton RW, *et al.* Pericarditis. *Lancet.* 2004;**363**:717–27
5. Imazio M, *et al.* Good prognosis for pericarditis with and without myocardial involvement: Results from a multicenter prospective cohort study. *Circulation.* 2013:2013 May 2024. [Epub ahead of print] PubMed PMID: 23709669.
6. Imazio M, *et al.* Colchicine in addition to conventional therapy for acute pericarditis: results of the COchicine for acute PEricarditis (COPE) trial. *Circulation.* 2005;**112**:2012–16
7. Ashikhmina EA, *et al.* Pericardial effusion after cardiac surgery: Risk factors, patient profiles, and contemporary management. *Ann Thorac Surg.* 2010;**89**:112–8
8. Maisch B, *et al.* Guidelines on the diagnosis and management of pericardial diseases executive summary; the Task Force on the diagnosis and management of pericardial diseases of the European Society of Cardiology. *Eur Heart J.* 2004;**25**:587–610
9. Imazio M, *et al.* Colchicine as first-choice therapy for recurrent pericarditis: results of the CORE (COlchicine for REcurrent pericarditis) trial. *Arch Intern Med.* 2005;**165**:1987–91

Chapter 47

Pericardial effusion and cardiac tamponade

Pericardial effusion

Definition

Pericardial effusion refers to accumulation of pericardial fluid, blood, or lymph, in excess of the 15 to 50 mL that are normally found in the pericardium. The pericardial fluid, therefore, can be a transudate, typically occurring in patients with congestive heart failure, or an exudate, which contains a high concentration of proteins and fibrin and can occur with any type of pericarditis, severe infections, or malignancy. The size of effusions can be graded as: small (echo-free space in diastole <10 mm), moderate (10–20 mm), large (≥20 mm), or very large (≥20 mm and compression of the heart).[1] Pericardial effusions can occur with or without cardiac tamponade (Table 47.1).

Pathophysiology

The pressure–volume curve of the normal pericardium is a J-shaped curve. After an initial short shallow portion that allows the pericardium to stretch slightly in response to physiological events, such as changes in posture or volume status, with minimal pressure increase, then the pericardium does not allow further sudden increases of the volume without a marked increase in the intrapericardial pressure. Thus, a slowly accumulating pericardial fluid may allow pericardial distention till the accumulation of 1–2 L of pericardial fluid without the development of cardiac tamponade, whereas a sudden increase of pericardial volume of 100–200 mL, as in haemopericardium, may elevate pericardial pressure to 20–30 mmHg with acute cardiac tamponade.[2]

Clinical settings

Aetiology of pericardial effusion is presented in Table 47.1 (see also acute pericarditis).

Idiopathic chronic pericardial effusion is defined as a collection of pericardial fluid that persists for more than 3 months and has no apparent cause. It is well tolerated for long periods in most patients, but severe tamponade can develop unexpectedly at any time.[3] Large idiopathic chronic effusions (>3 months) have a 30–35% risk of progression to cardiac tamponade.[3] Thus, large pericardial

Table 47.1 Aetiology of pericardial effusion in reported series

Condition	Reported frequency (%)
Idiopathic	7–48
Neoplasia	13–23
Infection	2–27
Connective tissue disease	5–12
Metabolic	6–12
Iatrogenic	0–16

Imazio M, *et al.* Controversial issues in the management of pericardial diseases. Circulation. 2010;**121**:916–28.

effusions (>20 mm) should be drained if they persist for more than a month or if there is right- sided collapse.

Moderate pericardial effusions without tamponade in the setting of **myocardial infarction** may indicate subacute ventricular wall rupture and carry the risk of late true wall rupture[4] (see Chapter 28 on MI).

Neoplasia-associated effusion is seen with lung cancer, breast cancer, melanoma, lymphomas, and leukaemias.[1] Primary tumours, such as mesothelioma, are rare. Intrapericardial instillation of cytostatic/sclerotic agents may be needed. However, approximately 75% of pericardial effusions in patients with malignancies are caused by other causes, such as radiation or opportunistic infections.

Presentation

Symptoms vary according to the speed of pericardial fluid accumulkation and aetiology of the effusion. The patients may be asymptomatic or complain of dysnoea on exertion and fatigue. Nausea (diaphragm), dysphagia (oesophagus), hoarshness (recurrent laryngeal nerve), and hiccups (phrenic nerve) that have been described with large effusions are very rare nowadays.

Physical examination

Usually, physical signs are not specific but quite heart sounds, and elevated jugular venous pressure may be seen. Pulsus paradoxus is typically a sign of tamponade.

Investigations

Most effusions are detected by echocardiography. CT and CMR may allow detection of loculated effusions, pericardial thickening and masses. In the absence of tamponade, pericardiocentesis is indicated if purulent, tuberculous, or neoplastic pericarditis is suspected. Routine analyses to performed on pericardial fluid are presented in Table 47.2.

Therapy

Underlying disease may be detected in up to 60% of cases and therapy is therefore specific.[2] When the diagnosis is unclear or idiopathic and inflammatory markers are elevated, aspirin (750–1000 mg tds) or a NSAID such as ibuprofen (600 mg tds) for 1–2 weeks is given. Combination of aspirin or a NSAID for 2–4 weeks with colchicine (0.5 mg bd for weight ≥70 kg and od for <70 kg) for 3–6 months is considered for recurrent cases, while corticosteroids at low to moderate doses (prednisone 0.2–0.5 mg/kg/day) for 2–4 weeks may be given for specific indications such as systemic inflammatory diseases and pregnancy.[2] Intrapericardial triamcinolone has also been tried in resistant cases.[2]

Pericardiocentesis alone frequently results in the resolution of large **idiopathic** effusions, but recurrence is common. Pericardiectomy should be considered only in highly symptomatic recurrences resistant to medical therapy, and in cases of chronic permanent constriction.[1,2] If smaller pericardial effusions recur and the patient remains asymptomatic without hemodynamic compromise, regular follow-up is recommended. **Subcritical uremic tamponade** often responds to intensified renal dialysis, but if this approach is unsuccessful, drainage is required. When recurrent pericardial effusions are related to **chylopericardium**, the underlying etiology may be thoracic duct obstruction, requiring surgical treatment.[4] In **neoplastic** pericardial disease, pericardial window by open surgery or thoracoscopy, balloon pericardiotomy, and sclerotic local therapy may be needed.

Table 47.2 Routine analyses performed on pericardial fluid

Analysis	Test	Aetiology or feature
General chemistry	Specific gravity >1015, protein level >3 g/dL, protein fluid/serum ratio >0.5, LDH >200 mg/dL, fluid/serum ratio >0.6[a] Glucose, blood cell count	Exudate
Cytology	Cytology (higher volumes of fluid, centrifugation, and rapid analysis improve diagnostic yield)	Cancer
Biomarkers	Tumour markers (i.e. CEA >5 ng/mL or CYFRA 21-1 >100 ng/mL) Adenosine deaminase >40 U/L, IFN-gamma	Cancer
Polymerase chain reaction (PCR)	PCR for specific infectious agents (i.e. TBC)	TBC
Microbiology	Acid-fast bacilli stainging, mycobacterium cultures, aerobic, and anaerobic cultures	TBC Other bacteria

LDH, lactate dehydrogenase; TBC, tuberculosis.

[a] These chemical features have been especially validated for pleural fluid and not pericardial fluid, although generally used also for pericardial effusion.

Imazio M, *et al* Management of pericardial effusion. *Eur Heart J*. 2013;**34**:1186–97.

Cardiac tamponade

Definition

Cardiac tamponade is a life-threatening, slow or rapid compression of the heart due to the pericardial accumulation of fluid, pus, blood, clots, or gas, as a result of effusion, trauma, or rupture of the heart.[5] Occurrences of tamponade can be acute, subacute, regional, or characterized by low pressure.

Pathophysiology

The true filling pressure is the myocardial transmural pressure, which is intracardiac minus pericardial pressure. The increased intrapericardial pressure equals or exceeds the pressure in the right heart chambers, leading to reduced chamber diastolic compliance and impaired filling, collapse of the right atrium and ventricle during diastole and diminished cardiac output. Expansion of the RV is limited to the interventricular septum, resulting in bulging of the RV into the LV, reduced LV compliance and decreased filling of the LV during inspiration (ventricular interdependence). Maximal pericardial pressure in tamponade occurs during end-diastole, when RA volume is minimal. When fluid collection is slow, the pericardium can stretch to accommodate a large volume with minimum compromise of cardiac function, partly due to systemic neurohumoral responses that compensate for reduced cardiac filling. Thus, intrapericardial hemorrhage from wounds or cardiac rupture occurs in the context of a relatively stiff pericardium and quickly overwhelms the pericardial capacity to stretch before most compensatory mechanisms can be activated, whereas in the case of a slow increase in pericardial volume as a result of inflammation, 2 liters or more may accumulate before critical, life-threatening tamponade occurs.[5]

Clinical settings

Pericarditis Tamponade is reported in about 15% of patients with idiopathic pericarditis but in as many as 60% of those with neoplastic, tuberculous, or purulent pericarditis.[6]

Myocardial infarction When pericardial effusion in a parasternal short-axis view exceeds 10 mm in the setting of myocardial infarction, the risk of free wall rupture is high, and pericardial aspiration for measurement of haematocrit in the effusion is useful.[7] Pericardial effusion indicates increased mortality in this setting, and early pericardiocentesis may be lifesaving.

Iatrogenic In the current era, invasive cardiac procedures that require anticoagulation and left atrial access using trans-septal puncture have become one of the most common causes of acute tamponade.[8] Its incidence is not exactly known, but it is estimated 1–6% (Table 47.3). In iatrogenic cardiac perforation, the development and perforation of tamponade depends on the state of anticoagulation, LV and PA pressures, and chamber perforated. RA perforation in the absence of anticoagulation may be well tolerated. LA perforation is more serious because trans-septal access involves anticoagulation, and LA pressure is higher than the RA pressure. RV (RV wall ≥4 mm), and especially LV (LV wall ≥10 mm), perforation may be tolerated, unless severe pulmonary hypertension or aortic stenosis pre-exist, respectively.[8]

Post-operative tamponade is more frequent after valve surgery than CABG and may be seen early or late (5 days to 2 weeks) after the operation. Reported incidence of post-operative pericardial effusions is 1.5% and of tamponade 0.7%.[9] Later, after cardiac surgery, the pericardium may be adherent to the myocardium and thus prevent the development of tamponade; however, this is the case universally, and posterior localized effusion that may not be accessible to pericardiocentesis may be seen.

Presentation

Presentation depends on the type and severity of tamponade. Patients are usually weak and faint with tachypnoea and possibly chest pain. The initial symptom may be also one of the complications of tamponade, such as renal failure or right

Table 47.3 Incidence of iatrogenic tamponade

Procedure	Incidence (%)	Timing
Atrial fibrillation ablation	1–6	During procedure, rarely later
Pacemakers	1.7	Within 7 days of the procedure
ICD	3.8	Within 30 days of the procedure
Percutaneous mitral valvuloplasty	4	During procedure, rarely later
LA appendage occlusion	1.8–3	During procedure
PFO closure	1.5	During procedure
PCI	0.2	During procedure, rarely later

Holmes DR Jr, *et al*. Iatrogenic pericardial effusion and tamponade in the percutaneous intracardiac intervention era. *JACC Cardiovasc Interv*. 2009;**2**:705–717.

upper quadrant pain due to hepatic congestion. Cardiac tamponade should also be considered in patients in cardiogenic shock, especially if they have increased jugular venous pressure or pulseless electrical activity.

Physical examination

Systemic arterial hypotension, tachycardia, quiet heart sounds, elevated jugular venous pressure, and pulsus paradoxus are the hallmarks of cardiac tamponade. However, most physical signs are not specific.

Systemic arterial hypotension is the rule, but aortic pressure may increase in the early stages of acute tamponade in hypertensive patients due to sympathetic response to pericardial irritation.[5] Patients may also be normotensive, with low pressure tamponade in patients with hypovolaemia or systemic disease.

Tachycardia may not be present in patients with uraemia or hypothyroidism. Bradycardia due to vasovagal reaction may also be initially seen, especially in iatrogenic tamponade.

Heart sounds are quiet, but patients with pre-existing cardiomegaly and anterior or apical pericardial adhesions may have active pulsations.

JVP is usually elevated, with preservation of the x descent but absence of the y descent. However, in acute haemopericardium, there is insufficient time for blood volume to increase, and JVP pulsations may be exaggerated without distension.

Pulsus paradoxus (>10 mmHg fall in systolic pressure during inspiration) may also be seen with pulmonary embolism, chronic obstructive pulmonary disease, constriction, and rarely in pregnancy. Conditions that can impede the detection of pulsus paradoxus in tamponade are: pericardial adhesions, marked left or right ventricular hypertrophy, severe AR, and ASD.

Pericardial rub can be heard in inflammatory effusions.

Kussmaul sign (JVP elevation during inspiration) can be seen but unusually in the absence of pericardial constriction.

Investigations

ECG may show low QRS voltage (<0.5 V in limb leads) and signs of pericarditis. Electrical alternans, defined as the alteration of QRS complex amplitude or axis between beats, are specific for cardiac tamponade, especially when combined with P wave alteration.[5]

Chest X-ray shows cardiomegaly with effusions >250 mL.

Echocardiography reveals diastolic collapse of the RA and early diastolic collapse of the RV when the intrapericardial pressure exceeds intracavitary pressure (Figure 47.1). RA collapse may also be seen in patients with hypovolaemia, but persistence of RA collapse for more than one-third of the cardiac cycle is highly sensitive and specific for tamponade. During inspiration, the interventricular septum bulges into the LV due to increased systemic venous return to the RV and limited expansion of the RV free wall. With expiration, the transmitral pressure gradient increases, and systemic venous return decreases with reversal of diastolic flow in the hepatic veins.

Left atrial collapse is very specific but not sensitive for tamponade.[4]

The inferior vena cava is dilated, with less than a 50% diameter reduction during inspiration.

When cardiac tamponade is due to aortic dissection or cardiac free wall rupture, a coagulated mass may be seen within the pericardium.

Cardiac CT or **transoesophageal echocardiography** can diagnose loculated pericardial effusions or haematoma, especially after cardiac surgery, not detectable by transthoracic echocardiography.

Cardiac catheterization, if performed, reveals inspiratory increase of the right and concomitant decrease of the left pressure, progressively increasing RA prressure and intracardiac diastolic pressure equilibration (15–30 mmHg).

Therapy

The presence of haemodynamic compromise requires urgent pericardiocentesis or surgical removal of pericardial fluid.

For **pericardiocentesis**, the needle is usually inserted between the xiphoid process and the left costal margin at a 15-degree angle to bypass the costal margin, and then its hub is depressed so that the point is aimed toward the left shoulder and is advanced slowly until fluid is aspirated. Ideally, this should be done in the catheterization laboratory or under echocardiographic guidance and with concomitant administration of IV saline. Attaching an electrode to the needle may provide misleading results. For prolonged drainage, an angiographic pigtail catheter may be left in the pericardium until the amount of fluid drained is <50 mL/day. Pericardiocentesis is relatively contraindicated in tamponade due to aortic dissection which represents a surgical emergency.

Surgical drainage is preferable in patients with intrapericardial bleeding or with clotted pericardium.

In hypotensive patients, rapid **volume expansion** with saline or dextran should be provided, especially if the systolic blood pressure is <100 mm Hg.[10] In patients without hypotension and hypovolaemia, fluid infusion may precipitate tamponade.[5]

Inotropic support is controversial since inotropic stimulation of the heart is often already maximal in tamponade.

Mechanical ventilation with positive airway pressure should be avoided because it further decreases cardiac

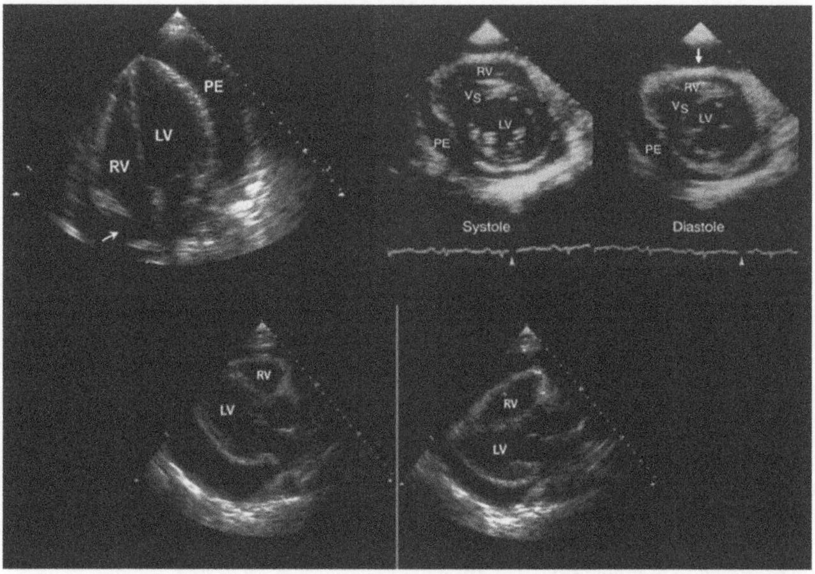

Figure 47.1 Two-dimensional echocardiographic features of cardiac tamponade. A: Apical 4-chamber view showing late diastolic collapse of the right atrium (RA, arrow). Persistence of RA collapse for more than one-third of the cardiac cycle is highly sensitive and specific for tamponade. B: Early diastolic collapse (arrow) of the right ventricle (RV) is specific for tamponade. C: Parasternal long-axis views showing the swinging motion of the heart within the pericardial cavity of a large pericardial effusion; the swinging motion is responsible for the electrocardiographic manifestation termed electrical alternans.

LV, left ventricle; PE, pericardial effusion; VS, ventricular septum.

Khandaker MH, *et al*. Pericardial disease: diagnosis and management. *Mayo Clin Proc* 2010; **85**:572–593.

output. In patients with cardiac arrest and a large amount of pericardial fluid, external cardiac compression has little or no value because there is little room for additional filling and because, even if systolic pressure rises, diastolic pressure falls and, in doing so, reduces coronary perfusion pressure.[5]

References

1. Maisch B, *et al.* Guidelines on the diagnosis and management of pericardial diseases executive summary; the Task Force on the diagnosis and management of pericardial diseases of the European Society of Cardiology. *Eur Heart J.* 2004;**25**:587–10
2. Imazio M, Adler Y. Management of pericardial effusion. *Eur Heart J.* 2013;**34**:1186–97
3. Sagrista-Sauleda J, *et al.* Long-term follow-up of idiopathic chronic pericardial effusion. *N Engl J Med.* 1999;**341**:2054–9
4. Khandaker MH, *et al.* Pericardial disease: diagnosis and management. *Mayo Clin Proc.* 2010;**85**:572–93
5. Spodick DH. Acute cardiac tamponade. *N Engl J Med.* 2003;**349**:684–90
6. Lange RA, *et al.* Clinical practice. Acute pericarditis. *N Engl J Med.* 2004;**351**:2195–202
7. Figueras J, *et al.* Hospital outcome of moderate to severe pericardial effusion complicating ST elevation acute myocardial infarction. *Circulation.* 2010;**122**:1902–9
8. Holmes DR, Jr., *et al.* Iatrogenic pericardial effusion and tamponade in the percutaneous intracardiac intervention era. *JACC Cardiovasc Interv.* 2009;**2**:705–17
9. Ashikhmina EA, *et al.* Pericardial effusion after cardiac surgery: risk factors, patient profiles, and contemporary management. *Ann Thorac Surg.* 2010;**89**:112–18
10. Sagrista-Sauleda J, *et al.* Hemodynamic effects of volume expansion in patients with cardiac tamponade. *Circulation.* 2008;**117**:1545–9

Chapter 48

Constrictive pericarditis

Definition

Constrictive pericarditis is due to fibrous thickening and/or calcification of the pericardial sac, with resultant abnormal diastolic filling with raised filling pressures.

Aetiology

Idiopathic, **cardiac surgery**, and **mediastinal radiation therapy** are the main causes in the western world whereas **tuberculosis** is a major cause in immunosuppressed patients and, especially, in developing countries. More rare causes of constrictive pericarditis include **connective tissue disorders**, **neoplasias**, **asbestosis**, **sarcoidosis**, **trauma**, **drugs**, and **uraemic pericarditis**. Constrictive pericarditis is a relatively rare complication of viral or idiopathic acute pericarditis (<0.5%) but, in contrast, is relatively frequent for specific aetiologies, especially **bacterial**.[1]

Pathophysiology

In constrictive pericarditis, diastolic filling is restricted by a non-compliant, inflamed, scarred, or calcified pericardium after an initial expansion of the myocardium. This results in dissociation of intracardiac and intrathoracic pressures during respiration and interdependence of ventricular filling. On inspiration, intrathoracic pressure decreases but is not transmitted to the left atrium. A reduced pulmonary vein to left atrium pressure gradient produces a fall in flow into the left atrium and left ventricle. Decreased left ventricular filling during diastole allows more room for right ventricular filling, which leads to a septal shift and an increase in right-sided inflow. The exact opposite sequence occurs in expiration.[2] Rapid completion of ventricular filling in early diastole may result in the typical ventricular diastolic waveform of dip and plateau (square root sign) configuration and resembles restrictive cardiomyopathy. Increased ventricular interdependence and discordant changes in LV and RV systolic pressures during respiration are features of pericardial constriction (Figures 48.1 and 48.2).

Presentation

Patients usually present with symptoms and signs of right heart failure, such as increased JVP and peripheral oedema. Symptoms of left ventricular failure, such as dyspnoea on exertion, may also appear. A history of pericarditis, cardiac surgery, or irradiation may be derived within the previous 3–12 months. Rarely, constriction may appear within days after cardiac surgery.

Physical examination

JVP is elevated with a prominent y descent (Friedrich's sign) in sinus rhythm.

Kussmaul sign, i.e. a rise or failure of JVP to decrease with inspiration, may be present and typically occurs in constrictive pericarditis.

Pericardial knock may be present but is difficult to distinguish from an S_3. Both coincide with the nadir of the y descent.

Hepatomegaly (pulsatile liver may be felt), **ascites**, **pleural effusions**, and significant **exercise intolerance** are seen in progressed disease.

Investigations

Chest X-ray reveals pericardial calcification in 25% of patients with constrictive pericarditis and is not associated with a specific aetiology. However, pericardial thickening and calcification is generally less prominent in non-tuberculous constriction.[3]

ECG shows non-specific ST-T changes and, perhaps, low voltage QRS. Conduction abnormalities are more common in restrictive cardiomyopathy.

Echocardiography

- **Increased pericardial thickness** may be present (not necessarily) and can be better appreciated by transoesophageal echocardiography.
- **Abnormal ventricular septal motion**.

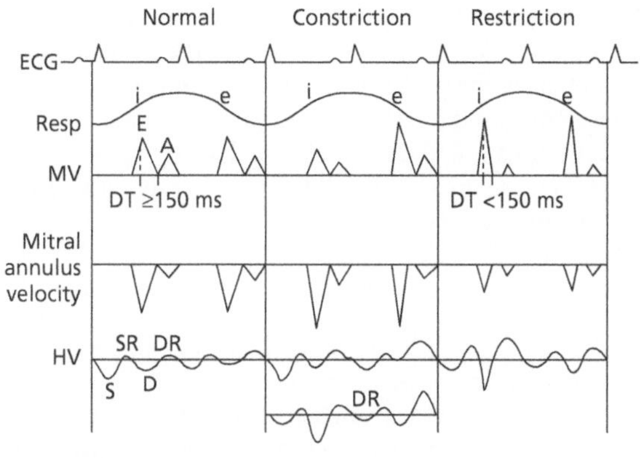

Figure 48.1 Schematic diagram of Doppler echocardiographic features in constrictive pericarditis vs restrictive cardiomyopathy. Schematic illustration of Doppler velocities from mitral inflow (MV), mitral annulus velocity, and hepatic vein (HV). Electrocardiographic (ECG) and respirometer (Resp) recordings indicating inspiration (i) and expiration (e) are also shown.

A, atrial filling; D, diastolic flow; DR, diastolic flow reversal; DT, deceleration time; E, early diastolic filling; S, systolic flow; SR, systolic flow reversal. Stippled areas under the curve represent flow reversal.
Khandaker MH, *et al.* Pericardial disease: diagnosis and management. *Mayo Clin Proc* 2010; **85**:572–593.

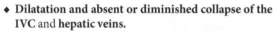

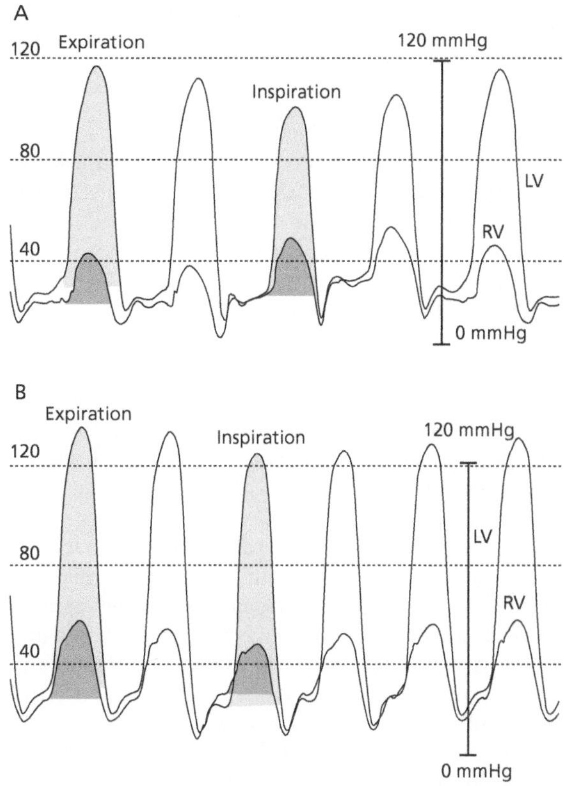

Figure 48.2 Ventricular interdependence and respiratory variation in ventricular filling in constrictive pericarditis and restrictive cardiomyopathy. Both conditions have early rapid filling and elevation and end-equalization of the left ventricular (LV) and right ventricular (RV) pressures at end expiration. A: Discordant pressure change between the LV and RV in constrictive pericarditis. During inspiration, there is an increase in the area of the RV pressure curve (orange shaded area) compared with expiration. The area of the LV pressure curve (yellow shaded area) decreases during inspiration as compared with expiration. Ejection time also varies with respiration in opposite directions in LV and RV. B: Concordant pressure change between the LV and RV in restrictive cardiomyopathy. During inspiration, there is a decrease in the area of the RV pressure curve (orange shaded area) as compared with expiration. The area of the LV pressure curve (yellow shaded area) is unchanged during inspiration as compared with expiration.

Khandaker MH, *et al.* Pericardial disease: diagnosis and management. *Mayo Clin Proc* 2010; **85**:572–593.

- **Dilatation and absent or diminished collapse of the IVC** and **hepatic veins.**
- **Preserved or increased early diastolic filling** (medial mitral annulus early diastolic velocity—E), which is an important distinction from restrictive cardiomyopathy in which the E is diminished with a cut-off value of 7 cm/s.[4] The velocity of propagation of early ventricular inflow from colour M-mode and the early mitral annular velocity from tissue Doppler imaging are markers of myocardial relaxation, and are typically normal in constrictive pericarditis.
- **Increased hepatic vein flow reversal with expiration,** reflecting the ventricular interaction and the dissociation of the intracardiac and intrathoracic pressures.

Cardiac catheterization

Volume challenge may be needed for full expression of haemodynamic signs.

Prominent x descent (occasionally absent) and y descents on the atrial waveform may produce M or W waveforms. One of the most reliable diagnostic criteria is the ratio of RV to LV systolic area during inspiration and expiration (Figure 48.2).[5]

Cardiac CT and cardiac MR

They can demonstrate increased pericardial thickness (>4 mm) and calcification. Up to 20% of patients do not have thickened pericardium.[6] High sensitivity and specificity have been reported for CMR.[3]

Differential diagnosis

Differentiation from **restrictive cardiomyopathy** is presented in Table 37.4 in Chapter 37 on restrictive cardiomyopathy. Thickened pericardium, significant respiratory variation in transmitral, pulmonary vein, and tricuspid inflows, and preserved indices of myocardial relaxation (velocity of propagation and early mitral annular velocity) are characteristics of pericarditis. In certain cases, endomyocardial biopsy or explorative thoracotomy may still be necessary for a definitive diagnosis. **Tricuspid regurgitation**, usually due to a pacemaker or ICD lead impinging on the tricuspid valve, may result in right heart failure and equalization of diastolic pressures simulating constrictive pericarditis. If echocardiography cannot establish the diagnosis, simultaneous recordings of LV and RV pressures in the catheter laboratory reveals that, on inspiration, the difference between RV and LV EDP becomes more prominent in TR.[7]

Therapy

Medical therapy is palliative by means of removing fluid by diuretics. In chronic constrictive pericarditis, surgical complete pericardiectomy is necessary and should be undertaken before calcification occurs but is associated with an operative mortality of up to 6%.[8,9] Advanced age, NYHA class, and, especially, history of radiation are predictors of a poor outcome.[10] In a subset of patients in whom constriction is due to reversible inflammation, it may resolve after 2 or 3 months, either spontaneously or with treatment with anti-inflammatory agents and/or steroids (**transient constrictive pericarditis**). In patients with effusion in the context of constriction (**effusive-constrictive pericarditis**), evacuation of the pericardium may, in some cases, result in resolution of the restrictive physiology.[11] Patients with systemic inflammation, as detected by cardiac MRI and biomarkers, such as ESR and CRP, may respond to anti-inflammatory medication.[12]

References

1. Imazio M, *et al.* Risk of constrictive pericarditis after acute pericarditis. *Circulation.* 2011;**124**:1270–5
2. Hatle LK, *et al.* Differentiation of constrictive pericarditis and restrictive cardiomyopathy by Doppler echocardiography. *Circulation.* 1989;**79**:357–70
3. Troughton RW, *et al.* Pericarditis. *Lancet.* 2004;**363**: 717–27
4. Rajagopalan N, *et al.* Comparison of new Doppler echocardiographic methods to differentiate constrictive pericardial heart disease and restrictive cardiomyopathy. *Am J Cardiol.* 2001;**87**:86–94
5. Talreja DR, *et al.* Constrictive pericarditis in the modern era: novel criteria for diagnosis in the cardiac catheterization laboratory. *J Am Coll Cardiol.* 2008;**51**:315–19
6. Khandaker MH, *et al.* Pericardial disease: diagnosis and management. *Mayo Clin Proc.* 2010;**85**:572–93
7. Jaber WA, *et al.* Differentiation of tricuspid regurgitation from constrictive pericarditis: novel criteria for diagnosis in the cardiac catheterisation laboratory. *Heart.* 2009;**95**:1449–54
8. Bertog SC, *et al.* Constrictive pericarditis: etiology and cause-specific survival after pericardiectomy. *J Am Coll Cardiol.* 2004;**43**:1445–52
9. Schwefer M, *et al.* Constrictive pericarditis, still a diagnostic challenge: comprehensive review of clinical management. *Eur J Cardiothorac Surg.* 2009;**36**:502–10
10. Ling LH, *et al.* Constrictive pericarditis in the modern era: evolving clinical spectrum and impact on outcome after pericardiectomy. *Circulation.* 1999;**100**:1380–6
11. Sagrista-Sauleda J, *et al.* Effusive-constrictive pericarditis. *N Engl J Med.* 2004;**350**:469–75
12. Feng D, *et al.* Cardiac magnetic resonance imaging pericardial late gadolinium enhancement and elevated inflammatory markers can predict the reversibility of constrictive pericarditis after anti-inflammatory medical therapy: a pilot study. *Circulation.* 2011;**124**:1830–7

Part IX

Tachyarrhythmias

Relevant guidelines

SVT

ACC/AHA/ESC 2003 guidelines on SVT

ACC/AHA/ESC guidelines for the management of patients with supraventricular arrhythmias—executive summary. *Circulation*. 2003;**108**:1871–909.

PACES/HRS 2012 statement on WPW syndrome

PACES/HRS expert consensus statement on the management of the asymptomatic young patient with a Wolff–Parkinson–White (WPW, ventricular preexcitation) electrocardiographic pattern: developed in partnership between the Pediatric and Congenital Electrophysiology Society (PACES) and the Heart Rhythm Society (HRS). *Heart Rhythm*. 2012;**9**:1006–24.

ESC 2011 guidelines on pregnancy

ESC guidelines on the management of cardiovascular diseases during pregnancy. *Eur Heart J*. 2011;**32**:3147–97.

AF

ACCF/AHA 2013 guidelines on AF

Management of patients with atrial fibrillation (compilation of 2006 ACCF/AHA/ESC and 2011 ACCF/AHA/HRS recommendations): A report of the American College of Cardiology/American Heart Association Task Force on practice guidelines. *J Am Coll Cardiol*. 2013;**61**:1935–44

HRS/EHRA 2011 consensus statement on genetic testing

HRS/EHRA expert consensus statement on the state of genetic testing for the channelopathies and cardiomyopathies. *Europace*. 2011;**13**:1077–109.

ACCF/AHA 2013 guideline on heart failure

2013 ACCF/AHA Guideline for the Management of Heart Failure. *JACC* 2013; doi: 10.1016/j.jacc.2013.05.019

ACCF/AHA guidelines on UA-NSTEMI 2012

2012 ACCF/AHA Focused Update Incorporated Into the ACCF/AHA 2007 Guidelines for the Management of Patients With Unstable Angina/Non–ST-Elevation Myocardial Infarction. *JACC* doi.org/10.1016/j.jacc.2013.01.014

AHA/ASA 2013 guidelines for acute ischemic stroke

Guidelines for the early management of patients with acute ischemic stroke: a guideline for healthcare professionals from the American Heart Association/American Stroke Association. *Stroke*. 2013;**44**:870–947.

HRS/EHRA/ECAS 2012 expert consensus statement on catheter and surgical ablation

HRS/EHRA/ECAS expert consensus statement on catheter and surgical ablation of atrial fibrillation: recommendations for patient selection, procedural techniques, patient management and follow-up, definitions, endpoints, and research trial design. *Europace*. 2012;**14**:528–606.

ESC 2010 guidelines on AF

Guidelines for the management of atrial fibrillation: the Task Force for the management of atrial fibrillation of the European Society of Cardiology (ESC). *Eur Heart J*. 2010;**31**: 2369–429.

ESC on AF 2012 update on AF

2012 focused update of the ESC guidelines for the management of atrial fibrillation: an update of the 2010 ESC guidelines for the management of atrial fibrillation. *Europace*. 2012;**14**:1385–413.

ESC 2012 guidelines on heart failure

ESC guidelines for the diagnosis and treatment of acute and chronic heart failure 2012. *Eur Heart J*. 2012;**33**:1787–847.

ESC 2011 guidelines

ESC guidelines on the management of cardiovascular diseases during pregnancy. *Eur Heart J*. 2011;**32**:3147–97.

VT

ACC/AHA ESC 2006 guidelines on ventricular arrhythmias

ACC/AHA ESC 2006 guidelines for management of patients with ventricular arrhythmias and the prevention of sudden cardiac death. *Circulation*. 2006;**114**:e385–484.

ACCF/AHA/HRS 2012 guidelines for device-based therapy of cardiac rhythm abnormalities

2012 ACCF/AHA/HRS focused update incorporated into the ACCF/AHA/HRS 2008 guidelines for device-based therapy of cardiac rhythm abnormalities. *J Am Coll Cardiol*. 2013;**61**:e6–75.

ACCF/HRS/AHA/ASE/HFSA/SCAI/SCCT/SCMR 2013 appropriate use criteria

ACCF/HRS/AHA/ASE/HFSA/SCAI/SCCT/SCMR 2013 appropriate use criteria for implantable cardioverter-defibrillators and cardiac resynchronization therapy. *J Am Coll Cardiol*. 2013; doi:10.1016/j.jacc.2012.12.017

AHA 2010 guidelines for cardiopulmonary resuscitation

2010 American Heart Association guidelines for cardiopulmonary resuscitation and emergency cardiovascular care. *Circulation*. 2010;**122**(18 Suppl 3): Part 1: executive summary: S640–56, Part 6: electrical therapies: S06–719, Part 8: adult advanced cardiovascular life support: S729–67, Part 10: acute coronary syndromes: S787–817.

ACCF/AHA 2013 guideline on heart failure.

ACCF/AHA 2013 Guideline for the Management of Heart Failure. *JACC* 2013; doi: 10.1016/j.jacc.2013.05.019

ESC 2011 guidelines on pregnancy

ESC guidelines on the management of cardiovascular diseases during pregnancy. *Eur Heart J*. 2011;**32**:3147–97.

EHRA/HRS 2009 expert consensus on catheter ablation of ventricular arrhythmias

EHRA/HRS expert consensus on catheter ablation of ventricular arrhythmias. *Europace*. 2009;**11**:771–817.

ESC 2012 guidelines on heart failure

ESC guidelines for the diagnosis and treatment of acute and chronic heart failure 2012. *Eur Heart J*. 2012;**33**:1787–847.

Chapter 49

Classification of tachyarrhythmias, mechanisms of arrhythmogenesis, and acute management

Definitions and classification

Definitions

The term **tachyarrhythmia** (Greek *tachy* = fast, and *arrhythmia* = rhythm disturbance) is used to describe conditions in which the heart rate exceeds the conventional number of 100 bpm, either in response to metabolic demand or other stimuli or due to disease. The term **tachycardia** requires more than 3 (or 5) consecutive beats, otherwise, we are talking about premature beats or extrasystoles. A tachycardia is called **sustained** when lasting more than 30 s, **paroxysmal** when it starts and stops abruptly, and **incessant** or **permanent** when it occurs most of the time with annoying perseverance. The term **chronic** refers to incessant tachycardias which occur on a long-term basis and may result in cardiac dilatation and impairment of ventricular contractility.

Classification of arrhythmias

Traditionally, tachyarrhythmias have been classified as **ventricular** or **supraventricular**. The term supraventricular has been used to describe all kinds of tachycardias, apart from ventricular tachycardias, and has, therefore, included tachycardias, such as atrioventricular nodal reentry or atrioventricular reentry due to accessory connections. In Table 49.1, we propose a more rational classification. From a clinical point of view, tachyarrhythmias can also be classified as narrow or wide QRS tachycardias, depending on the QRS duration during the arrhythmia (Table 49.2). Although a detailed electrophysiological study is usually necessary for a definite diagnosis and localization of the focus of the tachycardia, the 12-lead ECG can provide information for the differential diagnosis of most of these rhythms.

Table 49.1 Classification of tachyarrhythmias

Atrial arrhythmias
Sinus tachycardia
Physiological sinus tachycardia
Inappropriate sinus tachycardia
Sinus reentrant tachycardia
Atrial tachycardia
Focal atrial tachycardia
Multifocal atrial tachycardia
Macro-reentrant tachycardia
Isthmus-dependent atrial flutter
Non-isthmus-dependent atrial flutter
Atrial fibrillation
Atrioventricular junctional arrhythmias
Atrioventricular nodal reentrant tachycardia
Non-paroxysmal junctional tachycardia
Focal junctional tachycardia
Non-reentrant atrioventricular nodal tachycardia
Atrioventricular arrhythmias
Atrioventricular reentrant tachycardia
Ventricular arrhythmias
Monomorphic ventricular tachycardia
Accelerated idioventricular rhythm
Polymorphic ventricular tachycardia
Pleomorphic ventricular tachycardia
Bidirectional ventricular tachycardia
Torsade de pointes
Ventricular flutter
Ventricular fibrillation

Classification of antiarrhythmic drugs

The Vaughan-Williams classification, as modified by Singh and Harrison (Table 49.3), of the antiarrhythmic agents is outdated and oversimplistic but more practical than that proposed by the Sicilian Gambit.[1] Most drugs have additional modes of action.

Electrophysiological mechanisms of arrhythmogenesis

The action potential

Cardiac electrical activity starts by the spontaneous excitation of 'pacemaker cells' in the sinoatrial node in the right atrium and spreads through sinoatrial exit pathways (see Chapter 62 on bradyarrhythmias). By travelling through intercellular gap junctions (cell-to-cell connections), the excitation wave depolarizes adjacent atrial myocytes, ultimately resulting in excitation of the atria. The excitation wave then propagates via the atrioventricular node and the Purkinje fibres to the ventricles where ventricular myocytes are depolarized, resulting in excitation of the ventricles. Depolarization of each atrial or ventricular myocyte is represented by the initial action potential (AP) upstroke

Table 49.2 Differential diagnosis of tachyarrhythmias

Narrow QRS (<120 ms) tachycardias
Regular
Physiological sinus tachycardia
Inappropriate sinus tachycardia
Sinus reentrant tachycardia
Focal atrial tachycardia
Atrial flutter
Atrial fibrillation with AV block and a junctional escape rhythm
Atrioventricular nodal reentrant tachycardia
Non-paroxysmal or focal junctional tachycardia
Orthodromic atrioventricular reentrant tachycardia
Idiopathic ventricular tachycardia (especially fascicular VT)
Irregular
Atrial fibrillation
Atrial flutter with varying block
Multifocal atrial tachycardia
Wide QRS tachycardias
Regular
Atrial fibrillation with infrahisian escape rhythm
Antidromic atrioventricular reentrant tachycardia
Atrioventricular junctional reentrant tachycardia with bystander accessory pathway
Any of the regular tachycardias in the development of aberration
Ventricular arrhythmias
Accelerated idioventricular rhythm
Monomorphic (or pleomorphic) ventricular tachycardia
Ventricular flutter
Irregular
Any of the following conducted with aberration:
Atrial fibrillation
Atrial flutter with varying block
Polymorphic VT
Torsade de pointes
Ventricular fibrillation

Table 49.3 Vaughan-Williams classification

Class I	Fast Na+ channel blockers (slowing of conduction)
	IA (quinidine, procainamide)
	IB (lidocaine)
	IC (propafenone, flecainide)
Class II	Beta-blockers
Class III	Repolarization K+ channel blockers (prolongation of repolarization) (amiodarone,* ibutilide, dofetilide, vernakalant, bretylium, sotalol)
Class IV	Calcium channel blockers (non-dihydropyridine: verapamil, diltiazem)

* Amiodarone exhibits effects of all classes.

where the negative resting membrane potential depolarizes to positive voltages (Figure 49.1).[2] The action potential is produced by transmembrane flow of ions (**inward depolarizing currents, mainly through Na^+ and Ca^{2+} channels,** and **outward repolarizing currents, mainly through K^+ channels**). The resting potential of atrial and ventricular myocytes during AP **phase 4** (resting phase) is stable and negative (−85 mV) due to the high conductance of the potassium channels. Excitation by electrical impulses from adjacent cells activates the inward Na^+ current that depolarizes myocytes rapidly (**phase 0**). Transient outward K^+ current (**phase 1**) creates a notch during the early phase of repolarization (I_{to}). Balance of the inward depolarizing L-type Ca^{2+} current ($I_{Ca\text{-}L}$) and outward rectifier K^+ currents (slow-I_{Ks}, rapid-I_{Kr}, and ultra-rapid-I_{Kur}) forms a plateau phase (phase 2). Deactivation (closing) of the inward current $I_{Ca\text{-}L}$ and increase of the outward currents creates **phase 3**, with final repolarization mainly due to potassium efflux through the inward rectifier I_{K1} channels, and the membrane potential returns to its resting potential (phase 4). The pacemaker current (I_f) contributes to action potential generation in the sinus node and significantly determines heart rate.[3] It is called the funny current because it displays unusual gating properties. I_f is a mixed Na+/K+ current, which conducts an inward current during phases 3 and 4 and may underlie slow membrane depolarization in cells with pacemaker activity (i.e. cells with I_f and little, or no, I_{K1}). I_f activation is accelerated by intracellular cyclic adenosine monophosphate (cAMP) levels, thus regulated by sympathetic and parasympathetic activity, which control synthesis and degradation of intracellular cAMP, respectively.

Opening and closing (gating) of ion channels enable transmembrane ion currents that consist of proteins called pore-forming alpha (α)-subunits and accessory beta (β)-subunits. Terminology of genes encoding for these proteins describes their function. For example, the gene encoding the alpha-subunit of the cardiac sodium channel is called SCN5A: sodium channel, type 5, alpha-subunit. The alpha-subunit is termed Nav 1.5: Na^+ channel family, subfamily 1, member 5, and V means that channel gating is regulated by transmembrane voltage changes (voltage-dependent) (Table 49.4).[1] Polymorphisms of SCN5A and SCN10A are associated with slow conduction and QRS duration prolongation and, consequently, future development of cardiac arrhythmias.[4] For a detailed description of acquired diseases due to mutations of these genes affecting the action potential, see Chapter 56 on genetic channelopathies and Chapter 62 on bradyarrhythmias.

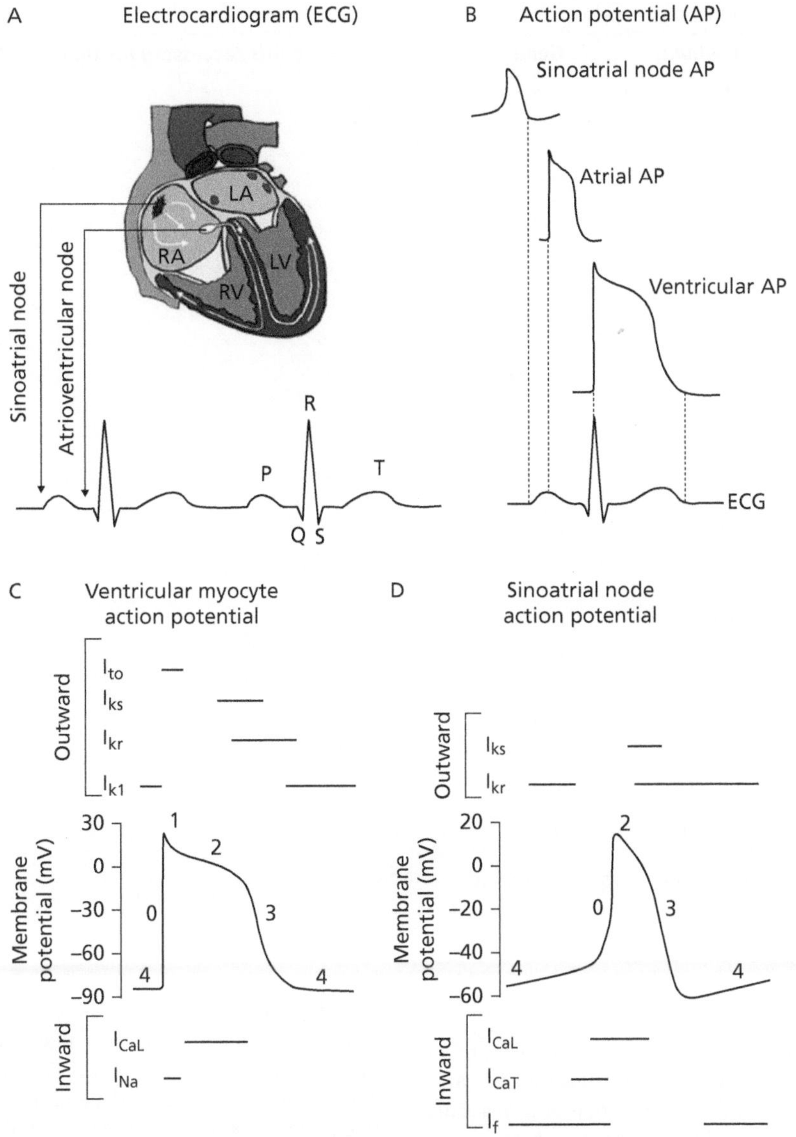

Figure 49.1 Cardiac electrical activity. A: Schematic representation of the electrical conduction system and its corresponding signal on the surface electrocardiogram (ECG). B: Relationship between ECG and action potentials (APs) of myocytes from different cardiac regions. C, D: Schematic representation of inward and outward currents that contribute to action potential formation in sinoatrial node and ventricular myocytes. The QT interval indicates the duration of ventricular depolarization and repolarization, which is caused by transmembrane flow of ions (e.g. inward depolarizing currents, mainly through Na^+ and Ca^{2+} channels, and outward repolarizing currents, mainly through K^+ channels). Initial depolarization of cardiac myocytes through gap junctions (cell-to-cell connections) activates the inward Na^+ current that depolarizes myocytes rapidly (phase 0). Transient outward K^+ current (phase 1) creates a notch during the early phase of repolarization (Ito). Balance of the inward depolarizing Ca^{2+} current (ICa-L) and outward rectifier K^+ currents (IKs and IKr) forms a plateau phase (phase 2). Deactivation of the inward current and increase of the outward current (IKs, IKr, IK1) complete repolarization (phase 3), and the membrane potential returns to its resting potential (phase 4).

Amin AS, *et al*. Cardiac ion channels in health and disease. *Heart Rhythm*. 2010;**7**:117–26.

Table 49.4 Genes encoding ion channels

Current	α-subunit	Gene	β-subunit(s)/accessory proteins	Gene
I_{Na}	$Na_v1.5$	*SCN5A*	β1	*SCN1B*
			β2	*SCN2B*
			β3	*SCN3B*
			β4	*SCN4B*
$I_{to,fast}$	$K_v4.3$	*KCND3*	MiRP1	*KCNE2*
			MiRP2	*KCNE3*
			KChIPs	Multiple genes
			DPP6	*DPP6*
$I_{to,slow}$	$K_v1.4$	*KCNA4*	$K_vβ1$	*KCNB1*
			$K_vβ2$	*KCNB2*
			$K_vβ3$	*KCNB3*
			$K_vβ4$	*KCNB4*
$I_{Ca,L}$	$Ca_v1.2$	*CACNA1C*	$Ca_vβ2$	*CACNB2*
			$Ca_vα2δ1$	*CACNA2D1*
$I_{Ca,T}$	$Ca_v3.1$	*CACNA1G*		
	$Ca_v3.2$	*CACNA1H*		
I_{Kur}	$K_v1.5$	*KCNA5*	$K_vβ1$	*KCNAB1*
			$K_vβ2$	*KCNAB2*
I_{Kr}	$K_v11.1$	*KCNH2*	MiRP1	*KCNE2*
I_{Ks}	Kv7.1	*KCNQ1*	minK	*KCNE1*
I_{K1}	Kir2.1	*KCNJ2*		
I_f (pacemaker current)	HCN1–4	*HCN1–4*		

Amin AS, *et al.* Cardiac ion channels in health and disease. *Heart Rhythm.* 2010;**7**:117–26.

Mechanisms of arrhythmias

Although the initiation of tachycardias is a complex process depending on the interaction of several factors, the main mechanisms responsible for the initiation of tachycardias are thought to be cell membrane hyperexcitability, i.e. enhanced automaticity or triggered activity and reduction in cell-to-cell electrical coupling, resulting in conduction block and reentry.[5] **Abnormal automaticity** is due to the maximum diastolic potential spontaneously becoming less negative (−40 to −60 mV; phase 4 of the AP). This is usually secondary to infarction, tissue stretch, and drugs. **Triggered activity** is caused by early after-depolarizations or delayed after-depolarizations, i.e. depolarizing oscillations in membrane voltage introduced by one or more preceding action potentials. **Early after-depolarizations** (i.e. occurring during phase 3 of the action potential) may be due to electrolyte disturbances, such as hypokalaemia, hypomagnesaemia, antiarrhythmic drugs (class Ia and class III), sympathetic stimulation, hypoxia, and hypercapnia. Typically, they occur in the long QT syndrome. **Delayed after-depolarizations** (i.e. after complete repolarization of the action potential) may be due to calcium overload, digoxin, catecholamines, and artificial pacing. Automatic and triggered arrhythmias depend on cell membrane hyperexcitability which is driven primarily by L-type calcium channels and/or adrenergic receptor stimulation.[6] A key molecule in membrane depolarizations (and in the generation of a delayed after-depolarization) is the electrogenic sodium-calcium exchanger, which allows diastolic calcium leak from the sarcoplasmic reticulum (Figure 49.2).[7]

Reentry denotes circulation of a wave of depolarization which is initiated when:

- Two functionally distinct pathways are present.
- Unidirectional block is induced in one pathway, for example, by a premature stimulus or by a physiological tachycardia.
- Sufficient slow conduction exists to allow recovery of excitability in the blocked pathway and permit retrograde conduction over that pathway and completion of the circuit.

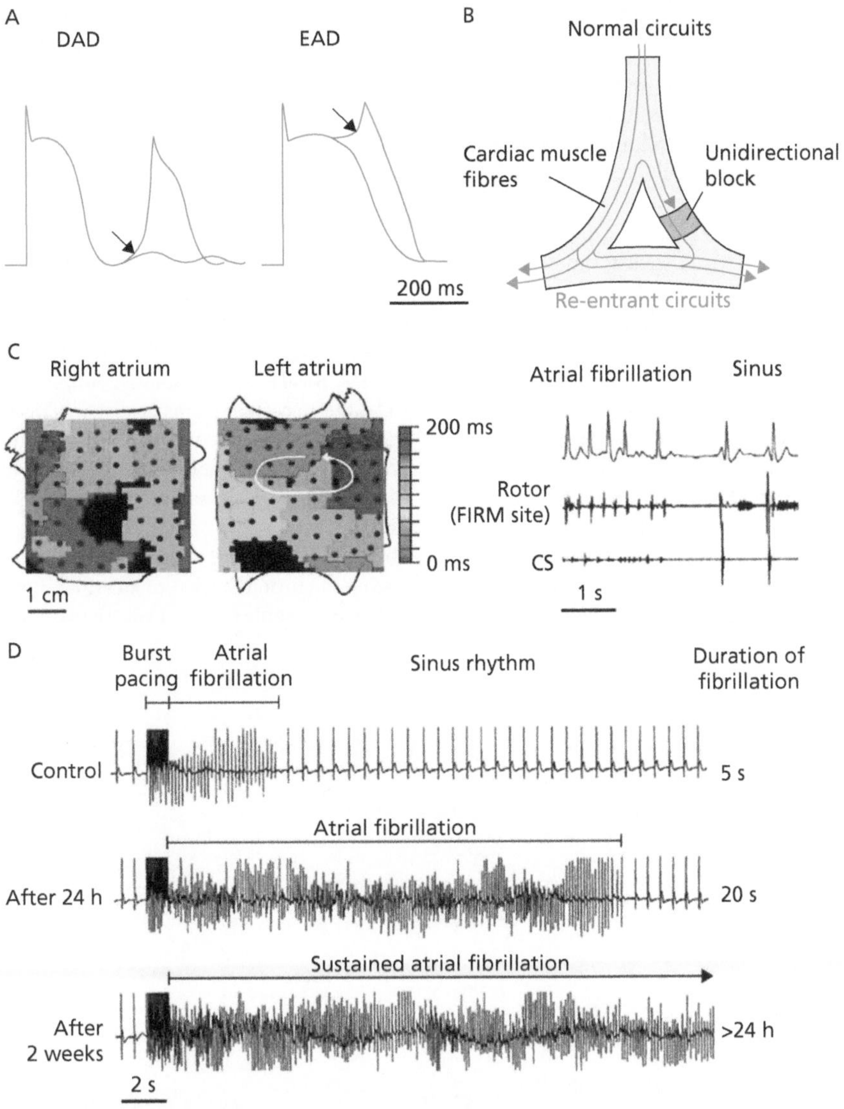

Figure 49.2 Conventional physiological mechanisms of arrhythmia. After-depolarizations are membrane depolarizations that occur late in or after the completion of the action potential. Delayed after-depolarizations (DADs) occur after full repolarization and early after-depolarizations (EADs) during late repolarization. (B) Circus movement reentry is characterized by an activation pattern that travels along a preferred anatomical structure to reactivate previously excited tissue. Such reentry is dependent on unidirectional block and is supported by slow conduction and short refractory periods. (C) Acute termination of atrial fibrillation (AF) to sinus rhythm by FIRM (focal impulse and rotor modulation) ablation. Left: left atrial rotor with counterclockwise activation (red to blue) and disorganized right atrium during AF in a 60-year old man. Right: FIRM ablation at left atrial rotor terminated AF to sinus rhythm in less than 1 min, with ablation artefact recorded at centre of rotor. The patient is AF-free on implanted cardiac monitor after more than 1 year. The demonstration of spiral waves and their functional importance in human AF potentially provides a widely applicable rational approach to AF ablation. (D) AF-induced changes (remodelling) that promote AF. Work done in paced goats provides strong evidence for an evolution of the substrate. In control goats, high-frequency burst pacing induced only 5 s of AF whereas, after 24 h of artificially maintained AF, the duration increased to 20 s. After 2 weeks, episodes of fibrillation lasted more than 24 h.

Grace AA, Roden DM. Systems biology and cardiac arrhythmias. *Lancet*. 2012;**380**:1498–508.

Reentrant mechanisms can be conventionally classified as:

- **Anatomical** due to defined loop. There is a large excitable gap between the crest and tail of impulse, i.e. properly timed stimuli can capture the circuit and reset the tachycardia. Typical examples are the atrioventricular reentrant tachycardias due to accessory atrioventricular connections.
- **Functional** due to altered cellular electrophysiological properties of myocardial tissue, such as functional barriers of conduction block or decremental conduction, leading to propagation failure. Functional reentry is exemplified by the 'leading circle' hypothesis which may be important in atrial fibrillation. In this model, the reentrant pathway is the shortest possible one and is determined on an instantaneous basis by refractoriness ahead of the activation wavefront. The cycle length, therefore, is determined only by refractoriness, and the excitable gap is as short as possible, independent of the cycle length. Functional circuits can also result in patterns, such as spirals or scrolls, that have been implicated in both atrial and ventricular fibrillation.[8]
- **Anisotropic** due to changes in microanatomical structures, such as cellular coupling and fibre orientation heterogeneity, which lead to anisotropic conduction or spatial inhomogeneity of refractoriness. The length of the circular pathway is determined by electrophysiological-anatomical changes, and there may be an excitable gap. This kind of reentry can be seen after myocardial infarctions.

There is evidence that more than 90% of the clinical tachycardias are due to reentrant mechanisms. Typical examples of reentry are tachycardias associated with the Wolff–Parkinson–White syndrome, the AV junctional reentry tachycardias, atrial flutter, and, most probably, atrial fibrillation. In addition, certain forms of sustained monomorphic ventricular tachycardia, such as VT in patients with coronary artery disease and bundle branch reentry in cases of dilated cardiomyopathy, demonstrate reentrant circuit with fully excitable gap. Anisotropic reentry appears to play an important role in ventricular tachycardias occurring in the setting of chronic healed myocardial infarcts. Torsades de pointes and some forms of ventricular tachycardia compli-

Table 49.5 ACC/AHA/ESC 2004 GL on SVT. Recommendations for acute management of haemodynamically stable and regular tachycardia

Narrow QRS complex tachycardia (SVT)	Vagal manoeuvres	I-B
	Adenosine	I-A
	Verapamil, diltiazem	I-A
	Beta-blockers	IIb-C
	Amiodarone	IIb-C
	Digoxin	IIb-C
Wide QRS complex tachycardia		
SVT + BBB		See above
Pre-excited SVT/AF	Flecainide‡	I-B (not in reduced LVEF)
	Ibutilide	I-B (not in reduced LVEF)
	Procainamide	I-B (not in reduced LVEF)
	DC cardioversion	I-C
Wide QRS complex tachycardia of unknown origin	Procainamide	I-B (not in reduced LVEF)
	Sotalol	I-B (not in reduced LVEF)
	Amiodarone	I-B
	DC cardioversion	I-B
	Lidocaine	IIb-B
	Adenosine	IIb-C (caution in severe coronary artery disease)
	Beta-blockers	III-C (first-line therapy in RVOT VT)
	Verapamil	III-B (first-line therapy in fascicular VT)
Wide QRS complex tachycardia of unknown origin in patients with poor LV function	Amiodarone DC cardioversion, lidocaine	I-B

All drugs are given IV.
ACC/AHA/ESC 2003 guidelines for the management of patients with supraventricular arrhythmias. Circulation. 2003; **108**:1871–909.

cating coronary artery disease are due to after-depolarization-induced triggered activity.

Reentrant mechanisms are postulated when programmed stimulation demonstrates that the tachycardia behaves in a manner similar to that of reentry. Thus, easy induction and termination by programmed stimulation, as well as entrainment of the tachycardia, usually indicate a reentrant mechanism. Tachycardias due to triggered activity may also be initiated and terminated by pacing and may be distinguished from reentrant ones because, progressively, more premature stimulation may cause progressively faster triggered activity. Usually, distinction from reentry is difficult. Arrhythmias due to abnormal automaticity occur spontaneously or in response to isoprenaline and are not induced by programmed stimulation.

Acute management of tachyarrhythmias

Physical examination is unremarkable in the absence of tachycardia. The presence of irregular cannon A waves and/or irregular variation in S_1 intensity during tachycardia suggest a ventricular origin of the tachycardia.

Regular arrhythmia suggests AVRT, AVNRT or other junctional tachycardia, AT, atrial flutter, or VT (Table 49.5).

Irregular arrhythmia suggests AF, multifocal AT, or atrial flutter with variable AV conduction (Table 49.5).

ECG In the absence of tachycardia, the presence of pre-excitation establishes the diagnosis of Wolff–Parkinson–White syndrome. Patients with atrial flutter, AVNRT, or AVRT due to a concealed accessory pathway have normal resting ECG.

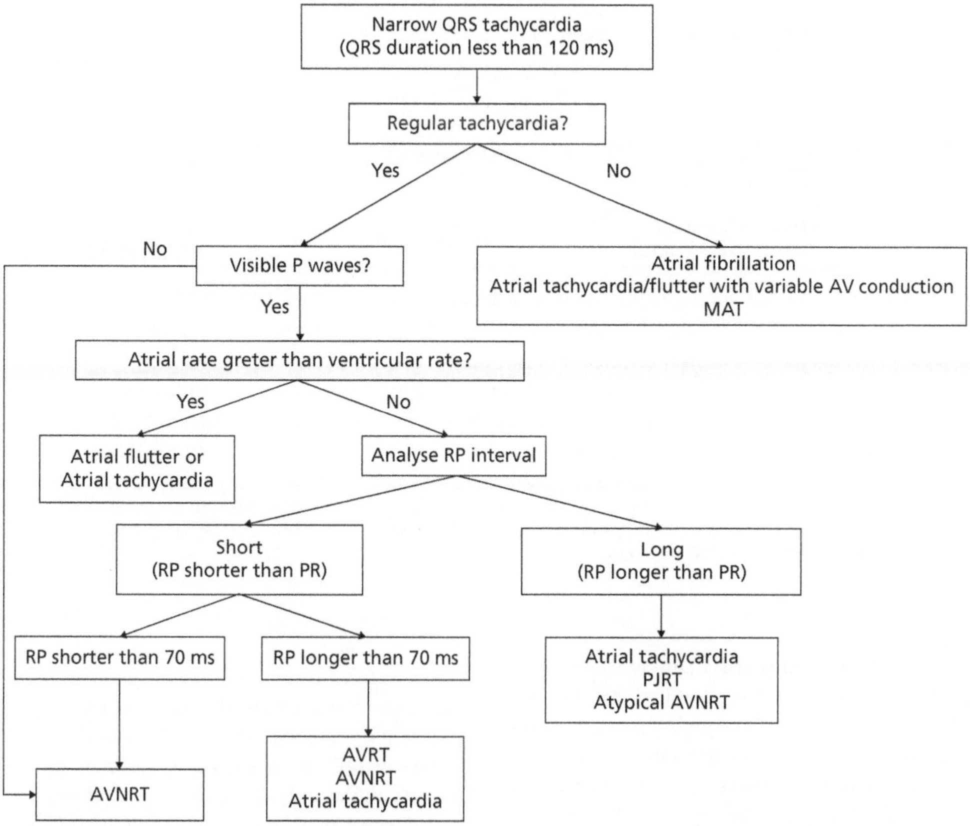

Figure 49.3 Differential diagnosis for narrow QRS tachycardia. Patients with focal junctional tachycardia may mimic the pattern of slow-fast AVNRT and may show AV dissociation and/or marked irregularity in the junctional rate.

AV indicates atrioventricular; AVNRT, atrioventricular nodal reciprocating tachycardia; AVRT, atrioventricular reciprocating tachycardia; MAT, multifocal atrial tachycardia; ms, milliseconds; PJRT, permanent form of junctional reciprocating tachycardia due to slowly conducting accessory pathway; QRS, ventricular activation on ECG. ACC/AHA/ESC 2003 guidelines for the management of patients with supraventricular arrhythmias. *Circulation*. 2003;**108**:1871–909.

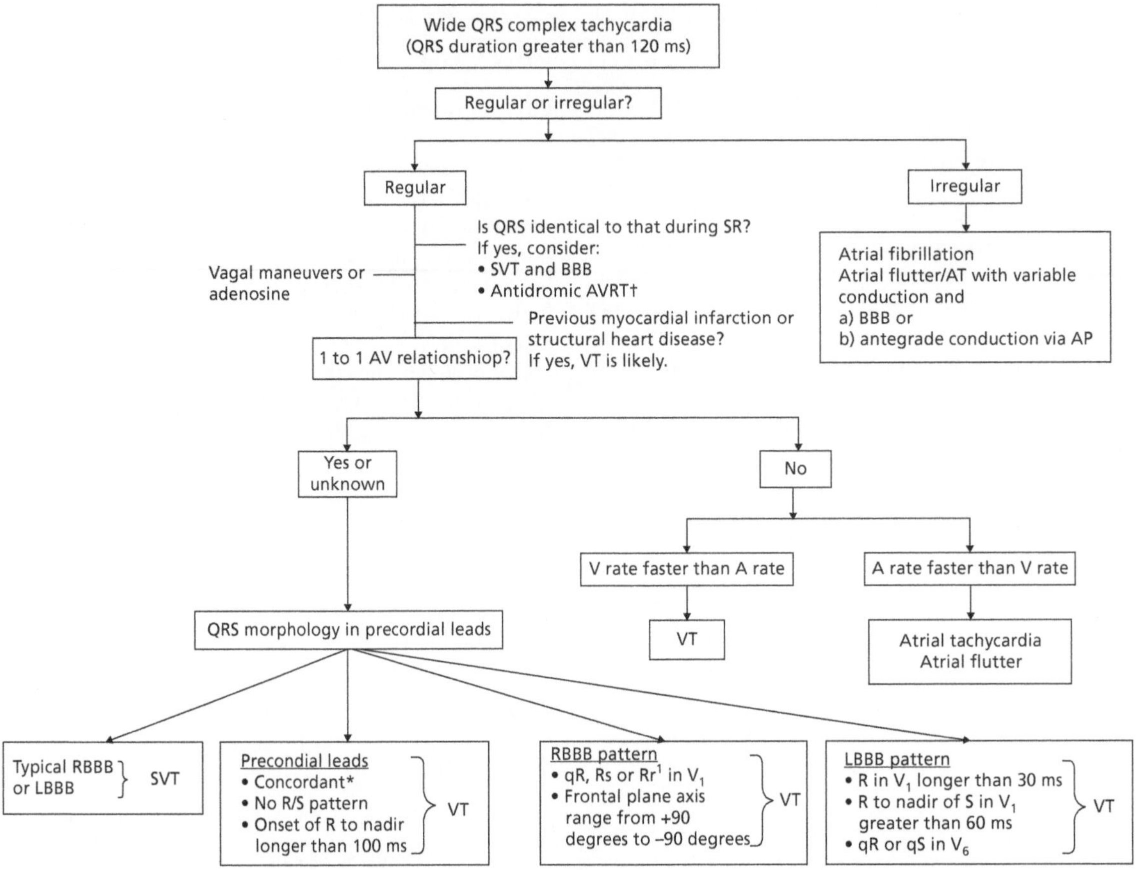

Figure 49.4 Differential diagnosis for wide QRS complex tachycardia (more than 120 ms). A QRS conduction delay during sinus rhythm, when available for comparison, reduces the value of QRS morphology analysis. Adenosine should be used with caution when the diagnosis is unclear because it may produce VF in patients with coronary artery disease and AF with a rapid ventricular rate in pre-excited tachycardias. *Concordant indicates that all precordial leads show either positive or negative deflections. Fusion complexes are diagnostic of VT. †In pre-excited tachycardias, the QRS is generally wider (i.e. more pre-excited) compared with sinus rhythm.

A indicates atrial; AP, accessory pathway; AT, atrial tachycardia; AV, atrioventricular; AVRT, atrioventricular reciprocating tachycardia; BBB, bundle branch block; LBBB, left bundle branch block; ms, milliseconds; QRS, ventricular activation on ECG; RBBB, right bundle branch block; SR, sinus rhythm; SVT, supraventricular tachycardias; V, ventricular; VF, ventricular fibrillation; VT, ventricular tachycardia. ACC/AHA/ESC 2003 guidelines for the management of patients with supraventricular arrhythmias. *Circulation*. 2003;**108**:1871–909.

Narrow QRS (<120 ms) tachycardia Differential diagnosis should address conditions described in Table 49.2 and Figure 49.3. Apart from SVT, VT of high septal origin and fascicular tachycardias may also have a narrow QRS.

Wide QRS (>120 ms) tachycardia Differential diagnosis between SVT and VT is presented in Table 49.2 and Figure 49.4 and in Chapter 55 on VT.

Wearable or **implantable loop recorders** are more useful in detecting tachycardia episodes than Holter monitoring.[8]

Electrophysiologic evaluation is usually required for a definitive diagnosis.

Therapy

The acute management depends on the haemodynamic condition of the patient (Figure 49.5 and Table 49.5).[9]

In **narrow QRS tachycardia**, vagal manoeuvres, such as Valsalva, unilateral carotid massage, and facial immersion in cold water, may be tried to terminate the tachycardia.

Adenosine, a naturally occurring nucleoside with a short-lived negative dromotropic effect on the AV node, given in rapid IV doses up to 0.25 mg/kg, will terminate or reveal most supraventricular tachycardias (Figure 49.6). Adenosine does not affect most ventricular tachycardias, with the exception of some

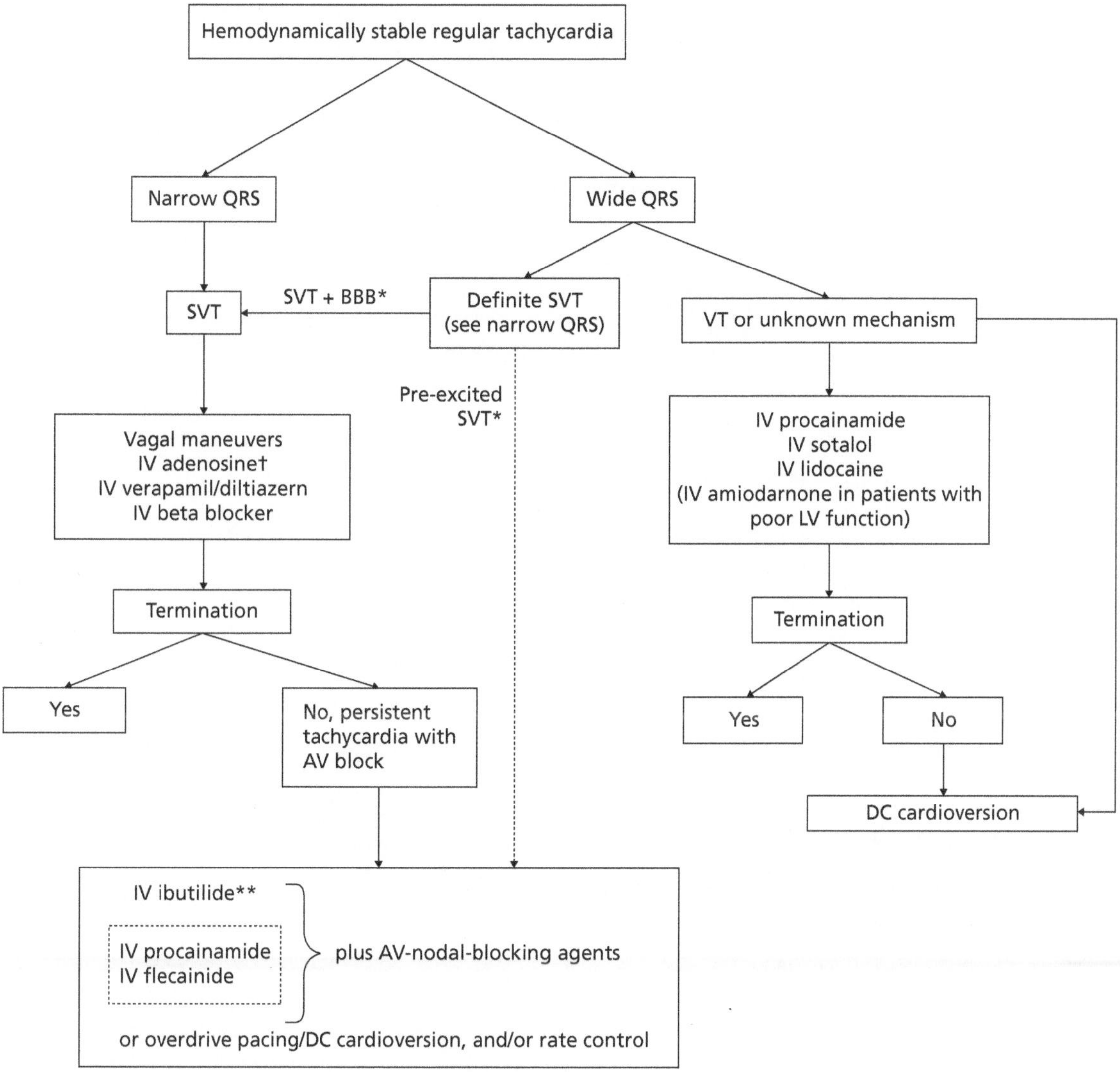

Figure 49.5 Acute management of patients with haemodynamically stable and regular tachycardia.

*A 12-lead ECG during sinus rhythm must be available for diagnosis. †Adenosine should be used with caution in patients with severe coronary artery disease and may produce AF, which may result in rapid ventricular rates for patients with pre-excitation. **Ibutilide is especially effective for patients with atrial flutter but should not be used in patients with EF less than 30% due to increased risk of polymorphic VT.

AF indicates atrial fibrillation; AV, atrioventricular; BBB, bundle branch block; DC, direct current; IV, intravenous; LV, left ventricle; QRS, ventricular activation on ECG; SVT, supraventricular tachycardia; VT, ventricular tachycardia.

ACC/AHA/ESC 2003 guidelines for the management of patients with supraventricular arrhythmias. *Circulation*. 2003; **108**:1871–909.

forms associated with apparently normal hearts, and can, therefore, be used as a diagnostic agent.[10] AF may be caused (1–5%) but is usually transient. Adenosine is contraindicated in severe bronchial asthma. Its action is antagonized by theophylline and potentiated by dipyridamole and carbamazepine.[9] Verapamil should not be used in this way because of the considerable incidence of life-threatening hypotension which is associated with its administration in ventricular tachycardia.

Acute management of **wide QRS tachycardia** depends on the haemodynamic condition of the patient. Patients should be treated as described in Chapter 55 on VT, unless there is documentation of NSVT. Haemodynamically unstable patients require immediate DC cardioversion.

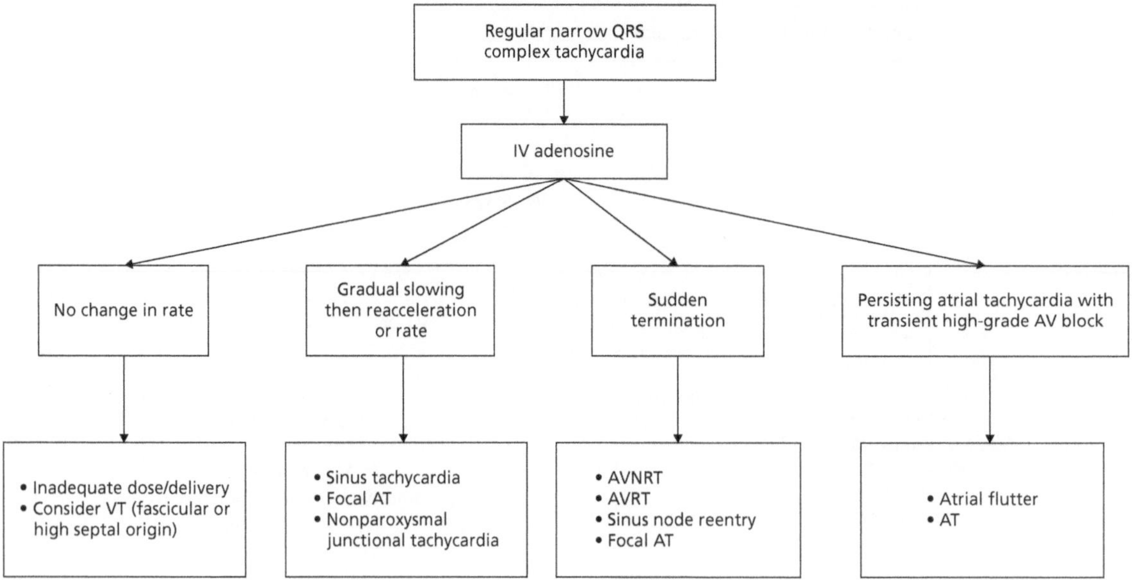

Figure 49.6 Responses of narrow complex tachycardias to adenosine.

AT indicates atrial tachycardia; AV, atrioventricular; AVNRT, atrioventricular nodal reciprocating tachycardia; AVRT, atrioventricular reciprocating tachycardia; IV, intravenous; QRS, ventricular activation on ECG; VT, ventricular tachycardia. ACC/AHA/ESC 2003 guidelines for the management of patients with supraventricular arrhythmias. *Circulation*. 2003;**108**:1871–909.

References

1. Katritsis D, *et al.* Antiarrhythmic drug classifications and the clinician: a gambit in the land of chaos. *Clin Cardiol.* 1994;**17**:142–8
2. Amin AS, *et al.* Cardiac ion channels in health and disease. *Heart Rhythm*. 2010;**7**:117–26
3. Verkerk AO, *et al.* Pacemaker current (i(f)) in the human sinoatrial node. *Eur Heart J*. 2007;**28**:2472–8
4. Ritchie MD, *et al.* Genome- and phenome-wide analysis of cardiac conduction identifies markers of arrhythmia risk. *Circulation*. 2013 Mar; [Epub ahead of print]
5. Rubart M, *et al.* Genesis of cardiac arrhythmias: electrophysiological considerations. In Libby P, Bonow RO, Mann DL, Zipes DP: Braunwald's Heart Disease. pp. 727–62, Saunders 2008.
6. Rokita AG, *et al.* New therapeutic targets in cardiology: arrhythmias and Ca2+/calmodulin-dependent kinase II (CAMKII). *Circulation*. 2012;**126**:2125–39
7. Grace AA, *et al.* Systems biology and cardiac arrhythmias. *Lancet*. 2012;**380**:1498–508
8. Zimetbaum P, *et al.* Ambulatory arrhythmia monitoring: choosing the right device. *Circulation*. 2010;**122**: 1629–36
9. Blomstrom-Lundqvist C, *et al.* ACC/AHA/ESC guidelines for the management of patients with supraventricular arrhythmias—executive summary. A report of the American College of Cardiology/American Heart Association Task Force on practice guidelines and the European Society of Cardiology Committee for practice guidelines (writing committee to develop guidelines for the management of patients with supraventricular arrhythmias) developed in collaboration with NASPE-Heart Rhythm Society. *J Am Coll Cardiol*. 2003;**42**:1493–531
10. Griffith MJ LN, Ward DE, Camm AJ. Adenosine in the diagnosis of broad complex tachycardias. *Lancet* 1988;**1**: 672–5.

Chapter 50

Classification, epidemiology, and presentation of supraventricular tachycardias

Definitions and classification

Usually, paroxysmal supraventricular tachycardia (SVT) denotes arrhythmias other than atrial fibrillation and ventricular tachycardias. This definition is inaccurate as discussed in Chapter 50 on classification of tachycarrhythmias but traditionally used. Figure 50.1 presents the mechanisms of supraventricular tachycardias.

Epidemiology of SVT

The prevalence of SVT is 2.25/1000 persons and the incidence 35/100 000 person-years (MESA study).[1] Thus, there are approximately 89 000 new cases/year and 570 000 persons with SVT in the United States. Mean age at presentation is 37 to 45 years,[1,2] and the incidence and prevalence of SVTs increase with age, with a risk of arrhythmia more than five times greater in persons >65 years than in those <65 years old.[1] Age of tachycardia onset is lower for atrioventricular reentrant tachycardia (AVRT) due to accessory pathway than atrioventricular nodal reentrant tachycardia (AVNRT). In a recent study on 1754 patients undergoing catheter ablation, AVNRT was the main aetiology (56%), followed by AVRT (27%) and atrial tachycardia (AT, 17%).[2] The proportion of AVRT in both sexes decreased with age whereas AVNRT and AT increased. The majority of patients with AVRT were men (55%) whereas the majority of patients with AVNRT and AT were women (70% and 62%, respectively). Atrial flutter has an incidence of 0.09%, and 58% of the patients have AF (MESA study).[3] Its incidence increases with age, from 5/100 000 for those less than 50 years to 587/100 000 over 80 years of age, and is 2.5 times more common in men than in women. The risk of developing atrial flutter increases 3.5 times in subjects with heart failure and 1.9 times ($p < 0.001$) in subjects with chronic obstructive pulmonary disease. Atrial flutter is usually associated with heart disease, such as heart failure (16%) or chronic obstructive lung disease (12%) whereas an apparently normal heart is found in <2% of patients.[3]

Presentation of SVT

Patients present due to paroxysms of regular or irregular palpitations with a characteristically sudden onset and offset that occur mostly in daylight, which may be associated with fatigue, light-headedness, dyspnoea, chest discomfort, and presyncope. Syncope and cardiac arrest are rare (<15%), usually denote underlying structural heart disease or AF in the presence of a conducting accessory pathway, and may be due to rapid heart rate or vasomotor factors.[4,5] Polyuria is due to release of atrial natriuretic peptide in response to increased atrial pressure, and vagal manoeuvres usually interrupt the tachycardia. Patients may also present with AF that has been initiated by the SVT and which usually,[6,7] but not invariably,[8] is eliminated by ablation of the SVT itself.

SVT in congenital heart disease

ASD and PFO

Surgical repair of ASD before the 25 years of age has been shown to reduce the incidence of arrhythmias, such as atrial flutter and fibrillation (AF), but patients over age 40 years may remain at risk of atrial arrhythmias.[9,10] Up to 68% of patients who present with preoperative AF may remain in AF after successful ASD closure[11] whereas, in patients over 40 years old, post-operative AF develops in 8–23% over the next 7 to 10 years.[9,10] More data exist in patients subjected to transcatheter closure of ASD that has been found beneficial, regardless of age.[11] New-onset AF occurs in 7% of patients after transcatheter PFO closure and 12% of patients with underlying ASD over the next 20 months.[12] A history of previous arrhythmia and age >40 years at closure are associated with increased incidence of AF.[13–15] Usually, patients with pre-existing persistent AF remain in AF after device closure of their ASD[11] whereas, in 45–67% of the patients, resolution of paroxysmal atrial arrhythmias may be seen.[16] Thus, ASD is associated with an increased incidence of AF, regardless of therapy, especially in patients >40 years. Transcatheter ASD closure may trigger early transient arrhythmias; persistent AF is unlikely to be affected, but paroxysmal arrhythmias may improve, although the likelihood decreases with age. Catheter ablation in experienced centres is recommended (Table 50.1). If ASD does not require closure on haemodynamic grounds, closure is unlikely to abolish flutter or AF. Post-surgical flutters require electroanatomic mapping for defining the isthmus since they can be CTI- or non-CTI-dependent or both.

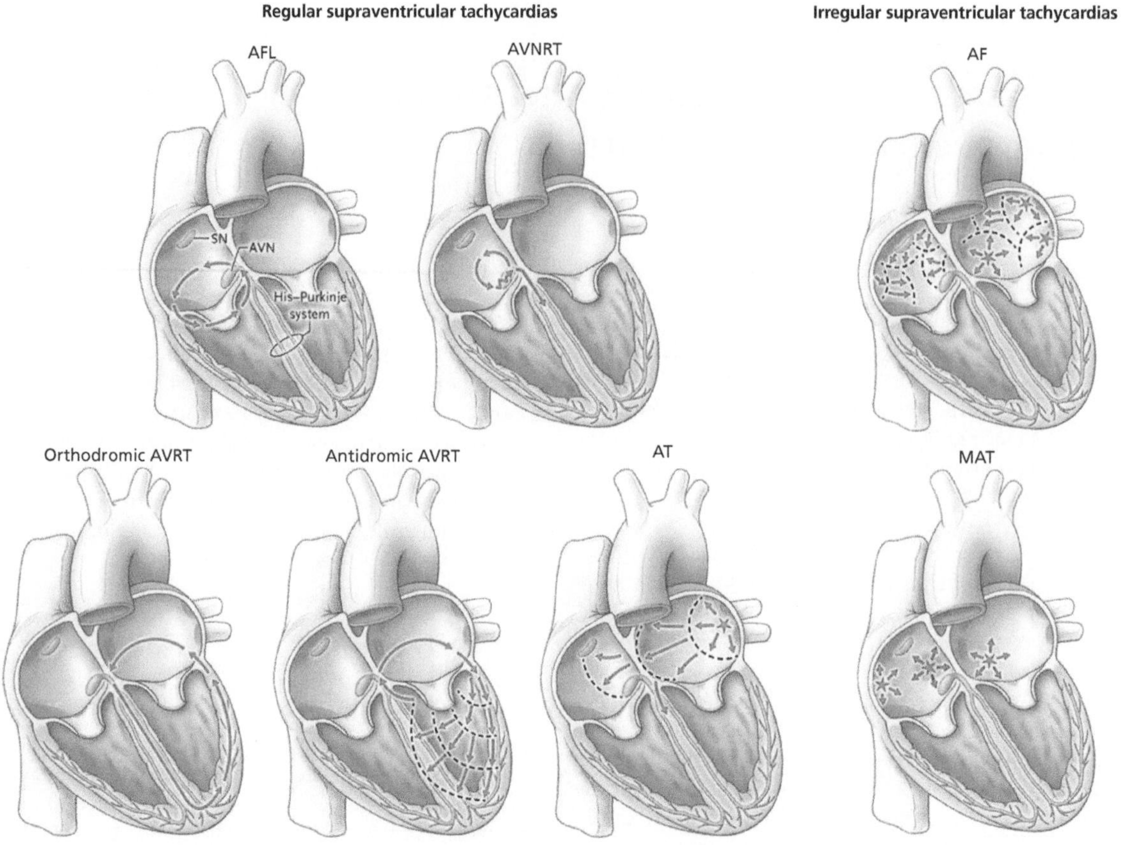

Figure 50.1 Mechanisms of supraventricular tachycardia.

AFL, atrial flutter; AVNRT, atrioventricular nodal reentrant tachycardia; AVRT, atrioventricular reentrant tachycardia; AT, atrial tachycardia. MAT, multifocal AT, Link MS. *N Engl J Med* 2012;**367**:1438–1448.

Table 50.1 ACC/AHA/ESC 2003 GL on SVT. Recommendations for treatment of SVTs in adults with congenital heart disease

Failed antiarrhythmic drugs and symptomatic		
Repaired ASD	Catheter ablation in an experienced centre	I-C
Mustard or Senning repair of transposition of the great vessels	Catheter ablation in an experienced centre	I-C
Unrepaired asymptomatic ASD not haemodynamically significant	Closure of the ASD for treatment of the arrhythmia	III-C
Unrepaired haemodynamically significant ASD with atrial flutter	Closure of the ASD combined with ablation of the flutter isthmus	I-C
PSVT and Ebstein's anomaly with haemodynamic indications for surgical repair	Surgical ablation of accessory pathways at the time of operative repair of the malformation at an experienced centre	I-C

ACC/AHA/ESC guidelines for the management of patients with supraventricular arrhythmias-executive summary. *Circulation*. 2003;**108**:1871–909.

Tetralogy of Fallot

Approximately 10% of patients develop incisional or CTI-dependent atrial flutter within the next 35 years after repair.[17] There is usually RBBB in the resting ECG of the majority of patients, and SVT are conducted with RBBB aberration, but this pattern also occurs in 25% of VT in this setting. Development of atrial flutter can be an indication of worsening ventricular function and tricuspid regurgitation, and reassessment for surgical revision may be indicated.

Table 50.2 ESC GL on pregnancy 2011

Management of supraventricular tachycardia (SVT)	
For acute conversion of paroxysmal SVT, vagal manoeuvre followed by IV adenosine.	I-C
Immediate electrical cardioversion for acute treatment of any tachycardia with haemodynamic instability.	I-C
For long-term management of SVT, oral digoxin[1] or metoprolol/propranolol.[2]	I-C
For acute conversion of paroxysmal SVT, IV metoprolol or propranolol.	IIa-C
For long-term management of SVT, oral sotalol[3] or encainide[4] if digoxin or a beta-blocking agent fails.	IIa-C
For acute conversion of paroxysmal SVT, IV verapamil.	IIb-C
For long-term management of SVT, oral propafenone or procainamide as a last option if other suggested agents fail and before amiodarone[3] is used.	IIb-C
For long-term management of SVT, oral verapamil for rate regulation if the other AV nodal blocking agents fail.	IIb-C
Atenolol[2] should not be used for any arrhythmia.	III-C

1: AV nodal blocking agents should not be used in patients with pre-excitation on resting ECG.
2: Beta-blocking agents should be used with caution in the first trimester.
3: Class III drugs should not be used in cases with prolonged QTc.
4: Consider AV nodal blocking agents in conjunction with flecainide and propafenone for certain atrial tachycardias.
ESC on Pregnancy 2011. ESC Guidelines on the management of cardiovascular diseases during pregnancy. *Eur Heart J*. 2011;**32**:3147–97.

Ebstein's anomaly

Accessory AV and atriofascicular pathways occur in up to 25% of patients and are more often right-sided and multiple than in patients without the disorder.[18,19] AF, atrial flutter, and AT may also occur. RBBB is usually present and, in the presence of a right-sided accessory pathway, ventricular pre-excitation can mask the ECG evidence of RBBB. LBBB tachycardias can be due to antidromic AVRT or conduction over a bystander accessory pathway. Depending on the severity of the malformation and the arrhythmia, SVT can produce cyanosis and severe symptoms or sudden death due to rapid conduction to the ventricles during AF or atrial flutter when an accessory pathway is present. Preoperative (success rates 75–89%, with recurrence in 30–35%)[20,21] or surgical ablation are recommended in the presence of SVT to avoid recurrent arrhythmias and instability in the perioperative period.

Fontan repairs

Incisional-related atrial flutter or AF occurs in up to 57% of patients, depending on the particular type of repair.[22] Catheter ablation is cumbersome due to multiple circuits and should be attempted only at experienced centres.[23]

SVT in pregnancy

Premature atrial beats are observed in up to 50% of pregnant women and are benign. Exacerbations of SVT occur in 20–40% of them.[24] Adenosine and electrical cardioversion are not contraindicated (Table 50.2). Digoxin is safe but of limited value. Catheter ablation may be performed during the second trimester, ideally with the aid of electroanatomic mapping that reduces exposure to radiation. Treatment of cases of atrial tachycardia during pregnancy is generally more challenging with respect to their drug-resistant nature, tendency to be persistent, and their association with structural heart disease. Rate control, using beta-blocking agents and/or digitalis, should be used to avoid tachycardia-induced cardiomyopathy. Prophylactic antiarrhythmic drug therapy includes flecainide, propafenone, or sotalol for patients with definite symptoms. Detailed comments on the drug use in pregnancy are presented in Appendix 3.

Therapy of SVT

This is discussed in individual Chapters. Catheter ablation offers now a means of permanent therapy for most kinds of SVT. Permanent pacing is now recommended only for symptomatic recurrent SVT that is reproducibly terminated by pacing when catheter ablation and/or drugs fail to control it, provided no rapid accessory pathway is present (see Chapter 65).[25]

References

1. Orejarena LA, *et al.* Paroxysmal supraventricular tachycardia in the general population. *J Am Coll Cardiol.* 1998;**31**:150–7
2. Porter MJ, *et al.* Influence of age and gender on the mechanism of supraventricular tachycardia. *Heart Rhythm.* 2004;**1**:393–6
3. Granada J, *et al.* Incidence and predictors of atrial flutter in the general population. *J Am Coll Cardiol.* 2000;**36**:2242–6
4. Leitch JW, *et al.* Syncope associated with supraventricular tachycardia. An expression of tachycardia rate or vasomotor response? *Circulation.* 1992;**85**:1064–71
5. Wood KA, *et al.* Frequency of disabling symptoms in supraventricular tachycardia. *Am J Cardiol.* 1997;**79**:145–9

6. Haissaguerre M, *et al.* Frequency of recurrent atrial fibrillation after catheter ablation of overt accessory pathways. *Am J Cardiol.* 1992;**69**:493–7
7. Sauer WH, *et al.* Atrioventricular nodal reentrant tachycardia in patients referred for atrial fibrillation ablation: response to ablation that incorporates slow pathway modification. *Circulation.* 2006;**114**:191–5
8. Centurion OA, *et al.* Mechanisms for the genesis of paroxysmal atrial fibrillation in the Wolff–Parkinson–White syndrome: intrinsic atrial muscle vulnerability vs electrophysiological properties of the accessory pathway. *Europace.* 2008;**10**:294–302
9. Attie F, *et al.* Surgical treatment for secundum atrial septal defects in patients >40 years old. A randomized clinical trial. *J Am Coll Cardiol.* 2001;**38**:2035–42
10. Konstantinides S, *et al.* A comparison of surgical and medical therapy for atrial septal defect in adults. *N Engl J Med.* 1995;**333**:469–73
11. Murphy JG, *et al.* Long-term outcome after surgical repair of isolated atrial septal defect. Follow-up at 27 to 32 years. *N Engl J Med.* 1990;**323**:1645–50
12. Humenberger M, *et al.* Benefit of atrial septal defect closure in adults: impact of age. *Eur Heart J.* 2011;**32**:553–60
13. Giardini A, *et al.* Long-term incidence of atrial fibrillation and flutter after transcatheter atrial septal defect closure in adults. *Int J Cardiol.* 2009;**134**:47–51
14. Silversides CK, *et al.* Predictors of atrial arrhythmias after device closure of secundum type atrial septal defects in adults. *Am J Cardiol.* 2008;**101**:683–7
15. Spies C, *et al.* Incidence of atrial fibrillation following transcatheter closure of atrial septal defects in adults. *Am J Cardiol.* 2008;**102**:902–6
16. Wilson NJ, *et al.* Transcatheter closure of secundum atrial septal defects with the amplatzer septal occluder in adults and children—follow-up closure rates, degree of mitral regurgitation and evolution of arrhythmias. *Heart Lung Circ.* 2008;**17**:318–24
17. Gatzoulis MA, *et al.* Risk factors for arrhythmia and sudden cardiac death late after repair of Tetralogy of Fallot: a multicentre study. *Lancet.* 2000;**356**:975–81
18. Delhaas T, *et al.* A multicenter, long-term study on arrhythmias in children with Ebstein anomaly. *Pediatr Cardiol.* 2010;**31**:229–33
19. Hebe J. Ebstein's anomaly in adults. Arrhythmias: diagnosis and therapeutic approach. *Thorac Cardiovasc Surg.* 2000;**48**:214–19
20. Cappato R, *et al.* Radiofrequency current catheter ablation of accessory atrioventricular pathways in Ebstein's anomaly. *Circulation.* 1996;**94**:376–83
21. Reich JD, *et al.* The pediatric radiofrequency ablation registry's experience with Ebstein's anomaly. Pediatric Electrophysiology Society. *J Cardiovasc Electrophysiol.* 1998;**9**:1370–7
22. Ghai A, *et al.* Outcomes of late atrial tachyarrhythmias in adults after the Fontan operation. *J Am Coll Cardiol.* 2001;**37**:585–92
23. Blomstrom-Lundqvist C, *et al.* ACC/AHA/ESC guidelines for the management of patients with supraventricular arrhythmias—executive summary. A report of the American College of Cardiology/American Heart Association Task Force on practice guidelines and the European Society of Cardiology Committee for practice guidelines (writing committee to develop guidelines for the management of patients with supraventricular arrhythmias) developed in collaboration with NASPE-Heart Rhythm Society. *J Am Coll Cardiol.* 2003;**42**:1493–531
24. Regitz-Zagrosek V, *et al.* ESC guidelines on the management of cardiovascular diseases during pregnancy: The Task Force on the management of cardiovascular diseases during pregnancy of the European Society of Cardiology (ESC). *Eur Heart J.* 2011;**32**:3147–97
25. 2012 ACCF/AHA/HRS focused update incorporated into the ACCF/AHA/HRS 2008 guidelines for device-based therapy of cardiac rhythm abnormalities. *J Am Coll Cardiol.* 2013;**61**:e6–75

Chapter 51

Atrial tachycardias

Atrial and junctional premature beats

Atrial premature beats

Atrial premature beats (APBs) are common in the healthy population, and their prevalence increases with age, history of cardiovascular disease, and BNP levels.[1] Although they have not been associated with sudden or non-sudden cardiac death,[1,2] frequent APBs (≥30 per hour or runs of ≥30 beats) may trigger AF and thus may be associated with a poor prognosis in terms of death or stroke.[3] They may also trigger SVT in the presence of a suitable background. Non-conducted APBs are a common cause of unexpected pauses. They can arise anywhere in the atria, including the sinus node. An APB is characterized by an abnormally shaped atrial depolarization wave which occurs prior to the next anticipated sinus beat. Several electrocardiographic leads may be needed to distinguish the different P wave shape, and, in the rare case of sinus node premature beats, the P wave will be identical. The post-extrasystolic cycle is typically less than compensatory due to penetration and resetting of the sinus node by the premature depolarization, but suppression of the sinus node automaticity may also occur and result in pauses equal to, or longer than, the sinus cycle. Intraventricular conduction may be normal or aberrant whereas the PR interval is marginally longer than that of normal sinus rhythm due to atrioventricular nodal delay. This especially occurs in the rare case of interpolated APBs which do not depolarize the sinus node and do not affect the sinus rate. Blocked premature beats may masquerade as pauses or bradycardias when P waves are not seen. The T wave of those beats that precede a pause should be carefully inspected to detect any 'hidden' premature P wave. Apart from age and cardiovascular disease, other potential causes of APBs are hypertension, pulmonary disease, such as bronchial carcinoma and pneumonia, hyperthyroidism, alcohol abuse, illicit drugs, and anxiety states. **Therapy** is directed towards avoidance or correction of the offending cause. Caffeine in moderate doses is well tolerated.[4] In symptomatic patients, beta-blockers are useful.

Junctional premature beats

Premature beats probably arise from the AV junction and conduct antegradely to the ventricles and retrogradely to the atria. There are, therefore, inverted retrograde P (negative in inferior leads and positive in aVR), the timing of which, relative to the QRS complex, depends on the exact origin of the beat and the conduction times to the atria and the ventricles. The retrograde P may occur immediately before, during, or following the QRS complex, which itself may display various degrees of aberration. Concealed His bundle extrasystoles may simulate first- or second-degree AV block, but they can also be associated with conduction disease.[5]

Physiological sinus tachycardia

Definition

Sinus tachycardia is defined as a non-paroxysmal increase in sinus rate to more than 100 bpm, in keeping with the level of physical, emotional, pathological, or pharmacologic stress.[6]

Aetiology and pathophysiology

Common causes are presented in Table 51.1. It is due to physiological influences on individual pacemaker cells and from an anatomical shift in the site of origin of atrial depolarization superiorly within the sinus node.

Diagnosis

In normal sinus rhythm, the P wave on a 12-lead ECG in adults is positive in leads I, II, and aVF and V_3 to V_6. It is negative in aVR and V_1 and V_2. In sinus tachycardia, P waves have a normal contour, but a larger amplitude may develop and the wave may become peaked.

Table 51.1 Causes of physiological sinus tachycardia

Anxiety-emotional stress
Pyrexia
Anaemia
Acidosis
Hypoxia
Hypovolaemia
Infection
Hyperthyroidism
Phaeochromocytoma
Stimulants
Alcohol, caffeine, nicotine
Drugs
Salbutamol, aminophylline, thyroxine, atropine, catecholamines, doxorubicin, adriamycin, daunorubicin
Recreational/illicit drugs
Amphetamines, cocaine, cannabis, ecstacy

Therapy

Elimination of the offending cause is mandatory. If additional symptomatic treatment is required, beta-blockers are the agents of choice, and, when contraindicated, verapamil or diltiazem may be used.

Inappropriate sinus tachycardia

Definition

Inappropriate sinus tachycardia is a fast sinus rhythm (>100 bpm) at rest or minimal activity that is out of proportion with the level of physical, emotional, pathological, or pharmacologic stress.[6]

Pathophysiology

Enhanced automaticity of the sinus node or increased sympathetic drive is the postulated mechanisms.

Presentation

Mean age of presentation is 38 years, and women are mainly affected. Symptoms may vary from palpitations (or even no symptoms at all) to presyncope.

Diagnosis

It is based on:

- The presence of a **persistent sinus tachycardia** (heart rate >100 bpm) during the day, with excessive rate increase in response to activity, and nocturnal normalization of rate as confirmed by a 24-hour Holter recording.

- The tachycardia (and symptoms) is usually **non-paroxysmal**, with P wave morphology and endocardial activation identical to sinus rhythm.
- Exclusion of a secondary systemic cause (e.g. **hyperthyroidism, physical deconditioning**) and postural orthostatic tachycardia syndrome (**POTS**). In POTS, there is a persistent increase in heart rate by >30 bpm or a rate >20 bpm within 10 min of changing from a supine to an upright position, in the absence of orthostatic hypotension.[7]

Therapy

Beta-blockers, verapamil, and diltiazem, with or without benzodiazepines, are usually effective (Table 51.2). Catheter modification of the sinus node is moderately effective (60%), but the benefits may be short-term and can be complicated by the need of permanent pacing in 10% of the patients.[7,8] Narrowing of the SVC and phrenic nerve palsy may also occur. Ivabradine, a specific sinus node I_f current inhibitor, is also promising.[9]

Sinus reentrant tachycardia

Definition

Sinus nodal reentrant tachycardia is due to reentry within the sinus node, with or without involvement of the perisinus atrial tissue. Up to 27% of focal AT are actually due to sinus nodal reentry. Usually, underlying cardiac disease exists.[6]

Diagnosis

It is based on:

- The tachycardia is **paroxysmal**.
- P wave morphology is almost **identical to sinus rhythm**.
- Endocardial atrial activation is similar to that of sinus rhythm.
- Induction and/or termination of the arrhythmia occurs with premature atrial stimuli.

Table 51.2 ACC/AHA/ESC 2003 GL on SVT

Recommendations for treatment of inappropriate sinus tachycardia		
Medical	Beta-blockers	I-C
	Verapamil, diltiazem	IIa-C
Interventional	Catheter ablation, sinus node modification/elimination*	IIb-C

* Used as a last resort.
ACC/AHA/ESC guidelines for the management of patients with supraventricular arrhythmias-executive summary. *Circulation*. 2003;**108**:1871–909.

- Termination occurs with **vagal manoeuvres or adenosine**.
- Induction of the arrhythmia is independent of atrial or AV nodal conduction time.

Therapy

Vagal manoeuvres or adenosine may be used for acute therapy. Beta-blockers, verapamil, and diltiazem may be tried for long-term control. In non-responders, catheter ablation is usually successful.[10]

Focal atrial tachycardia

Definition

Focal atrial tachycardia (AT) is characterized by a P wave rate of >250/min, although it can be <200/min, and an isoelectric interval between P waves (Figures 51.1 and 51.2).

Pathophysiology

Atrial activation originates from a discrete focus (<2 cm in diameter) with centrifugal spread.[11] Focal AT accounts for up to 10% of SVT referred for ablation.[12] Micro-reentry, abnormal automaticity, and triggered activity are the postulated mechanism, although electroanatomic abnormalities that may be detected in patients with focal AT are in support of micro-reentry, particularly in the elderly.[13] In childhood, the lack of effectiveness of DC cardioversion

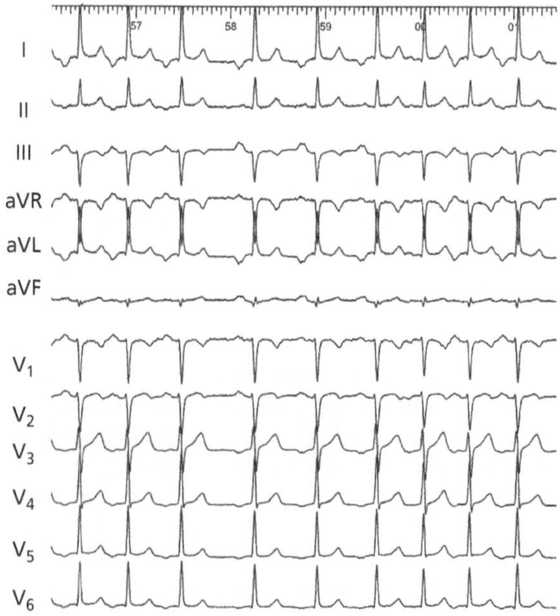

Figure 51.1 Left atrial tachycardia. Morphology of P waves in V_1 suggests a left PV origin.

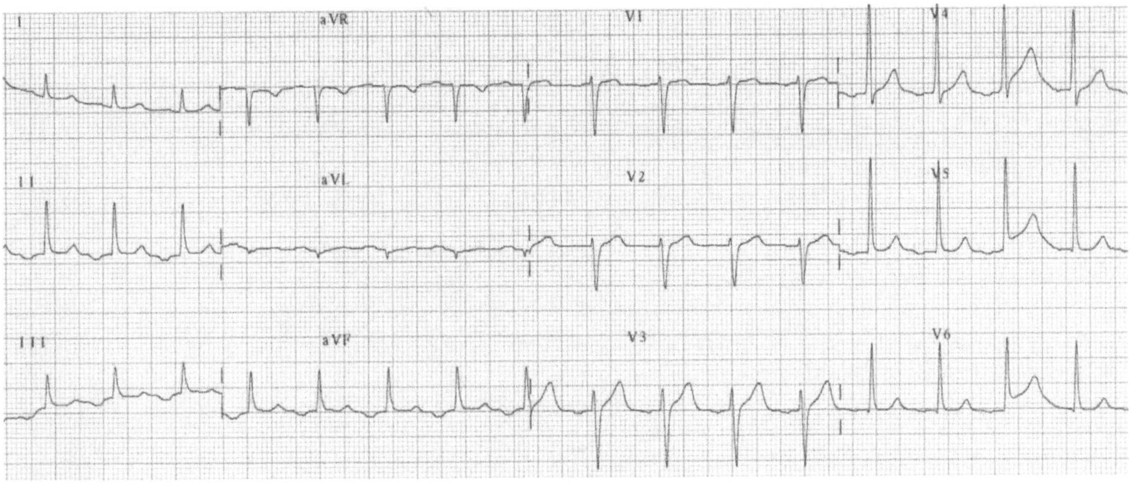

Figure 51.2 Atrial tachycardia originating at the CS ostium. Note negative P waves in inferior leads and V_1.

suggests abnormal automaticity as the underlying mechanism. Focal AT, as opposed to multifocal AT, is usually not associated with underlying heart disease, and the prognosis is benign, unless tachycardia-induced cardiomyopathy develops.

Presentation

Onset of episodes may occur at any age, from birth to old age. Palpitations are of substantial variation in duration, with **sudden increases and decreases in rate**. There is usually an **abrupt onset and termination** with bursts of activity. The clinical course is variable, and spontaneous remission is common.[14]

Diagnosis

- Classically, the P wave for focal AT is described as distinct with an intervening **isoelectric interval**, in contrast to a continuous undulation typical of macro-reentry tachycardia. However, an isoelectric interval may not be identifiable during accelerated heart rates and/or in the presence of atrial disease, resulting in slowing of conduction.
- Focal AT is characterized by a **change in P wave morphology** and dissociation between the atrium and ventricular response. The foci of focal AT mainly occur along the crista terminalis (>30%), tricuspid annulus and coronary sinus ostium, mitral annulus, perinodal or para-Hisian region, ostia of the pulmonary veins, left-sided septum, and near the aortic coronary cusps. The morphology of P wave may assist in identifying the tachycardia origin.[15,16] Foci arising from the superior crista terminalis display a negative or positive-negative P wave in lead V_1 or P wave may be indistinguishable from that during the sinus rhythm. A positive or negative-positive biphasic P wave in V_1 and negative in lead I indicate a left atrial focus. P waves from right PV foci are narrow and uniphasic whereas, from the left PV, broad and notched in lead V_1. CS ostium foci produce P waves negative in the inferior leads and positive in aVL and aVR.
- The distinction between focal AT and AVNRT or AVRT can be made by analysing the R-P relationship on the surface ECG. Typically, focal AT is associated with **a long and variable R-P relationship**. However, focal AT can show a short R-P relationship at higher rates and increased AV node conduction. Atypical AVNRT and a concealed accessory pathway with slow retrograde conduction may demonstrate a long R-P interval, but the R-P interval is typically constant.

The diagnosis of focal AT can only be established with certainty at the electrophysiology laboratory.

Therapy

Antiarrhythmic therapy (flecainide, sotalol, amiodarone) are partially effective in controlling symptoms (Table 51.3). Catheter ablation is the treatment of choice for patients, with success rates ranging from 40 to 90%.[17]

Multifocal atrial tachycardia

Multifocal atrial tachycardia is an irregular tachycardia characterized by three or more different P wave morphologies at different rates. The arrhythmia is most commonly associated with underlying **pulmonary disease** but may result from **metabolic or electrolyte derangements** or, rarely now, by **digitalis toxicity**. Calcium channel blockers and correction of the underlying disorder are the main therapeutic means. There is no role for DC cardioversion, antiarrhythmic drugs, or ablation.[6]

Table 51.3 ACC/AHA/ESC GL on SVT 2003. Recommendations for treatment of focal atrial tachycardia*

Acute treatment**		
A. Conversion		
Haemodynamically unstable patient	DC cardioversion	I-B
Haemodynamically stable patient	Adenosine	IIa-C
	Beta-blockers	IIa-C
	Verapamil, diltiazem,	IIa-C
	Procainamide,	IIa-C
	Flecainide/propafenone,	IIa-C
	Amiodarone, sotalol	IIa-C
B. Rate regulation (in absence of digitalis therapy)		
	Beta-blockers	I-C
	Verapamil, diltiazem	I-C
	Digoxin	IIb-C
Prophylactic therapy		
Recurrent symptomatic AT	Catheter ablation	I-B
	Beta blockers, calcium channel blockers	I-C
	Disopyramide*** Flecainide/propafenone (all combined with beta-blockers)	IIa-C
	Sotalol, amiodarone	IIa-C
Asymptomatic or symptomatic incessant AT	Catheter ablation	I-B
Non-sustained and asymptomatic	No therapy	I-C
	Catheter ablation	III-C

* Excluded are patients with multifocal atrial tachycardia in whom beta-blockers and sotalol are often contraindicated due to pulmonary disease.
** All listed drugs for acute treatment are administered intravenously.
*** Flecainide, propafenone, and disopyramide should not be used, unless they are combined with an AV nodal blocking agent.
AT indicates atrial tachycardia; DC, direct current;
ACC/AHA/ESC guidelines for the management of patients with supraventricular arrhythmias-executive summary. *Circulation*. 2003;**108**:1871–909.

Macro-reentrant atrial tachycardias (atrial flutters)

The mechanism of macro-reentrant atrial tachycardia is reentrant activation around a large central obstacle, generally several centimetres in diameter, at least in one of its dimensions. The central obstacle may consist of normal (i.e. cavotricuspid isthmus, CTI) or abnormal (i.e. postoperative scar) structures. The obstacle can be fixed, functional, or a combination of each. There is no single point of origin of activation, and atrial tissues outside the circuit are activated from various parts of the circuit.[11]

Isthmus-dependent atrial flutter

Isthmus-dependent flutter refers to circuits involving the CTI. The circuit is around the tricuspid annulus and contains a propagating wavefront and an excitable gap. The crista terminalis and Eustachian ridge are the functional posterior barriers, and the tricuspid annulus the anterior barrier. In approximately 60% of patients, there is underlying disease, such as COPD, pneumonia, myocardial ischaemia, or cardiac or pulmonary surgery.

Definitions and classification

The most common patterns include a tachycardia showing a **counterclockwise** rotation in the left anterior oblique view around the tricuspid valve (**typical atrial flutter**) (Figure 51.3). A less common pattern (10%) involves **clockwise** rotation around the tricuspid annulus (i.e. **reverse typical flutter**).[11] **Counterclockwise atrial flutter** is characterized electrocardiographically by dominant negative flutter waves in the inferior leads and a positive flutter deflection in lead V_1, with transition to a negative deflection in lead V_6 at rates of 250 to 350 bpm.

Clockwise isthmus-dependent flutter shows the opposite pattern (i.e. positive flutter waves in the inferior leads and wide, negative flutter waves in lead V_1, transitioning to positive waves in lead V_6).

Double-wave reentry is defined as a circuit in which two flutter waves simultaneously occupy the usual flutter pathway. This arrhythmia is transient, usually terminating within three to six complexes but may, on rare occasions, deteriorate into AF.

Lower-loop reentry is defined as a flutter circuit in which the reentry wavefront circulates around the inferior vena cava due to conduction across the crista terminalis.

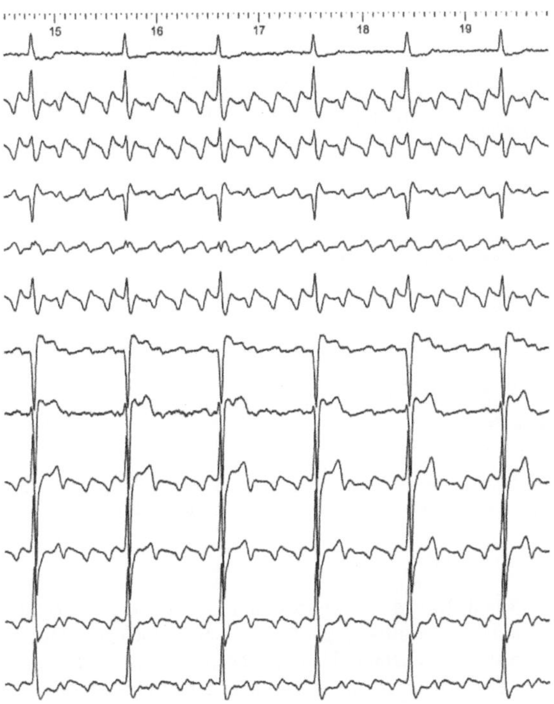

Figure 51.3 Typical atrial flutter with sawtooth P waves in inferior leads.

Table 51.4 ACC/AHA/ESC GL on SVT 2003. Recommendations for acute management of atrial flutter

Poorly tolerated flutter		
Conversion	DC cardioversion	I-C
Rate control	Beta-blockers Verapamil or diltiazem	IIa-C
	Digitalis (especially in HF) Amiodarone	IIb-C
Stable flutter		
Conversion	Atrial or transoesophageal pacing	I-A
	DC cardioversion	I-C
	Ibutilide (not in low LVEF)	IIa-A
	Flecainide, propafenone, procainamide (all with beta blockers)	IIb-A
	Sotalol	IIb-C
	Amiodarone	IIb-C
Rate control	Diltiazem or verapamil	I-A
	Beta-blockers	I-C
	Digitalis (especially in HF)	IIb-C
	Amiodarone	IIb-C

Cardioversion should be considered only if the patient is anticoagulated (INR = 2–3), the arrhythmia is less than 48 hours in duration, or the TOE shows no atrial clots.
ACC/AHA/ESC guidelines for the management of patients with supraventricular arrhythmias-executive summary. *Circulation*. 2003;**108**:1871–909.

Atrial flutter may present with unusual ECG patterns, and confirmation of isthmus involvement can be made only by entrainment pacing of the CTI during electrophysiological studies. It should be noted, however, that a long post-pacing interval may be due to delayed conduction and does not exclude isthmus-dependent flutter.[18] Regardless of the circuit, arrhythmias dependent on CTI conduction are amenable to isthmus ablation.

Presentation

Patients present with **sudden-onset palpitations, dyspnoea**, or **chest pain**. More insidious symptoms, such as fatigue and worsening of heart failure, may also occur. The typical sawtooth ECG patterns described in Definitions and classification may or may not be present. Usually, there is a **2:1 AV conduction**, with a resultant ventricular rate of approximately 150 beats/min. **Varying block** produces an irregular rhythm whereas 1:1 conduction may lead to haemodynamic instability.

Therapy

In emergencies, DC cardioversion (<50 J) is indicated (Table 51.4). Otherwise, ibutilde IV or overdrive pacing are used. For acute rate control, diltiazem IV is effective as verapamil but with a lower incidence of hypotension.[6] Atrial flutter lasting >48 h requires anticoagulation. No antiarrhythmic therapy is of proven efficacy for long-term rhythm control, and catheter ablation is the current treatment of choice, offering a >90% success rate and 10% recurrence (Table 51.5).[19,20] Although a <0.6% mortality has been reported in earlier studies,[20] no deaths are seen in recent trials.[21]

Non-isthmus-dependent atrial flutter

Lesion-related macro-reentry may be right or left atrial and is following repair of congenital defect (usually ASD), mitral valve surgery, maze procedures, or left atrial ablation for AF.

Right atrial free wall macro-reentry without atriotomy has also been described.[11]

Conduction delays within the circuit can prolong the atrial tachycardia cycle length, making it overlap with the classical focal atrial tachycardia range (>400 ms cycle length). Incisional macro-reentrant AT may also coexist with isthmus-dependent flutter or incorporate the CTI, thus resulting in multiple reentry circuits, and may respond to isthmus ablation.[22] Electroanatomic mapping and catheter ablation of the circuit are usually required for long-term therapy.[23]

Table 51.5 ACC/AHA/ESC 2003. Recommendations for long-term management of atrial flutter

First episode and well-tolerated atrial flutter	Cardioversion alone	I-B
	Catheter ablation	IIa-B
Recurrent and well-tolerated atrial flutter	Catheter ablation	I-B
	Dofetilide	IIa-C
	Amiodarone, sotalol	IIb-C
	Flecainide, propafenone, quinidine, procainamide, disopyramide (all with beta-blockers and not in structural heart disease)	IIb-C
Poorly tolerated atrial flutter	Catheter ablation	I-B
Atrial flutter appearing after use of class IC agents or amiodarone for treatment of AF	Catheter ablation	I-B
	Stop current drug and use another	IIa-C
Symptomatic, non-CTI-dependent flutter after failed antiarrhythmic drug therapy	Catheter ablation	IIa-B

Catheter ablation of the AV junction and insertion of a pacemaker should be considered if catheter ablative cure is not possible and the patient fails drug therapy.
ACC/AHA/ESC guidelines for the management of patients with supraventricular arrhythmias-executive summary. *Circulation*. 2003;**108**:1871–909.

References

1. Conen D, *et al.* Premature atrial contractions in the general population: frequency and risk factors. *Circulation.* 2012;**126**:2302–8
2. Cheriyath P, *et al.* Relation of atrial and/or ventricular premature complexes on a two-minute rhythm strip to the risk of sudden cardiac death (the Atherosclerosis Risk In Communities [ARIC] Study). *Am J Cardiol.* 2011;**107**:151–5
3. Binici Z, *et al.* Excessive supraventricular ectopic activity and increased risk of atrial fibrillation and stroke. *Circulation.* 2010;**121**:1904–11
4. Pelchovitz DJ, *et al.* Caffeine and cardiac arrhythmias: a review of the evidence. *Am J Med.* 2011;**124**:284–9
5. Ameen A, *et al.* His bundle extrasystoles revisited: the great electrocardiographic masquerader. *Pacing Clin Electrophysiol.* 2011;**34**:e56–9
6. Blomstrom-Lundqvist C, *et al.* ACC/AHA/ESC guidelines for the management of patients with supraventricular arrhythmias—executive summary. A report of the American College of Cardiology/American Heart Association Task Force on practice guidelines and the European Society of Cardiology Committee for practice guidelines (writing committee to develop guidelines for the management of patients with supraventricular arrhythmias) developed in collaboration with NASPE-Heart Rhythm Society. *J Am Coll Cardiol.* 2003;**42**:1493–531
7. Olshansky B, *et al.* Inappropriate sinus tachycardia. *J Am Coll Cardiol.* 2012;**61**:793–801
8. Killu AM, *et al.* Refractory inappropriate sinus tachycardia successfully treated with radiofrequency ablation at the arcuate ridge. *Heart Rhythm.* 2012;**9**:1324–7
9. Cappato R, *et al.* Clinical efficacy of ivabradine in patients with inappropriate sinus tachycardia: a prospective, randomized, placebo-controlled, double-blind, crossover evaluation. *J Am Coll Cardiol.* 2012;**60**:1323–9
10. Goya M, *et al.* Radiofrequency catheter ablation for sinoatrial node reentrant tachycardia: electrophysiologic features of ablation sites. *Jpn Circ J.* 1999;**63**:177–83
11. Saoudi N, *et al.* A classification of atrial flutter and regular atrial tachycardia according to electrophysiological mechanisms and anatomical bases; a Statement from a Joint Expert Group from the Working Group of Arrhythmias of the European Society of Cardiology and the North American Society of Pacing and Electrophysiology. *Eur Heart J.* 2001;**22**:1162–82
12. Porter MJ, *et al.* Influence of age and gender on the mechanism of supraventricular tachycardia. *Heart Rhythm.* 2004;**1**:393–6
13. Rosso R, *et al.* Focal atrial tachycardia. *Heart.* 2010;**96**:181–5
14. Poutiainen AM, *et al.* Prevalence and natural course of ectopic atrial tachycardia. *Eur Heart J.* 1999;**20**:694–700
15. Gonzalez-Torrecilla E, *et al.* EGC diagnosis of paroxysmal supraventricular tachycardias in patients without preexcitation. *Ann Noninvasive Electrocardiol.* 2011;**16**:85–95
16. Kistler PM, *et al.* P wave morphology in focal atrial tachycardia: development of an algorithm to predict the anatomic site of origin. *J Am Coll Cardiol.* 2006;**48**:1010–17
17. Anguera I, *et al.* Outcomes after radiofrequency catheter ablation of atrial tachycardia. *Am J Cardiol.* 2001;**87**:886–90
18. Vollmann D, *et al.* Misleading long post-pacing interval after entrainment of typical atrial flutter from the cavotricuspid isthmus. *J Am Coll Cardiol.* 2012;**59**:819–24
19. Natale A, *et al.* Prospective randomized comparison of antiarrhythmic therapy versus first-line radiofrequency ablation in patients with atrial flutter. *J Am Coll Cardiol.* 2000;**35**:1898–904
20. Spector P, *et al.* Meta-analysis of ablation of atrial flutter and supraventricular tachycardia. *Am J Cardiol.* 2009;**104**:671–7
21. Bohnen M, *et al.* Incidence and predictors of major complications from contemporary catheter ablation to treat cardiac arrhythmias. *Heart Rhythm.* 2011;**8**:1661–6
22. Chan DP, *et al.* Importance of atrial flutter isthmus in postoperative intra-atrial reentrant tachycardia. *Circulation.* 2000;**102**:1283–9
23. Delacretaz E, *et al.* Multi atrial maco-re-entry circuits in adults with repaired congenital heart disease: entrainment mapping combined with three-dimensional electroanatomic mapping. *J Am Coll Cardiol.* 2001;**37**:1665–76

Chapter 52

Atrial fibrillation

Definitions and classification

Atrial fibrillation (AF) is a supraventricular tachyarrhythmia characterized by uncoordinated atrial activation without effective atrial contraction.[1–5] On the ECG, there is replacement of consistent P waves by rapid oscillations or fibrillatory waves that vary in amplitude, shape, and timing (when visible, usually in lead V_1, the atrial length is variable and <200 ms, i.e. >300 bpm), associated with an irregular ventricular response.[1] QRS complexes may also be of variable amplitude. Regular R-R intervals are possible in the presence of AV block or coexistent AV junctional or ventricular tachycardia.

Paroxysmal AF is defined as recurrent AF (≥2 episodes) self-terminating within 7 days. Usually, self-termination occurs within 48 h. After this, the likelihood of spontaneous conversion is low.

Persistent AF is present when an AF episode either lasts longer than 7 days or requires termination by cardioversion, either with drugs or by direct current cardioversion.

Long-standing persistent AF is AF that has lasted for ≥1 year.

Permanent AF refers to the situation when the presence of the arrhythmia is accepted by the patient and physician. Hence, rhythm control interventions are, by definition, not pursued in patients with permanent AF. Should a rhythm control strategy be adopted, the arrhythmia is redesignated as 'long-standing persistent AF'.[1,4]

Silent AF, i.e. asymptomatic AF, is discovered at a routine medical or following a complication and may present as any of the temporal forms of AF.

Lone (idiopathic) AF has been variously defined but generally applies to young individuals (under 60 years of age) without clinical or echocardiographic evidence of cardiopulmonary disease, including hypertension. Its prevalence is not exactly known, with reports varying from 10 to 30% among patients with AF.[6,7]

Although, in certain cases, AF is vagally mediated (i.e. after meals or habitual aerobic training) whereas, in others, it follows sympathetic overactivity, the terms **vagal** and **adrenergic** AF are oversimplifications since the balance between sympathetic and parasympathetic influences is as important as absolute tone.

Epidemiology

AF is the most common sustained arrhythmia in humans and affects 1–2% of the general population worldwide. It affects up to 3 and 6 million people in the United States and Europe, respectively,[8–10] while in Asian countries its incidence is slightly lower.[11,12] It is also expected that these figures will increase up to 2.5-fold during the next 50 years.[6,7,10,13] The prevalence of AF increases with age, from approximately 2% in the general population to 5–15% at 80 years.[6,8] Whites are more often affected than blacks, while the overall number of men and women with AF is about equal.[4] The lifetime risk of developing AF has been calculated as 20–25% in those who have reached the age of 50,[10,14] and appears higher in recent studies. [10] The incidence of early-onset AF in persons <50 years is 0.62 cases per 1000 person-years for men and 0.19 cases per 1000 person-years for women.[6]

The presence of AF accounts for a 50% (men) to 90% (women) increased risk for overall mortality over 40 years follow-up in the Framingham Heart Study, thus diminishing the female advantage in survival.[15] AF is also associated with significant morbidity, including a 2- to 7-fold increased risk for stroke (average 5% per year), a 2- to 3-fold increased risk for dementia, and a tripling of risk for heart failure.[16–18] In the Framingham Study, the percentage of strokes attributable to AF increases steeply from 1.5% at 50–59 years of age to 23.5% at 80–89 years of age.[18] Approximately 20% of all strokes are due to AF,[1] and paroxysmal AF carries the same stroke risk as permanent or persistent AF.[19] Undiagnosed, silent AF is a probable cause of cryptogenic strokes.[20] Data from the ARIC study indicate that incident AF is associated with an increased risk of sudden and non-sudden cardiac death in the general population.[21] In a recent report on a large Swedish registry of 272,186 patients, AF was an independent risk factor of all-cause mortality. The highest relative risk of mortality was seen in women and in the youngest patients compared with controls.[22]

AF and its associated morbidity represent a significant socio-economic burden on the healthcare system. Direct cost estimates range from $2000 to 14 200 per patient-year in the USA and from €450 to 3000 in Europe.[21] This is comparable with other chronic conditions, such as diabetes. In the USA, AF hospitalizations alone cost approximately $6.65 billion in 2005.[23]

Patients with AF or heart failure have a significantly higher risk of post-operative mortality than patients with coronary artery disease, and even minor procedures carry a risk higher than previously appreciated.[24]

Table 52.1 Causes of AF

Systemic hypertension
Ageing
Heart failure
Valve disease
Obesity
Coronary artery disease
Diabetes mellitus
Chronic obstructive pulmonary disease
Chronic renal disease
Cardiomyopathies
Congenital heart disease (mainly ASD)
Post-operative (cardiac, pulmonary, or oesophageal)
Pulmonary hypertension (pulmonary embolism)
Pericarditis
Myocarditis
Intracardiac tumours or thrombi
Primary or metastatic disease in, or adjacent to, the atrial wall
Phaeochromocytoma
Chemotherapy agents
Hyperthyroidism
Subarachnoid haemorrhage
Non-haemorrhagic, major stroke
Metabolic syndrome
Sleep apnoea
Alcohol abuse
Hypomagnesaemia
Familial
Psoriasis
Long-term vigorous exercise
Sick sinus syndrome
AF as a result of ventricular pacing
Lone AF

Aetiology

Causes of AF are presented in Table 52.1. **Hypertension** is the most common cause of AF encountered in clinical practice.[4] Approximately 30% of patients with heart failure or valve disease have AF. Patients with coronary artery disease, diabetes, or COPD are at higher risk for AF (15–20%). Diastolic dysfunction presents a potentially important link between many common risk factors, such as hypertension, age, obesity, and diabetes, and the development of AF.[25] Postulated mechanisms of risk are increased atrial afterload, atrial myocyte stretching, and atrial wall stress. Chronic kidney disease and albuminuria,[26] metabolic syndrome,[27] and alcohol consumption [28] are associated with an increased prevalence of AF in adults. Thyroid disease is less common than previously thought. ASDs are associated with increased incidence of AF, regardless of treatment, and transcatheter ASD closure may trigger early transient arrhythmias; persistent AF is unlikely to be affected, but paroxysmal arrhythmias may improve, although that likelihood decreases with age >40 years.[29–31] Chemotherapy agents, such as anthracylines (at a rate of 2–10%), melphalan (7–12%), and cisplatin (12–32%), particularly with intrapericardial use, may cause AF.[32] Parental AF increases the future risk for offspring AF,[33] and a family history of AF is associated with substantial risk of lone AF,[34] thus supporting a genetic susceptibility to developing the arrhythmia. Mutations associated with AF are presented in Table 56.1 of Chapter 56 on genetic channelopathies). Mutations that cause loss of function of the sodium channel (such as in **SCN5A** and **10A genes**), gain of function of the potassium channels (**KCN genes**), or affect **connexins** or the **atrial natriuretic peptide**, as well as others, are mainly responsible, but account, for less than 5% of the disease.[35–38] Approximately 20% of patients with AF carry a common single nucleotide polymorphism on chromosome 4q25 that is associated with a lack of response to antiarrhythmic therapy for rhythm control.[39] Moderate to severe sleep apnoea is associated with a fourfold increase in the risk of AF.[40] Psoriasis is associated with increased risk of AF and ischaemic stroke.[41] Exercise intensity has a U-shaped relationship with AF.[42] Long-term vigorous exercise may predispose to AF (2–10 times more prevalent in active athletes),[43] but light to moderate physical activities, particularly leisure time activity and walking, are associated with significantly lower AF incidence in older adults.[42] Low serum magnesium is associated with the development of AF, even in persons without cardiovascular disease.[44]

Pathophysiology

Structural remodelling of the atria due to heart disease, atrial wall stretch, genetic causes, or other non-identified mechanisms results in electrical dissociation between muscle bundles and local conduction heterogeneities that facilitate the initiation and perpetuation of AF through multiple mechanisms.[45] Structural atrial abnormalities consist of areas of patchy fibrosis, enhanced connective tissue deposits juxtaposed with normal atrial fibres, inflammatory changes, intracellular substrate accumulation, and disruption of cell coupling at gap junctions with remodelling of connexins (i.e. transmembrane ion channel proteins in the gap junctions).[46] Connexin gene variants are associated with AF, and connexin gene transfer in animal studies has prevented AF.[47] Fibrosis and inflammatory changes have also been documented in patients with lone AF.[48] After the onset of AF, changes of atrial electrophysiological properties and mechanical function occur within days (>24 h). Shortening of the atrial effective refractory period results from abbreviation of the atrial action potential duration, which is caused by a decrease in the calcium channel current (I_{Ca}) and an increase in the potassium channel current (I_{K1}) and the constitutively active acetylcholine-sensitive current (I_{KACh}).[46,49] Restoration of sinus rhythm results in recovery of normal atrial refractoriness within a few days. Downregulation of the Ca^{2+} inward current and impaired release of Ca^{2+} from intracellular Ca^{2+} stores cause loss of contractility and increased compliance with subsequent atrial dilation. Electrical remodelling of the atria is, therefore, perpetuated by AF itself in a way that 'AF begets AF'.[49] A fast fibrillatory rate is associated with worse prognosis in patients without structural heart disease due to adverse atrial remodelling and prolonged episodes, but, in patients with heart failure, a low fibrillatory rate indicates poor prognosis probably due to adverse remodelling and atrial fibrosis.[50]

Electrophysiologic mechanisms

The initiation and perpetuation of AF requires both triggers for its onset and a substrate for its maintenance.

Focal electrical activity, contributing to the initiation and perhaps perpetuation of AF, has been identified at pulmonary veins (PV) ostia.[51] Due to shorter refractory periods, as well as abrupt changes in myocyte fibre orientation, the PV left atrial junctions have a stronger potential to initiate and perpetuate atrial tachyarrhythmias.[52] Mechanisms of focal activity might involve increased local automaticity, triggered activity, and micro-reentry (Figure 52.1). Apart from the PVs, other cardiac veins and certain areas of the posterior left atrial wall may have a profibrillatory role.[53] Localized anisotropic reentry, leading to rotors with a high dominant frequency, and fibrillatory conduction may also play a role in maintaining AF.[54] Elimination of these rotors and AF nests may be one of the mechanisms for the efficacy of real-time frequency analysis or complex fractionated electrogram-guided ablation.[55]

According to the **multiple wavelet hypothesis**, proposed by Moe and colleagues, AF is perpetuated by continuous conduction of several independent wavelets propagating through the atrial musculature in a seemingly chaotic manner. Fibrillation wavefronts continuously undergo wavefront-waveback interactions, resulting in wavebreak and the generation of new wavefronts, while block, collision, and fusion of wavefronts tend to reduce their number. As long as the number of wavefronts does not decline below a critical level, the multiple wavelets will sustain the arrhythmia.

Areas rich in **autonomic innervation** may be the source of activity that triggers AF. Ablation of the adjacent area of the ligament of Marshall has yielded moderate success in eliminating episodes of PAF.[56] Ganglionated plexi that can be identified around the circumference of the left atrial PV junction may also contribute to induction and perpetuation of AF.[53] These plexi are usually located 1–2 cm outside the PV ostia, they mediate both sympathetic and parasympathetic activity, and their ablation (autonomic denervation) has been found efficacious when added to antral PV isolation.[57]

These mechanisms are not mutually exclusive and may coexist at various times. While, in most patients with paroxysmal AF, localized sources of the arrhythmia can be identified, such attempts are often not successful in patients with persistent or permanent AF. This can be interpreted within the context of the multifactorial aetiology of AF.

Haemodynamic consequences

Loss of atrial contraction and atrioventricular synchrony, irregular ventricular response, rapid heart rate, and impaired coronary arterial blood flow affect the haemodynamic function during AF. Loss of atrial contraction, especially when diastolic filling is impaired, may reduce cardiac output up to 15%.[4] Irregular ventricular response affects both myocardial contractility and coronary flow. Rapid ventricular rates may compromise coronary flow and exacerbate MR. A persistently elevated ventricular rate (>130 bpm) is also a known cause of tachycardia-induced cardiomyopathy (see Chapter 40).[58] Ventricular response is limited by the intrinsic refractoriness of AV node and its atrial inputs and is being affected by concealed conduction to the node and autonomic tone. AF is also a cause of functional MR due to atrial dilatation.[59]

Thromboembolism

Thrombotic material in AF usually arises in the left atrial appendage due to decreased flow and stasis, possible endothelial dysfunction, and a hypercoagulable state, as indicated by increased fibrinogen, D-dimer, thromboglobulin, and platelet factor 4 levels.[4] The morphology of the left atrial appendage on MRI may affect the risk of stroke.[60] Both persistent and paroxysmal AF are causes of stroke, and subclinical episodes of AF are frequent in type 2 diabetic patients are associated with a significantly increased risk of silent cererbral infarcts and stroke.[61] Up to 25% of stroke in patients with AF are due to intrinsic cardiovascular diseases, such as hypertension, aortic atheromatosis, and LV dysfunction.[4] Prior embolic events, intracranial haemorrhage, myocardial infarction, vascular disease, and renal failure predict ischaemic stroke in AF, but thyroid disease (or hyperthyroidism) is not an independent risk factor for stroke.[62]

Diagnosis

Patients may present with palpitations or the arrhythmia may be an incidental finding. The 2012 ESC GL on AF recommend opportunistic screening for AF in patients ≥65 years of

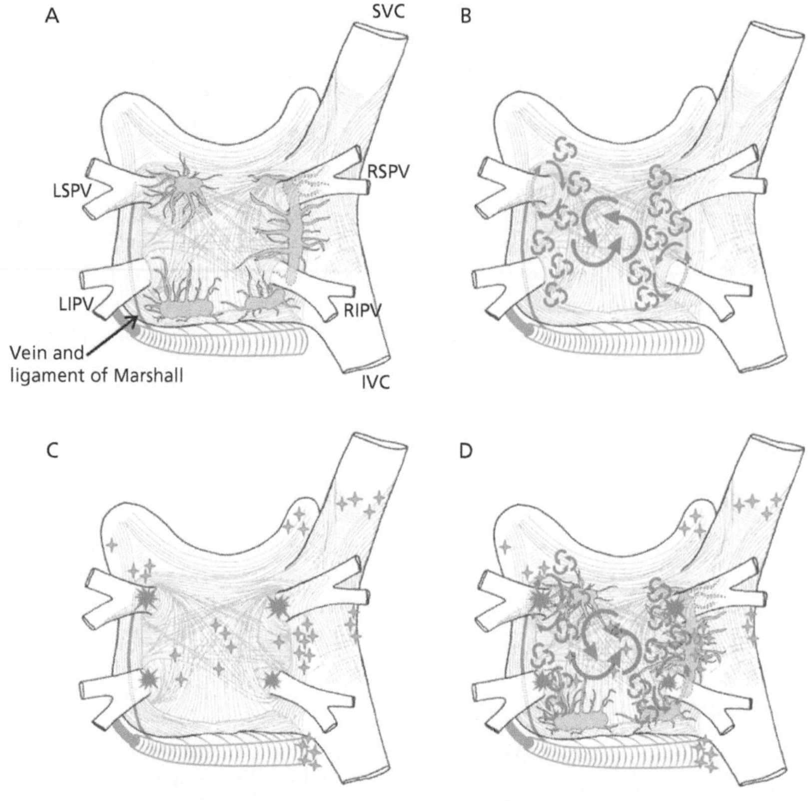

Figure 52.1 Structure and mechanisms of atrial fibrillation. (A) Schematic drawing of the left and right atria as viewed from the posterior. The extension of muscular fibres onto the PVs can be appreciated. Shown in yellow are the four major LA autonomic ganglionic plexi and axons (superior left, inferior left, anterior right, and inferior right). Shown in blue is the coronary sinus which is enveloped by muscular fibres which have connections to the atria. Also shown in blue is the vein and ligament of Marshall which travels from the coronary sinus to the region between the left superior PV and the LA appendage. (B) Large and small reentrant wavelets that play a role in initiating and sustaining AF. (C) Common locations of PV (red) and also the common sites of origin of non-PV triggers (shown in green). (D) Composite of the anatomical and arrhythmic mechanisms of AF.

Estes NA 3rd, *et al.* American Heart Association atrial fibrillation research summit: a conference report from the American Heart Association. *Circulation*. 2011;**124**:363–72.

age using pulse taking, followed by an ECG (I-B). Frequent atrial ectopy, atrial tachycardia, atrial flutter, and dual antegrade atrioventricular nodal conduction may present with rapid irregular R-R intervals and mimic AF. Most atrial tachycardias and flutters show longer atrial cycle lengths ≥200 ms, but patients on antiarrhythmic drugs may have slower atrial cycle lengths during AF. When the ventricular rate is fast, atrioventricular nodal blockade during the Valsalva manoeuvre, carotid massage, or intravenous adenosine administration can help to unmask atrial activity. Extremely rapid ventricular rates (> 200 bpm) suggest the presence of an accessory pathway or ventricular tachycardia.

Investigations

Complete **history** (including family and social history), **physical examination**, **12-lead ECG**, **blood pressure measurement**, **echocardiography**, and basic laboratory investigations (**full blood count; renal, liver, and thyroid function; electrolytes, including calcium and magnesium, glucose, and lipid profile**) are mandatory in every patient who presents with first detected AF. The quality of life of the patient should be also assessed, using either the EHRA[1] or the Canadian Cardiovascular Society[63] scales (EHRA I, asymptomatic; EHRA II, mild symptoms; EHRA III, severe symptoms; EHRA IV, disabling symptoms).

Additional tests in selected cases are:

- **Chest radiography** to exclude lung disease or before starting amiodarone
- **Ambulatory ECG monitoring** to document AF episodes and detect other initiating arrhythmia. A patch-type 7- to 14-day Holter or implantable loop recorder increases detection rate and is useful in the

investigation of cryptogenic stroke[64]

- **Six-minute walk test** or **treadmill exercise test** to assess rate control
- **Ischaemia testing** if coronary artery disease is suspected
- **Ambulatory blood pressure monitoring** in case of borderline hypertension
- **Transoesophageal echocardiography** to exclude left atrial appendage thrombus or mobile aortic plaques when cardioversion is planned
- **Electrophysiology study** when other supraventricular arrhythmia that initiates AF is suspected
- **Sleep study** when sleep apnoea is suspected
- **Genetic testing** is not indicated (Table 52.2).

Risk stratification

The main complications of AF are thromboembolism and impairment of LV function. Reduced LV function predisposes to thromboembolism and may evolve into tachycardiopathy. Baseline echocardiography, therefore, is essential for initial assessment of LA size and LVEF and follow-up. Arrhythmia-induced impairment of LV function should be considered with fast and persistently elevated ventricular rate (>130 bpm).[59]

Absolute stroke rates for non-anticoagulated patients vary between 1.5% and 10%, depending on the presence of risk factors. Prior stroke/TIA, advancing age, and hypertension have been consistently identified as independent risk factors for stroke in AF.[65,66] Left ventricular dysfunction, diabetes, renal failure, and female gender also increase the risk of thromboembolism.[63,64] Prior stroke/TIA is the most powerful risk factor and reliably confers a stroke risk averaging 10% per year.[66] Patients <60 years with lone AF have a very low cumulative stroke risk estimated to be 1.3% over 15 years.[1] The probability of stroke in young patients with lone AF appears to increase with advancing age or development of hypertension.

The simplest thromboembolic risk assessment scheme is the $CHADS_2$ score (cardiac failure, hypertension, age, diabetes, stroke (doubled)) risk index.[67] It has been recently revised as the CHA_2DS_2VASc score that is used by the recent ESC guidelines (Table 52.3).[68] These schemes apply to patients with any form of AF (paroxysmal, persistent, or permanent). N-terminal proBNP is often elevated in AF and independently associated with an increased risk for stroke and mortality, thus improving risk stratification beyond the CHA2DS2VASc score.[69]

Table 52.2 HRS/EHRA 2011 statement on genetic testing

State of genetic testing for atrial fibrillation	
Genetic testing is not indicated for atrial fibrillation at this time.	III
SNP genotyping, in general, and SNP rs2200733 genotyping at the 4q25 locus, in particular, for AF is not indicated at this time, based on the limited outcome data currently available	III

HRS/EHRA expert consensus statement on the state of genetic testing for the channelopathies and cardiomyopathies. *Europace*. 2011;**13**:1077–109.

Table 52.3 Risk of thromboembolism

$CHADS_2$ score	
Risk factor	**Score**
Heart failure	1
Hypertension	1
Age >75	1
Diabetes mellitus	1
Stroke/TIA/thromboembolism	2
$CHAD_2DS_2VASc$ score	
Risk factor	**Score**
Congestive heart failure/LV dysfunction	1
Hypertension	1
Age >75	2
Diabetes mellitus	1
Stroke/TIA/thromboembolism	2
Vascular disease (MI, peripheral artery disease, aortic plaque)	1
Age 65–74	1
Sex category (i.e. female sex)	1
Adjusted stroke rate according to CHA_2DS_2-VASc score	
Score	**Adjusted stroke rate (% per year)**
0	0
1	1.3
2	2.2
3	3.2
4	4.0
5	6.7
6	9.8
7	9.6
8	6.7
9	15.2

Previous stroke, TIA, systemic embolism, and age ≥75 years are considered major risk factors.

Therapy

Acute therapy

Direct current cardioversion is indicated in haemodynamic instability (Table 52.4) or when pharmacologic cardioversion has failed. Biphasic, R wave synchronized sho ck (at least 150–200 Joules to avoid repeated shocks and

Table 52.4 Direct current cardioversion of AF

ACCF/AHA 2013 GL on AF. Direct current cardioversion of atrial fibrillation and flutter	
Rapid ventricular rate does not respond to pharmacological measures in patients with ongoing myocardial ischaemia, symptomatic hypotension, angina, or HF.	I-C
Pre-excitation when very rapid tachycardia or haemodynamic instability.	I-B
Unacceptable symptoms without haemodynamic instability. Repeated direct current cardioversion attempts may be made following administration of antiarrhythmic medication.	I-C
Direct current cardioversion as part of a long-term management strategy for patients with AF (level of evidence: B).	IIa-B
Patient preference.	IIa-C
Frequent repetition of direct current cardioversion with short periods of sinus rhythm between relapses of AF, despite prophylactic antiarrhythmic drug therapy.	III-C
Digitalis toxicity or hypokalaemia.	III-C
ESC 2010 GL on AF. Recommendations for direct current cardioversion (DCC)	
Immediate DCC when a rapid ventricular rate does not respond promptly to pharmacological measures in patients with AF and ongoing myocardial ischaemia, symptomatic hypotension, angina, or heart failure.	I-C
Immediate DCC for patients with AF involving pre-excitation when rapid tachycardia or haemodynamic instability is present.	I-B
Elective DCC to initiate a long-term rhythm control management strategy.	IIa-B
Pre-treatment with amiodarone, flecainide, propafenone, ibutilide, or sotalol to enhance success of DCC and prevent recurrent AF.	IIa-B
Repeated DCC in highly symptomatic patients refractory to other therapy.	IIb-C
Pre-treatment with beta blockers, diltiazem, or verapamil for rate control, although the efficacy of these agents in enhancing success of DCC or preventing early recurrence of AF is uncertain.	IIb-C
DCC is contraindicated in patients with digitalis toxicity.	III-C

Management of patients with atrial fibrillation (compilation of 2006 ACCF/AHA/ESC and 2011 ACCF/AHA/HRS recommendations). *J Am Coll Cardiol.* 2013; **61**:1935–44.
Guidelines for the management of atrial fibrillation: The Task Force for the Management of Atrial Fibrillation of the European Society of Cardiology (ESC). *Eur Heart J.* 2010; **31**: 2369–2429.

occurrence of shock-induced VF) with anteroposterior electrode placement (at least 8 cm from a pacemaker battery, if present) is recommended.[70] To avoid thromboembolism (risk of 1–2%), a TOE should be performed to rule out atrial thrombi, unless AF is <48 h from a definite onset or adequate anticoagulation has been documented for 3 weeks (Figures 52.2 and 52.3). UFH (60 U/kg IV) or LMWH (1 mg/kg IV) are given before cardioversion. A pacing catheter or external pacing pads may be needed in patients with sick sinus syndrome or in elderly patients with structural heart disease. Ventricular arrhythmias (in digitalis intoxication or hypokalaemia) are rare. Pre-treatment with drugs, such as amiodarone, ibutilide, sotalol, flecainide, and propafenone, increases success rates (Table 52.5).[4]

Factors that predispose to AF recurrence are age, AF duration before cardioversion, number of previous recurrences, an increased LA size or reduced LA function, and the presence of coronary heart disease or pulmonary or mitral valve disease. Atrial ectopic beats with a long-short sequence, faster heart rates, and variations in atrial conduction also increase the risk of AF recurrence.

Pharmacological cardioversion is less effective than DC cardioversion. The same precautions for anticoagulation and thromboembolic risk prevention apply as in DC cardioversion. Drugs used are (Table 52.6):

- **Flecainide** (1.5–3 mg/kg IV over 10–20 min) or **propafenone** (2 mg/kg IV over 10 min) achieve SR in 67–92% and 41–91% of patients, respectively, within the next 6 h. They are both contraindicated in patients with coronary artery disease or impaired LV function, and are not effective in atrial flutter or persistent AF. They may prolong QRS duration with resultant ventricular tachycardia (and with flecainide, also the QT), and inadvertently increase the ventricular rate due to conversion to atrial flutter and 1:1 conduction to the ventricles.
- The **'pill-in-the pocket'** approach refers to oral flecainide (200–300 mg po) or propafenone (450–600 mg po) that may achieve SR in up to 45% of patients who present with <7 days AF.[71] They can also be used outside the hospital once treatment has proved safe in hospital for selected patients without sinus or AV node dysfunction, bundle branch block, QT interval prolongation, the Brugada syndrome, or structural heart disease, and especially previous MI. Before antiarrhythmic medication is initiated, a beta blocker or non-dihydropyridine calcium channel antagonist should be given to prevent rapid AV conduction in the event atrial flutter occurs (<0.2%).[1]
- **Ibutilide** is a class II agent blocking the rapid component of the rectifier potassium channel (I_{Kr}) and also activates the slow inward sodium current.[72] It is a moderately potent drug for acute conversion of AF (45–75%). It is given IV, 1 mg over 10 min in one or two doses, and achieves conversion within 90 min in 50% of patients. It prolongs the QTc by approximately 60 ms, and there is a 3.6% to 8.3% risk of torsades de pointes (watch for abnormal T-U waves or prominent QT prolongation). Co-administration of beta blockade may increase efficacy and diminish the proarrhythmic risk.[73] It is more effective in atrial flutter.
- **Amiodarone** (5 mg/kg IV over 1 h, followed by 50 mg/h for up to 24 h) achieves cardioversion in 40–60% of patients (80–90% with pre-treatment) but later than the other drugs. Hypotension and slow ventricular rate may be seen.
- **Dofetilide** is also a pure class III agent (selective Ikr blocking agent), that is moderately effective in cardio-

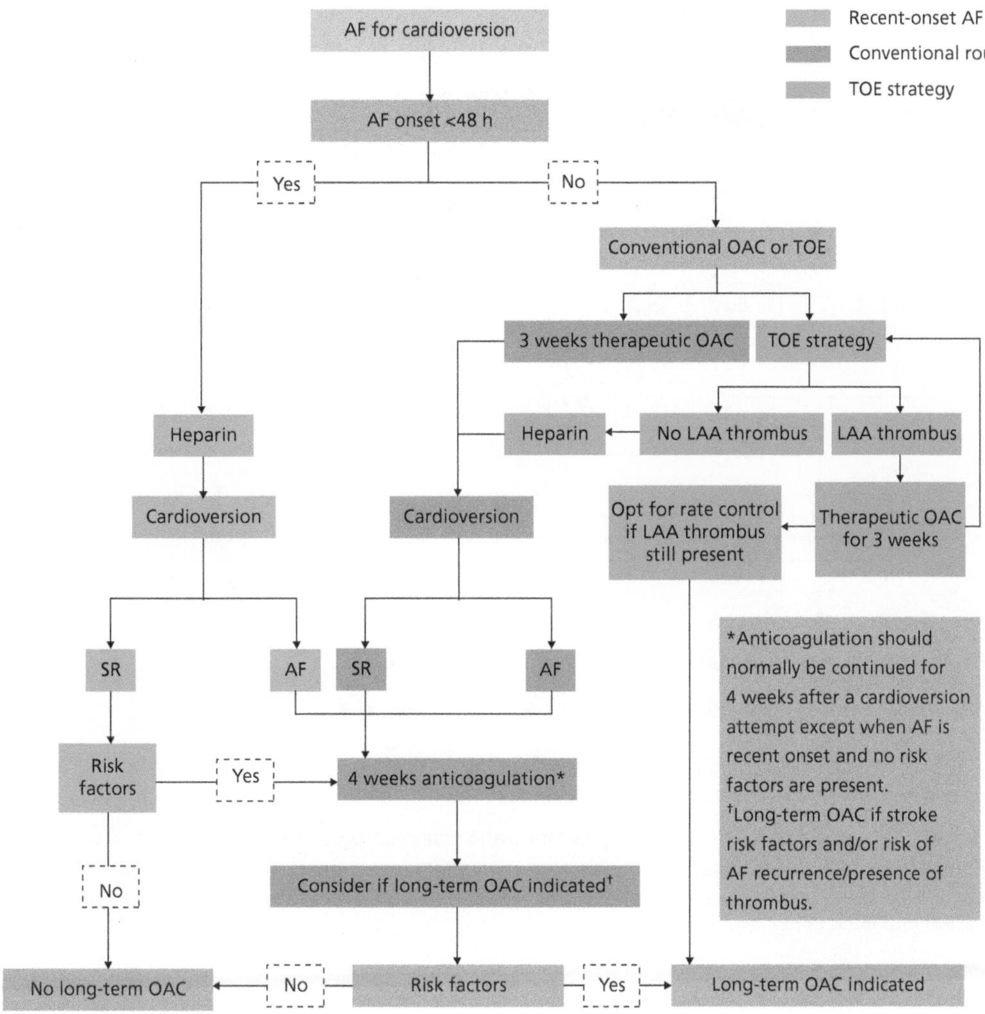

Figure 52.2 ESC 2010 GL on AF. Cardioversion of haemodynamically stable AF, the role of TOE-guided cardioversion, and subsequent anticoagulation strategy.

AF, atrial fibrillation; DCC, direct current cardioversion; LA, left atrium; LAA, left atrial appendage; OAC, oral anticoagulant; SR, sinus rhythm; TOE, transoesophageal echocardiography. Guidelines for the management of atrial fibrillation: The Task Force for the Management of Atrial Fibrillation of the European Society of Cardiology (ESC). *Eur Heart J* 2010; **31**: 2369–2429

verting AF or Afl to SR (30%) and significantly effective in maintaining SR for 1 year (60%).[74] It is given orally 500 mg bd and 250 or 125 mg bd with creatinine clearance <60 mL/min or 20–40 mL/min, respectively) and is also effective, even in AF >7 days in duration, but the response may be delayed. QTc prolongation also occurs, and there is a small, but not negligible, risk of proarrhythmia. Caution must be used when initiating dofetilide therapy to avoid torsade de pointes ventricular tachycardia, especially in patients with heart failure, hypertrophy, bradycardia, and female gender.

- **Vernakalant** blocks early activating potassium channels (IKur) and frequency-dependent sodium channels. It is relatively atrial-selective because the density of IKur channels is higher in the atria, and the effects on sodium channels are rate-dependent. In a dose of 3 mg/kg IV over 10 min, a second infusion of 2 mg/kg IV over 10 min after 15 min rest converts AF (of duration ≤7 days or ≤3 days after surgery) in up to 51% of patients within 90 min.[75] Vernakalant is contraindicated in patients with systolic blood pressure <100 mmHg, severe aortic stenosis, heart failure (class NYHA III and IV), ACS within the previous 30 days, or QT interval prolongation (uncorrected QT >440 ms).[5] Before its use, the patients should be adequately hydrated.

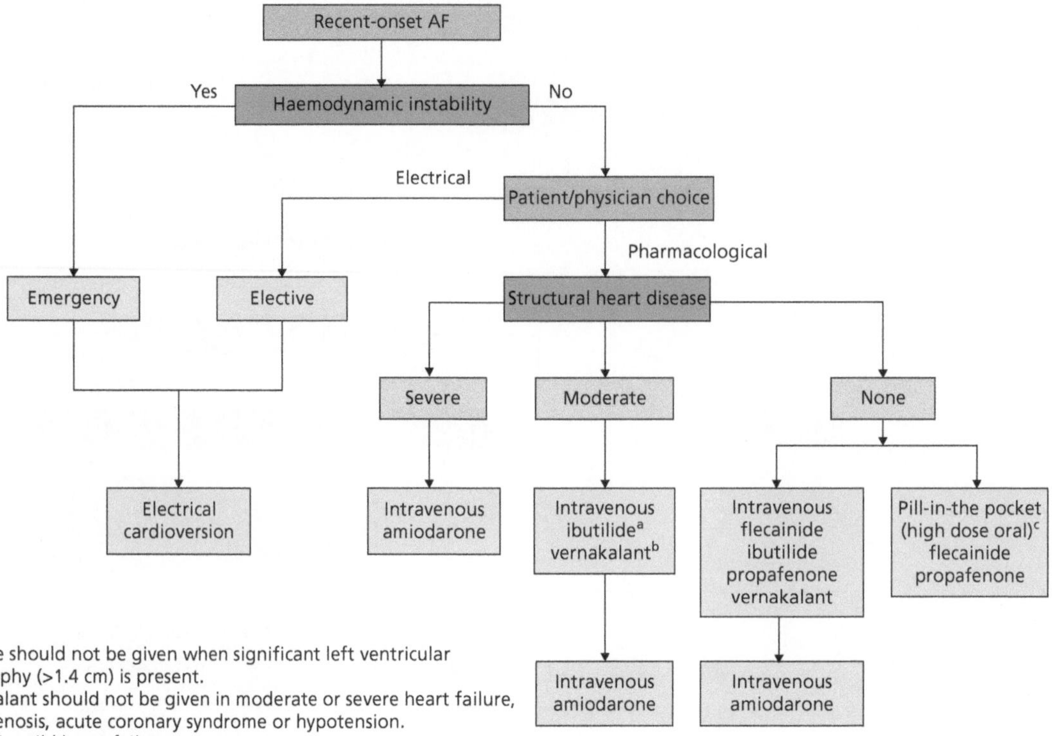

[1]Ibutilide should not be given when significant left ventricular hypertrophy (>1.4 cm) is present.
[b]Vernakalant should not be given in moderate or severe heart failure, aortic stenosis, acute coronary syndrome or hypotension. Caution in mild heart failure.
[c]Pill-in-the-pocet' technique—preliminary assessment in a medically safe environment and then used by the patient in the ambulatory setting.

Figure 52.3 ESC 2012 update on AF. Indications for electrical and pharmacological cardioversion, and choice of antiarrhythmic drugs for pharmacological cardioversion in patients with recent-onset AF.

2012 focused update of the ESC guidelines for the management of atrial fibrillation: an update of the 2010 ESC guidelines for the management of atrial fibrillation. *Europace*. 2012;**14**:1385–413.

Table 52.5 ACCF/AHA 2013 GL on AF

Pharmacological enhancement of direct current cardioversion	
Pre-treatment with amiodarone, flecainide, ibutilide, propafenone, or sotalol to enhance the success of direct current cardioversion and prevent recurrent AF.	IIa-B
Repeat cardioversion after AF relapse, following prophylactic administration of antiarrhythmic medication.	IIa-C
Beta blockers, disopyramide, diltiazem, dofetilide, procainamide, or verapamil in persistent AF	IIb-C
Out-of-hospital initiation of antiarrhythmic medications in patients without heart disease to enhance the success of cardioversion of AF.	IIb-C
Out-of-hospital administration of antiarrhythmic medications to enhance the success of cardioversion of AF in patients with certain forms of heart disease once the safety of the drug has been verified for the patient.	IIb-C

Management of patients with atrial fibrillation (compilation of 2006 ACCF/AHA/ESC and 2011 ACCF/AHA/HRS recommendations). *J Am Coll Cardiol*. 2013;**61**:1935–44.

Table 52.6 Pharmacological cardioversion of AF

ESC 2010 GL on AF and 2012 Update	
IV flecainide, propafenone, ibutilide, or vernakalant for cardioversion of recent-onset AF when pharmacological cardioversion is preferred and there is no structural heart disease.	I-A
IV amiodarone in patients with recent-onset AF and structural heart disease.	I-A
A single high oral dose of flecainide or propafenone (the 'pill-in-the-pocket' approach) in selected patients with recent-onset AF and no significant structural heart disease, provided this treatment has proven safe during previous testing in a medically secure environment.	IIa-B
Ibutilide in patients with recent-onset AF, structural heart disease, but without hypotension or manifest congestive heart failure. Serum electrolytes and the QTc interval must be within the normal range, and the patients must be closely monitored during, and for 4 h after, the infusion because of risk of proarrhythmia.	IIb-A
Vernakalant in AF ≤7 days and moderate structural heart disease (but without hypotension <100 mmHg, NYHA class III or IV heart failure, recent (<30 days) ACS, or severe aortic stenosis). It should be used with caution in patients with NYHA class I–II heart failure.	IIb-B
IV vernakalant for cardioversion of post-operative AF ≤3 days after cardiac surgery.	IIb-B
Digoxin.	III-A
Verapamil, sotalol, metoprolol.	III-B
Other beta-blocking agents and ajmaline are ineffective in converting recent-onset AF to sinus rhythm and are not recommended.	III-C
ACCF/AHA 2013 GL on AF.	
Flecainide, dofetilide, propafenone, or ibutilide.	I-A
Amiodarone.	IIa-A
Single oral bolus dose of propafenone or flecainide ('pill-in-the-pocket') outside the hospital once treatment has proved safe in hospital for selected patients without sinus or AV node dysfunction, bundle branch block, QT interval prolongation, the Brugada syndrome, or structural heart disease. Before antiarrhythmic medication is initiated, a beta blocker or non-dihydropyridine calcium channel antagonist should be given.	IIa-C
Amiodarone on an outpatient basis in patients with paroxysmal or persistent AF when rapid restoration of sinus rhythm is not necessary.	IIa-C
Quinidine or procainamide for pharmacological cardioversion.	IIb-C
Digoxin and sotalol may be harmful.	III-A
Quinidine, procainamide, disopyramide, and dofetilide should not be started out of hospital for conversion of AF.	III-B

Guidelines for the management of atrial fibrillation: The Task Force for the Management of Atrial Fibrillation of the European Society of Cardiology (ESC). *Eur Heart J.* 2010; **31**: 2369–2429.
Management of patients with atrial fibrillation (compilation of 2006 ACCF/AHA/ESC and 2011 ACCF/AHA/HRS recommendations). *J Am Coll Cardiol.* 2013; **61**:1935–44.

Peri-cardioversion anticoagulation In patients with AF <48 h from a definite onset, a bolus of UFH (5000 U IV) or LMWH (1 mg/kg IV) may be given, depending on underlying risk factors for thromboembolism. In the absence of such risk factors (CHA_2DS_2-VASc score 0), no oral anticoagulation is needed after cardioversion. In patients with AF >48 h or risk factors for thromboembolism, UFH (IV) or LMWH (IV or subcutaneous) are continued, together with oral anticoagulants, until the INR becomes 2–3 (for dosing, see CAD). Thereafter, anticoagulation is continued for 4 weeks, and then further anticoagulation depends on the presence of risk factors (Table 52.7).

Acute rate control When AF cannot be cardioverted or cardiovertion is contraindicated (i.e. presence of left atrial thrombus), acute rate control (80–100 bpm) can be accomplished by IV:

- **Beta blockers** (i.e. esmolol 0.5 mg/kg IV over 1 min, followed by 60–200 micrograms/kg/min, or metoprolol 2.5–5 mg bolus up to three doses), or
- **Non-dihydropyridine calcium antagonists** (diltiazem 0.25 mg/kg over 2 min, followed by 5–15 mg/h, or verapamil 0.075–0.15 mg/kg over 2 min).[1]

In the setting of heart failure or hypotension, **amiodarone** IV (150 mg over 10 min or 5 mg/kg IV over 1 h, and then followed by 50 mg/h) or **digitalis** (0.25–1.5 mg IV), under careful monitoring, may be used. In pre-excitation, only amiodarone, ibutilide, and class Ia are safe (see later). AF with slow ventricular rates may respond to atropine (0.5–2 mg IV), but temporary pacing may be required.

Chronic therapy

Rhythm vs rate control

Randomized control trials have failed to detect significant mortality and cardiovascular morbidity differences between patients with rate (i.e. controlling ventricular response with the patient in AF) vs rhythm (i.e. maintenance of SR) control achieved with antiarrhythmic medication (Table 52.8).[76–82] This is rather surprising, in view of the deleterious effects of AF, and has been mainly attributed to the proarrhythmic effects of drugs that may negate any benefits conferred by maintenance of SR.[83,84] In an extensive observational study, assessment of quality of life was also rather inadequate in most trials. In the J-RHYTHM trial, fewer patients requested changes of assigned treatment strategy in the rhythm control vs the

Table 52.7 Anticoagulation for cardioversion

ESC 2010 GL on AF and 2012 Update. Peri-cardioversion anticoagulation	
In AF of ≥48 h duration or when the duration of AF is unknown, OAC therapy (e.g. VKA with INR 2–3 or dabigatran) for ≥3 weeks prior to and for ≥4 weeks after cardioversion, regardless of the method (electrical or oral/IV pharmacological).	I-B
In patients with risk factors for stroke or AF recurrence, OAC therapy, whether with dose-adjusted VKA (INR 2–3) or a NOAC, should be continued lifelong, irrespective of the apparent maintenance of sinus rhythm following cardioversion.	I-B
For AF requiring immediate/emergency cardioversion because of haemodynamic instability, heparin (IV UFH bolus, followed by infusion, or weight-adjusted therapeutic dose LMWH) is recommended.	I-C
For patients with AF <48 h and at high risk of stroke, IV heparin or weight-adjusted therapeutic dose LMWH peri-cardioversion, followed by OAC with a VKA (INR 2.0–3.0) long-term.	I-B
As an alternative to anticoagulation prior to cardioversion, TOE-guided cardioversion to exclude thrombus in the left atrium or left atrial appendage.	I-B
For patients undergoing TOE-guided cardioversion who have no identifiable thrombus, cardioversion immediately after anticoagulation with heparin until OAC therapy has been established, which should be maintained for at least 4 weeks after cardioversion.	I-B
For patients undergoing a TOE-guided strategy in whom thrombus is identified, VKA (INR 2.0–3.0) for at least 3 weeks, followed by a repeat TOE to ensure thrombus resolution.	I-C
For atrial flutter undergoing cardioversion, anticoagulation is recommended as for patients with AF.	I-C
If thrombus resolution is evident on repeat TOE, cardioversion and OAC for 4 weeks or lifelong (if risk factors are present).	IIa-C
If thrombus remains on repeat TOE, an alternative strategy (e.g. rate control) may be considered.	IIb-C
For AF duration that is clearly <48 h and no thromboembolic risk factors.	IIb-C
ACCF/AHA 2013 GL on AF. Prevention of thromboembolism in patients with AF undergoing cardioversion	
In AF of 48 h duration, or longer, or when the duration of AF is unknown, anticoagulation (INR 2.0–3.0) for at least 3 wk prior to, and 4 wk after, cardioversion, regardless of the method (electrical or pharmacological) used to restore sinus rhythm.	I-B
In AF of >48 h duration requiring immediate cardioversion because of haemodynamic instability, heparin by IV bolus, followed by a continuous infusion to prolong the aPTT by 1.5 to 2. Thereafter, oral anticoagulation (INR 2.0–3.0) for at least 4 wk. Limited data support SC low molecular weight heparin in this indication.	I-C
In AF <48 h duration associated with haemodynamic instability (angina pectoris, MI, shock, or pulmonary oedema), cardioversion immediately without delay for prior initiation of anticoagulation.	I-C
During the first 48 h after onset of AF, the need for anticoagulation before and after cardioversion may be based on the patient's risk of thromboembolism.	IIa-C
TOE as an alternative to anticoagulation prior to cardioversion of AF.	IIa-B
For patients with no identifiable thrombus, cardioversion immediately after anticoagulation with unfractionated heparin, followed by a vitamin K antagonist for 4 weeks.	IIa-B
Limited data support SC low molecular weight heparin in this indication.	IIa-C
For patients in whom thrombus is identified by TOE, oral anticoagulation (INR 2.0–3.0) is reasonable for at least 3 wk prior to, and 4 wk after, restoration of sinus rhythm, and a longer period of anticoagulation may be appropriate, even after apparently successful cardioversion.	IIa-C
For patients with atrial flutter undergoing cardioversion, anticoagulation is according to the recommendations as for patients with AF.	IIa-C

Management of patients with atrial fibrillation (compilation of 2006 ACCF/AHA/ESC and 2011 ACCF/AHA/HRS recommendations). *J Am Coll Cardiol*. 2013; **61**:1935–44.

ESC on AF 2010. Guidelines for the management of atrial fibrillation: The Task Force for the Management of Atrial Fibrillation of the European Society of Cardiology (ESC). *Eur Heart J*. 2010; **31**: 2369–2429.

rate control group, which was accompanied by improvement in AF-specific quality of life scores.[80] Maintenance of SR also improved quality of life in the SAFE-T trial.[85] Finally, follow-up of most trials was relatively short. Superiority of rhythm control has been shown for certain patients groups. In the AFFIRM trial, patients ≥65 years and patients without a history of CHF had significantly better outcome with rate control therapy.[86] Improved survival with maintenance of sinus rhythm was also detected in the CHF-STAT (amiodarone in heart failure patients)[87,] nd DIAMOND (dofetilide in patients with LVEF <35%) [88] trials. In a recent extensive, observational trial, rhythm control therapy was associated with lower rates of stroke/TIA, particularly among patients with moderate and high risk of stroke.[89] In the ATHENA trial, the primary outcome (first hospitalization due to cardiovascular events or death) occurred in 734 patients (31.9%) in the dronedarone group and in 917 patients (39.4%) in the placebo group, with a hazard ratio for dronedarone of 0.76 (p <0.001). Cardiovascular mortality was also reduced by dronedarone (3.9% vs 2.7%; p = 0.003).[90] However, dronedarone is contraindicated in patients with heart failure[91] and in permanent AF (see Drugs for rhythm control).[92]

Recommendations are provided in Tables 52.9 and 52.10.

Table 52.8 Trials for rhythm control

Trial	Patients	Mean age (years)	Mean F-U (years)	Inclusion criteria	Primary outcome	P
PIAF (2000)	252	61.0	1.0	Persistent AF	Symptomatic improvement	0.32
AFFIRM (2002)	4060	69.7	3.5	Paroxysmal AF or persistent AF, age ≥65 years, or risk of stroke or death	All-cause mortality	0.08
RACE (2002)	522	68.0	2.3	Persistent AF or flutter for <1 years and 1–2 cardioversions over 2 years	Composite: cardiovascular death CHF, severe bleeding, pacemaker implantation, thromboembolic events, severe adverse effects of antiarrhythmic drugs	0.11
STAF (2003)	200	66.0	1.6	Persistent AF, LA size >45 mm, CHF NYHA II–IV, LVEF <45%	Composite: overall mortality, cerebrovascular complications	0.99
HOT CAFÉ (2004)	205	60.8	1.7	Persistent AF, age 50–75 years	Composite: death, thromboembolism, major haemorrhage	>0.71
AF-CHF (2008)	1376	66	3.1	CHF, LVEF ≤35%, history of AF	Cardiovascular death	0.59
J-RHYTHM (2009)	823	64.7	1.6	Paroxysmal AF	Composite: total mortality, cerebral infarction, systemic embolism, major bleeding, hospitalization for heart failure, or physical/psychological disability	0.012

Table 52.9 ESC 2010 GL on AF. Recommendations for rate and rhythm control of AF

Rate control as the initial approach in elderly patients with AF and minor symptoms (EHRA score 1)	I-A
Rate control throughout a rhythm control approach to ensure adequate control of the ventricular rate during recurrences of AF.	I-A
Rhythm control in patients with symptomatic (EHRA score ≥2) AF despite adequate rate control.	I-B
Rhythm control in AF-related heart failure for improvement of symptoms.	IIa-B
Rhythm control as an initial approach in young symptomatic patients in whom catheter ablation treatment has not been ruled out.	IIa-C
Rhythm control in AF secondary to a trigger or substrate that has been corrected (e.g. ischaemia, hyperthyroidism).	IIa-C

ESC on AF 2010. Guidelines for the management of atrial fibrillation: The Task Force for the Management of Atrial Fibrillation of the European Society of Cardiology (ESC). *Eur Heart J* 2010; **31**: 2369–2429.

Drugs for rate control

- **Beta blockers** (such as metoprolol 100–200 mg od slow release, bisoprolol 2.5–10 mg od, nebivol 2.5–5 mg, and carvedilol 3.125–25 mg bd) are the safest drugs.
- **Verapamil** (40 mg bd to 360 mg slow release) and **diltiazem** (60 mg tds to 360 mg slow release) are also safe but are contraindicated in heart failure.
- **Digoxin** (0.125–0.5 mg od) is only effective at rest. Life-threatening proarrhythmia may occur, especially with overdosing in the elderly. In a recent analysis of the AFFIRM study, digoxin was associated with a significant increase in all-cause mortality in patients with AF after correcting for clinical characteristics and co-morbidities, regardless of gender or of the presence or absence of HF.[93] This could be due to relatively high serum digoxin levels (≥1.0 ng/mL), required by the study for firma rate control. In another report, however, with very careful propensity score matching, no evidence of increased mortality with digoxin was found in patients with paroxysmal or persistent AF.[94]
- **Amiodarone** IV is the drug of choice (together with IV beta blockers) for slowing the ventricular rate in patients with acute coronary syndromes. In stable patients with AF, it should not be used for rate response due to its thyroid and pulmonary toxicity, unless all other drugs have failed.[4] Strict rate control (<80 bpm) has not been found superior to lenient rate control (<110 bpm),[95] and this recommendation is adopted by the ESC. The ACC/AHA/HRS accept this recommendation only for patients with LVEF >40% who do not have AF-related symptoms (Table 52.10).

AV nodal modification

In patients in whom drug or pulmonary vein ablation therapy has failed or there are signs of tachycardiopathy,

Table 52.10 Rate control of AF

ESC 2010 GL on AF. Acute rate control	
IV beta blockers or non-dihydropyridine calcium channel antagonists in the acute setting in the absence of pre-excitation to slow the ventricular response to AF, exercising caution in hypotension or heart failure.	I-A
IV digitalis or amiodarone in the acute setting to control the heart rate in concomitant heart failure or hypotension.	I-B
In pre-excitation, preferred drugs are class I antiarrhythmic drugs or amiodarone.	I-C
Beta blockers, non-dihydropyridine calcium channel antagonists, digoxin, and adenosine in pre-excited AF.	III-C
ESC 2010 GL on AF and 2012 Update. Drugs for long-term rate control of AF	
Beta blockers, non-dihydropyridine calcium channel antagonists, digitalis, or a combination thereof in paroxysmal, persistent, or permanent AF. Choice individualized and dose modulated to avoid bradycardia.	I-B
In activity-related symptoms, the adequacy of rate control should be assessed during exercise, and therapy should be adjusted to achieve a physiological chronotropic response and to avoid bradycardia.	I-C
In pre-excitation AF or in patients with a history of AF, preferred drugs are propafenone or amiodarone.	I-C
Initiate treatment with a lenient rate control protocol, aimed at a resting heart rate <110 bpm.	IIa-B
Adopt a stricter rate control strategy when symptoms persist or tachycardiomyopathy occurs, despite lenient rate control: resting heart rate <80 bpm and heart rate during moderate exercise <110 bpm. After achieving the strict heart rate target, assess safety with 24 h Holter monitor.	IIa-B
Digoxin in heart failure and LV dysfunction and in sedentary (inactive) patients.	IIa-C
Oral amiodarone when other measures are unsuccessful or contraindicated.	IIb-C
Digitalis as the sole agent to control the rate of ventricular response in paroxysmal AF.	III-B
Dronedarone is not recommended in patients with permanent AF.	III-B
ACC/AHA 2013 GL on AF. Pharmacological rate control during atrial fibrillation	
Beta blocker or non-dihydropyridine calcium channel antagonists.	I-B
IV beta blockers (esmolol, metoprolol, or propranolol) or non-dihydropyridine calcium channel antagonists (verapamil, diltiazem) in the absence of pre-excitation and with caution in patients with hypotension or HF.	I-B
IV digoxin or amiodarone in patients with AF and HF who do not have an accessory pathway.	I-B
In patients symptoms related to AF during activity, heart rate control should be assessed during exercise, adjusting pharmacological treatment to keep the rate in the physiological range.	I-C
Digoxin orally to control the heart rate at rest in patients with HF, LV dysfunction, or for sedentary individuals.	I-C
Digoxin and either a beta blocker or non-dihydropyridine calcium channel antagonist.	IIa-B
Ablation of the AV node or accessory pathway to control heart rate when pharmacological therapy is insufficient or associated with side effects.	IIa-B
IV amiodarone to control the heart rate in patients with AF when other measures are unsuccessful or contraindicated.	IIa-C
IV procainamide or ibutilide when electrical cardioversion is not necessary in patients with an accessory pathway.	IIa-C
Oral amiodarone, when beta blocker, non-dihydropyridine calcium channel antagonist, or digoxin, alone or in combination, cannot control the heart rate.	IIb-C
IV procainamide, disopyramide, ibutilide, or amiodarone for haemodynamically stable patients with AF conducting over an accessory pathway.	IIb-B
Catheter-directed ablation of the AV node when the rate cannot be controlled with pharmacological agents or tachycardia-mediated cardiomyopathy is suspected.	IIb-C

Management of patients with atrial fibrillation (compilation of 2006 ACCF/AHA/ESC and 2011 ACCF/AHA/HRS recommendations). *J Am Coll Cardiol*. 2013; **61**:1935–44.

ESC on AF 2010. Guidelines for the management of atrial fibrillation: The Task Force for the Management of Atrial Fibrillation of the European Society of Cardiology (ESC). *Eur Heart J*. 2010; **31**: 2369–2429.

AV nodal catheter ablation or modification, followed by **ventricular** or **biventricular pacing**, may be necessary (Table 52.11).[96,97] Septal RV or biventricular pacing if LVEF ≤35% are superior to apical RV pacing in this respect.[98] The increased risk of polymorphic VT and torsades that has been detected after complete AV nodal ablation (as opposed to modification) is probably transient, although 24-48 h monitoring may be needed.

Drugs for rhythm control

In a meta-analysis of 44 randomized trials with 11 322 patients, the efficacy of drugs, such as disopyramide, quinidine, flecainide, propafenone, amiodarone, dofetilide, and sotalol, for maintenance of SR was 40–60% per year. All drugs resulted in increased withdrawals due to side effects, and all, except amiodarone and propafenone, increased proarrhythmia. No drug reduced mortality whereas

Table 52.11 ESC 2010 GL on AF. Ablation of the AV node

ESC 2010 GL on AF	
When the rate cannot be controlled with pharmacological agents and when AF cannot be prevented by antiarrhythmic therapy or is associated with intolerable side effects and direct catheter-based or surgical ablation of AF is not indicated, has failed, or is rejected.	IIa-B
Patients with permanent AF and an indication for CRT (NYHA III or ambulatory class IV symptoms despite optimal medical therapy, LVEF <35%, QRS width ≥130 ms).	IIa-B
CRT non-responders in whom AF prevents effective biventricular stimulation and amiodarone is ineffective or contraindicated.	IIa-C
Biventricular stimulation after AV node ablation, in any type of AF and severely depressed LV function (LVEF ≤35%), and severe heart failure symptoms (NYHA III or IV).	IIa-C
When tachycardia-mediated cardiomyopathy is suspected and the rate cannot be controlled with pharmacological agents, and direct ablation of AF is not indicated, has failed, or is rejected.	IIb-C
Ablation of the AV node with consecutive implantation of a CRT device may be considered in permanent AF, LVEF ≤35%, and NYHA I or II symptoms on optimal medical therapy to control heart rate when pharmacological therapy is insufficient or associated with side effects.	IIb-C
Catheter ablation of the AV node without a prior trial of medication or catheter ablation for AF to control the AF and/or ventricular rate.	III-C
Recommendations for pacemakers after atrioventricular node ablation	
CRT pacemaker in any type of AF, moderately depressed LV function (LVEF ≤45%), and mild heart failure symptoms (NYHA II).	IIb-C
DDD pacemaker with mode-switch function in paroxysmal AF and normal LV function.	IIb-C
VVIR pacemaker in persistent or permanent AF and normal LV function.	IIb-C

ESC on AF 2010. Guidelines for the management of atrial fibrillation: The Task Force for the Management of Atrial Fibrillation of the European Society of Cardiology (ESC). *Eur Heart J.* 2010; **31**: 2369–2429.

disopyramide and quinidine drugs increased mortality.[84] In a subsequent meta-analysis, a trend for increased mortality was identified for sotalol and, possibly, amiodarone.[99]

- **Amiodarone** is the most effective drug,[100] but its long-term use is limited by its toxic effects, mainly on the thyroid, lungs, and liver (especially at doses >200 mg od). The possibility of a trend towards increased mortality with its long-term use has also been raised.[99] It is the drug of choice in heart failure NYHA III and IV (Figure 52.3). Proarrhythmia is rare, but QT monitoring is advisable (Table 52.12). Dosing is 800 mg po daily for 1 week (in one or two doses), followed by 600 mg daily for 1 week, 400 mg daily for 4 weeks, and then 200 mg od (alternatively, 600 mg od for 4 weeks, 400 mg po for 4 weeks, and then 200 mg od).
- **Dronedarone** (400 mg bd po) is less effective as well as less toxic than amiodarone at least over 1 year follow-up (dronedarone vs placebo in ADONIS and EURIDIS trials).[101] It reduces hospitalization due to paroxysmal AF or atrial flutter (ATHENA trial)[90] but is contraindicated in NYHA III or IV or recently decompensated (<4 weeks) heart failure (increased mortality in the ANROMEDA trial)[91] and in patients with permanent AF (PALLAS trial).[102] The PALLAS trial on patients with >2 years AF, 70% of whom had NYHA I–III heart failure, was stopped due to increased cardiovascular mortality by the drug.[102] Thus, dronedarone is not indicated in patients who cannot, or will not, be converted into normal sinus rhythm because it doubles the rate of cardiovascular death, stroke, and heart failure (FDA alert Dec 2011). It may cause creatinine levels elevation (2.5% of patients) and, very rarely, severe hepatic impairment. Although it mildly prolongs the QT, the risk of torsades is negligible.[99] It may be given in patients with recurrent AF for the maintenance of sinus rhythm (ESC 2012 I-A) and to reduce hospitalization for AF in patients in sinus rhythm with a history of non-permanent AF (FDA alert Dec 2011). Care is needed with concomitant administration of digoxin,[102] and this combination should be probably avoided.[5]
- **Beta blockers** (other than sotalol) are safe but modestly effective.
- **Sotalol** (80–160 mg bd po) A beta blocker with class III properties, at high doses, is equally effective with amiodarone in converting AF to SR (24% vs 27%, respectively) but less effective than maintaining SR (approximately 30% vs 47% at 1 year, respectively).[85] Sotalol should not be used in the presence of ventricular hypertrophy or significant repolarization abnormalities.[103] The main concern is proarrhythmia due to QT prolongation, and a trend towards increased mortality has been reported,[99,104] although not validated in all studies.[105] Careful monitoring of the QT is advisable and discontinuation of the drug when QT >500 ms (see VT).
- **Flecainide** (100–200 mg bd po) approximately doubles the likelihood of maintaining sinus rhythm. It is contraindicated in coronary artery disease and LV dysfunction and should be stopped if the QRS increases by >25% (risk of monomorphic VT). Concomitant administration of beta blockers reduces proarrhythmic risk and controls ventricular rate in case of conversion to atrial flutter.[106] Caution is necessary when using sodium channel blocking drugs as monotherapy in

Table 52.12 Adverse reactions to amiodarone

Reaction	Incidence (%)	Diagnosis	Management
Pulmonary	2	Cough and/or dyspnoea, especially with local or diffuse opacities on high-resolution CT scan and decrease in DLCO from baseline	Usually, discontinue drug; corticosteroids may be considered in more severe cases; occasionally, can continue drug if levels high and abnormalities resolve; rarely, continue amiodarone with corticosteroid if no other option
Gastrointestinal tract	30	Nausea, anorexia, and constipation	Symptoms may decrease with decrease in dose
	15–30	AST or ALT level greater than 2 times normal	If hepatitis considered, exclude other causes
	<3	Hepatitis and cirrhosis	Consider discontinuation, biopsy, or both to determine whether cirrhosis is present
Thyroid	4–22	Hypothyroidism	L-thyroxine
	2–12	Hyperthyroidism	Corticosteroids, propylthiouracil, or methimazole; may need to discontinue drug; may need thyroidectomy
Skin	<10	Blue discoloration	Reassurance; decrease in dose
	25–75	Photosensitivity	Avoidance of prolonged sun exposure; sunblock; decrease in dose
Central nervous system	3–30	Ataxia, paraesthesias, peripheral polyneuropathy, sleep disturbance, impaired memory and tremor	Often dose-dependent and may improve, or resolve, with dose adjustment
Ocular	<5	Halo vision, especially at night	Corneal deposits the norm; if optic neuropathy occurs, discontinue
	≤1	Optic neuropathy	Discontinue drug, and consult an ophthalmologist
	>90	Photophobia, visual blurring, and microdeposits	
Heart	5	Bradycardia and AV block	May need permanent cardiac pacing
	<1	Proarrhythmia	May need to discontinue the drug
Genitourinary	<1	Epididymitis and erectile dysfunction	Pain may resolve spontaneously

ALT, alanine aminotransferase; AST, aspartate aminotransferase; DLCO, diffusion capacity of carbon monoxide.

Goldschlager N, *et al.* A practical guide for clinicians who treat patients with amiodarone: 2007. *Heart Rhythm*. 2007;**4**:1250–9.

athletes with AF. These drugs may lead to (slow) atrial flutter, with 1:1 conduction to the ventricles during high sympathetic tone.[107] Short-term flecainide administration (4 weeks) after cardioversion is less effective than long-term treatment (80%) but can prevent recurrences of atrial fibrillation.[108]

- **Propafenone** (150–300 mg tds po) is safer and has a mild beta-blocking activity, but the same precautions as with flecainide should be taken.
- **Dofetilide** has also been found useful and safe in patients with AF and impaired LV function (DIAMOND trial) since mortality was not different compared to controls (>50% in 3 years).[109]

Recommendations for drug usage and complications are presented in Table 52.13 and Figures 52.4.

The primary goal of rhythm control drug therapy is to selectively prolong the refractory period in the atrium and avoid the risk of ventricular proarrhythmia. **Ranolazine** is an anti-ischaemic drug that was shown to reduce AF in the MERLIN-TIMI 36 trial. It blocks I_{Na}, I_{CaL}, and I_{Kr}, and it is postulated that the late sodium current contributes to the prolongation of the action potential duration associated with reduced I_{Kr} at slow heart rates.[110] Theoretically, inhibition of I_{Na} with ranolazine or vernakalant may reduce the risk of TDP associated with I_{Kr} inhibition by drugs, such as dofetilide or sotalol.[111] Combination therapy with amiodarone plus ranolazine or dronedarone plus ranolazine has been shown experimentally to have marked synergistic effects that result in atrium-selective blockade of sodium channels and suppression of AF.[111]

Anticoagulation

Adjusted-dose warfarin and antiplatelet agents, such as aspirin, reduce stroke by approximately 60% and 20%, respectively, in patients with AF.[112] In general, oral anticoagulation is preferred in patients with CHA_2DS_2VASc score ≥2 and no anticoagulation in patients with score 0 (Table 52.14 and Figure 52.5). In patients older than 75 years and especially women, oral anticoagulation is recommended, regardless of risk factors (ACC/AHA).[4]

Table 52.13 Rhythm control of AF

ESC 2010 GL on AF and 2012 Update. Drugs for rhythm control	
Depending on underlying heart disease	
Amiodarone	I-A
Dronedarone	I-A
Flecainide	I-A
Propafenone	I-A
d,l-sotalol	I-A
Amiodarone is more effective in maintaining sinus rhythm than sotalol, propafenone, flecainide (by analogy), or dronedarone.	I-A
But, because of its toxicity profile, should generally be used when other agents have failed or are contraindicated.	I-C
Amiodarone in severe heart failure, NYHA III and IV, or recently unstable (decompensation within the prior month) NYHA class II.	I-B
Dronedarone or flecainide or propafenone or sotalol for patients without significant structural heart disease.	I-A
Beta blockers for prevention of adrenergic AF.	I-C
Other antiarrhythmic drug is considered if one antiarrhythmic drug fails to reduce the recurrence of AF to a clinically acceptable level.	IIa-C
Dronedarone to reduce cardiovascular hospitalizations in patients with non-permanent AF and cardiovascular risk factors.	IIa-B
Beta blockers for rhythm (plus rate) control in patients with a first episode of AF.	IIa-C
Disopyramide in patients with vagally mediated AF.	IIb-B
Short-term (4 weeks) antiarrhythmic therapy after cardioversion may be considered in selected patients, e.g. those at risk for therapy-associated complications.	IIb-B
Dronedarone in patients with NYHA III and IV or with recently unstable (decompensation within the prior month) NYHA II heart failure.	III-B
Antiarrhythmic drug therapy for maintenance of sinus rhythm in patients with advanced sinus node disease or AV node dysfunction, unless they have a functioning permanent pacemaker.	III-C

2012 focused update of the ESC Guidelines for the management of atrial fibrillation: An update of the 2010 ESC Guidelines for the management of atrial fibrillation. Developed with the special contribution of the European Heart Rhythm Association. *Europace*. 2012;**14**:1385–413.

ACCF/AHA 2013 GL on AF. Maintenance of sinus rhythm	
Treatment of precipitating or reversible causes of AF.	I-C
Catheter ablation in experienced centres to maintain SR in patients with significantly symptomatic, paroxysmal AF who have failed treatment with an antiarrhythmic drug and have normal or mildly dilated left atria, normal or mildly reduced LV function, and no severe pulmonary disease.	I-A
Pharmacological therapy of AF to maintain sinus rhythm and prevent tachycardia-induced cardiomyopathy.	IIa-C
Infrequent, well-tolerated recurrence of AF as a successful outcome of antiarrhythmic drug therapy.	IIa-C
Outpatient initiation of antiarrhythmic drug therapy in patients with AF who have no associated heart disease when the agent is well tolerated.	IIa-C
In patients without structural or coronary heart disease, propafenone or flecainide, on an outpatient basis, in patients with paroxysmal AF who are in sinus rhythm at the time of drug initiation.	IIa-B
Sotalol in outpatients in sinus rhythm with little or no heart disease, prone to paroxysmal AF, if the baseline uncorrected QT interval is less than 460 ms, serum electrolytes are normal, and risk factors associated with class III drug-related proarrhythmia are not present.	IIa-C
Catheter ablation for symptomatic persistent AF.	IIa-A
Dronedarone to decrease the need for hospitalization in patients with paroxysmal AF or after conversion of persistent AF. It can be initiated during outpatient therapy.	IIa-B
Catheter ablation for symptomatic paroxysmal AF in patients with significant left atrial dilatation or with significant LV dysfunction.	IIb-A
Antiarrhythmic therapy with a particular drug for maintenance of sinus rhythm in patients with AF who have well-defined risk factors for proarrhythmia with that agent.	III-A
Pharmacological therapy for maintenance of sinus rhythm in patients with advanced sinus node disease or AV node dysfunction, unless they have a pacemaker.	III-C
Dronedarone in patients with class IV heart failure or patients who have had an episode of decompensated heart failure in the past 4 weeks, especially with LVEF <35%.	III-B

Management of patients with atrial fibrillation (compilation of 2006 ACCF/AHA/ESC and 2011 ACCF/AHA/HRS recommendations). *J Am Coll Cardiol*. 2013;**61**:1935–44

(Continued)

Table 52.13 (Continued)

ESC 2010 GL on AF. Suggested doses and main caveats for commonly used antiarrhythmic drugs

Drug	Dose	Main contraindications and precautions	ECG features prompting lower dose or discontinuation	AV nodal slowing
Disopyramide	100–250 mg tds	Contraindicated in systolic heart failure Caution when using concomitant therapy with QT-prolonging drugs	QT interval >500 ms	None
Flecainide	100–200 mg bd	Contraindicated if creatinine clearance <50 mg/mL, in coronary artery disease, reduced LV ejection fraction	QRS duration increase >25% above baseline	None
Flecainide XL	200 mg od	Caution in the presence of conduction system disease		
Propafenone	150–300 mg tds	Contraindicated in coronary artery disease, reduced LV ejection fraction	QRS duration increase >25% above baseline	Slight
Propafenone SR	225–425 mg bd	Caution in the presence of conduction system disease and renal impairment		
d.l-Sotalol	80–160 mg bd	Contraindicated in the presence of significant LV hypertrophy, systolic heart failure, pre-existing QT prolongation, hypokalaemia creatinine clearance <50 mg/mL. Moderate renal dysfunction requires careful adaptation of dose	QT interval >500 ms	Similar to high-dose beta blockers
Amiodarone	600 mg od for 4 weeks, 400 mg od for 4 weeks, then 200 mg od	Caution when using concomitant therapy with QT-prolonging drugs, heart failure. Dose of vitamin K antagonists and of digitoxin/digoxin should be reduced.	QT interval >500 ms	10–12 bpm in AF
Dronedarone	400 mg bd	Contraindicated in NYHA class III–IV or unstable heart failure, during concomitant therapy with QT-prolonging drugs, powerful CYP3A4 inhibitors, and creatinine clearance <30 mg/mL. Dose of digitoxin/digoxin should be reduced. Elevations in serum creatinine of 0.1–0.2 mg/dL are common and do not reflect reduced renal function.	QT interval >500 ms	10–12 bpm in AF

AF, atrial fibrillation; AV, atrioventricular; bpm, beats per minute; CYP, cytochrome P; ECG, electrocardiogram; LV, left ventricular; NYHA, New York Heart Association.

Guidelines for the management of atrial fibrillation: The Task Force for the Management of Atrial Fibrillation of the European Society of Cardiology (ESC). *Eur Heart J* 2010; **31**: 2369–2429.

The risk of bleeding is assessed by schemes, such as the HAS-BLED.[113] A score ≥3 indicates 'high risk' (Table 52.15). New anticoagulants are thrombin or factor Xa inhibitors and are now recommended for non-valvular AF as a potential alternative to warfarin. They carry a lower risk of intracranial haemorrhage (especially apixaban), no clear interactions with food, fewer interactions with medications, and no need for frequent laboratory monitoring and dose adjustments.[114–116] Main problems are the lack of antidotes and specific assays to measure anticoagulant effect. In patients taking warfarin, switching to a new agent is appropriate when the INR is <2. Mode of action of novel oral anticoagulants in the coagulation cascade is presented in Figure 52.6. A comparison of new anticoagulants is presented in Table 52.16.

Aspirin The evidence for effective stroke prevention with aspirin in AF is weak, as data indicate that the risk of major bleeding or intracranial haemorrhage with aspirin is not significantly different to that of oral anticoagulation, especially in the elderly.[5] Thus, aspirin for stroke prevention in AF should be limited to patients who refuse any form of oral anticoagulation.

Aspirin and clopidogrel offer increased protection compared to aspirin alone, albeit at an increased risk of major bleeding,[117] and is preferred when warfarin is contraindicated. Still, however, aspirin and clopidogrel offer less protection than warfarin (relative risk 1.44 for stroke, peripheral embolism, MI, and vascular death).[117] In patients who sustain an ischaemic stroke despite INR 2–3, targeting a higher INR should be considered (3–3.5), rather than adding an antiplatelet agent, since major bleeding risk starts at INR >3.5.[1]

Warfarin is superior to aspirin in the elderly (>75 years), offering a 52% reduction in yearly risk of stroke, intracranial

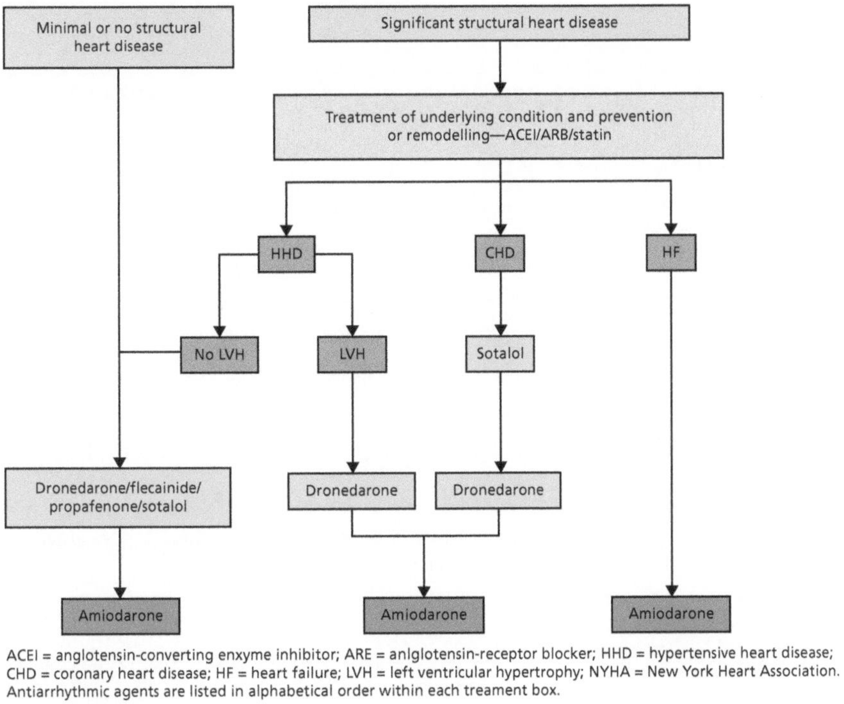

Figure 52.4 ESC 2012 update on AF. Choice of antiarrhythmic drug, according to underlying pathology.

2012 focused update of the ESC guidelines for the management of atrial fibrillation: an update of the 2010 ESC guidelines for the management of atrial fibrillation. *Europace*. 2012;**14**:1385–413.

Table 52.14 Prevention of thromboembolism

ESC 2012 Update on AF. Prevention of thromboembolism in non-valvular AF	
General	
Antithrombotic therapy for all patients with AF, except in those at low risk (lone AF, aged <65 years, or with contraindications).	I-A
The choice of the antithrombotic therapy should be based upon the absolute risks of stroke/thromboembolism and bleeding.	I-A
The CHA_2DS_2-VAS_c score is recommended as a means of assessing stroke risk in non-valvular AF.	I-A
In patients with a CHA_2DS_2-VAS_c score of 0 (i.e. aged <65 years with lone AF) who are at low risk, with none of the risk factors, no antithrombotic therapy.	I-B
In patients with a CHA_2DS_2-VAS_c score of ≥2, OAC therapy with: adjusted dose VKA (INR 2–3) or a direct thrombin inhibitor (dabigatran) or an oral factor Xa inhibitor (e.g. rivaroxaban, apixaban), unless contraindicated.	I-A
In patients with a CHA_2DS_2-VAS_c score of 1, OAC therapy with: adjusted dose VKA (INR 2–3) or a direct thrombin inhibitor (dabigatran) or an oral factor Xa inhibitor (e.g. rivaroxaban, apixaban), based upon an assessment of the risk of bleeding complications and patient preferences	IIa-A
No antithrombotic therapy in female patients who are aged <65 and have lone AF (but still have a CHA_2DS_2-VAS_c score of 1 by virtue of their gender)	IIa-B
When patients refuse the use of any oral anticoagulation (whether VKAs or NOACs), antiplatelet therapy should be considered, using combination therapy with aspirin 75–100 mg plus clopidogrel 75 mg daily (where there is a low risk of bleeding) or, less effectively, aspirin 75–325 mg daily.	IIa-B
Novel anticoagulants	
When dose-adjusted VKA (INR 2–3) cannot be used due to difficulties in keeping within therapeutic anticoagulation, experiencing side effects of VKAs, or inability to attend or undertake INR monitoring, one of the NOACs, either a direct thrombin inhibitor (dabigatran) or an oral factor Xa inhibitor (e.g. rivaroxaban, apixaban), is recommended.	I-B
Where OAC is recommended, one of the NOACs, either a direct thrombin inhibitor (dabigatran) or an oral factor Xa inhibitor (e.g. rivaroxaban, apixaban).	IIa-A

(Continued)

Table 52.14 (Continued)

Novel anticoagulants	
Where dabigatran is prescribed, a dose of 150 mg bd is preferred to 110 mg bd, with the latter dose recommended in:	IIa-B
Elderly patients aged ≥80	
Concomitant use of interacting drugs (e.g. verapamil)	
High bleeding risk (HAS-BLED score ≥3)	
Moderate renal impairment (CrCl 30–49 mL/min)	
Where rivaroxaban is being considered, a dose of 20 mg od is preferred to 15 mg od, with the latter dose recommended in:	IIa-C
High bleeding risk (HAS-BLED score ≥3)	
Moderate renal impairment (CrCl 30–49 mL/min)	
Annual baseline and subsequent regular assessment of renal function (by CrCl) in patients following initiation of any NOAC, but 2–3 times per year in those with moderate renal impairment.	IIa-B
NOACs (dabigatran, rivaroxaban, and apixaban) are not recommended in patients with severe renal impairment (CrCl <30 mL/min).	III-A
Bleeding	
Assessment of the risk of bleeding when prescribing antithrombotic therapy (whether with VKA, NOAC, aspirin/clopidogrel, or aspirin).	I-A
The HAS-BLED score should be considered to assess bleeding risk. A score ≥3 indicates 'high risk', and some caution and regular review is needed, following the initiation of antithrombotic therapy (with OAC or antiplatelet therapy).	IIa-A
Correctable risk factors for bleeding (e.g. uncontrolled blood pressure, labile INRs if the patient was on a VKA, concomitant drugs (aspirin, NSAIDs, etc.), alcohol, etc.) should be addressed.	IIa-B
Use of the HAS-BLED score should be used to identify modifiable bleeding risks but should not be used on its own to exclude patients from OAC therapy.	IIa-B
The risk of major bleeding with antiplatelet therapy (with aspirin-clopidogrel combination therapy, and especially in the elderly, also with aspirin monotherapy) should be considered as being similar to OAC.	IIa-B

OAC, oral anticoagulation with VKA (vitamin K antagonists). NOACs, new oral anticoagulants, i.e. dabigatran, rivarixaban, apixaban.
2012 focused update of the ESC Guidelines for the management of atrial fibrillation: An update of the 2010 ESC Guidelines for the management of atrial fibrillation. Developed with the special contribution of the European Heart Rhythm Association. *Europace*. 2012;**14**:1385–413.

ESC 2010 GL on AF. Prevention of thromboembolism in AF	
For patients with mechanical heart valves, the target intensity of anticoagulation with a VKA should be based on the type and position of the prosthesis, maintaining an INR of at least 2.5 in the mitral position and at least 2.0 for an aortic valve.	I-B
Antithrombotic therapy for patients with atrial flutter as for those with AF.	I-C
The selection of antithrombotic therapy should be considered using the same criteria, irrespective of the pattern of AF (i.e. paroxysmal, persistent, or permanent).	IIa-A
Interruption of VKA (with subtherapeutic anticoagulation for up to 48 h), without substituting heparin as 'bridging' anticoagulation therapy in patients **without** mechanical prosthetic heart valves or not at high risk for thromboembolism, and who are undergoing surgical or diagnostic procedures that carry a risk of bleeding.	IIa-C
'Bridging' anticoagulation with therapeutic doses of either LMWH or UFH during the temporary interruption of VKA therapy should be considered in patients with a mechanical prosthetic heart valve or at high risk for thromboembolism who are undergoing surgical or diagnostic procedures.	IIa-C
Following surgical procedures, resumption of VKA therapy at the 'usual' maintenance dose (without a loading dose) on the evening of (or the next morning after) surgery, assuming there is adequate haemostasis.	IIa-B
Re-evaluation at regular intervals of the benefits, risks, and need for antithrombotic therapy should be considered.	IIa-C
In patients with AF presenting with acute stroke or TIA, management of uncontrolled hypertension before antithrombotic treatment is started and cerebral imaging (CT or MRI) performed to exclude haemorrhage.	IIa-C
In the absence of haemorrhage, VKA should be considered ~2 weeks after stroke, but, in the presence of haemorrhage, anticoagulation should not be given.	IIa-C
In the presence of a large cerebral infarction, delaying the initiation of anticoagulation, given the risk of haemorrhagic transformation.	IIa-C
In patients with AF and an acute TIA, VKA as soon as possible in the absence of cerebral infarction or haemorrhage.	IIa-C
UFH or subcutaneous LMWH when surgical procedures require interruption of VKA for longer than 48 h in high-risk patients.	IIb-C

(Continued)

Table 52.14 (Continued)

ESC 2010 GL on AF. Prevention of thromboembolism in AF	
In patients who sustain ischaemic stroke or systemic embolism during treatment with usual intensity VKA (INR 2.0–3.0), raising the intensity of the anticoagulation to a maximum target INR of 3.0–3.5, rather than adding an antiplatelet agent.	IIb-C

* 'Major' risk factors are those associated with the highest risk for stroke patients with AF are prior thromboembolism (stroke, TIA, or systemic embolism), age ≥75 years, and rheumatic mitral stenosis. 'Clinically relevant non-major' risk factors include hypertension, heart failure, or moderate to severe LV dysfunction (ejection fraction 40% or less), and diabetes mellitus. Other 'clinically relevant non-major' risk factors include female sex, age 65–74 years, and vascular disease (myocardial infarction, complex aortic plaque, carotid disease, peripheral artery disease). This risk factor-based approach for non-valvular AF can also be expressed by the CHA2DS2-VASc score.

OAC, oral anticoagulant; TIA, transient ischaemic attack; VKA, vitamin K antagonist.

For prevention of thromboembolism in AF in the context of heart failure, see Chapter 31 on heart failure.

ESC on AF 2010. Guidelines for the management of atrial fibrillation: The Task Force for the Management of Atrial Fibrillation of the European Society of Cardiology (ESC). Eur Heart J 2010; 31: 2369–2429.

ACC/AHA GL on AF 2013. Prevention of thromboembolism	
Antithrombotic therapy for all patients with AF, except those with lone AF or contraindications.	I-A
The selection of the antithrombotic agent should be based upon the absolute risks of stroke and bleeding and the relative risk and benefit for a given patient.	I-A
For patients without mechanical heart valves at high risk of stroke, anticoagulant with a vitamin K antagonist to achieve INR 2.0–3.0, unless contraindicated. Highest risk: prior thromboembolism (stroke, TIA, or systemic embolism) and rheumatic mitral stenosis.	I-A
Vitamin K antagonist for patients with >1 moderate risk factor, i.e. age ≥75 years, hypertension, HF, LVEF ≤35% or fractional shortening <25%), and diabetes mellitus.	I-A
INR should be determined at least weekly during initiation of therapy and monthly when anticoagulation is stable.	I-A
Aspirin 81–325 mg daily as an alternative to vitamin K antagonists in low-risk patients or in those with contraindications to oral anticoagulation.	I-A
For patients with mechanical heart valves, the target INR should be based on the type of prosthesis (at least 2.5).	I-B
Antithrombotic therapy for patients with atrial flutter as for those with AF.	I-C
Dabigatran as an alternative to warfarin in patients with paroxysmal to permanent AF who do not have a prosthetic heart valve or haemodynamically significant valve disease, severe renal failure (creatinine clearance <15 mL/min), or advanced liver disease.	I-B
For non-valvular AF and age ≥75 years (especially in female patients), or hypertension, or HF, or impaired LV function, or diabetes mellitus, aspirin or a vitamin K antagonist, based on bleeding risk, compliance, and patient preferences.	IIa-A
For non-valvular AF and age 65–74 years and/or female gender, or CAD, aspirin or a vitamin K antagonist, based on bleeding risk, compliance, and patient preferences.	IIa-B
Select antithrombotic therapy using the same criteria, irrespective of the pattern (i.e. paroxysmal, persistent, or permanent) of AF.	IIa-B
In patients without mechanical prosthetic heart valves, interrupt anticoagulation for up to 1 wk without substituting heparin for surgical or diagnostic procedures that carry a risk of bleeding.	IIa-C
Re-evaluate the need for anticoagulation at regular intervals.	IIa-C
In patients ≥75 years at increased risk of bleeding, but without frank contraindications to anticoagulation, and in patients with moderate risk factors for thromboembolism who are unable to safely tolerate anticoagulation at INR 2.0–3.0, a lower INR target of 2.0 (range 1.6– 2.5) may be considered.	IIb-C
When surgical procedures require interruption of oral anticoagulant therapy for >1 wk in high-risk patients, UFH or LMWH subcutaneously (uncertain efficacy).	IIb-C
Following PCI or revascularization surgery in patients with AF, low-dose aspirin (<100 mg/d) and/or clopidogrel (75 mg/d) may be given concurrently with anticoagulation to prevent myocardial ischaemic events (increased risk of bleeding).	IIb-C
In PCI, anticoagulation may be interrupted to prevent bleeding at the site of peripheral arterial puncture but should be resumed after the procedure. Aspirin may be given temporarily during the hiatus with clopidogrel, 75 mg daily, plus warfarin (INR 2.0 to 3.0). Clopidogrel should be given for a minimum of 1 mo after implantation of a bare metal stent, at least 3 mo for a sirolimus-eluting stent, at least 6 mo for a paclitaxel-eluting stent, and 12 mo, or longer, in selected patients, following which warfarin may be continued as monotherapy.	IIb-C
Aspirin in patients <60 years without heart disease or risk factors for thromboembolism (lone AF).	IIb-C
In patients who sustain ischaemic stroke or systemic embolism during treatment with low-intensity anticoagulation (INR 2.0 to 3.0), raise INR to 3–5, instead of adding an antiplatelet agent.	IIb-C
Addition of clopidogrel to aspirin when anticoagulation with warfarin is unsuitable or not feasible.	IIb-B
Long-term anticoagulation with a vitamin K antagonist for primary prevention of stroke in patients <60 years without heart disease (lone AF) or any risk factors for thromboembolism.	III-C

Management of patients with atrial fibrillation (compilation of 2006 ACCF/AHA/ESC and 2011 ACCF/AHA/HRS recommendations). *J Am Coll Cardiol.* 2013;**61**:1935–44.

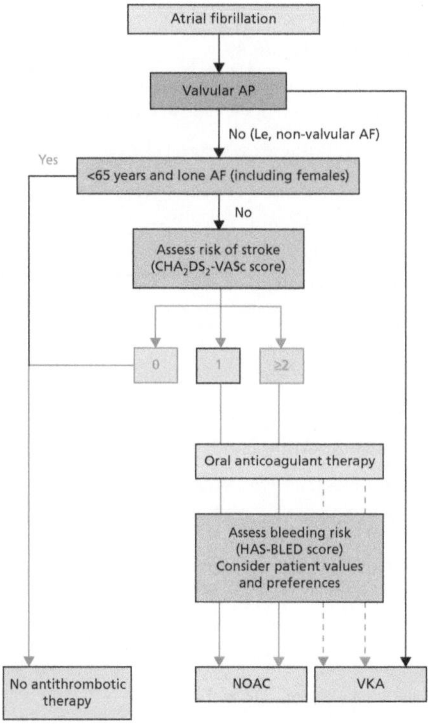

Antiplatelet therapy with aspirin plus clopidogrel, or—less effectively—aspirin only, should be considered in patients who refuse any OAC, or cannot tolerate anticoagulants for reasons unrelated to bleeding. If there are contraindications to OAC or antiplatelet therapy, left atrial appendage occlusion, closure or excision my be considered.
Colour: CHA$_2$DS$_2$-VASc; green = 0, blue = 1, red ≥2
Line: solid = best option; dashed = alternative option.
AF = atrial fibrillation; CHA$_2$DS$_2$-VASc = see text; HAS-BLED = see text;
NOAC = noverl oral anticoagulant; OAC = oral anticoagulant;
VKA = vitamin K antagonist.
[a]Includes rheumatic valvular disease and prosthetic valves.

Figure 52.5 ESC 2012 update on AF. Choice of anticoagulant.

2012 focused update of the ESC guidelines for the management of atrial fibrillation: an update of the 2010 ESC guidelines for the management of atrial fibrillation. *Europace*. 2012;**14**:1385–413.

Table 52.15 The HAS-BLED bleeding risk score

Letter	Clinical characteristic	Points awarded
H	Hypertension	1
A	Abnormal renal and liver function (1 point each)	1 or 2
S	Stroke	1
B	Bleeding	1
L	Labile INRs	1
E	Elderly (e.g. age >65 years)	1
D	Drugs or alcohol (1 point each)	1 or 2

Hypertension' is defined as systolic blood pressure >160 mmHg.
'Abnormal kidney function' is defined as the presence of chronic dialysis or renal transplantation or serum creatinine ≥200 mmol/L.
'Abnormal liver function' is defined as chronic hepatic disease (e.g. cirrhosis) or biochemical evidence of significant hepatic derangement (e.g. bilirubin >2 × upper limit of normal, in association with aspartate aminotransferase/alanine aminotransferase/alkaline phosphatase >3 × upper limit normal, etc.).
'Bleeding' refers to previous bleeding history and/or predisposition to bleeding, e.g. bleeding diathesis, anaemia, etc.
'Labile INRs' refers to unstable/high INRs or poor time in therapeutic range (e.g. <60%).
Drugs/alcohol use refers to concomitant use of drugs, such as antiplatelet agents, non-steroidal anti-inflammatory drugs, or alcohol abuse, etc.
Lip GY, *et al*. Comparative validation of a novel risk score for predicting bleeding risk in anticoagulated patients with atrial fibrillation. *J Am* Coll Cardiol. 2011;**57**:173–80.

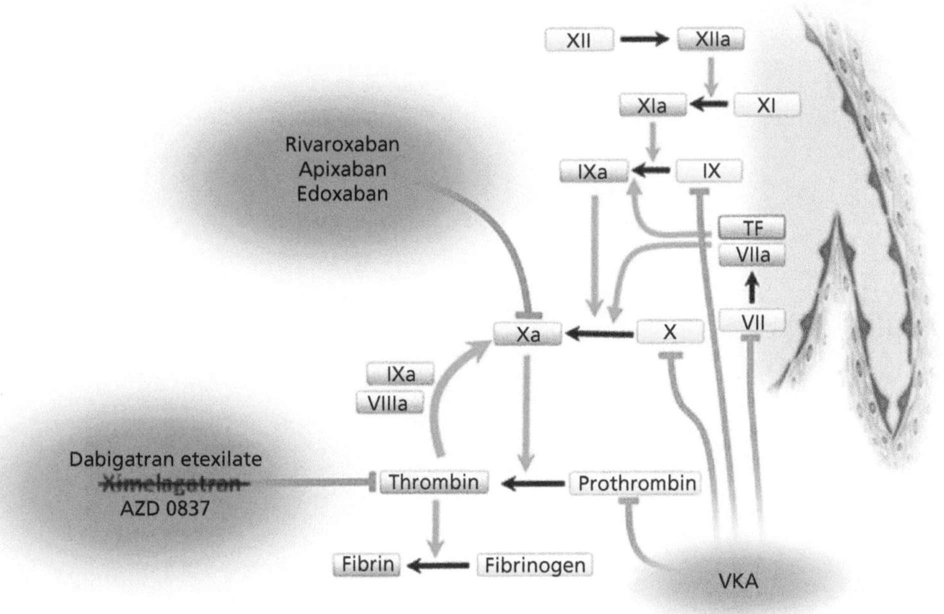

Figure 52.6 Point of action of novel oral anticoagulants in the coagulation cascade.

Steffel J, Braunwald E. Novel oral anticoagulants: focus on stroke prevention and treatment of venous thrombo-embolism: Licensed content author. *Eur Heart J*. 2011;**32**:1968–76.

haemorrhage, and peripheral embolism, (1.8% vs 3.8%), without a increased incidence of major haemorrhage (BAFTA trial).[118] Despite anticoagulation of more elderly patients with AF, intracerebral haemorrhage is considerably lower than in the past, ranging from 0.1 to 0.6%.[4] The risk increases with INR >3.5–4. Recommended INR values for AF are 2–3. Increased levels of coronary calcification has been recently reported in patients on long-term therapy with vitamin K antagonists.[119]

Novel oral anticoagulants are direct thrombin (dabigatran) or factor Xa (rivaroxaban, apixaban) inhibitors. Thrombin catalyses the final step in the coagulation cascade by converting fibrinogen to fibrin. Factor Xa, in conjuction with factor Va, mediates activation of prothrombin to thrombin. In patients with non-valvular AF, and without severe renal impairment (CrCl<25–30 mL/min), novel anticoagulants confer a reduced risk of stroke, mortality, and intracranial bleeding compared to warfarin,[120] without the need of regular monitoring of efficacy.[121] A practical guide by EHRA has been recently published and a web site has been created (www.NOACforAF.eu).[122]

Dabigatran etexilate is a pro-drug converted to the active direct thrombin (factor IIa) inhibitor dabigatran, independently of cytochrome P450, thus making drug and diet interactions less likely. In contrast to indirect thrombin inhibitors, such as heparin, dabigatran inhibits not only free thrombin, but also thrombin bound to fibrin.[114] In the RE-LY trial, 18 113 patients with **non-valvular AF** were randomized to warfarin (INR 2–3) or oral dabigatran 110 mg bd or 150 mg bd and were followed for 2 years.[123,] Eligible patients had at least one risk factor for stroke (previous stroke or TIA, LVEF <40%, and an age ≥75, or 65 to 74 years plus diabetes mellitus, hypertension, or coronary artery disease), with mean CHADS2 score of 2.1 and no severe stroke within 6 months or a creatinine clearance <30 mL per minute. Dabigatran was associated with yearly rates of stroke and systemic embolism that were similar (1.53%) with 110 mg bd, or lower (1.11%) with 150 mg bd, compared to those associated with warfarin (1.69%). Major haemorrhage per year was lower in the 110 mg dabigatran (2.71%) but similar (3.11%) in the 150 mg dose, compared to warfarin (3.36%). The rate of haemorrhagic stroke was 0.38% per year in the warfarin group, as compared with 0.12% per year with 110 mg of dabigatran (p <0.001), and 0.10% per year with 150 mg of dabigatran (p <0.001). Mortality rates per year were not different,

Table 52.16 Oral anticoagulants for AF

	Warfarin	Dabigatran	Rivaroxaban	Apixaban	Endoxaban
Dose	Variable od	150 or 110 bd	20 mg od	5 mg bd	30–60 mg od
Target	Vitamin K-dependent factors	Thrombin (factor II)	Factor Xa	Factor Xa	Factor Xa
Half-life	40 h	12–14 h	9–13 h	10–14 h	1–11 h
Renal clearance	0	80%	65%	25%	50%
Time to max inhibition	3–5 h	0.5–2 h	1–4 h	1–4 h	1–2 h
Anticoagulation monitoring	INR	Not required	Not required	Not required	Not required
Interactions	Multiple	Inhibitors of P-gp: verapamil, reduce dose; dronedarone: avoid; potent inducers of P-gp: avoid	Potent inhibitors of CYP3A4 and P-gp: avoid; Potent inducers of CYP3A4 and P-gp: use with caution	Potent inhibitors of CYP3A4 and P-gp: avoid; potent inducers of CYP3A4 and P-gp use with caution	Potent inhibitors of P-gp: reduce dose; potent inducers of P-gp: avoid
Antidote	Vitamin K	None	None	None (prothrombin complex concentrates?)	None (prothrombin complex concentrates?)

For antidotes of new anticoagulants, see text.
Potent inhibitors of CYP3A4 include antifungals (e.g. ketoconazole, intraconazole, voriconazole, posaconazole), chloramphenicol, clarithromycin, and protease inhibitors (e.g. ritonavir, atanazavir).
Potent CYP3A4 inducers include phenytoin, carbamazepine, phenobarbital, rifampicin, and St. John's wort (*Hypericum perforatum*).
CYP3A4 inhibitors are aczole antimycotic agents, HIV protease inhibitors.
P-glycoprotein (P-gp) inhibitors include verapamil, amiodarone, quinidine, clarithromycin, and grapefruit juice.
P-glycoprotein inducers include rifampicin, St. John's wort, carbamazepine, phenytoin, and trazodone.
Data from Granger CB, Armaganijan LV. Newer oral anticoagulants should be used as first-line agents to prevent thromboembolism in patients with atrial fibrillation and risk factors for stroke or thromboembolism. *Circulation*, 2012;**125**:159–64 and Siegal DM, Crowther MA. Acute management of bleeding in patients on novel oral anticoagulants. *Eur Heart J*. 2013; **34**: 489–98.

3.75%, 3.64%, and 4.13%, respectively. In 2010, the FDA approved dabigatran at a dose of 150 mg bd (creatinine clearance >30 mL/min) or 75 mg bd (creatinine clearance (15–30 mL/min). However, in the long-term RELY-ABLE trial, during 2.3 years of continued treatment with dabigatran, there was a higher rate of major bleeding with dabigatran 150 mg twice daily in comparison with 110 mg, and similar rates of stroke and death.[124] The European Medicines Agency (EMA) has approved both the 110 mg bd and 150 mg bd doses for non-valvular AF. The drug is also preferred to warfarin by the ESC [5] and CCS.[103] Elective cardioversion may be performed in patients taking dabigatran for at least 3 weeks.[5] In a recent analysis of data from the RE-LY trial, interruption of dabigatran (2 days) or warfarin (5 days) for allowance of surgery was not associated by a significant occurrence of stroke and systemic embolism, and major bleeding was not different in the two treatment groups.[63] Dabigatran is excreted via the kidneys, and no dosing recommendation is given for clearance <15 mL/min. In the elderly (>80 years old), a reduced dose is recommended (75 mg bd). It can be safely used together with aspirin.[123] Main side effect is dyspepsia and stomach pain (11%) and transaminase elevations 0.9–2%, although with a frequency similar to that caused by warfarin.[125] There is no evidence of liver toxicity as happened with ximelagartan. A trend in the RE-LY study towards more MIs in the dabigatran arm, as compared to warfarin, was not confirmed in a subsequent post hoc analysis.[126] A recent meta-analysis of seven trials, including the RE-LY, detected a higher risk of MI (1.19% vs 0.79%; p = 0.03),[127] and this was also observed in the recent RE-MEDY trial.[128] However, in the recent Danish Registry report (4,978 patients on dabigatran and 8,936 patients on warfarin), mortality, intracranial bleeding, pulmonary embolism,and myocardial infarction were lower with dabigatran, compared to warfarin. Stroke/systemic embolism, and major bleeding rates were similar in the two groups.[129] Exposure to dabigatran is higher, up to 2-fold, when it is co-administered with dronedarone and this combination is discouraged.[130] Verapamil and amiodarone, and quinidine, clarithromycin and erythromycin also increase levels of dabigatran, and its dose should be reduced in case of coadministartion.

Activated partial thromboplastin time (aPTT) and ***thrombin clotting time (TCT or thrombin time)*** may be

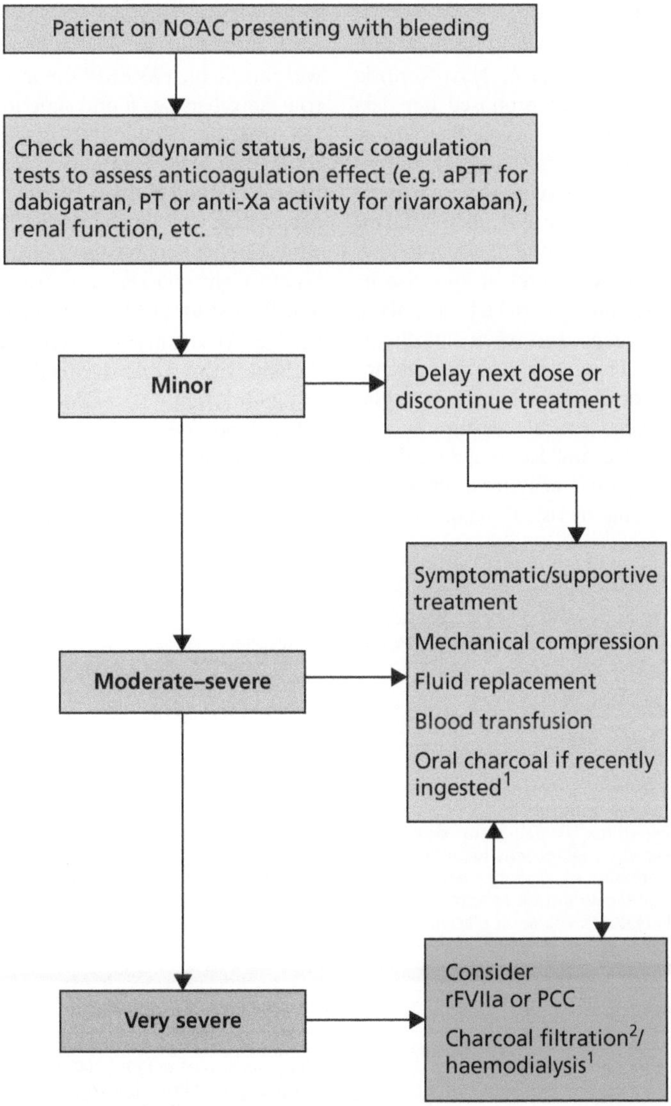

aPTT = activated partial thromboplastin time; NOAC = novel oral anticoagulant; PCC = prothrombin complex concentrate; PT = prothrombin time; rFVIIa = activated recombinant factor VII. [a]With dabigatran.

Figure 52.7 ESC 2012. Management of bleeding in patients taking novel oral anticoagulants.
2012 focused update of the ESC guidelines for the management of atrial fibrillation: an update of the 2010 ESC guidelines for the management of atrial fibrillation. *Europace*. 2012;**14**:1385–413.

used for assessment of anticoagulant action but not to guide dosage since the correlation is not linear. A normal aPTT indicates the absence of a significant dabigatran effect whereas an aPTT >2.5 times the control 8 to 12 hours after dabigatran dosing is suggestive of excess anticoagulant activity.[130,131] The ***Hemoclot direct thrombin inhibitor assay*** (HYPHEN BioMed) provides an accurate measure of dabigatran drug levels.[131]

There is no specific **antidote** to dabigatran, but a monoclonal antibody targeted against dabigatran is under development.[121] In emergencies, oral activated charcoal and renal dialysis may be tried (see also Perioperative anticoagulation).[132] Fresh ***frozen plasma, prothrombin complex concentrates*** (PCCs), or **activated PCC** (factor eight inhibitor bypassing activity—FEIBA, VH; Baxter, Vienna, Austria) may also be helpful (Figures 52.8 and

52.9, and Table 52.17).[131–133] Administration of aPCC (80U/kg) may be preferable to PCC (50 IU/kg).[121] Recombinant activated factor VII (rVIIa, NovoSeven, NovoNordisk, Bagsvaerd, Denmark) has also been proposed but data supporting its usefulness are lacking.[121] Note that, unlike the PCCs in Europe and Canada, which contain all four vitamin K-dependent procoagulant proteins, those currently available in the United States contain little, or no, factor VII.[131] Hemodialysis, oral charcoal within 2 hours following dabigatran ingestion, and desmopressin may also be tried in life-threatening conditions.[121] Packed red cells in anemia, platelet transfusions in patients receiving concurrent antiplatelet therapies, and fresh frozen in the presence of dilutional coagulopathy or disseminated intravascular coagulation, may also be tried as general measures.[121]

Apixaban is a highly selective oral factor Xa inhibitor. Apixaban reduced the risk of stroke or systemic embolism without significantly increasing the risk of major bleeding or intracranial haemorrhage in patients with non-valvular atrial fibrillation for whom vitamin K antagonist therapy was unsuitable (AVERROES trial).[134] In the ARISTOTLE trial, apixaban was found superior to warfarin in preventing stroke or systemic embolism, caused less bleeding, and resulted in lower mortality,[135] and this was true for both paroxysmal and persistent/permanent AF.[136] The used dose of apixaban was 5 mg bd, with a 2.5 mg bd dose for patients with ≥2 of the following criteria: age 80 years and older, body weight <60 kg, or a serum creatinine level of ≥1.5 mg/dL (133 μmol/L). A total of 18 201 patients with non-valvular AF and mean CHADS2 score 2.1 were included.[135] Patients with a stroke during the past 7 days or with a CrCl of <25 mL/min were excluded. The results showed a significant reduction of the primary outcome of stroke or systemic embolism from 1.60% per year in the warfarin group to 1.27% per year in the apixaban group. The rate of major bleeding was 3.09% per year for patients in the warfarin

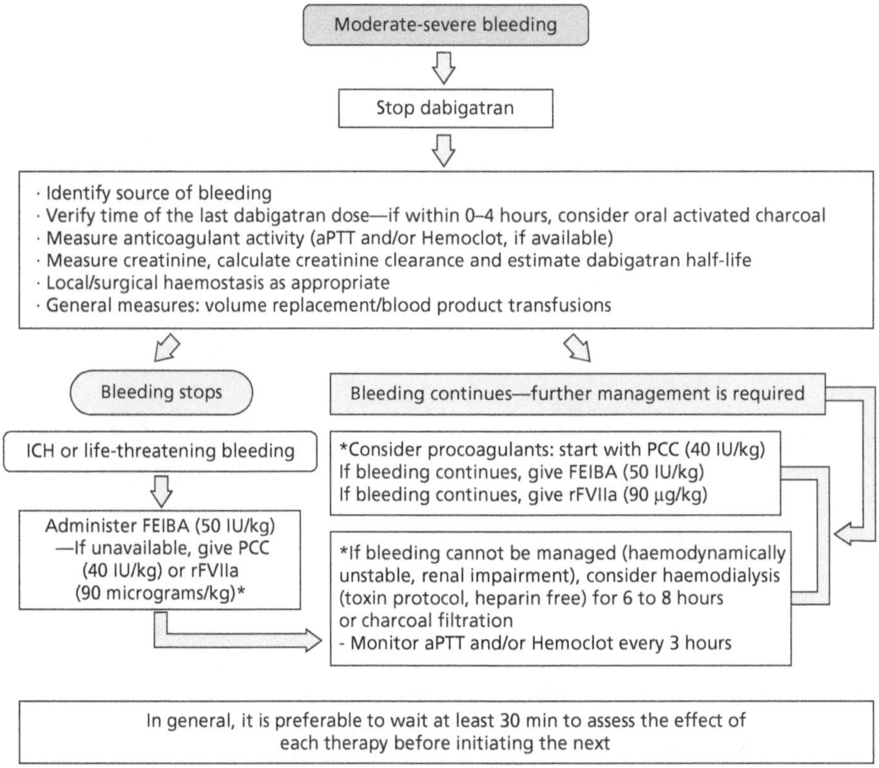

Figure 52.8 Proposed algorithm for management of moderate to severe bleeding and life-threatening bleeding episodes in patients treated with dabigatran. Recommendations are based on limited non-clinical data only.

PCC indicates prothrombin complex concentrates (non-activated); rFVIIa, recombinant activated factor VII; FEIBA, factor eight inhibitor bypassing activity. Moderate to severe bleeding indicates a reduction in haemoglobin ≥2 g/dL, transfusion of ≥2 U of red cells, or symptomatic bleeding in critical area (i.e. intraocular, intracranial, intraspinal, intramuscular with compartment syndrome, retroperitoneal, intra-articular, or pericardial bleeding). Life-threatening bleeding indicates symptomatic intracranial bleed, reduction in haemoglobin ≥5 g/dL, transfusion of ≥4 U of red cells, hypotension requiring inotropic agents, or bleeding requiring surgical intervention. Weitz JI, *et al.* Periprocedural management and approach to bleeding in patients taking dabigatran. *Circulation*. 2012;**126**:2428–32.

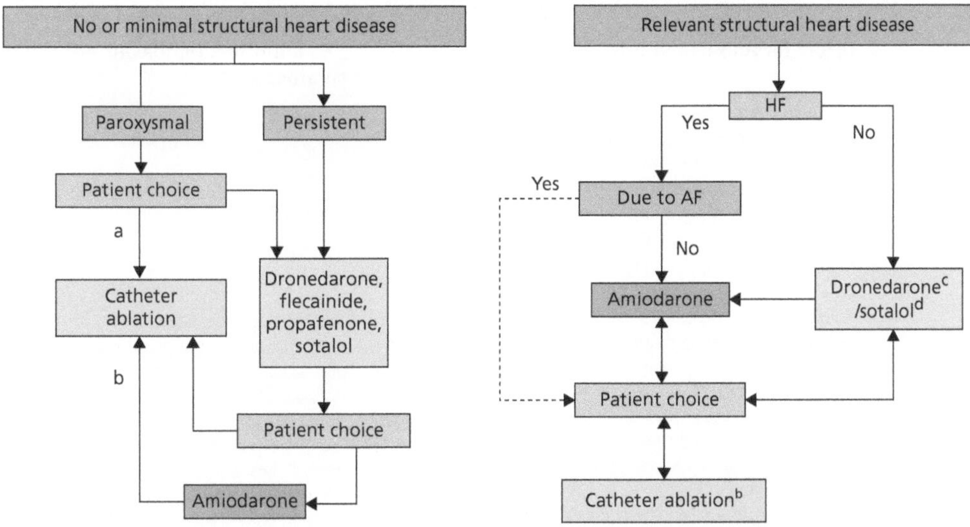

AF = atrial fibrillation; HF = heart failure. [a]Usually pulmonary vein isolation is appropriate. [b]More extensive left atrial ablation may be needed. [c]Caution with coronary heart disease. [d]Not recommended with left ventricular hypertrophy. Heart failure due to AF = tachcardiomyopathy.

Figure 52.9 ESC 2012. Antiarrhythmic drugs and/or left atrial ablation for rhythm control in AF.

2012 focused update of the ESC guidelines for the management of atrial fibrillation: an update of the 2010 ESC guidelines for the management of atrial fibrillation. *Europace*. 2012;**14**:1385–413.

group compared with 2.13% per year in the apixaban group (p <0.001). Rates of haemorrhagic stroke and intracranial bleeding were significantly lower in patients treated with apixaban than with warfarin (intracranial bleeding 0.33 per year vs 0.80% per year; p <0.001), and this was regardless of renal function.[137] Total mortality was 3.94% per year for warfarin compared with 3.52% per year for apixaban (p <0.047). The drug is metabolized in the liver via P450-dependent and -independent mechanisms, and 25% is excreted renally. Thus, apixaban is not recommended in patients receiving concomitant treatment with strong inhibitors of both CYP3A4 and P-glycoprotein, such as azole antimycotics and HIV protease inhibitors, and should also be used with caution in patients taking rifampicin, phenytoin, carbamazepine, and phenobarbital. There are limited clinical data on patients with a CrCl of 15 to 29 mL/min, and the drug is not recommended in patients with a CrCl of <15 mL/min. Apixaban is approved in Europe and Canada but has not been yet approved by the FDA for AF.

Prothrombin time, and especially ***anti-Xa assays***, may be used as rough estimates of the anticoagulant effect. Diltiazem results in increased apixabam levels.[130]

There are currently no specific **antidotes** for apixaban, but plasma-derived recombinant factor Xa are studied. [121] ***Prothrombin complex concentrates*** (50IU/kg) can be tried, and are probably preferred to aPCC (FEIBA).[121] Apixaban is not removed by dialysis, being protein bound. Packed red cells in anemia, platelet transfusions in patients receiving concurrent antiplatelet therapies, and fresh frozen in the presence of dilutional coagulopathy or disseminated intravascular coagulation, may also be tried as general measures.[121]

Rivaroxaban, an oral factor Xa inhibitor, in a single oral dose of 20 mg daily or 15 mg daily in patients with a creatinine clearance of 30 to 49 mL/min, was also not inferior to warfarin in patients with non-valvular AF for the prevention of stroke or systemic embolism and offered a lower rate of intracranial and fatal bleeding in high-risk patients with mean CHADS2 score of 3.5 (ROCKET AF).[138] However, there was a higher rate of gastrointestinal bleeding with rivaroxaban. The half-life of rivaroxaban is 7–11 hours, but factor Xa is inhibited for up to 24 hours, allowing once daily dosage. Its bioavailability increases with food. The drug is metabolized in the liver via P450-dependent and -independent mechanisms and is not recommended in patients receiving concomitant treatment with azole antimycotics and HIV protease inhibitors. Rivaroxaban is metabolized by the liver (33%) and excreted by the kidney (66%). There are limited data in CrCl 15–29 mL/min, and the drug is not recommended in patients with a CrCl of <15 mL/min. Clarithromycin and erythromycin also increase levels of rivaroxaban and its dose should be reduced in case of coadministartion. Rivaroxaban has been recently approved by the FDA and EMA for nonvalvular AF.

Prothrombin time, and especially ***anti-Xa assays***, may be used as rough estimates of the anticoagulant effect.[5]

No specific **antidotes** exist, but plasma-derived recombinant factor Xa are studied.[121] ***Prothrombin complex concentrates*** (50 IU/kg) are recommended for rivaroxaban,

Table 52.17 EHRA Practical Guide on the use of new oral anticoagulants. Possible measures in case of bleeding

	Direct thrombin inhibitors (dabigatran)	**FXa inhibitors (apibaxan, edoxaban, rivaroxaban)**
Non-life-threatening bleeding	Inquire last intake + dosing regimen Estimate normalization of haemostasis Normal renal function: 12–24 h CrCl 50–80 mL/min: 24–36 h CrCl 30–50 mL/min: 36–48 h CrCl <30 mL/min: ≥ 48 h Maintain diereses Local haemostatic measures Fluid replacement (colloids if needed) RBC substitution of necessary Platelet substitution (in case of thrombocytopenia ≤ 60 × 10^9/L or thrombopathy) Fresh frozen plasma as plasma expander (not as reversal agent) Tranexamic acid can be considered as adjuvans Desmopressin can be considered in special cases (coagulopathy or thrombopathy) Consider dialysis (preliminary evidence–65% after 4h) Charcoal haemoperfusion not recommended (no data)	Inquire last intake + dosing regimen Normalization of haemostatis: 12–24 h Local haemostatic measures Fluid replacement (colloids if needed) RBC substitution if necessary Platelet substitution (in case of thrombocytopenia ≤ 60 × 10^9/L or thrombopathy) Fresh frozen plasma as plasma expander (not as reversal agent) Tranexamic acid can be considered as adjuvans Desmopressin can be considered in special cases (coagulopathy or thrombopathy)
Life-threatening bleeding	All of the above Prothrombin complex concentrate (PCC) 25 U/kg (may be repeated once or twice) (but no clinical evidence) Activated PCC 50 IE/kg; max 200 IE/kg/day: no strong data about additional benefit over PCC. Can be considered before PCC if available Activated factor Vii (rFVIIa; 90 μg/kg) no data about additional benefit + expensive (only animal evidence)	All of the above Prothrombin complex concentrate (PCC) 25 U/kg (may be repeated once or twice) (but no clinical evidence) Activated PCC 50 IE/kg; max 200 IE/kg/day: no strong data about additional benefit over PCC. Can be considered before PCC if available Activated factor Vii (rFVIIa; 90 μg/kg) no data about additional benefit + expensive (only animal evidence)

RBC, red blood cells; CrCl, creatinine clearance; PCC, prothrombin complex concentrate

Heidbuchel H, *et al.* European Heart Rhythm Association Practical Guide on the use of new oral anticoagulants in patients with non-valvular atrial fibrillation. *Europace*. 2013;**15**:625–51.

and are probably preferred to aPCC (FEIBA).[139] Rivaroxaban is not removed by dialysis, being protein bound. Packed red cells in anemia, platelet transfusions in patients receiving concurrent antiplatelet therapies, and fresh frozen in the presence of dilutional coagulopathy or disseminated intravascular coagulation, may also be tried as general measures.[121]

Endoxaban, and betrixaban are other oral factor Xa inhibitor that have been found equivalent to warfarin in doses 30–60 mg od.[140,141]

Anticoagulation during acute coronary syndromes and PCI

Aspirin and clopidogrel are recommended in ACS and are considered mandatory for at least 4 weeks and 6–12 months after implantation of bare-metal stents (BMS) or drug-eluting stents (DES), respectively. In patients with a high risk of cardiovascular thrombotic complications (e.g. high GRACE or TIMI risk score), long-term therapy with warfarin (INR 2–2.5) may be combined with clopidogrel 75 mg daily (or, alternatively, aspirin 100 mg daily plus gastric protection) for 12 months.[142] In patients with AF, triple therapy (warfarin, aspirin, and clopidogrel) may be necessary but at an increased risk of bleeding. In a recent registry, the incidence rate of fatal or non-fatal bleeding per 100 person-years of therapy was 14.2 for triple therapy, 7–10.6 for dual therapy, and 6.6–7 for monotherapy, without a reduction in cardiovascular death, MI, or stroke.[143] PCI may be performed with concomitant heparin, aspirin, and clopidogrel, but IIb/IIIa inhibitors or bivalirudin should not be given if INR >2. If possible, DES should be avoided in patients on chronic anticoagulation and high HAS-BLED score, and triple therapy (INR 2–2.5) should be given for 4 weeks, followed by warfarin with either clopidogrel or aspirin for 12 months. In patients with HAS-BLED 0–2, DES may be used, and triple therapy is recommended for 6 months, followed by warfarin and clopidogrel or aspirin for 12 months (Tables 52.14 and 52.18). However, there has been evidence, that use of warfarin and clopidogrel without aspirin, might be safer in this setting.[145] PPIs may potentiate VKA-induced anticoagulation, resulting in increased INR values and bleeding risk, most likely due to facilitated gastric absorption of warfarin; thus carefull monitoring is required (see Chapter 27). Triple therapy with the use of newer anticoagulants is also associated with a substantially increased risk of bleeding,[146] as also happens with warfarin.

Table 52.18 PCI in patients on warfarin

ACC/AHA 2012 GL update on UA/NSTEMI. Recommendations for warfarin therapy	
Watch for bleeding, especially GI, and seek medical evaluation for evidence in patients on warfarin with aspirin and/or P2Y12 receptor inhibitor.	I-A
Warfarin without (INR 2.5 to 3.5) or with low-dose aspirin (81 mg od; INR 2.0 to 2.5), For patients at high coronary artery disease risk and low bleeding risk who do not require, or are intolerant of, P2Y12 receptor inhibitor.	IIb-B
A lower INR (e.g. 2.0 to 2.5) in patients with UA/NSTEMI managed with aspirin and a P2Y12 inhibitor.	IIb-C
ESC 2010 GL on AF. AF and ACS/PCI	
Following elective PCI in stable coronary artery disease, BMS should be considered and DES avoided, or strictly limited to, those clinical and/or anatomical situations (e.g. long lesions, small vessels, diabetes, etc.), where a significant benefit is expected when compared with BMS.	IIa-C
Following elective PCI, triple therapy (VKA, aspirin, clopidogrel) in the short term, followed by more long-term therapy (up to 1 year) with VKA plus clopidogrel 75 mg daily (or, alternatively, aspirin 75–100 mg daily, plus gastric protection with PPIs, H2 antagonists, or antacids).	IIa-C
Following elective PCI, clopidogrel in combination with VKA plus aspirin for a minimum of 1 month after implantation of a BMS, but longer with a DES (at least 3 months for a sirolimus-eluting stent and at least 6 months for a paclitaxel-eluting stent); following which VKA and clopidogrel 75 mg daily (or, alternatively, aspirin 75–100 mg daily, plus gastric protection with either PPIs, H2 antagonists, or antacids) should be considered, if required.	IIa-C
Following an ACS, with or without PCI, in patients with AF, triple therapy (VKA, aspirin, clopidogrel) in the short term (3–6 months), or longer in selected patients at low bleeding risk, followed by long-term therapy with VKA plus clopidogrel 75 mg daily (or, alternatively, aspirin 75–100 mg daily, plus gastric protection with PPIs, H2 antagonists, or antacids).	IIa-C
In anticoagulated patients at very high risk of thromboembolism, uninterrupted therapy with VKA as the preferred strategy and radial access used as the first choice, even during therapeutic anticoagulation (INR 2–3).	IIa-C
When VKA is given in combination with clopidogrel or low-dose aspirin, careful regulation of the anticoagulation dose intensity with an INR 2.0–2.5.	IIb-C
Following revascularization surgery in patients with AF, VKA plus a single antiplatelet drug in the initial 12 months, but this strategy has not been evaluated thoroughly and is associated with an increased risk of bleeding.	IIb-C
In patients with stable vascular disease (e.g. >1 year with no acute events), VKA monotherapy. Concomitant antiplatelet therapy should not be prescribed in the absence of a subsequent cardiovascular event.	IIb-C

2012 ACCF/AHA Focused Update Incorporated Into the ACCF/AHA 2007 Guidelines for the Management of Patients With Unstable Angina/Non–ST-Elevation Myocardial Infarction. *JACC* doi.org/10.1016/j.jacc.2013.01.014

ESC on AF 2010. Guidelines for the management of atrial fibrillation: The Task Force for the Management of Atrial Fibrillation of the European Society of Cardiology (ESC). *Eur Heart J*. 2010; **31**: 2369–2429.

In the RELY trial, addition of antiplatelet agents such as aspirin or clopidogrel or both was associated with higher risks of bleeding with either dabigatran or warfarin. The relative increase in the risk of major bleed was 1.6-fold on a single antiplatelet and 2.3-fold on double antiplatelets. However, the absolute risk of bleeding was lowest on dabigatran 110 mg bd.[147] Patients with AF in the absence of an acute coronary syndrome do not need additional aspirin.[5]

Perioperative anticoagulation

Warfarin Usually, surgical procedures require an INR of at least <1.5. Warfarin has a half-life of 36–42 h and should be stopped for 4–5 days before surgery. Bridging to UFH or LMWH is needed in patients with certain mechanical heart valves (see Chapter 22 on prosthetic heart valves). In urgent cases, oral or IV vitamin K (1–2 mg) may be considered. Although discontinuation of warfarin is usually advised in patients undergoing AF ablation, there is evidence that performance of the procedure without interruption of warfarin and with additional use of UFH (ACT >350) is safe and associated with less thrombotic complications.[148] In a recent meta-analysis, heparin bridging in patients receiving vitamin K antagonists for AF, prosthetic heart valves, or VTE conferred a >5-fold increased risk for bleeding whereas the risk of thromboembolic events was not significantly different between bridged and non-bridged patients.[149] The use of therapeutic dose LMWH was associated with an increased risk of bleeding compared with prophylactic or intermediate dose.[149]

New anticoagulants In general, discontinuation of new anticoagulants in patients with normal renal function is recommended 24h before procedures with a minor bleeding risk, and 48h in case of major bleeding risk.[122] For procedures with low haemorrhagic risk (dental extraction, skin biospsy, cataract surgery), a therapeutic window of 48 hours (last administration 24 hours before surgery and restart 24 hours after),[150] or even less (10 hours after last dosing),[131] is adequate. For procedures with moderate risk of bleeding (pacemaker/ICD implantation, colonoscopic resection of polyps), 1–2 days discontinuation of dabigatran is enough,[131] and, for procedures with high haemorrhagic risk, new anticoagulants should be stopped 3[131] to 5[149] days before surgery. Bridging with heparin has not been considered necessary,[146] but it should be used (UFH or LMWH) in high-risk cases, such as in patients with AF and a previous stroke.[150] Discontinuation of rivaroxaban in the ROCKET AF has been associated with a higher incidence of stroke compared to discontinuation of warfarin.[152] If urgent surgery or intervention is required, the risk of bleeding must be weighed against the clinical need for the procedure. Surgery or intervention should be deferred, if possible, until at least 12 h and ideally 24 h after the last dose. Perhaps shorter discontinuation windows are probably necessary wityh Xa inhibitors than with dabigatran.[151] Evaluation of common coagulation tests (aPTT for DTI; sensitive PT for FXa inhibitors) or of specific coagulation test (dTT for DTI; chromogenic assays for FXa inhibitors) can be considered but no clinical experience exists.[122] Non-specific antihaemorrhagic agents, such as recombinant human activated factor VIIa or prothrombin complex concentrates should probably not be given for prophylactic reversal due to their uncertain benefit-risk.[150] Reinitiation of these agents should be delayed 48–72 hours and once complete hemostasis is assured, since within 1 to 2 hours of reinitiation, the patient will be anticoagulated.

Management of stroke

Patients presenting within 4.5 h after the onset of ischaemic stroke should be considered for IV rt-PA (0.9 mg/kg, with 10% bolus, and the remainder over 60 min, maximum dose 90 mg). Either NECT or MRI is recommended before intravenous rtPA to exclude intracranial hemorrhage (absolute contraindication) and to determine whether CT hypodensity or MRI hyperintensity of ischemia is present.[153] Criteria are presented in Table 52.19. Of note, age >80 years is not an exclusion criterion.[154,155] However, fibrinolysis should be given only when possible within the first 3 hours in patients >80 years old, those taking oral anticoagulants regardless of INR, those with a baseline NIHSS score >25, those with imaging evidence of ischemic injury involving more than one third of the MCA territory, or those with a history of both stroke and diabetes mellitus.[153] Recently, tenecteplase (0.25 mg/kg, administered as a single bolus, with a maximum dose of 25 mg) was found superior to alteplase in patients subjected to thrombolysis within 6 h after the onset of ischaemic stroke.[156] In patients who present with stroke while taking new anticoagulants, if the aPTT is prolonged in a patient taking dabigatran (or the prothrombin time with an Xa inhibitor), it should be assumed that the patient is anticoagulated, and thrombolysis should not be administered.[5] Since dabigatran 150 mg bd resulted in a significant reduction in both ischaemic and haemorrhagic stroke, should the acute ischaemic stroke occur whilst the patient is taking rivaroxaban or apixaban (neither of which significantly reduced ischaemic stroke, compared with warfarin, in their respective trials), the use of dabigatran 150 mg bd instead may be reasonable.[5] Anticoagulants and antiplatelet agents should be withheld the first 24 h following fibrinolysis.[157] Recommendations for fibrinolysis and endovascular interventions in acute ischemic stroke have been recently provided.[158]

Catheter ablation

Left atrial catheter ablation (Figure 52.10 and Table 52.20) offers improved rates of SR maintenance and less complications compared to antiarrhythmic therapy.[159] In the MANTRA-PAF trial, 85% of ablated patients vs 71% medically treated patients with PAF were free of AF in 2 years (p = 0.004), but the cumulative burden of AF during that time was not significantly different on an intention-to-treat analysis (36% of patients initially assigned to medication eventually had ablation).[160] It may reduce functional MR with restoration of SR,[59] and, in patients with heart failure, pulmonary vein ablation is superior to AV nodal ablation and biventricular pacing.[161] Current catheter ablation strategies fall into two broad categories: ablation or isolation of focal triggers to prevent AF initiation through PV isolation and atrial substrate modification to impede AF perpetuation.[53] With these approaches, single-procedure 5-year success rates are approximately 40 to 50%. However, they offer approximately 60–80% freedom of AF in patients with paroxysmal AF subjected to a second (40%) or a third (10%) procedure.[162,163] PV isolation is achieved with PV antral ablation assisted by dedicated circumferential catheters or circumferential PV isolation with the assistance of electroanatomic mapping. Patients with persistent AF have lower success rates.[164] Additional linear lesions along the roof of the left atrium, connecting the superior aspects of the left and right upper PV isolation lesions, and along the region between the mitral annulus and the left inferior PV (mitral isthmus) may improve clinical outcomes in patients with persistent AF.[165] Novel techniques targeting areas with fractionated atrial electrograms or the anatomical areas of the major ganglionated autonomic plexi are also in clinical trials, but results have not yet been consistent.[166–168]

Complications of catheter ablation occur in 4.5% of cases and are mainly dependent on the operator's experience and adopted techniques.[169–171] They are tamponade (1.3%), TIA (0.71%), stroke (0.23%), femoral vein pseudoaneurysm (0.93%), and atrio-oesophageal fistulae (0.04%). Post-operative neurocognitive dysfunction has also been reported and depends on ablation techniques and anticoagulation strategies.[172] The reported mortality with AF ablation is 0.15% and is mainly due to tamponade or atrio-oesophageal fistulae, stroke, and massive pneumonia. Pulmonary vein stenosis occurs with ostial ablation (1% incidence of stenosis that requires intervention)[160] but not with antral or circumferential lesions. Phrenic nerve injury, coronary artery occlusion, and air embolism are rare. Female gender and CHADS2 score of ≥2 are significant independent risk factors for complications.[173] Use of irrigated tip catheters, with continuous fluid administration through catheter sheaths, meticulous anticoagulation with UFH without interruption of oral anticoagulation therapy, and avoidance of posterior wall lesions in the presence of a CT-assessed atrial-oesophageal distance <2 mm are necessary.[174] The use of an open irrigation ablation catheter and administration of UFH without interrupting warfarin may reduce the risk of periprocedural stroke without increasing the risk

Table 52.19 AHA/ASA 2013. AHA/ASA 2013 GL on acute ischaemic stroke. Inclusion and exclusion characteristics of patients with ischemic stroke who could be treated with IV rtPA within 3 hours from symptom onset

Inclusion criteria
Diagnosis of ischaemic stroke causing measurable neurological deficit
Onset of symptoms <3 h before beginning treatment
Aged ≥18 years
Exclusion criteria
Significant head trauma or prior stroke in previous 3 months
Symptoms suggest subarachnoid haemorrhage
Arterial puncture at non-compressible site within previous 7 days
History of previous intracranial haemorrhage
Recent intracranial or intraspinal surgery
Elevated blood pressure (systolic ≥185 mmHg or diastolic ≥110 mmHg)
Active internal bleeding
Acute bleeding diathesis, including, but not limited to:
Platelet count ≤100 000/mm³
Heparin received within 48 hours, resulting in abnormally elevated aPTT greater than the upper limit of normal
Current use of anticoagulant, with INR >1.7 or PT >15 s
Current use of direct thrombin inhibitors or direct factor Xa inhibitors with elevated sensitive laboratory tests (such as aPTT, INR, platelet count, and ECT; TT; or appropriate factor Xa activity assays)
Blood glucose concentration <50 mg/dL (2.7 mmol/L)
CT demonstrates multilobar infarction (hypodensity > 1/3 cerebral hemisphere)
Relative exclusion criteria
Recent experience suggests that under some circumstances—with careful consideration and weighting of risk to benefit—patients may receive fibrinolytic therapy despite 1 or more relative contraindications. Consider risk to benefit of IV rtPA administration carefully if any of these relative contraindications are present:
Only minor or rapidly improving stroke symptoms (clearing spontaneously)
Pregnancy
Seizure at onset with postictal residual neurological impairments
Major surgery or serious trauma within previous 14 days
Recent gastrointestinal or urinary tract hemorrhage (within previous 21 days)
Recent acute myocardial infarction (within previous 3 months)

The checklist includes some FDA-approved indications and contraindications for administration of IV rtPA for acute ischemic stroke. Recent guideline revisions have modified the original FDA-approved indications. A physician with expertise in acute stroke care may modify this list.
Onset time is defined as either the witnessed onset of symptoms or the time last known normal if symptom onset was not witnessed.
In patients without recent use of oral anticoagulants or heparin, treatment with IV rtPA can be initiated before availability of coagulation test results but should be discontinued if INR is >1.7 or PT is abnormally elevated by local laboratory standards.
In patients without history of thrombocytopenia, treatment with IV rtPA can be initiated before availability of platelet count but should be discontinued if platelet count is <100 000/mm.
aPTT indicates activated partial thromboplastin time; CT, computed tomography; ECT, ecarin clotting time;FDA, Food and Drug Administration; INR, international normalized ratio; IV, intravenous; PT, partial thromboplastin time; rtPA, recombinant tissue plasminogen activator; and TT, thrombin time.
Guidelines for the early management of patients with acute ischemic stroke: A Stroke Association guideline for healthcare professionals from the American Heart Association. *Stroke*. 2013:doi:10.1161/STR.1160b1013e318284056a

of pericardial effusion or other bleeding complications.[148] Periprocedural dabigatran use (150 mg bd), with the dose held on the morning of the procedure, increases the risk of bleeding or thromboembolic complications compared with uninterrupted warfarin therapy.[175] Dabigatran cessation 36 hours before the procedure and use of LMWH[176] or lower dabigatran doses (i.e. 110 bd) may be safer in this respect. Iatrogenic arrhythmias may occur in 4–20% of cases, depending on the method used for ablation.[177,178] Usually, they are macro-reentrant and respond to catheter ablation, although they do not always require repeat ablation.[177] Post-ablation left atrial arrhythmias are increased

Table 52.20 Recommendations for left atrial ablation

ESC 2012 GL on AF	
Paroxysmal AF in patients with symptomatic recurrences on antiarrhythmic drug therapy (amiodarone, dronedarone, flecainide, propafenone, sotalol) and who prefer further rhythm control therapy when performed by an electrophysiologist who has received appropriate training and is performing the procedure in an experienced centre.	I-A
Catheter ablation of AF should target isolation of the pulmonary veins.	IIa-A
Catheter ablation of AF should be considered as first-line therapy in selected patients with symptomatic paroxysmal AF as an alternative to antiarrhythmic drug therapy, considering patient choice, benefit, and risk.	IIa-B
When catheter ablation of AF is planned, continuation of oral anticoagulation with a VKA should be considered during the procedure, maintaining an INR close to 2.0.	IIa-B
When AF recurs within the first 6 weeks after catheter ablation, a watch-and-wait rhythm control therapy should be considered.	IIa-B

2012 focused update of the ESC Guidelines for the management of atrial fibrillation: An update of the 2010 ESC Guidelines for the management of atrial fibrillation. Developed with the special contribution of the European Heart Rhythm Association. *Europace*. 2012;**14**:1385–413.

HRS/EHRA/ECAS 2012 consensus statement	
Symptomatic AF refractory or intolerant to at least one class 1 or 3 antiarrhythmic medication	
Paroxysmal AF*	I-A
Persistent AF	IIa-B
Long-standing persistent AF	IIb-B
Symptomatic AF prior to initiation of antiarrhythmic drug therapy with a Class 1 or 3 antiarrhythmic agent	
Paroxysmal AF	IIa-B
Persistent or long-standing persistent AF	IIb-C

* Catheter ablation of symptomatic paroxysmal AF is considered a Class 1 indication only when performed by an electrophysiologist who has received appropriate training and is performing the procedure in an experienced centre.
2012 HRS/EHRA/ECAS Expert Consensus Statement on Catheter and Surgical Ablation of Atrial Fibrillation:recommendations for patient selection, procedural techniques, patient management and follow-up, definitions, endpoints, and research trial design. *Europace*. 2012;**14**:528–606.

with linear or fractionated electrogram ablation techniques. Warfarin is recommended for all patients for at least 2 months following an AF ablation procedure. Dabigatran may also be used. Decisions regarding the use of warfarin more than 2 months following ablation should be based on the patient's risk factors for stroke and not on the presence or type of AF. Discontinuation of warfarin therapy post-ablation is generally not recommended in patients who have a CHADS score ≥2.

Surgical ablation

Since its introduction, the MAZE procedure has gone through three modifications (Maze I, II, and III), using cut-and-sew techniques that ensure transmural lesions to isolate the PV, connect these dividing lines to the mitral valve annulus, and create electrical barriers in the RA that prevent macro-reentrant rhythms from becoming sustained. Success rates of around 70–95% have been reported.[179,180] Risks include death (less than 1% when performed as an isolated procedure), the need for permanent pacing (with right-sided lesions), recurrent bleeding requiring reoperation, impaired atrial transport function, delayed atrial arrhythmias (especially atrial flutter), and atrio-oesophageal fistula.[4] Variations of the MAZE procedure, using minimally invasive thoracoscopic approaches and radiofrequency or cryoablation energy, have also been successfully used. In patients with dilated left atrium and hypertension or failed prior catheter ablation, a minimally invasive approach has been found superior to catheter ablation in achieving freedom from left atrial arrhythmias after 12 months of follow-up but at a higher procedural adverse event rate.[179]

Surgical ablation of AF may also be considered in patients with symptomatic AF undergoing cardiac surgery, especially when mitral valve procedures are undertaken in experienced centres. Surgical ablation (PVI isolation and linear lesions), performed in patients with AF undergoing surgery for coronary artery or valve disease, improved the likelihood of SR but did not reduce total mortality, stroke rate, and the incidence of heart failure (PRAGUE-12).[181] The value of minimally invasive surgical ablation of AF without concomitant cardiac surgery in patients with symptomatic AF after failure of catheter ablation is not established (Table 52.21).

Left atrial appendage closure

The left atrial appendage is considered the main (but not the only) site of thrombus formation in AF. Recently,

Table 52.21 Recommendations for surgical ablation of AF

ESC 2010 GL on AF	
Surgical ablation of AF in patients with symptomatic AF undergoing cardiac surgery.	IIa-A
Surgical ablation of AF in patients with asymptomatic AF undergoing cardiac surgery if feasible with minimal risk.	IIb-C
Minimally invasive surgical ablation of AF without concomitant cardiac surgery in patients with symptomatic AF after failure of catheter ablation.	IIb-C
HRS/EHRA/ECAS 2012 consensus statement	
Indications for concomitant surgical ablation of AF	
Symptomatic AF refractory or intolerant to at least one Class 1 or 3 antiarrhythmic medication	
Paroxysmal, persistent, or long-standing persistent AF patients undergoing surgery for other indications.	IIa-C
Symptomatic AF prior to initiation of antiarrhythmic drug therapy with a class 1 or 3 antiarrhythmic agent.	
Paroxysmal or persistent AF patients undergoing surgery for other indications.	IIa-C
Long-standing persistent AF patients undergoing surgery for other indications.	IIb-C
Indications for stand-alone surgical ablation of AF	
Symptomatic AF refractory or intolerant to at least one class 1 or 3 antiarrhythmic medication	
Paroxysmal, persistent, or long-standing persistent AF patients who have failed one, or more, attempts at catheter ablation or who have not failed catheter ablation but prefer a surgical approach.	IIb-C
Symptomatic AF prior to initiation of antiarrhythmic drug therapy with a class 1 or 3 antiarrhythmic agent paroxysmal, persistent, or long-standing persistent AF.	III-C

Guidelines for the management of atrial fibrillation: the Task Force for the management of atrial fibrillation of the European Society of Cardiology (ESC). *Eur Heart J*. 2010; **31**: 2369–429.
HRS/EHRA/ECAS expert consensus statement on catheter and surgical ablation of atrial fibrillation: recommendations for patient selection, procedural techniques, patient management and follow-up, definitions, endpoints, and research trial design. *Europace*. 2012; **14**:528–606.

minimally invasive epicardial techniques and interventional trans-septal techniques have been developed for occlusion of the appendage orifice to reduce the stroke risk. Data on the safety and efficacy of this approach are rather insufficient. In the recent PROTECT AF trial, left appendage closure with the Watchman device was noninferior to ongoing warfarin therapy with regard to prevention of stroke, systemic embolism, and cardiovascular death. However, the closure arm sustained an increased number of procedure-related safety events, mainly pericardial tamponade and procedure-related stroke.[182] The 2012 ESC guidelines consider percutaneous closure in patients with a high stroke risk and contraindications for long-term oral anticoagulation (ESC IIb-B).[5] Surgical excision of the LAA may be considered in patients undergoing open heart surgery (ESC IIb-C).[5]

Atrial pacing

Atrial-based pacing is associated with a lower risk of AF and stroke than ventricular-based pacing in patients requiring pacemakers for bradyarrhythmias, but the value of pacing as a primary therapy for prevention of recurrent AF has not been proven.[183] Pacing in the interatrial septum, instead of the appendage, as well as anti-tachycardia algorithms for suppression of ectopic activity have produced promising results,[184,185] but the evidence is still inconclusive. There are no hard data to support the use of biatrial or multisite right atrial pacing for prevention of AF.

Upstream therapy

Upstream therapy to prevent or delay myocardial remodelling associated with hypertension, heart failure, or inflammation (e.g. after cardiac surgery) may deter the development of new AF (primary prevention) or, once established, its rate of recurrence or progression to permanent AF (secondary prevention) (Table 52.22).[186]

ACEIs/ARBs There has been compelling evidence supporting the role of RAAS in the genesis and perpetuation of AF. Experimental studies have demonstrated the beneficial effects of ACEIs and ARBs on AF prevention; however, clinical studies on the efficacy of such therapeutic interventions have produced variable results, depending on the clinical background of treated patients.[187] In patients with heart failure and/or LV hypertrophy, ACEIs and ARBs appear particularly useful for primary prevention of AF. Although meta-analyses of secondary prevention trials also suggest significant risk reduction after cardioversion with the use of ACEIs and ARBs, no effect was detected in large secondary prevention trials.[188,189] These agents are indicated for primary prevention in patients with hypertension or heart failure, but their value in secondary prevention is unproven.

Despite experimental evidence for a potential role of **statins**, **omega fatty acids**, and **steroids**, their clinical value is not proven.[190,191] Another potential target for drug therapy is endothelin-1, which modulates calcium recycling and promotes fibroblast proliferation.[40]

Table 52.22 ESC GL on AF 2010 upstream therapy. Recommendations for secondary prevention of AF with 'upstream' therapy

Pre-treatment with ACEIs and ARBs in patients with recurrent AF and receiving antiarrhythmic drug therapy.	IIb-B
ARBs or ACEIs for prevention of recurrent paroxysmal AF or in patients with persistent AF undergoing electrical cardioversion in the absence of significant structural heart disease if these agents are indicated for other reasons (e.g. hypertension).	IIb-B
Recommendations for primary prevention of AF with 'upstream' therapy	
ACEIs and ARBs in patients with heart failure and reduced ejection fraction.	IIa-A
ACEIs and ARBs in patients with hypertension, particularly with LV hypertrophy.	IIa-B
Statins after CABG, isolated or in combination with valvular interventions.	IIa-B
Statins in patients with underlying heart disease, particularly heart failure.	IIb-B
Upstream therapies with ACEIs, ARBs, and statins for primary prevention of AF in patients without cardiovascular disease.	III-C

Guidelines for the management of atrial fibrillation: The Task Force for the Management of Atrial Fibrillation of the European Society of Cardiology (ESC). *Eur Heart J* 2010; **31**: 2369–2429.

AF in specific conditions

Post-operative AF

AF is the most common complication after cardiac surgery, 30% after CABG, 40% after valve surgery, and 50% after combined CABG and valve surgery, with a peak incidence of post-operative AF between post-operative days 2 and 4.[1] Anticoagulation is necessary for AF persisting longer than 48 h (Table 52.23). **Beta blocker** therapy is most effective when provided both before and after cardiac surgery; [192,193] withdrawal of beta blockers is a significant risk factor for the development of post-operative AF and should be avoided. Treatment should be started at least 1 week before surgery with a beta 1 blocker without intrinsic sympathomimetic activity. Prophylactic **amiodarone** started orally before the operation also decreases the incidence of post-operative AF and reduces the incidence of stroke in most,[193,194] but not all, studies.[92] **IV magnesium** and **steroids** have also been beneficial.[192,193] **Colchicine** (1 mg bd the third post-op day, followed by 0.5 mg bd (0.25 bd in patients <70 kg)) for 1 month reduced the incidence of AF by 45% (COPPS substudy).[197] Use of **statins** has also been found to reduce post-operative AF.[198] There is also limited evidence that routine of atrial or biatrial pacing reduces AF.[199]

Acute coronary syndromes

AF occurs in 2–21% of patients with ACS and indicates increased in-hospital and long-term mortality (see Chapter 28),[200] particularly when occurring >30 days after MI.[198] Recommendation for the management of AF are presented in Table 52.24. Recommendations on anticoagulation are provided in Tables 52.14 and 52.17.

Heart failure

AF constitutes a strong and independent risk factor for the development of heart failure, and both conditions frequently coexist, partly because of common risk factors.[202] Beta blockers are the cornerstone of therapy in patients with systolic heart failure and confer a 27% reduction in the incidence of new-onset AF.[203] The rhythm control strategy has not been shown to be superior to rate control in heart failure patients with AF.[82] However, catheter ablation may lead to improvement in LV function, exercise tolerance, and quality of life in selected patients and is superior to AV nodal ablation and biventricular pacing.[161] It is also preferable to a rate-control strategy with beta blockers and/or digoxin by means of symptoms and neurohormonal status.[204]

Recommendations are provided in Table 31.15 (Chapter 31 on heart failure).

Valve disease

AF is frequently seen in mitral and progressed aortic valve disease. Paroxysmal or persistent AF constitutes an indication for percutaneous or surgical intervention in mitral valve disease (Table 52.25).

Hyperthyroidism

AF occurs in 10–25% of patients, with hyperthyoidism especially in men and the elderly.[4] Treatment is aimed primarily at restoring a euthyroid state, which may be associated with a spontaneous reversion to sinus rhythm. If a rhythm control strategy is selected, thyroid function should be normalized prior to cardioversion to reduce the risk of recurrence (Table 52.25). Amiodarone may cause both hyper- and hypothyroidism. Hypothyroidism typically occurs within the first 1–24 months, and the prevalence is as high as 22%, especially in patients with anti-thyroid antibodies (Table 52.26).[205] There are two types of amiodarone-induced hyperthyroidism: type I, where there is an excess iodide-induced production of T4 and T3; and type II, where there is a destructive thyroiditis with a transient excess release of T4 and T3 and, later, reduced thyroid function.[4] Although amiodarone may be continued when hypothyroidism has been successfully treated with replacement therapy, it is necessary to discontinue amiodarone if hyperthyroidism develops. Thyrotoxicosis may also occur after cessation of amiodarone therapy.

Table 52.23 Post-operative AF

ESC 2010 GL on AF. Prevention of post-operative AF	
Oral beta blockers for patients undergoing cardiac surgery in the absence of contraindications.	I-A
If used, beta blockers (or other oral antiarrhythmic drugs for AF management) are to be continued until the day of surgery.	I-B
Restoration of sinus rhythm by DCC in patients who develop post-operative AF and are haemodynamically unstable.	I-B
Ventricular rate control in patients with AF without haemodynamic instability.	I-C
Preoperative administration of amiodarone as prophylactic therapy for patients at high risk for post-operative AF.	IIa-A
Unless contraindicated, antithrombotic/anticoagulation medication for post-operative AF considered when the duration of AF is >48 h.	IIa-A
If sinus rhythm is restored successfully, anticoagulation for a minimum of 4 weeks but more prolonged in the presence of stroke risk factors.	IIa-B
Antiarrhythmic medications for recurrent or refractory post-operative AF in an attempt to maintain sinus rhythm.	IIa-C
Sotalol after cardiac surgery but is associated with risk of proarrhythmia.	IIb-A
Biatrial pacing after cardiac surgery.	IIb-A
Corticosteroids after cardiac surgery but are associated with risk.	IIb-B
ACCF/AHA 2013 GL on AF. Post-operative AF	
Unless contraindicated, oral beta blocker to prevent post-operative AF for patients undergoing cardiac surgery.	I-A
AV nodal blocking agents to achieve rate control in patients who develop post-operative AF.	I-B
Preoperative administration of amiodarone in patients undergoing cardiac surgery.	IIa-A
Cardioversion with ibutilide or direct current in patients who develop post-operative AF.	IIa-B
Antiarrhythmic medications in an attempt to maintain SR in patients with recurrent or refractory post-operative AF.	IIa-B
Antithrombotic medication in patients who develop post-operative AF, as recommended for non-surgical patients.	IIa-B
Prophylactic administration of sotalol for patients undergoing cardiac surgery.	IIb-B

Guidelines for the management of atrial fibrillation: the Task Force for the management of atrial fibrillation of the European Society of Cardiology (ESC). *Eur Heart J*. 2010; **31**: 2369–429.
Management of patients with atrial fibrillation (compilation of 2006 ACCF/AHA/ESC and 2011 ACCF/AHA/HRS recommendations): A report of the American College of Cardiology/American Heart Association Task Force on practice guidelines. *J Am Coll Cardiol*. 2013; **61**:1935–44.

Table 52.24 AF in acute coronary syndromes

ESC 2010 GL on AF. AF in acute coronary syndromes	
DCC for patients with severe haemodynamic compromise or intractable ischaemia or when adequate rate control cannot be achieved with pharmacological agents.	I-C
IV amiodarone to slow a rapid ventricular response.	I-C
IV beta blockers to slow a rapid ventricular response.	I-C
IV non-dihydropyridine calcium antagonists (verapamil, diltiazem) to slow a rapid ventricular response if no clinical signs of heart failure.	IIa-C
IV digoxin to slow a rapid ventricular response in heart failure.	IIb-C
Administration of flecainide or propafenone.	III-B
ACCF/AHA 2013 GL on AF. Acute myocardial infarction	
Direct current cardioversion in severe haemodynamic compromise or intractable ischaemia or when adequate rate control cannot be achieved with pharmacological agents.	I-C
IV amiodarone to slow a rapid ventricular response to AF and improve LV function.	I-C
IV beta blockers and non-dihydropyridine calcium antagonists to slow a rapid ventricular response in the absence of LV dysfunction, bronchospasm, or AV block.	I-C
Unfractionated heparin by continuous IV infusion or intermittent SC to prolong the aPTT 1.5–2.0 times, unless contraindications to anticoagulation exist.	I-C
IV digitalis to slow a rapid ventricular response and improve LV function in severe LV dysfunction and HF.	IIa-C
Class IC antiarrhythmic drugs in patients with AF in the setting of acute MI.	III-C

Guidelines for the management of atrial fibrillation: the Task Force for the management of atrial fibrillation of the European Society of Cardiology (ESC). *Eur Heart J*. 2010; **31**: 2369–429.
Management of patients with atrial fibrillation (compilation of 2006 ACCF/AHA/ESC and 2011 ACCF/AHA/HRS recommendations): A report of the American College of Cardiology/American Heart Association Task Force on practice guidelines. *J Am Coll Cardiol*. 2013; **61**:1935–44.

Table 52.25 ESC 2010 GL on AF. AF in valvular disease

OAC therapy (INR 2.0–3.0) in patients with mitral stenosis and AF (paroxysmal, persistent, or permanent).	I-C
OAC therapy (INR 2.0–3.0) in patients with AF and clinically significant mitral regurgitation.	I-C
Percutaneous mitral balloon valvotomy for asymptomatic patients with moderate or severe mitral stenosis and suitable valve anatomy who have new-onset AF in the absence of LA thrombus.	IIa-C
Early mitral valve surgery in severe mitral regurgitation, preserved LV function, and new-onset AF, even in the absence of symptoms, particularly when valve repair is feasible.	IIa-C

Guidelines for the management of atrial fibrillation: the Task Force for the management of atrial fibrillation of the European Society of Cardiology (ESC). *Eur Heart J*. 2010; **31**: 2369–429.

Table 52.26 Hyperthyroidism

ESC 2010 GL on AF. AF in hyperthyroidism	
Antithrombotic therapy, based on the presence of other stroke risk factors in patients with active thyroid disease.	I-C
Beta blocker to control the rate of ventricular response in patients with AF complicating thyrotoxicosis, unless contraindicated.	I-C
When a beta blocker cannot be used, a non-dihydropyridine calcium channel antagonist (diltiazem or verapamil) to control the ventricular rate in thyrotoxicosis.	I-C
If a rhythm control strategy is desirable, it is necessary to normalize thyroid function prior to cardioversion, as otherwise the risk of relapse remains high.	I-C
Once a euthyroid state is restored, recommendations for antithrombotic prophylaxis are the same as for patients without hyperthyroidism.	I-C
ACCF/AHA 2013 GL on AF. Hyperthyroidism	
A beta blocker is recommended to control the rate of ventricular response in patients with AF complicating thyrotoxicosis, unless contraindicated.	I-B
A non-dihydropyridine calcium channel antagonist (diltiazem or verapamil) when a beta blocker cannot be used,	I-B
Oral anticoagulation (INR 2.0 to 3.0), as recommended for AF patients with other risk factors for stroke.	I-C
Once a euthyroid state is restored, recommendations for antithrombotic prophylaxis are the same as for patients without hyperthyroidism.	I-C

Guidelines for the management of atrial fibrillation: the Task Force for the management of atrial fibrillation of the European Society of Cardiology (ESC). *Eur Heart J*. 2010; **31**: 2369–429.
Management of patients with atrial fibrillation (compilation of 2006 ACCF/AHA/ESC and 2011 ACCF/AHA/HRS recommendations): A report of the American College of Cardiology/American Heart Association Task Force on practice guidelines. *J Am Coll Cardiol*. 2013; **61**:1935–44.

Wolff–Parkinson–White syndrome

The incidence of SCD in patients with the Wolff–Parkinson–White syndrome ranges from 0 to 0.6% per year.[1] Markers of increased risk are short R-R intervals during pre-excited AF (<250 ms), a history of symptomatic tachycardia, the presence of multiple APs, or Ebstein's anomaly (see Chapter 54). AV nodal blocking agents are contraindicated in WPW syndrome (Table 52.27).

Hypertrophic cardiomyopathy

Patients with hypertrophic cardiomyopathy (HCM) are at greater risk of developing AF compared with the general population, and around 20–25% develop AF, with an annual incidence of 2%.[1] AF is associated with increased risk for mortality, stroke, and severe functional disability, particularly in patients with outflow obstruction, ≤50 years of age, or those developing chronic AF.[206] A rhythm control strategy with catheter ablation seems preferable.[207] Additional antiarrhythmic drugs may be necessary, and amiodarone or disopyramide may be reasonable, although no controlled studies are available. Fast AF may also predispose to haemodynamic collapse and VF, and electrical or pharmacological cardioversion is indicated in the absence of atrial thrombus in patients presenting with acute-onset AF. When myectomy is considered, addition of MAZE-III procedure may also eliminate AF without increased perioperative mortality (Table 52.28).

Chronic obstructive pulmonary disease

AF is common in patients with chronic lung disease and has adverse prognostic implications in the context of acute exacerbations associated with hypoxia. Treatment of the underlying pulmonary disease and correction of metabolic imbalance are the primary considerations, as antiarrhythmic therapy and electrical cardioversion are likely to be ineffective until respiratory decompensation has been corrected. Multifocal atrial tachycardia is common in severe COPD and may be mistaken for AF. Agents used to relieve bronchospasm, such as theophylline and beta-adrenergic agonists, may precipitate AF, and controlling the rate of ventricular response may be difficult in this situation. Non-selective beta blockers, propafenone, and adenosine are generally contraindicated in patients with bronchospasm, and non-dihydropyridine calcium channel antagonists are the preferred alternative (Table 52.29). Beta 1 selective blockers (e.g. nebivolol, bisoprolol, and metoprolol), in small doses, are also tolerated and effective.[208]

Other conditions

AF in GUCH, valve disease, and genetic channelopathies is discussed in the relevant chapters.

Table 52.27 WPW syndrome

ESC 2010 GL on AF. AF in WPW syndrome	
Catheter ablation of an overt AP in patients with AF to prevent SCD	I-A
Immediate referral to an experienced ablation centre of patients who survived SCD and have evidence of overt AP conduction.	I-C
Catheter ablation for patients with high-risk professions (e.g. pilots, public transport drivers) and overt, but asymptomatic, AP conduction on the surface ECG.	I-B
Catheter ablation in patients at high risk of developing AF in the presence of an overt, but asymptomatic, AP on the surface ECG.	I-B
Catheter ablation of the AP in asymptomatic patients with evidence of an overt AP only after a full explanation and careful counselling.	IIa-B
ACCF/AHA 2013 GL on AF. Wolff–Parkinson–White (WPW) pre-excitation syndromes	
Catheter ablation of the accessory pathway, particularly in patients with syncope due to rapid heart rate or those with a short bypass tract refractory period.	I-B
Immediate direct current cardioversion to prevent VF in patients with a short anterograde bypass tract refractory period in whom AF occurs with haemodynamic instability.	I-B
IV procainamide or ibutilide to restore SR in patients without haemodynamic instability in association with a wide QRS complex on the ECG (≥120 ms) or with a rapid pre-excited ventricular response.	I-C
IV flecainide or DC cardioversion when very rapid ventricular rates occur, involving conduction over an accessory pathway.	IIa-B
IV quinidine, procainamide, disopyramide, ibutilide, or amiodarone to haemodynamically stable patients with AF involving conduction over an accessory pathway.	IIb-B
IV digitalis glycosides or non-dihydropyridine calcium channel antagonists in patients with pre-excited ventricular activation during AF.	III-B

Guidelines for the management of atrial fibrillation: the Task Force for the management of atrial fibrillation of the European Society of Cardiology (ESC). *Eur Heart J*. 2010; **31**: 2369–429.
Management of patients with atrial fibrillation (compilation of 2006 ACCF/AHA/ESC and 2011 ACCF/AHA/HRS recommendations): A report of the American College of Cardiology/American Heart Association Task Force on practice guidelines. *J Am Coll Cardiol*. 2013; **61**:1935–44.

Table 52.28 Hypertrophic cardiomyopathy

ESC 2010 GL on AF. AF in hypertrophic cardiomyopathy	
Restoration of sinus rhythm by DCC or pharmacological cardioversion in patients with HCM presenting with recent-onset AF.	I-B
OAC therapy (INR 2.0–3.0) in patients with HCM who develop AF, unless contraindicated.	I-B
Amiodarone (or, alternatively, disopyramide plus beta blocker) to achieve rhythm control and to maintain sinus rhythm in patients with HCM.	IIa-C
Catheter ablation of AF in patients with symptomatic AF refractory to pharmacological control.	IIa-C
Ablation procedures (with concomitant septal myectomy if indicated) in patients with HCM and refractory AF.	IIa-C
ACCF/AHA 2013 GL on AF. Hypertrophic cardiomyopathy	
Oral anticoagulation (INR 2.0 to 3.0) in patients who develop AF, as for other patients at high risk of thromboembolism.	I-B
Antiarrhythmic medications to prevent recurrent AF. Disopyramide with a beta blocker or non-dihydropyridine calcium channel antagonist or amiodarone alone is preferred (insufficient data).	IIa-C

Guidelines for the management of atrial fibrillation: the Task Force for the management of atrial fibrillation of the European Society of Cardiology (ESC). *Eur Heart J*. 2010; **31**: 2369–429.
Management of patients with atrial fibrillation (compilation of 2006 ACCF/AHA/ESC and 2011 ACCF/AHA/HRS recommendations): A report of the American College of Cardiology/American Heart Association Task Force on practice guidelines. *J Am Coll Cardiol*. 2013; **61**:1935–44.

Athletes

The intensity of physical activity displays a U-shaped relationship with incident AF, which may indicate that the positive antiarrhythmic effects of physical activity are partially negated when exercise is too strenuous.[42,43] For practical purposes, only the pill-in-the pocket approach and catheter ablation are acceptable treatment options (Table 52.30).

AF in pregnancy

AF is rare during pregnancy in women without previously detected AF and without pre-existing heart disease.[1,4] In patients with previously diagnosed AF, 52% experience new episodes during pregnancy. AF during pregnancy is well tolerated in most patients without congenital or valvular disease, but more fetal complications occur in those women who develop arrhythmias during pregnancy.

Rate control drugs Beta blockers cross the placenta and are associated with various adverse effects, including intrauterine growth retardation, neonatal respiratory depression, bradycardia, and hypoglycaemia, especially if treatment is initiated early in pregnancy (i.e. 12–24 weeks). A meta-analysis in patients with hypertension assessing risks of beta receptor blockers in pregnancy found a borderline increase in 'small for gestational age' infants.[209] No association with low weight for gestational age has been

Table 52.29 Pulmonary disease

ESC 2010 GL on AF. AF in pulmonary disease	
Correction of hypoxaemia and acidosis as initial management for patients who develop AF during an acute pulmonary illness or exacerbation of chronic pulmonary disease.	I-C
DCC in patients with pulmonary disease who become haemodynamically unstable as a consequence of AF.	I-C
A non-dihydropyridine calcium channel antagonist (diltiazem or verapamil) to control the ventricular rate in patients with obstructive pulmonary disease who develop AF.	IIa-C
Beta 1 selective blockers (e.g. bisoprolol), in small doses, as an alternative for ventricular rate control.	IIa-C
Theophylline and beta-adrenergic agonist agents in bronchospastic lung disease.	III-C
Non-selective beta blockers, sotalol, propafenone, and adenosine in obstructive lung disease.	III-C

2011 ACCF/AHA/HRS focused update on the management of patients with atrial fibrillation (Updating the 2006 Guideline). *J Am Coll Cardiol*. 2011;**57**:223–42.

ACCF/AHA 2013 GL on AF. Pulmonary diseases	
Correction of hypoxaemia and acidosis for patients who develop AF.	I-C
A non-dihydropyridine calcium channel antagonist (diltiazem or verapamil) to control the ventricular rate.	I-C
Direct current cardioversion in patients who become haemodynamically unstable as a consequence of AF.	I-C
Theophylline and beta-adrenergic agonist agents in patients with bronchospastic lung disease who develop AF.	III-C
Beta blockers, sotalol, propafenone, and adenosine.	III-C

Management of patients with atrial fibrillation (compilation of 2006 ACCF/AHA/ESC and 2011 ACCF/AHA/HRS recommendations): A report of the American College of Cardiology/American Heart Association Task Force on practice guidelines. *J Am Coll Cardiol*. 2013; **61**:1935–44.

Table 52.30 ESC 2010 GL on AF. Recommendations for AF in athletes

When a 'pill-in-the-pocket' approach with sodium channel blockers is used, sport cessation for as long as the arrhythmia persists and until 1–2 half-lives of the antiarrhythmic drug used have elapsed.	IIa-C
Isthmus ablation in competitive or leisure time athletes with documented atrial flutter, especially when therapy with flecainide or propafenone is intended.	IIa-C
Where appropriate, AF ablation to prevent recurrent AF in athletes.	IIa-C
When a specific cause for AF is identified in an athlete (such as hyperthyroidism), it is not recommended to continue participation in competitive or leisure time sports until correction of the cause.	III-C
It is not recommended to allow physical sports activity when symptoms due to haemodynamic impairment (such as dizziness) are present.	III-C

Guidelines for the management of atrial fibrillation: the Task Force for the management of atrial fibrillation of the European Society of Cardiology (ESC). *Eur Heart J*. 2010; **31**: 2369–429.

found for labetalol (started after the 6th week of gestation) as opposed to atenolol (see Hypertension). Digoxin crosses the placenta freely, and digitalis intoxication in the mother has been associated with fetal death. Oral verapamil and diltiazem are most probably safe (Table 52.32). Sotalol, flecainide, or propafenone are second-choice drugs.

Drugs for atrial fibrillation conversion IV ibutilide or flecainide is usually effective and may be considered, although the experience during pregnancy is limited.[210,211] Amiodarone may cause neonatal hypothyroidism (9% of newborns), hyperthyroidism, goiter, and growth retardation. All drugs should, if possible, be avoided during the period of organogenesis in the first trimester of pregnancy.

Direct current cardioversion Several case reports have demonstrated successful cardioversion of maternal AF, without harm to the fetus. Prior anticoagulation or TOE exclusion of left atrial thrombus is mandatory when AF is >48 h, and anticoagulation is maintained for 4 weeks. In AF <48 h, one IV UH or LMWH is given pericardioversion. Energy requirements in pregnant and non-pregnant women are similar.

Anticoagulation is recommended in patients with ≥2 risk points of the $CHADS_2$ score or 2 risk points of the CHA_2DS_2VASC score.[211] Vitamin K antagonists can be teratogenic in up to 7% of fetuses and, in many cases, should be substituted with UFH or LMWH for the first trimester.[211] Warfarin may be used in the second trimester at an only slightly elevated teratogenic risk. Warfarin crosses the placenta freely, and the fetus may be overdosed, even when the mother is in the therapeutic INR range. LMWH does not cross the placenta barrier and has been used for treatment and prophylaxis of venous thromboembolism during pregnancy without adverse fetal effects. Perhaps the most practical policy is to recommend subcutaneous administration of weight-adjusted therapeutic doses of LMWH during the first trimester and during the last

Table 52.31 Pregnancy

ESC 2010 GL on AF. AF in pregnancy	
DCC can be performed safely at all stages of pregnancy and is recommended in patients who are haemodynamically unstable due to AF and whenever the risk of ongoing AF is considered high for the mother or for the fetus.	I-C
Protection against thromboembolism throughout pregnancy in AF patients with a high thromboembolic risk; the choice of agent (heparin or warfarin) according to the stage of pregnancy.	I-C
Oral VKA is from the second trimester until 1 month before expected delivery.	I-B
Subcutaneous LMWH during the first trimester and during the last month of pregnancy. Alternatively, UFH to prolong the aPTT to 1.5 times the control.	I-B
Beta blocker or a non-dihydropyridine calcium channel antagonist if rate control is necessary. During the first trimester of pregnancy, the use of beta blockers must be weighed against the potential risk of negative fetal effects.	IIa-C
IV flecainide or ibutilide if arrhythmia conversion is mandatory and DCC considered inappropriate in haemodynamically stable patients with structurally normal hearts.	IIb-C
Digoxin if rate control is indicated and beta blockers or non-dihydropyridine calcium channel antagonists are contraindicated.	IIb-C
ACCF/AHA 2013 GL on AF. AF in pregnancy	
Digoxin, a beta blocker, or a non-dihydropyridine calcium channel antagonist to control the rate of ventricular response.	I-C
Direct current cardioversion in pregnant patients who become haemodynamically unstable due to AF.	I-C
Protection against thromboembolism throughout pregnancy for all patients with AF (except those with lone AF and/or low thromboembolic risk).	I-C
Therapy (anticoagulant or aspirin) should be chosen according to the stage of pregnancy.	
Heparin during the first trimester and last month of pregnancy for patients with AF and risk factors for thromboembolism. Unfractionated heparin IV to prolong the aPTT 1.5 to 2 times or SC 10 000–20 000 units every 12 h to prolong the mid-interval (6 h after injection) aPTT 1.5 times control.	IIb-C
SC LMWH during the first trimester and last month of pregnancy (limited data).	IIb-C
Oral anticoagulant during the second trimester for pregnant patients with AF at high thromboembolic risk.	IIb-C
Quinidine or procainamide to achieve pharmacological cardioversion in haemodynamically stable patients who develop AF.	IIb-C

Guidelines for the management of atrial fibrillation: the Task Force for the management of atrial fibrillation of the European Society of Cardiology (ESC). *Eur Heart J*. 2010; **31**: 2369–429.
Management of patients with atrial fibrillation (compilation of 2006 ACCF/AHA/ESC and 2011 ACCF/AHA/HRS recommendations): A report of the American College of Cardiology/American Heart Association Task Force on practice guidelines. *J Am Coll Cardiol*. 2013; **61**:1935–44.

month of pregnancy (Table 52.31). The new oral thrombin antagonists, such as dabigatran, have shown fetotoxicity with high doses and should not be used.[211]

References

1. Camm AJ, *et al.* Guidelines for the management of atrial fibrillation: the Task Force for the Management of Atrial Fibrillation of the European Society of Cardiology (ESC). *Europace*. 2010;**12**:1360–420
2. Wann LS, *et al.* 2011 ACCF/AHA/HRS focused update on the management of patients with atrial fibrillation (update on Dabigatran): a report of the American College of Cardiology Foundation/American Heart Association Task Force on practice guidelines. *Circulation*. 2011;**123**:1144–50
3. Wann LS, *et al.* 2011 ACCF/AHA/HRS focused update on the management of patients with atrial fibrillation (Updating the 2006 Guideline): a report of the American College of Cardiology Foundation/American Heart Association Task Force on Practice Guidelines. *J Am Coll Cardiol*. 2011;**57**:223–42
4. Fuster V, *et al.* 2011 ACCF/AHA/HRS focused updates incorporated into the ACC/AHA/ESC 2006 guidelines for the management of patients with atrial fibrillation: a report of the American College of Cardiology Foundation/American Heart Association Task Force on practice guidelines. *Circulation*. 2011;**123**:e269–367
5. Camm AJ, *et al.* 2012 focused update of the ESC Guidelines for the management of atrial fibrillation: an update of the 2010 ESC Guidelines for the management of atrial fibrillation. Developed with the special contribution of the European Heart Rhythm Association. *Eur Heart J*. 2012;**33**:2719–47
6. Miyasaka Y, *et al.* Secular trends in incidence of atrial fibrillation in Olmsted County, Minnesota, 1980 to 2000, and implications on the projections for future prevalence. *Circulation*. 2006;**114**:119–25
7. Nieuwlaat R, *et al.* Atrial fibrillation management: a prospective survey in ESC member countries: the Euro Heart Survey on Atrial Fibrillation. *Eur Heart J*. 2005;**26**:2422–34
8. Davis RC, *et al.* Prevalence of atrial fibrillation in the general population and in high-risk groups: the ECHOES study. *Europace*. 2012;**14**:1553–59
9. Go AS, *et al.* Prevalence of diagnosed atrial fibrillation in adults: national implications for rhythm management and stroke prevention: the AnTicoagulation and Risk Factors in Atrial Fibrillation (ATRIA) Study. *JAMA*. 2001;**285**:2370–5
10. Wilke T, *et al.* Incidence and prevalence of atrial fibrillation: An analysis based on 8.3 million patients. *Europace*. 2013;**15**:486–93
11. Ohsawa M, *et al.* Rapid increase in estimated number of persons with atrial fibrillation in Japan: an analysis from

national surveys on cardiovascular diseases in 1980, 1990 and 2000. *J Epidemiol.* 2005;**15**:194–6
12. Zhou Z, *et al.* An epidemiological study on the prevalence of atrial fibrillation in the Chinese population of mainland China. *J Epidemiol.* 2008;**18**:209–16
13. Naccarelli GV, *et al.* Increasing prevalence of atrial fibrillation and flutter in the United States. *Am J Cardiol.* 2009;**104**:1534–9
14. Lloyd-Jones DM, *et al.* Lifetime risk for development of atrial fibrillation: the Framingham Heart Study. *Circulation.* 2004;**110**:1042–46
15. Benjamin EJ, *et al.* Impact of atrial fibrillation on the risk of death: the Framingham Heart Study. *Circulation.* 1998;**98**:946–52
16. Knecht S, *et al.* Atrial fibrillation in stroke-free patients is associated with memory impairment and hippocampal atrophy. *Eur Heart J.* 2008;**29**:2125–32
17. Santangeli P, *et al.* Atrial fibrillation and the risk of incident dementia: a meta-analysis. *Heart Rhythm.* 2012;**9**:1761–8
18. Wolf PA, *et al.* Atrial fibrillation as an independent risk factor for stroke: the Framingham Study. *Stroke.* 1991;**22**:983–8
19. Hart RG, *et al.* Stroke with intermittent atrial fibrillation: incidence and predictors during aspirin therapy. Stroke Prevention in Atrial Fibrillation Investigators. *J Am Coll Cardiol.* 2000;**35**:183–7
20. Friberg L, *et al.* Stroke in paroxysmal atrial fibrillation: report from the Stockholm Cohort of Atrial Fibrillation. *Eur Heart J.* 2010;**31**:967–75
21. Chen Y, *et al.* Atrial fibrillation and the risk of sudden cardiac death: the atherosclerosis risk in communities study and cardiovascular health study. *JAMA Intern Med.* 2013;**173**:29–35
22. Andersson T, *et al.* All-cause mortality in 272 186 patients hospitalized with incident atrial fibrillation 1995–2008: a Swedish nationwide long-term case–control study. *Eur Heart J.* 2013;**34**:1061–7
23. Wolowacz SE, *et al.* The cost of illness of atrial fibrillation: a systematic review of the recent literature. *Europace.* 2011;**13**:1375–85
24. van Diepen S, *et al.* Mortality and readmission of patients with heart failure, atrial fibrillation, or coronary artery disease undergoing noncardiac surgery: an analysis of 38 047 patients. *Circulation.* 2011;**124**:289–96
25. Rosenberg MA, *et al.* Diastolic dysfunction and risk of atrial fibrillation: a mechanistic appraisal. *Circulation.* 2012;**126**:2353–62
26. Alonso A, *et al.* Chronic kidney disease is associated with the incidence of atrial fibrillation: the Atherosclerosis Risk in Communities (ARIC) study. *Circulation.* 2011;**123**:2946–53
27. Tanner RM, *et al.* Association of the metabolic syndrome with atrial fibrillation among United States adults (from the REasons for Geographic and Racial Differences in Stroke [REGARDS] Study). *Am J Cardiol.* 2011;**108**:227–32
28. Kodama S, *et al.* Alcohol consumption and risk of atrial fibrillation: a meta-analysis. *J Am Coll Cardiol.* 2011;**57**:427–36
29. Humenberger M, *et al.* Benefit of atrial septal defect closure in adults: impact of age. *Eur Heart J.* 2011;**32**:553–60
30. Silversides CK, *et al.* Predictors of atrial arrhythmias after device closure of secundum type atrial septal defects in adults. *Am J Cardiol.* 2008;**101**:683–7
31. Spies C, *et al.* Incidence of atrial fibrillation following transcatheter closure of atrial septal defects in adults. *Am J Cardiol.* 2008;**102**:902–6
32. Guglin M, *et al.* Introducing a new entity: chemotherapy-induced arrhythmia. *Europace.* 2009;**11**:1579–86
33. Fox CS, *et al.* Parental atrial fibrillation as a risk factor for atrial fibrillation in offspring. *JAMA.* 2004;**291**:2851–5
34. Oyen N, *et al.* Familial aggregation of lone atrial fibrillation in young persons. *J Am Coll Cardiol.* 2012;**60**:917–21
35. Ackerman MJ, *et al.* HRS/EHRA expert consensus statement on the state of genetic testing for the channelopathies and cardiomyopathies: this document was developed as a partnership between the Heart Rhythm Society (HRS) and the European Heart Rhythm Association (EHRA). *Europace.* 2011;**13**:1077–109
36. Ellinor PT, *et al.* Meta-analysis identifies six new susceptibility loci for atrial fibrillation. *Nat Genet.* 2012;**44**:670–5
37. Judge DP. The complex genetics of atrial fibrillation. *J Am Coll Cardiol.* 2012;**60**:1182–4
38. Ritchie MD DJ, *et al.* Genome- and phenome-wide analysis of cardiac conduction identifies markers of arrhythmia risk. *Circulation.* 2013 Mar 2015; [Epub ahead of print]
39. Parvez B, *et al.* Symptomatic response to antiarrhythmic drug therapy is modulated by a common single nucleotide polymorphism in atrial fibrillation. *J Am Coll Cardiol.* 2012;**60**:539–45
40. Estes NA, 3rd, *et al.* American Heart Association atrial fibrillation research summit: a conference report from the American Heart Association. *Circulation.* 2011; **124**:363–72
41. Ahlehoff O, *et al.* Psoriasis and risk of atrial fibrillation and ischaemic stroke: a Danish Nationwide Cohort Study. *Eur Heart J.* 2012;**33**:2054–64
42. Mozaffarian D, *et al.* Physical activity and incidence of atrial fibrillation in older adults: The cardiovascular health study. *Circulation.* 2008;**118**:800–7
43. Aizer A, *et al.* Relation of vigorous exercise to risk of atrial fibrillation. *Am J Cardiol.* 2009;**103**:1572–7
44. Khan AM, *et al.* Low serum magnesium and the development of atrial fibrillation in the community: the Framingham Heart Study. *Circulation.* 2013;**127**:33–8
45. Wakili R, *et al.* Recent advances in the molecular pathophysiology of atrial fibrillation. *J Clin Invest.* 2011;**121**:2955–68
46. Allessie M, *et al.* Electrical, contractile and structural remodelling during atrial fibrillation. *Cardiovasc Res.* 2002;**54**:230–46
47. Kato T, *et al.* Connexins and atrial fibrillation: filling in the gaps. *Circulation.* 2012;**125**:203–6
48. Frustaci A, *et al.* Histological substrate of atrial biopsies in patients with lone atrial fibrillation. *Circulation.* 1997;**96**:1180–4
49. Wijffels MC, *et al.* Atrial fibrillation begets atrial fibrillation. A study in awake chronically instrumented goats. *Circulation.* 1995;**92**:1954–68
50. Platonov PG, *et al.* Low atrial fibrillatory rate is associated with poor outcome in patients with mild to moderate heart failure. *Circ Arrhythm Electrophysiol.* 2012;**5**:77–83

51. Haissaguerre M, *et al.* Spontaneous initiation of atrial fibrillation by ectopic beats originating in the pulmonary veins. *N Engl J Med.* 1998;**339**:659–66
52. Kumagai K, *et al.* Electrophysiologic properties of pulmonary veins assessed using a multielectrode basket catheter. *J Am Coll Cardiol.* 2004;**43**:2281–9
53. Katritsis D, *et al.* Catheter ablation of atrial fibrillation the search for substrate-driven end points. *J Am Coll Cardiol.* 2010;**55**:2293–8
54. Mandapati R, *et al.* Stable microreentrant sources as a mechanism of atrial fibrillation in the isolated sheep heart. *Circulation.* 2000;**101**:194–9
55. Calkins H, *et al.* 2012 HRS/EHRA/ECAS Expert Consensus Statement on Catheter and Surgical Ablation of Atrial Fibrillation: recommendations for patient selection, procedural techniques, patient management and follow-up, definitions, endpoints, and research trial design. *Europace.* 2012;**14**:528–606
56. Katritsis D, *et al.* Identification and catheter ablation of extracardiac and intracardiac components of ligament of marshall tissue for treatment of paroxysmal atrial fibrillation. *J Cardiovasc Electrophysiol.* 2001;**12**:750–8
57. Armour JA, *et al.* Gross and microscopic anatomy of the human intrinsic cardiac nervous system. *Anat Rec.* 1997;**247**:289–98
58. Pappone C, *et al.* Pulmonary vein denervation enhances long-term benefit after circumferential ablation for paroxysmal atrial fibrillation. *Circulation.* 2004;**109**:327–34
59. Grogan M, *et al.* Left ventricular dysfunction due to atrial fibrillation in patients initially believed to have idiopathic dilated cardiomyopathy. *Am J Cardiol.* 1992;**69**:1570–3
60. Gertz ZM, *et al.* Evidence of atrial functional mitral regurgitation due to atrial fibrillation: reversal with arrhythmia control. *J Am Coll Cardiol.* 2011;**58**:1474–81
61. Di Biase L, *et al.* Does the left atrial appendage morphology correlate with the risk of stroke in patients with atrial fibrillation? Results from a multicentre study. *J Am Coll Cardiol.* 2012;**60**:531–8
62. Friberg L, *et al.* Evaluation of risk stratification schemes for ischaemic stroke and bleeding in 182 678 patients with atrial fibrillation: the Swedish Atrial Fibrillation cohort study. *Eur Heart J.* 2012;**33**:1500–10
63. Healey JS, *et al.* Periprocedural bleeding and thromboembolic events with dabigatran compared with warfarin: results from the Randomized Evaluation of Long-Term Anticoagulation Therapy (RE-LY) randomized trial. *Circulation.* 2012;**126**:343–8
64. Mittal S, *et al.* Ambulatory external electrocardiographic monitoring: focus on atrial fibrillation. *J Am Coll Cardiol.* 2011;**58**:1741–9
65. Hughes M, *et al.* Stroke and thromboembolism in atrial fibrillation: a systematic review of stroke risk factors, risk stratification schema and cost effectiveness data. *Thromb Haemost.* 2008;**99**:295–304
66. Stroke risk in atrial fibrillation working group. Independent predictors of stroke in patients with atrial fibrillation: a systematic review. *Neurology.* 2007;**69**:546–54
67. Gage BF, *et al.* Validation of clinical classification schemes for predicting stroke: results from the National Registry of Atrial Fibrillation. *JAMA.* 2001;**285**:2864–70
68. Lip GY, *et al.* Refining clinical risk stratification for predicting stroke and thromboembolism in atrial fibrillation using a novel risk factor-based approach: the euro heart survey on atrial fibrillation. *Chest.* 2010;**137**:263–72
69. Hijazi Z, *et al.* NT-PROBNP for risk assessment in patients with atrial fibrillation: Insights from the aristotle trial. *J Am Coll Cardiol.* 2013; doi:10.1016/j.jacc.2012.1011.1082
70. Kirchhof P, *et al.* Anterior-posterior versus anterior-lateral electrode positions for external cardioversion of atrial fibrillation: a randomised trial. *Lancet.* 2002;**360**:1275–9
71. Alboni P, *et al.* Outpatient treatment of recent-onset atrial fibrillation with the 'pill-in-the-pocket' approach. *N Engl J Med.* 2004;**351**:2384–91
72. Murray KT. Ibutilide. *Circulation.* 1998;**97**:493–7
73. Fragakis N, *et al.* Acute beta-adrenoceptor blockade improves efficacy of ibutilide in conversion of atrial fibrillation with a rapid ventricular rate. *Europace.* 2009;**11**:70–4
74. Singh S, *et al.* Efficacy and safety of oral dofetilide in converting to and maintaining sinus rhythm in patients with chronic atrial fibrillation or atrial flutter: the symptomatic atrial fibrillation investigative research on dofetilide (SAFIRE-D) study. *Circulation.* 2000;**102**:2385–90
75. Camm AJ, *et al.* A randomized active-controlled study comparing the efficacy and safety of vernakalant to amiodarone in recent-onset atrial fibrillation. *J Am Coll Cardiol.* 2011;**57**:313–21
76. Wyse DG, *et al.* A comparison of rate control and rhythm control in patients with atrial fibrillation. *N Engl J Med.* 2002;**347**:1825–33
77. Hohnloser SH, *et al.* Rhythm or rate control in atrial fibrillation – Pharmacological Intervention in Atrial Fibrillation (PIAF): a randomised trial. *Lancet.* 2000;**356**:1789–94
78. Carlsson J, *et al.* Randomized trial of rate-control versus rhythm-control in persistent atrial fibrillation: the Strategies of Treatment of Atrial Fibrillation (STAF) study. *J Am Coll Cardiol.* 2003;**41**:1690–6
79. Van Gelder IC, *et al.* A comparison of rate control and rhythm control in patients with recurrent persistent atrial fibrillation. *N Engl J Med.* 2002;**347**:1834–40
80. Ogawa S, *et al.* Optimal treatment strategy for patients with paroxysmal atrial fibrillation: J-RHYTHM Study. *Circ J.* 2009;**73**:242–8
81. Opolski G, *et al.* Rate control vs rhythm control in patients with nonvalvular persistent atrial fibrillation: the results of the Polish How to Treat Chronic Atrial Fibrillation (HOT CAFE) Study. *Chest.* 2004;**126**:476–86
82. Roy D, *et al.* Rhythm control versus rate control for atrial fibrillation and heart failure. *N Engl J Med.* 2008;**358**:2667–77
83. Corley SD, *et al.* Relationships between sinus rhythm, treatment, and survival in the Atrial Fibrillation Follow-Up Investigation of Rhythm Management (AFFIRM) Study. *Circulation.* 2004;**109**:1509–13
84. Lafuente-Lafuente C, *et al.* Antiarrhythmic drugs for maintaining sinus rhythm after cardioversion of atrial fibrillation: a systematic review of randomized controlled trials. *Arch Intern Med.* 2006;**166**:719–28
85. Singh BN, *et al.* Amiodarone versus sotalol for atrial fibrillation. *N Engl J Med.* 2005;**352**:1861–72.

86. Curtis AB, *et al.* Clinical factors that influence response to treatment strategies in atrial fibrillation: the Atrial Fibrillation Follow-up Investigation of Rhythm Management (AFFIRM) study. *Am Heart J.* 2005;**149**:645–9
87. Deedwania PC, *et al.* Spontaneous conversion and maintenance of sinus rhythm by amiodarone in patients with heart failure and atrial fibrillation: observations from the veterans affairs congestive heart failure survival trial of antiarrhythmic therapy (CHF-STAT). The Department of Veterans Affairs CHF-STAT Investigators. *Circulation.* 1998;**98**:2574–9
88. Pedersen OD, *et al.* Does conversion and prevention of atrial fibrillation enhance survival in patients with left ventricular dysfunction? Evidence from the Danish Investigations of Arrhythmia and Mortality ON Dofetilide/(DIAMOND) study. *Card Electrophysiol Rev.* 2003;**7**:220–4
89. Tsadok MA, *et al.* Rhythm versus rate control therapy and subsequent stroke or transient ischaemic attack in patients with atrial fibrillation. *Circulation.* 2012;**126**:2680–7
90. Hohnloser SH, *et al.* Effect of dronedarone on cardiovascular events in atrial fibrillation. *N Engl J Med.* 2009;**360**:668–78
91. Kober L, *et al.* Increased mortality after dronedarone therapy for severe heart failure. *N Engl J Med.* 2008;**358**:2678–87
92. Mathew JP, *et al.* A multicentre risk index for atrial fibrillation after cardiac surgery. *JAMA.* 2004;**291**:1720–9
93. Whitbeck MG, *et al.* Increased mortality among patients taking digoxin—analysis from the affirm study. *Eur Heart J.* 2013;**34**:1481–88
94. Gheorghiade M, *et al.* Lack of evidence of increased mortality among patients with atrial fibrillation taking digoxin: Findings from post hoc propensity-matched analysis of the affirm trial. *Eur Heart J.* 2013;**34**:1489–97
95. Van Gelder IC, *et al.* Lenient versus strict rate control in patients with atrial fibrillation. *N Engl J Med.* 2010;**362**:1363–73
96. Chatterjee NA, *et al.* Atrioventricular nodal ablation in atrial fibrillation: a meta-analysis and systematic review. *Circ Arrhythm Electrophysiol.* 2012;**5**:68–76
97. Ganesan AN, *et al.* Role of AV nodal ablation in cardiac resynchronization in patients with coexistent atrial fibrillation and heart failure a systematic review. *J Am Coll Cardiol.* 2012;**59**:719–26
98. Brignole M, *et al.* Cardiac resynchronization therapy in patients undergoing atrioventricular junction ablation for permanent atrial fibrillation: a randomized trial. *Eur Heart J.* 2011;**32**:2420–9
99. Freemantle N, *et al.* Mixed treatment comparison of dronedarone, amiodarone, sotalol, flecainide, and propafenone, for the management of atrial fibrillation. *Europace.* 2011;**13**:329–45
100. Roy D, *et al.* Amiodarone to prevent recurrence of atrial fibrillation. Canadian trial of atrial fibrillation investigators. *N Engl J Med.* 2000;**342**:913–20
101. Singh BN, *et al.* Dronedarone for maintenance of sinus rhythm in atrial fibrillation or flutter. *N Engl J Med.* 2007;**357**:987–99
102 Connolly SJ, *et al.* Dronedarone in high-risk permanent atrial fibrillation. *N Engl J Med.* 2011;**365**:2268–76
103. Gillis AM, *et al.* Canadian cardiovascular society atrial fibrillation guidelines 2010: rate and rhythm management. *Can J Cardiol.* 2011;**27**:47–59
104. Southworth MR, *et al.* Comparison of sotalol versus quinidine for maintenance of normal sinus rhythm in patients with chronic atrial fibrillation. *Am J Cardiol.* 1999;**83**:1629–32
105. Andersen SS, *et al.* Antiarrhythmic therapy and risk of death in patients with atrial fibrillation: a nationwide study. *Europace.* 2009;**11**:886–91
106. Myerburg RJ, *et al.* Reversal of proarrhythmic effects of flecainide acetate and encainide hydrochloride by propranolol. *Circulation.* 1989;**80**:1571–9
107. Heidbuchel H, *et al.* Recommendations for participation in leisure-time physical activity and competitive sports of patients with arrhythmias and potentially arrhythmogenic conditions. Part II: ventricular arrhythmias, channelopathies and implantable defibrillators. *Eur J Cardiovasc Prev Rehabil.* 2006;**13**:676–86
108. Kirchhof P, *et al.* Short-term versus long-term antiarrhythmic drug treatment after cardioversion of atrial fibrillation (Flec-SL): a prospective, randomised, open-label, blinded endpoint assessment trial. *Lancet.* 2012;**380**:238–46
109. Pedersen OD, *et al.* Efficacy of dofetilide in the treatment of atrial fibrillation-flutter in patients with reduced left ventricular function: A Danish investigations of arrhythmia and mortality on dofetilide (diamond) substudy. *Circulation.* 2001;**104**:292–6
110. Scirica BM, *et al.* Effect of ranolazine, an antianginal agent with novel electrophysiological properties, on the incidence of arrhythmias in patients with non ST-segment elevation acute coronary syndrome: results from the Metabolic Efficiency With Ranolazine for Less Ischemia in Non ST-Elevation Acute Coronary Syndrome Thrombolysis in Myocardial Infarction 36 (MERLIN-TIMI 36) randomized controlled trial. *Circulation.* 2007;**116**:1647–52
111. Zimetbaum P. Antiarrhythmic drug therapy for atrial fibrillation. *Circulation.* 2012;**125**:381–9
112. Hart RG, *et al.* Meta-analysis: Antithrombotic therapy to prevent stroke in patients who have non-valvular atrial fibrillation. *Ann Intern Med.* 2007;**146**:857–67
113. Lip GY, *et al.* Comparative validation of a novel risk score for predicting bleeding risk in anticoagulated patients with atrial fibrillation: the HAS-BLED (Hypertension, Abnormal Renal/Liver Function, Stroke, Bleeding History or Predisposition, Labile INR, Elderly, Drugs/Alcohol Concomitantly) score. *J Am Coll Cardiol.* 2011;**57**:173–80
114. De Caterina R, *et al.* New oral anticoagulants in atrial fibrillation and acute coronary syndromes: ESC Working Group on Thrombosis-Task Force on Anticoagulants in Heart Disease position paper. *J Am Coll Cardiol.* 2012;**59**:1413–25
115. Dentali F, *et al.* Efficacy and safety of the novel oral anticoagulants in atrial fibrillation: a systematic review and meta-analysis of the literature. *Circulation.* 2012;**126**:2381–91
116. Granger CB, *et al.* Newer oral anticoagulants should be used as first-line agents to prevent thromboembolism in patients with atrial fibrillation and risk factors for stroke or thromboembolism. *Circulation.* 2012;**125**:159–64; discussion 164
117. Connolly S, *et al.* Clopidogrel plus aspirin versus oral anticoagulation for atrial fibrillation in the Atrial fibrillation Clopidogrel Trial with Irbesartan for prevention of Vascular Events (ACTIVE W): a randomised controlled trial. *Lancet.* 2006;**367**:1903–12

118. Mant J, *et al.* Warfarin versus aspirin for stroke prevention in an elderly community population with atrial fibrillation (the Birmingham Atrial Fibrillation Treatment of the Aged Study, BAFTA): a randomised controlled trial. *Lancet.* 2007;**370**:493–503
119. Weijs B, *et al.* Patients using vitamin K antagonists show increased levels of coronary calcification: an observational study in low-risk atrial fibrillation patients. *Eur Heart J.* 2011;**32**:2555–62
120. Miller CS, *et al.* Meta-analysis of efficacy and safety of new oral anticoagulants (dabigatran, rivaroxaban, apixaban) versus warfarin in patients with atrial fibrillation. *Am J Cardiol.* 2012;**110**:453–60
121. Siegal DM, *et al.* Acute management of bleeding in patients on novel oral anticoagulants. *Eur Heart J.* 2013; **34**:489–98
122. Heidbuchel H, *et al.* Ehra practical guide on the use of new oral anticoagulants in patients with non-valvular atrial fibrillation: Executive summary. *Eur Heart J.* 2013; doi: 10.1093/eurheartj/eht1134
123. Connolly SJ, *et al.* Dabigatran versus warfarin in patients with atrial fibrillation. *N Engl J Med.* 2009;**361**:1139–51
124. Connolly SJ, *et al.* The long-term multicenter observational study of dabigatran treatment in patients with atrial fibrillation (RELY-ABLE) study. *Circulation.* 2013;**128**:237–43
125. Ezekowitz MD, *et al.* Dabigatran with or without concomitant aspirin compared with warfarin alone in patients with non-valvular atrial fibrillation (PETRO Study). *Am J Cardiol.* 2007;**100**:1419–26
126. Hohnloser SH, *et al.* Myocardial ischemic events in patients with atrial fibrillation treated with dabigatran or warfarin in the RE-LY (Randomized Evaluation of Long-Term Anticoagulation Therapy) trial. *Circulation.* 2012;**125**:669–76
127. Uchino K, *et al.* Dabigatran association with higher risk of acute coronary events: meta-analysis of noninferiority randomized controlled trials. *Arch Intern Med.* 2012;**172**: 397–402
128. Schulman S, *et al.* Extended use of dabigatran, warfarin, or placebo in venous thromboembolism. *N Engl J Med.* 2013;**368**:709–18
129. Larsen TB, *et al.* Efficacy and safety of dabigatran etexilate and warfarin in 'real world' patients with atrial fibrillation: A prospective nationwide cohort study. *J Am Coll Cardiol.* 2013; doi: 10.1016/j.jacc.2013.1003.1020
130. Independent predictors of stroke in patients with atrial fibrillation: A systematic review. *Neurology.* 2007; **69**:546–54
131. Weitz JI, *et al.* Periprocedural management and approach to bleeding in patients taking dabigatran. *Circulation.* 2012;**126**:2428–32
132. van Ryn J, *et al.* Dabigatran etexilate—a novel, reversible, oral direct thrombin inhibitor: interpretation of coagulation assays and reversal of anticoagulant activity. *Thromb Haemost.* 2010;**103**:1116–27
133. Marlu R, *et al.* Effect of non-specific reversal agents on anticoagulant activity of dabigatran and rivaroxaban: a randomised crossover ex vivo study in healthy volunteers. *Thromb Haemost.* 2012;**108**:217–24
134. Connolly SJ, *et al.* Apixaban in patients with atrial fibrillation. *N Engl J Med.* 2011;**364**:806–17
135. Granger CB, *et al.* Apixaban versus warfarin in patients with atrial fibrillation. *N Engl J Med.* 2011;**365**:981–92
136. Al-Khatib SM, *et al.* Outcomes of apixaban vs. warfarin by type and duration of atrial fibrillation: Results from the aristotle trial. *Eur Heart J.* 2013; [Epub ahead of print]
137. Hohnloser SH, *et al.* Efficacy of apixaban when compared with warfarin in relation to renal function in patients with atrial fibrillation: insights from the ARISTOTLE trial. *Eur Heart J.* 2012;**33**:2821–30
138. Patel MR, *et al.* Rivaroxaban versus warfarin in non-valvular atrial fibrillation. *N Engl J Med.* 2011;**365**:883–91
139. Eerenberg ES, *et al.* Reversal of rivaroxaban and dabigatran by prothrombin complex concentrate: a randomized, placebo-controlled, crossover study in healthy subjects. *Circulation.* 2011;**124**:1573–9
140. Weitz JI, *et al.* Randomised, parallel-group, multicentre, multinational phase 2 study comparing edoxaban, an oral factor Xa inhibitor, with warfarin for stroke prevention in patients with atrial fibrillation. *Thromb Haemost.* 2010;**104**:633–41
141. Connolly SJ, *et al.* Betrixaban compared with warfarin in patients with atrial fibrillation: Results of a phase 2, randomized, dose-ranging study (EXPLORE-XA). *Eur Heart J.* 2013 Mar 13; [Epub ahead of print]
142. Lip GY, *et al.* Antithrombotic management of atrial fibrillation patients presenting with acute coronary syndrome and/or undergoing coronary stenting: executive summary – a Consensus Document of the European Society of Cardiology Working Group on Thrombosis, endorsed by the European Heart Rhythm Association (EHRA) and the European Association of Percutaneous Cardiovascular Interventions (EAPCI). *Eur Heart J.* 2010;**31**:1311–18
143. Lamberts M, *et al.* Bleeding after initiation of multiple antithrombotic drugs, including triple therapy, in atrial fibrillation patients following myocardial infarction and coronary intervention: a nationwide cohort study. *Circulation.* 2012;**126**:1185–93
144. Dewilde WJ, *et al.* Use of clopidogrel with or without aspirin in patients taking oral anticoagulant therapy and undergoing percutaneous coronary intervention: An open-label, randomised, controlled trial. *Lancet.* 2013;**381**:1107–15
145. Lamberts M, *et al.* Oral anticoagulation and antiplatelets in atrial fibrillation patients after myocardial infarction and coronary intervention. *J Am Coll Cardiol.* 2013; [Epub ahead of print]
146. Komocsi A, *et al.* Use of new-generation oral anticoagulant agents in patients receiving antiplatelet therapy after an acute coronary syndrome: systematic review and meta-analysis of randomized controlled trials. *Arch Intern Med.* 2012;**172**:1537–45
147. Dans AL, *et al.* Concomitant use of antiplatelet therapy with dabigatran or warfarin in the randomized evaluation of long-term anticoagulation therapy (RE-LY) trial. *Circulation.* 2013;**127**:634–40
148. Di Biase L, *et al.* Periprocedural stroke and management of major bleeding complications in patients undergoing catheter ablation of atrial fibrillation: the impact of periprocedural therapeutic international normalized ratio. *Circulation.* 2010;**121**:2550–6

149. Siegal D, *et al.* Periprocedural heparin bridging in patients receiving vitamin K antagonists: systematic review and meta-analysis of bleeding and thromboembolic rates. *Circulation.* 2012;**126**:1630–9
150. Sie P, *et al.* Surgery and invasive procedures in patients on long-term treatment with direct oral anticoagulants: thrombin or factor-Xa inhibitors. Recommendations of the Working Group on Perioperative Haemostasis and the French Study Group on Thrombosis and Haemostasis. *Arch Cardiovasc Dis.* 2011;**104**:669–76
151. Wysokinski WE, *et al.* Periprocedural bridging management of anticoagulation. *Circulation.* 2012;**126**:486–90
152. Patel MR, *et al.* Outcomes of discontinuing rivaroxaban compared with warfarin in patients with nonvalvular atrial fibrillation: analysis from the ROCKET AF trial (Rivaroxaban nce-daily, Oral, direct factor Xa inhibition Compared with Vitamin K antagonism for prevention of stroke and Embolism Trial in atrial fibrillation). *J Am Coll Cardiol.* 2013;**61**:651–8
153. Jauch EC, *et al.* Guidelines for the early management of patients with acute ischemic stroke: A Stroke Association guideline for healthcare professionals from the American Heart Association. *Lancet.* 2013; doi: 10.1161/STR.1160b1013e318284056a
154. Rothwell PM, *et al.* Medical treatment in acute and long-term secondary prevention after transient ischaemic attack and ischaemic stroke. *Lancet.* 2011;**377**:1681–92
155. Wechsler LR. Intravenous thrombolytic therapy for acute ischaemic stroke. *N Engl J Med.* 2011;**364**:2138–46
156. Parsons M, *et al.* A randomized trial of tenecteplase versus alteplase for acute ischaemic stroke. *N Engl J Med.* 2012;**366**:1099–107
157. Guidelines for the prevention of stroke in patients with stroke or transient ischemic attack. *Stroke.* 2011;**42**:227–76
158. Guidelines for the early management of patients with acute ischaemic stroke: A guideline for healthcare professionals from the American Heart Association/American Stroke Association. *Stroke.* 2013;**44**:870–947
159. Noheria A, *et al.* Catheter ablation vs antiarrhythmic drug therapy for atrial fibrillation: a systematic review. *Arch Intern Med.* 2008;168:581–6
160. Cosedis Nielsen J, *et al.* Radiofrequency ablation as initial therapy in paroxysmal atrial fibrillation. *N Engl J Med.* 2012;**367**:1587–95
161. Khan MN, *et al.* Pulmonary-vein isolation for atrial fibrillation in patients with heart failure. *N Engl J Med.* 2008;**359**:1778–85
162. Ouyang F, *et al.* Long-term results of catheter ablation in paroxysmal atrial fibrillation: lessons from a 5-year follow-up. *Circulation.* 2010;**122**:2368–77
163. Weerasooriya R, *et al.* Catheter ablation for atrial fibrillation: are results maintained at 5 years of follow-up? *J Am Coll Cardiol.* 2011;**57**:160–6
164. Elayi CS, *et al.* Atrial fibrillation termination as a procedural endpoint during ablation in long-standing persistent atrial fibrillation. *Heart Rhythm.* 2010;**7**:1216–23
165. O'Neill MD, *et al.* Long-term follow-up of persistent atrial fibrillation ablation using termination as a procedural endpoint. *Eur Heart J.* 2009;**30**:1105–12
166. Dixit S, *et al.* Randomized ablation strategies for the treatment of persistent atrial fibrillation: RASTA study. *Circ Arrhythm Electrophysiol.* 2012;**5**:287–94
167. Katritsis DG, *et al.* Rapid pulmonary vein isolation combined with autonomic ganglia modification: a randomized study. *Heart Rhythm.* 2011;**8**:672–8
168. Nademanee K, *et al.* A new approach for catheter ablation of atrial fibrillation: mapping of the electrophysiologic substrate. *J Am Coll Cardiol.* 2004;**43**:2044–53
169. Bohnen M, *et al.* Incidence and predictors of major complications from contemporary catheter ablation to treat cardiac arrhythmias. *Heart Rhythm.* 2011;**8**:1661–6
170. Cappato R, *et al.* Prevalence and causes of fatal outcome in catheter ablation of atrial fibrillation. *J Am Coll Cardiol.* 2009;**53**:1798–803
171. Cappato R, *et al.* Updated worldwide survey on the methods, efficacy, and safety of catheter ablation for human atrial fibrillation. *Circ Arrhythm Electrophysiol.* 2010;**3**:32–8
172. Medi C, *et al.* Subtle post-procedural cognitive dysfunction following atrial fibrillation ablation. *J Am Coll Cardiol.* 2013 May 15. doi:pii: S0735-1097(13)01882-2. 10.1016/j.jacc.2013.03.073.
173. Hoyt H, *et al.* Complications arising from catheter ablation of atrial fibrillation: temporal trends and predictors. *Heart Rhythm.* 2011;**8**:1869–74
174. Martinek M, *et al.* Identification of a high-risk population for esophageal injury during radiofrequency catheter ablation of atrial fibrillation: procedural and anatomical considerations. *Heart Rhythm.* 2010;**7**:1224–30
175. Lakkireddy D, *et al.* Feasibility and safety of dabigatran versus warfarin for periprocedural anticoagulation in patients undergoing radiofrequency ablation for atrial fibrillation: results from a multicentre prospective registry. *J Am Coll Cardiol.* 2012;**59**:1168–74
176. Winkle RA, *et al.* The use of dabigatran immediately after atrial fibrillation ablation. *J Cardiovasc Electrophysiol.* 2012;**23**:264–8
177. Katritsis D, *et al.* Atrial arrhythmias following ostial or circumferential pulmonary vein ablation. *J Interv Card Electrophysiol.* 2006;**16**:123–30
178. Wasmer K, *et al.* Incidence, characteristics, and outcome of left atrial tachycardias after circumferential antral ablation of atrial fibrillation. *Heart Rhythm.* 2012;**9**:1660–6
179. Boersma LV, *et al.* Atrial fibrillation catheter ablation versus surgical ablation treatment (FAST): a 2-centre randomized clinical trial. *Circulation.* 2012;**125**:23–30
180. Fragakis N, *et al.* Surgical ablation for atrial fibrillation. *Europace.* 2012;**14**:1545–52
181. Budera P, *et al.* Comparison of cardiac surgery with left atrial surgical ablation vs. Cardiac surgery without atrial ablation in patients with coronary and/or valvular heart disease plus atrial fibrillation: final results of the PRAGUE-12 randomized multicentre study. *Eur Heart J.* 2012;**33**:2644–52
182. Reddy VY, *et al.* Percutaneous left atrial appendage closure for stroke prophylaxis in patients with atrial fibrillation: 2.3-year follow-up of the PROTECT AF (Watchman left atrial appendage system for embolic PROTECTion in patients with Atrial Fibrillation) trial. *Circulation.* 2013;720–9

183. Knight BP, *et al.* Role of permanent pacing to prevent atrial fibrillation: science advisory from the American Heart Association Council on Clinical Cardiology (Subcommittee on Electrocardiography and Arrhythmias) and the Quality of Care and Outcomes Research Interdisciplinary Working Group, in collaboration with the Heart Rhythm Society. *Circulation.* 2005;**111**:240–3
184. Carlson MD, *et al.* A new pacemaker algorithm for the treatment of atrial fibrillation: results of the Atrial Dynamic Overdrive Pacing Trial (ADOPT). *J Am Coll Cardiol.* 2003;**42**:627–33
185. Padeletti L, *et al.* Combined efficacy of atrial septal lead placement and atrial pacing algorithms for prevention of paroxysmal atrial tachyarrhythmia. *J Cardiovasc Electrophysiol.* 2003;**14**:1189–95
186. Savelieva I, *et al.* Upstream therapies for management of atrial fibrillation: review of clinical evidence and implications for European Society of Cardiology guidelines. Part I: primary prevention. *Europace.* 2011;**13**:308–28
187. Zografos T, *et al.* Inhibition of the renin-angiotensin system for prevention of atrial fibrillation. *Pacing Clin Electrophysiol.* 2010;**33**:1270–85
188. Disertori M, *et al.* Valsartan for prevention of recurrent atrial fibrillation. *N Engl J Med.* 2009;**360**:1606–17
189. Yusuf S, *et al.* Irbesartan in patients with atrial fibrillation. *N Engl J Med.* 2011;**364**:928–38
190. Kowey PR, *et al.* Efficacy and safety of prescription omega-3 fatty acids for the prevention of recurrent symptomatic atrial fibrillation: a randomized controlled trial. *JAMA.* 2010;**304**:2363–72
191. Rahimi K, *et al.* Effect of statins on atrial fibrillation: collaborative meta-analysis of published and unpublished evidence from randomised controlled trials. *BMJ.* 2011;**342**:d1250
192. Bradley D, *et al.* Pharmacologic prophylaxis: American College of Chest Physicians guidelines for the prevention and management of postoperative atrial fibrillation after cardiac surgery. *Chest.* 2005;**128**:39S–47S
193. Burgess DC, *et al.* Interventions for prevention of postoperative atrial fibrillation and its complications after cardiac surgery: a meta-analysis. *Eur Heart J.* 2006;**27**: 2846–57
194. Bagshaw SM, *et al.* Prophylactic amiodarone for prevention of atrial fibrillation after cardiac surgery: a meta-analysis. *Ann Thorac Surg.* 2006;**82**:1927–37
195. Ho KM, *et al.* Benefits and risks of corticosteroid prophylaxis in adult cardiac surgery: a dose-response meta-analysis. *Circulation.* 2009;**119**:1853–66
196. Miller S, *et al.* Effects of magnesium on atrial fibrillation after cardiac surgery: a meta-analysis. *Heart.* 2005;**91**:618–23
197. Imazio M, *et al.* Colchicine reduces postoperative atrial fibrillation: results of the Colchicine for the Prevention of the Postpericardiotomy Syndrome (COPPS) atrial fibrillation substudy. *Circulation.* 2011;**124**:2290–5
198. Bhave PD, *et al.* Statin use and post-operative atrial fibrillation after major noncardiac surgery. *Heart Rhythm.* 2012;**9**:163–9
199. Archbold RA, *et al.* Atrial pacing for the prevention of atrial fibrillation after coronary artery bypass graft surgery: a review of the literature. *Heart.* 2004;**90**:129–33
200. Schmitt J, *et al.* Atrial fibrillation in acute myocardial infarction: a systematic review of the incidence, clinical features and prognostic implications. *Eur Heart J.* 2009;**30**:1038–45
201. Jabre P, *et al.* Atrial fibrillation and death after myocardial infarction: a community study. *Circulation.* 2011;**123**:2094–100
202. Darby AE, *et al.* Management of atrial fibrillation in patients with structural heart disease. *Circulation.* 2012;**125**:945–57
203. Nasr IA, *et al.* Prevention of atrial fibrillation onset by beta-blocker treatment in heart failure: a meta-analysis. *Eur Heart J.* 2007;**28**:457–62
204. Jones DG, *et al.* A randomized trial to assess catheter ablation versus rate control in the management of persistent atrial fibrillation in heart failure (ARC-HF). *J Am Coll Cardiol.* 2013; doi: 10.1016/j.jacc.2013.1001.1069
205. Goldschlager N, *et al.* A practical guide for clinicians who treat patients with amiodarone: 2007. *Heart Rhythm.* 2007;**4**:1250–9
206. Olivotto I, *et al.* Impact of atrial fibrillation on the clinical course of hypertrophic cardiomyopathy. *Circulation.* 2001;**104**:2517–24
207. Di Donna P, *et al.* Efficacy of catheter ablation for atrial fibrillation in hypertrophic cardiomyopathy: impact of age, atrial remodelling, and disease progression. *Europace.* 2010;**12**:347–55
208. Hawkins NM, *et al.* Heart failure and chronic obstructive pulmonary disease the quandary of beta-blockers and beta-agonists. *J Am Coll Cardiol.* 2011;**57**:2127–38
209. Magee LA, *et al.* Risks and benefits of beta-receptor blockers for pregnancy hypertension: overview of the randomized trials. *Eur J Obstet Gynecol Reprod Biol.* 2000;**88**:15–26
210. Kockova R, *et al.* Ibutilide-induced cardioversion of atrial fibrillation during pregnancy. *J Cardiovasc Electrophysiol.* 2007;**18**:545–7
211. Regitz-Zagrosek V, *et al.* ESC Guidelines on the management of cardiovascular diseases during pregnancy: the Task Force on the Management of Cardiovascular Diseases during Pregnancy of the European Society of Cardiology (ESC). *Eur Heart J.* 2011;**32**:3147–97

Chapter 53

Atrioventricular junctional tachycardias

Atrioventricular nodal reentrant tachycardia

Definition

Atrioventricular nodal reentrant tachycardia (AVNRT) denotes reentry in the area of the AV node. Several models have been proposed to explain the mechanism of the arrhythmia in the context of the complex anatomy of the AV node and its atrial extension.[1,2]

Epidemiology

AVNRT represents the most common regular supraventricular arrhythmia in the human.[3] The arrhythmia is more prevalent in women.

Pathophysiology

The concept of dual AV nodal pathways as the substrate for AVNRT dates from 1956 when Moe and colleagues demonstrated evidence of a dual AV conduction system in dogs. It was postulated that a dual conduction system was present, one having a faster conduction time and longer refractory period (fast pathway), the other having a slower conduction time and shorter refractory period (slow pathway) (Figure 53.1). At a critical coupling interval, the premature impulse blocks in the faster pathway and conducts in the, still excitable, slow pathway, causing a sudden jump in the AV conduction time. Following that, the impulse returns to the atria, supposedly via the fast pathway which has then recovered, and an atrial echo beat or sustained tachycardia results (Figure 53.2).[1] Denes and colleagues, in 1973, ascribed episodes of paroxysmal supraventricular tachycardia to AV node reentry due to the presence of dual atrioventricular nodal pathways and, using His bundle recordings and the atrial extrastimulus method, demonstrated sudden prolongation of the AH interval in a patient with dual atrioventricular nodal pathways (so-called atrioventricular conduction jumps).[1] In approximately 5% of patients with AV nodal reentry, antegrade conduction is thought to proceed over the fast pathway and retrograde conduction over the slow pathway and may result in an atypical form of AVNRT that may be incessant (Figure 53.3). In these patients, antegrade conduction curves are not discontinuous. This pattern of conduction as well as the incessant nature can also be seen in the presence of concealed septal accessory pathways with decremental properties.[3]

The concept of longitudinally dissociated dual AV nodal pathways that conduct around a central obstacle with proximal and distal connections can provide explanations for many aspects of the electrophysiological behaviour of these tachycardias, but several obscure points remain. These pathways have not been demonstrated histologically, the exact circuit responsible for the reentrant tachycardia is unknown, and critical questions still remain unanswered. Consequently, several attempts to provide a reasonable hypothesis based on anatomic or anisotropic models have appeared.[4,5] There has been considerable evidence that the right and left inferior extensions of the human AV node and the atrio-nodal inputs they facilitate may provide the anatomic substrate of the slow pathway,[6,7] and a comprehensive model of the tachycardia circuit for all forms of atrioventricular nodal reentrant tachycardia based on the concept of atrio-nodal inputs has been proposed (Figure 53.4 a,b,c).[1] Still, however, the exact circuit of AVNRT remains elusive.

Presentation

Reentrant atrioventricular tachycardias tend to appear first in youth, and the attacks recur throughout life as **regular palpitations of sudden onset and offset**. Occasionally, certain events, such as physical exercise, emotional upset, indigestion, or alcohol consumption, precipitate attacks. Polyuria, probably indicating increased ANP levels, may be present during or after a prolonged attack. AVNRT may result in AF that usually, although not invariably, is eliminated following catheter ablation of AVNRT.[8]

ECG morphologies

Typically, AVNRT is a narrow complex tachycardia, i.e. QRS duration less than 120 ms (Figure 53.2), unless an aberrant conduction, which is usually of the RBBB type, or a previous conduction defect exists. Tachycardia-related ST depression, as well as RR interval variation, may be seen. RR alternans may be seen but are more common in AVRT.

In the **typical form** of AVNRT (also called slow-fast AVRNT), abnormal (retrograde) P waves are constantly related to the QRS and, in the majority of cases, are indiscernible or very close to the QRS complex (RP/RR <0.5). Thus, P waves are either masked by the QRS complex or seen as a small terminal P' wave that is not present during sinus rhythm (Figure 53.5).

In the **atypical form** of AVNRT, P waves are clearly visible before the QRS, i.e. RP/PR >0.75 denoting a **'long RP tachycardia'**, and are negative or shallow in leads II, III, aVF, and V_6 but positive in V_1 (Figure 10)

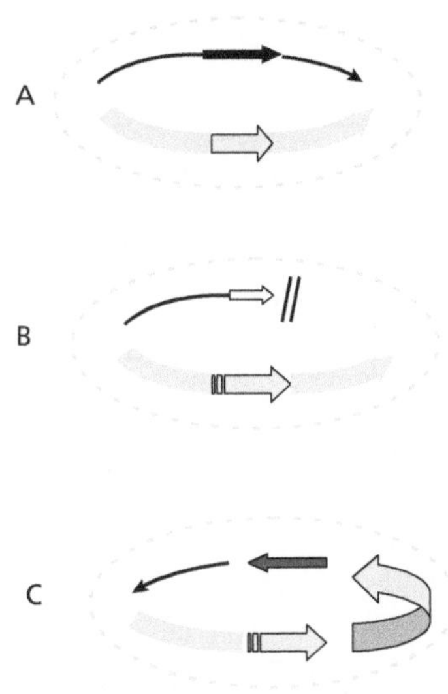

Figure 53.1 Theoretical depiction of the AV nodal reentrant circuit. During sinus rhythm, the impulse penetrates both the fast and slow pathways (A). A premature beat results in conduction block of the fast pathway and propagation through the slow pathway (B). An earlier impulse encounters more delay in the slow pathway in a way that the blocked fast pathway has recovered when the now retrograde impulse arrives and tachycardia begins (C).

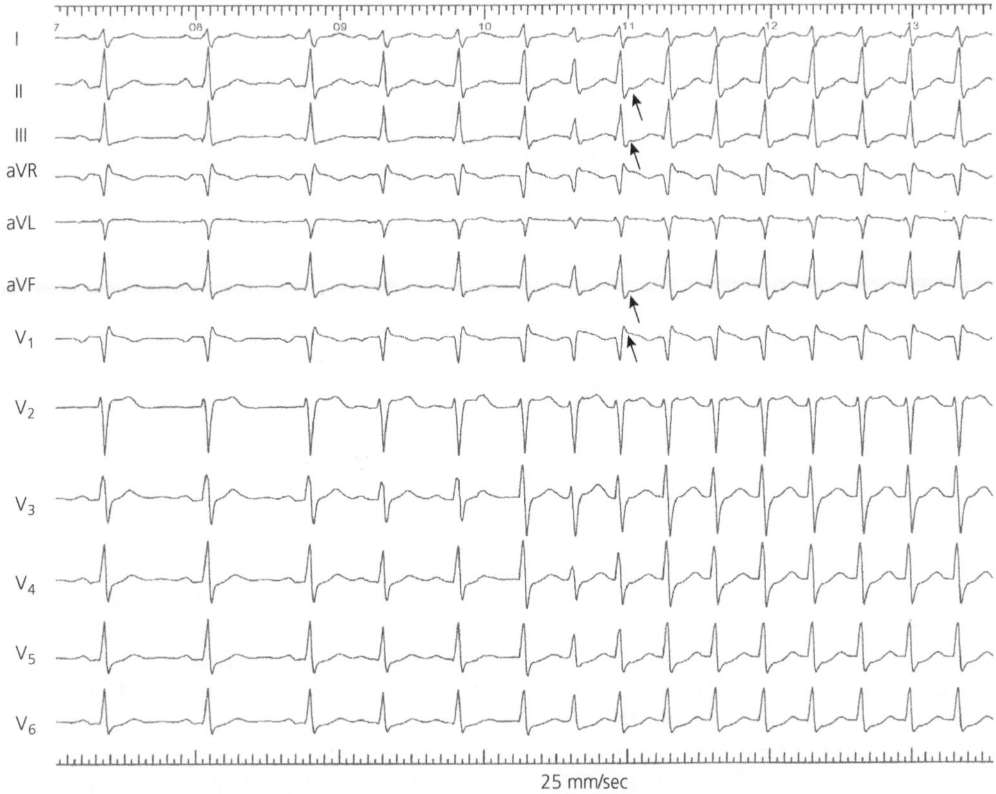

Figure 53.2 Induction of typical AVNRT by atrial ectopy. The first three beats are sinus beats. The next two are atrial ectopics conducted with a short PR (apparently over the fast pathway). The next atrial ectopic is conducted with a prolonged PR over the slow pathway, due to antegrade block of the fast pathway, and initiates AVNRT by returning retrogradely through the fast pathway that has recovered. Retrograde P waves are more prominent in lead V_1 and especially the inferior leads (arrows).
Katritsis DG, Camm AJ. Atrioventricular nodal reentrant tachycardia, *Circulation*. 2010;**122**:831–40.

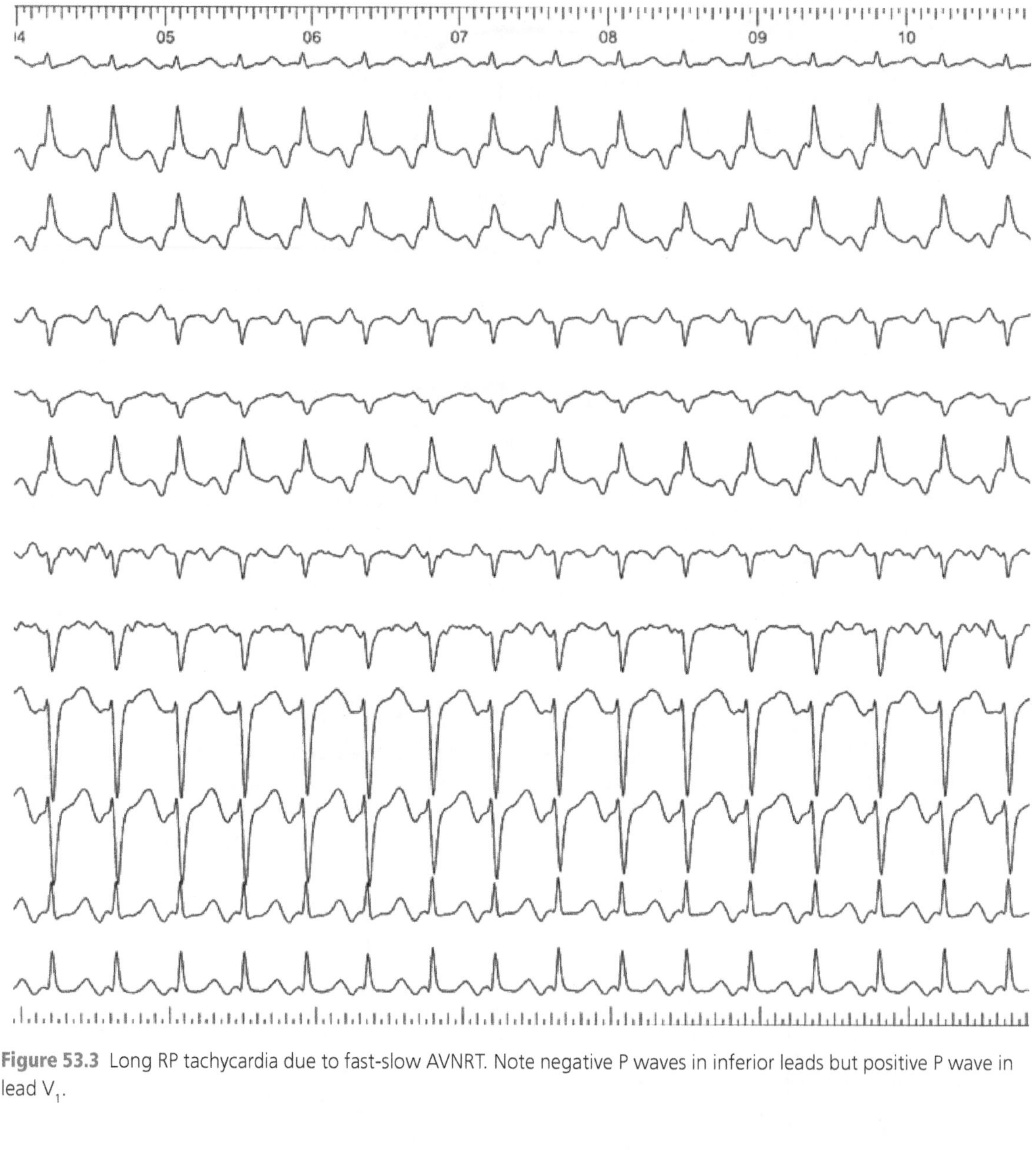

Figure 53.3 Long RP tachycardia due to fast-slow AVNRT. Note negative P waves in inferior leads but positive P wave in lead V_1.

Other causes of long RP tachycardia are presented in Table 53.1.

Although AV dissociation is usually not seen, it can occur since neither the atria nor the ventricles are necessary for the reentry circuit. If the tachycardia is initiated by atrial ectopic beats, the initial (ectopic) P wave usually differs from the subsequent (retrograde) P waves (Figure 53.2).

Electrophysiologic classification

The recognition of the fact that AVNRT may present with atypical retrograde atrial activation has made diagnosis of the arrhythmia, as well as classification attempts, more complicated. Heterogeneity of both fast and slow conduction patterns has been well described, and all forms of AVNRT may display anterior, posterior, and middle, or even left, atrial retrograde activation patterns (Table 53.2a).

Typical AVNRT

In the **slow-fast form** of AVNRT, the onset of atrial activation appears prior to, at the onset of, or just after the QRS complex, thus maintaining an atrial-His/His-atrial ratio (AH/HA) >1 (Figure 53.5). The VA interval measured from the onset of ventricular activation on surface ECG to the earliest deflection of the atrial activation in the His

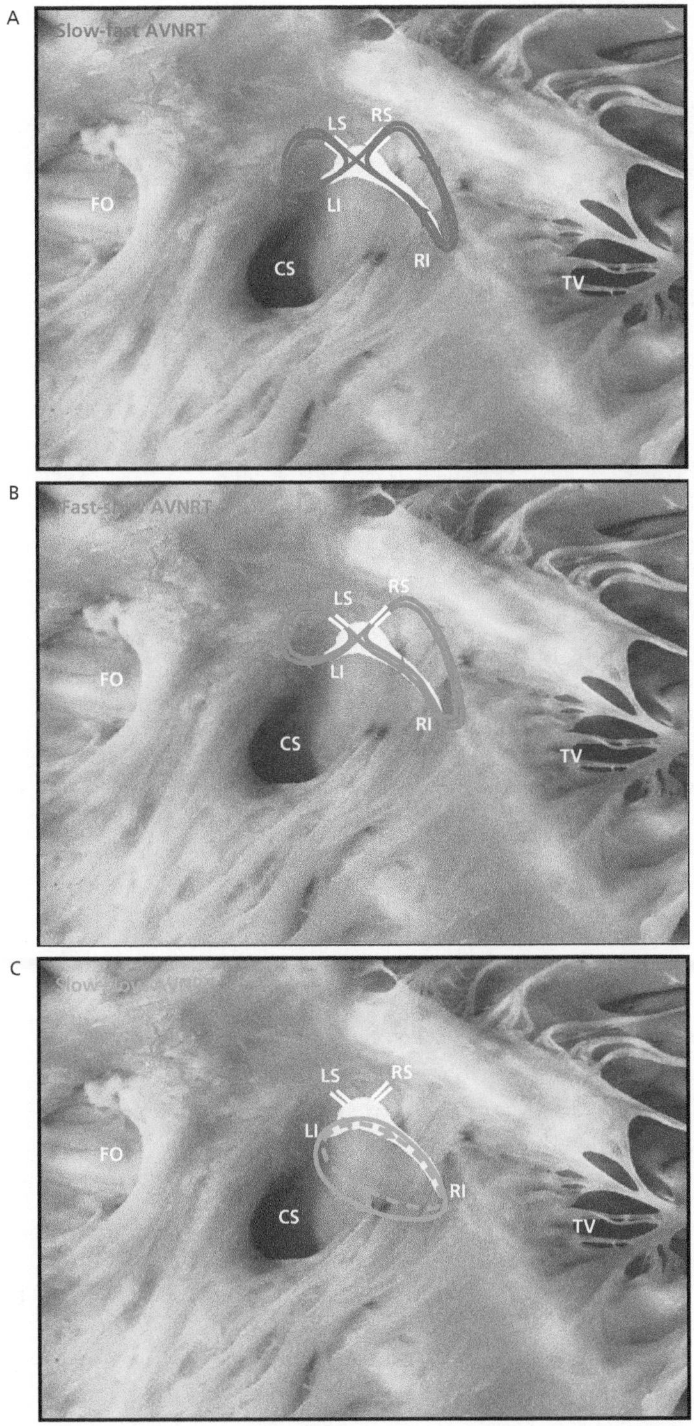

Figure 53.4a–c Proposed circuit of slow-fast AVNRT. Right- or left-sided circuits may occur with antegrade conduction through the inferior inputs (slow pathway conduction) and retrograde conduction through the superior inputs (fast pathway conduction). A: slow-fast AVNRT. Conduction is antegrade through the inferior inputs (slow pathway) and retrograde through the anterior inputs (fast pathway). B: fast-slow AVNRT. Conduction antegradely through the anterior inputs (fast pathway) and retrogradely through the inferior inputs (slow pathway). C: slow-slow AVNRT. Conduction antegradely and retrogradely through the inferior inputs (slow pathway).
Katritsis DG, Becker A. The atrioventricular nodal reentrant tachycardia circuit: a proposal. *Heart Rhythm*. 2007;**4**:1354–60.

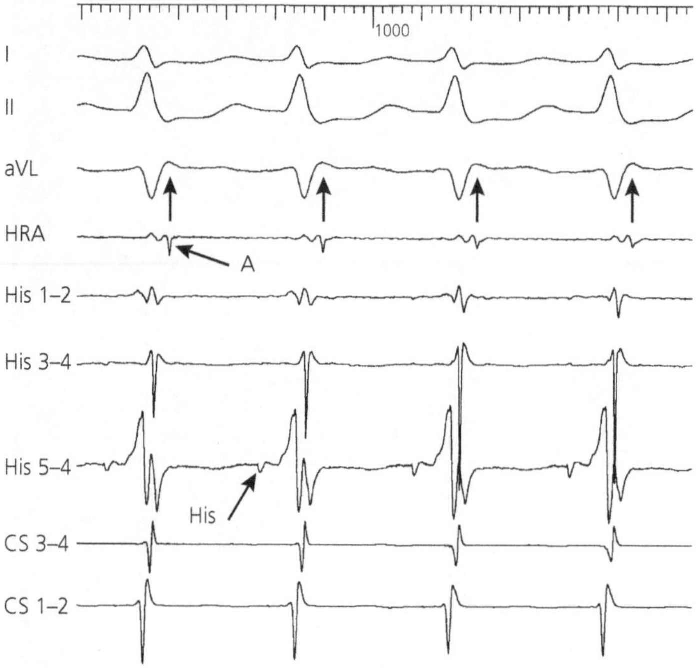

Figure 53.5 Electrograms during slow-fast AVNRT. The H-A interval (as measured from the A on the HRA electrode to the His on the His bundle electrode) is longer than the H-A. Small P waves at the end of QRS correspond to retrograde atrial conduction (arrows). I: ECG lead II, lead II of the surface ECG; aVL, lead aVL of the surface ECG; HRA, high right atrium; His, His bundle; CS, coronary sinus; A, atrial electrogram; His: His bundle electrogram.

Table 53.1 Long RP tachycardias

1. Sinus tachycardia
2. Atrial tachycardia
3. Atrioventricular nodal reentrant tachycardia (fast-slow or slow-slow variety)
4. Atrioventricular reentrant tachycardia due to slowly conducting concealed accessory pathways
5. Non-paroxysmal junctional tachycardia with 1:1 retrograde conduction

Table 53.2 Classification of AVNRT types. Variable earliest retrograde atrial activation has been described for all types. a: Conventional classification

	AH/HA	VA (His)	Usual ERAA
Typical AVNRT			
Slow-fast	>1	<60 ms	RHis, CS os, LHis
Atypical AVNRT			
Fast-slow	<1	>60 ms	CS os, LRAS, dCS
Slow-slow	>1	>60 ms	CS os, dCS

AH, atrial to His interval; HA, His to atrium interval; VA, interval measured from the onset of ventricular activation on surface ECG to the earliest deflection of the atrial activation in the His bundle electrogram; ERAA, earliest retrograde atrial activation; RHis, His bundle electrogram recorded from the right septum; LHis, His bundle electrogram recorded from the left septum; LRAS, low right atrial septum; CS os, ostium of the coronary sinus; dCS, distal coronary sinus.

Katritsis DG, Camm AJ. Atrioventricular nodal reentrant tachycardia, *Circulation*. 2010;**122**:831–40.

(Continued)

Table 53.2 (Continued)

b: New proposed classification

	HA	VA (His)	AH/HA
Typical AVNRT	≤70 ms	≤60 msec	>1
Atypical AVNRT	>70 ms	>60 msec	Variable

Atypical AVNRT has been traditionally classified as fast-slow (HA>70 ms, VA>60, AH/HA<1, and AH<200 ms) or slow-slow (HA>70 ms, VA>60 ms, AH/HA>1, and AH>200 ms). Not all of these criteria are always met and atypical AVNRT may not be sub-classified accordingly.

AH: atrial to His interval, HA: His to atrium interval, VA: interval measured from the onset of ventricular activation on surface ECG to the earliest deflection of the atrial activation on the His bundle electrogram.

Katritsis DG, Josephson ME. Classification of electrophysiological types of atrioventricular nodal re-entrant tachycardia: a reappraisal. *Europace*. 2013 Apr 23. [Epub ahead of print].

bundle electrogram is ≤60. Although, typically, the earliest retrograde atrial activation is being recorded at the His bundle electrogram, careful mapping studies have demonstrated that posterior, or even left, septal fast pathways may occur in up to 7.6% in patients with typical AVNRT.[9–11]

Atypical AVNRT

Atypical AVNRT is seen in approximately 5% of all AVNRT cases. It is traditionally classified as fast-slow or slow-slow, but criteria used are not unanimously accepted. In the **fast-slow form** of AVNRT, retrograde atrial electrograms begin well after ventricular activation with an AH/HA ratio <1, indicating that retrograde conduction is slower than antegrade conduction. The AH interval is less than 185–200 msec. The VA interval, measured from the onset of ventricular activation on surface ECG to the earliest deflection of the atrial activation in the His bundle electrogram, is >60 ms. Earliest retrograde atrial activation is traditionally reported at the base of the triangle of Koch, near the coronary sinus ostium. Detailed mapping of retrograde atrial activation in large series of patients, however, has produced variable results, with eccentric atrial activation at the lower septum or even the distal coronary sinus.[11–13] In the **slow-slow form**, the AH/HA ratio is >1, and the AH interval > 200 msec, but the VA interval is >60 ms, suggesting that two slow pathways are utilized for both anterograde and retrograde activation. Earliest retrograde atrial activation is usually at the coronary sinus ostium, but variants of left-sided atrial retrograde activation (distal coronary sinus) have also been published.[3]

The distinction between "fast-slow" and "slow-slow" forms is probably of no practical significance. AVNRT can be classified as typical or atypical according to the HA interval or, when a His bundle electrogram is not reliably recorded, the VA interval measured on the His bundle recording electrode (Table 53.2b).[14]

Differential diagnosis

In the presence of a **narrow QRS tachycardia**, AVNRT should be differentiated from **atrial tachycardia** or **orthodromic atrioventricular reentrant tachycardia** (AVRT) due to an accessory pathway.

When a wide QRS tachycardia is encountered and ventricular tachycardia is excluded, the possible diagnoses are **AVNRT or atrial tachycardia with aberrant conduction** due to bundle branch block, **AVNRT with a bystanding accessory pathway**, and **antidromic AVRT due to an accessory pathway**. Aberrant conduction, although rare, can be seen in AVNRT and is usually of the RBBB type. However, cases of LBBB have been reported.

AVNRT vs atrial tachycardia Exclusion of an atrial tachycardia on the 12-lead ECG is difficult, particularly with **peri-AV nodal atrial tachycardias** that, when reentrant, usually respond to adenosine and verapamil.[3]

AVNRT vs AVRT due to septal accessory pathways In case of relatively delayed retrograde conduction that allows the identification of retrograde P waves, ECG criteria can be applied for diagnosis. The presence of a pseudo R wave in lead V_1 or a pseudo S wave in leads II, III, and aVF has been reported to indicate anterior AVNRT with an accuracy of 100%. A difference of RP intervals in lead V_1 and III >20 ms was indicative of posterior AVNRT, rather than AVRT, due to a posteroseptal pathway.[15] ST elevation in aVR and marked repolarization changes during tachycardia suggest AVRT.[16] The documentation of pre-excited beats as well as AV dissociation, and the induction of bundle branch block during tachycardia may assist in the differential diagnosis. AV block or AV dissociation, although uncommon and short-lasting, may be seen in AVNRT and excludes the presence of an accessory pathway. Similarly, the development of bundle branch block, either spontaneously or after introduction of ventricular extrastimuli during AVNRT, does not change the AA or HH intervals. A significant change in the VA interval with the development of bundle branch block is diagnostic of orthodromic AVRT and localizes the pathway to the same side as the block.

AVNRT may display eccentric atrial activation, and septal pathways may have decremental conduction properties and concentric atrial activation, thus making even the electrophysiologic differential diagnosis challenging.

Table 53.3 ACC/AHA/ESC 2003 GL on SVT. Recommendations for long-term treatment of patients with recurrent AVNRT

Poorly tolerated AVNRT with haemodynamic intolerance	
Catheter ablation	I-B
Verapamil, diltiazem, beta-blockers, sotalol, amiodarone	IIa-C
Flecainide, propafenone (not in CAD/low LVEF)	IIa-C
Recurrent symptomatic AVNRT	
Catheter ablation	I-B
Verapamil	I-B
Diltiazem, beta-blockers	I-C
Digoxin (overridden by enhanced sympathetic tone)	IIb-C
Recurrent AVNRT unresponsive to beta-blockade or calcium channel blocker and patient not desiring RF ablation	
Flecainide, propafenone, sotalol	IIa-B
Amiodarone	IIb-C
AVNRT with infrequent or single episode in patients who desire complete control of arrhythmia	
Catheter ablation	I-B
Documented PSVT with only dual AV-nodal pathways or single echo beats demonstrated during electrophysiological study and no other identified cause of arrhythmia	
Verapamil, diltiazem, beta-blockers, flecainide, propafenone	I-C
Catheter ablation	I-B
Infrequent, well-tolerated AVNRT	
No therapy	I-C
Vagal manoeuvres	I-B
Pill-in-the-pocket	I-B
Verapamil, diltiazem, beta-blockers	I-B
Catheter ablation	I-B

ACC/AHA/ESC guidelines for the management of patients with supraventricular arrhythmias. *Circulation*. 2003;**108**:1871–909.

Table 53.4 ACC/AHA/ESC GL on SVT 2003. Recommendations for treatment of focal and non-paroxysmal junctional tachycardia syndromes

Focal junctional tachycardia	
Beta-blockers	IIa-C
Flecainide	IIa-C
Propafenone (paediatric pts)	IIa-C
Sotalol (paediatric pts)	IIa-C
Amiodarone (paediatric pts)	IIa-C
Catheter ablation	IIa-C
Non-paroxysmal junctional tachycardia	
Reverse digitalis toxicity	I-C
Correct hypokalaemia	I-C
Treat myocardial ischaemia	I-C
Beta-blockers, calcium channel blockers	IIa-C

ACC/AHA/ESC guidelines for the management of patients with supraventricular arrhythmias. *Circulation*. 2003;**108**:1871–909.

AVNRT with bystanding accessory pathways vs antidromic AVRT Antidromic AVRT, i.e. tachycardia utilizing the accessory pathway for antegrade conduction and the AV node for retrograde conduction, may be induced in approximately 6% of patients with accessory pathways located in the left or right free wall or the anterior septum at an adequate distance from the AV node. Mahaim atriofascicular pathways may give rise to AVRT or act as bystanders in AVNRT with LBBB morphology. Electrophysiologic evaluation is necessary for diagnosis.

Therapy

In acute episodes of AVNRT that do not respond to Valsalva manoeuvres, intravenous adenosine is the treatment of choice. Alternatively, a single dose of oral diltiazem (120 mg) and a beta-blocker (i.e. propranolol 80 mg) may be tried.[16] Chronic administration of antiarrhythmic drugs (such as beta-blockers, non-dihydropyridine calcium channel blockers, flecainide, or propafenone) may be ineffective in up to 50% of cases (Table 53.3).[3] Thus, catheter ablation is the current treatment of choice. Slow pathway ablation or modification is effective in both typical and atypical AVNRT. Usually, a combined anatomical and mapping approach is employed with ablation lesions delivered at the inferior or mid-part of the triangle of Koch, either from the right or the left septal side.[18,19] Multicomponent atrial electrograms or low amplitude potentials, although not specific for the identification of slow pathway conduction, are successfully used to guide ablation at these areas. This approach offers a success rate of 95%, is associated with a risk of 0.5–1% AV block, and has an approximately 4% recurrence rate. Although a <0.6% mortality has been reported in earlier studies,[20] no deaths are seen in recent trials.[21] Advanced age is not a contraindication for slow pathway ablation.[22] The pre-existence of first-degree heart block may carry a higher risk for late AV block and slow pathway modification, as opposed to complete elimination, and is probably preferable in this setting.[23]

Non-reentrant junctional tachycardias

Non-reentrant junctional tachycardias are rare, but should be recognized because catheter ablation conveys a higher risk of AV block than in AVNRT (5–10%) (Table 53.4).[24]
Non-paroxysmal junctional tachycardia was frequently diagnosed in the past as a junctional rhythm of gradual

onset and termination, with a rate between 70 and 130 beats/min, and was considered a typical example of digitalis-induced delayed after-depolarizations and triggered activity in the AV node. Myocardial ischaemia, hypokalaemia, COPD, and myocarditis are also associated conditions.

Focal junctional tachycardia occurs as a congenital arrhythmia or early after infant open heart surgery, but it can also be seen in adult patients with a structurally normal heart.[25,26] Aetiology is increased automaticity or triggered activity. The usual electrocardiographic finding is a narrow QRS tachycardia with AV dissociation. Occasionally, the tachycardia might be irregular, thus resembling atrial fibrillation.

Non-reentrant atrioventricular nodal tachycardia caused by simultaneous multiple nodal pathway conduction is an uncommon mechanism of AV nodal tachycardia and has been associated with repetitive retrograde concealment or 'linking' phenomena.[3] These are expressed in the form of ventricular pauses with consistent AV relationship after the pause.

References

1. Katritsis DG, *et al.* The atrioventricular nodal reentrant tachycardia circuit: a proposal. *Heart Rhythm.* 2007;**4**:1354–60
2. Kwaku KF, *et al.* Typical AVNRT—an update on mechanisms and therapy. *Card Electrophysiol Rev.* 2002;**6**:414–21
3. Katritsis DG, *et al.* Atrioventricular nodal reentrant tachycardia. *Circulation.* 2010;**122**:831–40
4. Mazgalev TN, *et al.* Anatomic-electrophysiological correlations concerning the pathways for atrioventricular conduction. *Circulation.* 2001;**103**:2660–7
5. Spach MS, *et al.* Initiating reentry: the role of nonuniform anisotropy in small circuits. *J Cardiovasc Electrophysiol.* 1994;**5**:182–209
6. Katritsis DG, *et al.* Retrograde slow pathway conduction in patients with atrioventricular nodal reentrant tachycardia. . *Europace* 2007;**9**:458–65
7. Katritsis DG, *et al.* Effect of slow pathway ablation in atrioventricular nodal reentrant tachycardia on the electrophysiologic characteristics of the inferior atrial inputs to the human atrioventricular node. *Am J Cardiol.* 2006;**97**:860–5
8. Sauer WH, *et al.* Atrioventricular nodal reentrant tachycardia in patients referred for atrial fibrillation ablation: response to ablation that incorporates slow-pathway modification. *Circulation.* 2006;**114**:191–5
9. Engelstein ED, *et al.* Posterior fast atrioventricular node pathways: implications for radiofrequency catheter ablation of atrioventricular node reentrant tachycardia. *J Am Coll Cardiol.* 1996;**27**:1098–1105
10. Katritsis DG, *et al.* Atrial activation during atrioventricular nodal reentrant tachycardia: studies on retrograde fast pathway conduction. *Heart Rhythm.* 2006;**3**:993–1000
11. Nam GB, *et al.* Left atrionodal connections in typical and atypical atrioventricular nodal reentrant tachycardias: activation sequence in the coronary sinus and results of radiofrequency catheter ablation. *J Cardiovasc Electrophysiol.* 2006;**17**:171–7
12. Hwang C, *et al.* Atypical atrioventricular node reciprocating tachycardia masquerading as tachycardia using a left-sided accessory pathway. *J Am Coll Cardiol.* 1997;**30**:218–25
13. Nawata H, *et al.* Heterogeneity of anterograde fast-pathway and retrograde slow-pathway conduction patterns in patients with the fast-slow form of atrioventricular nodal reentrant tachycardia: Electrophysiologic and electrocardiographic considerations. *J Am Coll Cardiol.* 1998;**32**:1731–40
14. Katritsis DG, Josephson ME. Classification of electrophysiological types of atrioventricular nodal re-entrant tachycardia: A reappraisal. *Europace.* 2013 Apr 23; [Epub ahead of print]
15. Tai CT, *et al.* A new electrocardiographic algorithm using retrograde P waves for differentiating atrioventricular node reentrant tachycardia from atrioventricular reciprocating tachycardia mediated by concealed accessory pathway. *J Am Coll Cardiol.* 1997;**29**:394–402
16. Gonzalez-Torrecilla E, *et al.* EGC diagnosis of paroxysmal supraventricular tachycardias in patients without preexcitation. *Ann Noninvasive Electrocardiol.* 2011;**16**:85–95
17. Alboni P, *et al.* Efficacy and safety of out-of-hospital self-administered single-dose oral drug treatment in the management of infrequent, well-tolerated paroxysmal supraventricular tachycardia. *J Am Coll Cardiol.* 2001;**37**:548–53
18. Kalbfleisch SJ, *et al.* Randomized comparison of anatomic and electrogram mapping approaches to ablation of the slow pathway of atrioventricular node reentrant tachycardia. *J Am Coll Cardiol.* 1994;**23**:716–23
19. Katritsis DG, *et al.* An approach to left septal slow pathway ablation. *J Interv Card Electrophysiol.* 2011;**30**:73–9
20. Spector P, *et al.* Meta-analysis of ablation of atrial flutter and supraventricular tachycardia. *Am J Cardiol.* 2009;**104**:671–7
21. Bohnen M, *et al.* Incidence and predictors of major complications from contemporary catheter ablation to treat cardiac arrhythmias. *Heart Rhythm.* 2011;**8**:1661–6
22. Rostock T, *et al.* Efficacy and safety of radiofrequency catheter ablation of atrioventricular nodal reentrant tachycardia in the elderly. *J Cardiovasc Electrophysiol.* 2005;**16**:608–10
23. Li YG, *et al.* Risk of development of delayed atrioventricular block after slow pathway modification in patients with atrioventricular nodal reentrant tachycardia and a pre-existing prolonged PR interval. *Eur Heart J.* 2001;**22**:89–95
24. Blomstrom-Lundqvist C, *et al.* ACC/AHA/ESC guidelines for the management of patients with supraventricular arrhythmias—executive summary. A report of the American College of Cardiology/American Heart Association Task Force on practice guidelines and the European Society of Cardiology Committee for practice guidelines (writing committee to develop guidelines for the management of patients with supraventricular arrhythmias) developed in collaboration with NASPE-Heart Rhythm Society. *J Am Coll Cardiol.* 2003;**42**:1493–531
25. Hamdan MH, *et al.* Role of invasive electrophysiologic testing in the evaluation and management of adult patients with focal junctional tachycardia. *Card Electrophysiol Rev.* 2002;**6**:431–5
26. Wren C. Incessant tachycardias. *Eur Heart J.* 1998;**19** Suppl E:E32–6, E54–39

Chapter 54

Atrioventricular reentrant tachycardias

Definitions

The anatomical basis for atrioventricular reentrant tachycardia (AVRT) is an abnormal connection (accessory pathway) between atrial and ventricular myocardium. One limb of the reentrant circuit is the AV node, and the other is the anomalous connection. The term **pre-excitation** refers to activation of the ventricle by an impulse arising in the atrium, earlier than would be expected if conduction occurred via the normal atrioventricular conduction pathway. The term was first used to describe electrocardiographic abnormalities in patients with typical **Wolff–Parkinson–White (WPW) syndrome**, i.e. short PR interval (<120 ms), prolonged QRS (>120 ms), with an initial delta wave and paroxysmal tachycardia (Figure 54.1).

Epidemiology

The Wolff–Parkinson–White syndrome is the second most common cause of paroxysmal supraventricular tachycardia in most parts of the world, and is the most common cause in China, being responsible for more than 70% of cases.[1] In Western countries, the prevalence of the Wolff–Parkinson–White syndrome is 0.1–0.3%, and there is 4-fold increase of this in family members of WPW patients.[1]

Pathophysiology

The atrioventricular connections (previously known as bundles of Kent), when fully operating, produce the typical **WPW syndrome.** Atrio-nodal bypass tracts (previously known as James fibres) are considered to result in the so-called **Lown–Ganong–Levine syndrome**, i.e. short PR and normal QRS, although there is no histologic evidence for the existence of this entity. Accessory pathways capable of conduction in the antegrade direction may produce pre-excitation during sinus rhythm, and the reentrant circuit can use either the AV node or the pathway as the antegrade limb. In the first case, the AVRT is called **orthodromic** and is narrow complex (Figure 54.2), unless showing RBBB or, less

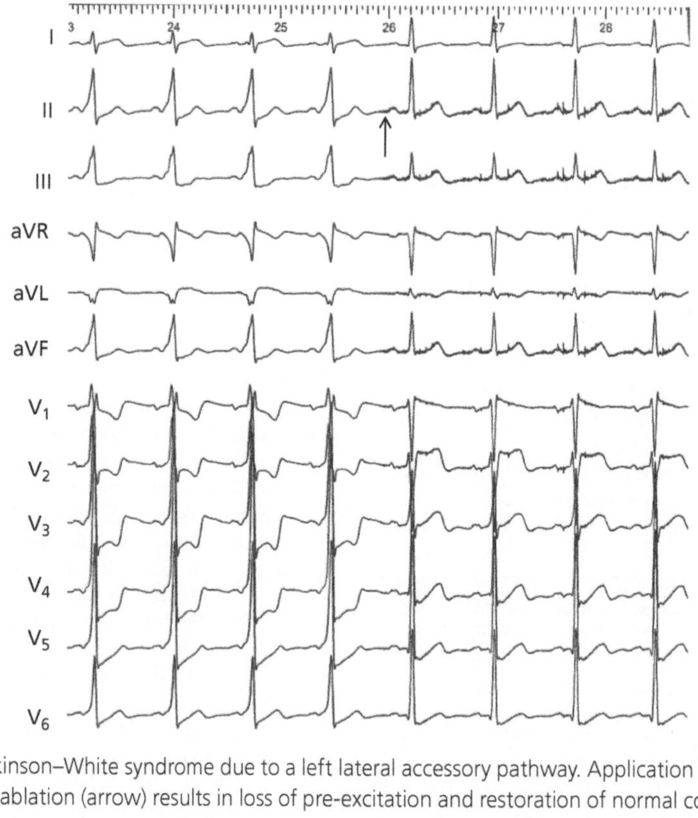

Figure 54.1 Wolff–Parkinson–White syndrome due to a left lateral accessory pathway. Application of radiofrequency energy during catheter ablation (arrow) results in loss of pre-excitation and restoration of normal conduction.

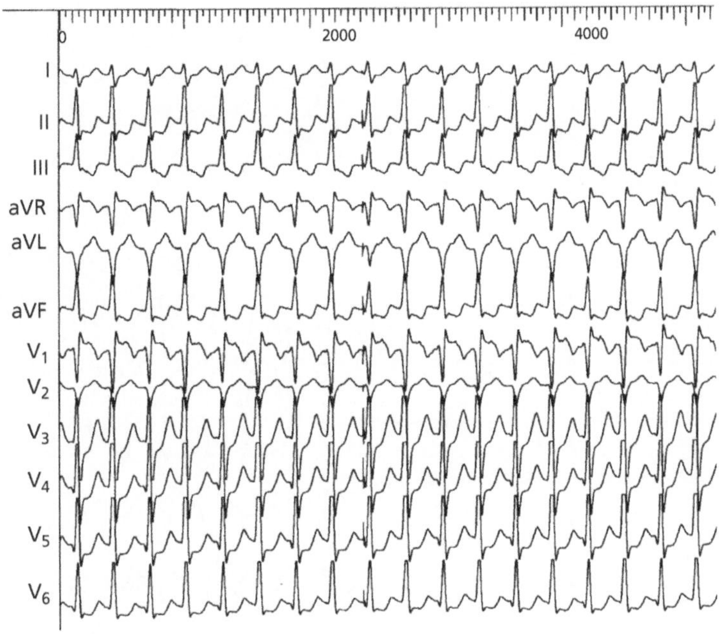

Figure 54.2 Orthodromic AVRT due to a concealed posteroseptal pathway.

usually, LBBB aberration. In the second case, the AVRT is **antidromic** and pre-excited, i.e. wide complex (Figure 54.3). Pre-excited AVRT, in which an accessory atrioventricular connection is used as the antegrade limb and the AV node or a second pathway serves as the retrograde limb of the circuit, has been clinically documented in less than 5% of patients with WPW syndrome and may be induced in less than 10% in the EP laboratory.[2] This usually happens in patients with multiple pathways or with free wall pathways located, at least, >4 cm from the AV node, although, in children, it may be seen even with septal pathways.[2] If the pathway conducts only in the retrograde direction, the so-called **concealed accessory pathway**, the ECG during sinus rhythm is normal and only orthodromic AVRT can be produced. Approximately 8% of accessory pathways display decremental antegrade or retrograde conduction. The term **permanent junctional reciprocating tachycardia** (PJRT) refers to orthodromic AVRT due to a slowly conducting, concealed, and usually septal pathway. There is incessant SVT, usually with negative P waves in the inferior leads and a long RP interval. **Mahaim** pathways are **atriofascicular** or (rarely) **nodoventricular** pathways, characterized by decremental conduction that results in gradual increase of the atrioventricular interval, simultaneous with the development of left bundle branch block. Antidromic and, rarely, orthodromic tachycardias may be induced with possible VA block in the case of a nodoventricular fibre.

Aetiology

Accessory pathways are a congenital disorder. Rarely, atrioventricular connections can be iatrogenic following a Fontan operation.[3] A missense mutation in the gene that encodes the gamma 2 regulatory subunit of AMP-activated protein kinase (PRKAG2) has been associated with ventricular pre-excitation and conduction disease.[4] A particular mutation in PRKAG2 has also been associated with Mahaim (nodoventricular fibres).[4] A novel form of WPW syndrome is associated with microdeletion in the region of gene BMP2 that encodes the bone morphogenetic protein-2, a member of the transformin growth factor (TGF-β) gene superfamily, and affects the development of annulus fibrosus. It is characterized by variable cognitive deficits, dysmorphic features, and prolonged AV conduction on atrial pacing.[4]

Presentation

Patients present due to **sudden onset and offset episodes of palpitations** or with **pre-excited AF** (ie, AF with wide-QRS–up to 30%). During AF, antegrade conduction over the accessory pathway results in a wide QRS complex tachyarrhythmia which may be mistaken for ventricular tachycardia. Up to 50% of patients with WPW syndrome are asymptomatic,[5] and diagnosis is made after an incidental ECG. Loss of antegrade conduction capacity occurs with time in up to 30% of patients,[5] but, when pre-excitation remains, the frequency of tachycardia increases with age.[6]

WPW predisposes to development of AF which may, or may not, be eliminated following ablation of the pathway.[7,8]

Diagnosis

Patients with concealed pathways, as well as some with Mahaim fibres, have completely normal resting ECG. Antegradely conducting pathways may produce the typical

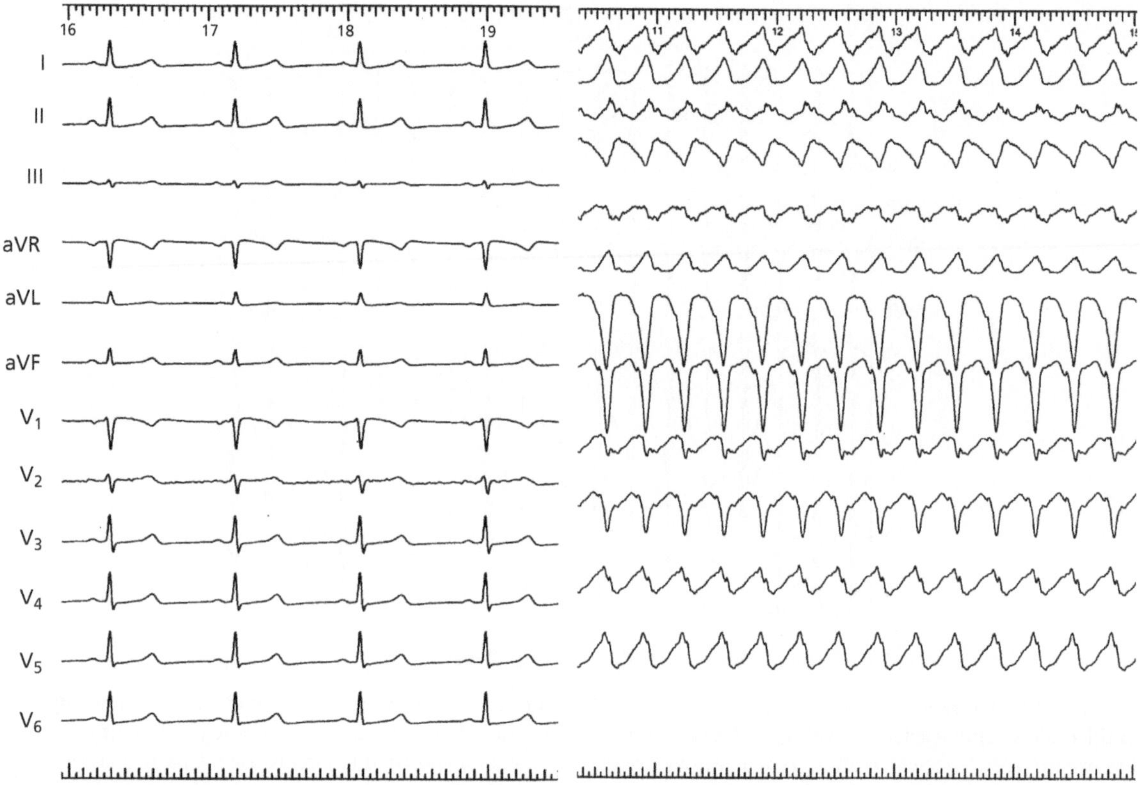

Figure 54.3 Antidromic AVRT due to an atriohisian Mahaim pathway. Note that ECG is normal during sinus rhythm (left panel).

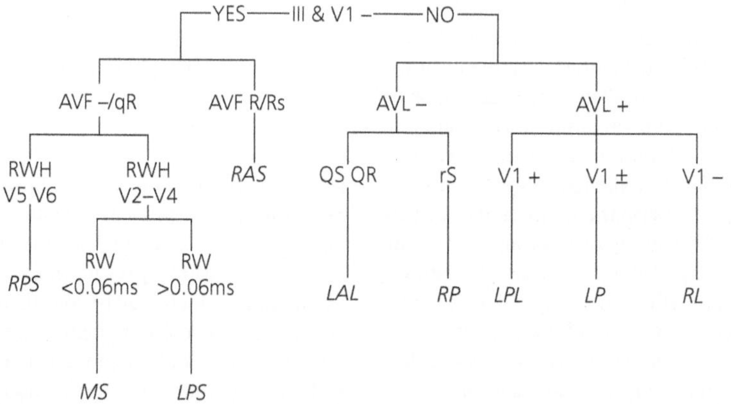

Figure 54.4 The St George's algorithm for localization of accessory pathways. +: positive QRS complex; -: negative QRS complex; ± = equiphasic QRS complex; LAL: left anterolateral; LP: left posterior; LPL: left posterolateral; LPS: left posteroseptal; MS: midseptal; RAS: right anteroseptal; RP = right posterior; RPS: right posteroseptal; RL = right lateral; RW: R wave width in V1; RWH: the highest R wave recorded in precordial leads.

Xie B, et al. Localization of accessory pathways from the 12-lead electrocardiogram using a new algorithm. *Am J Cardiol*. 1994;**74**:161–5.

WPW pattern or may be latent. Latent pathways, when conducting antegradely, may be revealed by infusion of adenosine or sometimes isoprenaline. In approximately 1.3% of cases of Wolff–Parkinson–White syndrome, more than one accessory pathway is present.[9] Left free wall pathways are the most common, followed by posteroseptal, right free wall, and anteroseptal. Right-sided pathways are found in 10% of patients with Ebstein's anomaly. Several guides for the localization of the pathway from the surface ECG have been proposed (Figure 54.4).[10]

Risk stratification in WPW syndrome

The clinical significance of pre-excitation is related to the common association with arrhythmias, such as atrioventricular reentrant tachycardias and atrial fibrillation. Atrial fibrillation associated with the WPW syndrome may be life-threatening, especially if the accessory pathway has a short refractory period, allowing a very rapid ventricular rate or resulting in ventricular fibrillation. The issues of risk stratification and need for catheter ablation still remain controversial. In patients with asymptomatic pre-excitation, the risk of sudden cardiac death is low, approximately 1.25/1000 person-years.[11] Symptomatic patients have a 7% risk of developing fast AF, with shortest pre-excited RR interval ≤250 ms, and a 1.4% risk of haemodynamic collapse or cardiac arrest resulting from ventricular fibrillation within the next 3–4 years.[12] A recent meta-analysis demonstrated a low incidence of life-threatening arrhythmia in patients with asymptomatic pre-excitation.[13]

Main methods of risk stratification are exercise testing to reveal potential disappearance of pre-excitation, and recording of shortest pre-excited RR interval (SPERRI) during AF (SPERRI <250 ms indicates high risk).[14] Additional risk factors are estimation of the antegrade refractory period of the pathway at electrophysiology study (<250 ms indicates high risk), the presence of male gender, young age, multiple accessory pathways, and inducibility of AVRT triggering AF.[11–13] The indications for catheter ablation of an overt AP in an asymptomatic patient are still controversial (especially in children), and each case should be addressed individually.[15–17] The 2012 PACES/HRS recommendations are presented in Table 54.1 and Figure 54.5.[14]

Therapy

In acute episodes of narrow QRS tachycardia that does not respond to Valsalva manoeuvres, intravenous adenosine is the treatment of choice. Alternatively, a single dose of oral diltiazem (120 mg) and a beta blocker (i.e. propranolol 80 mg) may be tried.[18] In wide QRS tachycardia, adenosine may also be given, but with caution, because it may produce AF with a rapid ventricular rate through a fast pathway. IV ibutilide, flecainide, or procainamide may be given. For long-term suppression beta blockers, propafenone or flecainide (in the absence of CAD) may be given, with a success rate <70% (Table 54.2). Catheter ablation is the treatment of choice in symptomatic or high-risk patients with WPW

Table 54.1. 2012 PACES/HRS Expert consensus Statement on the Management of Asymptomatic Young Patients with WPW

Recommendations for young asymptomatic patients (8–21 years) with WPW ECG pattern	
Exercise stress test. Clear and abrupt loss of preexcitation at physiological heart rates indicates a lower risk.	IIa-B/C
Invasive risk stratification (transesophageal or intracardiac) to assess the shortest preexcited R-R interval in AF in individuals whose noninvasive testing does not demonstrate clear and abrupt loss of preexcitation.	IIa-B/C
Young patients with a SPERRI<= 250 ms in AF are at increased risk for SCD. Consider catheter ablation, taking into account the procedural risk factors based on the anatomical location of the pathway.	IIa-B/C
Defer ablation in young patients with a SPERRI >250 ms in AF. Ablation may be considered at the time of diagnostic study if the location of the pathway and/or patient characteristics do not suggest that ablation may incur an increased risk of adverse events, such as AV block or coronary artery injury. Young patients initially deemed to be at low risk who subsequently develop cardiovascular symptoms such as syncope or palpitations, should then be considered symptomatic and may be eligible for catheter ablation.	IIa-C
Asymptomatic patients with a WPW ECG pattern and structural heart disease are at risk for both atrial tachycardia and AV reciprocating tachycardia, which may result in unfavorable hemodynamics. Ablation may be considered regardless of the anterograde characteristics of the accessory pathway.	IIb-C
Asymptomatic patients with a WPW ECG pattern and ventricular dysfunction secondary to dyssynchronous contractions may be considered for ablation, regardless of anterograde characteristics of the bypass tract.	IIb-C
Asymptomatic patients with a WPW ECG pattern may be prescribed attention-deficit/hyperactivity disorder (ADHD) medications. This recommendation follows the AHA Guidelines, which state that ADHD medications may be used in this setting after cardiac evaluation and with intermittent monitoring and supervision of a pediatric cardiologist	

Children ages 5–8 years may be placed in the "younger-observe" or "older-assess risk" categories based on provider preference and the specifics of the individual patient and his/her family.

SPERI: shortest pre-excited RR interval during AF. In the absence of AF, the shortest pre-excited RR interval determined by rapid atrial pacing is a reasonable surrogate.

PACES/HRS expert consensus statement on the management of the asymptomatic young patient with a Wolff–Parkinson–White (WPW, ventricular preexcitation) electrocardiographic pattern: developed in partnership between the Pediatric and Congenital Electrophysiology Society (PACES) and the Heart Rhythm Society (HRS). *Heart Rhythm*. 2012; **9**:1006–24.

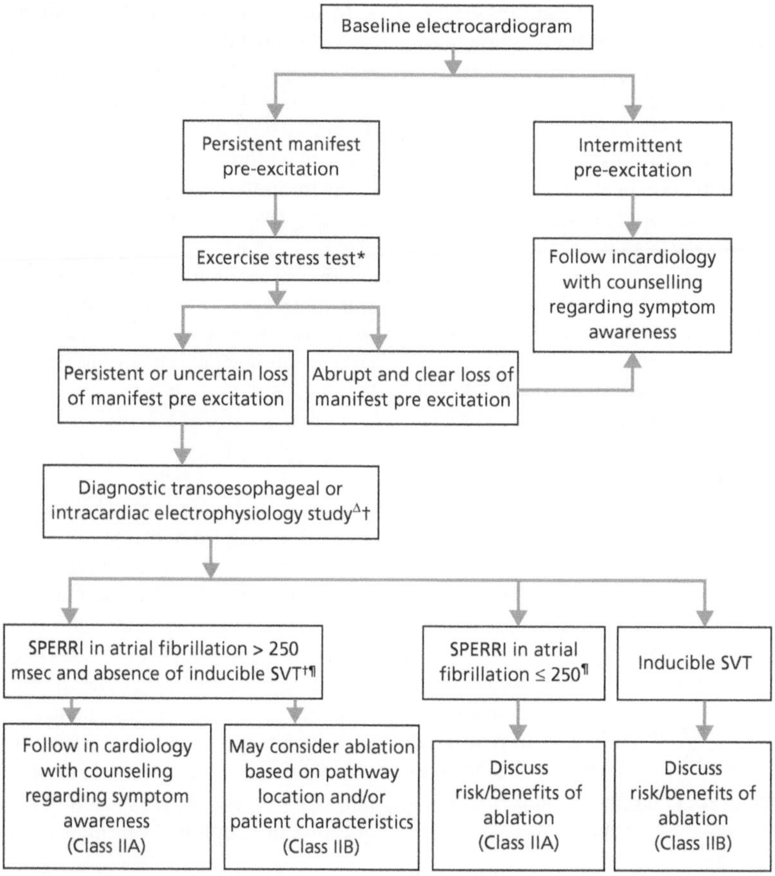

*Patients unable to perform an excercise stress test should undergo risk stratification with an EP study
Δ Prior to invasive testing, patients and the parents/guardians should be ccounselled to discuss the risks and benefits of proceeding with invasive studies, risks of observation only, and risks of medication strategy.
†Patients participating at moderate-high level competitive sports should be counseled with regards to risk-benefit of ablation (Class IIA) and follow the 36th Bethesda Conference Guidelines[6]
¶In the absence of inducible atrial fibrillation, the shortest pre-excited RR interval determined by rapid atrial pacing is a reasonable surrogate.

Figure 54.5 PACES/HRS management algorithm of patients with WPW.

PACES/HRS expert consensus statement on the management of the asymptomatic young patient with a Wolff-Parkinson-White (WPW, ventricular preexcitation) electrocardiographic pattern. *Heart Rhythm*. 2012; **9**:1006–24.

Table 54.2 ACC/AHA/ESC 2003 GL on SVT. Recommendations for long-term therapy of accessory pathway-mediated arrhythmias

WPW syndrome (pre-excitation and symptomatic arrhythmias), well tolerated	Catheter ablation	I-B
	Flecainide, propafenone sotalol, amiodarone, beta blockers	IIa-C
	Verapamil, diltiazem, digoxin	III-C
WPW syndrome (with AF and rapid-conduction or poorly tolerated AVRT)	Catheter ablation	I-B
AVRT, poorly tolerated (no pre-excitation)	Catheter ablation	I-B
	Flecainide, propafenone Sotalol, amiodarone	IIa-C
	Beta blockers	IIb-C
	Verapamil, diltiazem, digoxin	III-C

(Continued)

Table 54.2 (Continued)

Single or infrequent AVRT episode(s) (no pre-excitation)	None	I-C
	Vagal maneuvers	I-B
	Pill-in-the-pocket- verapamil, diltiazem, beta blockers	I-B
	Catheter ablation	IIa-B
	Sotalol, amiodarone	IIb-B
	Flecainide, propafenone	IIb-C
	Digoxin	III-C
Pre-excitation, asymptomatic	None	I-C
	Catheter ablation	IIa-B

ACC/AHA/ESC guidelines for the management of patients with supraventricular arrhythmias—executive summary. *Circulation*. 2003;**108**:1871–909.

syndrome (see Risk stratification). Success rate is 95% and complications, such as tamponade or AV block (septal pathways), <1%. A mortality 0–0.2% was usually reported,[19,20] but, in recent trials, perioperative mortality is 0%.[21,22]

References

1. Gollob MH, *et al.* Identification of a gene responsible for familial Wolff–Parkinson–White syndrome. *N Engl J Med.* 2001;**344**:1823–31
2. Katritsis D. Antidromic atrioventricular reentrant tachycardia. *Europace* (in press).
3. Hager A, *et al.* Congenital and surgically acquired Wolff–Parkinson–White syndrome in patients with tricuspid atresia. *J Thorac Cardiovasc Surg* 2005;**130**:48–53
4. Katritsis D. Progressive cardiac conduction disease. In Zipes DP, Jalife J. *Cardiac electrophysiology: from cell to bedside.* 6th edition (in press).
5. Klein GJ, *et al.* Longitudinal electrophysiologic assessment of asymptomatic patients with the Wolff–Parkinson–White electrocardiographic pattern. *N Engl J Med.* 1989;**320**:1229–33
6. Li CH, *et al.* The impact of age on the electrophysiological characteristics and different arrhythmia patterns in patients with Wolff–Parkinson–White syndrome. *J Cardiovasc Electrophysiol.* 2011;**22**:274–9
7. Centurion OA, *et al.* Mechanisms for the genesis of paroxysmal atrial fibrillation in the Wolff–Parkinson–White syndrome: intrinsic atrial muscle vulnerability vs electrophysiological properties of the accessory pathway. *Europace.* 2008;**10**:294–302
8. Haissaguerre M, *et al.* Frequency of recurrent atrial fibrillation after catheter ablation of overt accessory pathways. *Am J Cardiol.* 1992;**69**:493–7
9. Colavita PG, *et al.* Frequency, diagnosis and clinical characteristics of patients with multiple accessory atrioventricular pathways. *Am J Cardiol.* 1987;**59**:601–6
10. Xie B, *et al.* Localization of accessory pathways from the 12-lead electrocardiogram using a new algorithm. *Am J Cardiol.* 1994;**74**:161–5
11. Munger TM, *et al.* A population study of the natural history of Wolff–Parkinson–White syndrome in Olmsted County, Minnesota, 1953–89. *Circulation.* 1993;**87**:866–73
12. Pappone C, *et al.* Risk of malignant arrhythmias in initially symptomatic patients with Wolff–Parkinson–White syndrome: results of a prospective long-term electrophysiological follow-up study. *Circulation.* 2012;**125**:661–8
13. Obeyesekere MN, *et al.* Risk of arrhythmia and sudden death in patients with asymptomatic preexcitation: a meta-analysis. *Circulation.* 2012;**125**:2308–15
14. Cohen MI, *et al.* PACES/HRS expert consensus statement on the management of the asymptomatic young patient with a Wolff–Parkinson–White (WPW, ventricular pre-excitation) electrocardiographic pattern: developed in partnership between the Pediatric and Congenital Electrophysiology Society (PACES) and the Heart Rhythm Society (HRS). Endorsed by the governing bodies of PACES, HRS, the American College of Cardiology Foundation (ACCF), the American Heart Association (AHA), the American Academy of Pediatrics (AAP), and the Canadian Heart Rhythm Society (CHRS). *Heart Rhythm.* 2012;**9**:1006–24
15. Pappone C, *et al.* Radiofrequency ablation in children with asymptomatic Wolff–Parkinson–White syndrome. *N Engl J Med.* 2004;**351**:1197–205
16. Pappone C, *et al.* A randomized study of prophylactic catheter ablation in asymptomatic patients with the Wolff–Parkinson–White syndrome. *N Engl J Med.* 2003;**349**:1803–11
17. Wellens HJ. Should catheter ablation be performed in asymptomatic patients with Wolff–Parkinson–White? When to perform catheter ablation in asymptomatic patients with a Wolff–Parkinson–White electrocardiogram. *Circulation.* 2005;**112**:2201–7; discussion 2216
18. Alboni P, *et al.* Efficacy and safety of out-of-hospital self-administered single-dose oral drug treatment in the management of infrequent, well-tolerated paroxysmal supraventricular tachycardia. *J Am Coll Cardiol.* 2001;**37**:548–53
19. Blomstrom-Lundqvist C, *et al.* ACC/AHA/ESC guidelines for the management of patients with supraventricular arrhythmias—executive summary. A report of the American College of Cardiology/American Heart Association Task Force on practice guidelines and the European Society of Cardiology Committee for practice guidelines (writing committee to develop guidelines for the management of patients with supraventricular arrhythmias) developed in collaboration with NASPE-Heart Rhythm Society. *J Am Coll Cardiol.* 2003;**42**:1493–531
20. Spector P, *et al.* Meta-analysis of ablation of atrial flutter and supraventricular tachycardia. *Am J Cardiol.* 2009;**104**:671–7
21. Bohnen M, *et al.* Incidence and predictors of major complications from contemporary catheter ablation to treat cardiac arrhythmias. *Heart Rhythm.* 2011;**8**:1661–6
22. Sacher F, *et al.* Wolff–Parkinson–White ablation after a prior failure: a 7-year multicentre experience. *Europace.* 2010;**12**:835–41

Chapter 55

Ventricular arrhythmias

Definitions and classification

Definitions

Ventricular tachycardia (VT) is usually defined a tachycardia (rate >100 beats/min) with three, or more, consecutive beats that originate from the ventricles, independent of atrial or AV nodal conduction.[1,2]

Accelerated idioventricular rhythm denotes a ventricular rhythm <100 beats/min.

Sustained ventricular tachycardia lasts >30 s (unless requiring termination because of haemodynamic collapse) whereas **non-sustained tachycardia** terminates spontaneously within 30 s.

Monomorphic ventricular tachycardia has only one morphology during each episode (Figure 55.1).

Multiple monomorphic ventricular tachycardia has more than one morphology at different times.

Pleomorphic ventricular tachycardia has more than one morphologically distinct QRS complex occurring during the same episode of VT, but the QRS is not continuously changing. In patients with implantable defibrillators (ICD), pleomorphic VT, as well as multiple morphologies, indicate increased risk.[3]

In **polymorphic** ventricular tachycardia, there is a constant change in QRS configuration, indicating a changing ventricular activation sequence, at a heart rate <333 bpm (cycle length 180 ms). Rapid polymorphic ventricular tachycardia cannot be easily distinguished from ventricular fibrillation.

Bidirectional ventricular tachycardia is a rare form of tachycardia with two alternating morphologies, usually right bundle branch block with alternating left and right axis deviation. Typically occurs in digitalis intoxication, cathecholaminergic polymorphic ventricular tachycardia, and several other conditions that predispose cardiac myocytes to delayed after-depolarizations (DADs) and triggered activity.[4]

Incessant VT denotes haemodynamically stable VT lasting hours.

VT storm indicates very frequent episodes of VT, more than three episodes in 24 h, monomorphic or polymorphic, requiring cardioversion.[5]

Torsades de pointes are a form of polymorphic ventricular tachycardia with characteristic beat-by-beat changes (twisting around the baseline) in the QRS complex.

Ventricular flutter indicates a monomorphic, regular ventricular arrhythmia (cycle length variability ≤30 ms), with no isoelectric interval between QRS complexes.

Ventricular fibrillation is rapid, usually more than 333 bpm (cycle length ≤180 ms), grossly irregular ventricular rhythm with marked variability in QRS cycle length, morphology, and amplitude. Fine VF is low amplitude VF that can be perceived as asystole.

Pathophysiology

Electrophysiology

Ventricular tachycardia may be focal or macro-reentrant.

Focal VT has a point source of earliest ventricular activation, with a spread of activation away in all directions from that site. The mechanism can be triggered activity, automaticity, microreentry, or focal endocardial breakthrough from an epicardial reentry circuit.

Triggered activity due to early after-depolarizations is implicated in the initiation of polymorphic tachycardias in the **long QT syndromes** (see Chapter 57). Triggered activity due to delayed after-depolarizations is the mechanism of **idiopathic outflow tract tachycardias**.[6] Delayed after-depolarizations are caused by intracellular calcium overload by factors, such as increases in heart rate, beta-adrenergic stimulation, and digitalis, with subsequent activation of the Na/Ca exchanger (see also Chapter 49). Beta-adrenergic effects are mediated through a cAMP-induced increase in intracellular calcium and are antagonized by adenosine, which reduces cAMP. Termination of idiopathic ventricular outflow tract tachycardias by an intravenous bolus of adenosine or infusion of calcium channel blockers or by vagotonic manoeuvres is consistent with triggered activity as the likely mechanism for some of these tachycardias. These tachycardias can be difficult to induce at electrophysiology testing; rapid burst pacing and/or isoproterenol infusion is often required.

Automaticity that is provoked by adrenergic stimulation (not triggered) or disease processes that diminish cell-to-cell coupling may less commonly cause focal VT.[1] This type of VT may become incessant under stress or during isoproterenol administration but cannot be initiated or terminated by programmed electrical stimulation; it can sometimes be suppressed by calcium channel blockers or beta blockers. Automaticity from damaged Purkinje fibres has been suggested as a mechanism for catecholamine-sensitive, focal origin VT.[7] Automaticity can also occur in partially depolarized myocytes, as has been shown for VTs

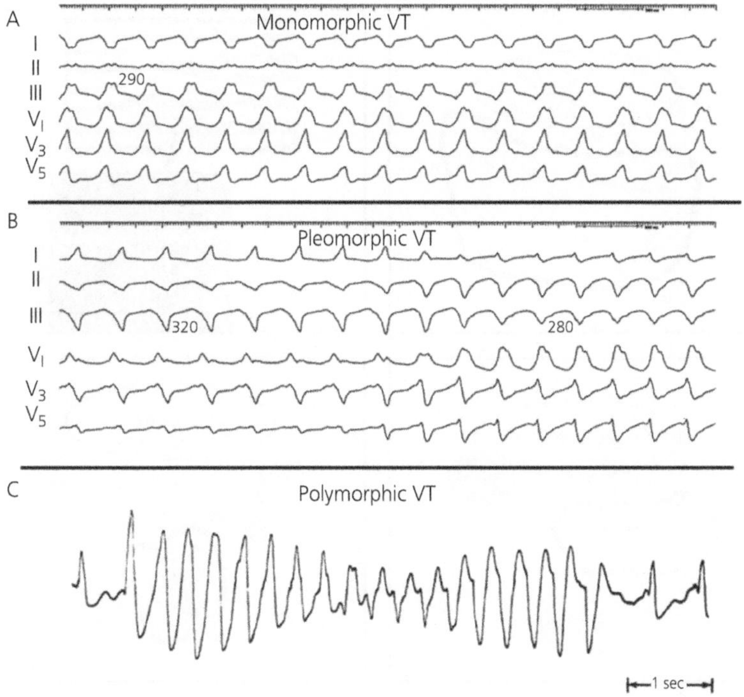

Figure 55.1 Types of VT. EHRA/HRS Expert Consensus on Catheter Ablation of Ventricular Arrhythmias. *Europace*. 2009;**11**:771–817.

during the early phase of myocardial infarction as well as in some patients with ventricular scars.[1] Automatic premature beats may, in addition, initiate reentrant VTs.

Macro-reentry refers to reentry circuits that can be defined over several centimetres and are due to myocardial scars secondary to a myocardial infarction or other disease process. Reentry around a myocardial scar (scar-related reentry), characterized by regions of slow conduction and anatomical or functional unidirectional conduction block at some point in the reentry path, is the cause of the majority of monomorphic VT seen in patients with heart disease.[7] Myocardial scar is identified from low-voltage regions on ventricular voltage maps, areas with fractionated electrograms, unexcitability during pace mapping, evidence of scar on myocardial imaging, or from an area of known surgical incision. Prior MI is the most common cause, but scar-related VT also occurs in cardiomyopathies and after cardiac surgery for congenital heart disease or valve replacement. Evidence supporting reentry includes initiation and termination by programmed stimulation (although this does not exclude triggered activity), demonstrable entrainment or resetting with fusion, and continuous electrical activity that cannot be dissociated from VT by extrastimuli.

Following MI, there is ion channel remodelling and regional reductions in I_{Na} and I_{Ca} within the scar, reduced coupling between myocytes by increased collagen and alterations in gap junction distribution and function, and intervening patchy fibrosis resulting in a zigzag pattern of transverse conduction.[2] Thus, scar remodelling contributes to the formation of channels and regions where conduction time is prolonged, facilitating reentry. Unidirectional conduction block may occur after a properly timed extra-beat; it is probably mostly functional, rather than fixed, and is present only during tachycardia when the refractory period of the tissue exceeds the tachycardia cycle length or maintained by collision of excitation waves. Functional conduction block can occur in figure-of-eight type of reentry circuits. Many reentry circuits contain a protected isthmus or channel of variable length, isolated by arcs of conduction block (Figure 55.2).[8] Critical isthmus sites (not necessarily corresponding to voltage map channels identified by electroanatomical mapping)[9] defined by concealed entrainment, i.e. no change of QRS morphology, S-QRS interval <70% of the VT cycle length, and a post-pacing interval—VT cycle length difference ≤30 ms, or pacing mapping with paced QRS morphology similar to that during VT and S-QRS interval >40 ms, are typically located within the dense scar (bipolar electrogram voltage <0.5 mV). Circuit exit sites, defined by local activation coincident with the onset of the QRS, are observed in the infarct border zone as described by voltage mapping. Multiple

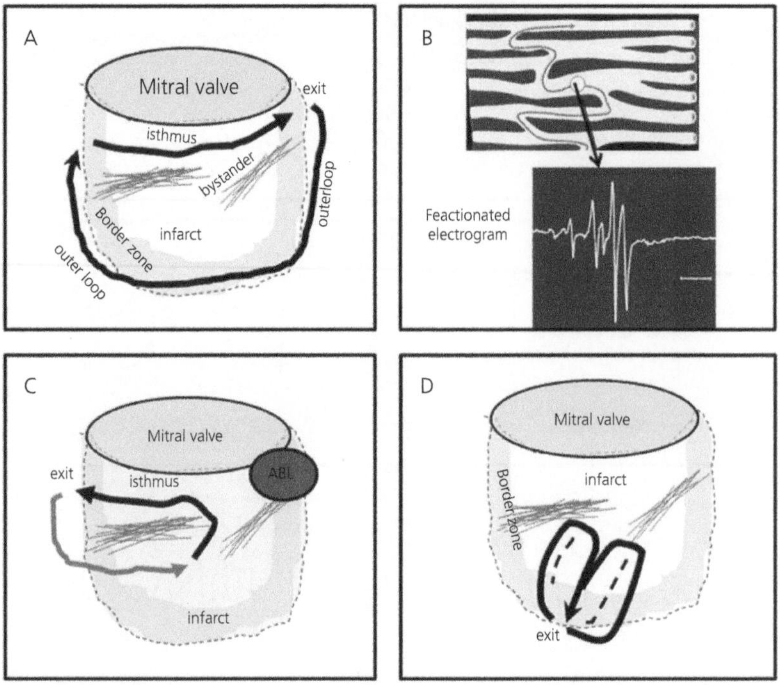

Figure 55.2 Theoretical reentry circuits related to an inferior wall infarct scar are shown. (A) A large inferior wall infarct designated by the dashed line and shaded border zone. Areas of dense fibrosis define an isthmus along the mitral annulus. A large reentry circuit uses this isthmus and exits at the lateral aspect of the scar. An outer loop propagates along the border to re-enter the isthmus at the medial aspect. Note that this circuit could potentially revolve in the opposite direction as well (not shown), producing VT with a different QRS morphology. Bystander regions are present as well. (B) The anatomical basis of slow conduction that facilitates reentry is shown. Fibrosis (dark bands) separates muscle bundles, creating circuitous paths for conduction. Electrograms from these regions have a fractionated appearance, indicating asynchronous activation of myocyte bundles. (C) The effect of ablation (Abl) at the exit for the VT. **VT–1** is interrupted, but other potential reentry paths are present that can allow other VTs. (D) A functionally defined figure-of-eight type of reentry circuit, in which the central isthmus is defined by functional block (dashed lines).

EHRA/HRS Expert Consensus on Catheter Ablation of Ventricular Arrhythmias. *Europace*. 2009;**11**:771–818

VT morphologies are usually inducible in the same patient, often related to multiple reentry circuits. The majority of reentrant circuits are located in the subendocardium, but subepicardial or intramyocardial reentry may also occur.

Macro-reentry through the bundle branches occurs in patients with slowed conduction through the His-Purkinje system and is usually associated with severe left ventricular (LV) dysfunction due to dilated cardiomyopathy, valvular heart disease, and, less often, ischaemic heart disease. The necessary condition for bundle branch reentry seems to be prolonged conduction in the His-Purkinje system, and this is reflected in the HV interval which is prolonged during sinus rhythm and prolonged, or equal to the baseline sinus rhythm, during VT. The circuit involves the right and left brunch bundles, with antegrade conduction occurring most of the times through the RB. The His bundle is activated as a bystander, and the HV interval is equal to, or greater than, that during sinus rhythm. HH interval variation usually precedes any VV interval variation in contrast to what happens in microreentrant ventricular tachycardia with retrograde activation of the His bundle.

Left ventric ular, fascicular, verapamil-sensitive VT occurs in patients without structural heart disease. The mechanism is reentry that appears to involve a portion of the LV Purkinje fibres, most often in the region of the left posterior fascicle, giving rise to a characteristic right bundle branch block (RBBB) superior axis QRS configuration and a QRS duration that is only slightly prolonged. [10,11]

Ventricular fibrillation

The mechanism of VF remains elusive, and both reentrant (caused by multiple wavelets, mother rotor, or a combination of both) and focal mechanisms (rapidly firing focus initiated by triggered activity or automaticity) have been implicated.[12] Rapid pacing-induced VF generally is attributed to reentrant mechanisms. Ischaemia, drugs, and genetic defects that prolong repolarization and alter intracellular calcium promote polymorphic ventricular arrhythmias degenerating to VF. In certain cases, focal mechanisms may be involved in VF initiation and maintenance.

Presentation

The clinical presentation of ventricular arrhythmias depends on the haemodynamic disturbance they produce. Rapid tachycardias, longlasting tachycardias, poor left ventricular function, and atrioventricular dissociation tend to contribute to haemodynamic collapse which may present as **presyncope**, **syncope**, or **sudden death**. When cardiac output and blood pressure are maintained and when the episodes are short-lived, the arrhythmia may present as recurrent palpitations, breathlessness, or chest pain. Occasionally, patients are completely **asymptomatic** during tachycardia. A history of ischaemic heart disease or congestive heart failure in men older than 35 years suggests that a wide QRS tachycardia is probably ventricular in origin.[13]

Physical examination

Low blood pressure, heart failure, and cardiogenic shock may be present as signs of haemodynamic distress.

Atrioventricular dissociation (apparent by a changeable pulse pressure or by Doppler assessment of flow in the ascending aorta[14]).

Irregular cannon waves in the jugular venous pulse.

Variable first heart sound may be seen if retrograde ventriculoatrial block is present.

None of these signs will be present if there is retrograde ventriculoatrial conduction which is present in 20–30% of cases. In this situation, atrial systole coincident with ventricular systole may produce **regular cannon waves**.

ECG morphologies

- With **monomorphic VT**, the ECG displays a wide QRS (>120 ms) tachycardia. Narrow QRS may be seen in fascicular VT, bundle branch reentry VT, and septal myocardial VT due to their origin within, or in close proximity to, the His-Purkinje network. Prior MI, idiopathic VT, and cardiomyopathies (more often dilated and ARVD) are the most common causes.
- **Polymorphic VT** may be seen in ischaemic heart disease with or without heart failure, cardiomyopathies, inherited channelopathies, such as Brugada syndrome and cathecholaminergic polymorphic VT, and congenital or acquired (drug-associated) long QT syndrome.
- Marked QT interval prolongation and the morphologically distinctive **torsades de pointes** occur in three common settings: in congenital LQTS, in drug-associated QTS, and in patients with advanced conduction system disease that has progressed to heart block.
- **Polymorphic VT storm** in a patient with coronary disease is strongly suggestive of acute myocardial ischaemia; pauses may occur prior to polymorphic VT, even in the absence of QT prolongation. Usually, severe underlying heart disease is present. More rarely, VT storm can occur (e.g. in Brugada syndrome, LQTS, catecholaminergic VT, or in drug overdose) in patients who have a structurally normal heart.

Differential diagnosis of wide QRS tachycardia

The differential diagnosis is between supraventricular tachycardia (AVRT or AVNRT) with aberrant (bundle branch block) conduction, AVNRT with a bystander accessory pathway, antidromic (pre-excited) AVRT, fast atrial fibrillation conducted over an accessory pathway, and electrolyte-induced QRS widening (Table 49.2 of Chapter 49).

Several morphologic criteria have been described and the 12-lead electrocardiogram may provide an accurate diagnosis of monomorphic VT in most but not all circumstances (Table 55.1 and Figures 55.3 to 55.5).[15–18] However, most of the existing morphologic criteria favouring ventricular tachycardia have been noted to be present in a substantial number of patients with intraventricular conduction defect during sinus rhythm.[19]

The following features are easily assessed:

- **Atrioventricular dissociation** may be seen as independent atrial activity, especially in lead II, or as 2:1 or 3:1 retrograde block with a P wave following every second or third QRS complex. Intermittent capture of the ventricles by conduction from the independent atrial activity will produce fusion beats (slightly premature with a shape intermediate between sinus and tachycardia morphologies) due to a depolarization of the ventricles, partially by the tachycardia beat and partially by the sinus beat, or capture beats (premature beats with a morphology of conducted beats) due to complete depolarization of the ventricles by the sinus beat. However, because ventricular tachycardia may show 1:1 retrograde conduction to the atrium, the presence of atrioventricular association cannot exclude the diagnosis of ventricular tachycardia.
- **Concordant negativity or concordant positivity** in all chest leads is also suggestive of VT.
- The absence of an RS complex in all precordial leads is highly specific for the diagnosis of ventricular tachycardia. If an RS complex is present in one or more precordial leads, the longest **RS interval (beginning of the R wave to the deepest part of the S wave) >100 ms** is highly

Table 55.1 Diagnosis of VT

Kindwall *et al.* criteria
1. R wave >30 ms in V_1 or V_2
2. Q wave in V_6
3. Onset of QRS to the nadir of S >60 ms in V_1 or V_2
4. Notching on the downstroke of the S wave in V_1 or V_2
Brugada *et al.* algorithm
RS in all precordial leads?
Yes: VT
No: RS interval (beginning of the R wave to the deepest part of the S wave) >100 ms?
Yes: VT
No: AV dissociation?
Yes: VT
No: apply the following conventional criteria:
RBBB morphology
V1 Monophasic R or QS or RS: VT
Triphasic QRS suggests SVT
V6 Monophasic R or QS or QR: VT
R > S: SVT
LBBB morphology
V1 or V2 Monophasic R >30 ms or >60 ms to nadir S, notched S or QS or RS: VT
Triphasic QRS: SVT
V6 Monophasic R, QS, or QR: VT
Monophasic R: SVT
Vereckei *et al.* algorithm
aVR
Initial R wave?
Yes: VT
No: Initial R or Q wave >40 ms?
Yes: VT
No: Notch on the descending limb of a negative onset and predominantly negative QRS?
Yes: VT
No: $v_i/v_t \leq 1$?
Yes: VT
No: SVT

v_i/v_t is the ventricular activation velocity ratio by measuring the vertical excursion in millivolts recorded on the ECG during the initial (v_i) and terminal (v_t) 40 ms of the QRS complex.

specific for ventricular tachycardia (Figure 55.3).[15]

- **A QRS complex >0.14 s in RBBB-like** tachycardia or **>0.16 s in LBBB-like** morphology, with regular RR intervals and with a left axis or an axis between −90 and +180, especially in the presence of a narrow, normal axis QRS during sinus rhythm, is suggestive of VT.
- In lead aVR: presence of an initial R wave, or width of an initial r or q wave >40 ms, or notching on the initial downstroke of a predominantly negative QRS complex suggest VT. If none of these criteria is present, then a v(i)/v(t) ≤ 1 (Figure 55.4) suggests VT.[18]
- An **R wave peak time (RWPT) ≥50 ms** in lead II (from the isoelectric line to the point of first change in polarity) suggests VT (Figure 55.5).[17]
- A triphasic RSR' with R' > R and the S wave extending beyond the baseline in lead V_1 favours the diagnosis of supraventricular tachycardia (SVT).

When the tachycardia has been terminated, further information can be gained from the 12-lead ECG in sinus rhythm. If bundle branch block is present, but with a different morphology or axis to that during tachycardia, the tachycardia is likely to be ventricular in origin. If delta waves are present and they have the same polarity as the QRS complexes of tachycardia, the diagnosis is most probably that of Wolff–Parkinson–White syndrome with antidromic AVRT or atrial fibrillation. An irregular, wide QRS tachycardia with ventricular rates faster than 200 bpm, especially in the younger patient with no previous history of ischaemic heart disease, should always raise the question of pre-excited atrial fibrillation.

Adenosine, given in rapid IV doses up to 0.25 mg/kg, will terminate or reveal most supraventricular tachycardias. Adenosine does not affect most ventricular tachycardias, with the exception of some forms associated with apparently normal hearts, and can, therefore, be used as a diagnostic agent.[20] Verapamil should not be used in this way because of the considerable incidence of life-threatening hypotension which is associated with its administration in ventricular tachycardia.

Acute therapy of ventricular arrhythmias

Cardiac arrest

Ventricular tachycardia or fibrillation was thought to be the most common cause of out-of-hospital cardiac arrest, accounting for approximately three-quarters of cases, the remaining 25% caused by bradyarrhythmias or asystole.[1,21] More recent studies suggest that the incidence of ventricular fibrillation or pulseless ventricular tachycardia as the first recorded rhythm in out-of-hospital cardiac arrest has declined to less than 30% in the past several decades.[22–24] Most patients (80%) with a cardiac arrest have demonstrable coronary artery disease, but less than half of all of them seem to have suffered an acute myocardial infarction,[25] and the use of thrombolysis during advanced life support for out-of-hospital cardiac arrest did not improve outcome.[26] VT/VF accounts for 67% of cardiac arrests in post-MI patients.[27]

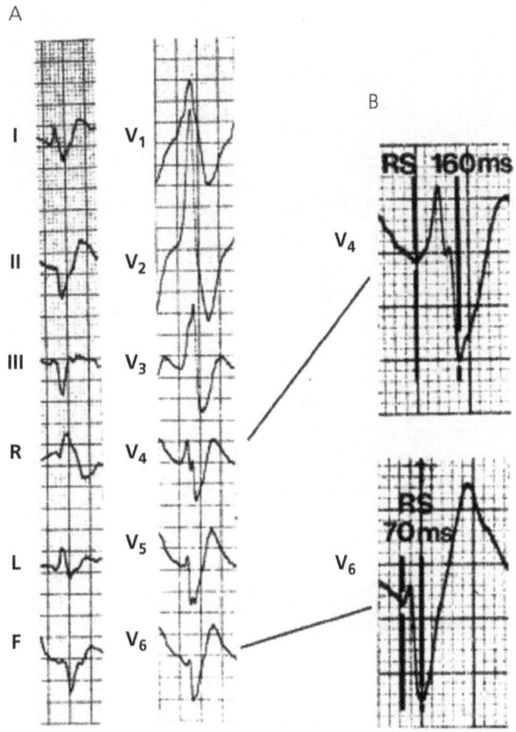

Figure 55.3 RS interval (enlarged in the right panel) measures 160 msec in lead V, and 70 msec in lead V6. Thus, the longest RS interval is more than 100 msec and diagnostic of ventricular tachycardia.

Brugada P *et al*. A new approach to the differtential diagnosis of a regular tachycardia with a wide QRS complex. *Circulation* 1991; **83**:1649.

A rapid response time is the major determinant of survival, and extracorporeal membrane oxygenation plus intra-arrest PCI of acutely occluded coronary arteries are associated with improved outcomes in patients unresponsive to conventional CPR.[28] Figure 55.6 presents the new 2010 AHA guidelines for CPR and emergency care.[29]

Important changes compared to previous (2005) AHA guidelines are:

- The basic life support (BLS) sequence of steps 'A-B-C' (Airway, Breathing, Chest compressions) has been changed to 'C-A-B' (Chest compressions, Airway, Breathing) for adults and paediatric patients.
- A universal compression-ventilation ratio of 30:2 performed by lone rescuers for victims of all ages.
- For most adults with out-of-hospital cardiac arrest, bystander CPR with chest compression only (**hands-only CPR**) appears to achieve outcomes similar to those of conventional CPR (compressions with rescue breathing). The predicted steep decline in arterial oxygen saturation does not occur until many minutes after the start of resuscitation, and the volume of oxygen in the lungs is relatively great when arrest occurs suddenly. In addition, initial reperfusion with hypoxaemic blood may result in fewer injurious oxygen free radicals and less reperfusion injury. Thus, continuous chest compression without active ventilation has been shown to result in a survival rate similar to that with chest compression with rescue breathing, avoids risks associated with mouth-to-mouth contact, and is recommended when CPR is performed by a bystanding layperson.[30–32] Recently, a study that analyzed 2 randomized clinical trials of 2500 cardiac arrest events involving dispatcher-assisted CPR instruction, demonstrated that chest compression alone was associated with even a better 5-year prognosis in comparison with standard CRP (compression plus recue breathing).[33] Survival with continuous chest compression is better among patients whose arrests were due to cardiac causes and among patients whose initial cardiac rhythm was ventricular tachycardia or fibrillation, rather than asystole or electromechanical dissociation.
- Chest compressions should be of adequate rate (at least **100/minute**) and of adequate depth of at least 2 inches (**5 cm**) in adults.
- Atropine is no longer recommended for routine use in the management of pulseless electrical activity/asystole.

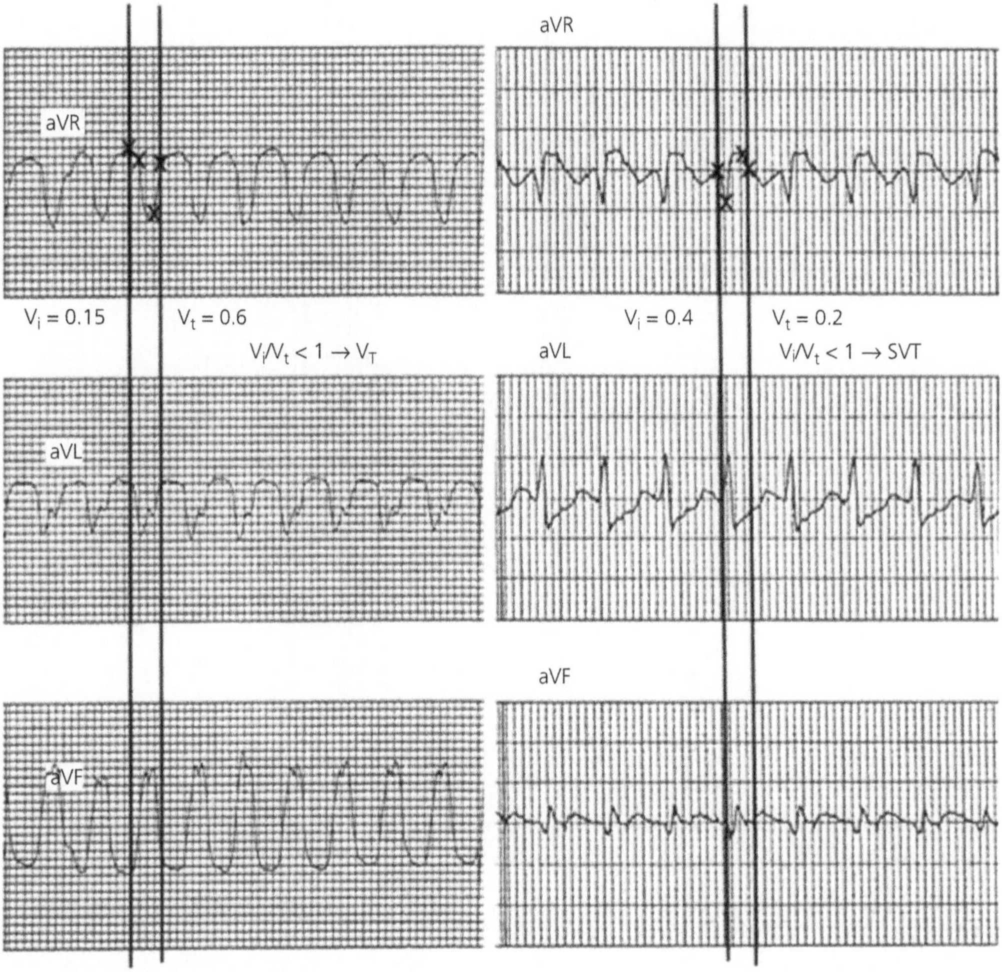

Figure 55.4 Use of V_i/v_t criterion in the fourth step of the new aVR algorithm. In both panels, the crossing points of the *vertical lines* with the QRS contour in lead aVR show the onset and end of the QRS complex in lead aVR. The crossing points and initial and terminal 40 ms of the chosen QRS complex are marked by *small crosses*. **Left:** During the initial 40 ms of the QRS, the impulse traveled vertically 0.15 mV; therefore, $v_i = 0.15$. During the terminal 40 ms of the QRS, the impulse traveled vertically 0.6 mV; therefore, $v_t = 0.6$. Thus, $v_i/v_t < 1$ yields a diagnosis of ventricular tachycardia (VT). **Right:** $v_i = 0.4$ and $v_t = 0.2$, determined the same way as in the left panel; thus, $v_i/v_t > 1$ suggests a diagnosis of supraventricular tachycardia (SVT).

Vereckei A, *et al*. New algorithm using only lead aVR for differential diagnosis of wide QRS complex tachycardia. *Heart Rhythm*. 2008;**5**:89–98.

The ACC/ESC guidelines are also presented in Table 55.2.

In case of suspected or definite ACS, recommendations are provided in Figure 55.7. Subsequent care should be implemented, as indicated in guidelines for ACS/MI (see Chapters 27 and 28).

Induction of therapeutic **hypothermia (32°C to 34°C) for 12 to 24 hours** after resuscitation from a ventricular tachycardia or ventricular fibrillation arrest has been shown to improve survival and neurological recovery.[34]

Monomorphic VT, polymorphic VT, torsade de pointes, incessant VT, and VT storm

Acute management is presented in Table 55.3. The value of lidocaine is now refuted while adenosine may be used in monomorphic VT, especially when the diagnosis of VT is not certain. The prognostic value of electrical storm is rather debatable, most probably depending on the underlying heart condition.[5,35,36] Catheter ablation may be useful for the short-term management of VT storm.[37]

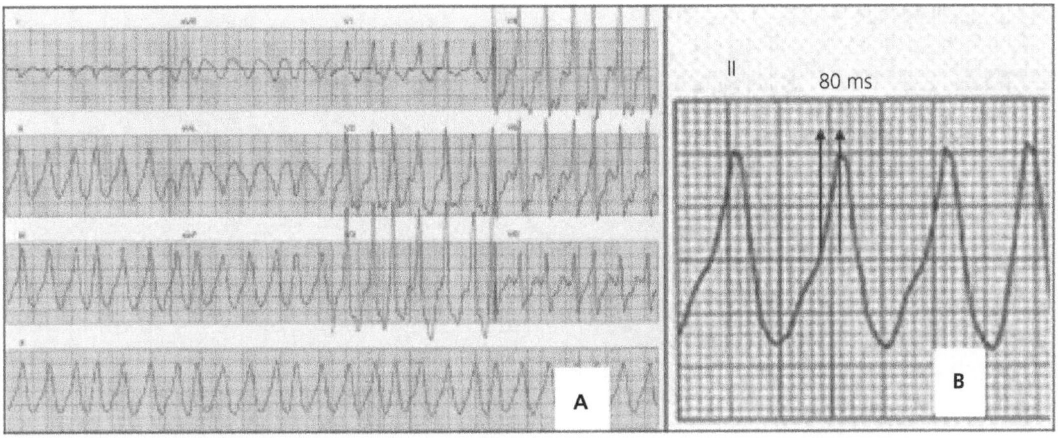

Figure 55.5 A: Twelve-lead ECG from a patient with ventricular tachycardia. **B:** Magnified lead II from panel A. R-wave peak time (RWPT) was ≥ 50 ms (RWPT duration 80 ms).

Pava LF, *et al.* R-wave peak time at DII: a new criterion for differentiating between wide complex QRS tachycardias. *Heart Rhythm*. 2010;**7**:922–6.

Risk stratification

Resting 12-lead ECG

ECG during tachycardia is essential for differential diagnosis. **ECG during sinus rhythm** after interruption of tachycardia may reveal signs of ischaemic heart disease, conduction defects, electrolyte disturbances, and syndromes of inherited arrhythmias (Brugada syndrome, ARVD, long QT syndrome). QRS duration >120 ms, ST-T abnormalities, and QT >440 ms or <400 ms have all been associated with increased mortality.[38]

Laboratory tests

Complete blood count, cardiac enzymes, serum electrolytes (including magnesium), creatinine, BUN, and liver and thyroid function tests should be checked.[39] Additional specific tests, such as iron studies and HIV, should also be obtained when clinically indicated.

Transthoracic echocardiography

Thansthoracic echocardiography may detect signs of cardiomyopathy, ARVC and other structural abnormalities, and impaired LV function. There has been overwhelming evidence that, in patients with heart disease in general, left ventricular ejection fraction is the major determinant of cardiac and total mortality.[2] The results of several studies, including the SCD-HeFT and MACAS, have also established the importance of **LVEF** as the most critical prognostic factor in patients with ischaemic or non-ischaemic LV dysfunction and NSVT.[40,41] However, analysis of arrhythmic death in patients enrolled in the MUSTT has shown that patients whose only factor is EF ≤30% have a predicted 2-year arrhythmic death risk ≤5% and the risk of sudden death in patients with coronary disease may depend on multiple variables in addition to LVEF.[42]

Exercise testing

Apart from demonstration of ischaemia, exercise tasting may also be helpful in patients with long QT syndrome, exercise-triggered RVOT tachycardia, and cathecholaminergic polymorphic VT (Table 55.4). NSVT induced by treadmill exercise testing, aimed at evaluating presumed long QT syndrome, suggests cathecholaminergic polymorphic VT, rather than long QT syndrome.[43] Although life-threatening arrhythmias may occur in up to 2% of individuals subjected to the test, exercise is recommended since it is better to expose arrhythmias under controlled circumstances.[1]

Other tests for myocardial ischaemia

Functional tests, such as myocardial perfusion and stress echocardiography, are required to demonstrate myocardial ischaemia. Acute myocardial ischaemia is an established cause of polymorphic ventricular rhythms.[44] The association of monomorphic ventricular tachycardia, a substrate-dependent arrhythmia, with acute ischaemia is less well characterized, but ischaemia may induce monomorphic ventricular tachycardia in the presence of a myocardial scar.[45]

Coronary angiography

It is mandatory in any patient with a life-threatening ventricular arrhythmia or aborted sudden death.[1]

Cardiac magnetic resonance

CMR imaging with delayed hyperenhancement has been used for detecting an arrhythmogenic substrate in patients with underlying LV dysfunction.[46] In this respect, cardiac

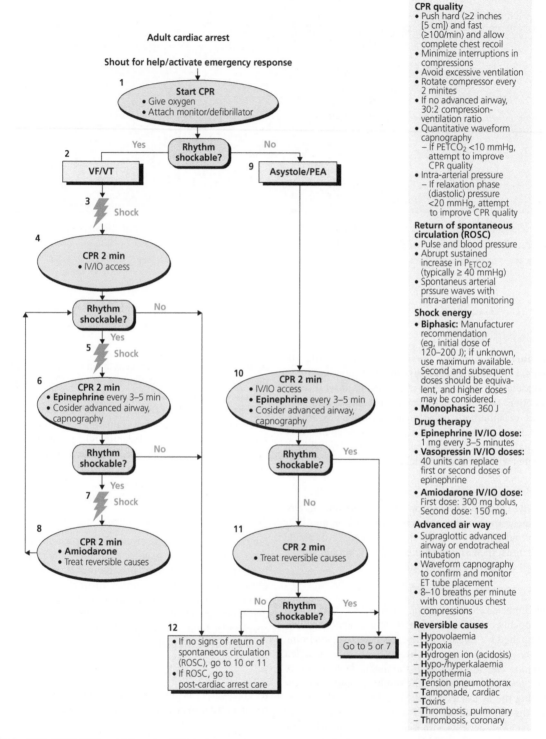

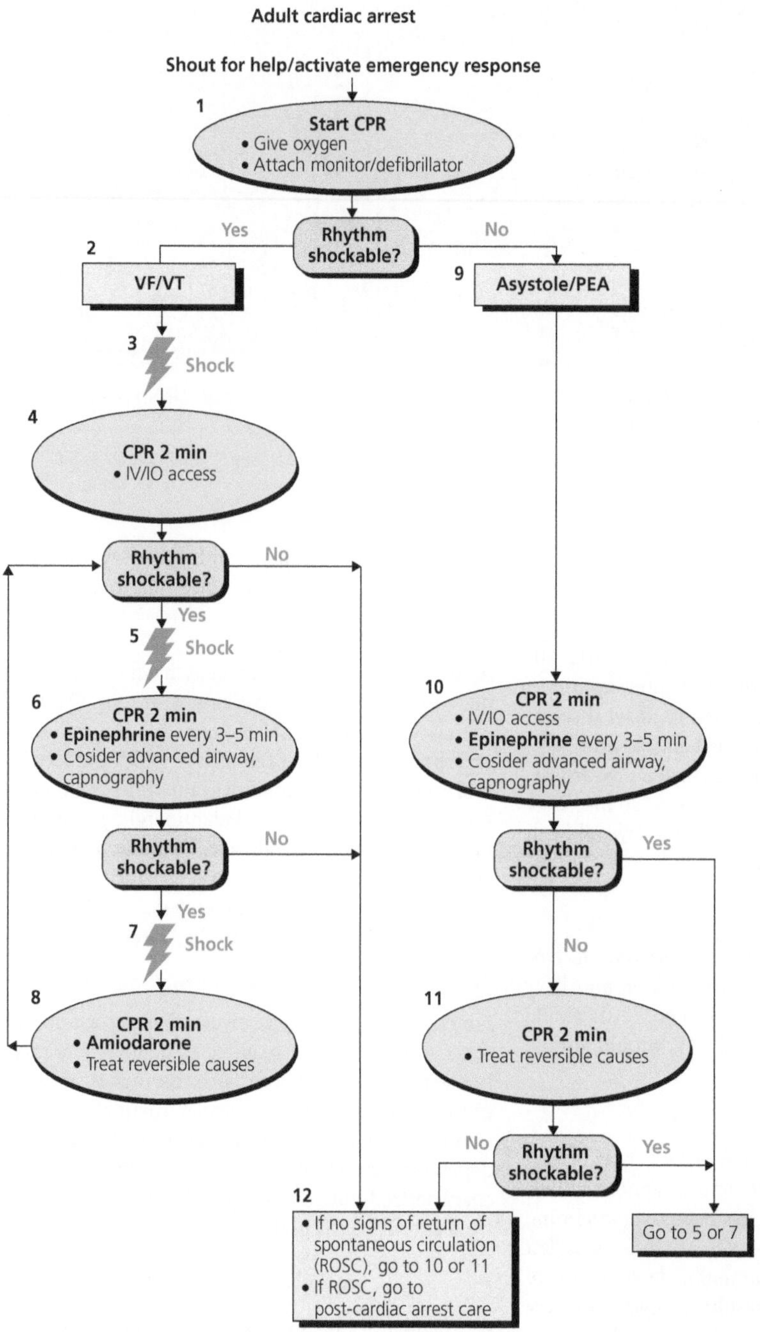

CPR quality
- Push hard (≥2 inches [5 cm]) and fast (≥100/min) and allow complete chest recoil
- Minimize interruptions in compressions
- Avoid excessive ventilation
- Rotate compressor every 2 minites
- If no advanced airway, 30:2 compression-ventilation ratio
- Quantitative waveform capnography
  - If $PETCO_2$ <10 mmHg, attempt to improve CPR quality
- Intra-arterial pressure
  - If relaxation phase (diastolic) pressure <20 mmHg, attempt to improve CPR quality

Return of spontaneous circulation (ROSC)
- Pulse and blood pressure
- Abrupt sustained increase in P_{ETCO2} (typically ≥ 40 mmHg)
- Spontaneus arterial prssure waves with intra-arterial monitoring

Shock energy
- **Biphasic:** Manufacturer recommendation (eg, initial dose of 120–200 J); if unknown, use maximum available. Second and subsequent doses should be equivalent, and higher doses may be considered.
- **Monophasic:** 360 J

Drug therapy
- **Epinephrine IV/IO dose:** 1 mg every 3–5 minutes
- **Vasopressin IV/IO doses:** 40 units can replace first or second doses of epinephrine
- **Amiodarone IV/IO dose:** First dose: 300 mg bolus, Second dose: 150 mg.

Advanced air way
- Supraglottic advanced airway or endotracheal intubation
- Waveform capnography to confirm and monitor ET tube placement
- 8–10 breaths per minute with continuous chest compressions

Reversible causes
- **H**ypovolaemia
- **H**ypoxia
- **H**ydrogen ion (acidosis)
- **H**ypo-/hyperkalaemia
- **H**ypothermia
- **T**ension pneumothorax
- **T**amponade, cardiac
- **T**oxins
- **T**hrombosis, pulmonary
- **T**hrombosis, coronary

Figure 55.6 2010 AHA guidelines for CPR and emergency care.

2010 American Heart Association Guidelines for Cardiopulmonary Resuscitation and Emergency Cardiovascular Care. *Circulation*. 2010;**122**(18 Suppl 3): Part 1: executive summary: S640–56, Part 6: electrical therapies: S06–719, Part 8: adult advanced cardiovascular life support: S729–67, Part 10: acute coronary syndromes: S787–817.

Table 55.2 ACC/AHA/ESC 2006 GL on VA. Management of cardiac arrest

Activation of a response team.	I-B
Immediate cardiopulmonary resuscitation (CPR).	I-A
Immediate shock in or out-hopsital setting (if AED available).	I-C
IV amiodarone when recurrences occur after a maximally defibrillating shock (generally 360 J for monophasic defibrillators).	I-B
Follow the algorithms contained in the documents on CPR developed by AHA/ILCOR/ERC.*	I-C
Management of hypoxia, electrolyte disturbances, mechanical factors, and volume depletion.	I-C
A brief (<90 to 180 s) period of CPR prior to attempting defibrillation for response times ≥5 min.	IIa-B
A single precordial thump by healthcare professional providers when responding to a witnessed cardiac arrest.	IIb-C

* ILCOR, International Liaison Committee on Resuscitation; ERC, European Resuscitation Council.

ACC/AHA/ESC 2006 Guidelines for Management of Patients With Ventricular Arrhythmias and the Prevention of Sudden Cardiac Death. *Circulation*. 2006;**114**: e385–484.

MRI is also useful in ARVC (see Cardiomyopathies), sarcoidosis, and other infiltrative myopathies[47] and has also been shown to help in risk stratification of hypertrophic cardiomyopathy.[48]

Ambulatory electrocardiography

Holter monitoring is valuable for detecting NSVT (Table 55.4). Although previous studies have detected NSVT as a predictor of arrhythmic mortality, in the era of reperfusion and beta blockers, NSVT does not carry independent predictive power in identifying patients with ischaemic or dilated cardiomyopathy at risk of sudden cardiac death, particularly in multivariate analyses when confounders, such as LVEF, are taken into account.[49–53] In non-ST elevation acute coronary syndrome, NSVT occurring beyond 48 hours after admission indicates an increased risk of sudden death.[54] In patients with HOCM and, most probably, in patients with inherited channelopathies, detection of NSVT on Holter predicts arrhythmia episodes.[55] The use of Holter for evaluation of treatment is limited since the suppression of frequent ventricular ectopy or NSVT by class IC antiarrhythmic drugs or amiodarone does not imply a favourable diagnosis. (CAST and CAST II and CHF-STAT).[56–58]

T wave alternans

T wave alternans are thought to reflect dispersion of repolarization and have been shown to predict future arrhythmic events better than SAECG and QRS duration.[59] In patients with reduced LV function (LVEF <40%) and NSVT, microvolt T wave alternans has also predicted unstable ventricular tachyarrhythmias better than electrophysiology testing and LVEF <30%.[60] However, although TWA predicted higher total mortality in a MADIT II-like population, the risk of tachyarrhythmic events did not differ according to TWA results.[61] The ABCD (Alternans Before Cardioverter-Defibrillator) study was the first trial to use micro-TWA to guide prophylactic ICD insertion in patients with LVEF <40% and NSVT. Risk stratification strategies using non-invasive TWA versus invasive EPS were comparable at 1 year, with very low positive and very high negative predictive values, and complementary when applied in combination. [62] Thus, strategies employing TWA, EPS, or both might identify subsets of patients least likely to benefit from ICD insertion. Data from patients with ICD have also suggested that variability of TWA is greater before spontaneous VT/VF recordings.[63]

Assessment of autonomic tone

Heart rate variability (HRV) has been identified as an independent risk factor for arrhythmic mortality in post-myocardial infarction patients.[64] Depressed baroreflex sensitivity has also been independently associated with an increased cardiac mortality and sudden death after MI and with a higher predictive power than heart rate variability.[65] However, in the beta-blocking era, the common arrhythmia risk variables, particularly the autonomic and standard ECG markers, such as QRS duration and QT dispersion, have limited predictive power in identifying patients at risk of sudden cardiac death.[66] In patients with non-ischaemic cardiomyopathy, results on the value of heart rate variability have been conflicting.[41,67] Heart rate turbulence and deceleration capacity are newer non-invasive measures of cardiac autonomic regulation under study.[68]

Signal-averaged electrocardiography

Although, in survivors of myocardial infarction, an abnormal SAECG has been associated with increased risk of arrhythmic and total mortality, its value for risk stratification purposes is not established, especially in patients treated with thrombolysis or beta blockers.[69] In patients presenting with unexplained syncope, the presence of late potentials is a good predictor of induction of sustained ventricular tachycardia.[70] However, its positive predictive value in this setting is low (<30%), as opposed to high negative predictive value (90%). Thus, a negative SAECG might obviate the need for further investigations when the suspicion of a ventricular arrhythmia is low, but, in the case of a high suspicion of ventricular arrhythmia, a negative SAECG is

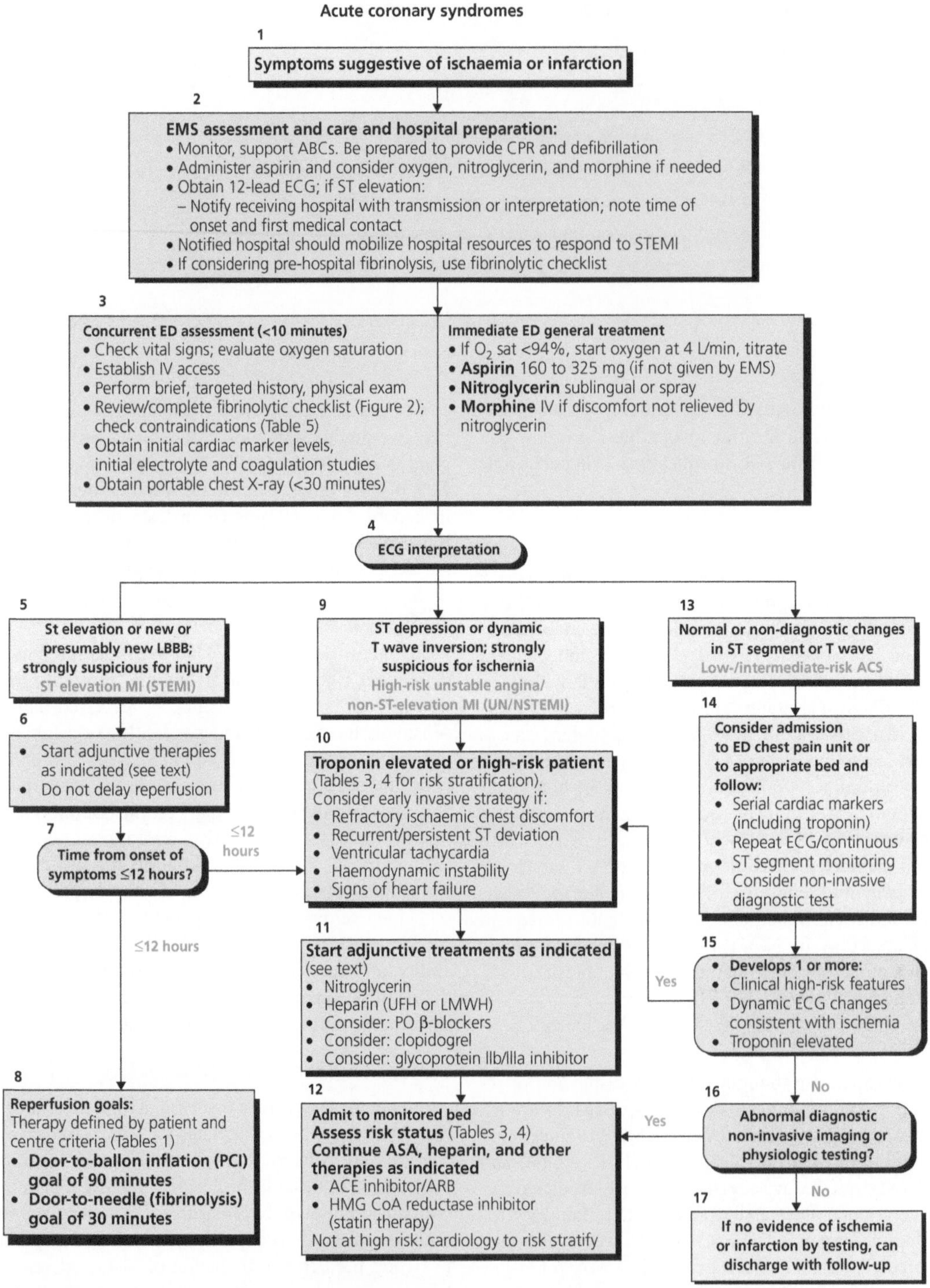

Figure 55.7 2010 AHA guidelines for CPR and emergency care in cardiac arrest due to a suspected acute coronary syndrome.

2010 American Heart Association Guidelines for Cardiopulmonary Resuscitation and Emergency Cardiovascular Care. Circulation. 2010;**122**(18 Suppl 3): Part 1: executive summary: S640–56, Part 6: electrical therapies: S06–S719, Part 8: adult advanced cardiovascular life support: S729–67, Part 10: acute coronary syndromes: S787–817.

Table 55.3 ACC/AHA/ESC 2006 GL on VA. Management of ventricular arrhythmias

Sustained monomorphic ventricular tachycardia	
Wide QRS tachycardia should be presumed to be VT if the diagnosis is unclear.	I-C
DC cardioversion with appropriate sedation in sustained monomorphic VT with haemodynamic compromise.	I-C
IV procainamide (or ajmaline in some European countries) for stable sustained monomorphic VT.	IIa-B
IV amiodarone in sustained monomorphic VT that is haemodynamically unstable, refractory to conversion with countershock, or recurrent despite procainamide or other agents.	IIa-C
Pacing termination of sustained monomorphic VT refractory to cardioversion or frequently recurrent despite antiarrhythmic medication.	IIa-C
IV lidocaine for stable sustained monomorphic VT specifically associated with acute myocardial ischaemia or infarction.	IIb-C
Calcium channel blockers, such as verapamil and diltiazem, in wide QRS complex tachycardia of unknown origin, especially in patients with a history of myocardial dysfunction.	III-C
Repetitive monomorphic ventricular tachycardia	
IV amiodarone, beta blockers, and IV procainamide (or sotalol or ajmaline in Europe) for repetitive monomorphic VT in the context of coronary disease and idiopathic VT.	IIa-C
Polymorphic VT	
DC cardioversion with appropriate sedation for sustained polymorphic VT with haemodynamic compromise.	I-B
IV beta blockers for recurrent polymorphic VT, especially if ischaemia is suspected or cannot be excluded.	I-B
IV loading with amiodarone for recurrent polymorphic VT in the absence of congenital or acquired LQTS.	I-C
Urgent angiography with a view to revascularization for patients with polymorphic VT when myocardial ischaemia cannot be excluded.	I-C
IV lidocaine for treatment of polymorphic VT specifically associated with acute myocardial ischaemia or infarction.	IIb-C
Torsades de pointes	
Withdrawal of offending drugs and correction of electrolyte abnormalities.	I-A
Acute and long-term pacing for torsades de pointes due to heart block and symptomatic bradycardia.	I-A
IV magnesium sulfate for LQTS and few episodes of torsades de pointes. Magnesium is not likely to be effective in patients with a normal QT interval.	IIa-B
Acute and long-term pacing for recurrent pause-dependent torsades de pointes.	IIa-B
Beta blockade combined with pacing as acute therapy for patients with torsades de pointes and sinus bradycardia.	IIa-C
Isoproterenol as temporary treatment in recurrent pause-dependent torsades de pointes without congenital LQTS.	IIa-B
Potassium repletion to 4.5–5 mmol/L for torsades de pointes.	IIb-B
IV lidocaine or oral mexiletine in LQT3 and torsades de pointes.	IIb-C
Incessant ventricular tachycardia	
Revascularization and beta blockade followed by IV procainamide or amiodarone for recurrent or incessant polymorphic VT due to acute myocardial ischaemia.	I-C
IV amiodarone or procainamide followed by VT ablation in frequently recurring or incessant monomorphic VT.	IIa-B
IV amiodarone and intravenous beta blockers, separately or together, in VT storm.	IIb-C
Overdrive pacing or general anaesthesia for frequently recurring or incessant VT.	IIb-C
Spinal cord modulation for frequently recurring or incessant VT.	IIb-C

ACC/AHA/ESC 2006 Guidelines for Management of Patients With Ventricular Arrhythmias and the Prevention of Sudden Cardiac Death. *Circulation*. 2006;**114**:e385–484.

Table 55.4 ACC/AHA/ESC 2006 GL on VA. Investigations in patients with ventricular arrhythmias

Exercise testing recommendations	
Adult patients who have an intermediate or greater probability of having CHD by age, gender, and symptoms to provoke ischaemic changes or ventricular arrhythmias.	I-B
Exercise testing, regardless of age, in known or suspected exercise-induced ventricular arrhythmias, including catecholaminergic VT.	I-B
To evaluate response to medical or ablation therapy in known exercise-induced ventricular arrhythmias.	IIa-B
In low probability of CHD by age, gender, and symptoms.	IIb-C
Isolated premature ventricular complexes (PVCs) in middle-aged or older patients without other evidence.	IIb-C

(Continued)

Table 55.4 (Continued)

Ambulatory electrocardiography	
To clarify the diagnosis by detecting arrhythmias, QT interval changes, T wave alternans (TWA), or ST changes, to evaluate risk, or to judge therapy.	I-A
When symptoms are sporadic, to establish whether or not they are caused by transient arrhythmias.	I-B
Implantable recorders in sporadic symptoms suspected to be related to arrhythmias, such as syncope when a symptom-rhythm correlation cannot be established by conventional diagnostic techniques.	I-B
Electrocardiographic techniques and measurements	
TWA to improve the diagnosis and risk stratification of patients with ventricular arrhythmias or who are at risk for developing life-threatening ventricular arrhythmias.	IIa-A
Signal-averaged ECG (SAECG), heart rate variability (HRV), baroflex sensitivity, and heart rate turbulence.	IIb-B
Left ventricular function and imaging	
Patients suspected of having structural heart disease.	I-B
Patients with dilated, hypertrophic, or RV cardiomyopathies, AMI survivors, or relatives of patients with inherited disorders associated with sudden cardiac death.	I-B
Exercise testing with an imaging modality (echocardiography or nuclear perfusion [single photon emission computed tomography (SPECT)]) to detect silent ischaemia in intermediate probability of CHD by age, symptoms, and gender and less reliable ECG assessment because of digoxin use, LVH, greater than 1 mm ST segment depression at rest, WPW syndrome, or LBBB.	I-B
Pharmacological stress testing with an imaging modality (echocardiography or myocardial perfusion SPECT) to detect silent ischaemia in intermediate probability of CHD by age, symptoms, and gender and physical inability to perform a symptom limited exercise test.	I-B
MRI, cardiac computed tomography (CT), or radionuclide angiography when echocardiography does not provide accurate assessment of LV and RV function and/or evaluation of structural changes.	IIa-B
Coronary angiography in patients with life-threatening ventricular arrhythmias or in survivors of SCD, who have an intermediate or greater probability of having CHD by age, symptoms, and gender.	IIa-C
LF imaging can be useful in patients undergoing biventricular pacing.	IIa-C

ACC/AHA ESC 2006 Guidelines for Management of Patients With Ventricular Arrhythmias and the Prevention of Sudden Cardiac Death. *Circulation*. 2006;**114**:e385–484.

not sufficient evidence for exclusion of non-sustained or sustained ventricular tachycardia as the cause of syncope. In patients with DCM, SAECG does not predict sudden death,[41] but, in arrhythmogenic right ventricular dysplasia, SAECG can identify those with more extensive disease and a propensity for inducible ventricular tachycardia at PES and is now considered a minor diagnostic criterion (see Cardiomyopathies).

Electrophysiology testing

Electrophysiology testing may be required for establishment of initial diagnosis in patients presenting with non-sustained ventricular rhythms (Table 55.5). For EP testing in syncope, see also Chapter 66 on syncope. Indications include the need for differential diagnosis from SVT with aberration, AF in the context of an accessory pathway or other forms of aberration, drug testing for the diagnosis of the Brugada syndrome, and programmed electrical stimulation for induction of VT.

Induction of sustained arrhythmia by programmed electrical stimulation (PES) still retains a predictive power in ischaemic patients with impaired LV function. In ischaemic patients with NSVT, the induction of sustained ventricular tachycardia is associated with a 2- to 3-fold increased risk of arrhythmia-related death.[71] In patients with reduced LVEF (<40%) and NSVT, inducibility of sustained monomorphic ventricular tachycardia at baseline PES is associated with a 2-year actuarial risk of sudden death or cardiac arrest of 50% compared to a 6% risk in patients without inducible ventricular tachycardia.[72] Analysis of patients enrolled in the MUSTT, as well as of those in the registry, revealed that non-inducible patients have a significantly lower risk of cardiac arrest or sudden death compared to inducible patients at 2 and 5 years (12% vs 24% and 18% vs 32%, respectively).[73] Still, however, as these results indicate, patients with non-inducible sustained VT are not free of risk of sudden death. The MUSTT Investigators have further analysed the relation of ejection fraction and inducible ventricular tachyarrhythmias to mode of death in 1791 patients enrolled in MUSTT who did not receive antiarrhythmic therapy. Total and arrhythmic mortality were higher in patients with an ejection fraction <30% than in those whose ejection fractions were 30% to 40%. The relative

Table 55.5 ACC/AHA/ESC 2006 GL on VA

Electrophysiological testing in patients with coronary heart disease	
Patients with remote MI and symptoms suggestive of ventricular tachyarrhythmias, including palpitations, presyncope, and syncope.	I-B
Patients with CHD to guide and assess the efficacy of VT ablation.	I-B
Patients with CHD for the diagnostic evaluation of wide QRS complex tachycardias of unclear mechanism.	I-C
Risk stratification in patients with remote MI, NSVT, and LVEF equal to ≤40%.	IIa-B
Electrophysiological testing in patients with syncope	
Patients with syncope of unknown cause with impaired LV function or structural heart disease.	I-B
Bradyarrhythmias or tachyarrhythmias are suspected, but non-invasive diagnostic studies are not conclusive.	IIa-B

ACC/AHA ESC 2006 Guidelines for Management of Patients With Ventricular Arrhythmias and the Prevention of Sudden Cardiac Death. *Circulation*. 2006;**114**:e385–484.

contribution of arrhythmic events to total mortality was significantly higher in patients with inducible tachyarrhythmia and among patients with an ejection fraction ≥30%. This study, therefore, suggested that the major utility of electrophysiological testing may be restricted to patients having an **ejection fraction between 30% and 40%**.[74] The prognostic significance of VT inducibility appears to be similar to that of VT induced by one, two, or three extrastimuli.[75] These results should be considered in the context of evidence from analysis of stored ICD data that have shown that there is little association between spontaneous and induced ventricular arrhythmias.[76] Furthermore, in these early studies, the use of beta blockers was suboptimal. There has been some recent evidence that programmed stimulation performed early (9 days) after MI in patients with LVEF ≤40% might identify patients at high risk for arrhythmic death.[77]

In the ischaemic patient with relatively preserved left ventricular function (LVEF >40%), the role of PES is not established. Inducible monomorphic VT, however, indicates consideration of catheter ablation and, if needed, ICD while inducibility of VF may be a non-specific sign, especially if three extrastimuli are used.[78] However, further investigations for ischaemia, cardiomyopathies, or inherited channelopathies may be appropriate. The prognostic usefulness of programmed stimulation in patients with non-ischaemic dilated cardiomyopathy, including those with NSVT, remains controversial.[79,80] There has been some evidence that inducibility of ventricular arrhythmias,[81] and especially polymorphic VT or VF,[82] indicates increased likelihood of subsequent ICD therapies and might be considered as useful risk stratifier.

Inducible sustained monomorphic or polymorphic VT is an independent risk factor for subsequent events in patients with repaired tetralogy of Fallot[83] and sarcoidosis.[84]

Long-term therapy

It depends on the underlying substrate and mechanism of arrhythmia, and details are provided in the next section. General principles are:

- Management of any identifiable underlying disorder (i.e. heart failure, significant ischaemia, etc.) is essential. **Beta blockers, ACEIs, ARBs**, and **statins** have been shown in many studies to reduce mortality and sudden cardiac death.[85] **Antiplatelet therapy** in the SOLVD trial was also associated with reduced incidence of sudden cardiac death.[86] Although there has been evidence that omega-3 fatty acids may reduce life-threatening arrhythmic events, results have not been consistent.[87,88] Fatty acid supplementation currently has a Class IIb-B recommendation. Statins should be used in all patients with CAD. They do not reduce the risk of VTs or cardiac arrest but result in a 11% reduction in the risk of SCD, presumably by preventing coronary events.[89]
- **Smoking** is strongly discouraged, and abstinence from **alcohol** is recommended in cases where there is a suspected correlation between alcohol intake and ventricular arrhythmias.
- Correction of **hypokalaemia** and **hypomagnesaemia** are useful. Intravenous magnesium prolongs sinus node recovery time, reduces automaticity, and homogenizes transmural ventricular repolarization. It has been reported to be useful in preventing atrial fibrillation and ventricular arrhythmias after cardiac and thoracic surgery; in reducing the ventricular response in acute-onset atrial fibrillation, including for patients with Wolff–Parkinson–White syndrome; in the treatment of digoxin-induced supraventricular and ventricular arrhythmias, multifocal atrial tachycardia, and polymorphic ventricular tachycardia or ventricular fibrillation from drug overdoses. Intravenous magnesium is, however, not useful in monomorphic ventricular tachycardia and shock-resistant ventricular fibrillation.[90,91]
- With the exception of beta blockers, no currently available antiarrhythmic agent has been shown in randomized clinical trials to reduce mortality in patients with ventricular arrhythmias or to prevent sudden cardiac death in patients prone to arrhythmias.[92,93]

Implantable cardioverter-defibrillators (ICD) remain the only means to reduce mortality in patients prone to life-threatening ventricular arrhythmias (primary prevention) with clinical life-threatening ventricular arrhythmias (secondary prevention). The ACCF/AHA 2012 general indications for ICD are presented in Table 55.6. Additional indications in patients with heart failure, post-MI, cardiomyopathies, and genetic channelopathies are discussed in the relevant chapters.[94]

In general an ICD is indicated in:

- **Survivors of cardiac arrest due to VF or haemodynamically unstable sustained VT**
- **Structural heart disease and spontaneous sustained VT**
- **Syncope of undetermined origin with, haemodynamically significant sustained VT or VF induced at electrophysiological study**
- **Ischaemic (>40 days post-MI) or dilated cardiomyopathy and LVEF ≤35% and NYHA II/III**
- **Ischaemic (>40 days post-MI) cardiomyopathy and LVEF ≤30% and NYHA I**
- **Post-MI (>48 h) sustained VT/VF, not due to transient or reversible ischaemia, re-infarction, or metabolic abnormalities**
- **Post-MI (>40 days) LVEF <40%, NSVT, and inducible VF/VT**
- **Sustained VT and normal ventricular function, cardiomyopathies and risk factors for sudden death, and genetic channelopathies with syncope.**

Other indications in specific clinical settings are discussed under Clinical forms of VT.

- **Amiodarone with beta blockers** may be considered in patients who do not meet the criteria for an ICD. This combination is preferred to sotalol due to its proarrhythmic potential.[95] In patients with ICD, **sotalol** may be used for reduction of the number of shocks in the absence of severely depressed LV function.[96] **Celivarone**, a non-iodinated analogue of amioadarone, has also been promising in preventing ICD interventions.[97]
- **Catheter ablation** is indicated in bundle branch reentry and idiopathic VT. In other forms of VT, such as monomorphic VT or VT storm in ischaemic patients who already have an ICD, ablation (endocardial or epicardial) [98–103] may also reduce the number of ICD shocks (Table 55.7). In ischaemic patients, all inducible VT are ablated in 38–72% of them, with a procedure-related mortality of 0.5% and 12–50% recurrence rate within the next year.[1] In non-ischaemic patients, acute success in eliminating inducible VT is 55–89%, with VT recurrence of 16–63% and with the outcome depending on the underlying heart disease.[104] Compared with patients with non-ischaemic dilated cardiomyopathy, patients with arrhythmogenic RV cardiomyopathy had better outcomes and patients with sarcoidosis had worse outcomes.[104]

Clinical forms of ventricular arrhythmias

Premature ventricular beats and non-sustained VT in normal subjects

In asymptomatic, apparently healthy persons, Holter recordings in older studies have revealed a frequency of NSVT, ranging from 0 to 3%, but get more frequent with age. The prognostic significance of PVCs and NSVT in normal subjects is not established.[52] Recent data from the ARIC study, however, indicate that subjects with PVCs are significantly more likely to die from SCD, despite not having any known history of cardiovascular disease. This effect appears to be additive when APCs occur concurrently.[105] When detected during exercise, and especially at recovery, NSVT indicates increased cardiovascular mortality within the next decades.[106,107] In trained athletes, NSVT commonly occurs during ambulatory Holter electrocardiography[108] and is most probably benign when suppressed by exercise. NSVT in athletes without structural heart disease is considered part of the 'athlete's heart syndrome' and has no adverse prognostic significance, provided conditions, such as hypertrophic cardiomyopathy, early repolarization syndrome (J wave and/or QRS slurring), and other genetic channelopathies, are excluded (see Arrhythmias in athletes).

Therapy

Specific antiarrhythmic drug therapy is not indicated for PVCs or NSVT (Table 55.8 and Figure 55.8). In symptomatic cases, beta 1 selective blockers may be given. Catheter ablation may also be tried in drug-resistant, frequent monomorphic VPBs.[2]

Idiopathic VT

Idiopathic VT indicates VT that occurs in the absence of clinically apparent structural heart disease. Approximately two-thirds of idiopathic VT originate in the RV and the rest in the LV (Figure 55.9).

Ventricular outflow tract tachycardias

Idiopathic ventricular outflow arrhythmias usually present in the form of **repetitive uniform PVCs, repetitive monomorphic NSVT** (that usually disappears as the heart rate increases with exercise), and **paroxysmal sustained monomorphic VT** (that is usually exercise-provoked). They mainly (approximately 80%) arise in the Right ventricular outflow tract (RVOT), and rarely below it, and

Table 55.6 ACCF/AHA 2012 GL on device therapy

Indications for ICD	
Cardiac arrest due to VF or unstable VT and no reversible cause	I-A
Structural heart disease and spontaneous sustained VT (stable or unstable)	I-B
Syncope of undetermined origin with inducible hemodynamically significant sustained VT at EPS	I-B
Ischemic (>40 days post-MI) or nonischemic cardiomyopathy, LVEF≤35%, NYHA II/III	I-A
Ischemic cardiomyopathy, >40 days post-MI, LVEF≤30%, NYHA I	I-A
Non-sustained VT due to prior MI, LVEF <40% and inducible VF or sustained VT at EPS	I-B
Unexplained syncope, significant LV dysfunction, and nonischemic cardiomyopathy	IIa-C
Sustained VT and normal or near-normal LV function	IIa-C
HCM and one or more risk factors for SCD	IIa-C
ARVD/C and one or more risk factors for SCD	IIa-C
LQTS and syncope and/or sustained VT on beta blockers	IIa-C
Non hospitalized patients awaiting transplantation	IIa-C
Brugada syndrome and syncope or documented VT	IIa-C
CPVT and syncope and/or sustained VT on beta blockers	IIa-C
Cardiac sarcoidosis, giant cell myocarditis, or Chagas disease	IIa-C
Non-ischemic cardiomyopathy, LVEF≤35%, NYHA I	IIb-C
LQTS and risk factors for sudden death	IIb-C
Syncope and advanced structural heart disease	IIb-C
Familial cardiomyopathy associated with sudden death	IIb-C
LV noncompaction	IIb-C
ICD therapy is not indicated for patients who do not have a reasonable expectation of survival with an acceptable functional status for at least 1 year, even if they meet ICD implantation criteria specified in the Class I, IIa, and IIb recommendations above	III-C
Incessant VT or VF	III-C
Significant psychiatric illnesses that may be aggravated by implantation or preclude follow-up	III-C
NYHA IV patients with drug-refractory congestive heart failure who are not candidates for cardiac transplantation or CRT-D	III-C
Syncope of undetermined cause without inducible ventricular tachyarrhythmias and without structural heart disease	III-C
VF or VT amenable to surgical or catheter ablation (eg, atrial arrhythmias associated with the Wolff-Parkinson-White syndrome, RVOT or LVOT VT, idiopathic VT, or fascicular VT in the absence of structural heart disease).	III-C
Ventricular tachyarrhythmias due to a completely reversible disorder in the absence of structural heart disease (eg, electrolyte imbalance, drugs, or trauma)	III-B

2012 ACCF/AHA/HRS focused update incorporated into the ACCF/AHA/HRS 2008 guidelines for device-based therapy of cardiac rhythm abnormalities. *J Am Coll Cardiol*. 2013; **61**:e6–75.

10–15% from the LVOT and are, most probably, due to triggered activity secondary to cAMP-mediated delayed afterdepolarizations.[6] Defects of connexins (proteins involved in cell-to-cell connections) may also be responsible.[109] Inducibility of sustained monomorphic VT (adenosine-sensitive) is possible with concomitant administration of isoprenaline in <50% of the cases of outflow tract tachycardias. **Right ventricular outflow tract (RVOT)** tachycardias produce a LBBB pattern with inferior axis and R/S transition at or beyond V_3. R/S transmission beyond V_4 and notching in the inferior leads indicates a free wall, rather than septal site, of origin, and a positive R wave in lead I posterior, rather than anterior, septal and free wall sites.[110] **Left ventricular outflow tract (LVOT)** tachycardias may produce a RBBB morphology with inferior axis and R/S transition at V_1 or V_2 due to the more posterior location of LVOT compared to RVOT.[111] If the R/S transition is in V_3, the tachycardia may originate from either the RVOT (usually) or the LVOT. A V_2 transition ratio ≥0.60 predicts LVOT origin.[112] This is calculated by measuring R wave (initial deflection to intersection of the isoelectric line) and S wave (lowest point to isoelectric line) durations in ms during VT and SR: $(R/R + S)_{VT}$ divided by $R/R + S)_{SR}$.

Ventricular outflow tract tachycardias originating above the semilunar valves usually arise at the coronary cusps.[110] They have a variable QRS morphology, depending on the site of origin: tachycardias originating in the **left coronary cusp** have a QRS morphology consistent with an M or a W pattern in lead V_1; tachycardias originating in the **right coronary cusp** or the **left ventricular side of the septum** may have an LBBB pattern; and tachycardias arising from the commissure between the left and right

Table 55.7 EHRA/HRS 2009 expert consensus on catheter ablation of ventricular arrhythmias. Indications for catheter ablation of ventricular tachycardia

Patients with structural heart disease (including prior MI, dilated cardiomyopathy, ARVC/D)
Catheter ablation of VT is recommended
For symptomatic sustained monomorphic VT (SMVT), including VT terminated by an ICD, that recurs despite antiarrhythmic drug therapy or when antiarrhythmic drugs are not tolerated or not desired*
For control of incessant SMVT or VT storm that is not due to a transient reversible cause
For patients with frequent PVCs, NSVTs, or VT that are presumed to cause ventricular dysfunction
For bundle branch reentrant or interfascicular VTs
For recurrent sustained polymorphic VT and VF that is refractory to antiarrhythmic therapy when there is a suspected trigger that can be targeted for ablation
Catheter ablation should be considered
In patients who have one or more episodes of SMVT despite therapy with one of more class I or III antiarrhythmic drugs*
In patients with recurrent SMVT due to prior MI who have LV ejection fraction >0.30 and expectation for 1 year of survival and is an acceptable alternative to amiodarone therapy*
In patients with haemodynamically tolerated SMVT due to prior MI who have reasonably preserved LV ejection fraction (>0.35), even if they have not failed antiarrhythmic drug therapy*
Patients without structural heart disease
Catheter ablation of VT is recommended for patients with idiopathic VT
For monomorphic VT that is causing severe symptoms
For monomorphic VT when antiarrhythmic drugs are not effective, not tolerated, or not desired
For recurrent sustained polymorphic VT and VF (electrical storm) that is refractory to antiarrhythmic theraphy when there is a suspected trigger that can be targeted for ablation
VT catheter ablation is contraindicated
In the presence of a mobile ventricular thrombus (epicardial ablation may be considered)
For asymptomatic PVCs and/or NSVT that are not suspected of causing or contributing to ventricular dysfunction
For VT due to transient, reversible causes, such as acute ischaemia, hyperkalaemia, or drug-induced torsade de pointes

* This recommendation for ablation stands, regardless of whether VT is stable or unstable or multiple VTs are present.
ARVC/D, arrhythmogenic right ventricular cardiomyopathy/dysplasia; ICD, implantable cardioverter-defibrillator; MI, myocardial infarction; VT, ventricular tachycardia; VF, ventricular fibrillation.

EHRA/HRS Expert Consensus on Catheter Ablation of Ventricular Arrhythmias. *Europace*. 2009;**11**:771–817.

cusps display a QS morphology in lead V_1, with notching on the downward deflection and precordial transition in V_3. LBBB morphology with an R wave in V_1 and large R waves in the inferior leads suggests the pulmonary artery as site of origin. Catheter ablation is the treatment of choice. Rarely (<10%), there can also be an **epicardial** site of origin (prominent r in V_1, delayed QRS onset to maximal deflection interval).[113,114]

Fascicular tachycardias

Idiopathic left ventricular tachycardias may also be due to reentry within the Purkinje network; they are verapamil- (but not adenosine-) sensitive and may originate within one of the fascicles of the left bundle branch. Usually, the posterior fascicle is involved, resulting in a tachycardia with RBBB and left axis deviation (90%), but cases with inferior axis due to anterior or high septal fascicular origin may also occur.[10,115]

Other sites of origin

Tachycardias may also originate in the **AV annuli**, either in the tricuspid (LBBB pattern) or the mitral annulus (RBBB pattern or RS in V_1 and monophasic R or RS in V_2–V_6). Tachycardias from the **papillary muscles** have a focal (no reentrant) mechanism not involving the Purkinje network but, usually, the posterior papillary muscle, and present with RBBB morphology. Tachycardias may also originate around the **His bundle** or in the **intraventricular septum** (LBBB with inferior axis).[116]

Prognosis and therapy

NSVT originating from the RVOT may occasionally cause syncope, although the risk of death is very low. However, malignant ventricular arrhythmias and sudden death may occur in patients with RVOT ectopic activity.[117–119] Short cycle length during NSVT and history of syncope have

Table 55.8 Specific management of NSVT

Clinical setting	Investigations	Therapy
Idiopathic NSVT	EP testing differentiates from ARVC	Beta blockers, calcium channel blockers; RF ablation if inducible sustained VT, progressively reduced LVEF, or symptoms
Arrhythmogenic ventricular cardiomyopathy	Value of EP testing not established NSVT indicates intermediate arrhythmic risk (<2% per year)	Not established. Perhaps amiodarone or sotalol; ICD frequently considered
Hypertension, valve disease	No need for specific management	Optimal antihypertensive therapy, including beta blockers
Non-STE ACS, NSVT >48 h after admission	Meticulous ischaemia testing	Revascularization and optimal medical therapy[1]
Acute MI, NSVT >24 h till predischarge	Routine for acute MI	Revascularization and optimal medical therapy
Previous MI with LVEF = 31–40%	Ischaemia testing, EP testing[2]	Revascularization and optimal medical therapy. If EP-inducible monomorphic VT or VF[3]: ICD[4]
Previous MI with LVEF ≤30% or LVEF ≤35% and NYHA II/III	Ischaemia testing. No EP needed [2]	Revascularization and optimal medical therapy ICD[4]
Asymptomatic CAD with EF >40%	Ischaemia testing	Revascularization and optimal medical therapy. No need for specific NSVT therapy
Syncope in CAD with EF >40%	Ischaemia testing, EP testing [2]	Revascularization and optimal medical therapy. If EP-inducible monomorphic VT or VF[3]: ICD
Non-ischaemic dilated cardiomyopathy	Value of EP testing not established	Optimal CCF therapy (medical and CRT if indicated). Ablation for bundle branch reentry. ICD for syncope or LVEF ≤30–35% and NYHA II/III
Hypertrophic cardiomyopathy	Evaluate additional risk factors:	Beta blockers, ICD, especially with frequent and prolonged (>10 beats) episodes of NSVT
	- Previous cardiac arrest	
	- Unexplained syncope	
	- Massive LV hypertrophy (≥30 mm)	
	- Hypotensive or attenuated blood pressure response to upright exercise	
Congenital heart disease (usually repaired Fallot)	EP testing	Predictive value of NSVT not established. Consider corrective surgery. If VT inducible: ablation and ICD
Long QT syndrome	Genotype analysis useful	Beta blockers, ICD if syncope despite beta blockers
Cathecholaminergic polymorphic VT	Value of EP testing not established	Beta blockers and perhaps calcium channel blockers. ICD if cardiac arrest
Brugada syndrome	Value of EP testing disputed	Possibly quinidine (more data needed). ICD if cardiac arrest

[1] Optimal medical therapy for NSVT in the setting of coronary artery disease is defined as administration of beta blockers (essential, unless absolutely contraindicated), aspirin, statins, and angiotensin-converting enzyme inhibitors or angiotensin receptor blockers.

[2] If conditions remain the same after indicated revascularization.

[3] Prognostic significance of inducible monomorphic VT induced by three extrastimuli is similar to that of VT induced by one or two extrastimuli. Monomorphic VT, as opposed to VF, usually does not respond to revascularization. VF induced by three extrastimuli may represent a non-specific response.

[4] ICD is recommended if indications exist at least 40 days after MI.

EP, electrophysiology study; ARVC, arrhythmogenic right ventricular cardiomyopathy; non-STE ACS, non-ST elevation acute coronary syndrome (non-STEMI or unstable angina); MI, myocardial infarction; LVEF, left ventricular ejection fraction; ICD, implantable cardioverter-defibrillator; CAD, coronary artery disease; CCF, congestive cardiac failure; CRT, cardiac resynchronization therapy.

Katritsis D, *et al.* Non-sustained ventricular tachycardia. *JACC* 2012;**60**:1993–2004

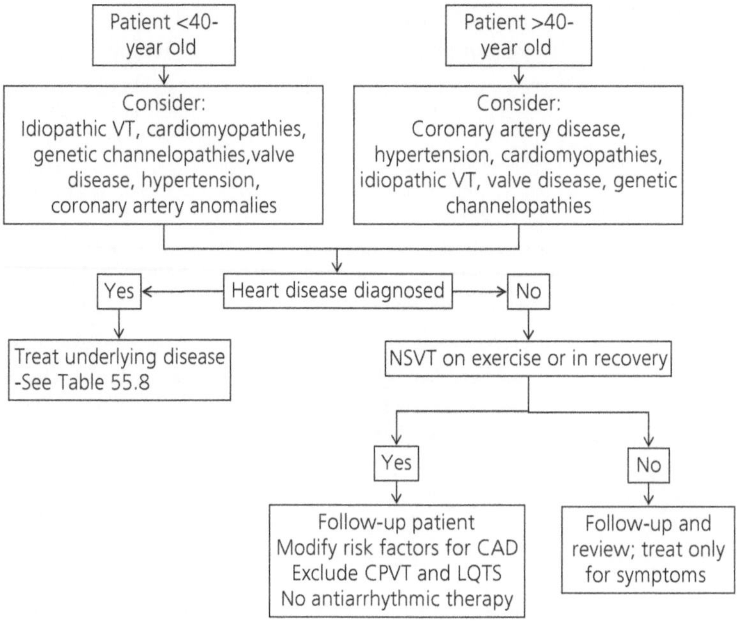

Figure 55.8 Clinical approach to the patient with NSVT.

CAD, coronary artery disease; CPVT, catecholaminergic polymorphic ventricular tachycardia; LQTS, long QT syndromes.
Katritsis D, *et al*. Non-sustained ventricular tachycardia. *JACC* 2012;**60**:1993–2004.

been proposed as predictors of coexistence of VF or polymorphic VT.[120]

Differentiation from ARVD (see Cardiomyopathies) is crucial, especially since, rarely, idiopathic VT may arise in the RV body, and subjects with RVOT VT may have subtle structural and functional abnormalities of the RVOT, as detected by magnetic resonance imaging.[121] QRS duration in lead I of >120 ms, earliest onset QRS in lead V_1, QRS notching, and a transition of V_5 predict the presence of ARVC (Figure 55.10).[122] The developed electrocardiographic scoring system to distinguish between idiopathic and ARVC VT,[123] is presentined in Table 38.3 of Chapter 38 on ARVC.

Catheter ablation is the treatment of choice for idiopathic VT, with success rates exceeding 80% for RVOT VT, and fascicular tachycardias (Table 55.9). Catheter ablation of tachycardias from the papillary muscles may be difficult due to the contraction of the muscle whereas success rates are lower with epicardial or intraseptal sites. There is no associated mortality, but there is a 1.7% risk of tamponade or pericardial effusion.[124,125] Calcium channel blockers and beta blockers may also be considered.

Ischaemic heart disease

Non-ST elevation acute coronary syndromes

Non-sustained VT is detected in 18–25% of patients 2 to 9 days after admission, and even short episodes of VT, lasting 4 to 7 beats, are independently associated with the risk of SCD over the subsequent year, especially when associated with myocardial ischaemia.[54] Earlier episodes within 48 hours after admission do not carry the same risk. In the EARLY ACS trial, the cumulative incidence of sustained VT/VF is 1.5%, with 60% of them occurring >48 h after enrollment.[126] Both early and late sustained VT/VF are associated with increased risk of death, even after adjustment for revascularization and LV function.[126] Appropriate revascularization as well as monitoring beyond 48 h are probably indicated in this setting.

Acute myocardial infarction

NSVT occurs in up to 75% of reperfused patients and, during the first 13[127] to 24 hours,[128] does not carry a prognostic significance. In-hospital NSVT following this period indicates increased in-hospital mortality. However, in patients who had a prior myocardial infarction treated with reperfusion and beta blockers, NSVT is not an independent predictor of long-term mortality when other covariates, such as left ventricular ejection fraction, are taken into account.[52]

Accelerated idioventricular rhythm, which characteristically follows myocardial infarction, tends to remain stable and usually does not give rise to ventricular fibrillation and does not require antiarrhythmic treatment.

Ventricular fibrillation during the acute phase (up to 48 h) indicates a high in-hospital mortality, but survivors do not have adverse prognosis.[129]

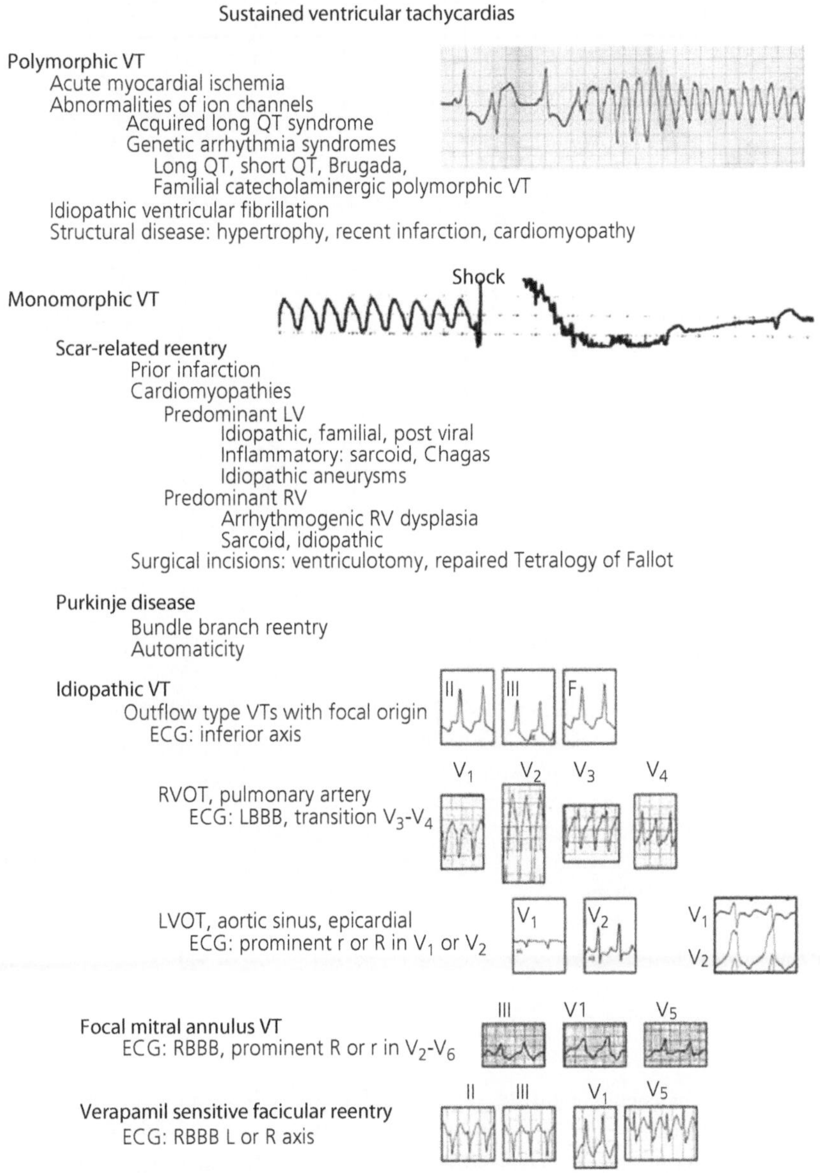

Sustained ventricular tachycardias
Polymorphic VT
Acute myocardial ischemia
Abnormalities of ion channels
Acquired long QT syndrome
Genetic arrhythmia syndromes
Long QT, short QT, Brugada,
Familial catecholaminergic polymorphic VT
Idiopathic ventricular fibrillation
Structural disease: hypertrophy, recent infarction, cardiomyopathy
Monomorphic VT
Shock
Scar-related reentry
Prior infarction
Cardiomyopathies
Predominant LV
Idiopathic, familial, post viral
Inflammatory: sarcoid, Chagas
Idiopathic aneurysms
Predominant RV
Arrhythmogenic RV dysplasia
Sarcoid, idiopathic
Surgical incisions: ventriculotomy, repaired Tetralogy of Fallot
Purkinje disease
Bundle branch reentry
Automaticity
Idiopathic VT
Outflow type VTs with focal origin
ECG: inferior axis
II
III
F
RVOT, pulmonary artery
ECG: LBBB, transition V3-V4
V1
V2
V3
V4
LVOT, aortic sinus, epicardial
ECG: prominent r or R in V1 or V2
V1
V2
Focal mitral annulus VT
ECG: RBBB, prominent R or r in V2-V6
III
V1
V5
Verapamil sensitive facicular reentry
ECG: RBBB L or R axis
II
III
V1
V5

Figure 55.9 ECG types of VT and most common causes are shown with characteristic ECG features of selected VTs.

Stevenson, W. G., Soejima K. Catheter ablation for ventricular tachycardia. *Circulation* 2007;**115**:2750–2760.

Sustained monomorphic VT indicates pre-existing scar.

Therapy Frequent VPBs and NSVT do not require antiarrhythmic drug therapy in the setting of an acute coronary syndrome. Electrolyte correction and oral beta blockers are useful.

Chronic IHD

Compared with the pre-reperfusion era, late ventricular tachyarrhythmias are now less common, but they are still documented in approximately 20% of patients with recent MI (more than 7 days) and EF <0.40 within the next 2 years.[49]

NSVT after discharge from MI, in the era of reperfusion and use of beta blockers, is not be an independent predictor of mortality, especially after ejection fraction is taken into account.[52] It may carry an adverse prognostic significance in patients with LVEF >35%.[53]

Monomorphic VT is usually due to scar-related reentry, and its incidence has been reduced from 3% to 1–2% in

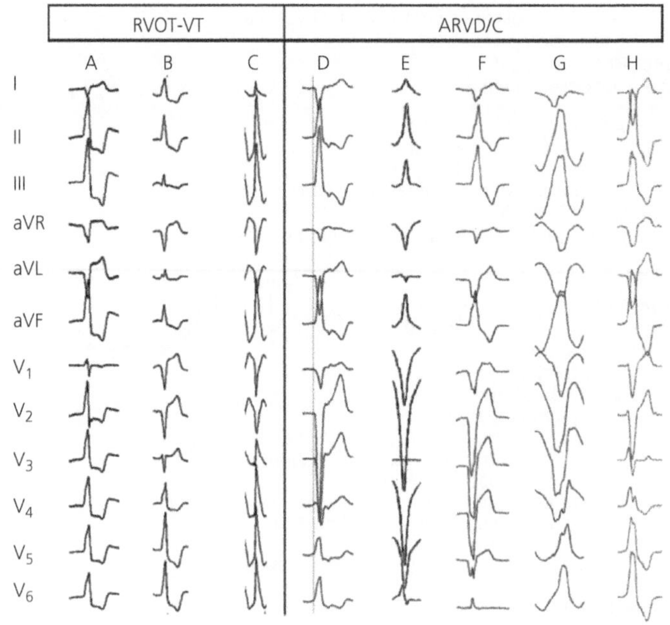

Figure 55.10 Differentiation between RVOT VT and ARVC. Twelve-lead electrocardiograms from patients with right ventricular outflow tract tachycardia (RVOT VT) (A to C) and arrhythmogenic right ventricular dysplasia/cardiomyopathy (ARVD/C) (D to H), showing characteristic features. (A) RVOT VT from an anterior septal location, showing precordial transition at V_2 and narrow QRS duration in lead I (78 ms). (B) RVOT VT originating superior to His bundle region, showing precordial transition at V_4, positive R wave in aVL, and narrow QRS in lead I (86 ms). (C) RVOT VT from a posterior septal location, showing precordial transition at V_3 and narrow QRS duration in lead I (118 ms). (D) ARVD/C ventricular tachycardia (VT), showing late precordial transition V_5, wide QRS duration in lead I (124 ms), and earliest onset QRS in V_1 (vertical line). (E) ARVD/C VT shows very late precordial transition in V_6 and wide QRS duration in lead I (126 ms). (F) ARVD/C VT shows very late precordial transition V_6 and wide QRS duration in lead I (150 ms). (G) ARVD/C VT shows late precordial transition in V_5, wide QRS duration in lead I (160 ms), and notching of the QRS (II, III, aVF, V_4 to V_6). (H) ARVD/C VT shows wide QRS duration in lead I (128 ms) and notching of the QRS (II, III, aVF, V_4 to V_6).

Hoffmayer KS, *et al*. Electrocardiographic comparison of ventricular arrhythmias in patients with arrhythmogenic right ventricular cardiomyopathy and right ventricular outflow tract tachycardia. *J Am Coll Cardiol*. 2011;**58**:831–8.

the reperfusion era. The QRS morphology during tachycardia may show either RBBB (origin of VT in the LV) or LBBB pattern (RV or septal origin) or may even be non-specific. Both RBBB and LBBB patterns can be seen in the same patient when the infarct scar involves the interventricular septum. Axis depends on the site of origin (apical origin has a superior axis while basal origin results in inferior axis) and may be 'undetermined'. Several algorithms have been published for identification of the exit site of post-infarction VT from the 12-lead ECG (Figure 55.11).[130]

Polymorphic VT or VF may be due to acute ischaemia (acute coronary syndrome or spasm) or in the context of scar-related VT that degenerates into VF (Figure 55.9).[21,44]

Therapy Monomorphic VT usually does not respond to revascularization.[131] Polymorphic VT or VF may, or may not, respond to revascularization (Table 55.10), and reassessment by means of LVEF and EPS if LVEF >35% is indicated 3 months after revascularization. [132,133] New-onset ventricular arrhythmias, especially VF occurring after the first 48 h of cardiac surery, are associated with increased long-term mortality, especially in older patients with reduced LV function.[134] Flecainide[57] and sotalol[95] increase mortality whereas amiodarone shows a trend towards reducing arrhythmia episodes but without significantly affecting total mortality (EMIAT and CAMIAT studies)[135,136] or even showing a trend towards increasing it.[137] Therefore, no antiarrhythmic drug is suitable for primary prevention of cardiac death, with exception for beta blockers which have been shown, in several studies, to reduce total and cardiac mortality in post-infarction patients, at least during the first year post-MI.[138]

Certain patients with NSVT, in the context of reduced LV function, need an ICD. In the MADIT study[139] on 196

Table 55.9 ACC/AHA/ESC 2006 GL on VA

Idiopathic ventricular tachycardia	
Catheter ablation in patients with structurally normal hearts with symptomatic, drug-refractory VT arising from the RV or LV or in those who are drug-intolerant or who do not desire long-term drug therapy.	I-C
EP testing in patients with structurally normal hearts with palpitations or suspected outflow tract VT.	IIa-B
Beta blockers and/or calcium channel blockers (and/or IC agents in RVOT VT) in patients with structurally normal hearts with symptomatic VT arising from the RV.	IIa-C
ICD implantation for sustained VT in patients with normal or near-normal ventricular function.	IIa-C

ACC/AHA ESC 2006 Guidelines for Management of Patients With Ventricular Arrhythmias and the Prevention of Sudden Cardiac Death. *Circulation*. 2006;**114**:e385–484.

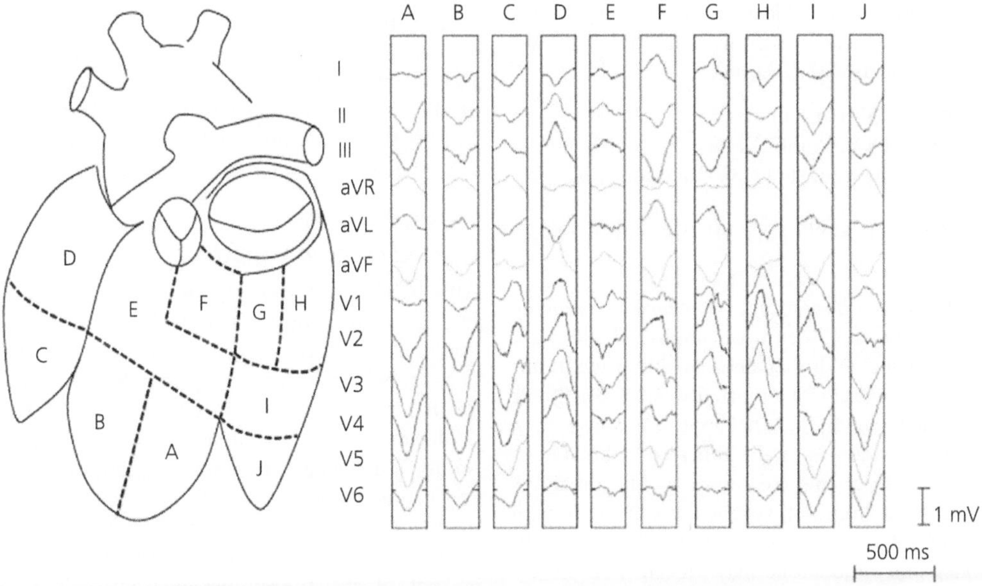

Figure 55.11 Localization of origin of post-infarct VT from the 12-lead ECG. Cardiac sections (left panel) and corresponding ECGs (right panel).

Yokokawa M, *et al.* Intramural idiopathic ventricular arrhythmias originating in the intraventricular septum: mapping and ablation. *Circ Arrhythm Electrophysiol*. 2012;**5**:258–63.

patients with prior MI, EF ≤35%, a documented episode of NSVT, and inducible and non-suppressible sustained VT, ICD yielded a 54% reduction in total mortality compared to conventional (mainly amiodarone) therapy during mean 27-month follow-up. The MUSTT enrolled 704 patients with coronary artery disease, asymptomatic NSVT, EF ≤40%, and inducible sustained VT.[140] The risk of cardiac arrest or death from arrhythmia among patients who received treatment with ICD was significantly lower than that among patients who did not receive ICDs (relative risk, 0.24; 95% confidence interval, 0.13–0.45; p <0.001). Subsequently, in the MADIT II on 1232 post-infarction patients with markedly depressed LV function (LVEF ≤30%), ICD resulted in 26% reduction of mortality over an 8-year follow-up, regardless of presence or absence of other risk stratifiers, including NSVT.[141] ICDs should be considered at least 40 days after MI in order to achieve reduction of total mortality (DINAMIT and IRIS studies)[142,143] and ≥3 months from a coronary revascularization procedure.[144] According to most published data, patients with a recent myocardial infarction do not benefit from ICD, especially when they have LVEF <25% and/or wide QRS,[145] but this is debatable.[146] However, both DINAMIT and IRIS had excluded patients with sustained ventricular arrhythmias during this period, and sudden cardiac death was reduced, despite no effect on overall mortality in the DINAMIT trial.[142] The recent ACC/AHA 2013 GL on STEMI now recommend ICD implantation in patients who develop sustained VT/VF more than 48 hours after STEMI, provided the arrhythmia is not due to transient or reversible ischaemia, re-infarction, or metabolic abnormalities (I-B).[147] Patients with an initially reduced LVEF who are possible candidates for ICD therapy should undergo re-evaluation of LVEF ≥40 days after discharge.[147] There has also been some evidence for a benefit of early ICD implantation if sustained monomorphic VT (CL ≥200 ms, lasting more than 10 s) is induced at electrophysiology study 9 days post-MI.[77] In addition, if new-onset VF occurs >48 h after cardiac surgery and no reversible cause can be found, ICD implantation may be considered earlier.[134] There have been concerns about the efficacy of ICD in women and the elderly.[148]

Other indications for **ICD implantation** in post-MI patients are presented in Table 55.5. In summary, ICD is indicated in patients who present with monomorphic VT or VF and for patients with IHD and:

- LVEF <30% and NYHA I, or
- LVEF <35% and NYHA II or III, or
- LVEF <40% in the context of NSVT and inducible VT at EPS, or
- Sustained VT/VF, >48 h after MI, and not due to a treatable cause.

Catheter ablation is also useful by means of reducing ICD discharges and can be now accomplished with electroanatomical mapping during sinus rhythm, even in unmappable tachycardias, with a mortality of 0.4–3% (Table 55.6).[101–103] Usually, an endocardial approach is necessary, and epicardial ablation is rarely indicated,[149] but recurrences in post-MI patients are common. Epicardial VT usually have delayed onset of ventricular activation, with a pseudodelta >34 ms and an RS >121 ms.[150] Alternatively, beta blockers and amiodarone may prevent ICD shocks and are more effective than sotalol in this respect but with a higher rate of complications.[96]

Heart failure

In patients with heart failure and LVEF <30–40%, the reported prevalence of NSVT is 30–80%.[52] Although the GESICA-GEMA investigators identified NSVT as an independent predictor of total mortality in patients with heart failure (35–40% IHD) and LVEF ≤35%,[151] in the CHF-STAT (70–75% IHD), after adjusting other variables and especially for LVEF, NSVT was not an independent predictor of sudden death or total mortality in patients with heart failure and LVEF <35-50%. [152] Similar results were published by the PROMISE investigators.[153] Only during the recovery period after exercise, frequent ventricular ectopy has been found to carry an adverse prognostic significance in patients with heart failure.[154] However, in a recent analysis of ICD interrogation data in the SCD-HeFT population, long runs of rapid rate NSVT were associated with subsequent appropriate ICD shocks and an increase in mortality.[155]

Therapy

In patients with heart failure (LVEF <35%), the GESICA study (516 patients of whom 75% with DCM) found **amiodarone** beneficial by means of reducing mortality and hospital admissions.[156] However, the much larger SCD-HeFT (2521 patienst, 52% ischaemic) indicated substantial benefit from ICD therapy in patients with low EF (<36%) and NYHA classes II and III. ICD therapy was associated with a decreased risk of death of 23% and an absolute decrease in mortality of 7.2 percentage points after 5 years in the overall population.[40] Dronedarone is detrimental in heart failure patients.[157] There has been some evidence (MADIT-CRT) that ventricular resynchronization may reduce episodes of VT or VF in patients who respond to it whereas non-responders may have a higher event rate.[158] LVEF values and QRS duration do not appear to directly modify the survival benefit of ICD in patients with baseline LVEF <35%.[145] Recommendations for ICD implantation are provided in Chapter 31 on heart failure.

Cardiomyopathies

Dilated cardiomyopathy

Although VT or VF are the most common cause of death in dilated cardiomyopathy (DCM), other causes, such as bradycardia, electromechanical dissociation, and pulmonary embolus account for up to 50% of sudden cardiac death in patients with advanced heart failure.[1,2] **NSVT** may be detected in 40–50% of patients with DCM, but results on its independent prognostic significance have been conflicting. LVEF and NSVT have been found significant predictors of arrhythmic events,[159] but, after medical stabilization with angiotensin-converting enzyme inhibitor and beta blocker, the number and length of NSVT runs did not increase the risk of MVA in patients with LVEF ≤0.35, as opposed to those with with LVEF >0.35.[160] In the Marburg Cardiomyopathy Study,[41] on univariate analysis, non-sustained VT and frequent ventricular premature beats showed a significant association with a higher arrhythmia risk, but, on multivariate analysis, only LVEF was found to be a significant predictor of major arrhythmic events. The combination of LVEF ≤30% and NSVT denoted an 8-fold higher risk for subsequent arrhythmic events, compared to LVEF ≤30% and no NSVT. There was a tendency for an increased risk of major arrhythmic events for patients without beta blockers. Signal-averaged ECG, baroreflex sensitivity, heart rate variability, and T wave alternans were not helpful for arrhythmia risk stratification.

The value of EP testing is debatable and is no longer recommended in this setting.[2] However, it may be useful in inducing a monomorphic VT that could be amenable to catheter ablation and as a risk stratifier since inducibility of ventricular arrhythmias,[81] and especially polymorphic VT or VF,[82] indicates increased likelihood of subsequent ICD therapies. In approximately one-third of the cases of idiopathic dilated cardiomyopathy, and probably in a small percentage of ischaemic patients, VT is due to **bundle branch reentry**.[161] Bundle branch reentrant tachycardia may also occur in patients with intraventricular conduction defects as well as in the absence of any myocardial or valvular abnormality.[162] Although these tachycardias are usually unstable, the 12-lead ECG, when obtainable, may show either LBBB or RBBB pattern, depending on the orientation of activation of the bundle branches. The majority of VT in non-ischaemic cardiomyopathy arises near the superior and lateral perivalvular aortic and mitral regions, and many of them are epicardial in origin. Criteria for epicardial VTs are a q wave in lead 1, but not in inferior leads, and delayed onset and decline of the ventricular activation in precordial leads.[163]

Therapy

Catheter ablation is the treatment of choice in bundle branch reentry.

The role of ICD for primary prevention in DCM is controversial. There was significant reduction of sudden death and a trend for reduced mortality with ICD in patients with non-ischaemic heart failure and non-sustained VT (DEFINITE),[164] but these results were not reproduced in the AMIOVIRT study,[165] that failed to detect any difference between amiodarone and ICD in patients with DCM and NSVT, or the CAT study,[166] that reported no difference between ICD and controls in DCM. The value of amiodarone is controversial. Current indications for ICD are provided in Chapter 31 on heart failure.

Hypertrophic cardiomyopathy

In hypertrophic cardiomyopathy, 20 to 30% of patients may have **NSVT**.[52] Frequent and prolonged (>10 beats) episodes of non-sustained VT on Holter, as opposed to rare, brief episodes, indicate an increased risk of sudden death in HOCM, especially in young patients (<30 years).[55,167] Mortality rate is approximately 1% annually, with events usually occurring without warning, largely in asymptomatic or mildly symptomatic young patients, with no difference according to gender.[168] Risk stratification and indications for ICD are discussed in Chapter 36. Amiodarone has no longer a role.

Arrhythmogenic right ventricular cardiomyopathy

Diagnosis and treatment of this condition are discussed in Chapter 38. The main problem is with ARVD-associated VT that presents with inferior axis; in this case, the differential diagnosis with idiopathic VT is of clinical importance. Asymptomatic patients with ARVD and NSVT have a trend for an increased arrhythmic risk and a rate of appropriate ICD intervention of 3.7% per year.[169] Syncope predicts life-threatening ventricular arrhythmia, and EPS has low predictive accuracy for future arrhythmic events.[169]

Other cardiomyopathies

The association between infiltrative cardiomyopathies and ventricular arrhythmias and sudden death is well documented. Specific conditions are discussed in Chapter 37 on cardiomyopathies. Complex ventricular arrhythmias are common in **amyloidosis** (57% of patients have PVCs and 18% NSVT) and carry prognostic significance.[170] Cardiac **sarcoidosis** may present with non-sustained polymorphic or monomorphic VT that usually responds to steroids. Spontaneous development or EPS induction of sustained monomorphic VT is an ominous sign, and ICD may be indicated.[84] Patients with **Chagas' cardiomyopathy**, presenting with either sustained VT or NSVT, have a major risk for mortality in the presence of moderate LV systolic dysfunction (LVEF <40%).[171]

Congenital heart disease

The congenital heart defects that have been associated with the greatest risks of late sudden death are tetralogy of Fallot, D- and L-transposition of the great arteries, aortic stenosis, and functional single ventricle.[2] Ventricular extrasystolic activity can be detected with Holter monitoring in up to 50% of patients with **repaired tetralogy of Fallot**, and recent studies have detected 4 to 14% prevalence of sustained ventricular tachycardia.[83,172,173] Recommenda-

Table 55.10 ACCF/AHA/ESC 2012 GL on device therapy

Indications for ICD in children, adolescents, and patients with congenital heart disease*	
ICD* in the survivor of cardiac arrest after evaluation to define the cause of the event and to exclude any reversible causes.	I-B
Patients with symptomatic sustained VT who have undergone hemodynamic and electrophysiological evaluation. Catheter ablation or surgical repair may offer possible alternatives in carefully selected patients.	I-C
Patients with recurrent syncope of undetermined origin in the presence of either ventricular dysfunction or inducible ventricular arrhythmias at electrophysiological study.	IIa-B
Patients with recurrent syncope, complex congenital heart disease and advanced systemic ventricular dysfunction when thorough invasive and noninvasive investigations have failed to find a cause.	IIb-C

* For patients who have reasonable expectation of survival with a good functional status >1 year.

2012 ACCF/AHA/HRS focused update incorporated into the ACCF/AHA/HRS 2008 guidelines for device-based therapy of cardiac rhythm abnormalities. *J Am Coll Cardiol*. 2013;**61**:e6–75.

tions for the management of patients with congenital heart disease are presented in Table 55.10.

Valvular disease

In patients with valvular disease, the incidence of non-sustained ventricular tachycardia is considerable (up to 25% in aortic stenosis and in significant mitral regurgitation) and appears to be a marker of underlying left ventricular pathology.[174] In mitral valve prolapse, although complex ventricular arrhythmias have been detected in patients who underwent Holter monitoring before sudden death, multivariate analysis failed to identify ventricular arrhythmias (as opposed to NYHA class, AF, and LVEF) as an independent predictor of sudden death.[175,176] Recommendations for management are provided in Table 55.11 and the relevant chapters on valve disease.

Hypertension

In patients with arterial hypertension, non-sustained ventricular tachycardia is correlated to the degree of cardiac hypertrophy and subendocardial fibrosis.[177] Approximately 12–28% of patients with hypertension and left ventricular hypertrophy present with non-sustained ventricular tachycardia as opposed to 8% of patients with hypertension alone.[178]

Other conditions

Acute myocarditis may be complicated by conduction disturbances or ventricular arrhythmias (see Chapter 44). Giant cell myocarditis is a cause of monomorphic or polymorphic VT that is usually sustained and associated with high mortality. Recommendations for patients with **myocarditis,** as well as for **rheumatic heart disease** or **endocarditis**, are presented in Table 55.12.

Cardiovascular causes account for at least 40% of deaths in patients with **end-stage renal failure**, and 20% of these are sudden.[2] Arrhythmias often occur during haemodialysis sessions and for at least 4 to 5 h afterward. During this period, haemodynamic status and fluctuations in electrolytes, especially potassium, magnesium, and calcium, are likely to play a crucial role in triggering events and should be monitored carefully. Risk factors predisposing to ventricular arrhythmias include LVH, hypertension, anaemia, LV dysfunction, and underlying CAD (Table 55.13).

Patients with **neuromuscular disorders** may present with ventricular arrhythmias or conduction defects. Permanent pacemaker insertion may be considered for progressive muscular dystrophies, such as myotonic muscular dystrophy type 1 (Steinert's disease), limb-girdle (Erb's) dystrophy, and Kearns–Sayre syndrome with any degree of AV block (including first-degree AV block) with or without symptoms, because there may be unpredictable progression of AV conduction disease (see Chapter 54). However, patients with myotonic muscular dystrophy type 1, as well as certain lamin A/C (LMNA—a cause of limb-girdle dystrophy) and desmin mutation carriers, may also need ICD backup due to malignant ventricular arrhythmias.[179,180] Patients with lamin A/C mututations are prone to ventricular arrhythmias when at least two of the following independent risk factors are present: non-sustained ventricular tachycar-

Table 55.11 ACC/AHA/ESC 2006 GL on VA

Valvular heart disease	
Patients with ventricular arrhythmias should be evaluated and treated following current recommendations for each disorder.	I-C
The effectiveness of mitral valve repair or replacement to reduce the risk of SCD in patients with mitral valve prolapse, severe mitral regurgitation, and serious ventricular arrhythmias is not well established.	IIb-C

ACC/AHA ESC 2006 Guidelines for Management of Patients With Ventricular Arrhythmias and the Prevention of Sudden Cardiac Death. *Circulation*. 2006;**114**:e385–484.

Table 55.12 ACC/AHA/ESC 2006 GL on VA

Myocarditis, rheumatic heart disease, or endocarditis	
Temporary pacemaker insertion in patients with symptomatic bradycardia and/or heart block during the acute phase of myocarditis.	I-C
Acute aortic regurgitation associated with VT should be treated surgically, unless otherwise contraindicated (level of evidence: C).	I-C
Acute endocarditis complicated by aortic or annular abscess and AV block should be treated surgically, unless otherwise contraindicated.	I-C
ICD* in patients with life-threatening ventricular arrhythmias who are not in the acute phase of myocarditis.	IIa-C
ICD* in cardiac sarcoidosis, giant cell myocarditis, or Chagas' disease	IIa-C
Antiarrhythmic therapy in patients with symptomatic NSVT or sustained VT during the acute phase of myocarditis.	IIa-C
ICD during the acute phase of myocarditis.	III-C

* For patients who are receiving chronic optimal medical therapy and who have reasonable expectation of survival with a good functional status >1 year.
ACC/AHA ESC 2006 Guidelines for Management of Patients With Ventricular Arrhythmias and the Prevention of Sudden Cardiac Death. *Circulation*. 2006;**114**:e385–484.

Table 55.13 ACC/AHA/ESC 2006 GL on VA

End-stage renal failure	
The acute management of ventricular arrhythmias in end-stage renal failure should immediately address haemodynamic status and electrolyte (potassium, magnesium, and calcium) imbalance.	I-C
Life-threatening ventricular arrhythmias, especially in patients awaiting renal transplantation, should be treated conventionally, including the use of ICD* and pacemaker as required.	I-C

* For patients who are receiving chronic optimal medical therapy and who have reasonable expectation of survival with a good functional status >1 year.
ACC/AHA ESC 2006 Guidelines for Management of Patients With Ventricular Arrhythmias and the Prevention of Sudden Cardiac Death. *Circulation*. 2006;**114**:e385–484.

Table 55.14 ACC/AHA/ESC 2006 GL on VA

Electrolyte disturbances	
Potassium (and magnesium) salts in treating ventricular arrhythmias secondary to hypokalaemia (or hypomagnesaemia) resulting from diuretic use in patients with structurally normal hearts.	I-B
Maintain serum potassium levels >4.0 mmol/L in any patient with documented life-threatening ventricular arrhythmias and a structurally normal heart.	IIa-C
Maintain serum potassium levels >4.0 mmol/L in patients with acute MI.	IIa-B
Magnesium salts in the management of VT secondary to digoxin toxicity in patients with structurally normal hearts.	IIa-B

ACC/AHA ESC 2006 Guidelines for Management of Patients With Ventricular Arrhythmias and the Prevention of Sudden Cardiac Death. *Circulation*. 2006;**114**:e385–484.

dia, ejection fraction <45%, male sex, and non-missense mutations. [181]

Electrolyte disorders

Rapid hyperkalaemia, hypokalaemia (<3.5 mM), and hypomagnesaemia are all associated with ventricular arrhythmias and SCD in patients with MI or even with structurally normal hearts (some of whom may have underlying channelopathies) .[2] Hypomagnesaemia is associated with polymorphic VT or torsades de pointes. Hypokalaemia, with or without hypomagnesaemia, may be responsible for ventricular arrhythmias in subjects with hypertension and congestive cardiac failure treated with thiazide and/or loop diuretics, acute starvation, acute alcohol toxicity/withdrawal, and those with ventricular arrhythmias associated with digoxin and other Vaughan Williams class 1 antiarrhythmic drugs.[182]

Changes in the extracellular ionic concentrations of calcium required to produce EP changes that may contribute to ventricular arrhythmias are not encountered in clinical practice. Significant **hypocalcaemia** can prolong the QT interval. Occasionally, hyperparathyroidism can cause important **elevations in serum calcium** concentrations. Intracellular fluctuations in calcium concentration influenced by drugs (e.g. digitalis glycosides), exercise (e.g. catecholamines), and reperfusion following myocardial ischaemia can trigger life-threatening arrhythmias. The protective effects of beta blockade in the latter settings may, in part, be due to the inhibition of calcium influx into myocytes.

Recommendations for management are provided in Table 55.14.

Drug-induced arrhythmias

With the exception of beta blockers, all antiarrhythmic drugs are proarrhythmic. In addition, drug interactions may also cause arrhythmia by means of intervening with metabolism and pharmacokinetics, such as inhibition of CYP3A4 that metabolizes certain drugs or impairment of renal function and drug excretion, and by combining drugs of similar proarrhythmic action that was not apparent when each drug was used alone (macrolides with QT-prolonging antiarrhythmics).

Drug-induced long QT syndrome

Marked QT prolongation, often accompanied by the development of torsades de pointes, occurs in ≥1% of patients receiving QT-prolonging antiarrhythmic drugs and, much more rarely, in patients receiving non-cardiac agents with QT-prolonging potential (<0.01 to 0.1%).[183] QTc prolongation is also associated with an increased risk of stroke, independent of traditional risk factors.[184] Fluoroquinolones that are currently on the market, for example, present a very low risk of drug-induced torsades de pointes, with a frequency of this adverse event occurring at a rate of approximately 0.2 to 2.7 per million prescriptions.[185] Recently, however, a small absolute increase in cardiovascular deaths, which was most pronounced among patients with a high baseline risk of cardiovascular disease, was detected during 5 days of azithromycin therapy (47–245 additional cardiovascular deaths per million courses),[186] and in March 2013 and FDA warning was published regarding the use of azithromycin for patients who are already at risk for cardiovascular events. However, in recent study on Danish national health care young and middle-aged adults, azithromycin use was not associated with an increased risk of death from cardiovascular causes compared to Penicillin V.[187] Antidepressants citalopram, escitalopram, and amitriptyline are associated with increased risk for modest QT prolongation, although the avsolute magnitude of these effects is modest. Selective serotonin reuptake inhibitors such as sertraline may be associated with less risk.[188] While many drugs have been associated with isolated cases of torsades de pointes, Table 55.15 lists those generally recognized as having QT-prolonging potential. An up-to-date list is maintained at http://www.torsades.org and http://www.qtdrugs.org. Patients with classic LQTS mutations, but normal or borderline QTc intervals, are generally much more susceptible to QTc-prolonging medications compared with the general population, yet they may be difficult to detect before drug exposure. Most clinically relevant drug-related QTc prolongation occurs via inhibition of IKr, a potassium current mediated in humans by the ion channel KCNH2 encoded by the human ether-a-go-go-related gene (HERG), analogous to the genetic LQT2 form of the disease. Risk amplifiers for QT prolongation include female gender, age, hypokalaemia, hypomagnesaemia, bradycardia, and the presence of underlying structural heart disease, particularly ventricular hypertrophy and congestive heart failure, and concomitant administration of drugs, such as ketoconazole that are inhibitors of the cytochrome P4504A4 (CYP3A4) that metabolizes other drugs that may prolong QT.[183] Most cases of drug-induced TdP occur in the setting of substantial prolongation of the QTc interval, typically to values >500 ms, although QTc alone is a relatively poor predictor of arrhythmic risk in any individual patient.[189,190]

In clinical practice, care should be taken when combining class III antiarrhythmic agents with other drugs that prolong the QT. After initiation of a drug associated with TdP, ECG signs indicative of risk for arrhythmia include:[191]

- An increase in QTc from pre-drug baseline of 60 ms
- Marked QTc interval prolongation >500 ms
- T-U wave distortion that becomes more exaggerated in the beat after a pause
- Visible (macroscopic) T wave alternans
- New-onset ventricular ectopy, couplets, and non-sustained polymorphic ventricular tachycardia initiated in the beat after a pause.

A reasonable strategy is to document the QTc interval before and at least every 8 to 12 hours after the initiation, increased dose, or overdose of QT-prolonging drugs. Management is presented in Tables 55.15 and 55.16.

Table 55.15 Drug-induced long QT

Antiarrhythmic drugs
Class I (quinidine, disopyramide, procainamide, ajmaline)
Class III (sotalol, ibutilide, dofetilide)
Psychiatric drugs
Antipsychotic agents (thioridazine, mesoridazine, droperidol, pimozide, chlorpromazine, haloperidol)
Tricyclic antidepressants (citalopram)
Antibiotics
Quinolones*
Macrolides (azithromycin, erythromycin, clarithromycin)
Pentamidine, halofantrine, chloroquine
Other drugs
Cisapride, ketanserin
Coronary vasodilators (bepridil)
Methadone, cocainearsenic intoxication, cocaine
Arsenic intoxication

*Sparfloxacin, the most potent, has been withdrawn from the market. Ciprofloxacin is the safest quinolone in this respect.
Among cardiac drugs, indapamide and amiodarone may cause mild QT prolongation.
The antihistamines astemizole and terfenadine have been withdrawn from the market.

Table 55.16 ACC/AHA/ESC 2006 GL on VA. Management of drug-induced long QT syndrome

Removal of the offending agent in patients with drug-induced LQTS.	I-A
IV magnesium sulfate for patients who take QT-prolonging drugs and present with few episodes of torsades de pointes in which the QT remains long.	IIa-B
Atrial or ventricular pacing or isoproterenol for patients taking QT-prolonging drugs who present with recurrent torsades de pointes (level of evidence: B).	IIa-B
Potassium ion repletion to 4.5–5 mmol/L for patients who take QT-prolonging drugs and present with few episodes of torsades de pointes in whom the QT remains long.	IIb-C

ACC/AHA ESC 2006 guidelines for management of patients with ventricular arrhythmias and the prevention of sudden cardiac death. *Circulation*. 2006; **114**:e385–484.

Digitalis toxicity

In mild cases, discontinuation of the drug and maintenance of normal potassium levels is enough. Management of severe cases is presented in Table 55.17.

Sodium channel blockers

They delay depolarization and thus slow conduction and prolong the QRS. In the presence of ischaemia or scar, this may result in reentrant arrhythmias. The use of flecainide or encainide in the CAST was associated with a 3.6-fold increase in the risk of fatal arrhythmias in post-MI patients.[56] Genetic factors, such as a SCN5A polymorphism, may play a role in determining susceptibility to these effects. In addition to slowing of conduction velocity, sodium channel blocking drugs may also selectively abbreviate epicardial action potential duration, resulting in a transmural gradient of repolarization, elevation of the ST segment, and reentry.[183] Non-antiarrhythmic agents with sodium channel properties are tricyclic antidepressants, phenytoin, local anaesthetic agents, and drugs used to treat neuropathic pain. Recently, nortriptyline was found to increase the risk for SCA in the general population, in the presence of genetic and/or non-genetic factors that block the cardiac sodium channel.[192]

5-fluorouracil

5-fluorouracil causes lethal and potentially fatal arrhythmias, irrespective of underlying coronary disease during the acute infusion period, the vast majority occurring during the first administration.[193] Arrhythmias induced by this drug are mostly ischaemic in origin and usually occur in the context of coronary spasm produced by this drug.[194] Cardiac monitoring during the infusion period, especially the first, is recommended for all patients receiving 5-fluorouracil therapy. Symptoms, with or without corresponding ECG changes compatible with cardiac ischaemia, should lead to an immediate discontinuation of the infusion.

Anthracycline (doxorubicin, amrubicin)

Cardiotoxicity is dose-dependent, with intermittent high doses and higher cumulative doses increasing the risk of cardiomyopathy and lethal arrhythmias (see also Chapter 30). Risk factors include younger age, female gender, and use of trastuzimab.[195] This form of cardiomyopathy can occur acutely soon after treatment, within a few months of treatment, or many years later. VT, as opposed to AF, is rare.[185,186]

Recommendations for **transient arrhythmias from reversible causes** are presented in Table 55.18.

Ventricular arrhythmias in athletes

Vigorous exertion increases the incidence of acute coronary events in those who did not exercise regularly whereas habitual physical activity reduces the overall risk of myocardial infarction and SCD. The risk of SCD among athletes appears to exceed the risk in comparably aged populations.[196] The major causes of SCD in athletes are HCM (36%), coronary artery anomalies (19%), ARVC, and myocarditis.[2,197] Marathons and half-marathons are associated with a low overall risk of cardiac arrest and sudden death. Cardiac arrest, most commonly attributable to hypertrophic cardiomyopathy or atherosclerotic coronary disease, occurs primarily among male marathon participants.[197] ECG and echocardiographic screening programmes can reduce the incidence of SCD in professional athletes, although differentiation between adaptive LV chamber enlargement from mild forms of cardiomyopathy may be impossible.[198] Electroanatomical mapping-guided endomyocardial biopsy may be useful in identifying athletes with ARVC or myocarditis.[199] Many athletes with ICDs can engage in vigorous and competitive sports without physical injury or failure to terminate the arrhythmia despite the occurrence of both inappropriate and appropriate shocks.[200]

Sinus bradycardia, junctional rhythm, and Wenckebach AV conduction are commonly seen with endurance

Table 55.17 ACC/AHA/ESC 2006 GL on VA

Digitalis toxicity	
Antidigitalis antibody in sustained ventricular arrhythmias, advanced AV block, and/or asystole that are considered due to digitalis toxicity.	I-A
Patients with mild cardiac toxicity (e.g. isolated ectopic beats only) can be managed effectively with recognition, continuous monitoring of cardiac rhythm, withdrawal of digitalis, restoration of normal electrolyte levels (including serum potassium >4 mmol/L), and oxygenation.	IIa-C
Magnesium or pacing for severe toxicity (sustained ventricular arrhythmias, advanced AV block, and/or asystole).	IIa-C
Dialysis for the management of hyperkalaemia for severe toxicity (sustained ventricular arrhythmias; advanced AV block, and/or asystole).	IIb-C
Lidocaine or phenytoin not recommended for severe digitalis toxicity (sustained ventricular arrhythmias, advanced AV block, and/or asystole).	III-C

ACC/AHA ESC 2006 guidelines for management of patients with ventricular arrhythmias and the prevention of sudden cardiac death. *Circulation*. 2006; **114**:e385–484.

Table 55.18 ACC/AHA/ESC 2006 GL on VA

Transient arrhythmias of reversible cause	
Myocardial revascularization, when appropriate, in patients experiencing cardiac arrest due to VF or polymorphic VT in the setting of acute ischaemia or MI.	I-C
Unless electrolyte abnormalities are proved to be the cause, survivors of cardiac arrest due to VF or polymorphic VT in whom electrolyte abnormalities are discovered, in general, should be evaluated and treated in a manner similar to that of cardiac arrest without electrolyte abnormalities.	I-C
Patients with sustained monomorphic VT should be evaluated and treated in a manner similar to that of patients with VT without electrolyte abnormalities or antiarrhythmic drugs present. Antiarrhythmic drugs or electrolyte abnormalities should not be assumed to be the sole cause of sustained monomorphic VT.	I-B
Patients with polymorphic VT, in association with prolonged QT interval due to antiarrhythmic medications or other drugs, should be advised to avoid exposure to all agents associated with QT prolongation. A list of such drugs can be found on the websites http://www.qtdrugs.org and http://www.torsades.org.	I-B

ACC/AHA ESC 2006 guidelines for management of patients with ventricular arrhythmias and the prevention of sudden cardiac death. *Circulation*. 2006; **114**:e385–484.

Table 55.19 ACC/AHA/ESC 2006 GL on VA

Athletes	
Pre-participation history and physical examination, including family history of premature or SCD, and specific evidence of cardiovascular diseases, such as cardiomyopathies and ion channel abnormalities.	I-C
Athletes presenting with rhythm disorders, structural heart disease, or other signs or symptoms suspicious for cardiovascular disorders should be evaluated as any other patient but with recognition of the potential uniqueness of their activity.	I-C
Athletes presenting with syncope should be carefully evaluated to uncover underlying cardiovascular disease or rhythm disorder.	I-B
Athletes with serious symptoms should cease competition while cardiovascular abnormalities are being fully evaluated.	I-C
Twelve-lead ECG and possibly echocardiography may be considered as pre-participation screening for heart disorders in athletes.	IIb-B

ACC/AHA ESC 2006 guidelines for management of patients with ventricular arrhythmias and the prevention of sudden cardiac death. *Circulation*. 2006; **114**:e385–484.

training. Athletes with non-sustained and asymptomatic exercise-induced ventricular arrhythmias may participate in low-intensity competitive sports, provided that no structural heart disease has been demonstrated. Athletic activity and high-level training strongly predispose to early repolarization, and the incidence of SCD is 1:43 000 per year.[201] A higher prevalence of J wave and/or QRS slurring (but not of ST elevation) has been found among athletes with cardiac arrest/sudden death than in controls.[202] Recommendations for disqualification from high-intensity sports have been published (Table 55.19).[203] See also Chapter 81 on athlete's heart on Miscellaneous Topics.

Ventricular arrhythmias in pregnancy

VT may be related to elevated cathecholamines; post-partum cardiomyopathy should be ruled out, especially if VT occurs during the last 6 weeks or in the early post-partum period.[204] In women with the congenital long QT syndrome, the risk of cardiac arrest is greater during the post-partum period compared with before or during pregnancy.[205] All antiarrhythmic drugs cross the placenta. Selective beta blockers may be used. There are some concerns about low weight for gestational age when used before the 6th week of pregnancy. No association with low weight for gestational age has been found for labetalol (started after the 6th week of gestation) as opposed to atenolol. Sotalol and flecainide are also considered safe, but experience is limited. Amiodarone may be used, but fetal concentration is 20% of maternal concentration and may cause neonatal hypothyroidism (9% of newborns), hyperthyroidism, goitre, and growth retardation. Ideally, all antiarrhythmic drugs should be avoided during the first 8 weeks. In emergencies, immediate cardioversion is safe. IV procainamide, IV sotalol (with normal QT), or IV amiodarone may also be used. The presence of an ICD is not a contraindication for pregnancy.[2] Recommendations of the ESC are presented in Table 55.20. See also Chapter 84 and 85.

Table 55.20 ESC GL on pregnancy 2011

VT in pregnancy	
Implantation of an ICD, if clinically indicated, prior to pregnancy but is also recommended, whenever indicated, during pregnancy.	I-C
For long-term management of the congenital long QT syndrome, beta-blocking agents during pregnancy and also post-partum when they have a major benefit.	I-C
Oral metoprolol,[1,2] propranolol,[1,2] or verapamil[1,3] for long-term management of idiopathic sustained VT.	I-C
Immediate electrical cardioversion of VT for sustained, unstable, and stable VT.	I-C
Sotalol[4] or procainamide for acute conversion of sustained, haemodynamically stable and monomorphic VT.	IIa-C
Implantation of permanent pacemakers or ICDs (preferably one chamber) should be considered with echocardiographical guidance, especially if the fetus is beyond 8 weeks gestation.	IIa-C
IV amiodarone for acute conversion of sustained, monomorphic, haemodynamically unstable VT, refractory to electrical cardioversion or not responding to other drugs.	IIa-C
Oral sotalole,[4] encainide,[3] propafenone[3] for long-term management of idiopathic sustained VT if other drugs fail.	IIa-C
Catheter ablation in drug-refractory and poorly tolerated tachycardias.	IIb-C

[1] AV nodal blocking agents should not be used in patients with pre-excitation on resting ECG.
[2] Beta-blocking agents should be used with caution in the first trimester.
[3] Consider AV nodal blocking agents in conjunction with flecainide and propafenone for certain atrial tachycardias.
[4] Class III drugs should not be used in cases with prolonged QTc.
ESC Guidelines on the management of cardiovascular diseases during pregnancy. *Eur Heart J*. 2011;**32**:3147–97.

References

1. Aliot EM, *et al.* EHRA/HRS Expert Consensus on Catheter Ablation of Ventricular Arrhythmias: developed in a partnership with the European Heart Rhythm Association (EHRA), a Registered Branch of the European Society of Cardiology (ESC), and the Heart Rhythm Society (HRS); in collaboration with the American College of Cardiology (ACC) and the American Heart Association (AHA). *Europace*. 2009;**11**:771–817
2. Zipes DP, *et al.* ACC/AHA/ESC 2006 Guidelines for Management of Patients With Ventricular Arrhythmias and the Prevention of Sudden Cardiac Death: a report of the American College of Cardiology/American Heart Association Task Force and the European Society of Cardiology Committee for Practice Guidelines (writing committee to develop Guidelines for Management of Patients With Ventricular Arrhythmias and the Prevention of Sudden Cardiac Death): developed in collaboration with the European Heart Rhythm Association and the Heart Rhythm Society. *Circulation*. 2006;**114**:e385–484
3. Hadid C, *et al.* Incidence, determinants, and prognostic implications of true pleomorphism of ventricular tachycardia in patients with implantable cardioverter-defribillators: a substudy of the DATAS Trial. *Circ Arrhythm Electrophysiol*. 2011;**4**:33–42
4. Baher AA, *et al.* Bidirectional ventricular tachycardia: ping pong in the His-Purkinje system. *Heart Rhythm*. 2011;**8**:599–605
5. Credner SC, *et al.* Electrical storm in patients with transvenous implantable cardioverter-defibrillators: incidence, management and prognostic implications. *J Am Coll Cardiol*. 1998;**32**:1909–15
6. Kim RJ, *et al.* Clinical and electrophysiological spectrum of idiopathic ventricular outflow tract arrhythmias. *J Am Coll Cardiol*. 2007;**49**:2035–43
7. Stevenson WG, *et al.* Identification of reentry circuit sites during catheter mapping and radiofrequency ablation of ventricular tachycardia late after myocardial infarction. *Circulation*. 1993;**88**:1647–70

8. de Chillou C, *et al.* Isthmus characteristics of reentrant ventricular tachycardia after myocardial infarction. *Circulation.* 2002;**105**:726–31
9. Mountantonakis SE, *et al.* Relationship between voltage map "channels" and the location of critical isthmus sites in patients with post-infarction cardiomyopathy and ventricular tachycardia. *J Am Coll Cardiol.* 2013; doi: 10.1016/j.jacc.2013.1002.1031
10. Katritsis D, *et al.* Catheter ablation for successful management of left posterior fascicular tachycardia: an approach guided by recording of fascicular potentials. *Heart.* 1996;**75**:384–8
11. Lopera G, *et al.* Identification and ablation of three types of ventricular tachycardia involving the His-Purkinje system in patients with heart disease. *J Cardiovasc Electrophysiol.* 2004;**15**:52–8
12. Nash MP, *et al.* Evidence for multiple mechanisms in human ventricular fibrillation. *Circulation.* 2006;**114**:536–42
13. Baerman JM, *et al.* Differentiation of ventricular tachycardia from supraventricular tachycardia with aberration: value of the clinical history. *Ann Emerg Med.* 1987;**16**:40–3
14. Griffith MJ, *et al.* Ascending aorta doppler echocardiography in the diagnosis of broad complex tachycardia. *Am Heart J.* 1988;**116**:555–7
15. Brugada P, *et al.* A new approach to the differential diagnosis of a regular tachycardia with a wide QRS complex. *Circulation.* 1991;**83**:1649–59
16. Kindwall KE, *et al.* Electrocardiographic criteria for ventricular tachycardia in wide complex left bundle branch block morphology tachycardias. *Am J Cardiol.* 1988;**61**:1279–83
17. Pava LF, *et al.* R-wave peak time at DII: a new criterion for differentiating between wide complex QRS tachycardias. *Heart Rhythm.* 2010;**7**:922–6
18. Vereckei A, *et al.* New algorithm using only lead aVR for differential diagnosis of wide QRS complex tachycardia. *Heart Rhythm.* 2008;**5**:89–98
19. Alberca T, *et al.* Evaluation of the specificity of morphological electrocardiographic criteria for the differential diagnosis of wide QRS complex tachycardia in patients with intraventricular conduction defects. *Circulation.* 1997;**96**:3527–33
20. Griffith MJ LN, Ward DE, Camm AJ. Adenosine in the diagnosis of broad complex tachycardias. . *Lancet* 1988;**1** 672–5
21. Myerburg RJ, *et al.* Sudden cardiac death. Structure, function, and time-dependence of risk. *Circulation.* 1992;**85**:I2–10
22. Cobb LA, *et al.* Changing incidence of out-of-hospital ventricular fibrillation, 1980–2000. *JAMA.* 2002;**288**:3008–13
23. Nichol G, *et al.* Regional variation in out-of-hospital cardiac arrest incidence and outcome. *JAMA.* 2008;**300**:1423–31
24. Weisfeldt ML, *et al.* Ventricular tachyarrhythmias after cardiac arrest in public versus at home. *N Engl J Med.* 2011;**364**:313–21
25. Spaulding CM, *et al.* Immediate coronary angiography in survivors of out-of-hospital cardiac arrest. *N Engl J Med.* 1997;**336**:1629–33
26. Bottiger BW, *et al.* Thrombolysis during resuscitation for out-of-hospital cardiac arrest. *N Engl J Med.* 2008;**359**:2651–62
27. Ye S, *et al.* Circumstances and outcomes of sudden unexpected death in patients with high-risk myocardial infarction: implications for prevention. *Circulation.* 2011;**123**:2674–80
28. Kagawa E, *et al.* Should we emergently revascularize occluded coronaries for cardiac arrest?: rapid-response extracorporeal membrane oxygenation and intra-arrest percutaneous coronary intervention. *Circulation.* 2012;**126**:1605–13
29. 2010 American Heart Association guidelines for cardiopulmonary resuscitation and emergency cardiovascular care. *Circulation.* 2010;**122**(18 Suppl 3):Part 1: executive summary: S640–56, Part 648: adult advanced cardiovascular life support: S729–667, Part 610: acute coronary syndromes: S787–817.
30. Hupfl M, *et al.* Chest-compression-only versus standard cardiopulmonary resuscitation: a meta-analysis. *Lancet.* 2010;**376**:1552–7
31. Rea TD, *et al.* CPR with chest compression alone or with rescue breathing. *N Engl J Med.* 2010;**363**:423–33
32. Svensson L, *et al.* Compression-only CPR or standard CPR in out-of-hospital cardiac arrest. *N Engl J Med.* 2010;**363**:434–42
33. Dumas F, *et al.* Chest compression alone cardiopulmonary resuscitation is associated with better long-term survival compared with standard cardiopulmonary resuscitation. *Circulation.* 2013;**127**:435–41
34. Bernard SA, *et al.* Treatment of comatose survivors of out-of-hospital cardiac arrest with induced hypothermia. *N Engl J Med.* 2002;**346**:557–63
35. Exner DV, *et al.* Electrical storm presages nonsudden death: the antiarrhythmics versus implantable defibrillators (AVID) trial. *Circulation.* 2001;**103**:2066–71
36. Greene M, *et al.* Is electrical storm in icd patients the sign of a dying heart? Outcome of patients with clusters of ventricular tachyarrhythmias. *Europace.* 2000;**2**:263–9
37. Nayyar S, *et al.* Venturing into ventricular arrhythmia storm: A systematic review and meta-analysis. *Eur Heart J.* 2013;**34**:560–71
38. Goldberger JJ, *et al.* American Heart Association/american College of Cardiology Foundation/heart Rhythm Society scientific statement on noninvasive risk stratification techniques for identifying patients at risk for sudden cardiac death: a scientific statement from the American Heart Association Council on Clinical Cardiology Committee on Electrocardiography and Arrhythmias and Council on Epidemiology and Prevention. *Heart Rhythm.* 2008;**5**:e1–21
39. Britton KA, *et al.* Clinical problem-solving. The beat goes on. *N Engl J Med.* 2010;**362**:1721–6
40. Bardy GH, *et al.* Amiodarone or an implantable cardioverter-defibrillator for congestive heart failure. *N Engl J Med.* 2005;**352**:225–37
41. Grimm W, *et al.* Non-invasive arrhythmia risk stratification in idiopathic dilated cardiomyopathy: results of the Marburg Cardiomyopathy Study. *Circulation.* 2003;**108**:2883–91
42. Buxton AE, *et al.* Limitations of ejection fraction for prediction of sudden death risk in patients with coronary artery disease: lessons from the MUSTT study. *J Am Coll Cardiol.* 2007;**50**:1150–7
43. Horner JM, *et al.* Ventricular ectopy during treadmill exercise stress testing in the evaluation of long QT syndrome. *Heart Rhythm.* 2008;**5**:1690–4

44. Wolfe CL, *et al.* Polymorphous ventricular tachycardia associated with acute myocardial infarction. *Circulation.* 1991;**84**:1543–51
45. Furukawa T, *et al.* Arrhythmogenic effects of graded coronary blood flow reductions superimposed on prior myocardial infarction in dogs. *Circulation.* 1991;**84**:368–77
46. Iles L, *et al.* Myocardial fibrosis predicts appropriate device therapy in patients with implantable cardioverter-defibrillators for primary prevention of sudden cardiac death. *J Am Coll Cardiol.* 2011;**57**:821–8
47. Soejima K, *et al.* The work-up and management of patients with apparent or subclinical cardiac sarcoidosis: with emphasis on the associated heart rhythm abnormalities. *J Cardiovasc Electrophysiol.* 2009;**20**:578–83
48. O'Hanlon R, *et al.* Prognostic significance of myocardial fibrosis in hypertrophic cardiomyopathy. *J Am Coll Cardiol.* 2010;**56**:867–74
49. Bloch Thomsen PE, *et al.* Long-term recording of cardiac arrhythmias with an implantable cardiac monitor in patients with reduced ejection fraction after acute myocardial infarction: the Cardiac Arrhythmias and Risk Stratification After Acute Myocardial Infarction (CARISMA) study. *Circulation.* 2010;**122**:1258–64
50. Hofsten DE, *et al.* Prevalence and prognostic implications of non-sustained ventricular tachycardia in ST segment elevation myocardial infarction after revascularization with either fibrinolysis or primary angioplasty. *Eur Heart J.* 2007;**28**:407–14
51. Huikuri HV, *et al.* Prediction of sudden cardiac death after myocardial infarction in the beta-blocking era. *J Am Coll Cardiol.* 2003;**42**:652–8
52. Katritsis DG, *et al.* Non-sustained ventricular tachycardia. *J Am Coll Cardiol.* 2012;**60**:1993–2004
53. Makikallio TH, *et al.* Prediction of sudden cardiac death after acute myocardial infarction: role of Holter monitoring in the modern treatment era. *Eur Heart J.* 2005;**26**:762–9
54. Scirica BM, *et al.* Relationship between nonsustained ventricular tachycardia after non-ST-elevation acute coronary syndrome and sudden cardiac death: observations from the metabolic efficiency with ranolazine for less ischemia in non-ST-elevation acute coronary syndrome-thrombolysis in myocardial infarction 36 (MERLIN-TIMI 36) randomized controlled trial. *Circulation.* 2010;**122**:455–62
55. Monserrat L, *et al.* Non-sustained ventricular tachycardia in hypertrophic cardiomyopathy: an independent marker of sudden death risk in young patients. *J Am Coll Cardiol.* 2003;**42**:873–9
56. Effect of the antiarrhythmic agent moricizine on survival after myocardial infarction. The Cardiac Arrhythmia Suppression Trial II Investigators. *N Engl J Med.* 1992;**327**:227–33
57. Echt DS, *et al.* Mortality and morbidity in patients receiving encainide, flecainide, or placebo. The Cardiac Arrhythmia Suppression Trial. *N Engl J Med.* 1991;**324**:781–8
58. Singh SN, *et al.* Amiodarone in patients with congestive heart failure and asymptomatic ventricular arrhythmia. Survival trial of antiarrhythmic therapy in congestive heart failure. *N Engl J Med.* 1995;**333**:77–82
59. Verrier RL, *et al.* Microvolt T-wave alternans physiological basis, methods of measurement, and clinical utility – consensus guideline by International Society for Holter and Noninvasive Electrocardiology. *J Am Coll Cardiol.* 2011;**58**:1309–24
60. Amit G, *et al.* Microvolt T wave alternans and electrophysiologic testing predict distinct arrhythmia substrates: implications for identifying patients at risk for sudden cardiac death. *Heart Rhythm.* 2010;**7**:763–8
61. Chow T, *et al.* Does microvolt T-wave alternans testing predict ventricular tachyarrhythmias in patients with ischemic cardiomyopathy and prophylactic defibrillators? The MASTER (Microvolt T Wave Alternans Testing for Risk Stratification of Post-Myocardial Infarction Patients) trial. *J Am Coll Cardiol.* 2008;**52**:1607–15
62. Costantini O, *et al.* The ABCD (Alternans Before Cardioverter Defibrillator) Trial: strategies using T-wave alternans to improve efficiency of sudden cardiac death prevention. *J Am Coll Cardiol.* 2009;**53**:471–9
63. Swerdlow C, *et al.* Intracardiac electrogram T wave alternans/variability increases before spontaneous ventricular tachyarrhythmias in implantable cardioverter-defibrillator patients: a prospective, multi-centre study. *Circulation.* 2011;**123**:1052–60
64. Camm AJ, *et al.* Mortality in patients after a recent myocardial infarction: a randomized, placebo-controlled trial of azimilide using heart rate variability for risk stratification. *Circulation.* 2004;**109**:990–6
65. La Rovere MT, *et al.* Baroreflex sensitivity and heart rate variability in the identification of patients at risk for life-threatening arrhythmias: implications for clinical trials. *Circulation.* 2001;**103**:2072–7
66. Abildstrom SZ, *et al.* Heart rate versus heart rate variability in risk prediction after myocardial infarction. *J Cardiovasc Electrophysiol.* 2003;**14**:168–73
67. Rashba EJ, *et al.* Preserved heart rate variability identifies low-risk patients with nonischaemic dilated cardiomyopathy: Results from the DEFINITE trial. *Heart Rhythm.* 2006;**3**:281–6
68. Stein KM. Non-invasive risk stratification for sudden death: Signal-averaged electrocardiography, non-sustained ventricular tachycardia, heart rate variability, baroreflex sensitivity, and QRS duration. *Prog Cardiovasc Dis.* 2008;**51**:106–17
69. Bauer A, *et al.* Reduced prognostic power of ventricular late potentials in post-infarction patients of the reperfusion era. *Eur Heart J.* 2005;**26**:755–61
70. Winters SL, *et al.* Signal averaging of the surface QRS complex predicts inducibility of ventricular tachycardia in patients with syncope of unknown origin: a prospective study. *J Am Coll Cardiol.* 1987;**10**:775–81
71. Kowey PR, *et al.* Does programmed stimulation really help in the evaluation of patients with non-sustained ventricular tachycardia? Results of a meta-analysis. *Am Heart J.* 1992;**123**:481–5
72. Wilber DJ, *et al.* Electrophysiological testing and non-sustained ventricular tachycardia. Use and limitations in patients with coronary artery disease and impaired ventricular function. *Circulation.* 1990;**82**:350–8
73. Buxton AE, *et al.* Electrophysiologic testing to identify patients with coronary artery disease who are at risk for sudden death. Multicentre Unsustained Tachycardia Trial Investigators. *N Engl J Med.* 2000;**342**:1937–45
74. Buxton AE, *et al.* Relation of ejection fraction and inducible ventricular tachycardia to mode of death in patients with coronary artery disease: An analysis of patients enrolled in

the multicentre unsustained tachycardia trial. *Circulation.* 2002;**106**:2466–72
75. Piccini JP, *et al.* Mode of induction of ventricular tachycardia and prognosis in patients with coronary disease: the Multicenter UnSustained Tachycardia Trial (MUSTT). *J Cardiovasc Electrophysiol.* 2009;**20**:850–5
76. Monahan KM, *et al.* Relation of induced to spontaneous ventricular tachycardia from analysis of stored far-field implantable defibrillator electrograms. *Am J Cardiol.* 1999;**83**:349–53
77. Kumar S, *et al.* Electrophysiology-guided defibrillator implantation early after ST elevation myocardial infarction. *Heart Rhythm.* 2010;**7**:1589–97
78. Mittal S, *et al.* Significance of inducible ventricular fibrillation in patients with coronary artery disease and unexplained syncope. *J Am Coll Cardiol.* 2001;**38**:371–6
79. Brilakis ES, *et al.* Role of programmed ventricular stimulation and implantable cardioverter defibrillators in patients with idiopathic dilated cardiomyopathy and syncope. *Pacing Clin Electrophysiol.* 2001;**24**:1623–30
80. Grimm W, *et al.* Programmed ventricular stimulation for arrhythmia risk prediction in patients with idiopathic dilated cardiomyopathy and non-sustained ventricular tachycardia. *J Am Coll Cardiol.* 1998;**32**:739–45
81. Daubert JP, *et al.* Ventricular arrhythmia inducibility predicts subsequent ICD activation in nonischaemic cardiomyopathy patients: a DEFINITE substudy. *Pacing Clin Electrophysiol.* 2009;**32**:755–61
82. Rolf S, *et al.* Induction of ventricular fibrillation rather than ventricular tachycardia predicts tachyarrhythmia recurrences in patients with idiopathic dilated cardiomyopathy and implantable cardioverter defibrillator for secondary prophylaxis. *Europace.* 2009;**11**:289–96
83. Khairy P, *et al.* Value of programmed ventricular stimulation after tetralogy of Fallot repair: a multicentre study. *Circulation.* 2004;**109**:1994–2000
84. Mehta D, *et al.* Primary prevention of sudden cardiac death in silent cardiac sarcoidosis: role of programmed ventricular stimulation. *Circ Arrhythm Electrophysiol.* 2011;**4**:43–8
85. Alberte C, *et al.* Use of nonantiarrhythmic drugs for prevention of sudden cardiac death. *J Cardiovasc Electrophysiol.* 2003;**14**:S87–95
86. Dries DL, *et al.* Effect of antithrombotic therapy on risk of sudden coronary death in patients with congestive heart failure. *Am J Cardiol.* 1997;**79**:909–13
87. Finzi AA, *et al.* Effects of n-3 polyunsaturated fatty acids on malignant ventricular arrhythmias in patients with chronic heart failure and implantable cardioverter-defibrillators: A substudy of the Gruppo Italiano per lo Studio della Sopravvivenza nell'Insufficienza Cardiaca (GISSI-HF) trial. *Am Heart J.* 2011;**161**:338–43
88. Saravanan P, *et al.* Cardiovascular effects of marine omega-3 fatty acids. *Lancet.* 2010;**376**:540–50
89. Rahimi K, *et al.* Effect of statins on ventricular tachyarrhythmia, cardiac arrest, and sudden cardiac death: a meta-analysis of published and unpublished evidence from randomized trials. *Eur Heart J.* 2012;**33**:1571–81
90. Christiansen EH, *et al.* Dose-related cardiac electrophysiological effects of intravenous magnesium. A double-blind placebo-controlled dose-response study in patients with paroxysmal supraventricular tachycardia. *Europace.* 2000;**2**:320–6
91. Ho KM, *et al.* Use of intravenous magnesium to treat acute onset atrial fibrillation: a meta-analysis. *Heart.* 2007;**93**:1433–40
92. Ellison KE, *et al.* Effect of beta-blocking therapy on outcome in the Multicenter UnSustained Tachycardia Trial (MUSTT). *Circulation.* 2002;**106**:2694–9
93. Kamath GS, *et al.* The role of antiarrhythmic drug therapy for the prevention of sudden cardiac death. *Prog Cardiovasc Dis.* 2008;**50**:439–48
94. Epstein AE, *et al.* 2012 ACCF/AHA/HRS focused update incorporated into the ACCF/AHA/HRS 2008 Guidelines for device-based therapy of cardiac rhythm abnormalities. *J Am Coll Cardiol.* 2013;**61**:e6–75
95. Waldo AL, *et al.* Effect of d-sotalol on mortality in patients with left ventricular dysfunction after recent and remote myocardial infarction. The SWORD Investigators. Survival With Oral d-Sotalol. *Lancet.* 1996;**348**:7–12
96. Connolly SJ, *et al.* Comparison of beta blockers, amiodarone plus beta blockers, or sotalol for prevention of shocks from implantable cardioverter defibrillators: the OPTIC Study: a randomized trial. *JAMA.* 2006;**295**:165–71
97. Kowey PR, *et al.* Efficacy and safety of celivarone, with amiodarone as calibrator, in patients with an implantable cardioverter-defibrillator for prevention of implantable cardioverter-defibrillator interventions or death: the ALPHEE study. *Circulation.* 2011;**124**:2649–60
98. Carbucicchio C, *et al.* Catheter ablation for the treatment of electrical storm in patients with implantable cardioverter-defibrillators: Short- and long-term outcomes in a prospective single-center study. *Circulation.* 2008;**117**:462–469
99. Di Biase L, *et al.* Endo-epicardial homogenization of the scar versus limited substrate ablation for the treatment of electrical storms in patients with ischaemic cardiomyopathy. *J Am Coll Cardiol.* 2012;**60**:132–41
100. Jais P, *et al.* Elimination of local abnormal ventricular activities: a new end point for substrate modification in patients with scar-related ventricular tachycardia. *Circulation.* 2012;**125**:2184–96
101. Kuck KH, *et al.* Catheter ablation of stable ventricular tachycardia before defibrillator implantation in patients with coronary heart disease (VTACH): a multicentre randomised controlled trial. *Lancet.* 2010;**375**:31–40
102. Stevenson WG, *et al.* Irrigated radiofrequency catheter ablation guided by electroanatomical mapping for recurrent ventricular tachycardia after myocardial infarction: The multicentre thermocool ventricular tachycardia ablation trial. *Circulation.* 2008;**118**:2773–82
103. Reddy VY, *et al.* Prophylactic catheter ablation for the prevention of defibrillator therapy. *N Engl J Med.* 2007;**357**:2657–65.
104. Tokuda M, *et al.* Catheter ablation of ventricular tachycardia in nonischaemic heart disease. *Circ Arrhythm Electrophysiol.* 2012;**5**:992–1000
105. Cheriyath P, *et al.* Relation of atrial and/or ventricular premature complexes on a two-minute rhythm strip to the risk

of sudden cardiac death (the Atherosclerosis Risk in Communities [ARIC] study). *Am J Cardiol.* 2011;**107**:151–5
106. Frolkis JP, *et al.* Frequent ventricular ectopy after exercise as a predictor of death. *N Engl J Med.* 2003;**348**:781–90
107. Jouven X, *et al.* Long-term outcome in asymptomatic men with exercise-induced premature ventricular depolarizations. *N Engl J Med.* 2000;**343**:826–33
108. Biffi A, *et al.* Patterns of ventricular tachyarrhythmias associated with training, deconditioning and retraining in elite athletes without cardiovascular abnormalities. *Am J Cardiol.* 2011;**107**:697–703
109. Boukens BJ, *et al.* Developmental basis for electrophysiological heterogeneity in the ventricular and outflow tract myocardium as a substrate for life-threatening ventricular arrhythmias. *Circ Res.* 2009;**104**:19–31
110. Dixit S, *et al.* Electrocardiographic patterns of superior right ventricular outflow tract tachycardias: distinguishing septal and free-wall sites of origin. *J Cardiovasc Electrophysiol.* 2003;**14**:1–7
111. Prystowsky EN, *et al.* Ventricular arrhythmias in the absence of structural heart disease. *J Am Coll Cardiol.* 2012;**59**:1733–44
112. Betensky BP, *et al.* The V(2) transition ratio: a new electrocardiographic criterion for distinguishing left from right ventricular outflow tract tachycardia origin. *J Am Coll Cardiol.* 2011;**57**:2255–62
113. Suleiman M, *et al.* Ablation above the semilunar valves: when, why, and how? Part I. *Heart Rhythm.* 2008;**5**:1485–92
114. Suleiman M, *et al.* Ablation above the semilunar valves: when, why, and how? Part II. *Heart Rhythm.* 2008;**5**:1625–30
115. Ouyang F, *et al.* Electroanatomical substrate of idiopathic left ventricular tachycardia: unidirectional block and macroreentry within the Purkinje network. *Circulation.* 2002;**105**:462–9
116. Yokokawa M, *et al.* Intramural idiopathic ventricular arrhythmias originating in the intraventricular septum: mapping and ablation. *Circ Arrhythm Electrophysiol.* 2012;**5**:258–63
117. Bottoni N, *et al.* Sudden death in a patient with idiopathic right ventricular outflow tract arrhythmia. *J Cardiovasc Med (Hagerstown).* 2009;**10**:801–3
118. Noda T, *et al.* Malignant entity of idiopathic ventricular fibrillation and polymorphic ventricular tachycardia initiated by premature extrasystoles originating from the right ventricular outflow tract. *J Am Coll Cardiol.* 2005;**46**:1288–94
119. Viskin S, *et al.* The 'short-coupled' variant of right ventricular outflow ventricular tachycardia: a not-so-benign form of benign ventricular tachycardia? *J Cardiovasc Electrophysiol.* 2005;**16**:912–16
120. Shimizu W. Arrhythmias originating from the right ventricular outflow tract: how to distinguish 'malignant' from 'benign'? *Heart Rhythm.* 2009;**6**:1507–11
121. Carlson MD, *et al.* Right ventricular outflow tract ventricular tachycardia: detection of previously unrecognized anatomical abnormalities using cine magnetic resonance imaging. *J Am Coll Cardiol.* 1994;**24**:720–7
122. Hoffmayer KS, *et al.* Electrocardiographic comparison of ventricular arrhythmias in patients with arrhythmogenic right ventricular cardiomyopathy and right ventricular outflow tract tachycardia. *J Am Coll Cardiol.* 2011;**58**:831–838
123. Hoffmayer KS, *et al.* An electrocardiographic scoring system for distinguishing right ventricular outflow tract arrhythmias in patientswith arrhythmogenic right ventricular cardiomyopathy from idiopathic ventricular tachycardia. *Heart Rhythm.* 2012
124. Bohnen M, *et al.* Incidence and predictors of major complications from contemporary catheter ablation to treat cardiac arrhythmias. *Heart Rhythm.* 2011;**8**:1661–6
125. Schreiber D, *et al.* Ablation of idiopathic ventricular tachycardia. *Curr Cardiol Rep.* 2010;**12**:382–8
126. Piccini JP, *et al.* Sustained ventricular tachycardia and ventricular fibrillation complicating non-ST segment-elevation acute coronary syndromes. *Circulation.* 2012;**126**:41–9
127. Cheema AN, *et al.* Non-sustained ventricular tachycardia in the setting of acute myocardial infarction: tachycardia characteristics and their prognostic implications. *Circulation.* 1998;**98**:2030–6
128. Heidbuchel H, *et al.* Significance of arrhythmias during the first 24 hours of acute myocardial infarction treated with alteplase and effect of early administration of a beta blocker or a bradycardiac agent on their incidence. *Circulation.* 1994;**89**:1051–9
129. Volpi A, *et al.* Incidence and prognosis of early primary ventricular fibrillation in acute myocardial infarction – results of the Gruppo Italiano per lo Studio della Sopravvivenza nell'Infarto Miocardico (GISSI-2) database. *Am J Cardiol.* 1998;**82**:265–71
130. Yokokawa M, *et al.* Automated analysis of the 12-lead electrocardiogram to identify the exit site of postinfarction ventricular tachycardia. *Heart Rhythm.* 2012;**9**:330–4
131. Brugada J, *et al.* Coronary artery revascularization in patients with sustained ventricular arrhythmias in the chronic phase of a myocardial infarction: effects on the electrophysiologic substrate and outcome. *J Am Coll Cardiol.* 2001;**37**:529–33
132. Kelly P, *et al.* Surgical coronary revascularization in survivors of prehospital cardiac arrest: its effect on inducible ventricular arrhythmias and long-term survival. *J Am Coll Cardiol.* 1990;**15**:267–73
133. Natale A, *et al.* Ventricular fibrillation and polymorphic ventricular tachycardia with critical coronary artery stenosis: does bypass surgery suffice? J Cardiovasc Electrophysiol. 1994;**5**:988–94
134. El-Chami MF, *et al.* Ventricular arrhythmia after cardiac surgery: incidence, predictors, and outcomes. J Am Coll Cardiol. 2012;**60**:2664–71
135. Cairns JA, *et al.* Post-myocardial infarction mortality in patients with ventricular premature depolarizations. Canadian Amiodarone Myocardial Infarction Arrhythmia Trial Pilot Study. *Circulation.* 1991;**84**:550–7
136. Julian DG, *et al.* Randomised trial of effect of amiodarone on mortality in patients with left-ventricular dysfunction after recent myocardial infarction: EMIAT. European Myocardial Infarct Amiodarone Trial Investigators. *Lancet.* 1997;**349**:667–74
137. Elizari MV, *et al.* Morbidity and mortality following early administration of amiodarone in acute myocardial infarc-

tion. GEMICA study investigators, GEMA Group, Buenos Aires, Argentina. Grupo de Estudios Multicéntricos en Argentina. *Eur Heart J.* 2000;**21**:198–205
138. Viscoli CM, *et al.* Beta blockers after myocardial infarction: influence of first-year clinical course on long-term effectiveness. *Ann Intern Med.* 1993;**118**:99–105
139. Moss AJ, *et al.* Improved survival with an implanted defibrillator in patients with coronary disease at high risk for ventricular arrhythmia. Multicenter Automatic Defibrillator Implantation Trial Investigators. *N Engl J Med.* 1996;**335**:1933–40
140. Buxton AE, *et al.* A randomized study of the prevention of sudden death in patients with coronary artery disease. Multicenter Unsustained Tachycardia Trial Investigators. *N Engl J Med.* 1999;**341**:1882–90
141. Goldenberg I, *et al.* Long-term benefit of primary prevention with an implantable cardioverter-defibrillator: an extended 8-year follow-up study of the Multicenter Automatic Defibrillator Implantation Trial II. *Circulation.* 2010;**122**:1265–71
142. Hohnloser SH, *et al.* Prophylactic use of an implantable cardioverter-defibrillator after acute myocardial infarction. *N Engl J Med.* 2004;**351**:2481–8
143. Steinbeck G, *et al.* Defibrillator implantation early after myocardial infarction. *N Engl J Med.* 2009;**361**:1427–36
144. Theuns DA, *et al.* Effectiveness of prophylactic implantation of cardioverter-defibrillators without cardiac resynchronization therapy in patients with ischaemic or non-ischaemic heart disease: a systematic review and meta-analysis. *Europace.* 2010;**12**:1564–70
145. Katritsis DG, *et al.* Effect of left ventricular ejection fraction and qrs duration on the survival benefit of implantable cardioverter-defibrillators: meta-analysis of primary prevention trials. *Heart Rhythm.* 2013;**10**:200–6
146. Piccini JP, *et al.* Mortality benefits from implantable cardioverter-defibrillator therapy are not restricted to patients with remote myocardial infarction: an analysis from the Sudden Cardiac Death in Heart Failure Trial (SCD-HeFT). *Heart Rhythm.* 2011;**8**:393–400
147. O'Gara PT, *et al.* 2013 ACCF/AHA guideline for the management of ST-elevation myocardial infarction: a report of the American College of Cardiology Foundation/American Heart Association Task Force on Practice Guidelines. *J Am Coll Cardiol.* 2013;**61**:e78–140.
148. Katritsis DG, *et al.* Sudden cardiac death and implantable cardioverter defibrillators: two modern epidemics? *Europace.* 2012;**14**:787–94
149. Yoshiga Y, *et al.* Correlation between substrate location and ablation strategy in patients with ventricular tachycardia late after myocardial infarction. *Heart Rhythm.* 2012;**9**:1192–9
150. Berruezo A, *et al.* Electrocardiographic recognition of the epicardial origin of ventricular tachycardias. *Circulation.* 2004;**109**:1842–7
151. Doval HC, *et al.* Nonsustained ventricular tachycardia in severe heart failure. Independent marker of increased mortality due to sudden death. GESICA-GEMA Investigators. *Circulation.* 1996;**94**:3198–3203
152. Singh SN, *et al.* Prevalence and significance of nonsustained ventricular tachycardia in patients with premature ventricular contractions and heart failure treated with vasodilator therapy. Department of Veterans Affairs CHF STAT Investigators. *J Am Coll Cardiol.* 1998;**32**:942–7
153. Teerlink JR, *et al.* Ambulatory ventricular arrhythmias in patients with heart failure do not specifically predict an increased risk of sudden death. PROMISE (Prospective Randomized Milrinone Survival Evaluation) Investigators. *Circulation.* 2000;**101**:40–6
154. O'Neill JO, *et al.* Severe frequent ventricular ectopy after exercise as a predictor of death in patients with heart failure. *J Am Coll Cardiol.* 2004;**44**:820–6
155. Chen J, *et al.* Rapid rate non-sustained ventricular tachycardia found on ICD interrogation: Relationship of NSVT to outcomes in the SCD-HEFT trial. *J Am Coll Cardiol.* 2013; doi: 10.1016/j.jacc.2013.1002.1046
156. Doval HC, *et al.* Randomised trial of low-dose amiodarone in severe congestive heart failure. Grupo de Estudio de la Sobrevida en la Insuficiencia Cardiaca en Argentina (GESICA). *Lancet.* 1994;**344**:493–8
157. Kober L, *et al.* Increased mortality after dronedarone therapy for severe heart failure. *N Engl J Med.* 2008;**358**:2678–87
158. Barsheshet A, *et al.* Reverse remodeling and the risk of ventricular tachyarrhythmias in the MADIT-CRT (Multicenter Automatic Defibrillator Implantation Trial-Cardiac Resynchronization Therapy). *J Am Coll Cardiol.* 2011;**57**:2416–23
159. Iacoviello M, *et al.* Ventricular repolarization dynamicity provides independent prognostic information toward major arrhythmic events in patients with idiopathic dilated cardiomyopathy. *J Am Coll Cardiol.* 2007;**50**:225–31
160. Zecchin M, *et al.* Are non-sustained ventricular tachycardias predictive of major arrhythmias in patients with dilated cardiomyopathy on optimal medical treatment? *Pacing Clin Electrophysiol.* 2008;**31**:290–9
161. Caceres J, *et al.* Sustained bundle branch reentry as a mechanism of clinical tachycardia. *Circulation.* 1989;**79**: 256–270
162. Blanck Z, *et al.* Bundle branch reentry: a mechanism of ventricular tachycardia in the absence of myocardial or valvular dysfunction. *J Am Coll Cardiol.* 1993;**22**: 1718–22
163. Valles E, *et al.* ECG criteria to identify epicardial ventricular tachycardia in nonischaemic cardiomyopathy. *Circ Arrhythm Electrophysiol.* 2010;**3**:63–71
164. Kadish A, *et al.* Prophylactic defibrillator implantation in patients with nonischaemic dilated cardiomyopathy. *N Engl J Med.* 2004;**350**:2151–8
165. Strickberger SA, *et al.* Amiodarone versus implantable cardioverter-defibrillator:randomized trial in patients with nonischemic dilated cardiomyopathy and asymptomatic nonsustained ventricular tachycardia – AMIOVIRT. *J Am Coll Cardiol.* 2003;**41**:1707–12
166. Bansch D, *et al.* Primary prevention of sudden cardiac death in idiopathic dilated cardiomyopathy: the Cardiomyopathy Trial (CAT). *Circulation.* 2002;**105**:1453–8
167. Spirito P, *et al.* Prognosis of asymptomatic patients with hypertrophic cardiomyopathy and non-sustained ventricular tachycardia. *Circulation.* 1994;**90**:2743–7

168. Maron BJ. Contemporary insights and strategies for risk stratification and prevention of sudden death in hypertrophic cardiomyopathy. *Circulation*. 2010;**121**:445–56
169. Corrado D, *et al.* Prophylactic implantable defibrillator in patients with arrhythmogenic right ventricular cardiomyopathy/dysplasia and no prior ventricular fibrillation or sustained ventricular tachycardia. *Circulation*. 2010;**122**:1144–52
170. Palladini G, *et al.* Holter monitoring in AL amyloidosis: prognostic implications. *Pacing Clin Electrophysiol.* 2001;**24**:1228–33
171. Sarabanda AV, *et al.* Predictors of mortality in patients with Chagas' cardiomyopathy and ventricular tachycardia not treated with implantable cardioverter-defibrillators. *Pacing Clin Electrophysiol.* 2011;**34**:54–62
172. Gatzoulis MA, *et al.* Risk factors for arrhythmia and sudden cardiac death late after repair of tetralogy of Fallot: a multicentre study. *Lancet*. 2000;**356**:975–81
173. Khairy P, *et al.* Arrhythmia burden in adults with surgically repaired tetralogy of Fallot: a multi-institutional study. *Circulation*. 2010;**122**:868–75
174. Martinez-Rubio A, *et al.* Patients with valvular heart disease presenting with sustained ventricular tachyarrhythmias or syncope: results of programmed ventricular stimulation and long-term follow-up. *Circulation*. 1997;**96**:500–8
175. Grigioni F, *et al.* Sudden death in mitral regurgitation due to flail leaflet. *J Am Coll Cardiol.* 1999;**34**:2078–85
176. Kligfield P, *et al.* Arrhythmias and sudden death in mitral valve prolapse. *Am Heart J.* 1987;**113**:1298–307
177. McLenachan JM, *et al.* Ventricular arrhythmias in patients with hypertensive left ventricular hypertrophy. *N Engl J Med.* 1987;**317**:787–92
178. Pringle SD, *et al.* Significance of ventricular arrhythmias in systemic hypertension with left ventricular hypertrophy. *Am J Cardiol.* 1992;**69**:913–17
179. Groh WJ. Arrhythmias in the muscular dystrophies. *Heart Rhythm*. 2012;**9**:1890–5
180. Katritsis D. Progressive cardiac conduction disease. In: Zipes DP, Jalife J. *Cardiac electrophysiology: from cell to bedside*. 6th edition. Saunders. Philadelphia (in press).
181. Van Rijaingen IAW, *et al.* Risk factors for malignant ventricular arrhythmias in lamin a/c mutation carriers. A European cohort study. *J Am Coll Cardiol.* 2012;**59**:493–500
182. Podrid PJ. Potassium and ventricular arrhythmias. *Am J Cardiol.* 1990;**65**:33E-44E; discussion 52E
183. Heist EK, *et al.* Drug-induced arrhythmia. *Circulation*. 2010;**122**:1426–35
184. Soliman EZ, *et al.* Prolongation of QTc and risk of stroke: The REGARDS (REasons for Geographic and Racial Differences in Stroke) study. *J Am Coll Cardiol.* 2012;**59**:1460–7
185. Katritsis D, *et al.* Quinolones: cardioprotective or cardiotoxic. *Pacing Clin Electrophysiol.* 2003;**26**:2317–20
186. Ray WA, *et al.* Azithromycin and the risk of cardiovascular death. *N Engl J Med.* 2012;**366**:1881–90
187. Svanström H, *et al.* Use of azithromycin and death from cardiovascular causes. *N Engl J Med.* 2013;**368**:1704–12
188. Castro VM, *et al.* QT interval and antidepressant use: A cross sectional study of electronic health records. *BMJ*. 2013;**346**: doi: 10.1136bmj.f1288
189. Hondeghem LM. QT prolongation is an unreliable predictor of ventricular arrhythmia. *Heart Rhythm*. 2008;**5**:1210–2
190. Sauer AJ, *et al.* Clinical and genetic determinants of torsade de pointes risk. *Circulation*. 2012;**125**:1684–94
191. Drew BJ, *et al.* Prevention of torsade de pointes in hospital settings: a scientific statement from the American Heart Association and the American College of Cardiology Foundation. *J Am Coll Cardiol.* 2010;**55**:934–47
192. Bardai A, *et al.* Sudden cardiac arrest associated with use of a non-cardiac drug that reduces cardiac excitability: Evidence from bench, bedside, and community. *Eur Heart J.* 2013;**34**:1506–16
193. Robben NC, *et al.* The syndrome of 5-fluorouracil cardiotoxicity. An elusive cardiopathy. *Cancer*. 1993;**71**:493–509
194. Guglin M, *et al.* Introducing a new entity: chemotherapy-induced arrhythmia. *Europace*. 2009;**11**:1579–86
195. Lipshultz SE, *et al.* Female sex and drug dose as risk factors for late cardiotoxic effects of doxorubicin therapy for childhood cancer. *N Engl J Med.* 1995;**332**:1738–43
196. Maron BJ. Sudden death in young athletes. *N Engl J Med.* 2003;**349**:1064–75
197. Kim JH, *et al.* Cardiac arrest during long-distance running races. *N Engl J Med.* 2012;**366**:130–40
198. Corrado D, *et al.* Risk of sports: do we need a pre-participation screening for competitive and leisure athletes? *Eur Heart J.* 2011;**32**:934–44
199. Dello Russo A, *et al.* Concealed cardiomyopathies in competitive athletes with ventricular arrhythmias and an apparently normal heart: role of cardiac electroanatomicalal mapping and biopsy. *Heart Rhythm*. 2011;**8**:1915–22
200. Lampert R, *et al.* Safety of sports for athletes with implantable cardioverter-defibrillators: Results of a prospective, multinational registry. *Circulation*. 2013;**127**:2021–30
201. Harmon KG, *et al.* Incidence of sudden cardiac death in national collegiate athletic association athletes. *Circulation*. 2011;**123**:1594–600
202. Cappato R, *et al.* J wave, QRS slurring, and ST elevation in athletes with cardiac arrest in the absence of heart disease: marker of risk or innocent bystander? *Circ Arrhythm Electrophysiol.* 2010;**3**:305–11
203. Maron BJ, *et al.* Introduction: eligibility recommendations for competitive athletes with cardiovascular abnormalities-general considerations. *J Am Coll Cardiol.* 2005;**45**:1318–21
204. Regitz-Zagrosek V, *et al.* ESC Guidelines on the management of cardiovascular diseases during pregnancy: the Task Force on the Management of Cardiovascular Diseases during Pregnancy of the European Society of Cardiology (ESC). *Eur Heart J.* 2011;**32**:3147–97
205. Rashba EJ, *et al.* Influence of pregnancy on the risk for cardiac events in patients with hereditary long QT syndrome. LQTS Investigators. *Circulation*. 1998;**97**:451–6

Part X

Genetic channelopathies

Relevant guidelines

HRS/EHRA 2011 expert consensus statement on the state of genetic testing

HRS/EHRA expert consensus statement on the state of genetic testing for the channelopathies and cardiomyopathies. *Europace.* 2011;**13**:1077–109.

HRS/EHRA/APHRS 2013 Expert Consensus Statement on Inherited Arrhythmia

HRS/EHRA/APHRS Expert Consensus Statement on the Diagnosis and Management of Patients with Inherited Primary Arrhythmia Syndromes. *Europace* E-Pub.

ACCF/AHA/HRS 2012 for device-based therapy of cardiac rhythm abnormalities

2012 ACCF/AHA/HRS focused update incorporated into the ACCF/AHA/HRS 2008 guidelines for device-based therapy of cardiac rhythm abnormalities. *J Am Coll Cardiol.* 2013;**61**:e6–75

Chapter 56

Definitions of inherited arrhythmias

Definitions

Inherited arrhythmias comprise a group of disorders with inherited susceptibility to arrhythmias and conduction disturbances due to mutations in genes mainly encoding the Na^+ and K^+ channels and other arrhythmogenic mechanisms, such as those linked to Ca^{++} transport (Table 56.1 and Figure 56.1).[1] The majority of heritable cardiomyopathies and channelopathies are associated with disease susceptibility genes characterized by incomplete penetrance, i.e. low likelihood that the mutation will cause clinically recognizable disease. Thus, although these disease entities are monogenic, there is variable penetrance, which reflects the contribution by modifier genes, thus resulting in diverse phenotypes.[2] Usually, they are autosomal dominant, rather than autosomal recessive. Genetic testing has now emerged as a useful clinical tool for the diagnosis and risk stratification of genetic conditions, but distinguishing pathologic mutations from innocent genetic variants is not always straightforward. Currently, genetic testing may put the diagnosis in LQTS, CPVT, BrS, and HCM and may also facilitate risk stratification in LQTS and HCM.[3] According to the 2010 Consensus Statement of HRS/EHRA, genetic testing is recommended in cases with a sound clinical suspicion for the presence of a channelopathy or a cardiomyopathy when the positive predictive value of a genetic test is high (likelihood of positive result >40% and signal/noise ratio <10) (Table 56.2).[4] The conventional approach of genetic linkage analysis has been replaced with the newer approach of Genome Wide Association studies (GWAS), and Next Generation DNA Sequencing (NGS).[5] The application of high-throughput sequencing techniques such as whole genome and exome sequencing, as well as the possibility of sequencing of personal genomes, are exciting future advancements of this technology.[6,7]

The DNA among humans consists of the same nucleotide sequence, but normal variations in small sections of sequence or single nucleotides do exist among individuals (polymorphisms). Single nucleotide substitutions that occur with a measurable frequency (i.e. >0.5% allelic frequency) among a particular ethic population are called single-nucleotide **polymorphisms** whereas those that occur less frequently are termed **mutations**.

Glossary of terms and acronyms

Allele: One of several alternative versions of a particular gene. An allele can refer to a segment of DNA or even a single nucleotide. The normal version of genetic information is often considered the 'wildtype' or 'normal' allele. The vast majority of the human genome represents a single version of genetic information. Multiple alleles are when one phenotype is controlled by more than two alleles, but only a combination of two determines the phenotype. For example, blood group has three alleles A, B, and O, but people only have a two-allele phenotype.

Autosomal dominant: The situation in which the disease can be expressed, even when just one chromosome harbours the mutation.

Autosomal recessive: The situation in which the disease is expressed only when both chromosomes of a pair are abnormal.

Cascade testing: Procedure whereby all first-degree relatives of a genotype-positive index case are tested in concentric circles of relatedness. If one of the family members is genotype-positive, all his/her first-degree relatives should be tested, continuing this process to follow each genotype-positive family member.

Compound heterozygosity: More than one genetic defect in the same gene.

Digenic heterozygosity: More than one genetic defect in a second complementary gene.

Epigenetics: Mitotically and/or meiotically heritable variations of gene function that cannot be explained by changes of DNA sequence.

Expressivity: The level of expression of the phenotype. When the manifestations of the phenotype in individuals who have the same genotype are diverse, the phenotype is said to exhibit variable expressivity.

Genotype: A person's genetic or DNA sequence composition at a particular location in the genome.

Genotypic heterogeneity: Genetic variability among individuals with similar phenotypes.

Genotype-phenotype plasticity: The concept that the link between genotype and phenotype is subject to broad variability with, as yet, limited predictability.

Genome-wide association studies: Examination of many common genetic variants in individuals, with and without a disease trait, to identify a possible higher frequency (i.e. association) of single-nucleotide polymorphisms in people with the trait.

Haploinsufficiency: The situation in which an individual who is heterozygous for a certain gene mutation or hemizygous at a particular locus, often due to a deletion of the corresponding allele, is clinically affected because a single copy of the normal gene is incapable of providing sufficient protein production to assure normal function. This is an example of incomplete or partial dominance.

Table 56.1 Known channel mutations in genetic channelopathies. New mutations are continuously discovered. Most conditions are inherited in an autosomal dominant pattern, although both recessive (JLN, CPVT2) and X-linked patterns (BrS) have been described

Chromosomal locus	Gene	Protein	Current	Function	Syndrome	Phenotype
11p15.5	*KCNQ1*	*$K_v7.1$*	*IKs*	Loss of function	LQT1	Long QT
				Loss of function	JLN	Long QT, deafness
				Gain of function	SQT	Short QT
				Gain of function	AF	Atrial fibrillation
7q35-q36	*KCNH2*	*HERG*	*IKr*	Loss of function	LQT2	Long QT
				Gain of function	SQT	Short QT
				Gain of function	AF	Atrial fibrillation
3p21	*SCN5A*	*$Na_v1.5$*	*INa*	Gain of function	LQT3	Long QT
				Loss of function	BrS1	Brugada syndrome
				Loss of function	AF	Atrial fibrillation
				Loss of function	PCCD	Conduction defects
				Loss of function	SSS	Sick sinus syndrome
				Loss of function	DCM	Dilated cardiomyopathy
				Gain of function	MEPPC	Ventricular premature conductions
4q25-q27	*ANK2*	*Ankyrin B*	*INa-K, INa-Ca, I_{Na}*	Loss of function	LQT4	Long QT
						Atrial fibrillation
						CPVT
21q22.1-q22.2	*KCNE1*	*MinK*	*IKs*	Loss of function	LQT5	Long QT
				Loss of function	JLN	Long QT, deafness
				Loss of function	AF	Atrial fibrillation
21q22.1-q22.2	*KCNE2*	*MiRP1*	*IKr*	Loss of function	LQT6	Long QT
				Gain of function	AF	Atrial fibrillation
17q23.1-q24.2	*KCNJ2*	*Kir2.1*	*IK1*	Loss of function	LQT7	Long QT, AV block, potassium-sensitive periodic paralysis, hypoplastic mandible *(Andersen–Tawil syndrome)*
				Gain of function	SQT	Short QT
				Gain of function	AF	Atrial fibrillation
12p13.3	*CACNA1C*	*$Ca_v1.2$*	*ICa*	Gain of function	LQT8	Long QT, syndactyly, septal defects *(Timothy syndrome)*
				Loss of function	BrS	Brugada syndrome
				Loss of function	SQT	Short QT
3p24	*CAV3*	*Caveolin-3*	*INa*	Gain of function	LQT9	Long QT
11q23.3	*SCN4B*	*Navβ4*	*INa*	Gain of function	LQT10	Long QT

(*Continued*)

Table 56.1 (Continued)

Chromosomal locus	Gene	Protein	Current	Function	Syndrome	Phenotype
7q21-q22	*AKAP9*	*A-kinase anchorin (yotiao)*	*IKs*	Reduced due to loss of cAMP sensitivity	LQT11	Long QT
20q11.2	*SNTA1*	*α-1 syntrophin*	*INa*	Increased due to S-nitrosylation of SCN5A	LQT12	Long QT
11q23.3–24.3	*KCNJ5*	*Kir3.4 subunit*	*IKAch*	Loss of function	LQT13	Long QT
10p12.33	*CACNB2b*	*Ca_vbeta 2β*	*ICa*	Loss of function	SQT	Short QT
				Loss of function	BrS	Brugada syndrome
7q21-q22	*CACNA2D1*	*Ca_vα2δ-1*	*ICa*	Loss of function	SQT	Short QT
				Loss of function	BrS	Brugada syndrome
13p22.3	*GPD1L*	*glycerol-3-phosphate dehydrogenase 1-like*	*INa*	Reduced	BrS	Brugada syndrome
19q13.1	*SCN1B*	*Na_vβ1*	*INa*	Loss of function	BrS	Brugada syndrome
						Conduction disease
						Atrial fibrillation
11q13-q14	*KCNE3*	*Beta subunit*	*Ito, Iks*	Gain of function	BrS	Brugada syndrome
11q23.3	*SCN3B*	*Beta subunit*	*INa*	Loss of function	BrS	Brugada syndrome
15q24.1	*HCN4*	*HCN4*	*If*	Loss of function	BrS	Brugada syndrome
1p13.3	*KCND3*	*Kv4.3*	*Ito*	Gain of function	BrS	Brugada syndrome
12p11.23	*KCNJ8*	*α subunit*	*IKATP*	Gain of function	BrS	Brugada syndrome
					ERS	
17p13.1	*MOG1*	*MOG1 (RAN guanine nucleotide release factor 1*	*INa*	Impaired trafficking of channel	BrS	Brugada syndrome
3p14.3–21.2	*SLMAP*	*SLMAP*	*INa*	Impaired trafficking of channel	BrS	Brugada syndrome
Xq22.3	*KVNE5*	*β subunit*	*Ito*	Loss of function	BrS	Brugada syndrome
Xq22.3	*KVNE5*	*β subunit*	*Ito*	Loss of function	BrS	Brugada syndrome
3q29	*DLG1*	*synapse-associated 97*	*Junction functions*	*Reduced*	BrS	Brugada syndrome
1q42–43	*RyR2*	*Cardiac ryanodine receptor*	*Ca kinetics*	*Diastolic Ca release*	CPVT1	Catecholaminergic tachycardia bradycardia, AF, AV block, dilated cardiomyopathy
1p13–21	*CASQ2*	*Cardiac calsequestrin*	*Ca kinetics*	*Diastolic Ca release*	CPVT2	Catecholaminergic tachycardia
17q23	*KCNJ2*	*Kir2.1*	*Ik1*	*Loss of function*	CPVT3	Catecholaminergic tachycardia
14q32.11	*CALM1*	*Calmodulin 1*	*Ca kinetics*	*Binding to RyR2*	CPVT	Catecholaminergic tachycardia
6q22.31	*TRDN*	*Triadin*	*Ca kinetics*	*Binding to RyR2*	CPVT	Catecholaminergic tachycardia

JLN, Jervel and Lange-Nielsen syndrome; SSS, sick sinus syndrome; ERS, early repolarization syndrome; DCM, dilated cardiomyopathy; CPVT, catecholaminergic polymorphic VT; PCCD, progressive conduction system disease; MEPPC, multifocal ectopic Purkinje-related premature contractions. For current terminology see Chapter 49.

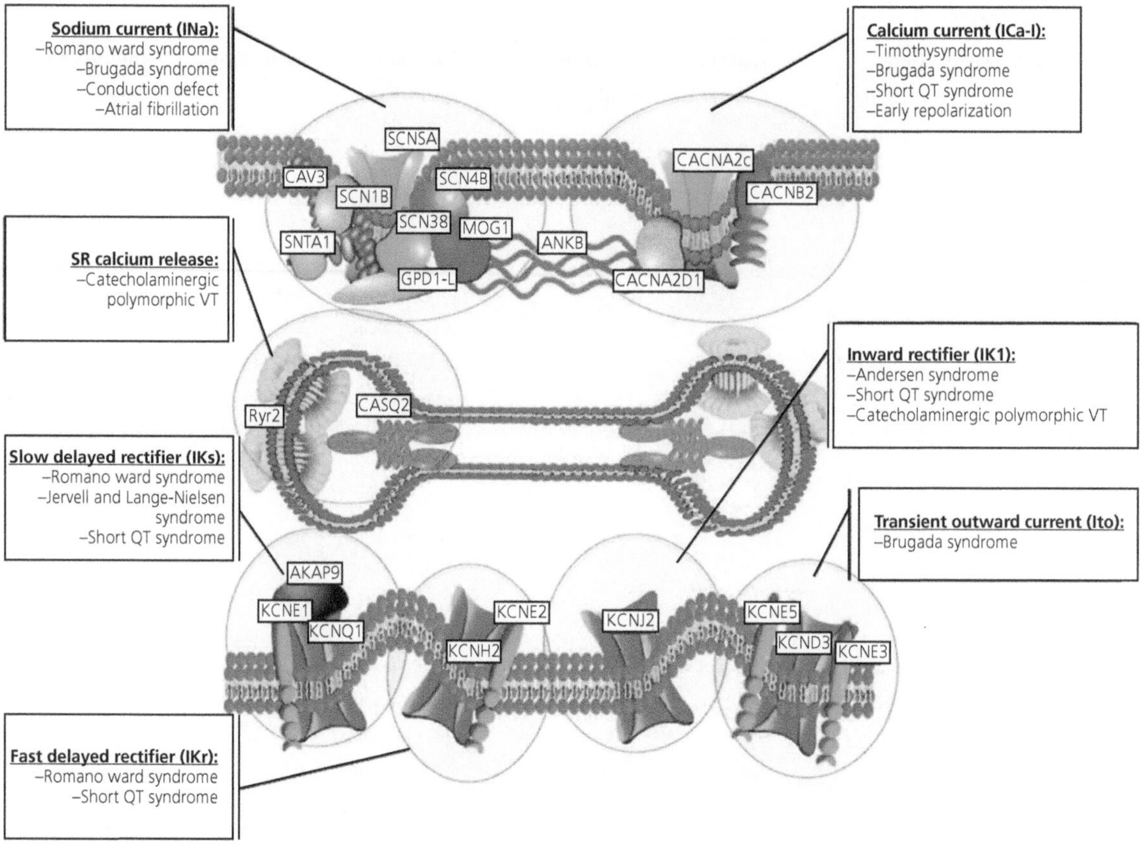

Figure 56.1 Genes associated with inherited arrhythmogenic diseases grouped by ion channel/function. SR, sarcoplasmic reticulum; VT, ventricular tachycardia.

Napolitano *et al*. Sudden cardiac death and genetic ion channelopathies: long QT, Brugada, short QT, catecholaminergic polymorphic ventricular tachycardia, and idiopathic ventricular fibrillation. *Circulation* 2012; **125**:2027–2034.

Heterozygote: An individual who has different alleles at a particular gene locus on homologous chromosomes (carrier of a single copy of the mutation).

Homozygote: An individual who has the same allele at a particular gene locus on homologous chromosomes (carrier of a double copy of the mutation).

Matrilinear inheritance: Women but not men transmit the disease to offspring (male or female), as happens with disease due to mitochondrial DNA mutations.

Modifier: Gene variants or environmental factors that are insufficient to cause observable disease on their own but which are capable of interacting with the disease gene to alter the phenotype.

Mutation: A change of the DNA sequence within the genome. A mutation considered in the context of a genetic disease usually refers to an alteration that causes a Mendelian disease whereas a genetic polymorphism refers to a common genetic variation observed in the general population.

Mutation—deletion/insertion: The removal (deletion) or addition (insertion) of nucleotides to the transcript that can be as small as a single nucleotide insertion/deletion or as large as several hundreds to thousands of nucleotides in length.

Mutation—disease-causing: A DNA sequence variation that represents an abnormal allele and is not found in the normal healthy population but exists only in the disease population and produces a functionally abnormal product.

Mutation—frameshift: Insertions or deletions occurring in the exon that alter the 'reading frame' of translation at the point of the insertion or deletion and produce a new sequence of amino acids in the finished product. Frameshift mutations often result in a different product length from the normal gene product by creating a new stop codon, which produces either a shorter or longer gene product, depending on the location of the new stop codon.

Mutation—germline: Heritable change in the genetic make-up of a germ cell (sperm or ovum) that, when transmitted to an offspring, is incorporated into every cell in the body.

Mutation—in-frame insertion/deletion: In-frame insertions and deletions occur when a multiple of three

Table 56.2 Yield and signal-to-noise associated with disease-specific genetic testing (HRS/EHRA statement 2011)

Disease	Yield of genetic test*	% of controls with a rare VUS#	Signal-to-noise (S:N) ratio+
LQTS	75% (80%)	4%	19:1
CPVT	60% (70%)	3%	20:1
BrS	20% (30%)	2% (just *SCN5A*)	10:1
CCD	Unknown	Unknown	Unknown
SQTS	Unknown	3%	Unknown
AF	Unknown	Unknown	Unknown
HCM	60% (70%)	~5% (unpublished data)	12:1
ACM/ARVC	60%	16%	4:1
DCM	30%	Unknown	Unknown
DCM + CCD	Unknown	4% (for SCN5A and LMNA)	Unknown
LVNC	17–41%	Unknown	Unknown
RCM	Unknown	Unknown	Unknown

* Yield of Genetic Test is a published/unpublished estimate, derived from unrelated cases with unequivocal disease phenotype. First number is the yield associated with the targeted major gene scan. The number in parentheses is the total yield when including all known disease-associated genes that have been included in commercial disease gene panels. When only a single percentage is provided, this represents the estimate from a comprehensive disease gene panel. These yield values represent estimates for whites with the particular disease phenotype. Evidence is lacking to establish point estimates for minority populations.
# % of controls with a rare variant of uncertain significance (VUS) represents a frequency of rare amino acid substitutions found in whites in the major disease-associated genes that, had it been found in a case, would have been reported as a 'possible disease-associated mutation.' This number does not include the frequency of rare genetic variants present in the minor disease-associated genes. Thus, it represents a lower point estimate for the potential false positive rate. A question mark indicates that an otherwise healthy
control population has not been systematically examined for the genes of interest. As with the Yield of Genetic Test, these estimates are derived for whites.
+ The signal-to-noise (S:N) ratio is derived by dividing the yield by the background rate of VUS in controls. This provides a sense of the positive predictive value of a 'positive' genetic test result.
HRS/EHRA 2011 expert consensus statement on the state of genetic testing for the channelopathies and cardiomyopathies, *Heart Rhythm*. 2011:1308–39.

nucleotides is affected and result in a single or multiple amino acids being removed or added without affecting the remainder of the transcript.

Mutation—missense: A single nucleotide substitution that results in the exchange of a normal amino acid in the protein for a different one.

Mutation—nonsense: A single nucleotide substitution resulting in a substitution of an amino acid for a stop codon. A nonsense mutation results in a truncated (shortened) gene product at the location of the new stop codon.

Mutation—somatic: Variants/mutations are said to be somatic if they occur in cells other than gametes. Somatic mutations cannot be transmitted to offspring.

Penetrance: The likelihood that a gene mutation will have any expression at all. In the situation in which the frequency of phenotypic expression is less than 100%, the genetic defect is said to be associated with reduced or incomplete penetrance.

Phenocopy: An individual who manifests the same phenotype (trait) as other individuals of a particular genotype but does not possess this genotype himself/herself.

Phenotype: A person's observed clinical expression of disease in terms of a morphological, biochemical, or molecular trait.

Phenotypic heterogeneity: Phenotypic variability among individuals with similar genotypes.

Polymorphism: Normal variations at distinct loci in the DNA sequence. The vast majority of the human genome represents a single version of genetic information. The DNA from one person is mostly made up of the same exact nucleotide sequence as another person. However, there are many small sections of sequence, or even single nucleotides, that differ from one individual to another.

Proband or index case or propositus: The first affected family member who seeks medical attention for a genetic disease.

Single-nucleotide polymorphism (SNP): A single nucleotide substitution that occurs with a measurable frequency (i.e. >0.5% allelic frequency) among a particular ethnic population(s).

SNP—non-synonymous: A single nucleotide substitution whereby the altered codon encodes for a different amino acid or terminates further protein assembly (i.e. introduces a premature stop codon).

SNP—synonymous: A single nucleotide substitution occurring in the coding region (exon), whereby the new codon still specifies the same amino acid.

X-linked inheritance: a recessive mode of inheritance in which a mutation in a gene on the X chromosome causes the phenotype to be expressed in males (who are necessarily hemizygous for the gene mutation) and in females who are homozygous for the gene mutation.

References

1. Leenhardt A, *et al.* Catecholaminergic polymorphic ventricular tachycardia. *Circ Arrhythm Electrophysiol.* 2012;**5**:1044–52
2. Golbus JR, *et al.* Population-based variation in cardiomyopathy genes. *Circ Cardiovasc Genet.* 2012;**5**:391–9
3. Tester DJ, *et al.* Genetic testing for potentially lethal, highly treatable inherited cardiomyopathies/channelopathies in clinical practice. *Circulation.* 2011;**123**:1021–37
4. Ackerman MJ, *et al.* HRS/EHRA expert consensus statement on the state of genetic testing for the channelopathies and cardiomyopathies: this document was developed as a partnership between the Heart Rhythm Society (HRS) and the European Heart Rhythm Association (EHRA). *Europace.* 2011;**13**:1077–109
5. Roberts R, *et al.* Genomics in cardiovascular disease. *J Am Coll Cardiol.* 2013; doi:10.1016/j.jacc.2012.1012.1054
6. Dewey FE, *et al.* DNA sequencing: clinical applications of new DNA sequencing technologies. *Circulation.* 2012;**125**:931–44
7. Schwartz P, *et al.* Impact of genetics on the clinical management of channelopathies. *J Am Coll Cardiol.* 2013;**62**:169–180

Chapter 57

Long QT syndrome

Definition

Inherited long QT syndrome (LQTS) is characterized by a prolonged QT interval, syncope, and sudden cardiac death due to ventricular tachyarrhythmias, typically torsades de pointes.[1]

Epidemiology

This genetic channelopathy has variable penetrance, and the estimated prevalence of clinically overt disease is approximately 1:2000 subjects.[2] Symptomatic patients without therapy have a high mortality rate, 21% within 1 year from the first syncope, but, with proper treatment, mortality is now ≈1% during a 15-year follow-up.[3]

Pathophysiology and genetics

The genetic basis of the LQTS is mutations or polymorphisms in genes encoding proteins that form ion channels affecting repolarization (Table 56.1 of Chapter 56). Nearly 1000 mutations have been identified in **13 distinct LQTS susceptibility genes**. Most of LQTS are due to loss-of-function mutations in the genes ***KCNQ1*** and ***KCNH2*** encoding for voltage-gated potassium channels that affect the repolarizing currents I_{Ks} (LQT1, 30–35% of all LQTS) and I_{Kr} (LQT2, 25–40% of all LQTS), respectively.[4–6] Up to 10% of LQTS are due to gain-of-function mutations of the gene ***SCN5A*** (I_{Na}-LQT3, mostly missense, i.e. single amino acid substitutions) encoding for the sodium channel. In patients with such mutations, the channel fails to close properly after initial depolarization, and continued leakage of sodium into the channel results in prolongation of the action potential. The location of a mutation within the cytoplasmic loop DNA sequence of the KCNQ1 gene may affect severity and risk of sudden death.[5] Nine minor LQTS susceptibility genes account for less than 5%, and up to 20% of congenital LQTS cases remain genotype-negative. Patients with LQTS, despite normal LVEF, have significantly longer contraction duration and greater indices of regional and transmural inhomogeneous contraction times, as assessed by strain echocardiography.[7]

The QT interval on the ECG represents the longest repolarization in the mid-myocardial M-cell region, i.e. a physiological transmural dispersion of repolarization. Gene mutations or medications that cause selective action potential prolongation in the M-cell region can lead to increased transmural repolarization gradients and thus create the conditions for functional reentry and subsequent torsades. A net decrease in repolarizing currents prolongs actions potentials in LQTS, and subsequently promotes the L-type Ca^{2+} current ($I_{Ca,L}$) and phase-2 early after-depolarizations.[1] Prolonged action potentials cause Ca^{2+} overload, leading to the activation of the inward Na^{+}-Ca^{2+} exchanger current that causes phase-3 early after-depolarizations. Early after-depolarizations (phase-2 and phase-3) and dispersion of repolarization contribute to torsades de pointes.[3] The trigger for TdP is thought to be a PVC that results from an early after-depolarization generated during the abnormally prolonged repolarization phase of the affected myocardium. A long preceding pause increases the amplitude of early after-depolarizations, which makes them more likely to reach the threshold necessary to produce a PVC or ventricular couplet (short-long-short RR intervals sequences mode of TdP onset). Torsades de pointes, therefore, is triggered by early after-depolarizations and can be maintained by repetitive, multifocal early after-depolarizations as well as reentry around shifting pathways.[8] Pause-dependent torsades de pointes is seen in LQT2 and perhaps LQT3, but not in LQT1, in which sympathetic activation is the usual trigger.[9] Sympathetic activity is an important modulator of the disorder and can further delay repolarization, induce early after-depolarizations, and trigger sudden arrhythmic death in patients with LQTS, especially LQT1. Patients with LQTS have an increased risk of AF.[10]

The classic LQTS is being transmitted as an autosomal dominant trait (initially described by **Romano and Ward**). A less common, but more severe, form is transmitted as an autosomal recessive disease (patients carry two abnormal LQT genes) and is associated with neurosensory deafness and higher risk of sudden death (**Jervell and Lange-Nielsen syndrome**).[3]

Presentation

The term 'torsades de pointes' was introduced by Dessertenne in 1866 when he described polymorphic ventricular tachycardia occurring in the setting of bradycardia due to complete heart block. Symptoms caused by this tachyarrhythmia range from dizziness and syncope to cardiac arrest and death in up to 16% of patients. Because torsades de pointes can cause seizures due to cerebral anoxia, LQTS is important to consider in patients with apparent drug-resistant seizure disorders. Both exercise (especially swimming) and emotional stress (sudden loud noise, anger) can trigger syncope in patients with LQTS, possibly via an increase in catecholamine concentrations. Pregnancy reduces the risk of cardiac events, but the risk increases in the 9-month period of post-partum, especially in patients with LQT2. β blockers reduce the occurrence of cardiac events post-partum. Specifically:

- **LQT1**: exercise (especially swimming), emotional stress
- **LQT2**: emotional stress, sudden noise
- **LQT3**: rest, sleep.

Diagnosis

QT prolongation The most important diagnostic and prognostic characteristic is QT interval prolongation (Figure 57.1), although it might not accurately predict the prognosis in LQT3 (Figure 57.2). The QT interval should be determined as a mean value derived from, at least, 3 to 5 heart beats and is measured from the beginning of the earliest onset of the QRS complex to the end of the T wave in leads II and V_5 or V_6, with the longest value being used. In situations in which the end of the T wave may be difficult to determine (e.g. biphasic or notched T waves, T waves with superimposed U waves), the end of the T wave can be determined by drawing a line from the peak of the T wave following the steepest T wave downslope. The intersection of this line with the isoelectric baseline is considered the end of the T wave (Figure 57.2).[11] In AF, the average of the QTc values of the shortest and longest R-R intervals is used. If the interval from R wave to the peak (or nadir) of the T wave is more than 50% of the R-R interval, there is an indication that it would be longer than the critical threshold of 500 ms if measured. The QT interval is usually corrected for heart rate because the QT interval shortens at fast heart

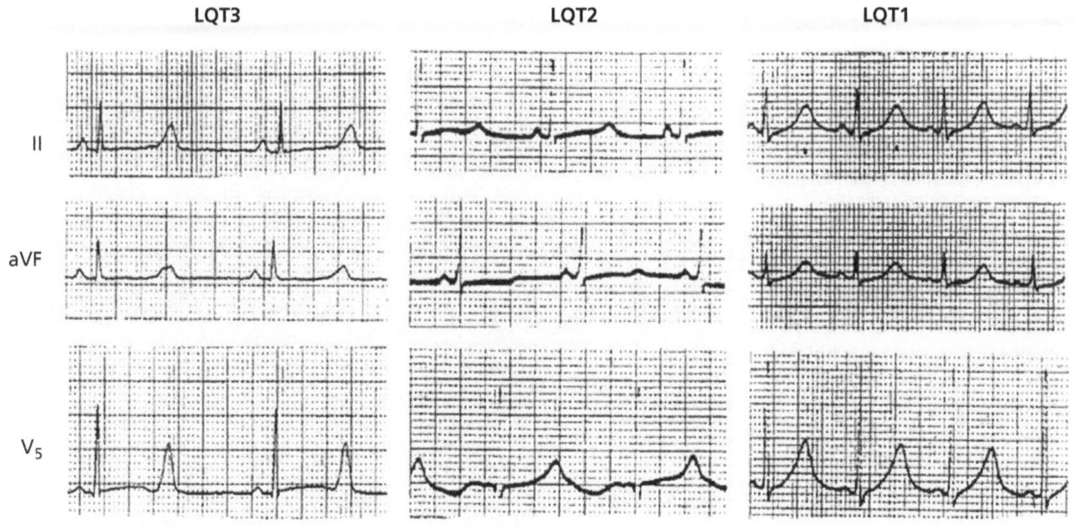

Figure 57.1 QT prolongation in the major three LQT syndromes T-wave morphology by LQTS genotype: LQT1: typical broad-based T-wave pattern (corrected QT [QTc] 570 ms); LQT2: typical bifid T-wave (QTc 583 ms); and LQT3: typical late-onset peaked/biphasic T-wave (QTc 573 ms).

Goldenberg I, Moss AJ. Long QT syndrome. *J Am Coll Cardiol*. 2008;**51**:2291–300.

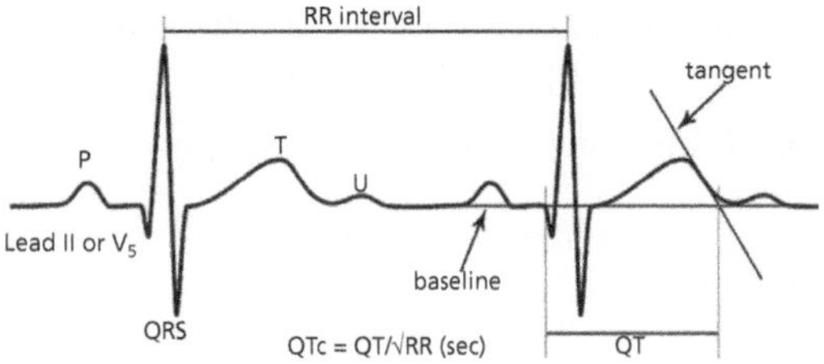

Figure 57.2 Measurement of the QT interval. A tangent is drawn to the steepest slope of the last limb of the T wave in lead II or V_5. The end of the T wave is the intersection of the tangent with the baseline. QT is heart rate corrected with Bazett's formula with use of the preceding RR interval.
Postema PG, *et al.* Accurate electrocardiographic assessment of the QT interval: teach the tangent. *Heart Rhythm.* 2008;**5**:1015–8.

rates and prolongs at slow heart rates. The Bazett formula (QTc = QT/√RR, with all intervals in seconds) remains the standard for clinical use, despite some limitations at particularly fast or slow heart rates, in which the formula may overcorrect or undercorrect, respectively. Various criteria have been proposed (Table 57.1),[2,5] but they carry a high specificity and low sensitivity.

Normal QTc values are <440 for age 1–15 years, <430 for adult males, and <450 ms for adult females.[3]

A **QTc value of ≥430 ms** distinguishes carriers from non-carriers (<430 ms), with a 72% sensitivity and 86% specificity.[12]

Increased **QT dispersion** (>100 ms), measured as the difference between the minimum and maximum QT intervals in the 12-lead ECG, indicates ventricular repolarization heterogeneity and is increased in symptomatic patients and reduced by beta blockers.

Prominent **U waves** and T-U complexes are frequently seen.

T-wave alternans, ie a beat-to-beat alternation in T-wave morphology, is a marker of high cardiac electrical instability. Notches on the T-wave are rather typical for LQT2 and are associated with a hogher proarrhythmia risk.[2]

Sinus bradycardia may be present, and **sinus pauses** are mainly seen in LQT3.

Response to exercise or catecholamine injection In healthy individuals, acute sympathetic stimulation increases inward Ca^{2+} currents, shortens the RR interval, and initially prolongs and then shortens the QT interval by activating the delayed rectifier K^+ current (slow component, I_{Ks}).

- LQT1: prolongation of both QT and QTc interval during and after cessation of exercise or catecholamine injection (paradoxical QT response)
- LQT2: initial prolongation followed by shortening of the QT and QTc and promotion of the notch on the descending T wave
- LQT3: shortening of the QT interval. The QTc is slightly prolonged at the peak effect of exercise and returns to baseline at steady state.

Table 57.1 HRA/EHRA/APHRS 2013 statement on inherited arrhythmia

Recommendations on LQTS Diagnosis
1. LQTS is diagnosed: a. In the presence of an LQTS risk score > 3.5 in the absence of a secondary cause for QT prolongation, *and/or* b. In the presence of an unequivocally pathogenic mutation in one of the LQTS genes, *or* c. In the presence of a QTc> 500 ms in repeated 12-lead ECG and in the absence of a secondary cause for QT prolongation.
2. LQTS can be diagnosed in the presence of a QTc between 480–499 ms in repeated 12-lead ECGs in a patient with unexplained syncope in the absence of a secondary cause for QT prolongation and in the absence of a pathogenic mutation.

HRS/EHRA/APHRS Expert Consensus Statement on the Diagnosis and Management of Patients with Inherited Primary Arrhythmia Syndromes. *Europace* E-Pub

The presence and genotype of LQTS can be established by **exercise testing** that may reveal features, such as inadequate QT shortening, postural T wave change, and exercise-related T wave notching.[13, 14] The post-recovery QTc may also be helpful. LQT1 patients begin the recovery period at a very prolonged QTc that decreases during recovery whereas the LQT2 patients begin recovery at a lower QTc that increases during recovery. At the end of recovery, a QTc cut-off value of 445 ms indicates LQTS while a start-of-recovery QTc >460 ms suggests LQT1 and <460 ms LQT2. [15] Symptomatic LQT1 patients have a greater heart rate reduction (≥17%) at the first minute of recovery phase from the peak heart rate during exercise when compared with asymptomatic LQT1 patients, regardless of the use of beta blockers. This does not occur in LQT2 and LQT3 patients. Thus, heart rate reduction immediately after exercise, a marker of vagal reflex response, can be used for risk stratification in LQT1.[16]

Other provocative tests are absence of QT shortening (but prominent QTc increase), with tachycardia induced by standing,[17] and QT prolongation (15%) by **adenosine** boluses of 6–24 mg.[18] Results from the Cardiac Arrest Survivors With Preserved Ejection Fraction Registry (CASPER) have shown that **epinephrine** challenge at doses of 0.05, 0.10, and 0.20 microgram/kg per minute may also disclose LQTS in unexplained cardiac arrest. A test is considered positive for long QT syndrome if the absolute QT interval is prolonged by ≥30 ms at 0.10 microgram/kg per minute and borderline if QT prolongation is 1 to 29 ms.[19]

Risk stratification

- A history of aborted **cardiac arrest** and/or ECG-documented episodes of **torsades de pointes**, particularly with β blocker treatment, indicates high risk. Children and adolescents who present after an episode of syncope should be considered to be at high risk of development of subsequent syncope episodes and fatal/near-fatal events, regardless of QTc duration.[20] Among symptomatic cases, the untreated 10-year mortality is approximately 50%.[6]

- High-risk patients usually have QTc intervals of, at least, **500 ms** and can also show **T wave alternans** (Table 57.2). There is no threshold of QTc prolongation at which TdP is certain to occur. However, there is a gradual increase in risk for TdP as the QTc increases, and a QTc >500 ms is associated with a 2- to 3-fold higher risk for TdP.[2]
- **LQT2 females** and **LQT3 males with QT >500 ms** are high-risk, independently of other factors.[21] Patients with LQT3 have a lower incidence of cardiac events but higher lethality than those with LQT1 and LQT2, and the risk may not be associated with prolongation of the QTc interval. Genetic testing is, therefore, useful in this respect. A risk stratification scheme has also been proposed for LQTS2: LQT2: females >13 years or males with mutations in the pore-loop region of KCNH2 and QTc ≥500 ms indicate intermediate risk while the presence of syncope in this category indicates high risk.[22]
- The presence of missense mutations in distinct functional domains of the KCNQ1 protein, the **S2-S3 and S4-S5 cytoplasmic loops** (C loops), is associated with a significantly increased risk for life-threatening cardiac events compared with other mutations, and these patients gain greater benefit when treated with β-blockers compared with patients having other KCNQ1 mutations independently of clinical risk factors.[23] Mutations in these regions are responsible for the condition in 7–15% of patients with LQT1.
- A family history of premature SCD is not an independent risk factor for subsequent lethal events in an affected individual.
- Two well-defined malignant variants are the **Jervell and Lange–Nielsen** syndrome and **LQT8.**[3]

Genetic testing

Apart from risk stratification purposes, genetic testing is useful for the identification of concealed LQTS because individuals with genetically proven LQTS may have a non-diagnostic QTc (Table 57.3).[4] However, no treatment decision should be influenced solely by either the genotype or the specific LQTS-causative mutation that was identified. In particular, a decision to implant an ICD prophylactically in an asymptomatic LQT3 host must include risk factors besides LQT3 genotype status.[4] Genetic testing should be considered for patients with drug-induced torsade, and a 12-lead ECG is recommended for first-degree relatives.

Specific LQTS types

LQT1 is the most common type of LQTS and is due to heterozygous gene mutations of *KCNQ1* (encoding the alpha subunit of the I_{Ks} channel). I_{ks} reduction increases transmural dispersion of repolarization and sensitivity to catecholamine stimulation. Mutations of *KCNQ1* reduce I_{Ks}, but I_{Kr} (i.e. the rapid component of the delayed rectifier K^+ current) could maintain a near-normal duration of action potentials, concealing LQT1. In this case, I_{Kr} blockade (e.g. by drugs) or inactivation (e.g. by hypokalaemia) can induce substantial QT prolongation and trigger torsades de pointes. Anti-adrenergic treatment is usually effective for LQT1.[1]

Table 57.2 Age-specific risk factors

Childhood (1–12 years) Beta blockers reduce risk by 73%
Prior syncope, especially recent (<2 years)
Male gender
QTc >500 ms
Adolescence (10–20 years) Beta blockers reduce risk by 64%
Prior syncope, especially recent (<2 years) and when ≥2 events
QTc >530 ms
Adulthood (18–40 years) Beta blockers reduce risk by 60%
QTc ≥500 ms
Prior syncope, especially recent (<2 years)
Female gender
Adulthood (41–60 years) Beta blockers may reduce risk
Recent syncope (<2 years)
LQT3 genotype
QTc >530 ms

Goldenberg I, Moss AJ. Long QT syndrome. *J Am Coll Cardiol*. 2008;**51**:2291–300.

Table 57.3 HRS/EHRS 2011 statement on genetic testing

Comprehensive or LQT1–3 (KCNQ1, KCNH2, and SCN5A) targeted LQTS genetic testing	
Any patient in whom a cardiologist has established a strong clinical index of suspicion for LQTS based on examination of the patient's clinical history, family history, and expressed electrocardiographic (resting 12-lead ECGs and/or provocative stress testing with exercise or catecholamine infusion) phenotype.	I
Any asymptomatic patient with QT prolongation in the absence of other clinical conditions that might prolong the QT interval (such as electrolyte abnormalities, hypertrophy, bundle branch block, etc., i.e. otherwise idiopathic) on serial 12-lead ECGs defined as QTc >480 ms (prepuberty) or >500 ms (adults).	I
Mutation-specific genetic testing is recommended for family members and other appropriate relatives, subsequently following the identification of the LQTS-causative mutation in an index case.	I
Any asymptomatic patient with otherwise idiopathic QTc values >460 ms (prepuberty) or >480 ms (adults) on serial 12-lead ECGs.	IIb

HRS/EHRA 2011 expert consensus statement on the state of genetic testing for the channelopathies and cardiomyopathies. *Heart Rhythm*. 2011 **8**:1308–39.

LQT2 is the second most common genotype of LQTS and is associated with reduced I_{Kr} by gene mutations (*KCNH2*) that encode the α subunit (HERG) of the I_{Kr} channel. Reduced I_{Kr} slows repolarization and increases the transmural dispersion of repolarization. I_{Kr} is unaffected by catecholamine stimulation.[1] Emotional stress and sudden loud noises can cause a rapid increase in heart rate from sympathetic discharge, which acutely prolongs the action potential before subsequent shortening by a slowed enhancement of I_{Ks}. Bradycardia reduces I_{Kr}, delays repolarization, and increases transmural dispersion. Although β blockers reduce cardiac events in patients with LQT2, they worsen bradycardia, resulting in more cardiac event than in patients with LQT1. Use of potassium treatment in LQT2 has shortened QT, reduced QT dispersion, normalized T waves, and suppressed torsades de pointes.

LQT3 results in cardiac events leading to sudden death, occurs usually at night or rest without arousal, and occasionally follows sympathetic stimulation. Typical ECG in LQT3 shows a flat, long ST segment with late appearance of a narrow peaked T wave. LQT3 is caused by *SCN5A* mutations that lead to gain-of-function of Na^+ channels via a late sustained current that prolongs the plateau phase of the action potential and produces long ST segments and late appearance of T wave in the ECG, which are LQT3 characteristics. β blocker treatment is less effective in LQT3, and treated patients still have more cardiac events (30%) than those with LQT1 and LQT2. Since the occurrence of cardiac events is not frequent in LQT3, it is unknown whether β blockers are useful. They can be used, unless it is clear that ventricular arrhythmias worsen, at which time Na^+ channel blockers can be added to the β blocker treatment.[1, 3]

Jervell and Lange-Nielsen syndrome occurs in 1–7% of patients with LQTS. Diagnosis is considered on the basis of the established diagnostic criteria for LQTS and on the presence of congenital neurosensory deafness. The first cardiac event often occurs in the first year of life, and 90% of patients have syncope during their early lifetime, usually induced by exercise and emotional stress. Subgroups at relatively lower risk for sudden death are females, patients with a QTc <550 ms, those without events in the first year of life, and those with mutations on KCNE1.[3] Beta blockers have limited efficacy, and early ICD implantation must be considered.

Therapy

Beta blockers should be administered to all intermediate- or high-risk affected individuals and considered in low-risk patients, unless there is a contraindication. β adrenergic blockade does not shorten QT at rest but suppresses cardiac events in LQT1 whereas the efficacy of β blockade is reduced in LQT2 and especially in LQT3. Targeting of the pathologic, LQT3-associated late sodium current with propranolol (as the preferred beta blocker) and the possible addition of mexiletine, flecainide, or ranolazine represents the preferred pharmacotherapeutic option for LQT3.[6,24] Potassium supplements shorten QT interval by increasing the I_{Kr} that is inversely regulated by the concentration of extracellular potassium. This approach has been proposed for LQT2, although it has the potential to shorten QT interval in all patients with, at least, one KCNH2 wildtype (functional) allele.[24] The problem is that, in the presence of normal renal function, the additional dietary potassium load typically may be excreted without clinically significant increases in serum potassium levels.

Implantable cardioverter defibrillators are indicated in cardiac arrest survivors and patients with recurrent syncope despite β blocker treatment and for primary prevention in high-risk patients, usually with β blockers (Table 57.4). Recent data suggest that ICDs were implanted in some LQTS patients whose high risk now appears questionable, and the following recommendations have been proposed for ICD implantation:[25, 26]

- Patients who have survived a cardiac arrest on therapy
- Many of those who have survived a cardiac arrest off therapy, except those with a reversible/preventable cause, but noting that, for most LQT1 grown-up patients, full-dose beta blockers might be sufficient
- Patients who continue to have syncope, despite full-dose beta blockade, whenever the option of left cardiac sympathetic denervation is either not available or is discarded after discussion with the patients
- Patients with two mutations who continue to have syncope despite beta blockade
- Asymptomatic patients with a QTc >550 ms who also manifest signs of high electric instability (e.g. T wave alternans) or other evidence of being at very high risk (e.g. very long sinus pauses that might favour early after-depolarizations)
- The identification of LQT2 or LQT3 genotypes does not, by itself, constitute an indication of ICD implantation.[27]

Left cardiac sympathetic denervation is considered in patients with recurrent syncope, despite beta-blocker therapy, and in patients who experience arrhythmia storms with an ICD but does not offer full protection. **Permanent pacing** may be needed for documented pause-dependent VT (Table 57.5). Although pacemaker implantation may reduce the incidence of symptoms in these patients, the long-term survival benefit is not proven. **RF ablation** of the torsade-triggering PVC has also been reported.[23] **Gene-specific** treatments are investigational.[3]

All LQTS patients should avoid drugs that block the I_{Kr} current (http://www.torsades.org) (see also Chapter 55 Drug Induced VT).

Restriction of physical activities depends on the type of LQTS.[24] Asymptomatic patients with short baseline QTc intervals should not be significantly restricted.[6] QTc >0.47 s in male subjects or QTc >0.48 s in female subjects is an indication for low-intensity only competitive sports (36th Bethesda Conference) while the ESC recommends

Table 57.4 Therapy of long QT syndrome

ACCF/AHA 2012 GL on Device therapy. Indications for ICD	
LQTS and syncope and/or sustained VT on beta blockers	IIa-C
2012 ACCF/AHA/HRS focused update incorporated into the ACCF/AHA/HRS 2008 guidelines for device-based therapy of cardiac rhythm abnormalities. *J Am Coll Cardiol*. 2013;**61**:e6–75.	
HRS/EHRA/APHRS 2013 statement on inherited arrhythmia. Recommendations on LQTS Therapeutic Interventions	
The following lifestyle changes are recommended in all patients with a diagnosis of LQTS:	I
a) Avoidance of QT prolonging drugs (www.qtdrugs.org)	
b) Identification and correction of electrolyte abnormalities that may occur during diarrhea, vomiting, metabolic conditions or imbalanced diets for weight loss.	
Beta-blockers for patients with a diagnosis of LQTS who are:	I
a) Asymptomatic with QTc > 470 ms, *and/or*	
b) Symptomatic for syncope or documented VT/VF.	
Left cardiac sympathetic denervation (LCSD) for high-risk patients with a diagnosis of LQTS in whom:	I
a) ICD therapy is contraindicated or refused, *and/or*	
b) Beta-blockers are either not effective in preventing syncope/arrhythmias, not tolerated, not accepted or contraindicated.	
ICD for patients with a diagnosis of LQTS who are survivors of a cardiac arrest.	I
All LQTS patients who wish to engage in competitive sports should be referred to a clinical expert for evaluation of risk.	I
Beta-blockers in patients with a diagnosis of LQTS who are asymptomatic with QTc < 470ms.	IIa
ICD in patients with a diagnosis of LQTS who experience recurrent syncopal events while on beta-blocker therapy.	IIa
LCSD in patients with a diagnosis of LQTS who experience breakthrough events while on therapy with beta-blockers/ICD.	IIa
Sodium channel blockers, as add-on therapy, for LQT3 patients with a QTc 500 ms who shorten their QTc by > 40 ms following an acute oral drug test with one of these compounds.	IIa
Except under special circumstances, ICD implantation is not indicated in asymptomatic LQTS patients who have not been tried on beta-blocker therapy.	III

HRS/EHRA/APHRS Expert Consensus Statement on the Diagnosis and Management of Patients with Inherited Primary Arrhythmia Syndromes. *Europace* E-Pub

recreational only sports in QTc >0.44 s in male subjects and QTc >0.46 s in female subjects.[28]

Recent data suggest that, low-risk patients, with genetically confirmed LQTS (especially not LQTS1) but with borderline QTc prolongation, no history of cardiac symptoms, and no family history of multiple sudden cardiac deaths (SCD), may be allowed to participate in competitive sports

Table 57.5 ACCF/AHA/HRS 2012 GL on device therapy

Recommendations for pacing to prevent tachycardia	
Permanent pacing for sustained pause-dependent VT, with or without QT prolongation.	I-C
Permanent pacing for high-risk patients with congenital long QT syndrome.	IIa-C
Permanent pacing for prevention of symptomatic, drug-refractory, recurrent AF in patients with coexisting SND.	IIb-B
Permanent pacing for frequent or complex ventricular ectopic activity without sustained VT in the absence of the long QT syndrome.	III-C
Permanent pacing for torsade de pointes VT due to reversible causes.	III-A

2012 ACCF/AHA/HRS focused update incorporated into the ACCF/AHA/HRS 2008 guidelines for device-based therapy of cardiac rhythm abnormalities. *J Am Coll Cardiol*. 2013;**61**:e6–75

in special cases after full clinical evaluation, utilization of appropriate LQTS therapy and when competitive activity is performed where automated external defibrillators are available and personnel trained in basic life support.[29,2]

References

1. Morita H, *et al.* The QT syndromes: long and short. *Lancet*. 2008;**372**:750–63
2. HRS/EHRA/APHRS expert consensus statement on the diagnosis and management of patients with inherited primary arrhythmia syndromes. *Europace* 2013. E-Pub
3. Schwartz PJ, *et al.* Long-QT syndrome: from genetics to management. *Circ Arrhythm Electrophysiol*. 2012;**5**:868–77
4. Ackerman MJ, *et al.* HRS/EHRA expert consensus statement on the state of genetic testing for the channelopathies and cardiomyopathies: this document was developed as a partnership between the Heart Rhythm Society (HRS) and the European Heart Rhythm Association (EHRA). *Europace*. 2011;**13**:1077–109
5. Goldenberg I, *et al.* Long QT syndrome. *J Am Coll Cardiol*. 2008;**51**:2291–300
6. Webster G, *et al.* An update on channelopathies: from mechanisms to management. *Circulation*. 2013;**127**:126–40
7. Haugaa KH, *et al.* Transmural differences in myocardial contraction in long-QT syndrome: mechanical consequences of ion channel dysfunction. *Circulation*. 2010;**122**:1355–63
8. Sauer AJ, *et al.* Clinical and genetic determinants of torsade de pointes risk. *Circulation*. 2012;**125**:1684–94
9. Tan HL, *et al.* Genotype-specific onset of arrhythmias in congenital long-QT syndrome: possible therapy implications. *Circulation*. 2006;**114**:2096–103
10. Johnson JN, *et al.* Prevalence of early-onset atrial fibrillation in congenital long QT syndrome. *Heart Rhythm*. 2008;**5**:704–9
11. Postema PG, *et al.* Accurate electrocardiographic assessment of the QT interval: teach the tangent. *Heart Rhythm*. 2008;**5**:1015–18
12. Hofman N, *et al.* Diagnostic criteria for congenital long QT syndrome in the era of molecular genetics: do we need a scoring system? *Eur Heart J*. 2007;**28**:1399
13. Modi S, *et al.* Sudden cardiac arrest without overt heart disease. *Circulation*. 2011;**123**:2994–3008

14. Wong JA, *et al.* Utility of treadmill testing in identification and genotype prediction in long-QT syndrome. *Circ Arrhythm Electrophysiol.* 2010;**3**:120–5
15. Chattha IS, *et al.* Utility of the recovery electrocardiogram after exercise: a novel indicator for the diagnosis and genotyping of long QT syndrome? *Heart Rhythm.* 2010;**7**:906–11
16. Crotti L, *et al.* Vagal reflexes following an exercise stress test: a simple clinical tool for gene-specific risk stratification in the long QT syndrome. *J Am Coll Cardiol.* 2012;**60**:2515–24
17. Viskin S, *et al.* The response of the QT interval to the brief tachycardia provoked by standing: a bedside test for diagnosing long QT syndrome. *J Am Coll Cardiol.* 2010;**55**:1955–61
18. Obeyesekere MN, *et al.* How to perform and interpret provocative testing for the diagnosis of Brugada syndrome, long-QT syndrome, and catecholaminergic polymorphic ventricular tachycardia. *Circ Arrhythm Electrophysiol.* 2011;**4**:958–64
19. Krahn AD, *et al.* Epinephrine infusion in the evaluation of unexplained cardiac arrest and familial sudden death: from the cardiac arrest survivors with preserved ejection fraction registry. *Circ Arrhythm Electrophysiol.* 2012;**5**:933–40
20. Liu JF, *et al.* Risk factors for recurrent syncope and subsequent fatal or near-fatal events in children and adolescents with long QT syndrome. *J Am Coll Cardiol.* 2011;**57**:941–50
21. Cerrone M, *et al.* Genetics of sudden death: focus on inherited channelopathies. *Eur Heart J.* 2011;**32**:2109–18
22. Migdalovich D, *et al.* Mutation and gender-specific risk in type 2 long QT syndrome: implications for risk stratification for life-threatening cardiac events in patients with long QT syndrome. *Heart Rhythm.* 2011;**8**:1537–43
23. Barsheshet A, *et al.* Mutations in cytoplasmic loops of the kcnq1 channel and the risk of life-threatening events: Implications for mutation-specific response to beta-blocker therapy in type 1 long-qt syndrome. *Circulation.* 2012;**125**:1988–96
24. Napolitano C, *et al.* Sudden cardiac death and genetic ion channelopathies: long QT, Brugada, short QT, catecholaminergic polymorphic ventricular tachycardia, and idiopathic ventricular fibrillation. *Circulation.* 2012;**125**:2027–34
25. Schwartz PJ, *et al.* Who are the long-QT syndrome patients who receive an implantable cardioverter-defibrillator and what happens to them?: data from the European Long-QT Syndrome Implantable Cardioverter-Defibrillator (LQTS ICD) registry. *Circulation.* 2010;**122**:1272–82
26. Tester DJ, *et al.* Effect of clinical phenotype on yield of long QT syndrome genetic testing. *J Am Coll Cardiol.* 2006;**47**:764–8
27. Garratt CJ, *et al.* Heart Rhythm UK position statement on clinical indications for implantable cardioverter defibrillators in adult patients with familial sudden cardiac death syndromes. *Europace.* 2010;**12**:1156–75
28. Pelliccia A, *et al.* Bethesda Conference #36 and the European Society of Cardiology Consensus recommendations revisited a comparison of U.S. and European criteria for eligibility and disqualification of competitive athletes with cardiovascular abnormalities. *J Am Coll Cardiol.* 2008;**52**:1990–6
29. Johnson JN, *et al.* Competitive sports participation in athletes with congenital long QT syndrome. *JAMA.* 2012;**308**:764–5

Chapter 58

Short QT syndrome

Definition

Short QT syndrome (SQTS) is characterized by abnormally short QT interval, with an increased propensity to atrial and ventricular arrhythmias and a high risk of sudden death.[1, 2] A short QT is defined as QT ≤360 ms at heart rates <60 bpm (QTc <350 ms for males and <360 ms for females).[2]

Aetiology

Gain-of-function mutations affecting the I_{Kr}, I_{Ks}, I_{K1}, and I_{Ca} currents are responsible for heterogenous repolarization and refractoriness (Figure 58.1 and Table 58.1). However, none of the known disease-associated genes has been shown to account for ≥5% of this disease.[3] Rufinamide, an antiepileptic drug, has been recently shown to significantly shorten the QT interval although not necessarily associated with significant clinical adverse effects.[4] Increasing doses of buproprion have also been found to significantly decrease QTc.[5]

Presentation

Patients often have permanent or paroxysmal **atrial fibrillation** (24%) and occasionally have **depression of the PR** interval. **Tall, peaked T waves** without flat ST segments and impaired rate-dependent QT shortening have been recorded (Figure 58.2). Triggers are adrenergic-dependent (exercise, loud noise), but events at rest have been reported.

Diagnosis

- Short QTc interval
- Syncope and/or family history of syncope

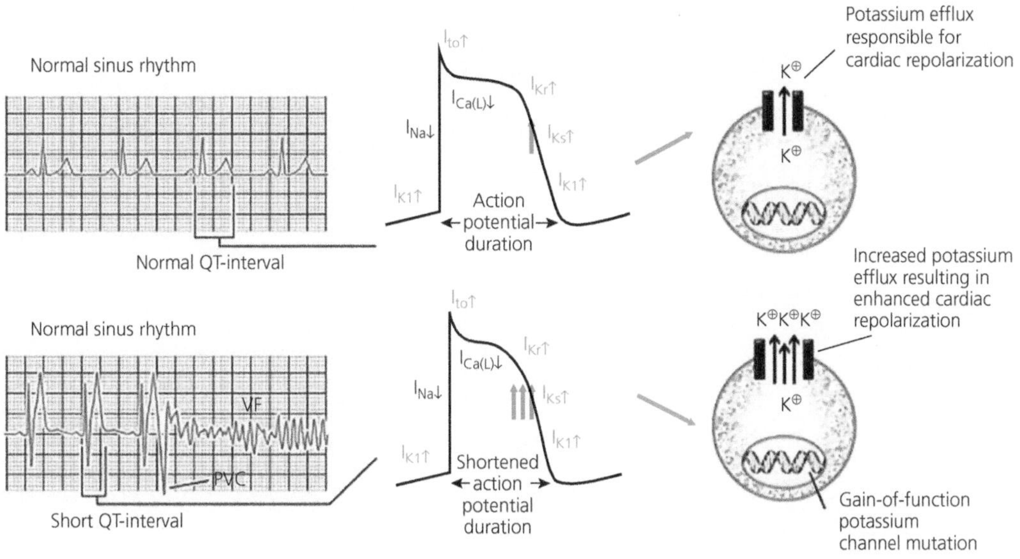

Figure 58.1 Cellular mechanism of short QT interval. A gain-of-function potassium channel mutation results in an increased efflux of potassium current from the cell, resulting in an acceleration of cardiomyocyte repolarization and a shortened action potential duration. Additional cellular mechanisms, possibly due to non-potassium channels, remain to be elucidated.

Gollob MH, *et al*. The short QT syndrome: proposed diagnostic criteria. *J Am Coll Cardiol*. 2011;**57**:802–12.

Table 58.1 Diagnosis of SQTS

HRA/EHRA/APHRS 2013. statement on inherited arrhythmia. Recommendations on Short QT Syndrome Diagnosis
SQTS is diagnosed in the presence of a QTc < 330 ms.
SQTS can be diagnosed in the presence of a QTc < 360 ms and one or more of the following:
a pathogenic mutation
family history of SQTS
family history of sudden death at age <40
survival of a VT/VF episode in the absence of heart disease.

HRS/EHRA/APHRS Expert Consensus Statement on the Diagnosis and Management of Patients with Inherited Primary Arrhythmia Syndromes. *Europace* E-Pub

- Episodes of VF or polymorphic VT and AF (AF and VF can be induced easily by programmed electrical stimulation)
- No obvious heart disease or extracardiac conditions that abbreviate QT interval
- Specific electrocardiographic and clinical diagnostic criteria have also been recently proposed.[6,7]
- Indications for genetic testing are presented in Table 58.2.

Secondary causes of a short QT include hyperkalaemia, hypercalcaemia, acidosis, cathecholamines, digitalis, rufinamide (a recently FDA-approved anticonvulsant), and hyperthermia. Ischaemia-induced activation of the K_{ATP} channel and parasympathetic activation of the KA-Ch channel (deceleration-dependent QT shortening) may also cause QT shortening.[2]

Therapy

It is poorly defined. The sensitivity of electrophysiology study for VF inducibility is about 50%, and non-inducibility does not rule out risk of SCD. Thus, **ICD** may be needed for primary and secondary prevention (Table 58.3); T wave oversensing may result in inappropriate shocks and requires careful programming. SCD may occur in young males with a Gollob score >5.[8] Females are less prone to arrhythmic events, probably due to estrogen induced QT prolongation. **Quinidine** can be efficacious in SQTS by prolonging the QT interval, normalizing the QT response to RR interval change and preventing cardiac events in some patients. It is proposed for children or patients refusing an ICD.[1] I_{Kr} blockers, such as sotalol, may fail to normalize the QT interval in patients with SQTS. Disopyramide and amiodarone might also be helpful, and propafenone is effective in preventing AF.[2]

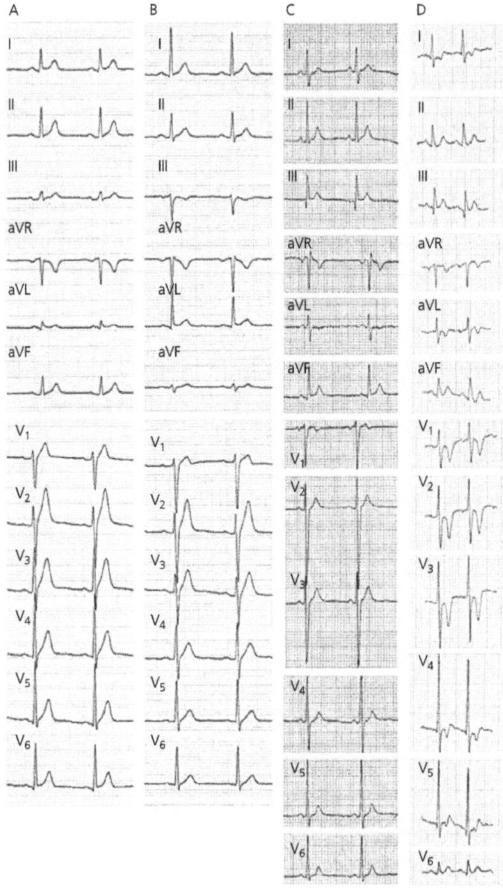

Figure 58.2 ECG of four patients with SQTS. A: 50 years, QTc 313, ms B: 39 years, QTc 311, ms C: 6 years, QTc 293, ms D: 35 months, QTc 324 ms. Heart rate is 143 bpm. The deep negative T waves in leads V_1–V_3 are the equivalent of the high peaked T waves in adult patients.

Giustetto C, *et al*. Short QT syndrome: clinical findings and diagnostic-therapeutic implications. *Eur Heart J* 2006; **27**: 2440–47.

Table 58.2 HRS/EHRA 2011 statement on genetic testing

State of genetic testing for short QT syndrome (SQTS)	
Mutation-specific genetic testing for family members and appropriate relatives following the identification of the SQTS-causative mutation in an index case.	I
Comprehensive or SQT1–3 (KCNH2, KCNQ1, and KCNJ2) targeted SQTS genetic testing may be considered for any patient in whom a cardiologist has established a strong clinical index of suspicion for SQTS based on examination of the patient's clinical history, family history, and electrocardiographic phenotype.	IIb

HRS/EHRA 2011 expert consensus statement on the state of genetic testing for the channelopathies and cardiomyopathies, *Heart Rhythm*. 2011 Aug;**8**(8):1308–39.

Table 58.3. HRA/EHRA/APHRS 2013

Expert Consensus Recommendations on Short QT Syndrome Therapeutic Interventions	
ICD implantation in symptomatic patients with a diagnosis of SQTS who:	I
a. Are survivors of a cardiac arrest and/or	
b. Have documented spontaneous sustained VT with or without syncope.	
ICD in asymptomatic patients with a diagnosis of SQTS and a family history of SCD.	IIb
Quinidine in asymptomatic patients with a diagnosis of SQTS and a family history of SCD.	IIb
Sotalol in asymptomatic patients with a diagnosis of SQTS and a family history of SCD.	IIb

HRS/EHRA/APHRS Expert Consensus Statement on the Diagnosis and Management of Patients with Inherited Primary Arrhythmia Syndromes. *Europace* E-Pub

References

1. Giustetto C, *et al.* Short QT syndrome: clinical findings and diagnostic-therapeutic implications. *Eur Heart J.* 2006;**27**:2440–7
2. Patel C, *et al.* Short QT syndrome: from bench to bedside. *Circ Arrhythm Electrophysiol.* 2010;**3**:401–8
3. Ackerman MJ, *et al.* HRS/EHRA expert consensus statement on the state of genetic testing for the channelopathies and cardiomyopathies: this document was developed as a partnership between the Heart Rhythm Society (HRS) and the European Heart Rhythm Association (EHRA). *Europace.* 2011;**13**:1077–109
4. Schimpf R, *et al.* Drug-induced QT-interval shortening following antiepileptic treatment with oral rufinamide. *Heart Rhythm.* 2012;**9**:776–81
5. Castro VM, *et al.* QT interval and antidepressant use: A cross sectional study of electronic health records. *BMJ.* 2013;**346**: doi: 10.1136bmj.f1288
6. HRS/EHRA/APHRS expert consensus statement on the diagnosis and management of patients with inherited primary arrhythmia syndromes. *Europace* 2013. E-Pub
7. Gollob MH, *et al.* The short QT syndrome: proposed diagnostic criteria. *J Am Coll Cardiol.* 2011;**57**:802–12
8. Villafane J, *et al.* Long-term follow-up of a pediatric cohort with short QT syndrome. *J Am Coll Cardiol.* 2013;**61**:1183–91

Chapter 59

Brugada syndrome

Definition

The Brugada syndrome is defined as ST segment elevation in the right precordial leads (V_1–V_3) that is unrelated to ischaemia, electrolyte disturbances, or structural heart disease, and a high incidence of sudden death due to ventricular arrhythmias.[1]

Epidemiology

The prevalence of the disease in the general population cannot be accurately assessed due to the dynamic nature of the ECG pattern that can fluctuate over time but is estimated to be 1/5000–10 000 inhabitants in the western world.[2, 3] It is 8–10 times more prevalent in males than in females.[4] The prevalence is probably higher in the Far Eastern countries (initially described as sudden unexplained death syndrome).[5] Inheritance in Brugada syndrome occurs as an autosomal dominant trait. In up to 60% of patients, the disease can be sporadic, i.e. absent in parents and other relatives. Patients with Brugada syndrome have an annual incidence of cardiac arrest between 1 and 2%.[6]

Genetics and pathophysiology

The pathophysiological mechanism of the Brugada syndrome remains elusive, and the ECG manifestations are solely the phenotype of a multitude of possible aetiologies.[7, 8] Genetic mutations in 15 genes that alter ion channel functions have been identified that may also affect the QT interval (Table 56.1 of Chapter 56). The first identified mutations were located in **SCN5A**, the gene encoding the α subunit of the cardiac sodium channel ($Na_v1.5$), leading to reduced cardiac sodium current (I_{Na}). According to the repolarization hypothesis, sodium loss-of-function conditions create an imbalance between outward and inward positive currents during phase 1, enhancing repolarization and resulting in the appearance of a particular notch in the action potential mediated by the transient outward potassium current (I_{to}). This gives rise to a transmural voltage gradient between the epicardium and endocardium, resulting in the characteristic ST segment elevation and propensity to ventricular arrhythmias, probably through phase 2 reentry mechanisms. The depolarization hypothesis underlines the role of conduction delay induced by SCN5A mutations, particularly in the RVOT.[1] The SCNA gene represents the majority of mutations (20–25%) identified in Brugada syndrome but has a low penetrance.[8, 9] Other mutations affecting calcium and potassium channels or acting through other mechanisms have also been described but are rare. Up to 300 mutations have been so far identified but can be found in less than 30% of patients, and, in the majority of Brugada syndrome cases, the aetiology remains unknown. Delayed onset of right ventricular contraction that that can be seen on echocardiography suggest that structural abnormalities are intrinsic to the syndrome and question its characterization as a mere channelopathy.[7] This notion was also supported by the recently reported efficacy of epicardial RVOT ablation in patients with Brugada syndrome.[10]

Presentation

The syndrome typically manifests during adulthood, with either detection of the **typical ECG pattern** or development of polymorphic **VT or VF** in 10–25% of patients during their lifetime.[3, 11] **SCD** may occur typically at rest or during sleeping and is precipitated by fever or the consumption of large meals, presumably due to glucose-induced insulin secretion that may enhance ST segment elevation.[12] Syncopal episodes, nocturnal agonal respiration, palpitations and chest discomfort may also occur. Patients may also be entirely asymptomatic, and approximately 20% of them develop supraventricular arrhythmias, such as **AF or atrial flutter, or sick sinus syndrome.** New-onset AF may be the first clinical manifestation of Brugada syndrome.[3]

Diagnosis

Diagnostic criteria are presented in Table 59.1. Conditions that are associated with ST segment elevation (Table 59.2) should be ruled out. A variety of drugs have also been reported to produce a Brugada-like ST segment elevation (Table 59.3), although it is not yet clear whether, or to what extent, a genetic predisposition may be involved.[3] Recent data suggest that lead V_3 does not yield diagnostic information; typical ECG changes in only one of V_1 or V_2 leads should be enough for diagnosis.[13]

Three repolarization patterns are described (Figure 59.1):

- **Type-1 ECG pattern** Coved ST segment elevation ≥2 mm followed by a negative T wave, with little or no isoelectric separation, in >1 right precordial lead (from V_1 to V_3), imitating incomplete right bundle branch block but without the typical widened S wave in the left lateral lead
- **Type-2 ECG pattern** ST segment elevation followed by a positive or biphasic T wave with a saddleback configuration

Table 59.1 Diagnosis of Brugada syndrome

HRAS/EHRA/APHRS 2013 statement on inherited arrhythmia
1. BrS is diagnosed in patients with ST segment elevation with type 1 morphology > 2 mm in > 1 lead among the right precordial leads V1,V2, positioned in the 2nd, 3rd or 4th intercostal space occurring either spontaneously or after provocative drug test with intravenous administration of Class I antiarrhythmic drugs.
2. BrS is diagnosed in patients with type 2 or type 3 ST segment elevation in > 1 lead among the right precordial leads V1,V2 positioned in the 2nd, 3rd or 4th intercostal space when a provocative drug test with intravenous administration of Class I antiarrhythmic drugs induces a type 1 ECG morphology

HRS/EHRA/APHRS Expert Consensus Statement on the Diagnosis and Management of Patients with Inherited Primary Arrhythmia Syndromes. *Europace* E-Pub

Table 59.2 Conditions that can lead to ST segment elevation in V_1–V_3

Atypical right bundle branch block
Hyperkalaemia
Hypercalcaemia
Hypothermia
Left ventricular hypertrophy
Early repolarization, especially in athletes
Acute pericarditis
Acute myocardial infarction (especially of RV)
Pulmonary embolism
Dissecting aortic aneurysm
Duchenne muscular dystrophy
Thiamine deficiency
Arrhythmogenic right ventricular cardiomyopathy
Pectus excavatum
Mechanical compression of the right ventricular outflow tract (mediastinal tumour or haemopericardium)

Table 59.3 Drug-induced Brugada-like ECG patterns

1. Antiarrhythmic drugs
Na+ channel blockers
Class IC drugs (flecainide, pilsicainide, propafenone)
Class IA drugs (ajmaline, procainamide, disopyramide, cibenzoline)
Ca^{2+} channel blockers, beta blockers
2. Nitrates
3. K^+ channel openers (nicorandil)
4. Psychotropic drugs
Tricyclic antidepressants (amitriptyline, nortriptyline, desipramine, clomipramine)
Tetracyclic antidepressants (maprotiline)
Phenothiazine (perphenazine, cyamemazine)
Selective serotonin reuptake inhibitors (fluoxetine)
5. Other drugs
Dimenhydrinate
Cocaine
Alcohol intoxication

Antzelevitch C, *et al.* Brugada syndrome: report of the second consensus conference: endorsed by the Heart Rhythm Society and the European Heart Rhythm Association. *Circulation*. 2005;**111**:659–70.

- **Type-3 ECG pattern** Right precordial ST segment elevation ≤1 mm with either a coved-type or a saddleback morphology.

The ECG typically fluctuates over time in Brugada patients and thus can change from type-1 to type-2 or type-3, or even be transiently normal. Vagal manoeuvres, heavy

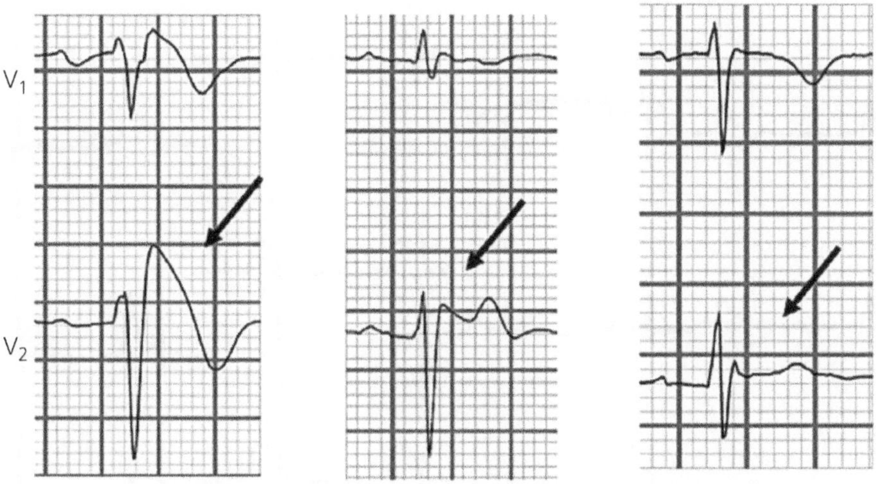

Figure 59.1 ECG abnormality diagnostic or suspected of Brugada syndrome. Type-1 ECG (coved-type ST segment elevation) is the only diagnostic ECG in Brugada syndrome and is defined as a J wave amplitude or an ST segment elevation of ≥2 mm or 0.2 mV at its peak (followed by a negative T wave, with little or no isoelectric separation). Type-2 ECG (saddleback-type ST segment elevation), defined as a J wave amplitude of ≥2 mm, gives rise to a gradually descending ST segment elevation (remaining ≥1 mm above the baseline), followed by a positive or biphasic T wave that results in a saddleback configuration. Type-3 ECG is a right precordial ST segment elevation (saddleback type, coved-type, or both) without meeting the aforementioned criteria.

Mizusawa Y, Wilde AA. Brugada syndrome. *Circ Arrhythm Electrophysiol*. 2012;**5**:606–16

meals, and beta blockers accentuate the ECG patterns. Only the coved-type ST segment elevation (type-1 ECG pattern) is diagnostic of the syndrome in the presence of clinical criteria described in Table 59.1. Mild prolongation of the PR interval may also be seen.

Patients displaying the characteristic type-2 or -3 ECG without further clinical criteria should be described as having Brugada ECG pattern and not Brugada syndrome, unless the administration of sodium channel blockers reveals a typical type-1 pattern. Brugada-like ECG can occasionally appear after direct current cardioversion or with the administration of certain drugs that probably should be avoided in diagnosed cases of the syndrome (Table 59.3), but it is not known whether a genetic predisposition is involved. Another confounding factor is the type of ST segment elevation encountered in well-trained athletes (Figure 59.2), which is distinguished by an upslope, rather than a downslope, pattern and by remaining largely unaffected by challenge with a sodium channel blocker (see also Chapter 81 on athlete's heart).

Pharmacological challenge. Drugs used are:

- Ajmaline 1 mg/kg over 5 min IV (probably the best for this purpose)
- Flecainide 2 mg/kg over 10 min IV or 400 mg po
- Procainamide 10 mg/kg over 10 min IV
- Pilsicainide 1 mg/kg over 10 min IV.

Placement of the right precordial leads in a superior position (up to the second intercostal space above normal, Figure 59.3) can increase the sensitivity of the ECG for detecting the Brugada phenotype in some patients, both in the presence or absence of a drug challenge.[14]

In young patients, it can be performed as a bedside test. A pacing electrode may be necessary in patients at high risk for AV block. The pharmacological test should be monitored with a continuous ECG recording and should be terminated when: (1) the diagnostic test is positive; (2) premature ventricular beats or other arrhythmias develop; (3) QRS widens to ≥130% of baseline. Isoproterenol is the antidote when required.

Sodium channel blockade may provoke the Brugada ECG pattern in conditions, such as ARVD and Chagas' disease.[6]

Echocardiography may reveal the delayed onset of right ventricular contraction that reflects delayed depolarization over the anterior aspect of the RVOT epicardium.

Exercise testing is useful for risk stratification.[15]

Genetic testing indications are presented in Table 59.4.[2] The yield of genetic testing is approximately 21% but approaches 40% for SCN5A-mediated BrS (BrS1) when the

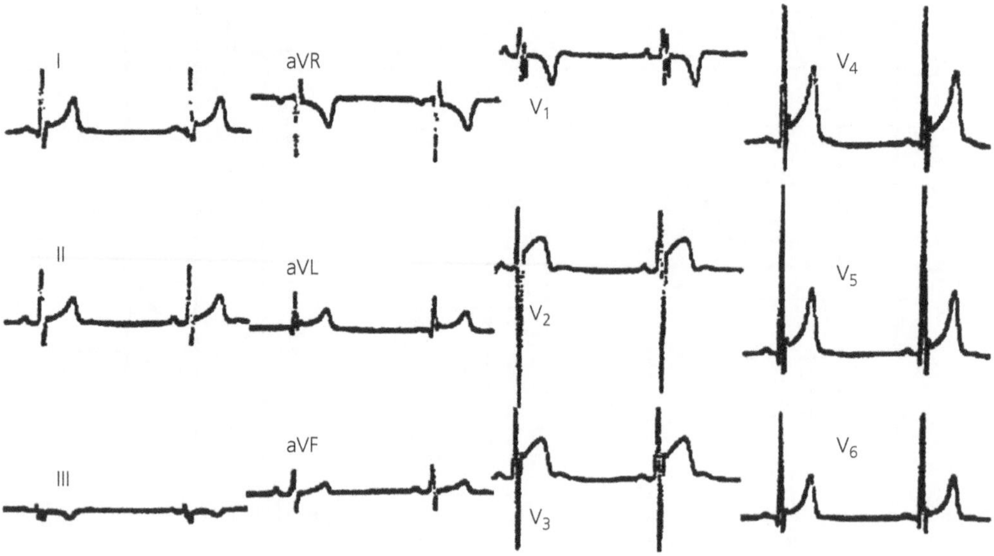

Figure 59.2 ECG of a well-trained, asymptomatic 24-year old soccer player. ST segment elevation is observed in V_2 to V_6 but with characteristics totally different from those seen in Brugada syndrome. A coved-type ST segment elevation is not observed. A rounded or upsloping ST elevation in seen in V_2 and V_3 whereas V_4 to V_5 show a pattern resembling that commonly encountered in early repolarization syndrome.

Antzelevitch C, *et al.* Brugada syndrome: report of the second consensus conference: endorsed by the Heart Rhythm Society and the European Heart Rhythm Association. *Circulation*. 2005;**111**:659–70.

PQ interval exceeds 200 ms.[9] Genetic test results should be interpreted in the context of the fact that 2% of healthy Caucasians and 5% of healthy non-white subjects also host rare missense SCN5A variants.[16]

Risk stratification

Previous history of syncope, a spontaneous type-1 ECG at baseline, and male gender have been shown to be related to the occurrence of cardiac events during follow-up.[17] The inducibility of ventricular arrhythmias during the EPS (class IIb indication) may also bear ominous prognosis,[17, 18] but this is disputed.[11, 19, 20] In the FINGER registry, inducibility of sustained ventricular arrhythmias was significantly associated with a shorter time to first arrhythmic event in the univariate analysis, but in the multivariate analysis, it did not predict arrhythmic events.[11] Recently, the PRELUDE registry reported their results on 208 patients followed for approximately 3 years. VT/VF inducibility was unable to identify high-risk patients, whereas the presence of a spontaneous type I ECG, history of syncope, ventricular effective refractory period <200 ms, and QRS fragmentation (Figure 59.4) were indicators of high risk.[20] VF may be induced in up to 9% of apparently healthy individuals when aggressive stimulation protocols are used.[3] The presence or absence of a family history of SCD does not carry prognostic ability.[21] Augmentation of ST segment elevation ≥0.05 mV in V_1 to V_3 leads, observed at early recovery (1 to 4 min) after treadmill exercise, has been reported to predict future arrhythmic events.[10] The prognostic significance of NSVT is not known, but syncope indicates high risk and could be due to sustained or long runs of non-sustained VT. The value of risk stratification in Brugada syndrome, in general, is low.[22]

Therapy

Cardiac arrest or syncope in the presence of a diagnostic ECG are indications for ICD (Table 59.5). Quinidine, a drug with I_{to} blocking properties, has been successfully tried, but the evidence for its widespread use is not sufficient.[23] Quinidine-induced diarrhoea is treated with cholestyramine.[1] Denopramine, colistazol, and bepridil have also been proposed for VF suppression.[1] Controversy exists about asymptomatic patients with a spontaneous type-1 ECG at baseline or after pharmacological challenge.[6, 10, 17, 18]

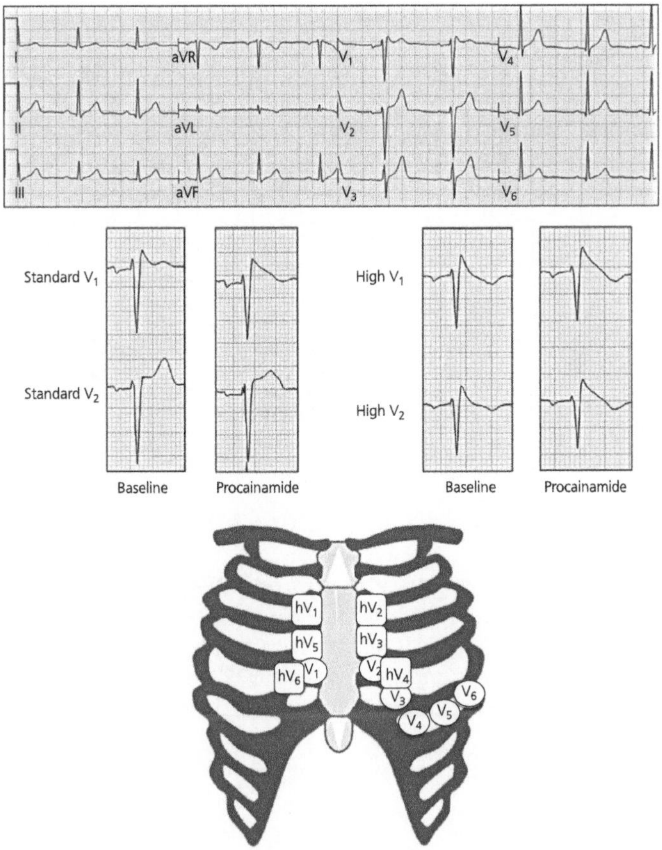

Figure 59.3 ECG series on a 55-year old man who presented with nocturnal cardiac arrest. The top panel shows the resting ECG with suspicious ST segments in V_1, consistent with a type-2 Brugada ECG. Procainamide infusion and high precordial lead placement unmask a type-1 Brugada ECG.

Modi S, Krahn AD. Sudden cardiac arrest without overt heart disease. *Circulation*. 2011;**123**:2994–3008

Table 59.4 HRS/EHRA 2011 statement on genetic testing

Stage of genetic testing for Brugada syndrome (BrS)	
Mutation-specific genetic testing for family members and appropriate relatives following the identification of the BrS-causative mutation in an index case.	I
Comprehensive or BrS1 (SCN5A) targeted BrS genetic testing for any patient in whom a cardiologist has established a clinical index of suspicion for BrS, based on examination of the patient's clinical history, family history, and expressed electrocardiographic (resting 12-lead ECGs and/or provocative drug challenge testing) phenotype.	IIa
Genetic testing is not indicated in the setting of an isolated type-2 or type-3 Brugada ECG pattern.	III

HRS/EHRA 2011 expert consensus statement on the state of genetic testing for the channelopathies and cardiomyopathies, *Heart Rhythm*. 2011 Aug;**8**(8):1308–39.

Catheter ablation over the epicardial RVOT has been recently reported to result in normalization of the Brugada ECG pattern and prevent clinical and inducible VT/VF.[9] Drugs that should be avoided in Brugada syndrome are listed on http://www.brugadadrugs.org.

Although a clear association between exercise and sudden death has not been established in Brugada syndrome, the ESC and the 36th Bethesda Conference recommend abstinence from **competitive sports.**[24] Recommendations to these patients should be better individualized. [8]

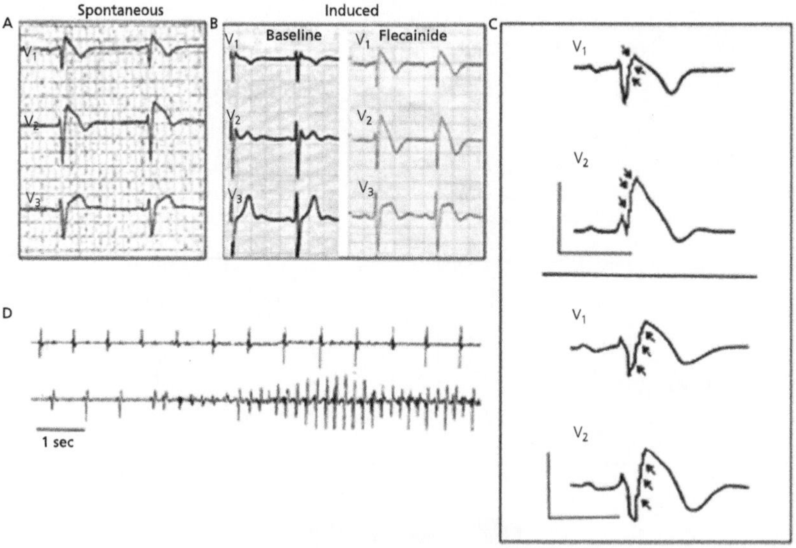

Figure 59.4 Examples of electrocardiographic (ECG) traces (A to C). (A) A 35-year old male patient with presenting spontaneous type-1 ECG. (B) A 30-year old male patient presenting with type-3 ECG (left panel), converted to type-1 after 2 mg/L intravenous flecainide (right panel). (C) V_1 and V_2 leads of two patients with spontaneous ST segment elevation presenting with QRS fragmentation at enrolment; arrows indicate the QRS peaks (calibration bars 10 mV/400 ms). (D) Implantable cardioverter-defibrillator-stored ventricular fibrillation in a PRELUDE (PRogrammed ELectrical stimUlation preDictive valuE) patient.

Priori SG, *et al.* Risk Stratification in Brugada Syndrome Results of the PRELUDE (PRogrammed ELectrical stimUlation preDictive valuE) Registry. *J Am Coll Cardiol.* 2012;**59**:37–45.

Table 59.5 Therapy of Brugada syndrome

ACCF/AHA 2012 GL on Device therapy. Indications for ICD	
Brugada syndrome and syncope or documented VT	IIa-C
2012 ACCF/AHA/HRS focused update incorporated into the ACCF/AHA/HRS 2008 guidelines for device-based therapy of cardiac rhythm abnormalities. *J Am Coll Cardiol* 2013;**1**:e6–75.	
HRAS/EHRA/APHRS 2013. Expert Consensus Recommendations on Brugada Syndrome 2013 statement on inherited arrhythmia. Therapeutic Interventions	
The following lifestyle changes are recommended in all patients: avoidance of drugs that may induce or aggravate ST segment elevation in right precordial leads (for example, visit Brugadadrugs.org), avoidance of excessive alcohol intake, immediate treatment of fever with antipyretic drugs.	I
ICD in patients who are survivors of a cardiac arrest, and/or have documented spontaneous sustained VT with or without syncope.	I
ICD implantation in patients with a spontaneous diagnostic Type I ECG and a history of syncope judged to be likely caused by ventricular arrhythmias.	IIa
Quinidine in patients and history of arrhythmic storms defined as more than two episodes of VT/VF in 24 hours. who qualify for an ICD but present a contraindication to the ICD or refuse it, and/or have a history of documented supraventricular arrhythmias that require treatment.	IIa
Isoproterenol infusion in suppressing arrhythmic storms	IIa
ICD implantation in patients who develop VF during programmed electrical stimulation (inducible patients).	IIb
Quinidine in asymptomatic patients with a spontaneous type 1 ECG.	IIb
Catheter ablation in patients with a history of arrhythmic storms or repeated appropriate ICD shocks.	IIb
ICD is not indicated in asymptomatic BrS patients with a drug induced type 1 ECG and on the basis of a family history of SCD alone.	III

HRS/EHRA/APHRS Expert Consensus Statement on the Diagnosis and Management of Patients with Inherited Primary Arrhythmia Syndromes. *Europace* E-Pub.

References

1. Mizusawa Y, *et al.* Brugada syndrome. *Circ Arrhythm Electrophysiol.* 2012;**5**:606–16
2. Ackerman MJ, *et al.* HRS/EHRA expert consensus statement on the state of genetic testing for the channelopathies and cardiomyopathies: this document was developed as a partnership between the Heart Rhythm Society (HRS) and the European Heart Rhythm Association (EHRA). *Europace.* 2011;**13**:1077–109
3. Antzelevitch C, *et al.* Brugada syndrome: report of the Second Consensus Conference: endorsed by the Heart Rhythm Society and the European Heart Rhythm Association. *Circulation.* 2005;**111**:659–70
4. HRS/EHRA/APHRS expert consensus statement on the diagnosis and management of patients with inherited primary arrhythmia syndromes. *Europace* 2013. E-Pub
5. Nademanee K, *et al.* Arrhythmogenic marker for the sudden unexplained death syndrome in Thai men. *Circulation.* 1997;**96**:2595–600
6. Napolitano C, *et al.* Sudden cardiac death and genetic ion channelopathies: long QT, Brugada, short QT, catecholaminergic polymorphic ventricular tachycardia, and idiopathic ventricular fibrillation. *Circulation.* 2012;**125**:2027–34
7. Hoogendijk MG, *et al.* The Brugada ECG pattern: a marker of channelopathy, structural heart disease, or neither? Toward a unifying mechanism of the Brugada syndrome. *Circ Arrhythm Electrophysiol.* 2010;**3**:283–90
8. Webster G, *et al.* An update on channelopathies: from mechanisms to management. *Circulation.* 2013;**127**:126–40
9. Crotti L, *et al.* Spectrum and prevalence of mutations involving BRS1- through BRS12-susceptibility genes in a cohort of unrelated patients referred for Brugada syndrome genetic testing: implications for genetic testing. *J Am Coll Cardiol.* 2012;**60**:1410–18
10. Nademanee K, *et al.* Prevention of ventricular fibrillation episodes in Brugada syndrome by catheter ablation over the anterior right ventricular outflow tract epicardium. *Circulation.* 2011;**123**:1270–9
11. Probst V, *et al.* Long-term prognosis of patients diagnosed with Brugada syndrome: results from the FINGER Brugada syndrome registry. *Circulation.* 2010;**121**:635–43
12. Nishizaki M, *et al.* Influence of meals on variations of ST segment elevation in patients with Brugada syndrome. *J Cardiovasc Electrophysiol.* 2008;**19**:62–8
13. Richter S, *et al.* Number of electrocardiogram leads displaying the diagnostic coved-type pattern in Brugada syndrome: a diagnostic consensus criterion to be revised. *Eur Heart J.* 2010;**31**:1357–64
14. Modi S, *et al.* Sudden cardiac arrest without overt heart disease. *Circulation.* 2011;**123**:2994–3008
15. Makimoto H, *et al.* Augmented ST-segment elevation during recovery from exercise predicts cardiac events in patients with Brugada syndrome. *J Am Coll Cardiol.* 2010;**56**:1576–84
16. Kapplinger JD, *et al.* An international compendium of mutations in the SCN5A-encoded cardiac sodium channel in patients referred for Brugada syndrome genetic testing. *Heart Rhythm.* 2010;**7**:33–46
17. Brugada J, *et al.* Determinants of sudden cardiac death in individuals with the electrocardiographic pattern of Brugada syndrome and no previous cardiac arrest. *Circulation.* 2003;**108**:3092–6
18. Delise P, *et al.* Risk stratification in individuals with the Brugada type 1 ECG pattern without previous cardiac arrest: usefulness of a combined clinical and electrophysiologic approach. *Eur Heart J.* 2011;**32**:169–76
19. Eckardt L, *et al.* Long-term prognosis of individuals with right precordial ST-segment-elevation Brugada syndrome. *Circulation.* 2005;**111**:257–63
20. Sarkozy A, *et al.* The value of a family history of sudden death in patients with diagnostic type I Brugada ECG pattern. *Eur Heart J.* 2011;**32**:2153–60
21. Priori SG, *et al.* Risk stratification in Brugada syndrome: results of the PRELUDE (PRogrammed ELectrical stimUlation preDictive valuE) registry. *J Am Coll Cardiol.* 2012;**59**:37–45
22. Raju H, *et al.* Low prevalence of risk markers in cases of sudden death due to Brugada syndrome relevance to risk stratification in Brugada syndrome. *J Am Coll Cardiol.* 2011;**57**:2340–5
23. Belhassen B, *et al.* Efficacy of quinidine in high-risk patients with Brugada syndrome. *Circulation.* 2004;**110**:1731–7
24. Pelliccia A, *et al.* Bethesda Conference #36 and the European Society of Cardiology consensus recommendations revisited a comparison of U.S. and European criteria for eligibility and disqualification of competitive athletes with cardiovascular abnormalities. *J Am Coll Cardiol.* 2008;**52**:1990–6

Chapter 60

Catecholaminergic polymorphic ventricular tachycardia

Definition

Catecholaminergic polymorphic ventricular tachycardia (CPVT) is VT that typically occurs on exercise, and episodes of provoked tachycardia are sustained or usually non-sustained.[1, 2] CPVT is one of the most lethal inherited channelopathies, with sudden death occurring in up to 30% of patients before age 40 in the absence of anti-adrenergic therapy.[1, 3] The estimated 4- and 8-year cardiac event rates were 33% and 58%, respectively, in a series of patients without β blockers.[1]

Epidemiology

The prevalence of CPVT is virtually unknown.[4]

Genetics and pathophysiology

CPVT is mainly due to mutations in the genes encoding the **cardiac ryanodine receptor (Ryr2)** channel (60% of patients—autosomal dominant inheritance) and calsequestrin that are involved in calcium kinetics (autosomal recessive inheritance). A locus on chromosome 7p14–p22 has also been reported, with an early-onset lethal form of recessive CPVT.[1] Triadine is a new gene involved in an autosomal recessive form of CPVT, and three new mutations in the triadin gene (*TRDN*), a protein that links RyR2 and CASQ2, were recently identified (Table 56.1).[1] Increased leak of Ca^{2+} from the sarcoplasmic reticulum triggers delayed after-depolarization and ultimately leads to CPVT.[5] Adrenergic stimulation increases spontaneous Ca^{2+} release, and this leak is amplified in the presence of CPVT mutations. There has been evidence that delayed after-depolarizations caused by calcium overload are a more common occurrence in Purkinje cells than in ventricular myocytes, and Purkinje cells are probably critical contributors to arrhythmic triggers.[1] Extended clinical phenotypes in patients with Ryr2 mutations and CPVT have been described with sinoatrial node and atrioventricular node dysfunction, atrial fibrillation, atrial standstill, and dilated cardiomyopathy.[6]

Presentation

QRS morphology suggests an outflow tract origin of the initiating beat in more than 50% of patients, and subsequent beats portray a polymorphic, or typically bidirectional, VT morphology.[7] They may originate from the LVOT and, less frequently, from the RVOT or the RV apex.[2]

Diagnosis

The resting ECG is normal (Table 60.1). NSVT, induced by treadmill exercise testing aimed at evaluating presumed long QT syndrome, suggests cathecholaminergic polymorphic VT rather than long QT syndrome.[8] Provocative testing with epinephrine (infusion of 0.05 microgram/kg/min and increased every 5 min to 0.1 and 0.2 microgram/kg/min for 5 min at each dose) induces VT in 80% of patients, but a negative test does not exclude the diagnosis.[9] Care should be taken since patient diagnosed with CPVT on the basis of the presence of bidirectional ventricular tachycardia on exercise have been identified as possessing KCNJ2 mutations, which are associated with the rarely lethal Andersen–Tawil syndrome (LQTS 7).[10] Polymorphic VT is usually not inducible by programmed ventricular stimulation.[1]

Therapy

All phenotypically and/or genotypically diagnosed CPVT patients should receive a **beta blocker without sympathomimetic activity in the highest tolerable dose**, such as nadolol in up to 1.8 mg/kg.[1] A possible exception might be asymptomatic patients >60 years of age who are

Table 60.1 HRS/EHRA/APHRS 2013 statement on inherited arrhythmia. CPVT diagnosis

CPVT is diagnosed in the presence of a structurally normal heart, normal ECG, and unexplained exercise or catecholamine induced bidirectional VT or polymorphic ventricular premature beats or VT in an individual <40 years of age.
CPVT is diagnosed in patients (index case or family member) who have a pathogenic mutation.
CPVT is diagnosed in family members of a CPVT index case with a normal heart who manifest exercise induced PVCs or bidirectional/polymorphic VT.
CPVT can be diagnosed in the presence of a structurally normal heart and coronary arteries, normal ECG, and unexplained exercise or catecholamine induced bidirectional VT or polymorphic ventricular premature beats or VT in an individual >40 years of age

HRS/EHRA/APHRS Expert Consensus Statement on the Diagnosis and Management of Patients with Inherited Primary Arrhythmia Syndromes. *Europace* E-Pub.

Table 60.2 Therapy of CPVT

ACCF/AHA 2012 GL on Device therapy. Indications for ICD	
CPVT and syncope and/or sustained VT on beta blockers	IIa-C

2012 ACCF/AHA/HRS focused update incorporated into the ACCF/AHA/HRS 2008 guidelines for device-based therapy of cardiac rhythm abnormalities. *J Am Coll Cardiol*. 2013;**61**:e6–75.

HRS/EHRA/APHRS 2013 statement on inherited arhythmia. CPVT therapeutic Interventions.	
The following lifestyle changes are recommended in all patients: limit/ avoid competitive sports; limit/avoid strenuous exercise; limit exposure to stressful environments.	I
Beta-blockers in all symptomatic patients	I
ICD in patients who experience cardiac arrest, recurrent syncope or polymorphic/ bidirectional VT despite optimal medical management, and/or left cardiac sympathetic denervation (LCSD).	I
Flecainide in addition to beta- blockers In patienys who experience recurrent syncope or polymorphic/ bidirectional VT while on betablockers.	IIa
Beta-blockers in carriers of a pathogenic CPVT mutation without clinical manifestations of CPVT (concealed mutation-positive patients).	IIa
LCSD in patients with a diagnosis of CPVT who experience recurrent syncope or polymorphic/bidirectional VT/ several appropriate ICD shocks while on beta-blockers, and in patients who are intolerant or with contraindication to beta-blockers.	IIb
ICD as a standalone therapy is not indicated in an asymptomatic patient	III
Electrical stimulation is not indicated in CPVT patients.	III

HRS/EHRA/APHRS Expert Consensus Statement on the Diagnosis and Management of Patients with Inherited Primary Arrhythmia Syndromes. *Europace* E-Pub.

Table 60.3 HRS/EHRA 2011 statement on genetic testing

State of genetic testing for catecholaminergic polymorphic ventricular tachycardia	
Comprehensive or CPVT1 and CVPT2 (RYR2 and CASQ2) targeted CPVT genetic testing is recommended for any patient in whom a cardiologist has established a clinical index of suspicion for CPVT, based on examination of the patient's clinical history, family history, and expressed electrocardiographic phenotype during provocative stress testing with cycle, treadmill, or catecholamine infusion.	I
Mutation-specific genetic testing for family members and appropriate relatives following the identification of the CPVT-causative mutation in an index case.	I

HRS/EHRA 2011 expert consensus statement on the state of genetic testing for the channelopathies and cardiomyopathies, *Heart Rhythm*. 2011 Aug;**8**(8):1308–39.

newly diagnosed by cascade screening. Participation in competitive sports is prohibited, and the use of sympathomimetic agents is contraindicated. Complete suppression of asymptomatic VPBs may to be mandatory, but the presence of couplets or more successive VPBs during exercise testing is associated with future arrhythmic events, suggesting intensifying the treatment in these cases. A carvedilol analogue, in combination with a non-selective beta blocker, such as metoprolol or bisoprolol, is also under study.[1] **Verapamil** may be added to beta blocker therapy.[11] **Flecainide** directly blocks RyR2 channels, prevents premature Ca^{2+} release, and reduces exercise-induced ventricular arrhythmias in patients with CPVT uncontrolled by conventional drug therapy.[12] Thus, the addition of flecainide (or probably propafenone) to beta blockers may be more effective.[13] ICD (with beta blockers) is recommended in patients with cardiac arrest or documented VT despite beta blocker therapy (Table 60.1). Left cardiac sympathetic denervation may also be helpful.[14] Indications for genetic testing are presented in Table 60.2. Catheter ablation of the bidirectional ventricular premature beats that trigger ventricular fibrillation may become an adjunctive therapy in patients with refractory CPVT,[15] but experience is limited. **Competitive exercise** is not allowed. Only recreational, low-intensity sports are permitted (see Chapter 81 on athlete's heart for sports classification).

References

1. Leenhardt A, *et al.* Catecholaminergic polymorphic ventricular tachycardia. *Circ Arrhythm Electrophysiol.* 2012; **5**:1044–52
2. Sy RW, *et al.* Arrhythmia characterization and long-term outcomes in catecholaminergic polymorphic ventricular tachycardia. *Heart Rhythm*. 2011;**8**:864–71
3. Cerrone M, *et al.* Genetics of sudden death: focus on inherited channelopathies. *Eur Heart J*. 2011;**32**:2109–18
4. HRS/EHRA/APHRS expert consensus statement on the diagnosis and management of patients with inherited primary arrhythmia syndromes. *Europace* 2013. E-Pub
5. Suetomi T, *et al.* Mutation-linked defective interdomain interactions within ryanodine receptor cause aberrant Ca2+ release leading to catecholaminergic polymorphic ventricular tachycardia. *Circulation*. 2011;**124**:682–94

6. Bhuiyan ZA, *et al.* Expanding spectrum of human RYR2-related disease: new electrocardiographic, structural, and genetic features. *Circulation.* 2007;**116**:1569–76
7. Napolitano C, *et al.* Diagnosis and treatment of catecholaminergic polymorphic ventricular tachycardia. *Heart Rhythm.* 2007;**4**:675–8
8. Horner JM, *et al.* Ventricular ectopy during treadmill exercise stress testing in the evaluation of long QT syndrome. *Heart Rhythm.* 2008;**5**:1690–4
9. Obeyesekere MN, *et al.* How to perform and interpret provocative testing for the diagnosis of Brugada syndrome, long-QT syndrome, and catecholaminergic polymorphic ventricular tachycardia. *Circ Arrhythm Electrophysiol.* 2011;**4**:958–64
10. Tester DJ, *et al.* Genetic testing for potentially lethal, highly treatable inherited cardiomyopathies/channelopathies in clinical practice. *Circulation.* 2011;**123**:1021–37
11. Rosso R, *et al.* Calcium channel blockers and beta-blockers versus beta-blockers alone for preventing exercise-induced arrhythmias in catecholaminergic polymorphic ventricular tachycardia. *Heart Rhythm.* 2007;**4**:1149–54
12. van der Werf C, *et al.* Flecainide therapy reduces exercise-induced ventricular arrhythmias in patients with catecholaminergic polymorphic ventricular tachycardia. *J Am Coll Cardiol.* 2011;**57**:2244–54
13. van der Werf C, *et al.* Therapeutic approach for patients with catecholaminergic polymorphic ventricular tachycardia: state of the art and future developments. *Europace.* 2012;**14**:175–83
14. Wilde AA, *et al.* Left cardiac sympathetic denervation for catecholaminergic polymorphic ventricular tachycardia. *N Engl J Med.* 2008;**358**:2024–9
15. Kaneshiro T, *et al.* Successful catheter ablation of bidirectional ventricular premature contractions triggering ventricular fibrillation in catecholaminergic polymorphic ventricular tachycardia with RYR2 mutation. *Circ Arrhythm Electrophysiol.* 2012;**5**:e14–17

Chapter 61

Early repolarization syndromes

Definition

Early repolarization is defined electrocardiographically by either a sharp well-defined positive deflection or notch immediately following a positive QRS complex at the onset of the ST-segment, or slurring at the terminal part of the QRS complex (J-waves or J-point elevation).[1] The early repolarization pattern has long been considered to be a benign ECG manifestation (6–13% in the general population) that is seen more commonly in young healthy men and athletes (22–44%). However, there has been evidence suggesting that the early repolarization pattern may be associated with a risk for VF, depending on the location of early repolarization, magnitude of the J wave, and degree of ST elevation.[1-3] The term **J wave syndromes** has been proposed to include cases previously labelled as idiopathic VF that display a prominent J wave and early repolarization.[2] **Inherited** J wave syndromes are usually due to mutations affecting the calcium or potassium channel (that have also have been associated with forms of SQTS and LQTS and Brugada syndrome) and have been classified to ERS type 1 (anterolateral J-wave abnormalities in I, V_4-V_6), ERS type 2 (inferior J-wave abnormalities in II, III, aVF), andERS 3 (J-wave abnormalities in all leads).[2] The Brugada syndrome (J-wave abnormalities in V_1-V_3) has also been considered as a J-wave syndrome,[2] (approximately 12% of patients display typical early repolarization abnormalities) but several pathophysiological differences exist between patients with early repolarization and typical Brugada syndrome.[1] **Acquired** J wave syndromes are ischaemia- or hypothermia-induced.[2] Thus, in the typical ER there is J point elevation (with or without a notch or frank J wave) in leads other than V_1 to V_3.

Genetics and pathophysiology

The J wave deflection occurring at the QRS-ST junction (also known as Osborn wave) was first described in 1953 and is seen in many conditions, such as acute ischaemia (especially in true posterior myocardial infarction), hypothermia, hypercalcaemia, brain injury, acidosis, and early repolarization syndromes. An increase in net repolarizing current, due to either a decrease of inward Na^+ or Ca^{2+} currents (I_{Na}, and $I_{Ca,L}$) or augmentation of outward currents, such as I_{to}, $I_{K\text{-}ATP}$, and $I_{K\text{-}ACh}$, lead to augmentation of the J wave or the appearance of ST segment elevation that is more prominent during slow heart rates.[2] Physiological heterogeneity of electrical properties and transmural gradients in ion channel distribution in the endocardial, mid-myocardial (M-cells), and epicardial layers result in regional differences in electrophysiological properties. Ventricular epicardial (particularly RV) and M-cells, but not endocardial action potentials, display a prominent phase 1 due to a large transient outward potassium current (I_{to}), giving rise to the typical spike-and-dome or notched configuration of the action potential and inscription of the J wave in the ECG. The degree of accentuation of the action potential notch leading to loss of the dome depends on the magnitude of I_{to}. When I_{to} is prominent, as it is in the right ventricular epicardium, an outward shift of current causes phase 1 of the action potential to progress to more negative potentials at which the L-type calcium current ($I_{Ca,L}$) fails to activate, leading to all-or-none repolarization and loss of the dome. Loss of the action potential dome usually is heterogeneous, resulting in marked abbreviation of the action potential at some sites but not at others. The dome then can propagate from regions where it is maintained to regions where it is lost, giving rise to local transmural reentry and closely coupled extrasystoles (phase 2 reentry). When the extrasystole occurs on the preceding T wave, it results in an R-n-T phenomenon that initiates polymorphic VT or VF.[2]

Clinical significance

The clinical significance of early repolarization has been questioned,[4] but there are data associating it with a propensity to sudden death.[5] In a large study on a community-based general population of 10 864 middle-aged subjects, an early-repolarization pattern, with J-point elevation of, at least, 0.1 mV in the inferior leads of a resting ECG, was associated with an increased risk of death from cardiac causes.[6] In addition, among patients with a history of idiopathic ventricular fibrillation, an increased prevalence of early repolarization (up to 23%) defined as an elevation of the QRS-ST junction of, at least, 0.1 mV from baseline in the inferior or lateral lead manifested as QRS slurring or notching, has been detected (Figure 61.1).[3,7] A horizontal/descending type (defined as ≤0.1 mV elevation of the ST segment within 100 ms after the J point) in the inferior leads may help to identify those individuals who are clearly at risk (Figures 61.2 and 61.3, and Table 61.1).[8,9]

However, several obscure points remain with this syndrome. An early repolarization pattern in the inferolateral leads occurs in 5% of apparently healthy individuals,[6,7] it

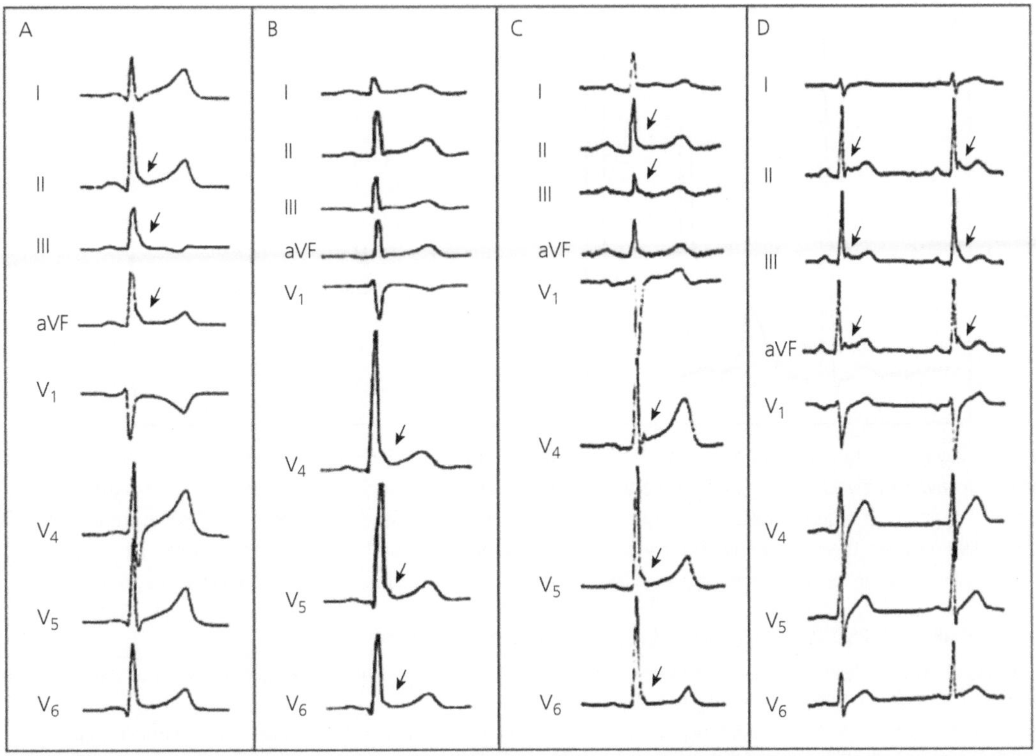

Figure 61.1 J-point elevation patterns. In each panel, early repolarization is evident in the varying patterns of QRS slurring or notching in inferolateral leads (arrows). Panel D shows a beat-to-beat fluctuation in this pattern.

Haissaguerre M, *et al*. Sudden cardiac arrest associated with early repolarization. *N Engl J Med* 2008;**358**:2016–2023.

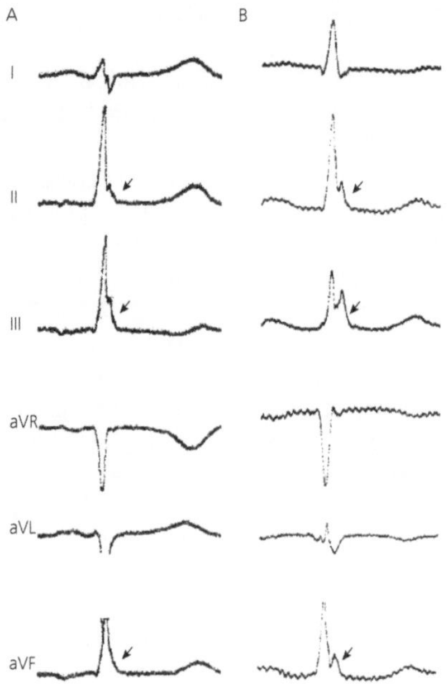

Figure 61.2 Horizontal/descending ST segment patterns from two subjects in the general population.

Tikkanen JT, *et al.* Early repolarization: electrocardiographic phenotypes associated with favorable long-term outcome. *Circulation*. 2011;**123**:2666–73.

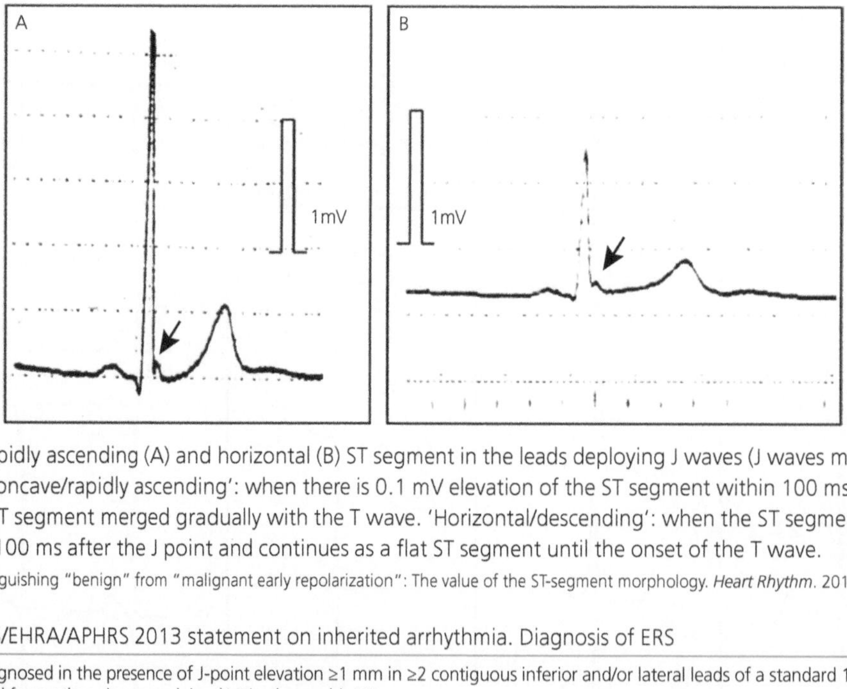

Figure 61.3 Rapidly ascending (A) and horizontal (B) ST segment in the leads deploying J waves (J waves marked with arrowhead). 'Concave/rapidly ascending': when there is 0.1 mV elevation of the ST segment within 100 ms after the J point and the ST segment merged gradually with the T wave. 'Horizontal/descending': when the ST segment elevation is 0.1 mV within 100 ms after the J point and continues as a flat ST segment until the onset of the T wave.

Rosso R, *et al.* Distinguishing "benign" from "malignant early repolarization": The value of the ST-segment morphology. *Heart Rhythm*. 2012;**9**:225–9.

Table 61.1 HRS/EHRA/APHRS 2013 statement on inherited arrhythmia. Diagnosis of ERS

ER syndrome is diagnosed in the presence of J-point elevation ≥1 mm in ≥2 contiguous inferior and/or lateral leads of a standard 12-lead ECG in a patient resuscitated from otherwise unexplained VF/ polymorphic VT
ER syndrome can be diagnosed in a SCD victim with a negative autopsy and medical chart review with a previous ECG demonstrating J-point elevation ≥1 mm in ≥2 contiguous inferior and/or lateral leads of a standard 12-lead ECG
ER pattern can be diagnosed in the presence of J-point elevation ≥1 mm in ≥2 contiguous inferior and/or lateral leads of a standard 12-lead ECG

HRS/EHRA/APHRS Expert Consensus Statement on the Diagnosis and Management of Patients with Inherited Primary Arrhythmia Syndromes. *Europace* E-Pub.

Table 61.2 HRA/EHRA/APHRS 2013 statement on inherited arrhythmia

ICD in patients who have survived a cardiac arrest.	I
Isoproterenol infusion for suppressing electrical storms.	IIa
Quinidine in addition to an ICD for secondary prevention of VF.	IIa
ICD in symptomatic family members of ER syndrome patients with a history of syncope in the presence of ST segment elevation >1mm in 2 or more inferior or lateral leads.	IIb
ICD in asymptomatic individuals who demonstrate a high-risk ER ECG pattern (high J-wave amplitude, horizontal/descending ST-segment) in the presence of a strong family history of juvenile unexplained sudden death with or without a pathogenic mutation.	IIb
ICD is not recommended asymptomatic patients with an isolated ER ECG pattern.	III

HRS/EHRA/APHRS Expert Consensus Statement on the Diagnosis and Management of Patients with Inherited Primary Arrhythmia Syndromes. *Europace* E-Pub.

may not be consistently seen, and even the horizontal/descending ST type was seen in 3% of controls.[8,9] In the ARIC study, J-point elevation was associated with an increased risk of SCD in whites and in females but not in blacks or males.[10] A pattern of J wave and/or QRS slurring (but not of ST elevation) has been associated with cardiac arrest/sudden death in athletes,[11] but many healthy athletes have early repolarization with a rapidly ascending pattern. For physiological ECG patterns in athletes, see Chapter 81 on athlete's heart. A high prevalence of early repolarization in short QT syndrome has also been reported.[12] Brugada syndrome is also characterized by J-point or ST segment elevation in the right precordial leads, and some patients may also have ER in the inferolateral leads. However, in Brugada syndrome, the ST segment elevation is augmented in the right precordial leads by sodium channel blockers whereas in ERS, the early repolarization pattern is usually attenuated.[13] The possibility that false tendons, i.e. discrete, fibromuscular structures that transverse the LV cavity, are related to the genesis of J waves has also been raised.[14] Finally, a large genome-wide association study has been unable to identify genetic variants associated with the pattern, possibly reflecting the phenotypic heterogeneity that exists among these individuals.[15] It seems, therefore, that the majority of individuals with ER are at no or minimal risk for arrhythmic events.[1]

Therapy

The risk stratification and optimum management of these patients are not well defined, and the recognition of the truly malignant forms is difficult (Table 61.2). Electrophysiology testing may be useful in patients with aborted sudden death but not in asymptomatic ones.[10] Patients with aborted sudden death in the absence of identifiable cause (idiopathic VF) are treated with ICD. Ablation of idiopathic VF, targeted to short coupled VPB that originate predominantly from the Purkinje system and the right ventricular outflow track and trigger VF, has also been reported.[16]

References

1. Obeyesekere MN, *et al.* A clinical approach to early repolarization. *Circulation*. 2013;**127**:1620–9
2. Antzelevitch C, *et al.* J wave syndromes. *Heart Rhythm*. 2010;**7**:549–58
3. Surawicz B, *et al.* Inappropriate and confusing electrocardiographic terms: J-wave syndromes and early repolarization. *J Am Coll Cardiol*. 2011;**57**:1584–6
4. Wu SH, *et al.* Early repolarization pattern and risk for arrhythmia death: a meta-analysis. *J Am Coll Cardiol*. 2013;**61**:645–50
5. Tikkanen JT, *et al.* Long-term outcome associated with early repolarization on electrocardiography. *N Engl J Med*. 2009;**361**:2529–37
6. Haissaguerre M, *et al.* Sudden cardiac arrest associated with early repolarization. *N Engl J Med*. 2008; **358**:2016–23
7. Derval N, *et al.* Prevalence and characteristics of early repolarization in the casper registry: Cardiac arrest survivors with preserved ejection fraction registry. *J Am Coll Cardiol*. 2011;**58**:722–8
8. Rosso R, *et al.* Distinguishing 'benign' from 'malignant early repolarization': the value of the ST-segment morphology. *Heart Rhythm*. 2012;**9**:225–9
9. Tikkanen JT, *et al.* Early repolarization: electrocardiographic phenotypes associated with favorable long-term outcome. *Circulation*. 2011;**123**:2666–73
10. Olson KA, *et al.* Long-term prognosis associated with J-point elevation in a large middle-aged biracial cohort: the ARIC Study. *Eur Heart J*. 2011;**32**:3098–106
11. Cappato R, *et al.* J wave, QRS slurring, and ST elevation in athletes with cardiac arrest in the absence of heart disease: marker of risk or innocent bystander? *Circ Arrhythm Electrophysiol*. 2010;**3**:305–11
12. Watanabe H, *et al.* High prevalence of early repolarization in short QT syndrome. *Heart Rhythm*. 2010;**7**:647–52
13. Kawata H, *et al.* Effect of sodium-channel blockade on early repolarization in inferior/lateral leads in patients with idiopathic ventricular fibrillation and Brugada syndrome. *Heart Rhythm*. 2012;**9**:77–83
14. Nakagawa M, *et al.* Electrocardiographic characteristics of patients with false tendon: possible association of false tendon with J waves. *Heart Rhythm*. 2012;**9**:782–8
15. Sinner MF, *et al.* A meta-analysis of genome-wide association studies of the electrocardiographic early repolarization pattern. *Heart Rhythm*. 2012;**9**:1627–34
16. Knecht S, *et al.* Long-term follow-up of idiopathic ventricular fibrillation ablation: a multicenter study. *J Am Coll Cardiol*. 2009;**54**:522–8

Part XI

Bradyarrhythmias

Relevant guidelines

ESC 2013 guidelines on pacing and cardiac resynchronization.

2013 ESC Guidelines on cardiac pacing and cardiac resynchronization therapy. *Eur Heart J* 2013. doi:10.1093/eurheartj/eht150.

ESC 2012 GL on heart failure

ESC guidelines for the diagnosis and treatment of acute and chronic heart failure 2012. Eur Heart J. 2012;**33**:1787–847

ACCF/AHA/HRS 2012 GL for device-based therapy of cardiac rhythm abnormalities

2012 ACCF/AHA/HRS focused update incorporated into the ACCF/AHA/HRS 2008 guidelines for device-based therapy of cardiac rhythm abnormalities. *J Am Coll Cardiol.* 2013;**61**:e6–75

HRS/EHRA 2011 expert consensus statement on the state of genetic testing

HRS/EHRA expert consensus statement on the state of genetic testing for the channelopathies and cardiomyopathies. *Europace.* 2011;**13**:1077–109.

AHA/ACCF/HRS 2009 recommendations for the standardization and interpretation of the electrocardiogram

AHA/ACCF/HRS recommendations for the standardization and interpretation of the electrocardiogram. Six parts have been published in 2009.

HRS/AACF 2012 statement on pacemaker device mode selection

HRS/ACCF Expert Consensus Statement on pacemaker device and mode selection. *Heart Rhythm.* 2012;**9**:1344–65.

HRS/EHRA/APHRS 2013 Expert Consensus Statement on Inherited Arrhythmia

HRS/EHRA/APHRS Expert Consensus Statement on the Diagnosis and Management of Patients with Inherited Primary Arrhythmia Syndromes. *Heart Rhythm.* 2012 E-Pub.

Chapter 62

The cardiac conduction system

Overview

The **sinus node** is a crescent-like, 2.5 mm long subepicardial structure with irregular margins. It is not insulated by a sheath of fibrous tissue, and there are multiple extensions to the atrial myocardium.[1] Pacemaker automaticity is due to spontaneous diastolic repolarization of phase 4 that generates rhythmic action potentials and determines the heart rate through various currents, including the I_f current (see Chapter 49 on mechanisms of arrhythmogenesis).[2] Depolarization spreads within the sinus node and then is transmitted to the atria via several specialized sinoatrial exit pathways.[3] Impulses arrive at the **AV node** that functions as a filter for ventricular protection from fast atrial rates as well as a backup pacemaker in case of sinus node dysfunction.[4] Conduction to the ventricles is then through the **bundle of His** which passes through the annulus fibrosus and penetrates the membranous intraventricular septum before separating into the left and right bundle branches at the superior margin of the muscular septum. The **right bundle** crosses the anterior part of the intraventricular septum and reaches the apex of the ventricle and the base of the anterior papillary muscle. The **left bundle** is anatomically less discrete and subdivides into the **anterior (superior)** and **posterior (inferior) fascicle**. Finally, the bundle branches ramify to produce the endocardial **Purkinje fibres** which activate the ventricles. Dense innervation of the sinus node and the conduction system by post-ganglionic adrenergic and cholinergic nerve terminals, determines sinus rate and AV conduction. The sinus nodal branch of the right coronary artery (sinus nodal branch may also originate from the proximal circumflex artery in up to 40% of cases) provides blood supply to the sinus node. In 85–90% of human hearts, the blood supply to the AV node (AV nodal artery) is provided by the distal RCA and by the left circumflex in the remainder. Septal branches of the LAD also provide blood to the upper muscular interventricular septum and the conduction system. The specialized cells of the cardiac conduction system have relatively poor contractility and express specialized ion channels and gap-junction proteins, such as connexins, that mediate electrical coupling with neighbouring cells.

Mutations that affect the cardiac conduction system and are associated with conduction disturbances are presented in Table 62.1.

Table 62.1 Genetic causes of conduction system disease

Gene	Protein	Conduction Defect	Associated Conditions	Mechanism
	Ion channels			
SCN5A	Nav1.5	AV conduction defect	Brugada syndrome, LQTS 3, sick sinus syndrome, bundle branch block	Slowing of conduction velocity and pacemaking rate, AF, dilated cardiomyopathy, tissue degeneration via TGF-beta 1
TRPM4	TRPM4	AV conduction defect	Possibly elevated density of TRPM4 channels disables action potential propagation down the Purkinje fibres	
SCN1B	Scn1b	Bundle branch block	Brugada syndrome	Slowing of conduction velocity mainly in Purkinje fibres
KCNJ2	Kir2.1	AV block, bundle branch block	Andersen–Tawil syndrome (LQTS 7)	Prolongation of action potential and slowing of pacemaking rate
HCN4	HCN4	Sick sinus syndrome	Reduction of pacemaker current I_f	
	Structural proteins			
GJA5	Connexin40	AV block, bradycardia	Ventricular arrhythmias	Defective coupling of conducting myocytes
ANK2	Ankyrin-B	Sick sinus syndrome	LQTS 4, AF, CPVT	Abnormal sinoatrial electrical activity due to dysfunction in ankyrin B-based trafficking pathways

(Continued)

Table 62.1 (Continued)

Gene	Protein	Conduction Defect	Associated Conditions	Mechanism
DES	Desmin	AV block	VT/VF, cardiomyopathy, skeletal myopathy	Desmin-positive aggregates and inability of mutated desmin to interact with cellular structures. Mitochondrial dysfunction
	Protein kinases			
PRKAG2	γ-2 subunit of AMP-activated protein kinase (AMPK)	Sinus bradycardia, AV block	Wolff–Parkinson–White syndrome Glycogen storage cardiomyopathy	Disruption of annulus fibrosus by glycogen-filled myocytes
DMPK	Myotonic dystrophy protein kinase	AV block, bundle branch block	VT/VF, cardiomyopthy Myotonic dystrophy type I	Toxic mutant RNA impairs conduction with various mechanisms
	TGF-β superfamily			
BMP2	Bone morphogenetic protein 2	AV block	Wolff–Parkinson–White syndrome, cognitive defects, dysmorphic features	Disruption of annulus fibrosus
	Transcription factors			
TBX5	Tbx5	Sinus bradycardia, AV block bundle branch block	Holt–Oram syndrome	Defective development and coupling of conducting myocytes
NKX2–5	Nkx2–5	AV block, bundle branch block	VSD, Fallot, subvalvar AS, pulmonary atresia	Defective development and coupling of conducting myocytes
	Nuclear membrane proteins			
LMNA	Lamin A/C	AV block,	VT/VF, cardiomyopathy Emery–Dreifuss muscular dystrophy Limb-girdle muscular dystrophy	Possibly, hyperactivation of mitogen-activated protein. kinase and interference with nucleus integrity and gap junctions
EMD	Emerin	AV block	VT/VF, Emery–Dreifuss muscular dystrophy	Mechanism poorly understood
	Lysosomal enzymes			
GLA	Alpha galactosidase (a-GALA)	AV block	Anderson–Fabry disease	Accumulation of glycosphingolipids
	Ca^{2+} handling proteins			
RYR2	Ryanodine receptor	Sick sinus syndrome, AV block	CPVT 1, AF, dilated cardiomyopathy	Altered calcium handling mechanism of bradycardia and block unknown
CASQ2	Calsequestrin	Sinus bradycardia	CPVT 2	Altered calcium handling Mechanism of bradycardia and block unknown

Katritsis DG. Progressive Conduction System Disease. In: Zipes DO, Jalife J. *Cardiac Electrophysiology. From Cell to Bedside*. 6th Edition. Saunders 2013.

References

1. Sanchez-Quintana D, *et al.* Sinus node revisited in the era of electroanatomical mapping and catheter ablation. *Heart.* 2005;**91**:189–94
2. Park DS, *et al.* The cardiac conduction system. *Circulation.* 2011;**123**:904–15
3. Fedorov VV, *et al.* Optical mapping of the isolated coronary-perfused human sinus node. *J Am Coll Cardiol.* 2010;**56**:1386–94
4. Kurian T, *et al.* Anatomy and electrophysiology of the human AV node. *Pacing Clin Electrophysiol.* 2010;**33**:754–62

Chapter 63

Sinus nodal disease

Sinus bradycardia

Definitions

Sinus rates <60 beats/min are defined as bradycardia.[1] It is common in young adults, particularly well-trained athletes. During sleep, the sinus rate may fall to 35 beats/min, with pauses up to 3 s, and is not considered abnormal.

Sinus arrhythmia usually refers to sinus cycle phasic variation that is related to the respiratory cycle and is normal in the youth. Non-respiratory sinus arrhythmia may be seen with digitalis toxicity.

Sinus arrest (sinus pauses) manifests itself as pauses, with the P-P interval containing the pause not being equal or multiple of the basic P-P interval.

In **sinoatrial exit block** (first-, second-, or third-degree), the atrium is not depolarized despite the sinus stimulus, and the duration of the pause is a multiple of the basic P-P interval.

Wandering pacemaker refers to a shift of the dominant pacemaker from the sinus node to other atrial focus, usually lower at the crista terminalis. It is a normal finding, especially in athletes.

Asymptomatic bradycardia does not require treatment, and no drugs increase the heart rate efficiently and safely. Pacing is considered only in the presence of bradycardia-induced low cardiac output state.

Aetiology

Intracranial and mediastinal tumours, severe hypoxia, hypothermia, myxoedema, Chagas' disease, mental depression, and drugs, such as beta blockers (orally or by conjunctival instillation for glaucoma), verapamil and diltiazem, amiodarone, propaphenone, and lithium, may cause sinus bradycardia. Transient sinus bradycardia occurs in 10–25% patients with acute MI (usually inferior) but is an ominous sign if it occurs following resuscitation from cardiac arrest.[5]

Sick sinus syndrome

Definition

Sick sinus syndrome (SSS) refers to any of the following conditions that may coexist:

- Persistent spontaneous bradycardia not caused by drugs with or without chronotropic incompetence, i.e. inability to achieve 85% of the age-predicted maximum heart rate on the treadmill[2]
- Sinus pauses either due to sinus arrest or exit block
- Combinations of sinus arrest with AV conduction disturbances
- Alternating episodes of bradycardia, usually following tachycardia (mostly AF).

Sinus nodal disease is the most common cause of bradyarrhythmias requiring pacing in the western world.[3]

Epidemiology

The prevalence of sinus node dysfunction in the USA has been estimated to be approximately 500 per million, with an incidence of 63 per million requiring pacemaker therapy. It accounts for 50% of implantation of permanent pacemakers.[4] SSS is primarily a disease of the elderly, with an average of 68 years of age.

Pathophysiology

Fibrotic or degenerative destruction of the sinus node, its atrial radiations and the surrounding nerves, and perhaps sinus nodal occlusion comprise the pathological basis of the disease.[5] Mutations associated with SSS are presented in Table 62.1 of Chapter 62.

Diagnosis

SSS is primarily a disease of the elderly. It is suspected when symptoms, such as light-headedness, fatigue, dizziness, and presyncope or syncope are related to bradycardia. Sinus nodal recovery time (SNRT) is derived from electrophysiology studies by pacing at the right atrium between 600 and 350 ms for 30–60 s. This is corrected for the underlying sinus cycle length (CSNRT = SNRT – SCL). Values >525 ms are considered abnormal and represent a specific, but highly insensitive, test for SSS. Abnormal head-up tilt testing or carotid sinus massage in the presence of normal CSNRT suggest a vasodepressor reflex, rather than SSS (see Chapter 66 on syncope).[6] Supraventricular tachycardia, including AF, occurs in approximately 50% of patients with sinus node dysfunction.[4]

Therapy

No drugs can effectively and safely increase the sinus rate. Indications for pacing are presented in Table 63.1.[7,8] Minimally symptomatic patients may be just followed up, unless atrial tachycardias necessitate the use of beta blockers. The natural history of SSS is variable, but the majority of patients who have experienced syncope due to sinus pause or bradycardia will have recurrent syncope.

Table 63.1 Pacing in SSS

ACCF/AHA/HRS 2012 GL on device-based therapy **Recommendations for permanent pacing in sinus node dysfunction (SND)**	
SND with documented symptomatic bradycardia, including frequent sinus pauses that produce symptoms	I-C
Symptomatic chronotropic incompetence	I-C
Symptomatic sinus bradycardia that results from required drug therapy	I-C
SND with heart rate <40 bpm when a clear association between significant symptoms consistent with bradycardia and the actual presence of bradycardia has not been documented	IIa-C
Syncope of unexplained origin when clinically significant abnormalities of sinus node function are discovered or provoked in EP studies	IIa-C
Minimally symptomatic patients with chronic heart rate <40 bpm while awake	IIb-C
SND in asymptomatic patients	III-C
SND in patients for whom the symptoms have been clearly documented to occur in the absence of bradycardia	III-C
SND with symptomatic bradycardia due to non-essential drug therapy	III-C

2012 ACCF/AHA/HRS focused update incorporated into the ACCF/AHA/HRS 2008 guidelines for device-based therapy of cardiac rhythm abnormalities. *J Am Coll Cardiol*. 2013;**61**:e6–75.

ESC 2013 GL on Pacing and CRT	
Indication for pacing in persistent bradycardia (sinus node disease)	
Pacing when symptoms can clearly be attributed to sinus bradycardia.	I-B
Pacing when symptoms are likely to be due to sinus bradycardia, even if the evidence is not conclusive.	IIb-C
Pacing in patients with sinus bradycardia which is asymptomatic or due to reversible causes.	III-C
Indication for pacing in intermittent documented bradycardia	
Pacing in patients affected by sinus node disease (including the tachy-brady form) who have the documentation of symptomatic bradycardia due to sinus arrest or sinus-atrial block.	I-B
Pacing in patients ≥40 years with recurrent, unpredictable reflex syncopes and documented symptomatic pause/s due to sinus arrest or AV block or the combination of the two.	IIa-B
Pacing in patients with history of syncope and documentation of asymptomatic pauses >6 s due to sinus arrest, or sinus-atrial block or AV block.	IIa-C
Pacing in reversible causes of bradycardia.	III-C

2013 ESC Guidelines on cardiac pacing and cardiac resynchronization therapy. *Eur Heart J* 2013. doi:10.1093/eurheartj/eht150.

The incidence of sudden death, however, is extremely low, and SSS, treated or untreated, does not affect survival. [11] The risk of developing AV block within the next 5 years is 3–35%.[7] At time of diagnosis, 40–70% of patients may have AF whereas the incidence of new AF in follow-up ranges from 4 to 22%.[3]

Choice of the pacemaker mode

Several trials on patients with SSS and/or AV block [9–14] have compared atrial or dual-chamber with ventricular pacing. Although results have not been consistent, atrial-based pacing reduces the incidence of atrial fibrillation and may modestly reduce stroke compared to ventricular pacing but does not improve survival or reduce heart failure or cardiovascular death.[15] However, ventricular desynchronization imposed by ventricular pacing, even when AV synchrony is preserved, has also been shown to increase the risk of heart failure and AF in patients with sinus nodal disease and normal baseline QRS duration.[16] DDDR pacing, with a very short atrioventricular interval and more than 99% ventricular pacing, has been reported to increase the incidence of atrial fibrillation when compared with DDDR pacing with automated features to minimize ventricular pacing by prolonging the atrioventricular interval.[17] In the recent DANPACE trial, AAIR pacing was associated with a higher incidence of paroxysmal AF and a 2-fold increased risk of pacemaker reoperation compared to DDDR pacing programmed with a moderately prolonged atrioventricular interval.[13] Low atrial septal pacing with dual-chamber pacemakers has been reported to reduce atrial fibrillation in sick sinus syndrome, but further experience is needed.[18] Atrial pacing may be arrhythmogenic,[19] and sublinical atrial arrhythmias in patients with a history of hypertension but no prior diagnosis of clinical atrial fibrillation, predispose to embolic events.[20] Indications for pacing and pacemaker mode selection are presented in Figures 63.1 and 63.2 and Table 63.2.

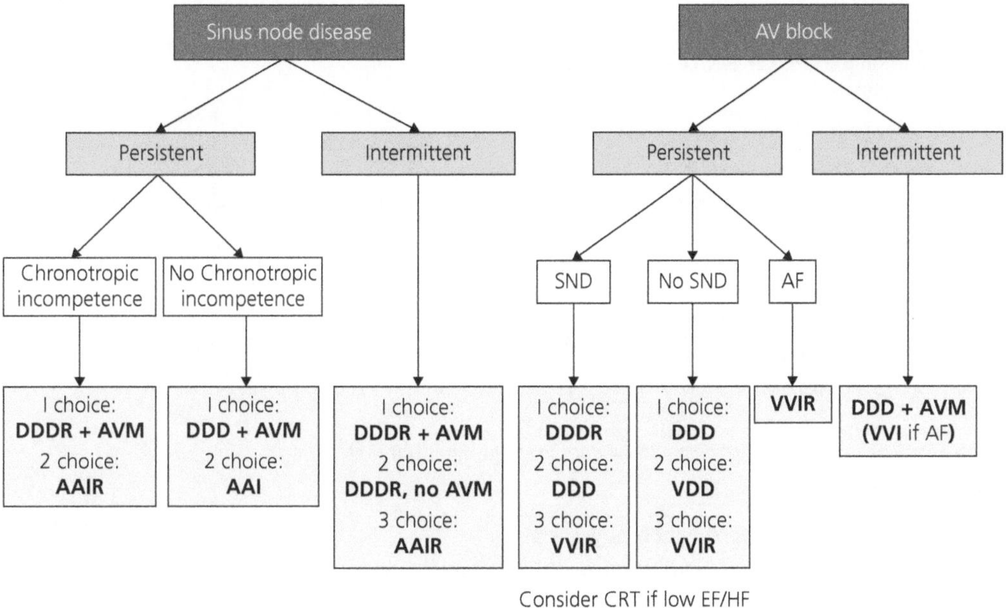

Figure 63.1 ESC 2013 GL on cardiac pacing and CRT. Optimal pacing mode in sinus node disease and AV block.

AF: atrial fibrillation; AV: atrioventricular; AVM: AV delay management, i.e. to prevent unnecessary right ventricular pacing by means of manual optimization of AV interval or programming of AV hysteresis; SND: sinus node disease.

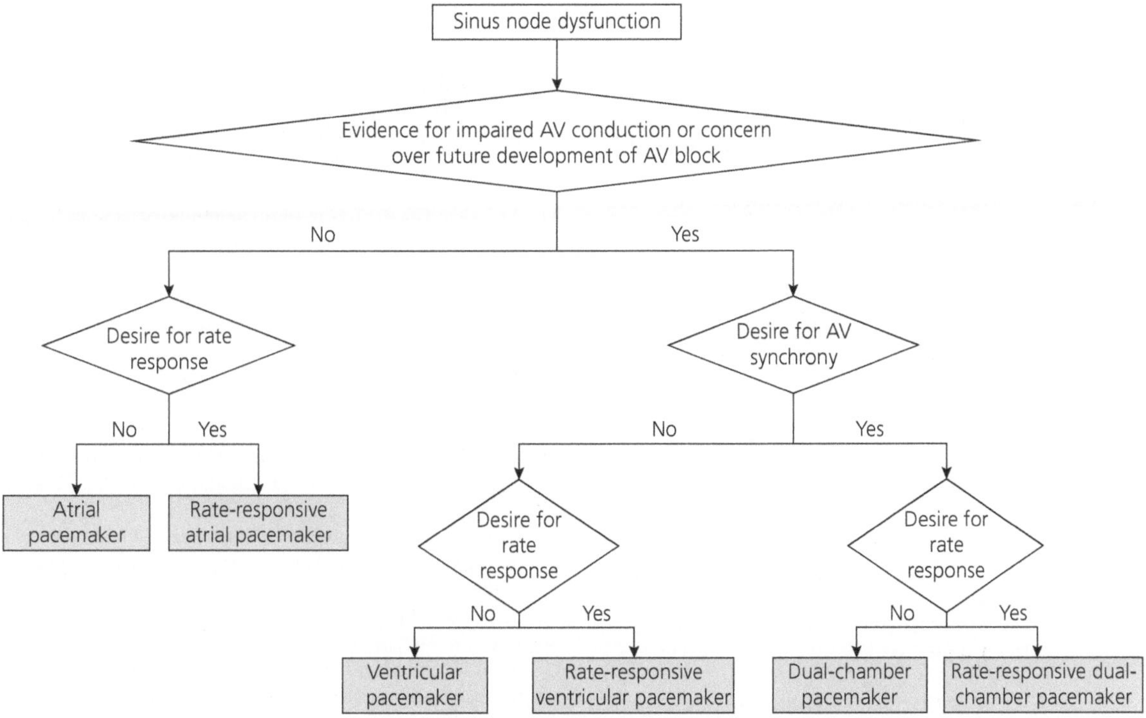

Figure 63.2 ACCF/AHA/HRS 2012 GL on device-based therapy of cardiac rhythm abnormalities. Pacing mode in sick sinus syndrome.

2012 ACCF/AHA/HRS focused update incorporated into the ACCF/AHA/HRS 2008 guidelines for device-based therapy of cardiac rhythm abnormalities. *J Am Coll Cardiol*. 2013;**61**:e6–75.

Table 63.2 Selection of pacing mode in SSS

HRS/AACF 2012 statement on pacemaker device mode section. Pacing mode selection in SSS	
DDD or AAI pacing is recommended over VVI pacing in patients with SND and intact AV conduction	I-A
DDD or AAI pacing is recommended over AAI pacing in patients with SND	I-B
Rate adaptive pacing in patients with significant symptomatic chronotropic incompetence, and its need should be re-evaluated during follow-up	IIa-C
In patients with SND and intact AV conduction, programming DDD pacemakers to minimize ventricular pacing can be useful for prevention of AF	IIa-B
AAI pacing may be considered in selected patients with normal AV and ventricular conduction	IIb-B
VVI pacing may be considered in instances where frequent pacing is not expected or the patient has significant co-morbidities	IIb-C
DDD or AAI pacing should not be used in patients in permanent or longstanding persistent AF where efforts to restore or maintain SR are not planned	III-C

HRS/ACCF Expert Consensus Statement on pacemaker device and mode selection. *Heart Rhythm*. 2012;**9**:1344–65.

ESC 2013 GL on Pacing and CRT	
Choice of pacing mode/programming in persistent bradycardia	
Dual-chamber PM with preservation of spontaneous AV conduction for reducing the risk of AF and stroke, avoiding pacemaker syndrome syndrome and improving quality of life.	I-A (vs VVI), I-B (vs AAI)
Rate response features should be adopted for patients with chronotropic incompetence, especially if young and physically active.	IIa-C
Choice of pacing mode in intermittent documented bradycardia	
Dual-chamber pacing with rate hysteresis is the preferred mode in reflex asystolic syncope in order to preserve spontaneous sinus rhythm.	I-C

2013 ESC Guidelines on cardiac pacing and cardiac resynchronization therapy. *Eur Heart J* 2013. doi:10.1093/eurheartj/eht150.

References

1. Olgin J, *et al.* Specific arrhythmias. In: Libby P, Bonow RO, Mann DL, Zipes DP. *Braunwald's Heart Disease*. pp. 863–931, Saunders, [CITY] 2008
2. Katritsis D, *et al.* Chronotropic incompetence: a proposal for definition and diagnosis. *Br Heart J*. 1993;**70**:400–2
3. Gillis AM, *et al.* HRS/ACCF expert consensus statement on pacemaker device and mode selection: developed in partnership between the Heart Rhythm Society (HRS) and the American College of Cardiology Foundation (ACCF) and in collaboration with the Society of Thoracic Surgeons. *Heart Rhythm*. 2012;**9**:1344–65
4. Go AS, *et al.* Heart disease and stroke statistics—2013 update: a report from the American Heart Association. *Circulation*. 2013;**127**:e6–245
5. Park DS, *et al.* The cardiac conduction system. *Circulation*. 2011;**123**:904–15
6. Alboni P, *et al.* Treatment of persistent sinus bradycardia with intermittent symptoms: are guidelines clear? *Europace*. 2009;**11**:562–4
7. 2012 ACCF/AHA/HRS focused update incorporated into the ACCF/AHA/HRS 2008 guidelines for device-based therapy of cardiac rhythm abnormalities. *J Am Coll Cardiol*. 2013;**61**:e6–75
8. Brignole M, *et al.* 2013 ESC Guidelines on cardiac pacing and cardiac resynchronization therapy. *Eur Heart J*. 2013. doi:10.1093/eurheartj/eht150
9. Lamas GA, *et al.* Quality of life and clinical outcomes in elderly patients treated with ventricular pacing as compared with dual-chamber pacing. Pacemaker selection in the elderly investigators. *N Engl J Med*. 1998;**338**:1097–104
10. Kerr CR, *et al.* Canadian trial of physiological pacing: effects of physiological pacing during long-term follow-up. *Circulation*. 2004;**109**:357–62
11. Andersen HR, *et al.* Long-term follow-up of patients from a randomised trial of atrial versus ventricular pacing for sick-sinus syndrome. *Lancet*. 1997;**350**:1210–16
12. Lamas GA, *et al.* Ventricular pacing or dual-chamber pacing for sinus-node dysfunction. *N Engl J Med*. 2002;**346**:1854–62
13. Nielsen JC, *et al.* A comparison of single-lead atrial pacing with dual-chamber pacing in sick sinus syndrome. *Eur Heart J*. 2011;**32**:686–96
14. Toff WD, *et al.* Single-chamber versus dual-chamber pacing for high-grade atrioventricular block. *N Engl J Med*. 2005;**353**:145–55
15. Healey JS, *et al.* Cardiovascular outcomes with atrial-based pacing compared with ventricular pacing: meta-analysis of randomized trials, using individual patient data. *Circulation*. 2006;**114**:11–17
16. Sweeney MO, *et al.* Adverse effect of ventricular pacing on heart failure and atrial fibrillation among patients with normal baseline QRS duration in a clinical trial of pacemaker therapy for sinus node dysfunction. *Circulation*. 2003;**107**:2932–7
17. Sweeney MO, *et al.* Minimizing ventricular pacing to reduce atrial fibrillation in sinus-node disease. *N Engl J Med*. 2007;**357**:1000–8

18. Verlato R, *et al.* Efficacy of low interatrial septum and right atrial appendage pacing for prevention of permanent atrial fibrillation in patients with sinus node disease: results from the Electrophysiology-guided PAcing Site Selection (EPASS) Study. *Circ Arrhythm Electrophysiol.* 2011;**4**:844–50
19. Elkayam LU, *et al.* The influence of atrial and ventricular pacing on the incidence of atrial fibrillation: a meta-analysis. *Pacing Clin Electrophysiol.* 2011;**34**:1593–9
20. Healey JS, *et al.* Subclinical atrial fibrillation and the risk of stroke. *N Engl J Med.* 2012;**366**:120–9

Chapter 64

Atrioventricular and intraventricular block

Atrioventricular block

Definitions

First-degree AV block is characterized by a PR interval >200 ms. A narrow QRS complex indicates that the block is most probably at the AV node whereas a wide QRS can be seen with block either at the node or His-Purkinje system.

Second degree-AV block is characterized by P waves not conducted to the ventricles.

Type I AV block (Mobitz I or Wenckebach) shows progressively increasing PR intervals until a P wave fails to be conducted to the ventricles. A narrow QRS type I block is almost always AV nodal whereas a type I block with bundle branch block is infranodal in 60% to 70% of cases. Type I AV block can be physiological in athletes, resulting from heavy physical training, and occasionally in young people. It may also be normally seen during sleep in patients with high vagal tone.[1]

Type II AV block (Mobitz II) shows **consecutive**, non-conducted P waves without visible changes in the PR interval (i.e. AV conduction time) before and after the blocked impulse, provided there is normal sinus rhythm. Block is infranodal at the His-Purkinje level.

Third-degree (complete) AV block No P wave is conducted to the ventricles, and ventricular contraction is maintained by an escape nodal or intra- or infra-Hisian rhythm.

Epidemiology

The prevalence of third-degree AV block in the general population is approximately 0.03%. The prevalence of first-degree AV block in NHANES III was 3.7%.[2]

Pathophysiology

Causes of conduction disease are presented in Table 64.1. **Progressive cardiac conduction disease (PCCD)** is diagnosed in the presence of unexplained progressive conduction abnormalities in young (<50 years) individuals with structurally normal hearts in the absence of skeletal myopathies especially if there is a family history of PCCD.[3] It was initially described by **Lenegre and Lev** who hypothesized that progressive conduction defects were due to a primary degenerative disease of unknown origin that was exaggerated by ageing. There has been now evidence that progressive conduction system disease has genetic and autoimmune origins.[3,4] Myocardial ischaemia and infarction, hypertension, inherited degenerative disease affecting the conduction system, sarcoidosis, rheumatic disorders (rheumatoid arthritis, scleroderma), congenital heart deformities, neuromuscular disorders, aortic stenosis, infections, such as Lyme disease and Chagas' disease, electrolyte abnormalities, myocarditis, endocarditis, cardiac surgery, sleep apnoea, and catheter ablation procedures may affect the conduction system and cause permanent of paroxysmal AV block. **Cardiac sarcoidosis** and a mild form of giant cell myocarditis are the causes for more than 25% of initially unexplained AV block in young and middle-aged adults. These patients are at high risk for adverse cardiac events.[5] **Lyme** is a common tickborne disease transmitted to humans through the bite of the Ixodes tick. The causative bacterium is *Borrelia burgdorferi*, and the disease is characterized by an early localized infection, with erythema migrans, fever, fatigue, headache, myalgias, and arthralgias, followed by early disseminated infection (occurring days to weeks later), with neurologic, musculoskeletal, or cardiovascular symptoms and multiple erythema migrans lesions. Late Lyme disease, with intermittent swelling and pain of one or more joints (especially knees), may also occur.[6] However, although Lyme borreliosis is the most common tickborne infectious disease in North America and in countries with moderate climates in Eurasia, Lyme carditis is rare. AV block may be seen during the acute course of the disease that involves the heart, with a clinical picture similar to acute rheumatic fever, and responds to antibiotics. Borrelia antibodies may be sought with Western blot in cases of otherwise unexplained acute AV block. Recurrent erythema migrans after antibiotic treatment is caused by reinfection rather than relapse of the original infection,[7] and persistent arthritis

Table 64.1 Causes of AV conduction disease

Myocardial ischaemia and infarction
Calcified valve disease
Aortic stenosis
Mitral annulus calcification
Electrolyte disturbances
Endocarditis
Myocarditis
Sleep apnoea
Cardiac valve and congenital surgery
Cardiac transplantation
Catheter ablation procedures
Drugs
Digitalis
Beta blockers
Verapamil, diltiazem
Amiodarone
Procainamide
Flecainide, propafenone
Doxorubicin
Methotrexate
Chloroquine
Infective disorders
Lyme borreliosis
Chagas' disease
Autoimmune disorders
Sarcoidosis
Rheumatoid arthritis
Systemic sclerosis
Ankylosing spondylitis (HLA B27)
Systemic lupus erythymatosus
Sjögren syndrome
Wegener's granulomatosis
Behçet's disease
Anti-Ro/SSA, anti-LA/SSA antibodies
Inherited
Isolated (progressive familial heart block type IA and IB)
Genetic arrhythmia syndromes (Brugada syndrome, long QT syndrome 3, arrhythmia-prone cardiomyopathy)
Congenital cardiac defects (Holt–Oram syndrome, non-syndromic cardiac defects)
Wolff–Parkinson–White syndrome and cardiomyopathy
Muscular dystrophies (myotonic dystrophy type 1, Emery–Dreifuss, limb girdle, desmin myopathy)
Anderson--Fabry disease

(*Continued*)

Table 64.1 (Continued)

Familial amyloidosis
Mucopolysaccharidosis IV
Kearns–Sayre syndrome
Malignancy (lymphomatous or solid tumour)

is probably due to infection-induced autoimmunity. Thus, prolonged antibiotic therapy for the so-called 'chronic Lyme disease' is not justified. **Mutations** associated with AV conduction disease are presented in Table 62.1. Up to 5% of AV conduction disease are due to SCN5A mutations.[8] **Vagally induced** AV block, i.e. by vomiting, is a benign phenomenon.

Syncope **(Stokes–Adams)** and death may occur due to complete heart block if an escape rhythm at a lower level than the site of block does not intervene.

Diagnosis

First-degree AV block

1. Atrial premature beats may produce prolonged PR intervals due to refractory fast pathway of the AV node.
2. Several drugs, such as beta blockers, non-dihydropyridine calcium channel blockers, flecainide, and amiodarone may prolong the PR interval.

Second-degree AV block

1. Non-conducted atrial premature beats may mimic AV block.
2. An apparent narrow QRS type II block may be a type I block with miniscule increments of the PR interval.
3. Concealed His bundle or ventricular extrasystoles confined to the specialized conduction system without myocardial depolarization can produce electrocardiographic patterns that mimic type I and/or type II block (pseudo-AV block). Occasionally, retrograde P waves may be present.
4. A pattern resembling a narrow QRS type II block, in association with an obvious type I pattern in the same recording, effectively rules out type II block because the coexistence of both types of narrow QRS block is exceedingly rare.[9]
5. Although the diagnosis of type II block is possible with an increasing sinus rate, the absence of sinus slowing is an important criterion of type II block, because a vagal surge can cause simultaneous sinus slowing and AV nodal block, which can superficially resemble type II block. Significant PR prolongation before and after block and prolonged PP intervals during ventricular asystole are indicative of vagal block that is a benign condition, rather than **paroxysmal AV block**, i.e. pause-dependent phase 4 AV block, that is potentially dangerous for syncope.[10]

6. The diagnosis of type II block cannot be established if the first post-block P wave is followed by a shortened PR interval or is not discernible.
7. A 2:1 AV block is not necessarily a type II block. It can be high-grade if the sinus rate is low or even normal response of the AV node to an atrial tachycardia or flutter.

Third-degree AV block

Unless the escape rhythm is lower than the sinus rate (and usually <45 bpm), complete AV block cannot be differentiated from AV dissociation.

Indications for electrophysiology study in second-degree AV block are presented in Table 64.2 and for genetic testing in progressive conduction disease in Table 64.3.

The value of adenosine or ATP testing for induction of latent AV block is not established.[11] However, there has been evidence that induction of cardiac pauses (due to AV block or sinoatrial block >10 s by an IV bolus of 20 mg ATP) indicates the need for DDD pacing.[12, 13] Adenosine may also be used, but its effects are not identical with those of ATP.[13]

Therapy

Marked **first-degree AV block** (PR 0.30 s or greater) can produce a clinical condition similar to that of the pacemaker syndrome. Clinical evaluation often requires a treadmill stress test because patients are more likely to become symptomatic with mild or moderate exercise when the PR interval cannot adapt appropriately. In patients with marked first-degree AV block with LV systolic dysfunction, it would seem prudent to consider a biventricular DDD device.[1] First-degree AV block during cardiac resynchronization therapy (CRT) predisposes to loss of ventricular resynchronization during biventricular pacing. This is because it favours the initiation of electrical 'desynchronization', especially in association with a relatively fast atrial rate and a relatively slow programmed upper rate. In patients with myotonic dystrophy type I and PR >200 ms, QRS >100 ms, or both, pacing is indicated when HV >70 ms, and improves survival.[14]

In **type I second-degree AV block**, the indications for permanent pacing are controversial, unless the conduction delay occurs below the AV node or there are symptoms. However, type I block is not usually benign in patients 45 years of age or older, and pacemaker implantation may be considered, even in the absence of symptomatic bradycardia or organic heart disease.[15] **Type II block** progresses to complete heart block, particularly when the QRS is wide, and infranodal blocks require pacing, regardless of form or symptoms.[16,17]

In **third-degree block**, pacing improves survival.[16,17]

Indications for permanent pacing and pacemaker mode selection are presented in Tables 64.4 and 64.5 and Figure 63.1.

Exercise-provoked distal atrioventricular block, if not due to acute ischaemia, has a poor prognosis and should be paced.[18]

Patients who develop complete atrioventricular block within 24 hours after **valve replacement**, which then

Table 64.2 Indications for invasive study of second-degree atrioventricular block

Asymptomatic type I second-degree AV block with bundle branch block
Asymptomatic advanced second-degree AV block with bundle branch block
Questionable diagnosis of type II block with a narrow QRS complex
Suspicion of concealed AV junctional or ventricular extrasystoles
Confirmation of bradycardia-dependent (phase 4) infranodal block in selected cases
Transient second-degree AV block with bundle branch block in patients with inferior myocardial infarction where the site of block is suspected to be in the His-Purkinje system rather than the AV node
Third-degree AV block with a fast ventricular rate

Modified from Barold SS, Hayes DL. Second-degree atrioventricular block: a reappraisal. *Mayo Clin Proc*. 2001;**76**:44–57.

Table 64.3 HRS/EHRA 2011

State of genetic testing for progressive cardiac conduction disease (CCD)	
Mutation-specific genetic testing for family members and appropriate relatives following the identification of the CCD-causative mutation in an index case.	I
Genetic testing for patients with either isolated CCD or CCD with concomitant congenital heart disease, especially when there is documentation of a positive family history of CCD.	IIb

HRS/EHRA expert consensus statement on the state of genetic testing for the channelopathies and cardiomyopathies. *Europace*. 2011;**13**:1077–109.

Table 64.4 Pacing in AV block

ACCF/AHA/HRS 2012 GL on device-based therapy	
Recommendations for acquired atrioventricular block in adults	
Third-degree and advanced second-degree AV block at any anatomicalal level associated with bradycardia with symptoms (including heart failure) or ventricular arrhythmias presumed to be due to AV block.	I-C
Third-degree and advanced second-degree AV block at any anatomicalal level associated with arrhythmias and other medical conditions that require drug therapy that results in symptomatic bradycardia.	I-C
Third-degree and advanced second-degree AV block at any anatomicalal level in awake, symptom-free patients in sinus rhythm, with documented periods of asystole ≥3.0 s or any escape rate <40 bpm, or with an escape rhythm that is below the AV node.	I-C
Third-degree and advanced second-degree AV block at any anatomicalal level in awake, symptom-free patients with atrial fibrillation and bradycardia with one or more pauses ≥5 s.	I-C
Third-degree and advanced second-degree AV block at any anatomical level after catheter ablation of the AV junction.	I-C
Third-degree and advanced second-degree AV block at any anatomical level associated with post-operative AV block that is not expected to resolve after cardiac surgery.	I-C
Third-degree and advanced second-degree AV block at any anatomical level associated with neuromuscular diseases with AV block, such as myotonic muscular dystrophy, Kearns–Sayre syndrome, Erb dystrophy (limb-girdle muscular dystrophy), and peroneal muscular atrophy, with or without symptoms.	I-B
Second degree AV block with associated symptomatic bradycardia, regardless of type or site of block.	I-B
Asymptomatic persistent third-degree AV block at any anatomical site with average awake ventricular rates ≥40 bpm if cardiomegaly or LV dysfunction is present or if the site of block is below the AV node.	I-B
Second- or third-degree AV block during exercise in the absence of myocardial ischaemia.	I-C
Persistent third-degree AV block with an escape rate >40 bpm in asymptomatic adult patients without cardiomegaly.	IIa-C
Asymptomatic second-degree AV block at intra- or infra-His levels found at electrophysiological study.	IIa-B
First- or second-degree AV block with symptoms similar to those of pacemaker syndrome or haemodynamic compromise.	IIa-B
Asymptomatic type II second-degree AV block with a narrow QRS (class I when type II second-degree AV block occurs with a wide QRS, including isolated RBBB).	IIa-B
Neuromuscular diseases, such as myotonic muscular dystrophy, Erb dystrophy (limb-girdle muscular dystrophy), and peroneal muscular atrophy with any degree of AV block (including first-degree AV block), with or without symptoms, because there may be unpredictable progression of AV conduction disease.	IIb-B
AV block in the setting of drug use and/or drug toxicity when the block is expected to recur, even after the drug is withdrawn.	IIb-B
Asymptomatic first-degree AV block.	III-B
Asymptomatic type I second-degree AV block at the supra-His (AV node) level or that which is not known to be intra- or infra-Hisian.	III-C
AV block that is expected to resolve and is unlikely to recur (e.g. drug toxicity, Lyme disease, or transient increases in vagal tone, or during hypoxia in sleep apnoea syndrome in the absence of symptoms).	III-B
2012 ACCF/AHA/HRS focused update incorporated into the ACCF/AHA/HRS 2008 guidelines for device-based therapy of cardiac rhythm abnormalities. *J Am Coll Cardiol*. 2013;**61**:e6–75	
ESC 2013 GL on Pacing and CRT	
First-degree AV block	
Permanent pacemaker implantation for patients with persistent symptoms similar to those of pacemaker atrioventricular block (PR >0.3 s).	IIa-C
Indication for pacing in persistent bradycardia	
Pacing with third- or second-degree type 2 acquired AV block irrespective of symptoms.	I-C
Pacing second-degree type 1 acquired AV block which causes symptoms or is found to be located at intra- or infra-His levels at EPS	IIa-C
Pacing in block or due to reversible causes.	III-C

(*Continued*)

Table 64.4 (Continued)

Indication for pacing in intermittent documented bradycardia	
Pacing in intermittent/paroxysmal intrinsic third- or second degree AV block (including AF with slow ventricular conduction).	I-C
Pacing in patients ≥40 years with recurrent, unpredictable reflex syncopes and documented symptomatic pause/s due to sinus arrest or AV block or the combination of the two.	IIa-B
Pacing in patients with history of syncope and documentation of asymptomatic pauses >6 s due to sinus arrest, or sinus-atrial block or AV block.	IIa-C
Pacing in reversible causes of bradycardia.	III-C
HRS/EHRA/APHRS 2013 Expert Consensus Statement on Inherited Arrhythmia	
Recommendations on Progressive Cardiac Conduction Disease	
Pacemaker implantation is recommended in patients with a diagnosis of PCCD and the presence of:	I
a) Intermittent or permanent third degree or high-grade AV block or	
b) Symptomatic Mobitz I or II second degree AV block.	
Pacemaker implantation can be useful in patients with a diagnosis of PCCD and the presence of bifascicular block with or without first degree AV block.	IIa
ICD implantation can be useful in adult patients diagnosed with PCCD with a mutation in the Lamin A/C gene with left ventricular dysfunction and/ or non-sustained VT.	IIa

HRS/EHRA/APHRS Expert Consensus Statement on the Diagnosis and Management of Patients with Inherited Primary Arrhythmia Syndromes. *Heart Rhythm* 2013. E-Pub

Table 64.5 Selection of pacing mode in AV block

HRS/AACF 2012 statement on pacemaker device mode section: Pacing mode selection in AV block	
DDD pacing is recommended in patients with AV block	I-C
CCI pacing is recommended as an acceptable alternative to DDD pacing in patients with AV block who have specific clinical situations that limit the benefits of DDD pacing (sedentary patients, significant medical co-morbidities, and technical issues, such as vascular access limitations)	I-B
DDD is recommended over VVI pacing in adult patients with AV block who have documented pacemaker syndrome	I-B
VDD pacing can be useful in patients with normal sinus node function and AV block (e.g. the younger patient with congenital AV block)	IIa-C
VVI pacing can be useful in patients with AV junction ablation for rate control of AF due to the high rate of progression to permanent AF	IIa-B
DDD pacing should not be used in patients with AV block in permanent or longstanding persistent AF in whom efforts to restore or maintain SR are not planned	III-C
HRS/ACCF Expert Consensus Statement on pacemaker device and mode selection. *Heart Rhythm*. 2012; **9**:1344–65.	
ESC 2013 GL on Pacing and CRT	
Choice of pacing mode/programming in persistent bradycardia	
In patients with sinus rhythm and acquired AV block, dual-chamber PM should be preferred to single chamber ventricular pacing for avoiding pacemaker syndrome and improving quality of life.	IIa-A
Ventricular pacing with rate-response function is recommended permanent AF and AV block.	I-C
Choice of pacing mode in intermittent documented bradycardia	
Preservation of spontaneous AV conduction is recommended.	I-B

2013 ESC Guidelines on cardiac pacing and cardiac resynchronization therapy. *Eur Heart J* 2013. doi:10.1093/eurheartj/eht150.

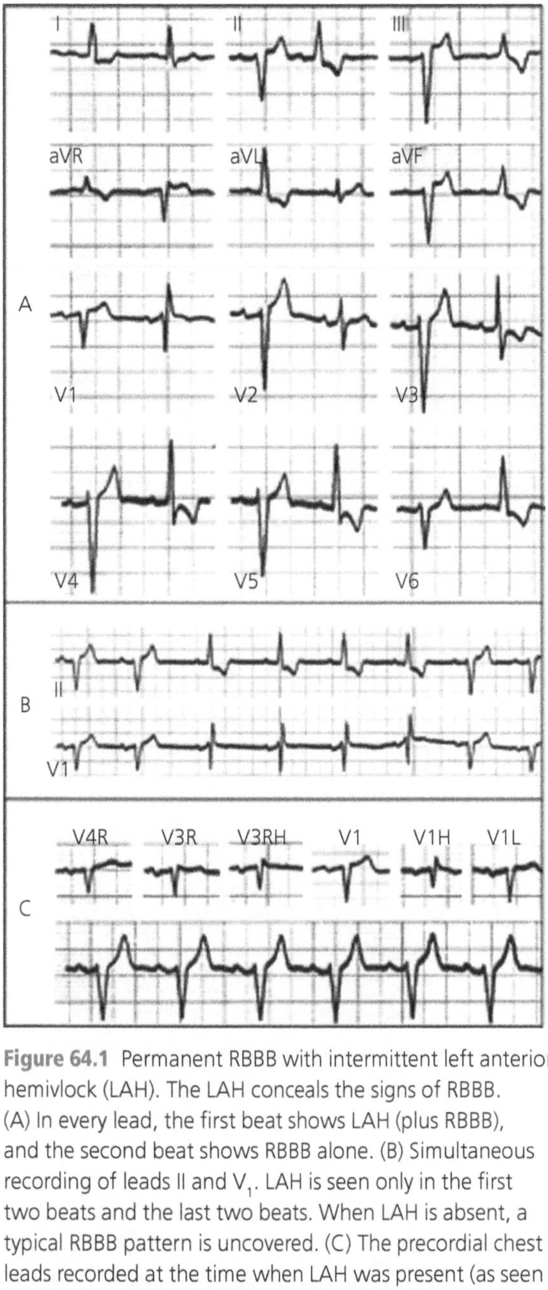

Figure 64.1 Permanent RBBB with intermittent left anterior hemivlock (LAH). The LAH conceals the signs of RBBB. (A) In every lead, the first beat shows LAH (plus RBBB), and the second beat shows RBBB alone. (B) Simultaneous recording of leads II and V_1. LAH is seen only in the first two beats and the last two beats. When LAH is absent, a typical RBBB pattern is uncovered. (C) The precordial chest leads recorded at the time when LAH was present (as seen in lead II) show the pattern of RBBB when V_3R and V_1 were recorded one intercostal space above the normal level (V_3RH and V_1H).

Elizari MV, *et al*. Hemiblocks revisited. *Circulation*. 2007;**115**:1154–63.

persisted for >48 hours, are unlikely to recover.[19] AV block occurs in 1–3% after operations for **congenital heart disease.**[17] Pacemaker implantation is recommended with persistent AV block for 7–10 days post-operatively. Endocardial leads, when feasible, are preferable to epicardial leads.[20]

Genetic therapies and the development of biological pacemakers by means of viral-based or stem cell-based gene delivery systems are a new exciting possibility for treating these patients.[21]

Atrioventricular dissociation

AV dissociation is independent beating of the atria and ventricles due to:

1. Slowing of the sinus rate which allows escape of a subsidiary or latent pacemaker
2. Acceleration of a latent pacemaker, as happens in non-paroxysmal AV junctional tachycardia or VT
3. Complete heart block with junctional or ventricular escape rhythm.

Intraventricular block

Definition

This is block at any level of the His-Purkinje system and is usually due to ischaemic heart disease and hypertension as well as the causes described in AV block. It may also be seen in apparently healthy persons. Definitions have been provided by the AHA/ACCF/HRS[22] (Table 64.6). Current criteria for LBBB include a QRS duration ≥120 ms, and this threshold is also used for CRT recommendations. However, certain patients may not have true complete LBBB but likely have a combination of left ventricular hypertrophy and left anterior fascicular block, and stricter criteria, such as a QRS duration ≥140 ms for men and ≥130 ms for women, along with mid-QRS notching or slurring in ≥2 contiguous leads, have been recently proposed.[23]

Left bundle branch block (LBBB) or **right bundle block (RBBB)** leads to interventricular dyssynchrony. The prevalence of bundle branch block increases from 1% at age 50 years to 17% at age 80 years, resulting in a cumulative incidence of 18%.[24]

RBBB may display normal axis or 180° (common type or Wilson block). Left or extreme right axis deviation suggest coexistent hemiblock. Both RBBB and incomplete RBBB are two to three times more common among men than women.[25] RBBB can be seen in hypertensives, and as opposed to LBBB, was considered not to be associated with increased mortality. There has been recent evidence, however, that complete RBBB (but not incomplete) is associated with increased cardiovascular risk and all-cause mortality.[26]

LBBB may display normal or, more often, left axis deviation that implies worse prognosis. Right axis deviation may be seen in dilated cardiomyopathy. Preexisting left bundle branch block in the absence of clinical evidence of heart disease is rare but carries a slightly increased mortality. The presence of an initial r wave of ≥1 mm in lead V_1

Table 64.6 AHA/ACC/HRS 2009 recommendations for standardization and interpretation of ECG (part III)

Criteria for intraventricular block

Complete RBBB

1. QRS duration ≥120 ms in adults, >100 ms in children ages 4 to 16 years, and <90 ms in children <4 years of age.
2. rsr′, rsR′, or rSR′ in leads V_1 or V_2. The R′ or r′ deflection is usually wider than the initial R wave. In a minority of patients, a wide, and often notched, R wave pattern may be seen in lead V_1 and/or V_2.
3. S wave of greater duration than R wave or >40 ms in leads I and V_6 in adults.
4. Normal R peak time in leads V_5 and V_6 but >50 ms in lead V_1.

Of the above criteria, the first three should be present to make the diagnosis. When a pure dominant R wave, with or without a notch, is present in V_1, criterion 4 should be satisfied.

Incomplete RBBB

Incomplete RBBB is defined by QRS duration 110–120 ms in adults, 90–100 ms in children 4 to 16 years of age, and 86–90 ms in children <8 years of age.

Other criteria are the same as for complete RBBB.

Complete LBBB

1. QRS duration ≥120 ms in adults, >100 ms in children 4 to 16 years of age, and >90 ms in children <4 years of age.
2. Broad notched or slurred R wave in leads I, aVL, V_5, and V_6 and an occasional RS pattern in V_5 and V_6 attributed to displaced transition of QRS complex.
3. Absent q waves in leads I, V_5, and V_6, but, in the lead aVL, a narrow q wave may be present in the absence of myocardial pathology.
4. R peak time >60 ms in leads V_5 and V_6 but normal in leads V_1, V_2, and V_3, when small initial r waves can be discerned in the above leads.
5. ST and T waves usually opposite in direction to QRS.
6. Positive T wave in leads with upright QRS may be normal (positive concordance).
7. Depressed ST segment and/or negative T wave in leads with negative QRS (negative concordance) are abnormal.
8. The appearance of LBBB may change the mean QRS axis in the frontal plane to the right, to the left, or to a superior, in some cases in a rate-dependent manner.

Incomplete LBBB

1. QRS duration 110–119 ms in adults, 90–100 ms in children 8 to 16 years of age, and 80–90 ms in children <8 years of age.
2. Presence of left ventricular hypertrophy pattern.
3. R peak time greater than 60 ms in leads V_4, V_5, and V_6.
4. Absence of q wave in leads I, V_5, and V_6.

Left anterior fascicular block

1. Frontal plane axis between –45° and –90°.
2. qR pattern in lead aVL.

Left anterior fascicular block

3. R peak time in lead aVL of 45 ms or more.
4. QRS duration less than 120 ms.

These criteria do not apply to patients with congenital heart disease in whom left axis deviation is present in infancy.

Left posterior fascicular block

1. Frontal plane axis 90°–180° in adults. Owing to the more rightward axis in children up to 16 years of age, this criterion should only be applied to them when a distinct rightward change in axis is documented.
2. rS pattern in leads I and aVL.
3. qR pattern in leads III and aVF.
4. QRS duration <120 ms.

AHA/ACCF/HRS recommendations for the standardization and interpretation of the electrocardiogram Part III: Intraventricular Conduction Disturbances, *Circulation* 2009;**119**:e235–40.

usually indicates intact left to right ventricular septal activation,[27] unless the r wave is due to a large septal scar.[28] Newly acquired LBBB is most often a hallmark of advanced hypertensive and/or ischaemic heart disease, and carries a 10-fold increase in mortality.[29] Patients with bifascicular or trifascicular conduction defects have a 4.9% cumulative incidence of high-degree AV block at 5 years (17% if they present with syncope).[30] A prolonged HV interval (>70 ms) may,[31] or may not,[30] indicate increased risk for development of advanced block. In patients with LVEF<35%, RBBB is associated with significantly greater scar size than LBBB and occlusion of a proximal LAD septal perforator causes RBBB. In contrast, LBBB is most commonly caused by nonischemic pathologies.[32]

Fascicular block (left anterior, LAH; or left posterior hemiblock, LPH) leads to intraventricular dyssynchrony. LAH (left axis deviation with Q in I and aVL) and LPH (right axis deviation with Q in inferior leads) may mimic or mask anterior or inferior myocardial infarction.

Left anterior hemiblock is more common in men and increases in frequency with advancing age (Figure 64.1). Evidence is presented regarding the relationship of spontaneous closure of ventricular septal defects, which may explain the finding of this and other conduction defects in young populations. Isolated left anterior hemiblock is a relatively frequent finding in subjects devoid of evidence of structural heart disease. Conversely, isolated **left posterior hemiblock** is a very rare finding; its prognostic significance is unknown and is commonly associated with right bundle branch block, and there is great propensity to develop complete atrioventricular block and Stoke–Adams seizures (Figure 64.2).[33]

Bifascicular block refers to LBBB or RBBB plus a hemiblock.

Trifascicular block refers to block of both the left and right bundles or to first-degree AV block with additional bifascicular block.

Atypical intraventricular conduction defects refer to wide QRS without any typical ECG pattern and usually occur in patients with ischaemic or non-ischaemic heart failure. Prolonged QRS duration in a standard 12-lead ECG is associated with increased mortality in a general population, with intraventricular conduction delay being most strongly associated with an increased risk of arrhythmic death.[34] Subjects with prolonged QRS durations, even without bundle branch block, are at increased risk for future pacemaker implantation. Such individuals may warrant monitoring for progressive conduction disease.[35]

Indications for permanent pacing are presented in Table 64.6.

Therapy

Pacing is indicated in the presence of syncope (Table 64.7 and Figure 64.3),[17] particularly in the presence of a prolonged HV interval. However, up to 14% of patients with

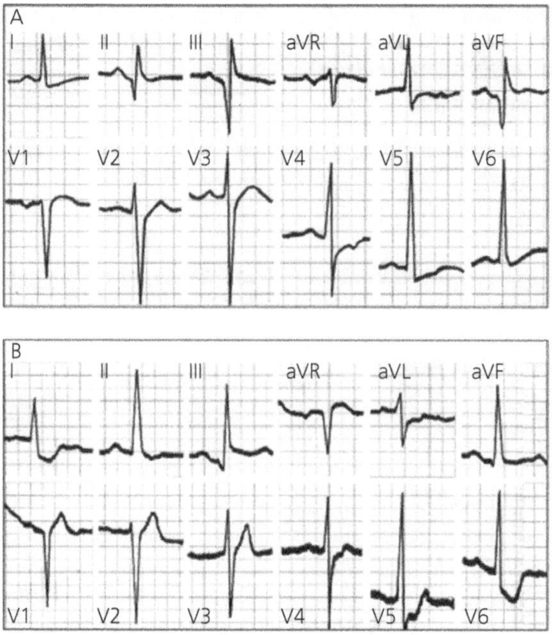

Figure 64.2 Transient left posterior hemiblock (LPH) caused by subepicardial inferior wall injury greatly conceals the pattern of inferior wall myocardial infarction in a 62-year old patient with unstable angina. (A) Clear-cut signs of inferior infarction. (B) During an episode of angina, the ECG shows a transient LPH, which almost completely conceals the signs of the inferior wall myocardial infarction.
Elizari MV, *et al*. Hemiblocks revisited. *Circulation*. 2007;**115**:1154–63.

BBB and preserved LV function may have induced SVT or VT at electrophysiology study.[36] In patients without syncope, the rate of progression to high-degree AV block is low, and there is no non-invasive technique with a high predictive value. An HV interval >100 ms or the demonstration of intra- or infra-Hisian block during incremental atrial pacing at a pacing rate >150 bpm is predictive for the development of high-grade AV block, but the sensitivity of these findings is low. Permanent pacing, apart from preventing future symptoms, however, has been found to have no beneficial effect on survival. Genetic therapies and biological pacemakers by means of viral-based or stem cell-based gene delivery systems are under study.[37]

Choice of pacing mode

DDD pacing has not been shown to offer reduced rates of cardiovascular death or stroke, or even quality of life, compared to VVI pacing.[38–40] However, there may be a significant reduction in the development of atrial fibrillation with physiological pacing,[38] although not in all trials,[40] as well as avoidance of pacemaker syndrome that may be seen in 5–25% of patients with VVI pacing. VDD pacing is a viable

Table 64.7 Pacing in chronic bifascicular block

ACCF/AHA/HRS 2012 GL on device-based therapy	
Recommendations for permanent pacing in chronic bifascicular block	
Advanced second-degree AV block or intermittent third-degree AV block.	I-B
Type II second-degree AV block.	I-B
Alternating bundle branch block.	I-C
Syncope not demonstrated to be due to AV block when other likely causes have been excluded, specifically VT.	IIa-B
Incidental finding at electrophysiological study of a markedly prolonged HV interval (≥100 ms) in asymptomatic patients.	IIa-B
Incidental finding at electrophysiological study of pacing-induced infra-His block that is not physiological.	IIa-B
Neuromuscular diseases, such as myotonic muscular dystrophy, Erb dystrophy (limb-girdle muscular dystrophy), and peroneal muscular atrophy with bifascicular block or any fascicular block, with or without symptoms.	IIb-C
Fascicular block without AV block or symptoms.	III-B
Fascicular block with first-degree AV block without symptoms.	III-B
ESC 2013 on pacing and CRT	
Indication for cardiac pacing in patients with BBB	
BBB, unexplained syncope and abnormal EPS	
Pacing in syncope, BBB and HV ≥70 ms, or second- or third-degree His-Purkinje block during incremental atrial pacing or with pharmacological challenge.	I-B
Alternating BBB	
Pacing is indicated in alternating BBB with or without symptoms.	I-C
BBB, unexplained syncope non diagnostic investigations	
Pacing in selected patients with unexplained syncope and BBB.	II-B
Asymptomatic BBB	
Pacing for BBB in asymptomatic patients.	III-B

2012 ACCF/AHA/HRS focused update incorporated into the ACCF/AHA/HRS 2008 guidelines for device-based therapy of cardiac rhythm abnormalities. *J Am Coll Cardiol.* 2013;**61**:e6–75.
2013 ESC Guidelines on cardiac pacing and cardiac resynchronization therapy. *Eur Heart J* 2013. doi:10.1093/eurheartj/eht150

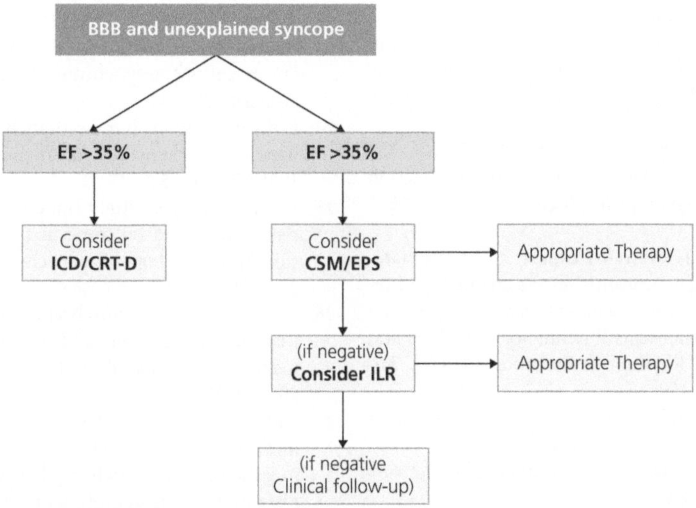

Figure 64.3 ESC GL on pacing and CRT.
Therapeutic algorithm for patients presenting with unexplained syncope and bundle branch block (BBB).
CRT-D: cardiac resynchronization therapy and defibrillator; CSM: carotid sinus massage; EF: ejection fraction; EPS: electrophysiological study; ICD: implantable cardioverter defibrillator; ILR: implantable loop recorder.

alternative to DDD pacing in patients with high-degree AV block and normal sinus node function, offering lower cost, high reliability, and abbreviated implantation time.[41,42] The main problem is the degradation of atrial sensing ability with time. Prolonged ventricular dyssynchrony induced by long-term RV apical pacing is associated with deleterious LV remodelling and deterioration of both LV diastolic and systolic function.[43,44] Non-apical RV pacing such as hisian, septal or RVOT pacing may be associated with improved LV function,[45] but the issue remains controversial.[46] Theoretically, a mid-septal positions should be the optimum site, at least in patients without a previous anteroseptal myocardial infarction. However, in a recent study on long-term pacing in children, RV apical pacing was found superior to RVOT, RV lateral and even septal pacing by means of affecting LV mechanical synchrony.[47] Biventricular pacing may be preferable in patients with reduced LVEF [48] (see Chapter 31 on CCF).

Recommendations for pacing mode selection are presented in Table 64.5.

References

1. Barold SS, *et al.* First-degree atrioventricular block. Clinical manifestations, indications for pacing, pacemaker management and consequences during cardiac resynchronization. *J Interv Card Electrophysiol.* 2006;**17**:139–52
2. Go AS, *et al.* Heart disease and stroke statistics—2013 update: a report from the American Heart Association. *Circulation.* 2013;**127**:e6–245
3. HRS/EHRA/APHRS expert consensus statement on the diagnosis and management of patients with inherited primary arrhythmia syndromes, *Europace* 2013, E-Pub
4. Katritsis D. Progressive cardiac conduction disease. In: Zipes DP, Jalife J. *Cardiac electrophysiology: from cell to bedside.* 6th edition. Saunders, Philadelphia (in press)
5. Kandolin R, *et al.* Cardiac sarcoidosis and giant cell myocarditis as causes of atrioventricular block in young and middle-aged adults. *Circ Arrhythm Electrophysiol.* 2011;**4**:303–9
6. Stanek G, *et al.* Lyme borreliosis. *Lancet.* 2012;**379**:461–73
7. Nadelman RB, *et al.* Differentiation of reinfection from relapse in recurrent Lyme disease. *N Engl J Med.* 2012;**367**:1883–90
8. Ackerman MJ, *et al.* HRS/EHRA expert consensus statement on the state of genetic testing for the channelopathies and cardiomyopathies: this document was developed as a partnership between the Heart Rhythm Society (HRS) and the European Heart Rhythm Association (EHRA). *Europace.* 2011;**13**:1077–109
9. Barold SS, *et al.* Second-degree atrioventricular block: a reappraisal. *Mayo Clin Proc.* 2001;**76**:44–57
10. Lee S, *et al.* Paroxysmal atrioventricular block. *Heart Rhythm.* 2009;**6**:1229–34
11. Brignole M, *et al.* Lack of correlation between the responses to tilt testing and adenosine triphosphate test and the mechanism of spontaneous neurally mediated syncope. *Eur Heart J.* 2006;**27**:2232–9
12. Brignole M, *et al.* Adenosine-induced atrioventricular block in patients with unexplained syncope: the diagnostic value of ATP testing. *Circulation.* 1997;**96**:3921–7
13. Flammang D, *et al.* Treatment of unexplained syncope: a multicenter, randomized trial of cardiac pacing guided by adenosine 5'-triphosphate testing. *Circulation.* 2012;**125**:31–6
14. Wahbi K, *et al.* Electrophysiological study with prophylactic pacing and survival in adults with myotonic dystrophy and conduction system disease. *JAMA.* 2012;**307**:1292–301
15. Shaw DB, *et al.* Is Mobitz Type I atrioventricular block benign in adults? *Heart.* 2004;**90**:169–74
16. 2012 ACCF/AHA/HRS focused update incorporated into the ACCF/AHA/HRS guidelines for device-based therapy of cardiac rhythm abnormalities *J Am Coll Cardiol.* 2013;**61**:e66–75
17. 2013 ESC guidelines on cardiac pacing and cardiac resynchronization therapy. *Eur Heart J.* 2013:doi:10.1093/eurheartj/eht1150
18. Chokshi SK, *et al.* Exercise-provoked distal atrioventricular block. *Am J Cardiol.* 1990;**66**:114–16
19. Kim MH, *et al.* Complete atrioventricular block after valvular heart surgery and the timing of pacemaker implantation. *Am J Cardiol.* 2001;**87**:649–51, A610
20. Walker F, *et al.* Long-term outcomes of cardiac pacing in adults with congenital heart disease. *J Am Coll Cardiol.* 2004;**43**:1894–901
21. Cho HC, *et al.* Biological therapies for cardiac arrhythmias: can genes and cells replace drugs and devices? *Circ Res.* 2010;**106**:674–85
22. Surawicz B, *et al.* AHA/ACCF/HRS recommendations for the standardization and interpretation of the electrocardiogram: part III: intraventricular conduction disturbances: a scientific statement from the American Heart Association Electrocardiography and Arrhythmias Committee, Council on Clinical Cardiology; the American College of Cardiology Foundation; and the Heart Rhythm Society: endorsed by the International Society for Computerized Electrocardiology. *Circulation.* 2009;**119**:e235–40
23. Strauss DG, *et al.* Defining left bundle branch block in the era of cardiac resynchronization therapy. *Am J Cardiol.* 2011;**107**:927–34
24. Eriksson P, *et al.* Bundle-branch block in a general male population: the study of men born 1913. *Circulation.* 1998;**98**:2494–500
25. Bussink BE, *et al.* Right bundle branch block: Prevalence, risk factors, and outcome in the general population: Results from the copenhagen city heart study. *Eur Heart J.* 2013;**34**:138–46
26. Eriksson P, *et al.* Bundle-branch block in middle-aged men: Risk of complications and death over 28 years. The primary prevention study in Göteborg, Sweden. *Eur Heart J.* 2005;**26**:2300–6
27. Padanilam BJ, *et al.* The surface electrocardiogram predicts risk of heart block during right heart catheterization in patients with preexisting left bundle branch block: implications for the definition of complete left bundle branch block. *J Cardiovasc Electrophysiol.* 2010;**21**:781–5
28. Wellens HJ. Is the left bundle branch really blocked when suggested by the electrocardiogram? *Europace.* 2012;**14**:619–20

29. Flowers NC. Left bundle branch block: a continuously evolving concept. *J Am Coll Cardiol.* 1987;**9**:684–97
30. McAnulty JH, *et al.* Natural history of 'high-risk' bundle-branch block: final report of a prospective study. *N Engl J Med.* 1982;**307**:137–43
31. Dhingra RC, *et al.* Significance of the HV interval in 517 patients with chronic bifascicular block. *Circulation.* 1981;**64**:1265–71
32. Strauss DG, *et al.* Right, but not left, bundle branch block is associated with large anteroseptal scar. *J Am Coll Cardiol.* 2013:doi:10.1016/j.jacc.2013.1004.1060
33. Elizari MV, *et al.* Hemiblocks revisited. *Circulation.* 2007;**115**:1154–63
34. Aro AL, *et al.* Intraventricular conduction delay in a standard 12-lead electrocardiogram as a predictor of mortality in the general population. *Circ Arrhythm Electrophysiol.* 2011;**4**:704–10
35. Cheng S, *et al.* Relation of QRS width in healthy persons to risk of future permanent pacemaker implantation. *Am J Cardiol.* 2010;**106**:668–72
36. Moya A, *et al.* Diagnosis, management, and outcomes of patients with syncope and bundle branch block. *Eur Heart J.* 2011;**32**:1535–41
37. Boink GJJ, *et al.* Hcn2/skm1 gene transfer into canine left bundle branch induces stable, autonomically responsive biological pacing at physiological heart rates. *J Am Coll Cardiol.* 2013;**61**:1192–1201
38. Lamas GA, *et al.* Quality of life and clinical outcomes in elderly patients treated with ventricular pacing as compared with dual-chamber pacing. Pacemaker selection in the elderly investigators. *N Engl J Med.* 1998;**338**:1097–104
39. Kerr CR, *et al.* Canadian trial of physiological pacing: effects of physiological pacing during long-term follow-up. *Circulation.* 2004;**109**:357–62
40. Toff WD, *et al.* Single-chamber versus dual-chamber pacing for high-grade atrioventricular block. *N Engl J Med.* 2005;**353**:145–55
41. Huang M, *et al.* Optimal pacing for symptomatic AV block: a comparison of VDD and DDD pacing. *Pacing Clin Electrophysiol.* 2004;**27**:19–23
42. Wiegand UK, *et al.* Cost-effectiveness of dual-chamber pacemaker therapy: does single lead VDD pacing reduce treatment costs of atrioventricular block? *Eur Heart J.* 2001;**22**:174–80
43. Fang F, *et al.* Deleterious effect of right ventricular apical pacing on left ventricular diastolic function and the impact of pre-existing diastolic disease. *Eur Heart J.* 2011;**32**:1891–99
44. Zhang XH, *et al.* New-onset heart failure after permanent right ventricular apical pacing in patients with acquired high-grade atrioventricular block and normal left ventricular function. *J Cardiovasc Electrophysiol.* 2008;**19**:136–41
45. Shimony A, *et al.* Beneficial effects of right ventricular non-apical vs. Apical pacing: A systematic review and meta-analysis of randomized-controlled trials. *Europace.* 2012;**14**:81–91
46. Varma N, *et al.* Alternative site pacing: accessing normal precordial activation: is it possible? *J Electrocardiol.* 2012;**45**:660–2
47. Janousek J, *et al.* Permanent cardiac pacing in children: Choosing the optimal pacing site: A multicenter study. *Circulation.* 2013;**127**:613–23
48. Chan JY, *et al.* Biventricular pacing is superior to right ventricular pacing in bradycardia patients with preserved systolic function: 2-year results of the PACE trial. *Eur Heart J.* 2013;**32**:2533–40

Chapter 65

Conduction disease in specific conditions

Recent myocardial infarction

In the reperfusion era, the incidence of AV block has decreased to 7%[1] whereas the incidence of bundle branch block remains at 5% (and an additional 18% as transient).[2] They both predict higher mortality. See also Chapter 28 on MI. Indications for permanent pacing (>14 days after MI) are presented in Table 65.1.

Congenital AV block

Congenital AV block may be immune (usually) or non-immune. Transplacental penetration of anti-Ro/SSA and anti-La/SSB ribonucleoprotein antibodies from the mother, who may have systemic lupus erythymatosus, systemic sclerosis, or Sjögren syndrome, or may even be entirely asymptomatic, into the fetal circulation is associated with congenital conduction disturbances. Half of these asymptomatic women develop symptoms of a rheumatic disease, most commonly arthralgias and xerophthalmia, but few develop lupus nephritis.[3] Anti-Ro/SSA antibodies may cross-react with T- and L-type calcium channels and the potassium channel hERG, and induce AV block.[4] Congenital complete heart block is the more severe manifestation of so-called 'neonatal lupus'. It occurs in approximately 2% of neonates whose mothers are positive for anti-Ro/SSA and anti-La/SSB, suggesting that additional genetic and environmental factors may also play a role in the development of block.[4, 5] It is typically detected *in utero* or within

Table 65.1 Pacing in MI

ESC 2013 on Cardiac Pacing and CRT	
Indications for permanent pacing in acute myocardial infarction	
In the rare cases in which AV block becomes permanent, cardiac pacing is indicated with the same recommendations presented in Table 64.4	I-C
Cardiac pacing is not indicated after resolution of high degree or complete AV block complicating the acute phase of myocardial infarction	III-B
ACCF/AHA/HRS 2012 GL on device-based therapy	
Recommendations for permanent pacing after the acute phase of myocardial infarction	
Persistent second-degree AV block in the His-Purkinje system with alternating bundle branch block or third-degree AV block within or below the His-Purkinje system after ST segment elevation myocardial infarction.	I-B
Transient advanced second- or third-degree infranodal AV block and associated bundle branch block. If the site of block is uncertain, an electrophysiological study may be necessary.	I-B
Persistent and symptomatic second- or third-degree AV block.	I-C
Persistent second- or third-degree AV block at the AV node level, even in the absence of symptoms.	IIb-B
Transient AV block in the absence of intraventricular conduction defects.	III-B
Transient AV block in the presence of isolated left anterior fascicular block.	III-B
New bundle branch block or fascicular block in the absence of AV block.	III-B
Persistent asymptomatic first-degree AV block in the presence of bundle branch or fascicular block.	III-B

2013 ESC Guidelines on cardiac pacing and cardiac resynchronization therapy. *Eur Heart J* 2013 .doi:10.1093/eurheartj/eht150.
2012 ACCF/AHA/HRS focused update incorporated into the ACCF/AHA/HRS 2008 guidelines for device-based therapy of cardiac rhythm abnormalities. *J Am Coll Cardiol.* 2013; **61**:e6–75.

the neonatal period (0–27 days after birth).[6] Of affected fetuses, 17.5% die, 30% *in utero*, and the cumulative probability of survival at 10 years for a child born alive is 86%, with a higher case fatality rate in non-white patients.[7] The risk of recurrence of complete heart block in a subsequent child is 10–18%.[8] A pacemaker is required in about 66% of cases in childhood, and eventually almost 100% of children will require one by adulthood.[9] Complete AV block is irreversible while incomplete AV block may be potentially reversible after fluorinated steroid therapy.[6] Maternal use of hydroxychloroquine is also associated with a reduced risk of recurrent cardiac manifestations.[10] Anti-Ro/SSA antibodies might also be pathogenic for the adult heart with second-degree AV block, sinus bradycardia, QT prolongation, and ventricular arrhythmias seen in adults.[6] The adult AV node is generally thought to be resistant to the damaging effect of anti-Ro (SSA) and anti-La (SSB) autoantibodies. However, anecdotal case reports suggest that heart block developing in adult SS patients may be associated with such concurrent autoantibodies. Congenital or childhood non-immune AV block may also occur. Recently, ECG screening in parents of children affected by idiopathic AV block revealed a high prevalence of conduction abnormalities, thus suggesting an inheritable trait.[11] Permanent pacing should avoid the right ventricular apex and prefer a septal position.[12] Indications for permanent pacing in congenital heart block, as well as in other congenital conditions, are presented in Table 65.2.

Sleep apnoea

Nasal continuous positive airway pressure (CPAP) therapy is effective in reducing sleep apnoea episodes whereas atrial overdrive pacing may not be.[13] Pacing may be needed in patients with symptomatic bradycardia despite CPAP, but its value is not established.[9]

Cardiac transplantation

Pacemaker requiring bradyarrhythmias occurr in 10% of patients after cardiac transplantation.[13] The bicaval surgical technique and young donor/recipient age are protective against a post-operative pacemaker requirement.[14] Following orthotopic heart transplantation, a degree of chronotropic incompetence is inevitable, but both sinus node and AV node functions improve during the first weeks after the operation.[15] The optimal timing for permanent pacing should be individualized (Table 64.3).[15] Late-onset AV block occurs in 2.4% of patients with orthotopic heart transplant or heart-lung transplant. AV block is predominantly intermittent and often does not progress to permanent AV block. There are no predictable factors for its onset.[16]

Pacing in pregnancy

For women who have a stable, narrow, complex junctional escape rhythm, PM implantation can be deferred until after

Table 65.2 Pacing in congenital heart disease

ESC 2013 GL on Cardiac Pacing and CRT	
Indications for pacing therapy in paediatric patients and congenital heart disease	
Congenital AV block	
Pacing in high degree and complete AV block in symptomatic patients and in asymptomatic patients with any of the following risk conditions: ventricular dysfunction, prolonged QTc interval, complex ventricular ectopy, wide QRS escape rhythm, ventricular rate <50 b.p.m., ventricular pauses >three-fold the cycle length of the underlying rhythm.	I-C
Pacing in asymptomatic patients with high degree and complete AV block in absence of the above risk conditions.	IIb-C
Postoperative AV block in congenital heart disease.	
Permanent pacing for advanced second degree or complete AV block persisting >10 days postoperatively.	I-B
Permanent pacing for persistent, asymptomatic bifascicular block (with or without PR prolongation) associated with transient, complete AV block.	IIa-C
Sinus node disease.	
Permanent pacing for symptomatic sinus node disease, including brady-tachy syndrome, when a correlation between symptoms and bradycardia is judged to be established.	I-C
Permanent pacing for asymptomatic resting heart rate <40 b.p.m. or ventricular pauses lasting >3 sec.	IIb-C
ACCF/AHA/HRS 2012 GL on device-based therapy	
Recommendations for permanent pacing in children, adolescents, and patients with congenital heart disease	
Advanced second- or third-degree AV block associated with symptomatic bradycardia, ventricular dysfunction, or low cardiac output.	I-C
SND with correlation of symptoms during age-inappropriate bradycardia. The definition of bradycardia varies with the patient's age and expected heart rate.	I-B
Post-operative advanced second- or third-degree AV block that is not expected to resolve or that persists at least 7 days after cardiac surgery.	I-B
Permanent pacemaker implantation is indicated for congenital third-degree AV block with a wide QRS escape rhythm, complex ventricular ectopy, or ventricular dysfunction.	I-B
Permanent pacemaker implantation is indicated for congenital third-degree AV block in the infant with a ventricular rate <55 bpm or with congenital heart disease and a ventricular rate <70 bpm.	I-C
Patients with congenital heart disease and sinus bradycardia for the prevention of recurrent episodes of intra-atrial reentrant tachycardia; SND may be intrinsic or secondary to antiarrhythmic treatment.	IIa-C
Congenital third-degree AV block beyond the first year of life with an average heart rate <50 bpm, abrupt pauses in ventricular rate that are 2 or 3 times the basic cycle length, or associated with symptoms due to chronotropic incompetence.	IIa-B
Sinus bradycardia with complex congenital heart disease with a resting heart rate <40 bpm or pauses in ventricular rate >3 s.	IIa-C
Ppatients with congenital heart disease and impaired haemodynamics due to sinus bradycardia or loss of AV synchrony.	IIa-C
Unexplained syncope in the patient with prior congenital heart surgery complicated by transient complete heart block with residual fascicular block after a careful evaluation to exclude other causes of syncope.	IIa-B
Transient post-operative third-degree AV block that reverts to sinus rhythm with residual bifascicular block.	IIb-C
Congenital third-degree AV block in asymptomatic children or adolescents with an acceptable rate, a narrow QRS complex, and normal ventricular function.	IIb-C
Asymptomatic sinus bradycardia after biventricular repair of congenital heart disease with a resting heart rate <40 bpm or pauses in ventricular rate >3 s.	IIb-C
Transient post-operative AV block with return of normal AV conduction in the otherwise asymptomatic patient.	III-B
Asymptomatic bifascicular block with or without first-degree AV block after surgery for congenital heart disease in the absence of prior transient complete AV block.	III-C
Asymptomatic type I second-degree AV block.	III-C
Asymptomatic sinus bradycardia with the longest relative risk interval <3 s and a minimum heart rate >40 bpm.	III-C

2013 ESC Guidelines on cardiac pacing and cardiac resynchronization therapy. *Eur Heart J* 2013. doi:10.1093/eurheartj/eht150.

2012 ACCF/AHA/HRS focused update incorporated into the ACCF/AHA/HRS 2008 guidelines for device-based therapy of cardiac rhythm abnormalities. *J Am Coll Cardiol.* 2013;**61**:e6–75.

delivery.[15] Complete heart block who exhibit with a slow, wide QRS complex escape rhythm needs permanent pacing. This can be performed safely, especially if the foetus is beyond 8 weeks' gestation using echo guidance (ESC 2013 GL on pacing, IIa-C) or, ideally, electro-anatomic navigation.

Other pacing indications

Pacing for **hypertrophic cardiomyopathy** is discussed in Chapter 36, and pacing for **tachyarrhythmias** is presented in Table 65.4.

Table 65.3 Pacing after cardiac transplantation

ESC 2013 GL on Cardiac Pacing and CRT.	
Pacing after cardiac surgery, transcatheter aortic valve implantation and heart transplantation	
High degree or complete AV block after cardiac surgery and TAVI	
A period of clinical observation up to 7 days is indicated in order to assess whether the rhythm disturbance is transient and resolves.	I-C
In case of complete AV block with low rate of escape rhythm this observation period can be shortened since resolution is unlikely.	
Sinus node dysfunction after cardiac surgery and heart transplantation	
A period of clinical observation from 5 days up to some weeks is indicated in order to assess if the rhythm disturbance resolves.	I-C
Chronotropic incompetence after heart transplantation	
Cardiac pacing for chronotropic incompetence impairing the quality of life late in the post-transplant period.	IIa-C
ACCF/AHA/HRS 2012 for device-based therapy of cardiac rhythm abnormalities	
Recommendations for pacing after cardiac transplantation	
Persistent inappropriate or symptomatic bradycardia not expected to resolve and for other class I indications for permanent pacing.	I-C
Relative bradycardia is prolonged or recurrent, which limits rehabilitation or discharge after post-operative recovery from cardiac transplantation.	IIb-C
Syncope after cardiac transplantation, even when bradyarrhythmia has not been documented.	IIb-C

2013 ESC Guidelines on cardiac pacing and cardiac resynchronization therapy. *Eur Heart J* 2013. doi:10.1093/eurheartj/eht150.

2012 ACCF/AHA/HRS focused update incorporated into the ACCF/AHA/HRS 2008 guidelines for device-based therapy of cardiac rhythm abnormalities. *J Am Coll Cardiol.* 2013;**61**:e6–75.

Table 65.4 Anti-tachycardia pacing

ACCF/AHA/HRS 2012 GL on device-based therapy	
Recommendations for permanent pacemakers that automatically detect and pace to terminate tachycardias	
Symptomatic recurrent supraventricular tachycardia that is reproducibly terminated by pacing when catheter ablation and/or drugs fail to control the arrhythmia or produce intolerable side effects.	IIa-C
Presence of an accessory pathway that has the capacity for rapid anterograde conduction.	III-C
ACCF/AHA/HRS 2012 GL on device-based therapy	
Recommendations for pacing to prevent tachycardia	
Sustained pause-dependent VT, with or without QT prolongation.	I-C
High-risk patients with congenital long QT syndrome.	IIa-C
Prevention of symptomatic, drug-refractory, recurrent atrial fibrillation in patients.	IIb-B
Frequent or complex ventricular ectopic activity without sustained VT in the absence of the long QT syndrome.	III-C
Torsade de pointes VT due to reversible causes.	III-A
Prevention of atrial fibrillation in patients without any other indication for pacemaker implantation.	III-B
ESC 2013 GL on Cardiac Pacing and CRT	
Prevention and termination of atrial tachyarrhymias is not a stand-alone indication for pacing	III-A

2013 ESC Guidelines on cardiac pacing and cardiac resynchronization therapy. *Eur Heart J* 2013. doi:10.1093/eurheartj/eht150.

2012 ACCF/AHA/HRS focused update incorporated into the ACCF/AHA/HRS 2008 guidelines for device-based therapy of cardiac rhythm abnormalities. *J Am Coll Cardiol.* 2013;**61**:e6–75.

References

1. Meine TJ, *et al.* Incidence, predictors, and outcomes of high-degree atrioventricular block complicating acute myocardial infarction treated with thrombolytic therapy. *Am Heart J.* 2005;**149**:670–74
2. Newby KH, *et al.* Incidence and clinical relevance of the occurrence of bundle-branch block in patients treated with thrombolytic therapy. *Circulation.* 1996;**94**:2424–8
3. Brucato A, *et al.* Pregnancy outcomes in patients with autoimmune diseases and anti-Ro/SSA antibodies. *Clin Rev Allergy Immunol.* 2011;**40**:27–41
4. Eisen A, *et al.* Arrhythmias and conduction defects in rheumatological diseases—a comprehensive review. *Semin Arthritis Rheum.* 2009;**39**:145–56
5. Lee HC, *et al.* Autoantibodies and cardiac arrhythmias. *Heart Rhythm.* 2011;**8**:1788–95
6. Brucato A, *et al.* Arrhythmias presenting in neonatal lupus. *Scand J Immunol.* 2010;**72**:198–204
7. Izmirly PM, *et al.* Maternal and fetal factors associated with mortality and morbidity in a multi-racial/ethnic registry of anti-SSA/Ro-associated cardiac neonatal lupus. *Circulation.* 2011;**124**:1927–35
8. Ambrosi A, *et al.* Development of heart block in children of SSA/SSB-autoantibody-positive women is associated with maternal age and displays a season-of-birth pattern. *Ann Rheum Dis.* 2012;**71**:334–40
9. 2012 ACCF/AHA/HRS focused update incorporated into the ACCF/AHA/HRS guidelines for device-based therapy of cardiac rhythm abnormalities. *J Am Coll Cardiol.* 2013;**61**:e6–75
10. Izmirly PM, *et al.* Maternal use of hydroxychloroquine is associated with a reduced risk of recurrent anti-SSA/Ro-antibody-associated cardiac manifestations of neonatal lupus. *Circulation.* 2012;**126**:76–82
11. Baruteau AE, *et al.* Parental electrocardiographic screening identifies a high degree of inheritance for congenital and childhood nonimmune isolated atrioventricular block. *Circulation.* 2012;**126**:1469–77
12. Fischbach PS, *et al.* Natural history and current therapy for complete heart block in children and patients with congenital heart disease. *Congenit Heart Dis.* 2007;**2**:224–34
13. Simantirakis EN, *et al.* Atrial overdrive pacing for the obstructive sleep apnea-hypopnea syndrome. *N Engl J Med.* 2005;**353**:2568–77
14. Cantillon DJ, *et al.* Long-term outcomes and clinical predictors for pacemaker-requiring bradyarrhythmias after cardiac transplantation: analysis of the UNOS/OPTN Cardiac Transplant Database. *Heart Rhythm.* 2010;**7**:1567–71
15. 2013 ESC Guidelines on cardiac pacing and cardiac resynchronization therapy *Eur Heart J.* 2013.doi:10.1093/eurheartj/eht150
16. Tay AE, *et al.* Permanent pacing for late-onset atrioventricular block in patients with heart transplantation: a single center experience. *Pacing Clin Electrophysiol.* 2011;**34**:72–5

Part XII

Syncope and sudden cardiac death

Relevant guidelines

Syncope

ESC/HRS 2009 guidelines on syncope

ESC, EHRA, HFA, HRS guidelines for the diagnosis and management of syncope (version 2009). *Eur Heart J.* 2009;**30**:2631–71.

AHA/ACCF 2006 statement on syncope

AHA/ACCF scientific statement on the evaluation of syncope. *Circulation.* 2006;**113**:316–27.

ACCF/AHA/HRS 2012 guidelines for device-based therapy of cardiac rhythm abnormalities

2012 ACCF/AHA/HRS focused update incorporated into the ACCF/AHA/HRS 2008 guidelines for device-based therapy of cardiac rhythm abnormalities. *J Am Coll Cardiol.* 2013;**61**:e6–75.

ESC 2013 guidelines on pacing and cardiac resynchronization

2013 ESC Guidelines on cardiac pacing and cardiac resynchronization therapy. *Eur Heart J.* 2013. doi:10.1093/eurheartj/eht150.

HRS/AACF statement on pacemaker device mode selection 2012

HRS/ACCF expert consensus statement on pacemaker device and mode selection: *Heart Rhythm.* 2012;**9**:1344–65.

Sudden cardiac death

ACC/AHA/ESC 2006 guidelines on ventricular arrhythmias and sudden cardiac death

ACC/AHA/ESC 2006 guidelines for management of patients with ventricular arrhythmias and the prevention of sudden cardiac death. *Circulation.* 2006;**114**:e385–484.

HRS/EHRA 2011 statement on genetic testing

HRS/EHRA expert consensus statement on the state of genetic testing for the channelopathies and cardiomyopathies. *Europace.* 2011;**13**:1077–109.

AHA 2010 guidelines for cardiopulmonary resuscitation

2010 American Heart Association guidelines for cardiopulmonary resuscitation and emergency cardiovascular care. *Circulation.* 2010;**122**(18 Suppl 3): Parts 1–16.

HRS/EHRA/APHRS 2013 Expert Consensus Statement on Inherited Arrhythmia

HRS/EHRA/APHRS Expert Consensus Statement on the Diagnosis and Management of Patients with Inherited Primary Arrhythmia Syndromes. *Heart Rhythm.* 2013.E-Pub.

Chapter 66

Syncope

Definition

Syncope is a transient loss of consciousness due to transient global cerebral hypoperfusion characterized by rapid onset, short duration, and spontaneous complete recovery.[1]

Epidemiology

The estimated incidence of self-reported syncope was 6.2 per 1000 person-years in the Framingham study. The age-adjusted incidence was 7.2 per 1000 person-years among both men and women.[2] In the United States, 1 to 2 million patients are evaluated for syncope annually; 3% to 5% of emergency department visits are for syncope evaluation, and 1% to 6% of urgent hospital admissions are for syncope.[3–4] There is a higher prevalence of first faints in patients between 10 and 30 years and after the age of 70.[1,2]

Classification

Table 66.1 presents the ESC/HRS classification of syncope.

Neurally mediated, or reflex, syncope is the commonest form of syncope and can be divided to vasodepressor, mixed, or cardioinhibitory types. Vasovagal syncope refers to 'common faint' that is mediated by emotion or orthostatic stress, is seen in young adults (about 1% of toddlers may have a form of vasovagal syncope), and may be preceded by prodromal symptoms of autonomic activation.[1] There is absence of heart disease, and syncope occurs after prolonged standing in crowded, hot places, during a meal or postprandial, with head rotation, pressure on carotid sinus, or after exertion. **Orthostatic hypotension** is defined by a fall >20 mmHg systolic and/or >10 mmHg diastolic in response to standing from the supine position within 3 minutes or during head-up tilt at 60 degrees (see Chapter 24 on hypertension) and is seen in ages over 40 years and typically in the elderly. 'Initial' (i.e. immediate decrease (>40 mmHg) and restoration of blood pressure) and 'delayed' (progressive decrease without bradycardic reflex) orthostatic hypotension seen in the elderly are atypical forms.[5] There may be a relationship with start of changes of dosage of vasodepressive drugs and presence of autonomic neuropathy or parkinsonism. **Postural orthostatic tachycardia syndrome (POTS)** is characterized by orthostatic intolerance associated with marked heart rate increases (>30 bpm or to >120 bpm). Dependent acrocyanosis of the legs that occurs with standing may be present and is characteristic of POTS.[6] The aetiology of this condition is still eluting and has been attributed to various forms of autonomic dysfunction, although in young ages a small-size heart in the context of reduced blood volume may also be responsible.[7]

Cardiac syncope is the second most common cause and is mostly due to arrhythmias, and less due to sick sinus or AV nodal disease (Stokes–Adams syndrome). Structural heart disease may cause syncope due to restricted cardiac output and inappropriate reflex vasodilation and arrhythmia.

Pathophysiology

Syncope is due to a fall in systemic blood pressure (systolic BP to 60 mmHg or lower), with resultant decrease in global cerebral blood flow that can be as short as 6–8 s.[1] Systemic BP is determined by cardiac output and total peripheral vascular resistance. A low peripheral resistance can be due to inappropriate reflex activity, causing vasodilatation and bradycardia, or to drug-induced, primary, and secondary autonomic nervous system failure. Low cardiac output can be due to reflex bradycardia, arrhythmia, structural heart disease (i.e. aortic stenosis or pulmonary embolus), and inadequate venous return due to volume depletion or venous pooling.

Presentation

Typically, syncope is brief and occurs without warning. Recovery is characterized by immediate restoration of appropriate behaviour and orientation. In some forms, however, prodromal symptoms (light-headedness, nausea, visual disturbances) may be present, and the episode may last longer, rarely even minutes. Minor injury, such as laceration and bruises, are reported in 29% of patients with syncope whereas fractures and motor vehicle accidents in 6% of patients. In older patients with syncope complicated by a severe trauma, carotid sinus syndrome is the most common cause.[8] Recurrent syncope has serious effects on quality of life, with psychological impairment occurring in up to 33% of patients. Indications of admission are shown in Figure 66.1.

Aetiologic diagnosis

The causes of syncope are highly age-dependent. Paediatric and young patients are most likely to have

Table 66.1 Classification of syncope (modified from ESC/HRS 2009 GL on syncope)

Reflex (neurally mediated syncope)
Vasovagal
Emotional distress (fear, pain, instrumentation, blood phobia)
Orthostatic stress
Situational
Cough, sneeze
GI stimulation (swallow, defecation, visceral pain)
Post-micturition
Post-exercise
Postprandial
Others (laughter, brass instrument playing, weightlifting)
Carotid sinus syncope
Atypical forms (no apparent trigger)
Orthostatic hypotension
Primary autonomic failure
Diabetes, amyloidosis, uraemia, spinal cord injuries
Secondary autonomic failure
Pure autonomic failure (Bradbury–Eggleston syndrome), multiple system atrophy (Shy–Drager syndrome)
Drug-induced orthostatic hypotension
Alcohol, vasodilators, diuretics, phenothiazines, antidepressants
Volume depletion
Haemorrhage, diarrhoea, vomiting
Cardiovascular syncope
Arrhythmia
Bradycardia (SSS, AV disease, PPM malfunction)
Tachycardia (SVT, VT, VF due to channelopathies)
Drug-induced arrhythmia
Structural disease
Cardiac (CAD, valve disease, HCM, cardiac tumours, tamponade, congenital coronary anomalies, prosthetic valve malfunction)
Others (PE, aortic dissection, pulmonary hypertension)

ESC, EHRA, HFA, HRS Guidelines for the diagnosis and management of syncope (version 2009). *Eur Heart J*. 2009;**30**:2631–71.

neurocardiogenic syncope, conversion reactions (psychiatric causes), and primary arrhythmic causes, such as genetic channelopathies and Wolff–Parkinson–White syndrome. In middle age, neurocardiogenic syncope remains the most frequent cause of syncope. Elderly patients have a higher frequency of syncope caused by obstructions to cardiac output, e.g. aortic stenosis and pulmonary embolus, arrhythmias resulting from underlying heart disease, orthostatic hypotension, and carotid sinus syndrome.[8–10] Initial evaluation, especially in multidisciplinary syncope units,[9] defines the cause of syncope in 23–50% of patient whereas diagnosis is not established in up to 40% of cases. Conditions incorrectly diagnosed as syncope are presented in Table 66.2, and diagnostic criteria are presented in Table 66.3. A careful history about the onset and end of the attack, the circumstances under which syncope occurred, and the medical background of the patient are crucial for diagnosis.[11] Pseudosyncope usually occurs without a recognizable trigger many times in a day and lasts longer than syncope (up to 15 minutes). Trauma is more common in pseudoseizures. The eyes are usually open in epileptic seizures and syncope but are usually closed in functional transient loss of consciousness. During tilt testing, the combination of apparent unconsciousness with loss of motor control, normal BP, HR, and EEG rules out syncope and most forms of epilepsy. Differentiation from epilepsy is presented in Table 66.4. Early impotence, disturbed micturition, and later parkinsonism and ataxia suggest autonomic failure.

Investigations

ECG It is necessary to exclude conditions of cardiovascular syncope as shown in Table 66.5. The ECG may display conduction disturbances (atrioventricular or intraventricular block), pre-excited complexes, or signs of cardiomyopathy or genetic channelopathies.

Electrocardiographic monitoring Indications are presented in Table 66.5. Implantable loop recorders (ILR) may be necessary in patients with unexplained falls, suspected AV block or VT, or unsuccessful treatment for suspected epilepsy.[12,13] A high incidence of bradyarrhythmias and asystole, i.e. convulsive cardioinhibitory reflex syncope, has been found with the use of ILR in patients previously diagnosed with epilepsy.[14] A classification of ECG recordings has been proposed (Table 66.6).

Echocardiography is necessary to diagnose structural disease and evaluate the LVEF.

TOE, **computed tomography**, or **magnetic resonance** may be needed in selected cases (suspicion of aortic dissection, pulmonary embolus, etc.).

Exercise testing is indicated in syncope during or after exertion (Table 66.7).

Tests for ischaemia are indicated in clinical suspicion of IHD.

Orthostatic challenge produces a displacement of blood from the thorax to the lower limbs, with resultant decrease in venous return and cardiac output. **Active standing** (Table 66.8) should be evaluated with sphygmomanometers. If more than four measurements per minute are necessary, continuous beat-to-beat non-invasive BP measurement can be used. **Tilt testing** reproduces a neurally mediated reflex and can also be positive in sick sinus syndrome (Table 66.9). It may be accelerated by provocative agents such as isoproterenol.

The ROSE rule	
Admit if <u>any</u> of the following are present:	
B	**B** NP level ≥ 300pg/ml
	B radycardia ≤50 in Emergency Depaertment or pre-hospital
R	**R** ectal examination showing fecal occult blood (if suspicion of gastrointestinal bleed)
A	**A** nemia – Hemoglobin ≤90 g/l
C	**C** hest pain associated with syncope
E	**E** CG showing Q wave (not in lead III)
S	**S** aturation ≤94% on room air

Figure 66.1 The ROSE rule.

Reed MJ, *et al*. The ROSE (risk stratification of syncope in the emergency department) study. *J Am Coll Cardiol*. 2010;**55**:713–21

Table 66.2 ESC/HRS 2009 GL on syncope. Conditions incorrectly diagnosed as syncope

Disorders with partial or complete loss of consciousness but without global cerebral hypoperfusion
Epilepsy
Metabolic disorders (hypoglycaemia, hypoxia, hyperventilation with hypocapnia)
Intoxication
Vertebrobasilar TIA
Disorders without impairment of consciousness
Cataplexy
Drop attacks
Falls
Functional (psychogenic pseudosyncope)
TIA of carotid origin

ESC, EHRA, HFA, HRS Guidelines for the diagnosis and management of syncope (version 2009). *Eur Heart J*. 2009;**30**:2631–71.

Table 66.3 ESC/HRS 2009 GL on syncope. Diagnostic criteria for syncope

Vasovagal if precipitated by emotional or orthostatic distress with typical prodrome	I-C
Situational if during or immediately after specific triggers (Table 66.1)	I-C
Orthostatic when it occurs after standing up and there is hypotension	I-C
Arrhythmia-related when:	I-C
Sinus bradycardia (<40 bpm) if awake or sinus pauses ≥3 s	
Mobitz II second- or third-degree AV block	
Alternating LBBB and RBBB	
VT or rapid SVT	
Polymorphic NSVT and long or short QT	
PPM or ICD malfunction with pauses	
Cardiac, ischaemia-related when syncope presents with ECG evidence of acute ischaemia with or without MI	I-C
Cardiovascular when syncope presents in patients with prolapsing atrial myxoma, severe AS, pulmonary hypertension, PE, or acute aortic dissection	I-C

ESC, EHRA, HFA, HRS Guidelines for the diagnosis and management of syncope (version 2009). *Eur Heart J*. 2009;**30**:2631–71.

Carotid sinus massage Diagnosis of CSS requires the reproduction of spontaneous symptoms during 10 s of sequential right and left CSM, performed supine and erect, under continuous monitoring of HR and periodic measurement of BP, permitting better evaluation of the vasodepressor component (Table 66.10). In up to 30% of patients, an abnormal reflex is present only in the upright position.

Electrophysiology study Sensitivity and specificity of EPS is not good,[1] and positive results occur predominantly in patients with structural heart disease.[15] Indications are presented in Table 66.11. Values of sinus node recovery time (SNRT) ≥1.6 s or of corrected SNRT ≥525 ms are defined as abnormal responses, but the prognostic value of SNRT is not well defined.[1] Although a history of syncope and prolonged HV interval increase the risk of subsequent AV block in patients with BBB, neither of these factors are associated with a higher risk of death as opposed to increasing age, congestive heart failure, and coronary artery disease.[16] Furthermore, the absence of these findings does not exclude the development of AV block, and the prognostic

Table 66.4 ESC/HRS 2009 GL on syncope. Epilepsy vs syncope

Clinical findings that suggest the diagnosis		
	Seizure likely	**Syncope likely**
Symptoms before the event	Aura (such as funny smell)	Nausea, vomiting, abdominal discomfort, feeling of cold sweating (neurally mediated) Light-headedness, blurring of vision
Findings during loss of consciousness (as observed by an eyewitness)	Tonic-clonic movements are usually prolonged, and their onset coincides with loss of consciousness Hemilateral clonic movement Clear automatisms, such as chewing or lip smacking or frothing at the mouth (partial seizure) Tongue biting Blue face	Tonic-clonic movements are always of short duration (<15 s), and they start after the loss of consciousness
Symptoms after the event	Prolonged confusion Aching muscles	Usually of short duration Nausea, vomiting, pallor (neurally mediated)
Other clinical findings of less value for suspecting seizure (low specificity)		
Family history		
Timing of the event (night)		
'Pins and needles' before the event		
Incontinence after the event		
Injury after the event		
Headache after the event		
Sleepy after the event		
Nausea and abdominal discomfort		

ESC, EHRA, HFA, HRS Guidelines for the diagnosis and management of syncope (version 2009). *Eur Heart J*. 2009;**30**:2631–71.

Table 66.5 ESC/HRS 2009 GL on syncope. Recommendations for electrocardiographic monitoring

Indications	
ECG features suggesting arrhythmic syncope (Table 66.1). Duration of monitoring according to risk and predicted recurrence rate:	I-B
Immediate in-hospital (in bed or telemetric) in high risk (see below)	I-C
Holter in very frequent syncope or pre syncope (≥1 per week)	I-B
Implantable loop recorder (ILR) in:	
Recurrent syncope of uncertain origin, absence of high risk, and high likelihood of recurrence within battery life	I-B
High-risk patients with comprehensive evaluation unable to indicate diagnosis or specific treatment	I-B
ILR should be considered before implantation of cardiac pacemaker in suspected reflex syncope presenting with frequent or traumatic syncopal episodes	IIa-B
External loop recorders in patients with intersymptom interval ≤4 weeks	IIa-B
Diagnostic criteria	
ECG monitoring is diagnostic when a correlation between syncope and arrhythmia is detected.	I-B
If no such correlation, ECG monitoring is diagnostic when periods of Mobitz 2nd or 3d degree AV block or a ventricular pause >3s (with the possible exception of young trained persons, during sleep, medicated pts, or rate-controlled AF), or rapid, prolonged SVT/VT are detected.	I-C
ECG documentation of pre-syncope without relevant arrhythmia is not an accurate Surrogate for syncope.	III-C
Asymptomatic arrhythmias (other than listed above) are not an accurate surrogate for syncope.	III-C
Sinus bradycardia (in the absence of syncope) is not an accurate surrogate for syncope.	III-C

ESC, EHRA, HFA, HRS Guidelines for the diagnosis and management of syncope (version 2009). *Eur Heart J*. 2009;**30**:2631–71.

Table 66.6 ESC/HRS 2009 GL on syncope. Classification of ECG recordings obtained with ILR, with their probable-related mechanism (adapted from ISSUE classification)

	Classification	Suggested mechanism
Type 1, asystole: R-R pause ≥3 s	Type 1A, sinus arrest: progressive sinus bradycardia or initial sinus tachycardia, followed by progressive sinus bradycardia until sinus arrest	Probably reflex
	Type 1B, sinus bradycardia plus AV block: progressive sinus bradycardia followed by AV block (and ventricular pause/s), with concomitant decrease in sinus rate, or sudden-onset AV block (and ventricular pause/s), with concomitant decrease in sinus rate	Probably reflex
	Type 1C, AV block: sudden-onset AV block (and ventricular pause/s), with concomitant increase in sinus rate	Probably intrinsic
Type 2, bradycardia: decrease in HR >30% or <40 bpm for >10 s		Probably reflex
Type 3, no or slight rhythm variations: variations in HR <30% and heart rate >40 bpm		Uncertain
Type 4, tachycardia: increase in heart rate >30% of >120 bpm	Type 4A, progressive sinus tachycardia	Uncertain
	Type 4B, atrial fibrillation	Cardiac arrhythmia
	Type 4C, SVT (except sinus)	Cardiac arrhythmia
	Type 4D, VT	Cardiac arrhythmia

AV, atrioventricular; bpm, beats per minute; ECG, electrocardiographic; HR, heart rate; ILR, implantable loop recorder; ISSUE, International Study on Syncope of Unknown Etiology; SVT, supraventricular tachycardia; VT, ventricular tachycardia.
ESC, EHRA, HFA, HRS Guidelines for the diagnosis and management of syncope (version 2009). *Eur Heart J.* 2009;**30**:2631–71.

Table 66.7 ESC/HRS 2009 GL on syncope. Exercise testing

Indications	
Syncope during or shortly after exertion	I-C
Diagnostic criteria	
Exercise testing is diagnostic when syncope is reproduced during or immediately after exercise in the presence of ECG abnormalities or severe hypotension	I-C
Exercise testing is diagnostic if Mobitz second- or third-degree AV block develops during exercise, even without syncope	I-C

ESC/HRS guidelines on syncope 2009. ESC, EHRA, HFA, HRS Guidelines for the diagnosis and management of syncope (version 2009). *Eur Heart J.* 2009;**30**:2631–71.

value of a pharmacologically prolonged HV interval to a value ≥120 ms without induction of AV block is uncertain. In patients with previous myocardial infarction and preserved LVEF (>40%), induction of sustained monomorphic VT is strongly predictive of the cause of syncope[17] whereas the induction of ventricular fibrillation may be a non-specific finding, particularly when three extrastimuli are used.[18] However, the absence of induction of ventricular arrhythmias identifies a group of patients at lower risk of arrhythmic syncope.[19] The adenosine triphosphate test is no longer recommended for the selection of patients for cardiac pacing.[1] However, there has been recent evidence that elderly patients with syncope of unknown origin and a positive ATP (20 mg IV bolus causing pause due to sinoatrial or atrioventricular block >10 s) may benefit from DDD pacing.[20]

Electroencephalography is indicated only when epilepsy is suspected (Table 66.12).

Brain imaging (CT or MRI) are not indicated unless based on a neurological evaluation.[1]

Carotid Doppler ultrasonography is rarely indicated since TIA related to carotid artery disease do not cause loss of consciousness.

Subclavian ultrasonography may detect 'steal' due to subclavian artery stenosis (usually left), but most cases are asymptomatic.

Table 66.8 ESC/HRS 2009 GL on syncope. Active standing

Indications	
Manual intermittent determination with sphygmomanometer of BP supine and during active standing for 3 min when orthostatic hypotension is suspected	I-B
Continuous beat-to-beat non-invasive pressure measurement in cases of doubt	IIb-C
Diagnostic criteria	
Symptomatic fall in systolic BP ≥20 mm Hg or diastolic BP ≥New10 mm Hg, or a decrease in systolic BP to <90 mm Hg	I-C
Asymptomatic fall in systolic BP ≥20 mm Hg or diastolic BP ≥New10 mm Hg, or a decrease in systolic BP to <90 mm Hg	IIa-C

ESC, EHRA, HFA, HRS Guidelines for the diagnosis and management of syncope (version 2009). *Eur Heart J.* 2009;**30**:2631–71.

Table 66.9 ESC/HRS 2009 GL on syncope. Tilt testing

Methodology	
Supine pre-tilt phase of at least 5 min when no venous cannulation is undertaken, and of at least 20 min when cannulation is undertaken	I-C
Tilt angle between 60 and 70°	I-B
Passive phase of a minimum of 20 min and a maximum of 45 min	I-B
For nitroglycerine, a fixed dose of 300–400mg sublingually is administered in the upright position	I-B
For isoproterenol, an incremental infusion rate from 1 up to 3 microNewgram/min in order to increase average heart rate by ~20–25% over baseline is recommended	I-B
Indications	
Unexplained single syncopal episode in high-risk settings (e.g. occurrence, or potential risk, of physical injury or with occupational implications), or recurrent episodes in the absence of organic heart disease, or in the presence of organic heart disease after cardiac causes of syncope have been excluded	I-B
To demonstrate susceptibility to reflex syncope to the patient	I-C
To discriminate between reflex and OH syncope	IIa-C
For differentiating syncope with jerking movements from epilepsy	IIb-C
For evaluating patients with recurrent unexplained falls	IIb-C
For evaluating patients with frequent syncope and psychiatric disease	IIb-C
Not recommended for assessment of treatment	III-B
Isoproterenol tilt testing is contraindicated in patients with ischaemic heart disease	III-C
Diagnostic criteria	
In patients without structural heart disease, the induction of reflex hypotension/bradycardia with reproduction of syncope or progressive OH (with or without symptoms) are diagnostic of reflex syncope and OH, respectively	I-B
In patients without structural heart disease, the induction of reflex hypotension/bradycardia without reproduction of syncope may be diagnostic of reflex syncope	IIa-B
In patients with structural heart disease, arrhythmia or other cardiovascular cause of syncope should be excluded prior to considering positive tilt results as diagnostic	IIa-C
Induction of loss of consciousness in absence of hypotension and/or bradycardia should be considered diagnostic of psychogenic pseudosyncope	IIa-C

ESC, EHRA, HFA, HRS Guidelines for the diagnosis and management of syncope (version 2009). *Eur Heart J.* 2009;**30**:2631–71.

Vertebral artery ultrasonography may reveal stenosis that usually causes focal signs and occulomotor palsies and possibly also loss of consciousness.

Psychiatric consultation may be needed (Table 66.13).

Risk stratification

The prognosis is good, provided that structural heart disease and genetic channelopathies are excluded

Table 66.10 ESC/HRS 2009 GL on syncope. Carotid sinus massage

Indications	
Pts >40 years with syncope of unknown aetiology after initial evaluation	I-B
Avoided in pts with previous TIA or stroke within the past 3 months and in pts with carotid bruits (unless Doppler excluded significant stenosis)	III-C
Diagnostic criteria	
Syncope is reproduced in the presence of asystole >3 s and/or fall in systolic BP>50 mm Hg	I-B

ESC, EHRA, HFA, HRS Guidelines for the diagnosis and management of syncope (version 2009). *Eur Heart J*. 2009;**30**:2631–71.

Table 66.11 ESC/HRS 2009 GL on syncope. Electrophysiology study

Indications	
In ischaemic heart disease when initial evaluation suggests an arrhythmic cause of syncope, unless there is already an established indication for ICD	I-B
In BBB when non-invasive tests have failed to make the diagnosis	IIa-B
In syncope preceded by sudden and brief palpitations when other non-invasive tests have failed to make the diagnosis	IIb-B
In Brugada syndrome, ARVC, and hypertrophic cardiomyopathy in selected cases	IIb-C
In selected cases of patients with high-risk occupations, in whom every effort to exclude a cardiovascular cause of syncope is warranted	IIb-C
Patients with normal ECG, no heart disease, and no palpitations	III-B
Diagnostic criteria	
EPS is diagnostic, and no additional tests are required in:	
Sinus bradycardia and prolonged CSNRT (>525 ms)	I-B
BBB and either a baseline HV interval of ≥New100ms, or second- or third-degree His-Purkinje block is demonstrated during incremental atrial pacing, or with pharmacological challenge	I-B
Induction of sustained monomorphic VT in patients with previous MI	I-B
Induction of rapid SVT which reproduces hypotensive or spontaneous symptoms	I-B
HV interval between 70 and 100 ms	IIa-B
Induction of polymorphic VT or VF in Brugada syndrome, ARVC, and patients resuscitated from cardiac arrest	IIb-B
Induction of polymorphic VT or VF in ischaemic cardiomyopathy or DCM cannot be considered a diagnostic finding	III-B

ESC, EHRA, HFA, HRS Guidelines for the diagnosis and management of syncope (version 2009). *Eur Heart J*. 2009;**30**:2631–71.

Table 66.12 ESC/HRS 2009 GL on syncope

Recommendations: neurological evaluation	
Patients in whom transient loss of consciousness is suspected to be epilepsy	I-C
When syncope is due to autonomic failure in order to evaluate the underlying disease	I-C
EEC, ultrasound of neck arteries, and brain CT or MRI are not indicated, unless a non-syncopal cause of transient loss of consciousness is suspected	III-B

ESC, EHRA, HFA, HRS Guidelines for the diagnosis and management of syncope (version 2009). *Eur Heart J*. 2009;**30**:2631–71.

(Table 66.14). The San Francisco Syncope Rule (history of congestive heart failure, Hematocrit <30%, abnormal ECG result [new changes or non-sinus rhythm], complaint of shortness of breath, and systolic blood pressure <90 mm Hg during triage) has a sensitivity of 96% and specificity 62% for predicting adverse outcomes.[20]

The ROSE rule has also shown high sensitivity and negative predictive value in the identification of high-risk patients with syncope.[21] In the EGSYS 2 trial, death of any cause occurred in 9.2% of patients with syncope during a mean follow-up of 614 days; 82% had an abnormal ECG and/or heart disease, and only 6 deaths (3%) occurred in patients without any apparent cardiac abnormality.[22]

Therapy

Reflex syncope

Avoiding precipitating factors, maintaining hydration, and non-pharmacological physical isometric counterpressure manoeuvres are the treatment of choice (Table 66.15).[23] Beta blockers are not generally effective,[24] although they may reduce syncope in patients >42 years.[20] The value of midodrine is questionable.[1] Selective serotonin reuptake inhibitors such as paroxetine may also be of value in refractory vasovagal syncope.[20] Pacing is not indicated in general.[25,26] It is effective in reducing recurrence of syncope in patients ≥40 years with severe asystolic neurally mediated syncope (syncope with ≥3 s asystole or ≥ 6 s asystole without syncope—ISSUE-3 trial).[27] It might be also considered in unresponsive patients over 40 years, with tilt-induced pure cardioinhibitory response, but its value is not established.[20, 28–30] If pacing is deemed necessary, a dual-chamber unit is implanted.[30] Carotid sinus massage causing a pause >3 s is also an indication for pacing (DDD or VVI)[30] in symptomatic patients (Table 66.15).

Orthostatic intolerance syndromes

The principal treatment strategy in drug-induced autonomic dysfunction is elimination of the offending agent. Expansion of extracellular volume is important (Table 66.16). In

Table 66.13 ESC/HRS 2009 GL on syncope

Psychiatric evaluation	
Patients in whom transient loss of consciousness is suspected to be psychogenic pseudosyncope	I-C
Tilt testing, preferably with concurrent EEG recording and video monitoring, for diagnosis of transient loss of consciousness mimicking syncope ('pseudosyncope') or epilepsy	IIb-C

ESC, EHRA, HFA, HRS Guidelines for the diagnosis and management of syncope (version 2009). *Eur Heart J*. 2009;**30**:2631–71.

Table 66.14 ESC/HRS 2009 GL on syncope. Risk stratification

Short-term high risk criteria which require prompt hospitalization or intensive evaluation
Severe structural or coronary artery disease (heart failure, low LVEF, or previous myocardial infarction)
Clinical or ECG features suggesting arrhythmic syncope
◆ Syncope during exertion or supine
◆ Palpitations at the time of syncope
◆ Family history of SCD
◆ Non-sustained VT
◆ Bifascicular block (LBBB or RBBB combined with left anterior or left posterior fascicular block) or other intraventricular conduction abnormalities with QRS duration ≥120 ms
◆ Inadequate sinus bradycardia (<50 bpm) or sinoatrial block in absence of negative chronotropic medications or physical training
◆ Pre-excited QRS complex
◆ Prolonged or short QT interval
◆ RBBB pattern with ST elevation in leads V_1–V_3 (Brugada pattern)
◆ Negative T waves in right precordial leads, epsilon waves, and ventricular late potentials suggestive of ARVC
Important co-morbidities
◆ Severe anaemia ◆ Electrolyte disturbance

ESC/HRS guidelines on syncope 2009. ESC, EHRA, HFA, HRS Guidelines for the diagnosis and management of syncope (version 2009). *Eur Heart J*. 2009;**30**:2631–71.

Table 66.15 Therapy of reflex syncope

ESC/HRS 2009 GL on syncope	
Treatment of reflex syncope	
Explanation of the diagnosis, provision of reassurance, and explanation of risk of recurrence in all patients	I-C
Isometric physical counterpressure manoeuvres in patients with prodrome	I-B
Cardiac pacing in patients with dominant cardioinhibitory CSS	IIa-B
Cardiac pacing in patients with frequent recurrent reflex syncope, age >40 years, and documended spontaneous cardioinhibitory response during monitoring	IIa-B
Midodrine in patients with vasovagal syncope refractory to lifestyle measures	IIb-B
Tilt training for education of patients, but long-term benefit depends on compliance	IIb-B
Cardiac pacing in patients with tilt-induced cardioinhibitory response with recurrent, frequent unpredictable syncope and age >40 after alternative therapy has failed	IIb-C
Cardiac pacing is not indicated in the absence of a documended cardioinhibitory reflex	III-C
Beta adrenergic blocking drugs are not indicated	III-A
ESC 2013 GL on Pacing and CRT	
Indication for pacing in intermittent documented bradycardia	
Pacing in patients ≥40 years with recurrent, unpredictable reflex syncopes and documented symptomatic pause/s due to sinus arrest or AV block or the combination of the two.	IIa-B
Dual-chamber pacing with rate hysteresis is the preferred mode in reflex asystolic syncope in order to preserve spontaneous sinus rhythm.	I-C
Indication for pacing in undocumented reflex syncope	
Carotid sinus syncope	
Pacing in patients with dominant cardioinhibitory carotid sinus syndrome and recurrent unpredictable syncope.	I-B
Tilt-induced cardioinhibitory syncope	
Pacing in patients with tilt-induced cardioinhibitory response with recurrent frequent unpredictable syncope and age >40 years after alternative therapy has failed.	IIb-B
Tilt-induced non-cardioinhibitory syncope	
Cardiac pacing in the absence of a documented cardioinhibitory reflex	III-B
Choice of pacing mode in undocumented reflex syncope	
Carotid sinus syncope	
Dual-chamber pacing is the preferred mode of pacing.	I-B
Tilt-induced cardioinhibitory syncope	
In cardioinhibitory vasovagal syncope, dual-chamber pacing is the preferred mode of pacing.	I-C
Lower rate and rate hysteresis should be programmed in order to achieve back-up pacing function which preserves native heart rhythm and AV conduction.	IIa-C
Choice of pacing mode in in intermittent documented bradycardia	
Preservation of spontaneous AV conduction is recommended	
Dual-chamber pacing with rate hysteresis is the preferred mode in reflex asystolic syncope in order to preserve spontaneous sinus rhythm	
ACCF/AHA/HRS 2012 GL for device-based therapy	
Recommendations for permanent pacing in hypersensitive carotid sinus syndrome and neurocardiogenic syncope	
Permanent pacing for recurrent syncope caused by spontaneously occurring carotid sinus stimulation and carotid sinus pressure that induces ventricular asystole >3 s	I-C
Permanent pacing for syncope without clear, provocative events and with a hypersensitive cardioinhibitory response of 3 s or longer	IIa-C
Permanent pacing for significantly symptomatic neurocardiogenic syncope associated with bradycardia documented spontaneously or at the time of tilt table testing	IIb-B
Permanent pacing for a hypersensitive cardioinhibitory response to carotid sinus stimulation without symptoms or with vague symptoms	III-C
Permanent pacing for situational vasovagal syncope in which avoidance behaviour is effective and preferred	III-C

ESC, EHRA, HFA, HRS guidelines for the diagnosis and management of syncope (version 2009). *Eur Heart J*. 2009;**30**:2631–71.

2013 ESC Guidelines on cardiac pacing and cardiac resynchronization therapy. *Eur Heart J*. 2013. doi:10.1093/eurheartj/eht150.

2012 ACCF/AHA/HRS focused update incorporated into the ACCF/AHA/HRS 2008 guidelines for device-based therapy of cardiac rhythm abnormalities. *J Am Coll Cardiol*. 2013; **61**:e6–75.

Table 66.16 ESC/HRS 2009 GL on syncope.

Treatment of orthostatic hypotension	
Adequate hydration and salt intake	I-C
Midodrine as adjunctive therapy if needed	IIa-B
Fludrocortisone as adjunctive therapy if needed	IIa-C
Physical counterpressure manoeuvres	IIb-C
Abdominal binders and/or support stockings to reduce venous pooling	IIb-C
Head-up tilt sleeping (>10°) to increase fluid volume	IIb-C

ESC, EHRA, HFA, HRS Guidelines for the diagnosis and management of syncope (version 2009). *Eur Heart J.* 2009;**30**:2631–71.

Table 66.17 ESC/HRS 2009 GL on syncope

Treatment of syncope due to cardiac arrhythmias	
Treatment should be appropriate to the cause	I-B
Cardiac pacing	
Sinus node disease with syncope demonstrated to be due to sinus arrest (symptom-ECG correlation) without a correctable cause	I-C
Sinus node disease with syncope and abnormal CSNRT	I-C
Sinus node disease with syncope and asymptomatic pauses ≥3 s (with the possible exceptions of young trained persons, during sleep, and in medicated patients)	I-C
Syncope and second-degree Mobitz II, advanced or complete AV block	I-B
Syncope, BBB, and positive EPS	I-B
Unexplained syncope and BBB	IIa-C
Unexplained syncope and sinus node disease with persistent sinus bradycardia, itself asymptomatic	IIb-C
Unexplained syncope without evidence of any conduction disturbance	III-C
Catheter ablation	
Symptom-arrhythmia ECG correlation in both SVT and VT in the absence of structural heart disease (with the exception of atrial fibrillation)	I-C
Syncope due to onset of rapid atrial fibrillation	IIb-C
Antiarrhythmic drug therapy	
Syncope due to onset of rapid AF	I-C
Symptom-arrhythmia ECG correlation in both SVT and VT when catheter ablation cannot be undertaken or has failed	IIa-C
Implantable cardioverter defibrillator	
Documented VT and structural heart disease	I-B
Sustained monomorphic VT is induced at EPS in patients with previous MI	I-B
Documended VT and inherited cardiomyopathies or channelopathies	IIa-B

ESC, EHRA, HFA, HRS Guidelines for the diagnosis and management of syncope (version 2009). *Eur Heart J.* 2009;**30**:2631–71.

Table 66.18 Indications for ICD

ESC/HRS 2009 GL on syncope. Indications for implantable cardioverter defibrillator (ICD) in patients with unexplained syncope and at high risk of sudden cardiac death	
In patients with ischaemic or non-ischaemic cardiomyopathy with severely depressed LVEF or HF, according to current guidelines for ICD-CRT.	I-A
In patients with non-ischaemic cardiomyopathy with several depressed LVEF or HF, according to current guidelines for ICD-cardiac resynchronization therapy implantation.	I-A
In hypertrophic cardiomyopathy, ICD therapy should be considered in patients at high risk. In non-high risk, consider ILR.	IIa-C
In right ventricular cardiomyopathy, ICD therapy should be considered in patients at high risk. In non-high risk, consider ILR.	IIa-C
In Brugada syndrome, ICD therapy should be considered in patients with spontaneous type I ECG. In the absence of spontaneous type I ECG, consider ILR.	IIa-B
In long QT syndrome, ICD therapy, in conjunction with beta blockers, should be considered in patients at risk. In non-high risk, consider ILR.	IIa-B
In patients with ischaemic or non-ischaemic cardiomyopathy without severely depressed LVEF or HF and negative programmed electrical stimulation. Consider ILR to help define the nature of unexplained syncope.	IIb-C
ACCF/AHA 2012 GL on device therapy. Indications for ICD*	
Patients with syncope of undetermined origin with clinically relevant, haemodynamically significant sustained VT or VF induced at electrophysiological study	I-B
Unexplained syncope, significant LV dysfunction, and non-ischaemic cardiomyopathy	IIa-C
Syncope and advanced structural heart disease	IIb-C
ICD is not indicated for syncope of undetermined cause without inducible ventricular tachyarrhythmias and without structural heart disease.	III-C

* For patients who are receiving chronic optimal medical therapy and who have reasonable expectation of survival with a good functional status >1 year.
CRT, cardiac resynchronization therapy; ILR; implantable loop recorder.
ESC, EHRA, HFA, HRS Guidelines for the diagnosis and management of syncope (version 2009). *Eur Heart J.* 2009; **30**:2631–71.

ACC/AHA/HRS 2008 guidelines for Device-Based Therapy of Cardiac Rhythm Abnormalities: executive summary. *Heart Rhythm.* 2008;**5**:934–55.

the absence of hypertension, patients should be instructed to take sufficient salt and water intake, targeting 2–3 L of fluids per day and 10 g of NaCl. Rapid cool water ingestion is reported to be effective in orthostatic intolerance and postprandial hypotension.[31] Midodrine (5–20 mg tds) [32] and fluorocortisone (0.1–0.3 mg od) may also be effective.

Cardiac arrhythmias

Recommendations for treatment are provided in Table 66.17. Cardiac pacing in sick sinus syndrome relieves symptoms but may not affect survival, and syncope recurs in 20% of patients.[1] Device malfunction and pacemaker syndrome should also be considered. ICD is indicated in patients with syncope of undetermined origin

Table 66.19 ESC/HRS 2009 GL on syncope. Recommendations for driving

Diagnosis	Group 1 (private drivers)	Group 2 (professional drivers)
Cardiac arrhythmias		
Cardiac arrhythmia, medical treatment	After successful treatment is established	After successful treatment is established
Pacemaker implant	After 1 week	After appropriate function is established
Successful catheter ablation	After successful treatment is established	After long-term success is confirmed
ICD implant	In general, low risk, restriction according to current recommendations	Permanent restriction
Reflex syncope		
Single/mild	No restrictions	No restriction, unless it occurred during high-risk activity*
Recurrent and severe*	After symptoms are controlled	Permanent restriction, unless effective treatment has been established
Unexplained syncope		
	No restrictions, unless absence of prodrome, occurrence during driving, or presence of severe structural heart disease	After diagnosis and appropriate therapy is established

Group 1: private drivers of motorcycles, cars, and other small vehicles with and without a trailer; group 2: professional drivers of vehicles over 3.5 tons or passenger-carrying vehicles exceeding eight seats, excluding the driver. Drivers of taxicabs, small ambulances, and other vehicles form an intermediate category between the ordinary private driver and the vocational driver and should follow local legislation.

* Neurally mediated syncope is defined as severe if it is very frequent or occurring during the prosecution of a 'high-risk' activity or recurrent or unpredictable in 'high-risk' patients.

ESC, EHRA, HFA, HRS Guidelines for the diagnosis and management of syncope (version 2009). *Eur Heart J*. 2009;**30**:2631–71.

with clinically relevant, haemodynamically significant sustained VT or VF induced at EPS, or in patients with syncope and advanced structural heart disease in whom thorough invasive and non-invasive investigations have failed to define a cause (Table 66.18).

Structural heart disease

Treatment is discussed in relevant chapters. ICD may be indicated (Table 66.18), and appropriate shocks in patients with heart failure are more likely in patients with syncope.[33] Of course, ICD reduces arrhythmic death but may not prevent syncope. Syncope is an ominous sign in hypertrophic cardiomyopathy, ARVC, and, most probably, genetic channelopathies, although not as much as documented cardiac arrest.[34]

Syncope in the elderly

The most common causes of syncope in the elderly are OH, reflex syncope, especially CSS, and cardiac arrhythmias.[1] Syncope occurring in the morning favours orthostatic hypotension. Symptoms, such as nausea, blurred vision, and sweating, are predictive of non-cardiac syncope whereas only dyspnoea is predictive of cardiac syncope in elderly people.[35] One-third of individuals over 65 years are taking three, or more, prescribed medications, which may cause, or contribute, to syncope. Their withdrawal reduces recurrences of syncope and falls.[36] Medication history should include the time relationship with the onset of syncope. History should include co-morbidity, association with physical frailty, and locomotor disability. Gait, balance instability, and slow protective reflexes are present in 20–50% of community-dwelling elderly. In these circumstances, moderate haemodynamic changes, insufficient to cause syncope, may result in falls.[36] Cognitive impairment is present in 5% of 65-year olds and 20% of 80-year olds. This may attenuate the patient's memory of syncope and falls.[1] Cardioinhibitory CSS is the recognized cause of symptoms in up to 20% of elderly patients with syncope. The elderly should be managed according to the identified cause.

Unexplained syncope

Pacing has not been shown to prevent recurrences in patients with unexplained falls, and ILR monitoring is probably the optimal diagnostic strategy.[29] The recent ESC recommendations are presented in Table 66.18.

Driving

Recommendations are provided in Table 66.19.

References

1. Moya A, *et al.* Guidelines for the diagnosis and management of syncope (version 2009). *Eur Heart J.* 2009;**30**:2631–71
2. Soteriades ES, *et al.* Incidence and prognosis of syncope. *N Engl J Med.* 2002;**347**:878–85
3. Kapoor WN. Evaluation and outcome of patients with syncope. *Medicine (Baltimore).* 1990;**69**:160–75
4. Salkani P, *et al.* Syncope. *Circulation.* 2013;**127**:1330–9

5. Freeman R. Clinical practice. Neurogenic orthostatic hypotension. *N Engl J Med*. 2008;**358**:615–24
6. Rai SR. Postural tachycardia syndrome (POTS). *Circulation*. 2013;**127**:2336–42
7. Fu Q, *et al.* Cardiac origins of the postural orthostatic tachycardia syndrome. *J Am Coll Cardiol*. 2010;**55**:2858–68
8. Bartoletti A, *et al.* Physical injuries caused by a transient loss of consciousness: main clinical characteristics of patients and diagnostic contribution of carotid sinus massage. *Eur Heart J*. 2008;**29**:618–24
9. Shen WK, *et al.* Syncope Evaluation in the Emergency Department Study (SEEDS): a multidisciplinary approach to syncope management. *Circulation*. 2004;**110**:3636–45
10. Strickberger SA, *et al.* AHA/ACCF scientific statement on the evaluation of syncope: from the American Heart Association Councils on Clinical Cardiology, Cardiovascular Nursing, Cardiovascular Disease in the Young, and Stroke, and the Quality of Care and Outcomes Research Interdisciplinary Working Group; and the American College of Cardiology Foundation: in collaboration with the Heart Rhythm Society: endorsed by the American Autonomic Society. *Circulation*. 2006;**113**:316–27
11. Hoefnagels WA, *et al.* Transient loss of consciousness: the value of the history for distinguishing seizure from syncope. *J Neurol*. 1991;**238**:39–43
12. Parry SW, *et al.* Implantable loop recorders in the investigation of unexplained syncope: a state of the art review. *Heart*. 2010;**96**:1611–16
13. Zimetbaum P, *et al.* Ambulatory arrhythmia monitoring: choosing the right device. *Circulation*. 2010;**122**:1629–36
14. Petkar S, *et al.* Prolonged implantable electrocardiographic monitoring indicates a high rate of misdiagnosis of epilepsy—REVISE study. *Europace*. 2012;**14**:1653–60
15. Linzer M, *et al.* Diagnosing syncope. Part 2: unexplained syncope. Clinical efficacy assessment project of the American College of Physicians. *Ann Intern Med*. 1997;**127**:76–86
16. McAnulty JH, *et al.* Natural history of 'high-risk' bundle-branch block: final report of a prospective study. *N Engl J Med*. 1982;**307**:137–43
17. Olshansky B, *et al.* Clinical significance of syncope in the electrophysiologic study versus electrocardiographic monitoring (ESVEM) trial. The ESVEM investigators. *Am Heart J*. 1999;**137**:878–86
18. Mittal S, *et al.* Significance of inducible ventricular fibrillation in patients with coronary artery disease and unexplained syncope. *J Am Coll Cardiol*. 2001;**38**:371–6
19. Link MS, *et al.* Long-term outcome of patients with syncope associated with coronary artery disease and a nondiagnostic electrophysiologic evaluation. *Am J Cardiol*. 1999;**83**:1334–7
20. Flammang D, *et al.* Treatment of unexplained syncope: a multicenter, randomized trial of cardiac pacing guided by adenosine 5'-triphosphate testing. *Circulation*. 2012;**125**:31–6
21. Ammirati F, *et al.* Permanent cardiac pacing versus medical treatment for the prevention of recurrent vasovagal syncope: A multicenter, randomized, controlled trial. *Circulation*. 2001;**104**:52–7
22. Reed MJ, *et al.* The ROSE (risk stratification of syncope in the emergency department) study. *J Am Coll Cardiol*. 2010;**55**:713–21
23. Ungar A, *et al.* Early and late outcome of treated patients referred for syncope to emergency department: the EGSYS 2 follow-up study. *Eur Heart J*. 2010;**31**:2021–6
24. van Dijk N, *et al.* Effectiveness of physical counterpressure manoeuvers in preventing vasovagal syncope: the physical counterpressure manoeuvres trial (PC-trial). *J Am Coll Cardiol*. 2006;**48**:1652–7
25. Sheldon R, *et al.* Prevention of syncope trial (POST): a randomized, placebo-controlled study of metoprolol in the prevention of vasovagal syncope. *Circulation*. 2006;**113**:1164–70
26. Connolly SJ, *et al.* Pacemaker therapy for prevention of syncope in patients with recurrent severe vasovagal syncope: second vasovagal pacemaker study (VPS II): a randomized trial. *JAMA*. 2003;**289**:2224–9
27. Raviele A, *et al.* A randomized, double-blind, placebo-controlled study of permanent cardiac pacing for the treatment of recurrent tilt-induced vasovagal syncope. The vasovagal syncope and pacing trial (SYNPACE). *Eur Heart J*. 2004;**25**:1741–8
28. Brignole M, *et al.* Pacemaker therapy in patients with neurally mediated syncope and documented asystole: third international study on syncope of uncertain etiology (ISSUE-3): a randomized trial. *Circulation*. 2012;**125**:2566–71
29. Brignole M, *et al.* 2013 ESC Guidelines on cardiac pacing and cardiac resynchronization therapy. *Eur Heart J*. 2013. doi:10.1093/eurheartj/eht150
30. 2012 ACCF/AHA/HRS focused update incorporated into the ACCF/AHA/HRS 2008 guidelines for device-based therapy of cardiac rhythm abnormalities. *J Am Coll Cardiol*. 2013;**61**:e6–75
31. Gillis AM, *et al.* HRS/ACCF expert consensus statement on pacemaker device and mode selection: developed in partnership between the Heart Rhythm Society (HRS) and the American College of Cardiology Foundation (ACCF) and in collaboration with the Society of Thoracic Surgeons. *Heart Rhythm*. 2012;**9**:1344–65
32. Schroeder C, *et al.* Water drinking acutely improves orthostatic tolerance in healthy subjects. *Circulation*. 2002;**106**:2806–11
33. Low PA, *et al.* Efficacy of midodrine vs placebo in neurogenic orthostatic hypotension. A randomized, double-blind multicenter study. Midodrine study group. *JAMA*. 1997;**277**:1046–51
34. Olshansky B, *et al.* Syncope predicts the outcome of cardiomyopathy patients: analysis of the SCD-HEFT study. *J Am Coll Cardiol*. 2008;**51**:1277–82
35. Sacher F, *et al.* Outcome after implantation of a cardioverter-defibrillator in patients with Brugada syndrome: a multicenter study. *Circulation*. 2006;**114**:2317–24
36. Galizia G, *et al.* Role of early symptoms in assessment of syncope in elderly people: results from the Italian group for the study of syncope in the elderly. *J Am Geriatr Soc*. 2009;**57**:18–23
37. van der Velde N, *et al.* Withdrawal of fall-risk-increasing drugs in older persons: effect on tilt-table test outcomes. *J Am Geriatr Soc*. 2007;**55**:734–9

Chapter 67

Sudden cardiac death

Definition

Sudden cardiac death (SCD) is usually defined as death of cardiac origin, occurring within 1 h from onset of symptoms.[1]

Epidemiology

Its incidence approximates 300–350,000 in the USA (0.1% to 0.2% of the population annually), and annually increases as a function of advancing age, being 100-fold less in adolescents and adults younger than 30 y (0.001%) than it is in adults older than 35 y.[1,2] A similar incidence occurs probably in Europe.[3] When the aetiologic definition is limited to coronary artery disease and its tachyarrhythmic burden, the estimate is <200,000 events per year.[4] Approximately 50% of all cardiac deaths are sudden, and this proportion remains the same despite the overall decrease in cardiovascular mortality over the last decades. The proportion of all natural deaths due to SCD is 13% whereas, if a '24 h from onset of symptoms' definition is used, it becomes 18.5%.[4] Analysis of data from the Department of Defense Cardiovascular Death Registry in the USA reveals that the incidence of sudden unexplained death is 1.2 per 100,000 person-years for persons 18–35 years of age, and 2.0 per 100,000 person-years for those >35 years of age.[5] Relatively higher numbers were provided by the King County (Washington) Cardiac Arrest Database: 2.1 (0–2 years of age), 0.61 (3–13 years of age), 1.44 (14–24 years of age), and 4.4 (25–35 years of age) per 100,000 person-years, respectively.[6]

The main problem with SCD is that the majority of out-of-hospital sudden cardiac arrests occur among either those patients in whom cardiac arrest is the first clinical expression of the underlying disease or those in whom disease was previously identified but classified as low-risk (Figure 67.1).[4] There is an inverse relationship between incidence and absolute numbers of events, indicating that a large portion of the total population burden emerges from subgroups with lower risk indexes (Figure 67.2),[4] thus making identification and prevention of future events particularly difficult.

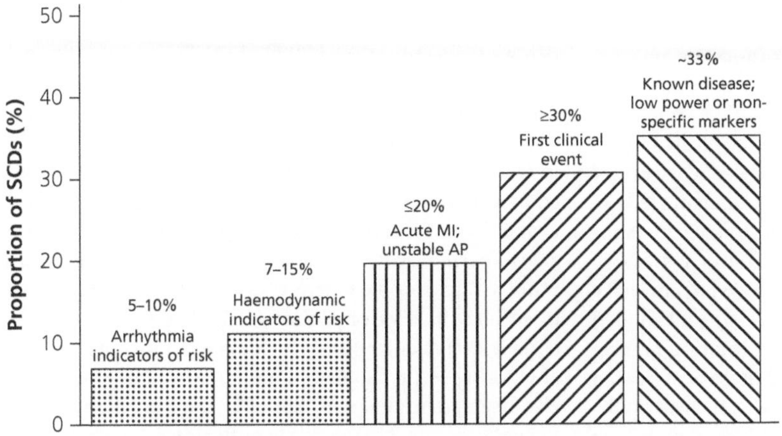

Figure 67.1 Clinical circumstance at the time of sudden cardiac arrest. The majority of out-of-hospital sudden cardiac arrests occur among either those patients in whom cardiac arrest is the first clinical expression of the underlying disease or those in whom disease was previously identified but classified as low risk. The high-risk subgroups that have achieved clinical attention, such as post-myocardial infarction (MI) patients at high risk for or who manifest life-threatening arrhythmias and those with haemodynamic abnormalities, including heart failure, constitute a smaller proportion of the total sudden cardiac death (SCD) burden (<25%). The remainder occurs during the evolution of acute coronary syndromes. AP indicates angina pectoris.

Myerburg RI, *et al.* Sudden cardiac death caused by coronary heart disease. *Circulation* 2012; **125**:1043–1052.

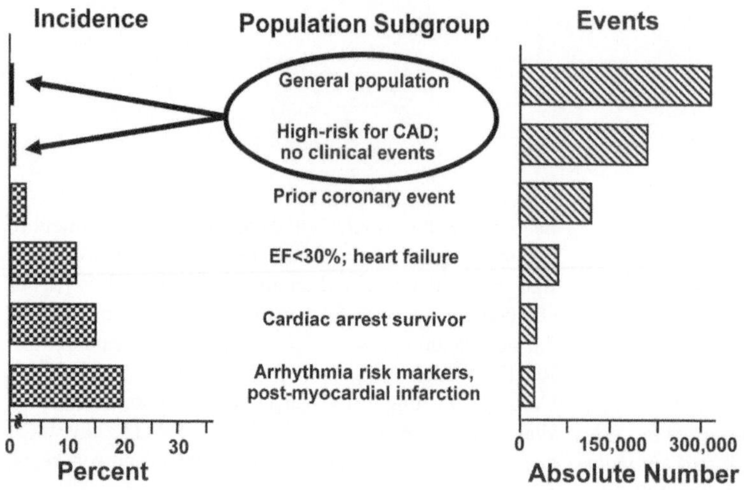

Figure 67.2 Incidence and total population burden of sudden cardiac death. Event rates are compared with total numbers of events for the general population and for specific subgroups with coronary artery disease (CAD). There is an inverse relationship between incidence and absolute numbers of events, indicating that a large portion of the total population burden emerges from subgroups with lower risk indexes, namely the general population and those with risk profiles for atherogenesis but free of events (circled).

EF indicates ejection fraction.

Myerburg RI, *et al*. Sudden cardiac death caused by coronary heart disease. *Circulation* 2012; **125**:1043–1052.

The incidence of **sports-related sudden death** in the general population is 3.6 to 5.6/100,000 persons per year.[7]

Aetiology

Coronary artery disease is the most common substrate underlying SCD in the western world (75–80%), and cardiomyopathies and genetic channelopathies account for most of the remainder (Table 67.1).[8] SCD accounts for 50% of all coronary artery disease-related deaths.[4] The incidence of SCD-related atherosclerotic coronary artery disease is 0.7 per 100,000 person-years in persons 18–35 year-old, whereas it becomes 13.7 per 100,000 person-years for those >35 years of age.[5] Females survivors of cardiac arrest are less likely to have underlying coronary artery disease (45%) whereas valve disease and dilated or arrhythmogenic cardiomyopathy are more common compared to men.[9] Following **acute MI** there is increased risk during the first months either due to tachyarrhythmias or other complications such as re-infarction or myocardial rupture,[10] and myocardial scar predisposes to monomorphic VT. However, although most patients with a cardiac arrest have demonstrable coronary artery disease, less than half seem to have suffered an acute myocardial infarction.[11,12] Only 38% of cardiac arrest survivors will develop evidence of myocardial infarction,[8] and the use of tenecteplase during advanced life support for out-of-hospital cardiac arrest did not improve outcome.[13] In the current era, **cardiomyopathy related to obesity or alcoholism** and **fibrotic cardiomyopathy** are the most common causes of non-ischaemic sudden cardiac death.[14] In patients with preserved ejection fraction (CASPER Registry), an aetiologic diagnosis was possible in approximately half of cardiac arrest survivors, the rest being considered cases of idiopathic VF presumambly due to intrinsic electric abnormalities, such as early repolarization.[15] **Idiopathic VF** is defined as a resuscitated cardiac arrest victim, preferably with documentation of VF, in whom known cardiac, respiratory, metabolic and toxicological etiologies have been excluded through clinical evaluation.[16] **Coronary spasm** is also a cause of cardiac arrest, particularly in male smokers with minimal or no pre-existing coronary artery disease.[17] A phenotype of **bileaflet mitral valve prolapse**, female sex, and frequent complex ventricular ectopy including PVC of outflow tract alternating with papillary muscle/fascicular origin, has also been associated with out of hospital cardiac arrest.[18] Recently, an association of **air pollution** (fine particulate matter with an aerodynamic diameter <2.5 μm and ozone) with out of hospital cardiac arrest was demonstrated.[19] SCD account for most cardiac and many non-AIDS natural deaths in HIV-infected patients.[20] **Lower socioeconomic status, depression, anxiety, social isolation, and acute emotional stress** have all been linked to an increase risk of SCD.[21,22] A **circadian variation** is documented with the peak incidence of SCD occurs in the morning hours

Table 67.1 Common causes of sudden cardiac arrest

Ischaemic heart disease
Myocardial infarction (including NSTEMI)
Anomalous coronary origin
Coronary spasm
Inherited channelopathies
Long QT syndrome
Short QT syndrome
Brugada syndrome
Early repolarization syndrome
Catecholaminergic polymorphic ventricular tachycardia
Cardiomyopathies
Alcoholic
Obesity-related
Fibrotic
Hypertrophic
ARVC
Myocarditis
Heart failure
LVEF <35%
Valve disease
Aortic stenosis
Congenital diseases
Tetralogy of Fallot
Other causes
Severe electrolyte disturbances
Massive pulmonary embolus
Vigorous activity in sedentary individuals
Acute psychosocial and economic stress

Kaltman JR, Thompson PD, Lantos J, *et al.* Screening for sudden cardiac death in the young: report from a national heart, lung, and blood institute working group. *Circulation*. 2011;**123**:1911–8.

from 6 am to noon (and is blunted by beta blockers) with a smaller peak in the late afternoon for out-of-hospital VF arrests, and is highest on Monday.[23,24]

In the young (<35 years), the most common cause of SCD is arrhythmias, mostly in the context of an apparently normal heart.[6,25] In particular, causes of SCD are congenital abnormalities (0–13 years of age), primary arrhythmia (14–24 years), and coronary artery disease (>25 years).[6] In 5–20% of cases a significant cardiac abnormality is not found at autopsy[5,25]

In **sports-related sudden death** in the general population a clear diagnosis is made in less than 25% of the cases, but is usually an acute coronary syndrome (75%).[26] In trained athletes, a diagnosis is usually made in up to 65% of the cases and is usually cardiovascular disease such as hypertrophic cardiomyopathy, congenital coronary anomalies, and genetic channelopathies, with blunt trauma, commotio cordis, and heat stroke being less frequent.[7,26,27] Recently, findings from the RACER initiative indicate that marathons and half-marathons are associated with a low overall risk of cardiac arrest or sudden death. However, event rates, most commonly attributable to hypertrophic cardiomyopathy or atherosclerotic coronary disease, have risen over the past decade among male marathon runners.[23] **Vigorous exertion**, can trigger cardiac arrest or SCD, especially in untrained persons, but habitual vigorous exercise diminishes the risk of sudden death during vigorous exertion.[28] Most studies have found inverse associations between regular physical activity and SCD.8 In untrained persons, although vigorous exercise may trigger SCD, most studies have found inverse associations between regular physical activity and SCD.[8]

Several studies have demonstrated a familial predisposition to SCD that may, or may not, be related to genetic channelopathies.[29–31] Still, however, the heritability of SCD remains poorly understood.

Pathophysiology

Mechanisms

Ventricular tachycardia or fibrillation was thought to be the most common cause of out-of-hospital cardiac arrest, accounting for approximately three-quarters of cases, the remaining 25% caused by bradyarrhythmias or asystole.[32,33] More recent studies suggest that the incidence of ventricular fibrillation or pulseless ventricular tachycardia as the first recorded rhythm in out-of-hospital cardiac arrest, has declined to less than 30% in the past several decades.[34–36] However, the majority of survivors are in the subgroup of persons whose initial rhythm is ventricular fibrillation or pulseless ventricular tachycardia.[35] Ventricular fibrillation is a cause of cardiac arrest and, if untreated, the arrhythmia is usually fatal, but spontaneous reversions to sinus rhythm have been recorded. Non-arrhythmic mechanisms such as myocardial rupture or aortic aneurysm rupture may also result in SCD.

Investigations in survivors

A full cardiac assessment is needed in cardiac arrest survivors. Patients presenting with ventricular fibrillation or sustained monomorphic ventricular tachycardia are at a considerable risk of recurrence, particularly in the presence of reduced left ventricular function. Studies of out-of-hospital cardiac arrest survivors, as well as of patients with sustained ventricular tachycardia, have shown that the actual incidence of sudden death at two years following the presenting arrhythmia varies from 15 to 30%. Up to 74% of patients with out-of-hospital cardiac arrest have VF recurrence during pre-hospital care, and the time in

VF is associated with worse outcome.[37] However, long-term survival among patients who have undergone rapid defibrillation after out-of-hospital cardiac arrest is similar to that among age-, sex-, and disease-matched patients who did not have out-of-hospital cardiac arrest, although only 40% of survivors had an ICD implanted.[38] Family members of young SCD victims are at increased risk for ventricular arrhythmias and ischemic heart disease. Screening of first-degree relatives, especially those <35-year old, is important.[39] When findings suggest cardiomyopathy or genetic channelopathy evaluation of family members is also necessary. Examination of relatives (cascade family screening) may have a significant diagnostic yield.[40] It should be noted, however, that no reported history of sudden death among the relatives of most young (aged<35 years) decedents may be identified.[25] Investigations of a genetic basis of SCD such as the candidate gene approach has explored the potential association between SCD in CAD and genes associated with genetic channelopathies, and genome-wide association studies are promising but of limited clinical value.[4]

The following tests are useful for establishing a diagnosis in SCD survivors:[17]

- ECG (ischaemia, MI, inherited channelopathies)
- Echocardiography (heart failure, cardiomyopathies, valve disease, congenital heart disease)
- Coronary angiography (coronary artery disease, congenital coronary anomalies, coronary spasm)

Table 67.2 HRS/EHRA 2011 statement on genetic testing

State of genetic testing for out-of-hospital cardiac arrest survivors	
In the survivor of an unexplained out-of-hospital cardiac arrest, genetic testing should be guided by the results of medical evaluation and is used for the primary purpose of screening at-risk family members for subclinical disease.	I
Routine genetic testing, in the absence of a clinical index of suspicion for a specific cardiomyopathy or channelopathy, is not indicated for the survivor of an unexplained out-of-hospital cardiac arrest.	III
State of post-mortem genetic testing in sudden unexplained death case (SUD/SIDS)	
For all SUDS and SIDS cases, collection of a tissue sample (5–10 mL whole blood in EDTA tube, blood spot card, or a frozen sample of heart, liver, or spleen) for subsequent DNA analysis/genetic testing. Mutation-specific genetic testing is recommended for family members and other appropriate relatives following the identification of a SUDS-causative mutation in the decedent.	I
In the setting of autopsy-negative SUDS, comprehensive or targeted (*RYR2, KCNQ1, KCNH2,* and *SCN5A*) ion channel genetic testing to establish probable cause and manner of death and to facilitate the identification of potentially at-risk relatives, if circumstantial evidence points toward a clinical diagnosis of LQTS or CPVT specifically (such as emotional stress, acoustic trigger, drowning as the trigger of death).	IIb

HRS/EHRA expert consensus statement on the state of genetic testing for the channelopathies and cardiomyopathies. *Europace*. 2011;**13**:1077–109.

Table 67.3 HRS/EHRA/APHRS 2013 Expert Consensus Statement on Inherited Arrhythmia

Recommendations on Idiopathic Ventricular Fibrillation	
Evaluation	
Genetic testing in IVF when there is a suspicion of a specific genetic diseasefollowing clinical evaluation of the IVF patient and/or family members.	IIa
Genetic screening of a large panel of genes in IVF patients in whom there is no suspicion of an inherited arrhythmogenic disease after clinical evaluation.	III
Therapeutic Interventions	
ICD implantation in patients with the diagnosis of IVF.	I
Antiarrhythmic therapy with quinidine inpatients with a diagnosis of IVF in conjunction with ICD implantation or when ICD implantation is contraindicated or refused.	IIb
Ablation of Purkinje potentials in patients with a diagnosis of IVF presenting with uniform morphology PVCs in conjunction with ICD implantation or when ICD implantation is contraindicated or refused.	IIb
If a first degree relative of an IVF victim presents with unexplained syncope and no identifiable phenotype following thorough investigation then after careful counseling an ICD implant may be considered.	IIb
Evaluation of Family Members	
Evaluation of first degree relatives of all IVF victims with resting ECG exercise stresstesting and echocardiography. Assessment of first degree relatives with history of palpitations arrhythmias or syncope should be prioritized.	I
Follow up clinical assessment in young family members I of IVF victims whomay manifest symptoms and /or signs of the disease at an older age and in all family members whenever additional SUDS or SUDI events occur.	I
Evaluation of first degree relatives of IVF victims with Holter and signal averaged ECGs cardiac MRI and provocative testing with Class Ic antiarrhythmic drugs.	IIa
Evaluation of first degree relatives of IVF victims with epinephrine infusion	IIb

HRS/EHRA/APHRS Expert Consensus Statement on the Diagnosis and Management of Patients with Inherited Primary Arrhythmia Syndromes. *Heart Rhythm.* 2013 E-Pub

- Exercise test (ischaemia, LQTS, CPVT)
- Electrophysiology testing (induction of arrhythmia, pharmacological provocation for Brugada, LQTS, CPVT)
- Cardiac MRI (ARVC, sarcoidosis, myocarditis, myocardial injury from coronary spasm)
- Genetic testing is indicated when an inherited phenotype is detected (ARVC, Brugada, CPVT, LQTS). Its role in phenotypically ambiguous or negative patients is not established since the differentiation between disease-causing mutations and irrelevant genetic variants is not always possible. Recommendations for genetic testing are presented in Tables 67.2 and 67.3
- Cardiac biopsy may also be needed in elusive cases.

A molecular autopsy may also be considered as part of the community forensic investigation to enhance prevention for other family members.[41] Thus, in cases of documented sudden cardiac death without an obvious cause, collection of appropriate blood (in EDTA, ie the purple-top tube to enable DNA extraction), and tissues for subsequent DNA analysis is advisable.[41] A forensic examination, including a toxicology screen, may establish the diagnosis in cases of traumatic, toxic, or cardiac causes, whereas a negative pathological examination, suggests a genetic channelopathy.[42] Postmortem MRI is also a valuable tool to non-invasively document pathological findings such as myocardial infarction or severe myocardial hypertrophy,[43] and postmortem computed tomography coronary angiography is now possible.[44] However, despite every effort nearly half of the causes of cardiac arrest will remain unexplained.[15]

Management of cardiac arrest

Specific recommendations for management are presented in Chapter 55 on tachyarrhythmias.

Defibrillators in public locations may reduce the incidence of sudden cardiac death only when they are accompanied by training programmes of the local population.[48]

References

1. Lloyd-Jones D, *et al.* Heart disease and stroke statistics—2010 update: a report from the American Heart Association. *Circulation.* 2010;**121**:e46–215
2. Kong MH, *et al.* Systematic review of the incidence of sudden cardiac death in the United States. *J Am Coll Cardiol.* 2011;**57**:794–801
3. de Vreede-Swagemakers JJ, *et al.* Out-of-hospital cardiac arrest in the 1990's: a population-based study in the Maastricht area on incidence, characteristics and survival. *J Am Coll Cardiol.* 1997;**30**:1500–5
4. Myerburg RJ, *et al.* Sudden cardiac death caused by coronary heart disease. *Circulation.* 2012;**125**:1043–52
5. Eckart RE, *et al.* Sudden death in young adults: an autopsy-based series of a population undergoing active surveillance. *J Am Coll Cardiol.* 2011;**58**:1254–61
6. Meyer L, *et al.* Incidence, causes, and survival trends from cardiovascular-related sudden cardiac arrest in children and young adults 0 to 35 years of age: a 30-year review. *Circulation.* 2012;**126**:1363–72
7. Chandra N, *et al.* Sudden cardiac death in young athletes: Practical challenges and diagnostic dilemmas. *J Am Coll Cardiol.* 2013;**61**:1027–40
8. Deo R, *et al.* Epidemiology and genetics of sudden cardiac death. *Circulation.* 2012;**125**:620–37
9. Albert CM, *et al.* Sex differences in cardiac arrest survivors. *Circulation.* 1996;**93**:1170–6
10. Pouleur AC, *et al.* Pathogenesis of sudden unexpected death in a clinical trial of patients with myocardial infarction and left ventricular dysfunction, heart failure, or both. *Circulation.* 2010;**122**:597–602
11. Farb A, *et al.* Sudden coronary death. Frequency of active coronary lesions, inactive coronary lesions, and myocardial infarction. *Circulation.* 1995;**92**:1701–9
12. Kannel WB, *et al.* Sudden coronary death: the Framingham Study. *Ann N Y Acad Sci.* 1982;**382**:3–21
13. Bottiger BW, *et al.* Thrombolysis during resuscitation for out-of-hospital cardiac arrest. *N Engl J Med.* 2008;**359**:2651–62
14. Hookana E, *et al.* Causes of nonischemic sudden cardiac death in the current era. *Heart Rhythm.* 2011;**8**:1570–5
15. Derval N, *et al.* Prevalence and characteristics of early repolarization in the CASPER registry: Cardiac arrest survivors with preserved ejection fraction registry. *J Am Coll Cardiol.* 2011;**58**:722–8
16. HRS/EHRA/APHRS Expert Consensus Statement on the Diagnosis and Management of Patients with Inherited Primary Arrhythmia Syndromes. *Heart Rhythm.* 2013, E-Pub
17. Modi S, *et al.* Sudden cardiac arrest without overt heart disease. *Circulation.* 2011;**123**:2994–3008
18. Sriram CS, *et al.* Malignant bileaflet mitral valve prolapse syndrome in patients with otherwise idiopathic out of hospital cardiac arrest. *J Am Coll Cardiol.* 2013; doi: 10.1016/j.jacc.2013.1002.1060
19. Ensor KB, *et al.* A case-crossover analysis of out-of-hospital cardiac arrest and air pollution. *Circulation.* 2013;**127**:1192–9
20. Tseng ZH, *et al.* Sudden cardiac death in patients with human immunodeficiency virus infection. *J Am Coll Cardiol.* 2012;**59**:1891–6
21. Empana JP, *et al.* Clinical depression and risk of out-of-hospital cardiac arrest. *Arch Intern Med.* 2006;**166**:195–200
22. Leor J, *et al.* Sudden cardiac death triggered by an earthquake. *N Engl J Med.* 1996;**334**:413–19
23. Arntz HR, *et al.* Diurnal, weekly and seasonal variation of sudden death. Population-based analysis of 24,061 consecutive cases. *Eur Heart J.* 2000;**21**:315–20
24. Kim JH, *et al.* Cardiac arrest during long-distance running races. *N Engl J Med.* 2012;**366**:130–40
25. Puranik R, *et al.* Sudden death in the young. *Heart Rhythm.* 2005;**2**:1277–82
26. Marijon E, *et al.* Sports-related sudden death in the general population. *Circulation.* 2011;**124**:672–81
27. Maron BJ, *et al.* Sudden deaths in young competitive athletes: Analysis of 1866 deaths in the United States. *Circulation.* 2009;**119**:1085–92

28. Albert CM, *et al.* Triggering of sudden death from cardiac causes by vigorous exertion. *N Engl J Med.* 2000; **343**:1355–61
29. Crotti L, *et al.* Torsades de pointes following acute myocardial infarction: evidence for a deadly link with a common genetic variant. *Heart Rhythm.* 2012;**9**:1104–12
30. Dekker LR, *et al.* Familial sudden death is an important risk factor for primary ventricular fibrillation: a case-control study in acute myocardial infarction patients. *Circulation.* 2006;**114**:1140–5
31. Jouven X, *et al.* Predicting sudden death in the population: the Paris Prospective Study I. *Circulation.* 1999;**99**:1978–83
32. Bayes de Luna A, *et al.* Ambulatory sudden cardiac death: mechanisms of production of fatal arrhythmia on the basis of data from 157 cases. *Am Heart J.* 1989;**117**:151–9
33. Myerburg RJ, *et al.* Sudden cardiac death. Structure, function, and time-dependence of risk. *Circulation.* 1992;**85**:I2–10
34. Cobb LA, *et al.* Changing incidence of out-of-hospital ventricular fibrillation, 1980–2000. *JAMA.* 2002;**288**: 3008–13
35. Nichol G, *et al.* Regional variation in out-of-hospital cardiac arrest incidence and outcome. *JAMA.* 2008;**300**:1423–31
36. Weisfeldt ML, *et al.* Ventricular tachyarrhythmias after cardiac arrest in public versus at home. *N Engl J Med.* 2011;**364**:313–21
37. Berdowski J, *et al.* Time in recurrent ventricular fibrillation and survival after out-of-hospital cardiac arrest. *Circulation.* 2010;**122**:1101–8
38. Bunch TJ, *et al.* Long-term outcomes of out-of-hospital cardiac arrest after successful early defibrillation. *N Engl J Med.* 2003;**348**:2626–33
39. Ranthe MF, *et al.* Risk of cardiovascular disease in family members of young sudden cardiac death victims. *Eur Heart J.* 2013;**34**:503–11
40. Hofman N, *et al.* Active cascade screening in primary inherited arrhythmia syndromes: does it lead to prophylactic treatment? *J Am Coll Cardiol.* 2010;**55**:2570–6
41. Semsarian C, *et al.* Key role of the molecular autopsy in sudden unexpected death. *Heart Rhythm.* 2012;**9**:145–50
42. Basso C, *et al.* Guidelines for autopsy investigation of sudden cardiac death. *Pathologica.* 2010;**102**:391–404
43. Jackowski C, *et al.* Postmortem cardiac 3t magnetic resonance imaging: Visualizing the sudden cardiac death? *J Am Coll Cardiol.* 2013; doi: 10.1016/j.jacc.2013.1001.1089
44. Michaud K, *et al.* Evaluation of postmortem MDCT and MDCT-angiography for the investigation of sudden cardiac death related to atherosclerotic coronary artery disease. *Int J Cardiovasc Imaging.* 2012;**28**:1807–22
45. Estes NA, 3rd. Predicting and preventing sudden cardiac death. *Circulation.* 2011;**124**:651–6

Part XIII

Implantable devices

Relevant guidelines

AHA 2010 scientific statement on cardiovascular implantable electronic device infections

Update on cardiovascular implantable electronic device infections and their management: a scientific statement from the American Heart Association. *Circulation*. 2010;**121**:458–77.

ESC 2009 guidelines on infective endocarditis

Guidelines on the prevention, diagnosis, and treatment of infective endocarditis (new version 2009): the Task Force on the Prevention, Diagnosis, and Treatment of Infective Endocarditis of the European Society of Cardiology (ESC). *Eur Heart J*. 2009;**30**:2369–413.

HRS/ASA 2011 expert consensus statement on the perioperative management of patients with implantable devices

The Heart Rhythm Society (HRS)/American Society of Anesthesiologists (ASA) Expert Consensus Statement on the perioperative management of patients with implantable defibrillators, pacemakers and arrhythmia monitors: facilities and patient management. *Heart Rhythm*. 2011;**8**:1114–54.

EHRA 2009 recommendations for driving by patients with ICDs

Consensus statement of the European Heart Rhythm Association: updated recommendations for driving by patients with implantable cardioverter defibrillators. *Europace*. 2009;**11**:1097–107.

ACC/AHA/HRS 2012 guidelines for device-based therapy of cardiac rhythm abnormalities

2012 ACCF/AHA/HRS focused update incorporated into the ACCF/AHA/HRS 2008 guidelines for device-based therapy of cardiac rhythm abnormalities. *J Am Coll Cardiol*. 2013;**61**:e6–75

AHA 2012 scientific statement on sexual activity and cardiovascular disease

Sexual activity and cardiovascular disease: a scientific statement from the American Heart Association. *Circulation*. 2012;**125**:1058–72.

ACCF/HRS/AHA/ASE/HFSA/SCAI/SCCT/SCMR 2013 appropriate use criteria

ACCF/HRS/AHA/ASE/HFSA/SCAI/SCCT/SCMR 2013 appropriate use criteria for implantable cardioverter-defibrillators and cardiac resynchronization therapy. *J Am Coll Cardiol*. 2013; doi:10.1016/j.jacc.2012.12.017

ESC 2013 guidelines on pacing and cardiac resynchronization

2013 ESC Guidelines on cardiac pacing and cardiac resynchronization therapy. *Eur Heart J*. doi:10.1093/eurheartj/eht150.

2012 EHRA/HRS expert consensus statement on cardiac resynchronization therapy in heart failure

2012 EHRA/HRS expert consensus statement on cardiac resynchronization therapy in heart failure: implant and follow-up recommendations and management. *Europace*. 2012;**14**:1236–86.

Chapter 68

Technical issues

Permanent pacemakers

Pacemaker modes

A 5-letter code is used to describe the pacemaker mode. The first letter refers to the chamber that is paced (**a**trium, **v**entricle, **d**ual); the second letter refers to the chamber sensed (**a**trium, **v**entricle, **d**ual); the third letter refers to the response to sensing (**i**nhibit, **t**rigger, **d**ual); the fourth letter indicates the presence or absence of rate modulation, and the fifth letter indicates multisite pacing (Table 68.1).[1] Thus, a VVI pacemaker is a ventricular-only pacemaker, a DDDR a dual-chamber pacemaker with rate response ability, a DDI pacemaker is a non-tracking dual-chamber pacemaker that paces both the atrium and the ventricle but does not respond to intrinsic sinus or atrial rate changes (no atrial synchronous pacing); that can be useful to avoid tracking atrial tachyarrhythmias. Single-chamber atrial or ventricular pacemakers sense myocardial signals emanating from the corresponding cardiac chamber and deliver a pacing stimulus if no signal is sensed at the programmed lower rate. Dual-chamber pacemakers sense and pace both the atrium and the ventricle. Depending on the particular clinical situation and programming, sensed events trigger or inhibit pacing. For example, in the DDD pacing mode and during atrioventricular sequential pacing, atrial pacing takes place at the lower rate limit. Atrial pacing triggers ventricular pacing once the programmed AV delay has timed out. Ventricular pacing is inhibited if a ventricular event is sensed before the end of the paced AV delay. If the atrial rate is faster than the programmed lower rate, atrial pacing is inhibited. After the sensed atrial signal, ventricular pacing would occur only if no ventricular event is sensed by the end of the programmed sensed AV delay.[2]

Rate response

In the presence of chronoropic incompetence, rate-adaptive pacemakers are useful.[3] These devices have special sensor(s) that, when triggered during exercise, increase the pacing rate. Most commonly used sensors monitor body movement by detecting vibration (activity sensor or accelerometer) (Table 68.2). More physiologic sensors detect changes in minute ventilation by measuring changes in thoracic impedance with ventilation or changes in QT interval that reflect sympathetic drive. Some pacemakers incorporate more than one sensor to limit disadvantages of individual sensors and enhance specificity without compromising sensitivity. A commonly used combination is an activity sensor combined with a QT interval sensor or a minute ventilation sensor. Careful programming by considering a short walk or exercise is often required to achieve optimal clinical results.[3]

Choice of pacemaker mode

Recommendations by the 2012 HRS/ACCF Expert Consensus Statement [4] are presented in Chapters 63–65.

Interrogation monitoring

Modern pacemakers are able to capture and store a wealth of information that may be helpful in clinical management, follow-up, and troubleshooting. Interrogation of the pacemaker will reveal recorded arrhythmias and programmed parameters, such as pacing mode and pacing rates, as well as battery and lead parameters. Recommendations on the frequency of in-office or remote monitoring of patients with implanted devices is provided in Table 68.3.

Pacemaker syndrome

Ventricular pacing without proper atrial synchronization (as happens with VVI pacing in the absence of AF) results in loss of the atrial contribution to ventricular filling, and atrial contraction may occur against closed AV valves. Thus, pacemaker syndrome develops and can lead to symptoms, such as dizziness, weakness, heart failure, and presyncope or syncope. It is usually manifests itself by prominent V waves in the JVP and predisposes the patient to the development of atrial fibrillation and increased incidence of stroke.[5]

Endless loop (ELT) or pacemaker-mediated tachycardia (PMT)

PMT is initiated by a premature ventricular stimulus that is conducted retrograde via the AV node to the atrium. The retrograde atrial signal then is sensed by the atrial channel and triggers pacing in the ventricle. Ventricular pacing causes retrograde conduction to the atria, and the PMT circuit is established. Most pacemakers have algorithms to recognize and terminate PMT. Alternatively, adjustment of AV delays or post-ventricular pacing atrial refractory periods (PVARP) are necessary. Pacemaker component failures are responsible for other unusual, but dangerous, causes of high pacing rate, such as runaway pacemaker and sensor-driven tachycardia.[2] Figure 68.1 presents an algorithm for evaluation of suspected pacemaker malfunction,

Table 68.1 The revised North American Society of Pacing and Electrophysiology (NASPE)/British Pacing and Electrophysiology Group (BPEG) generic code for antibradycardia, adaptive-rate, and multisite pacing

	I	II	III	IV	V
Category	Chamber(s) paced	Chamber(s) sensed	Response to sensing	Rate modulation	Multisite pacing
	O = None	O = None	O = None	O = None	O = None
	A = Atrium	A = Atrium	T = Triggered	R = Rate modulation	A = Atrium
	V = Ventricle	V = Ventricle	I = Inhibited		V = Ventricle
	D = Dual (A + V)	D = Dual (A + V)	D = Dual (T + I)	D = Dual (A + V)	
Manufacturers' designation only	S = Single (A or V)		S = Single (A or V)		

Bernstein AD, et al. The revised NASPE/BPEG generic code for antibradycardia, adaptive-rate, and multisite pacing. *Pacing Clin Electrophysiol*. 2002;**25**: 260–264.

Table 68.2 Commonly used sensors for heart rate modulation

	Technology	Advantage	Disadvantage
Activity sensor	Measures mechanical stress to piezoelectric material as a result of motion or acceleration	Simple; compatible with any device or lead; small energy requirement	Non-physiological estimate of exercise level and non-proportional response to exercise; environmental/external source interference
Minute ventilation sensor	Measures transthoracic impedance change between pacemaker lead and pulse generator	Compatible with any lead; measures physiological changes related to exercise; proportional response to exercise	Slow change at the beginning of exercise; has limitations in children or those with severe lung disease; subject to interference from certain medical equipment
QT interval-based sensors	Measures evoked QT interval changes as estimate of adrenergic tone	Measures physiological changes related to exercise; responds to mental stress	Interindividual variability; T wave sensing may vary; false response during ischaemia or presence of QT-prolonging medications; requires ventricular lead
Contractility sensors, impedance-based	Measures intracardiac impedance change during early ejection period as estimate of local contractility	Measures physiological changes related to exercise; proportional response to exercise; responds to mental stress	Requires ventricular lead; false response if local myocardial properties change (i.e. MI)
Contractility sensors, activity sensor-based	Measures peak endocardial acceleration as estimate of contractility and global LV function	Measures physiological changes related to exercise	Proprietary lead is required; limited long-term safety data

Kaszala K, Ellenbogen KA. Device sensing: sensors and algorithms for pacemakers and implantable cardioverter defibrillators. *Circulation*. 2010;**122**:1328–40.

and Table 68.4 presents an approach to common problems related to electromagnetic interference.

Biventricular pacing

Cardiac resynchronization therapy (CRT) is an integral component of modern heart failure therapy for patients with severe symptoms (NYHA class III or IV), LVEF ≤35%, and a wide QRS complex (>120 ms). Indications are discussed in Chapter 31 on CCF. The presence of LBBB and QRS >150 s are predictors of response,[6,7] and CRT may also reduce morbidity and mortality in patients with mildly symptomatic heart failure (NYHA class II).[8] Specific problems are implant failure due to inability to obtain LV pacing (7–10%), lead dislodgement (5–10%), and coronary sinus dissection (<1%).[8,9] Adverse events, such as failure to implant, pneumothorax, pocket haematoma, and infection, are significantly higher among patients subjected to CRT than ICD alone.[8,10] There are no significant differences in clinical outcomes or complication rates between upgrades of existing devices and *de novo* CRT procedures.[11] Recommendations on indications, as well as on lead placement and follow-up of devices, have been recently published.[12,13]

Implantable cardioverter-defibrillators

Secondary and primary prevention randomized trials to assess the impact of ICD are presented in Tables 68.5 and 68.6. Recommendations for ICD implantation are presented in relevant chapters.

Table 68.3 ACC/AHA/HRS 2012 update on device therapy. Minimum frequency of CIED in person or remote monitoring*

Type and frequency	Method
Pacemaker/ICD/CRT	
Within 72 h of CIED implantation	In person
2–12 wk post-implantation	In person
Every 3–12 mo for pacemaker/CRT-pacemaker	In person or remote
Every 3–6 mo for ICD/CRT-D	In person or remote
Annually until battery depletion	In person
Every 1–3 mo at signs of battery depletion	In person or remote
Implantable loop recorder	
Every 1–6 mo, depending on patient symptoms and indication	In person or remote
Implantable haemodynamic monitor	
Every 1–6 mo, depending on indication	In person or remote
More frequent assessment as clinically indicated	In person or remote

* More frequent in-person or remote monitoring may be required for all the above devices as clinically indicated.
CIED indicates cardiovascular implantable electronic device; CRT, cardiac resynchronization therapy; CRT-D, cardiac resynchronization therapy defibrillator; CRT-pacemaker, cardiac resynchronization therapy pacemaker; and ICD, implantable cardioverter-defibrillator.
2012 ACCF/AHA/HRS Focused Update of the 2008 Guidelines for Device-Based Therapy of Cardiac Rhythm Abnormalities. *J Am Coll Cardiol*. 2012.

ICD are the only means for preventing sudden cardiac death in certain clinical settings. However, repeat shocks may lead to worsening of heart failure and a decline in survival.[14,15] Several important points should be noted:

- In patients with documented sustained ventricular arrhythmias and/or cardiac arrest, implantable cardioverter-defibrillators (ICD) confer a survival benefit (secondary prevention of sudden cardiac death). In several clinical settings, this might be lost when modern medical therapy, including beta blockers, is implemented.[16]
- In patients without sustained ventricular arrhythmias or cardiac arrest, ICD confer a survival benefit (primary prevention of sudden cardiac death) only in high-risk patients with ischaemic cardiomyopathy and LVEF ≤35% due to a remote MI at least >40 days and especially >18 months, although this is debatable.[16]
- The benefits of ICD in the elderly, as well as in women, are not established. Elderly patients excibit increased mortality after ICD implantation, but rates of appropriate device shocks are similar across age groups.[17] In a recent report, one-third of 66,974 Medicare ICD recipients died within 3 years, reflecting a population with more advanced age and progressed heart failure than seen in trial populations for primary prevention ICD.[18]
- With current prices, ICD are definitely cost-effective only when used in high-risk patients without associated co-morbidities that limit the life expectancy to <10 years.[16]

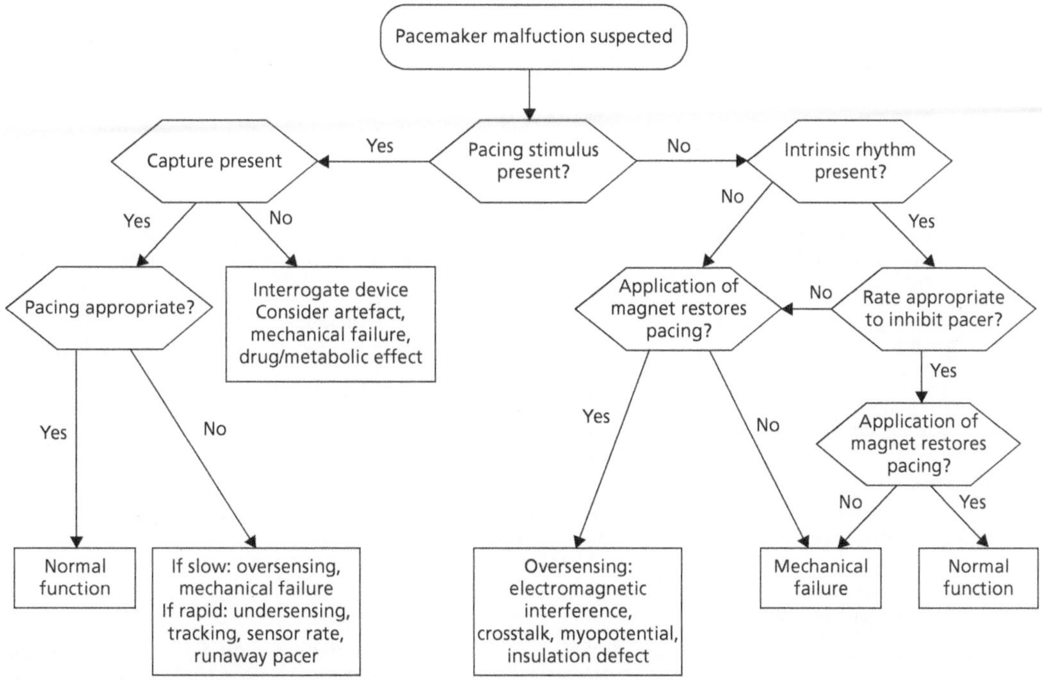

Figure 68.1 A guide for evaluating suspected pacemaker malfunction.
Kaszala K, *et al*. Contemporary pacemakers: what the primary care physician needs to know. *Mayo Clin Proc*. 2008; **83**:1170–86.

Table 68.4 Approach to common problems related to electromagnetic interference in patients with pacemakers

Problem	Solution
Cellular telephones	Keep telephone in contralateral pocket Place telephone over contralateral ear when talking
Household appliances (e.g. microwave oven, television, stereo, toaster, electric blanket)	No specific concerns
Dental office	No specific concerns
Theft detection equipment at stores	Do not loiter when passing through device
Magnetic resonance imaging	Absolute/relative contraindication, except when special precautions are used
Surgery (electrocautery)	Program device to asynchronous mode Alternative: place magnet over device during surgery. Place grounding pad away from the device. Monitor pulse pressure on telemetry. Check device after surgery
Transcutaneous electrical nerve stimulation	May need to programme pacemaker in asynchronous mode in some patients
Radiation therapy	Discuss with radiotherapist May need to move device in pacemaker-dependent patients
Direct current cardioversion	Place pads in anteroposterior position, at least 5 cm from the pulse generator Have programmer present; check device for increased pacing thresholds after cardioversion

Kaszala K, *et al*. Contemporary pacemakers: what the primary care physician needs to know. *Mayo Clin Proc*. 2008; **83**:1170–86.

Table 68.5 Major implantable cardioverter-defibrillator trials for primary prevention of sudden cardiac death

Study		Patients (n)	Inclusion criteria	Therapy	Hazard ratio	95% CI	P-value
AMIOVIRT	Amiodarone versus implantable cardioverter-defibrillator	103	NYHA I-III, DCM, asymptomatic NSVT, LVEF ≤0.35	ICD vs amiodarone	0.87	0.31–2.42	NS
CABG-Patch	Coronary artery bypass graft Patch	900	Scheduled for CABG, LVEF ≤0.35, positive SAECG	ICD vs standard medical therapy	1.07[1]	0.81–1.42	NS
CAT	Cardiomyopathy trial	104	NYHA II or III, DCM ≤ months, LVEF ≤0.30,	ICD vs standard medical therapy	0.83	0.45–1.82	NS
DEFINITE	Defibrillators in non-ischaemic cardiomyopathy treatment evaluation	458	DCM, LVEF ≤New0.35, PVCs or NSVT	ICD vs standard medical therapy	0.65[1] 0.20[2]	0.40–1.06 0.06–0.71	0.08 0.006
DINAMIT	Defibrillator in acute myocardial infarction trial	674	Recent MI, LVEF ≤0.35, impaired cardiac autonomic function	ICD vs standard medical therapy	1.08[1] 0.42[2]	0.76–1.55 0.22–0.83	NS 0.009
IRIS	Immediate risk stratification improves survival	898	Recent MI, LVEF ≤0.40, or NSVT	ICD vs standard medical therapy	1.04	0.81–1.35	NS
MADIT	Multicenter automatic defibrillator implantation trial	196	NYHA I–III, prior MI, LVEF ≤0.35, NSVT, and positive EPS	ICD vs standard medical therapy	0.46[1]	0.26–0.82	0.009
MADIT-II	Multicenter automatic defibrillator implantation trial-II	1232	Prior MI, LVEF ≤0.30	ICD vs standard medical therapy	0.69[1]	0.51–0.93	0.016
MUSTT	Multicenter unsustained tachycardia trial	351[3]	CAD, LVEF ≤0.40, NSVT, and positive EPS	ICD vs conventional antiarrhythmic therapy	0.40[1] 0.24[4]	0.27–0.59 0.13–0.45	<0.001 <0.001

(*Continued*)

Table 68.5 (Continued)

Study		Patients (n)	Inclusion criteria	Therapy	Hazard ratio	95% CI	P-value
SCD-HeFT	Sudden cardiac death in heart failure trial	1676[5]	NYHA II or III, LVEF ≤0.35, ischaemic and non-ischaemic cardiomyopathy	ICD plus standard medical therapy vs placebo plus standard medical therapy	0.77[1]	0.62–0.96	0.007

1: overall mortality; 2: death from arrhythmia; 3: group randomized to EPS-guided therapy with antiarrhythmic medications or ICDs (out of 704 patients in total); 4: cardiac arrest or death from arrhythmia; 5: ICD and placebo arms only (excluding amiodarone arm).
CI, confidence interval; NYHA, New York Heart Association; DCM, dilated cardiomyopathy; NSVT, non-sustained ventricular tachycardia; NS, non-significant (p >0.05); CABG, coronary artery bypass graft; LVEF, left ventricular ejection fraction; SAECG, signal-averaged electrocardiogram; PVC, premature ventricular complex; MI, myocardial infarction; EPS, electrophysiologic study; CAD, coronary artery disease.
Katritsis DG, Josephson ME. Sudden cardiac death and implantable cardioverter defibrillators: two modern epidemics? *Europace*. 2012;**14**:787–94.

Table 68.6 Major implantable cardioverter-defibrillator trials for secondary prevention of sudden cardiac death

Study		Patients (n)	Inclusion criteria	Therapy	Hazard ratio	95% CI	P-value
AVID	Antiarrhythmics versus implantable defibrillators	1016	VF or symptomatic SVT	ICD vs antiarrhythmic medical therapy	0.62[1]	0.43–0.82	<0.02
CASH	Cardiac arrest study Hamburg	288	Cardiac arrest survivors	ICD vs antiarrhythmic medical therapy	0.77[1] 0.42[2]	1.112[3] 0.721[3]	0.081[4] 0.005[4]
CIDS	Canadian implantable defibrillator study	659	Cardiac arrest, VF, or symptomatic VT	ICD vs amiodarone	0.82[1]	0.60–1.10	NS
DEBUT	Defibrillator vs beta blockers for unexplained death in Thailand	86	Cardiac arrest survivors	ICD vs beta blocker therapy	NA (0 vs 4 deaths)	NA	0.02
DUTCH		60	Prior MI, cardiac arrest survivors	ICD as first choice vs conventional strategy	0.27[5]	0.09–0.85	0.02

1: overall mortality; 2: sudden death 3: upper bound of 97.5% confidence interval; 4: one-tailed; 5: death, recurrent cardiac arrest, cardiac transplantation.
CI, confidence interval; VF, ventricular fibrillation; SVT, sustained ventricular tachycardia; VT, ventricular tachycardia; NA, not available; NS, non-significant (p >0.05); MI, myocardial infarction.
Recommendations for ICD implantation are presented in relevant chapters.
Katritsis DG, Josephson ME. Sudden cardiac death and implantable cardioverter defibrillators: two modern epidemics? *Europace*. 2012 Jun;**14**(6):787–94.

- Implant failure rates are 0.1%
- Mean battery longevity of an ICD is approcimately 5 years. In a recent study, devices implanted by Medtronic lasted the longest, followed by Guidant, with the shortest longevity in St Jude and Biotronik devices.[19]

Practical points regarding the choice and programming of ICD devices:[20]

- Single-coil integrated bipolar (or true bipolar) leads are recommended for primary prevention ICDs in order to reduce the odds of failure.
- Atrial or ventricular pacing, as well as rate-responsive pacing, should be avoided, if possible, to increase generator longevity and avoid disruption of normal ventricular conduction.
- Defibrillation testing is probably necessary only in secondary prevention and conditions associated with higher defibrillation thresholds (DFT), such as right-sided implants and amiodarone therapy.
- Strategies to avoid shocks with anti-tachycardia pacing and shorten shocked episode durations should be sought.
- Inappropriate ICD schocks nay cause myocardial damage and have been associated with increased mortality.[15] Recently, a specific programming policy has been found beneficial: between 170 and 199 bpm monitor-only zone is set up. This is followed by a therapy zone, beginning at 200 bpm after a 2.5 s monitoring delay and atrial discriminators turned on. In the therapy zone, anti-tachycardia pacing is implemented as appropriate and is followed by shock therapy if pacing did not terminate the detected arrhythmia (MADIT-RIT).[21]

References

1. Bernstein AD, *et al.* The revised NASPE/BPEG generic code for antibradycardia, adaptive-rate, and multisite pacing. North American Society of Pacing and Electrophysiology/ British Pacing and Electrophysiology Group. *Pacing Clin Electrophysiol.* 2002;**25**:260–64
2. Kaszala K, *et al.* Contemporary pacemakers: what the primary care physician needs to know. *Mayo Clin Proc.* 2008;**83**:1170–86
3. Kaszala K, *et al.* Device sensing: sensors and algorithms for pacemakers and implantable cardioverter defibrillators. *Circulation.* 2010;**122**:1328–40

4. Gillis AM, *et al.* HRS/ACCF expert consensus statement on pacemaker device and mode selection: developed in partnership between the Heart Rhythm Society (HRS) and the American College of Cardiology Foundation (ACCF) and in collaboration with the Society of Thoracic Surgeons. *Heart Rhythm.* 2012;**9**:1344–65
5. Camm AJ, *et al.* Ventricular pacing for sick sinus syndrome—a risky business? *Pacing Clin Electrophysiol.* 1990;**13**:695–9
6. Sipahi I, *et al.* Impact of QRS duration on clinical event reduction with cardiac resynchronization therapy: meta-analysis of randomized controlled trials. *Arch Intern Med.* 2011;**171**:1454–62
7. Bilchick KC, *et al.* Bundle-branch block morphology and other predictors of outcome after cardiac resynchronization therapy in Medicare patients. *Circulation.* 2010;**122**:2022–30
8. Adabag S, *et al.* Cardiac resynchronization therapy in patients with minimal heart failure: a systematic review and meta-analysis. *J Am Coll Cardiol.* 2011;**58**:935–41
9. Trohman RG, *et al.* Cardiac pacing: the state of the art. *Lancet.* 2004;**364**:1701–19
10. Bogale N, *et al.* The European Cardiac Resynchronization Therapy Survey: comparison of outcomes between *de novo* cardiac resynchronization therapy implantations and upgrades. *Eur J Heart Fail.* 2011;**13**:974–983
11. Landolina M, *et al.* Long-term complications related to biventricular defibrillator implantation: rate of surgical revisions and impact on survival: insights from the Italian Clinical Service Database. *Circulation.* 2011;**123**:2526–35
12. Daubert JC, *et al.* 2012 EHRA/HRS expert consensus statement on cardiac resynchronization therapy in heart failure: implant and follow-up recommendations and management. *Europace.* 2012;**14**:1236–86
13. Tracy CM, *et al.* 2012 ACCF/AHA/HRS focused update of the 2008 guidelines for device-based therapy of cardiac rhythm abnormalities: a report of the American College of Cardiology Foundation/American Heart Association Task Force on practice guidelines. *J Am Coll Cardiol.* 2012;**60**:1297–313
14. Dorian P, *et al.* Mechanisms underlying the lack of effect of implantable cardioverter-defibrillator therapy on mortality in high-risk patients with recent myocardial infarction: insights from the Defibrillation IN Acute Myocardial Infarction Trial (DINAMIT). *Circulation.* 2010;**122**:2645–52
15. Poole JE, *et al.* Prognostic importance of defibrillator shocks in patients with heart failure. *N Engl J Med.* 2008;**359**:1009–17
16. Katritsis DG, *et al.* Sudden cardiac death and implantable cardioverter defibrillators: two modern epidemics? *Europace.* 2012;**14**:787–94
17. Yung D, *et al.* Survival after implantable cardioverter-defibrillator implantation in the elderlyr. *Circulation.* 2013;**127**:2383–2392
18. Chen C-Y, *et al.* Impact of baseline heart failure burden on post-implantable cardioverter-defibrillator mortality among medicare beneficiaries. *JACC.* 2013;**61**:2142–2150
19. Thijssen J, *et al.* Implantable cardioverter-defibrillator longevity under clinical circumstances: An analysis according to device type, generation, and manufacturer. *Heart Rhythm.* 2012;**9**:513–9
20. Sweeney MO. The implantable cardioverter-defibrillator minimalist: an approach to patient follow-up and management of implantable defibrillators. *Circulation.* 2012;**126**:369–77
21. Moss AJ, *et al.* Reduction in inappropriate therapy and mortality through ICD programming. *N Engl J Med.* 2012;**367**:2275–83

Chapter 69

Complications of implantable devices

Implantation-related complications

The incidence of complications following implantation of permanent pacemakers and ICD is 3–12%, and ICD or biventricular pacemakers implantation carries an in-hospital mortality of 0.05%.[1-3] Chronic heart failure as an indication, inexperienced operators, CRT or DDD devices, and passive fixation atrial leads are independent risk factors for lead complications.[4]

Pneumothorax occurs in 1.5% after subclavian puncture.

Haematomas of the pocket requiring evacuation occur in 1–2% of implants. Pocket haematoma is after lead dislodgement, the second more frequent complication of device implantation.[5]

Deep venous thrombosis/venous occlusion, air embolism, and perforation of cardiac chambers are rare complications. Venous thrombosis leading to SVC syndrome may be seen in 0–6% of patients, but asymptomatic pulmonary embolism may be detected in up to 20% of patients. Mobile thrombi on device leads can be detected in up to 30% of patients with intracardiac echocardiography, but their clinical significance is not known.[6] Increasing age predicts worsening outcomes in the elderly, but the absolute rates are modest, even in nonagenarians, and comorbidity is a stronger predictor of complications following implantation of permanent pacemakers.[7]

Device-related infections

They now occur in <1% of implants and is higher with ICD than pacemakers.[7–11] One-year mortality is 17–24%.[10,13] The majority of patients (up to 60%) present with localized infection involving the device pocket, and the rest with bloodstream infection, with or without evidence of inflammation of the device pocket.[10,12] A negative transoesophageal echo does not rule out lead infection. Intarcardiac echocardiography is superior to transoesophageal echocardiography in detecting intracardiac vegetations, especially around the tricuspid valve, in this respect.[14] Renal failure, haematoma formation, poor wound healing, and implantation of devices with multiple leads are risk factors. Although several studies have identified device revision or replacement as a risk factor for infection, the REPLACE registry showed a low rate of major infection (0.8%).[11] Perioperative antibiotic prophylaxis (i.e. cefazolin) reduces the risk of device-related infections.8 Main causes are staphylococci (60–80% and up to half of them methicillin-resistant). Gram-negative bacilli and polymicrobial infections are rare (<15%). Infections due to coagulase-negative staphylococci usually have an indolent presentation whereas *S. aureus* infections, particularly those complicated by bloodstream infection or infective endocarditis, develop more rapidly, with more severe systemic manifestations. Device infection will be confirmed in 35% or more of patients with bacteraemia due to staphylococcal species whereas its likelihood is lower (20% or less) in patients with bacteraemia caused by non-staphylococcal Gram-positive cocci or by Gram-negative bacilli. A single blood culture that is positive for coagulase-negative staphylococci usually represents contamination rather than infection; multiple blood cultures that are positive for coagulase-negative staphylococci should prompt consideration of a device-related infection, even if there are no other suggestive symptoms or signs.[8] In patients with left ventricular assist devices, device infection occurs in 22% of patients per year despite the use of newer, smaller devices, and affects mortality. Staphylococci are the most common pathogen (approximately 50%), but pseudomonas or other Gram-negative bacteria cause up to 30% of infections.[15]

Therapy

Aspiration of the pocket should be avoided because it could result in infection. If the pocket has to be surgically explored, deep tissue and lead tip, rather than swab, cultures are obtained. Device removal is not required for superficial or incisional-only infection at the pocket size if there is no involvement of the device. Seven to ten days of oral antibiotic therapy with anti-staphylococcal activity is recommended. However, if localized pocket infection is established or blood cultures become positive, early and complete removal of the device and leads is necessary.[8,16] Biofilm formation on the leads without obvious vegetations is a distinct possibility and precludes eradication of the infection without system extraction. The high frequency of leads extracted in patients with findings limited to the pocket indicates that the spread of the infection from the pocket site is common, and complete removal of the device is usually necessary to prevent relapse. In established pocket infection, IV vancomycin should be given, pending culture results, and therapy should last up to 14 days if there is no evidence of infective endocarditis. A new device should be implanted in the contralateral side at least 72 hours after the infected device has been removed. Clinical manifestations of pocket infection are present in the majority of patients with early lead-associated endocarditis. However, late lead-associated endocarditis (>6 months after device implantation) should be considered in any patient who presents with fever, bloodstream infection, or signs of sepsis, even if the device pocket appears uninfected. Prompt recognition and management may improve outcomes.[14] Development of lead vegetations >2 cm in diameter may require surgical removal to avoid pulmonary embolism. In patients too sick to be subjected to lead extraction, a conservative approach may be adopted by extensive resection of infected and non-viable tissue, mechanical and chemical sterilization of all remaining hardware and local antibiotics by a closed irrigation system, and oral antibiotics upon discharge.[18,19] The AHA and ESC recommendations for management of infections are presented in Table 69.1 and a management algorithm in Figure 69.1.

Device implantation in the anticoagulated patient

In patients on chronic anticoagulation, continuation of warfarin in patients with $CHADS_2$ score ≥2 or interruption of warfarin in low-risk patients (maintain an INR<3 or <3.5 for patients with mechanical valves) is preferable to bridging with unfractionated or LMWH and interruption 12–18 h before the procedure.[20–22] It has been postulated that, during minor surgery, haemostasis is primarily dependent on capillary and platelet function as opposed to the coagulation cascade itself, and antithrombotics that interfere with the former (e.g. heparin and antiplatelet drugs), as well as antiplatelet agents, are less well tolerated than those that do not[23] Another explanation is the concept of an "anticoagulant stress test." That is, if patients undergo surgery while receiving full-dose anticoagulation therapy, any excessive bleeding will be detectable and appropriately managed while the wound is still open.[22]

Reimplantation

Lead complications are the main reason for reoperation after implantation of pacemakers or cardiac

Table 69.1 Management of device-related infections

AHA 2010 scientific statement on cardiovascular implantable electronic device infections	
Recommendations for diagnosis of CIED infection and associated complications	
All patients should have at least two sets of blood cultures drawn at the initial evaluation before prompt initiation of antimicrobial therapy for CIED infection.	I-C
Generator-pocket tissue Gram's stain and culture and lead-tip culture should be obtained when the CIED is explanted.	I-C
Patients with suspected CIED infection, who either have positive blood cultures or who have negative blood cultures but have had recent antimicrobial therapy before blood cultures were obtained, should undergo TOE for CIED infection or valvular endocarditis.	I-C
All adults suspected of having CIED-related endocarditis should undergo TOE to evaluate the left-sided heart valves, even if transthoracic views have demonstrated lead-adherent masses.	I-B
In paediatric patients with good views, transthoracic echocardiography may be sufficient.	
Patients should seek evaluation for CIED infection by cardiologists or infectious disease specialists if they develop fever or bloodstream infection for which there is no initial explanation.	IIa-C
Percutaneous aspiration of the generator pocket should not be performed as part of the diagnostic evaluation of CIED infection.	III-C
Recommendations for antimicrobial management of CIED infection	
Choice of antimicrobial therapy should be based on the identification and *in vitro* susceptibility results of the infecting pathogen.	I-B
Duration of antimicrobial therapy should be 10 to 14 days after CIED removal for pocket-site infection.	I-C
Duration of antimicrobial therapy should be at least 14 days after CIED removal for bloodstream infection.	I-C
Duration of antimicrobial therapy should be at least 4 to 6 weeks for complicated infection (i.e. endocarditis, septic thrombophlebitis, or osteomyelitis, or if bloodstream infection persists despite device removal and appropriate initial antimicrobial therapy.	I-C
Recommendations for removal of infected CIED	
Complete device and lead removal for all patients with definite CIED infection, as evidenced by valvular and/or lead endocarditis or sepsis.	I-A
Complete device and lead removal is recommended for all patients with CIED pocket infection, as evidenced by abscess formation, device erosion, skin adherence, or chronic draining sinus without clinically evident involvement of the transvenous portion of the lead system.	I-B
Complete device and lead removal is recommended for all patients with valvular endocarditis without definite involvement of the lead(s) and/or device.	I-B
Complete device and lead removal is recommended for patients with occult staphylococcal bacteraemia.	I-B
Complete device and lead removal is reasonable in patients with persistent, occult Gram-negative bacteraemia despite appropriate antibiotic therapy.	IIa-B
CIED removal is not indicated for a superficial or incisional infection without involvement of the device and/or leads.	III-C
CIED removal is not indicated for relapsing bloodstream infection due to a source other than a CIED and for which long-term suppressive antimicrobials are required.	III-C
Recommendations for new CIED implantation after removal of an infected CIED	
Each patient should be evaluated carefully to determine whether there is a continued need for a new CIED.	I-C
The replacement device implantation should not be ipsilateral to the extraction site. Preferred alternative locations include the contralateral side, the iliac vein, and epicardial implantation.	I-C
When positive before extraction, blood cultures should be drawn after device removal and should be negative for at least 72 hours before new device placement is performed.	IIa-C
New transvenous lead placement should be delayed for at least 14 days after CIED system removal when there is evidence of valvular infection.	IIa-C
Recommendations for use of long-term suppressive antimicrobial therapy	
Long-term suppressive therapy should be considered for patients who have CIED infection and who are not candidates for complete device removal.	IIb-C
Long-term suppressive therapy should not be administered to patients who are candidates for infected CIED removal.	III-C
Recommendations for antimicrobial prophylaxis at the time of CIED placement	
Prophylaxis with an antibiotic that has *in vitro* activity against staphylococci should be administered. If cefazolin is selected for use, then it should be administered IV within 1 hour before incision; if vancomycin is given, then it should be administered IV within 2 hours before incision.	I-A
Recommendations for antimicrobial prophylaxis for invasive procedures in patients with CIEDs	
Antimicrobial prophylaxis is not recommended for dental or other invasive procedures not directly related to device manipulation to prevent CIED infection.	III-C
Recommendations to avoid microbiological studies in cases of CIED removal for non-infectious reasons	

Table 69.1 (Continued)

Routine microbiological studies should not be conducted on CIEDs that have been removed for non-infectious reasons.	III-B
ESC 2009 GL on infective endocarditis. Management of cardiac device-related IE (CDRIE)	
Principles of treatment	
Prolonged antibiotic therapy and device removal in definite CDRIE.	I-B
Device removal when CDRIE is suspected on the basis of occult infection without other apparent source of infection.	IIa-C
Device extraction in patients with native or prosthetic valve endocarditis and no evidence of associated device infection.	IIb-C
Mode of device removal	
Percutaneous extraction, even in patients with large (>10 mm) vegetations.	I-B
Surgical extraction if percutaneous extraction is incomplete or impossible or in severe destructive tricuspid endocarditis.	IIa-C
Surgical extraction in patients with very large (>25 mm) vegetations.	IIb-C
Reimplantation	
Reassessment of the need of reimplantation.	I-B
Reimplantation postponed, if possible, to allow a few days or weeks of antibiotic therapy.	IIa-B
Temporary pacing is not recommended.	III-C
Prophylaxis	
Routine antibiotic prophylaxis before device implantation.	I-B

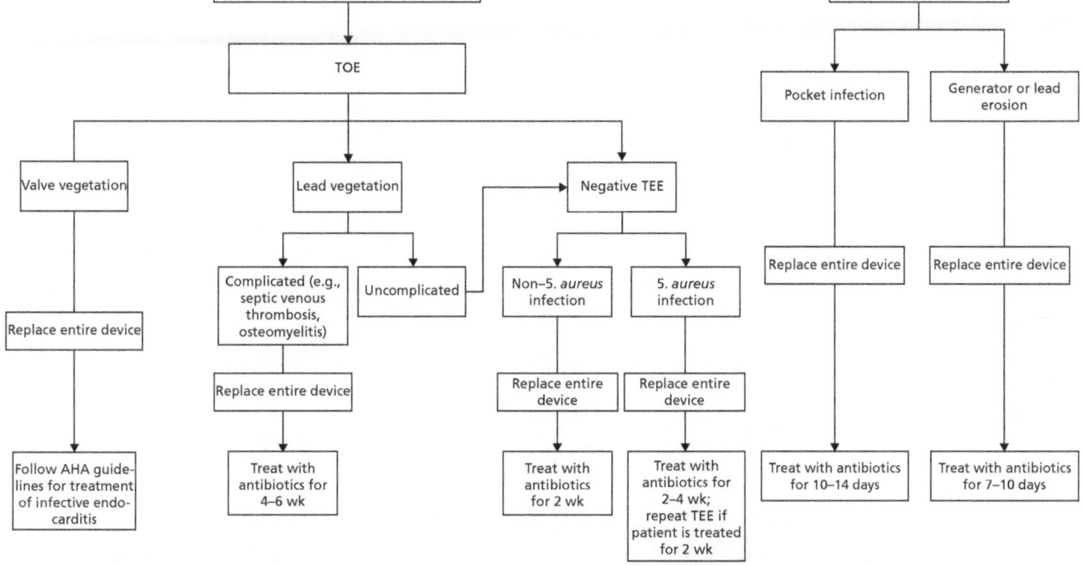

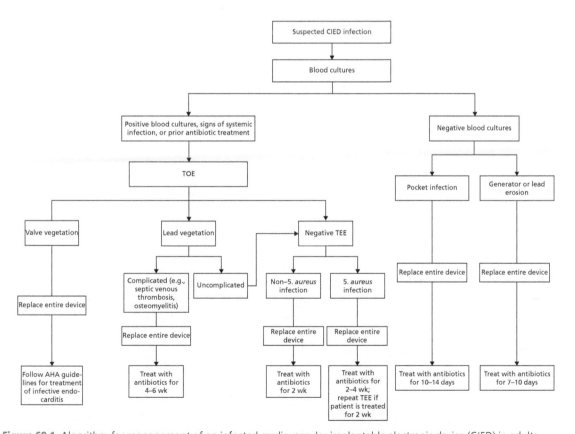

Figure 69.1 Algorithm for management of an infected cardiovascular implantable electronic device (CIED) in adults.

AHA, American Heart Association; TOE, transoesophageal echocardiography.

Baddour LM, *et al.* Clinical practice. Infections of cardiovascular implantable electronic devices. *N Engl J Med.* 2012;**367**:842–9.

resynchronization therapy devices.[4,24] Sprint Fidelis (Medtronic) and Riata (St Jude Medical) defibrillator leads have a failure rate at 2.6–2.7% per year and have been removed from the market. Fracture of a pace-sense conductor is the most widely studied failure mode of the Sprint Fidelis. Fractures of high voltage conductors are much less common; but, unlike pace-sense conductor fractures, may result in failed defibrillation.[25] Patients with an ICD-CRT have a significantly higher Fidelis fracture rate than patients with an ICD [26]

The Riata and Riata ST ICD leads are prone to high-voltage failures that have resulted in death. These failures appeared to have been caused by insulation defects that resulted in short circuiting between high-voltage components.[27] Early extraction of Riata leads with externalized conductors may be resonable to avoid the potential for large organized thrombus formation that has been recently described.[28]

Lead dislodgment for primary implantation is approximately 0.8–1% per procedure-year for pacemakers and ICDs, and 3% for CRT.[29]

Lead extraction, more than 4–6 months after implantation, requires extensive experience and can be accomplished in 90% of cases with the use of various dedicated devices. It is associated with a 12% complication rate, including 0.8% mortality.[17]

Pacemaker and ICD generator replacements are associated with a notable complication risk (1–2% and 4–6%, respectively), particularly those with lead additions.[30] Pacemaker reuse, although not allowed in most countries, is an interesting opportunity for elimination of resources waste.[31] Pacemaker reuse has an overall low rate of infection and device malfunction, but there is a higher rate of device malfunction as compared with new device implantation.[32]

Strategies for avoiding complications, as well as the optimum management of patients with electronic devices during and after medical and surgical procedures, have been described.[32,33]

Perioperative management of patients with devices

The HRS has recently published a statement on the issue.[34] Main points are presented in Tables 69.2–69.5.

Table 69.2 HRS/ASA 2011 consensus statement on the perioperative management of patients with implantable devices

Problems that can occur during medical procedures
• Bipolar electrosurgery does not cause EMI, unless it is applied directly to a CIED
• EMI from monopolar electrosurgery is the most common problem incurred during surgical procedures
- Pacemakers may have oversensing and be inhibited when exposed to EMI
- ICDs and pacemakers with anti-tachycardia function may be inhibited or may falsely detect arrhythmias when exposed to EMI
- Device reset occurs infrequently with electrosurgery
- Electrosurgery applied below the umbilicus is much less likely to cause PM or ICD interference than when applied above the umbilicus
- Pulse generator damage from electrosurgery can occur but is uncommon
- Impedance-based rate-responsive systems may go to upper rate behaviour with electrosurgery exposure
- Risk mitigation strategies can be effective
- Keeping the current path away from CIED diminishes the potential for adverse interaction with the CIED
- Using bipolar electrosurgery whenever possible
- Minimizing the length of monopolar electrosurgery bursts to 5 s or less
• Lead tissue interface damage from external current is considered an unlikely risk
• Cardioversion can cause reset of the CIED
• RF ablation can cause all of the interactions that monopolar electrosurgery can cause but may have a more significant risk profile due to the prolonged exposure to current
• Therapeutic radiation is the most likely source of EMI to result in CIED reset
• ECT has rarely been reported to cause EMI during the stimulus, but the more common problem with EMI may be the extreme sinus tachycardia that occurs with the seizure, prompting a need to review tachycardia therapy zones in ICDs
• GI procedures that use electrosurgery may result in interference
• TENS units can result in EMI

ICD, implantable cardioverter defibrillator; EMI, electromagnetic interference; CIED, cardiovascular implantable electronic device; RF, radio frequency; ECT, electroconvulsive therapy; TUNA, transurethral needle ablation; TURP, transurethral resection of the prostate; TENS, transcutaneous electrical nerve stimulation; CRT-P, cardiac resynchronization therapy pacemaker; CRT-D, cardiac resynchronization therapy defibrillator.
The Heart Rhythm Society (HRS)/American Society of Anesthesiologists (ASA) Expert Consensus Statement on the perioperative management of patients with implantable defibrillators, pacemakers and arrhythmia monitors: facilities and patient management. *Heart Rhythm*. 2011;**8**:1114–54.

Table 69.3 HRS/ASA 2011 consensus statement on the perioperative management of patients with implantable devices

Preoperative recommendations
• The procedure team must advise the CIED team about the nature of the planned procedure.
• he CIED team will provide guidance in the form of a prescription to the procedure team for the management of the CIED.
• General principles guiding this prescription include the acknowledgement that:
- Inactivation of ICD detection is not a universal requirement for all procedures.
- Rendering pacemakers asynchronous in pacemaker-dependent patients is not a universal requirement of all procedures.
- Pacemakers that need to be protected from inhibition may be made asynchronous by programming or by placement of a magnet applied over the pulse generator, provided the pulse generator is accessible.
- ICD arrhythmia detection can be suspended by placement of a magnet over the pulse generator, provided the pulse generator is accessible.
- A magnet placed over an ICD generator will not render pacemaker function in an ICD asynchronous.
- Inactivation of ICD detection is recommended for all procedures using monopolar electrosurgery or RF ablation above the umbilicus.
- Rendering a pacemaker asynchronous in a pacemaker-dependent patient is preferable for most procedures above the umbilicus.
- In pacemaker patients, no reprogramming is usually needed if the electrosurgery is applied below the level of the umbilicus.
• All patients with pacemakers undergoing elective surgery should have had a device check as part of routine care within the past 12 months that identifies the required elements specified below.
• All patients with ICDs undergoing elective surgery should have had a device check as part of routine care within the past 6 months.

The Heart Rhythm Society (HRS)/American Society of Anesthesiologists (ASA) Expert Consensus Statement on the perioperative management of patients with implantable defibrillators, pacemakers and arrhythmia monitors: facilities and patient management. *Heart Rhythm*. 2011;**8**:1114–54.

Table 69.4 HRS/ASA 2011 consensus statement on the perioperative management of patients with implantable devices

Approach to emergent/urgent procedures
Identify the type of device
• ICD, pacemaker, CRT-ICD, or CRT-pacemaker. Options for help in identification are:
- Evaluate the medical record
- Examine the patient registration card
- Telephone the company to clarify device type
- Examine the chest radiograph
Determine if the patient is pacing
• Obtain a 12-lead electrocardiogram or rhythm strip documentation
• If there are pacemaker spikes in front of all, or most, P waves and/or QRS complexes, assume pacemaker dependency
Pacemaker dependent?#
—**Yes:** pacemaker (not ICD): Use short electrosurgical bursts; place magnet over device for procedures above umbilicus or extensive electrosurgery, and have magnet immediately available for procedures below umbilicus
— Monitor patient with plethysmography or arterial line
— Transcutaneous pacing and defibrillation pads placed anterior/posterior
— Evaluate the pacemaker before leaving a cardiac-monitored environment
— **Yes:** ICD or CRT-D*: Place magnet over device to suspend tachyarrhythmia detection; use short electrosurgical bursts†
— Monitor patient with plethysmography or arterial line
— Transcutaneous pacing and defibrillation pads placed anterior/posterior
— Evaluate the ICD before leaving a cardiac-monitored environment
— **No:** pacemaker (not ICD): Have magnet immediately available
— Monitor patient with plethysmography or arterial line
— Transcutaneous pacing and defibrillation pads placed anterior/posterior
— Evaluate the pacemaker before leaving a cardiac-monitored environment
—**No:** ICD or CRT-D: Place magnet over device to suspend tachyarrhythmia detection; use short electrosurgery bursts†

(*Continued*)

Table 69.4 (Continued)

— Monitor patient with plethysmography or arterial line
— Transcutaneous pacing and defibrillation pads placed anterior/posterior
— Evaluate the ICD before leaving a cardiac-monitored environment
Contact CIED team
• A member of the CIED team should be contacted as soon as feasible
- Provide preoperative recommendations for CIED management if time allows
- Contact manufacturer representative to assist in interrogation of device pre- and/or post-operative (under the direction of a physician knowledgeable in CIED function and programming)
-Perform or review post-operative interrogation

* A magnet placed over an ICD (or CRT-ICD) will not result in asynchronous pacemaker function. This can only be accomplished by reprogramming of ICDs (or CRT-ICDs) capable of this feature (majority of newer devices implanted).

† Long electrosurgery application (>5 s and/or frequent close spaced bursts) may result in pacemaker inhibition, causing haemodynamic risk in a pacemaker-dependent patient. Long electrosurgery application in close proximity to the device generator may rarely result in power on reset or Safety Core™ programming.

Pacemaker dependency is defined as absence of a life-sustaining rhythm without the pacing system.

The Heart Rhythm Society (HRS)/American Society of Anesthesiologists (ASA) Expert Consensus Statement on the perioperative management of patients with implantable defibrillators, pacemakers and arrhythmia monitors: facilities and patient management. *Heart Rhythm*. 2011;**8**:1114–54.

Table 69.5 HRS/ASA 2011 consensus statement on the perioperative management of patients with implantable devices

Recommendations for the intraoperative monitoring of patients with CIEDs
• External defibrillation equipment is required in the OR and immediately available for all patients with pacemakers or ICDs having surgical and sedation procedures or procedures where EMI may occur
• All patients with ICDs deactivated should be on a cardiac monitor and, during surgery, should have immediate availability of defibrillation
• Some patients may need to have pads placed prophylactically during surgery (e.g. high-risk patients and patients in whom pad placement will be difficult due to surgical site)
• All patients with pacemakers or ICDs require plethysmographic or arterial pressure monitoring for all surgical and sedation procedures
• Use an ECG monitor with a pacing mode set to recognize pacing stimuli
• Pacemakers may be made asynchronous, as needed, with either a magnet application or reprogramming, provided that the pulse generator is accessible
• ICD detection may be suspended by either magnet application, as needed, or reprogramming, provided that the pulse generator is accessible
• During the placement of central lines using the Seldinger technique from the upper body, caution should be exercised to avoid causing false detections and/or shorting the RV coil to the SVC coil
• Because of interactions with monitoring, ventilation, and other impedance monitoring operative devices, inactivating minute ventilation sensors can be considered
• Keep a magnet immediately available for all patients with a CIED who are undergoing a procedure that may involve EMI

The Heart Rhythm Society (HRS)/American Society of Anesthesiologists (ASA) Expert Consensus Statement on the perioperative management of patients with implantable defibrillators, pacemakers and arrhythmia monitors: facilities and patient management. *Heart Rhythm*. 2011;**8**:1114–54.

Table 69.6 Private driving with ICD

AHA/HRS	
Primary prevention	**Secondary prevention (or shock from ICD implanted for primary prevention)**
Until recovery from implantation	6 months (at least 1 week)
EHRA	
	Restriction for private driving
ICD implantation for secondary prevention	3 months
ICD implantation for primary prevention	4 weeks
After appropriate ICD therapy	3 months
After inappropriate ICD therapy	Until measures to prevent inappropriate therapy are taken

(Continued)

Table 69.6 (Continued)

After replacement of the ICD	1 week
After replacement of the lead system	4 weeks
Patients refusing ICD for primary prevention	No restriction
Patients refusing ICD implantation for secondary prevention	7 months

2012 EHRA/HRS expert consensus statement on cardiac resynchronization therapy in heart failure: implant and follow-up recommendations and management. *Europace*. 2012;**14**:1236–86.

Table 69.7 ESC 2013 GL on cardiac pacing and CRT

Magnetic resonance in patients with implanted cardiac devices	
In patients with **conventional cardiac devices**, MR at 1.5 T can be performed with a low risk of complications if appropriate precautions are taken.	IIb-B
In patients with **MR-conditional PM systems**, MR at 1.5 T can be done safely following manufacturer instructions.	IIa-B

MRI: magnetic resonance imaging; PM: pacemaker.

2013 ESC Guidelines on cardiac pacing and cardiac resynchronization therapy. *Eur Heart J*. doi:10.1093/eurheartj/eht150.

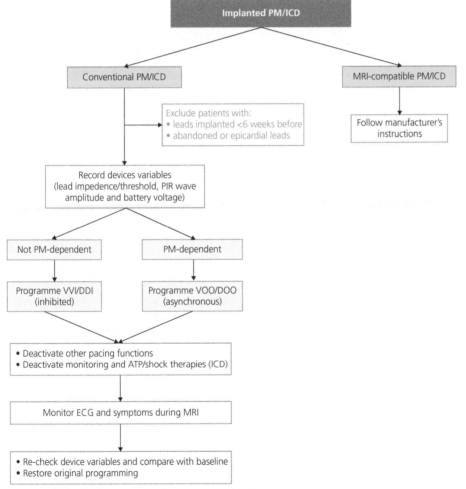

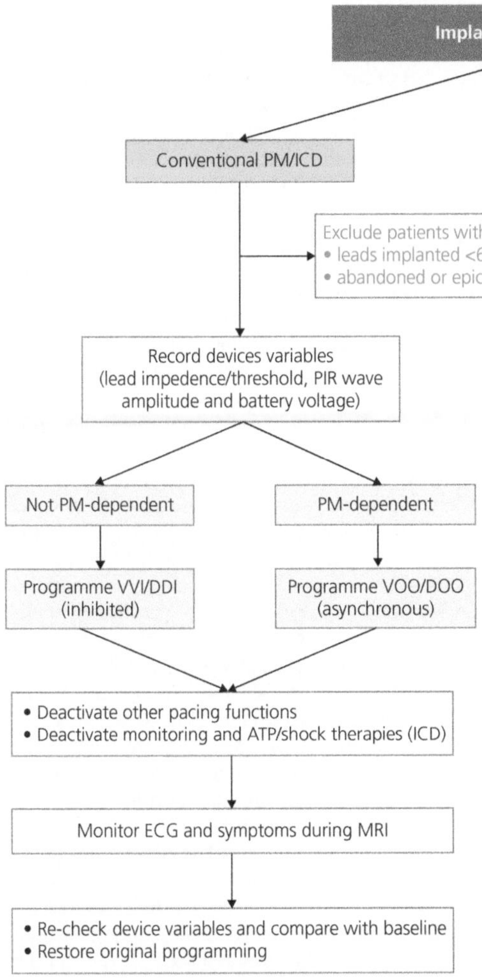

Figure 69.2 ESC 2013 GL on cardiac pacing and CRT.

Safety precautions for magnetic resonance imaging (MRI) in patients with conventional cardiac devices.

ATP: anti-tachycardiac pacing; ECG: electrocardiogram; ICD: implantable cardioverter defibrillator; PM: pacemaker.

Magnetic resonance imaging

Up to 75% of patients with implanted devices may need an MRI in the future, and this can now be performed in scanners with up to 1.5 T under certain circumstances.[35] The ESC has recently published the following recommendations (Table 69.7, and Figure 69.2);

- Exclude patients with leads that have not matured (,6 weeks since implantation, during which the leads are prone to spontaneous dislodgement) and those with epicardial and abandoned leads (which are prone to heating).
- Programme an asynchronous pacing mode in pacemaker-dependent patients to avoid inappropriate inhibition of pacing due to detection of electromagnetic interference.
- Use an inhibited pacing mode for patients without pacemaker dependence, to avoid inappropriate pacing due to tracking of electromagnetic interference.
- Deactivate other pacing functions (magnet, rate, noise, PVC, ventricular sense, AF response) in order to ensure that sensing of electromagnetic interference does not lead to unwarranted pacing.
- Deactivate tachyarrhythmia monitoring and therapies (ATP/ shock) to avoid delivery of unwarranted therapies.

Driving and sexual activity

Driving is allowed 4 weeks after permanent pacemaker implantation.[36] Following ICD implantation, professional driving is not allowed.[36,37] Private driving is allowed as indicated in Table 69.6. Similar recommendations were offered by a recent study.[38] Sexual activity is reasonable for patients with an ICD used for secondary prevention, in whom moderate physical activity (>3–5 METS) does not precipitate ventricular tachycardia or fibrillation, and who do not receive frequent multiple appropriate shocks (AHA 2012 on sexual activity and cardiovascular disease IIa-C).[39]

References

1. Adabag S, *et al.* Cardiac resynchronization therapy in patients with minimal heart failure: a systematic review and meta-analysis. *J Am Coll Cardiol.* 2011;**58**:935–41
2. Trohman RG, *et al.* Cardiac pacing: the state of the art. *Lancet.* 2004;**364**:1701–19
3. Ellenbogen KA, *et al.* Complications arising after implantation of DDD pacemakers: the most experience. *Am J Cardiol.* 2003;**92**:740–1
4. Kirkfeldt RE, *et al.* Risk factors for lead complications in cardiac pacing: a population-based cohort study of 28,860 Danish patients. *Heart Rhythm.* 2011;**8**:1622–8
5. Pakarinen S, *et al.* Short-term implantation-related complications of cardiac rhythm management device therapy: a retrospective single-centre 1-year survey. *Europace.* 2010;**12**:103–8
6. Supple GE, *et al.* Mobile thrombus on device leads in patients undergoing ablation: identification, incidence, location, and association with increased pulmonary artery systolic pressure. *Circulation.* 2011;**124**:772–8
7. Mandawat A, *et al.* Safety of pacemaker implantation in nonagenarians: An analysis of the healthcare cost and utilization project-nationwide inpatient sample. *Circulation.* 2013;**127**:1453–65
8. Baddour LM, *et al.* Clinical practice. Infections of cardiovascular implantable electronic devices. *N Engl J Med.* 2012;**367**:842–9
9. Baddour LM, *et al.* Update on cardiovascular implantable electronic device infections and their management: a scientific statement from the American Heart Association. *Circulation.* 2010;**121**:458–77
10. Tarakji KG, *et al.* Cardiac implantable electronic device infections: presentation, management, and patient outcomes. *Heart Rhythm.* 2010;**7**:1043–7
11. Uslan DZ, *et al.* Cardiovascular implantable electronic device replacement infections and prevention: results from the REPLACE registry. *Pacing Clin Electrophysiol.* 2012;**35**:81–7
12. Uslan DZ, *et al.* Permanent pacemaker and implantable cardioverter defibrillator infection: a population-based study. *Arch Intern Med.* 2007;**167**:669–75
13. Nagpal A, *et al.* Microbiology and pathogenesis of cardiovascular implantable electronic device infections. *Circ Arrhythm Electrophysiol.* 2012;**5**:433–41
14. Narducci ML, *et al.* Usefulness of intracardiac echocardiography for the diagnosis of cardiovascular implantable electronic device-related endocarditis. *J Am Coll Cardiol.* 2013; [Epub ahead of print]
15. Gordon RI, *et al.*, the Ventricular Assist Device Infection Study Group. rospective, multicenter study of ventricular assist device infections. *Circulation.* 2013;**127**:691–703
16. Le KY, *et al.* Impact of timing of device removal on mortality in patients with cardiovascular implantable electronic device infections. *Heart Rhythm.* 2011;**8**:1678–85
17. Greenspon AJ, *et al.* Timing of the most recent device procedure influences the clinical outcome of lead-associated endocarditis results of the MEDIC (Multicenter Electrophysiologic Device Infection Cohort). *J Am Coll Cardiol.* 2012;**59**:681–7
18. Glikson M. Conservative treatment of pacemaker pocket infection: Is it a viable option? *Europace.* 2013;**15**:474–5
19. Lopez JA. Conservative management of infected pacemaker and implantable defibrillator sites with a closed antimicrobial irrigation system. *Europace.* 2013;**15**:541–5
20. Cano O, *et al.* Evaluation of a new standardized protocol for the perioperative management of chronically anticoagulated patients receiving implantable cardiac arrhythmia devices. *Heart Rhythm.* 2012;**9**:361–7
21. Cheng A, *et al.* Continuation of warfarin during pacemaker or implantable cardioverter-defibrillator implantation: a randomized clinical trial. *Heart Rhythm.* 2011;**8**:536–40
22. Birnie DH, *et al.* Pacemaker or defibrillator surgery without interruption of anticoagulation. *N Engl J Med.* 2013; doi: 10.1056/NEJMoa1302946
23. Brinker J. Device surgery in the anticoagulated patient: the Goldilocks principle. *Heart Rhythm.* 2012;**9**:368–9

24. Kalahasty G, *et al.* Management of the patient with implantable cardioverter-defibrillator lead failure. *Circulation*. 2011;**123**:1352–4
25. Koneru JN, *et al.* Diagnosis of high voltage conductor fractures in sprint fidelis leads. *Heart Rhythm*. 2013; doi: pii: S1547-5271(1513)00170-00177
26. Parkash R, *et al.* Sprint fidelis lead fractures in patients with cardiac resynchronization therapy devices: Insight from the resynchronization/defibrillation for ambulatory heart failure (RAFT) study. *Circulation*. 2012;**126**:2928–34
27. Hauser RG, *et al.* Deaths caused by the failure of Riata and Riata ST implantable cardioverter-defibrillator leads. *Heart Rhythm*. 2012;**9**:1227–35
28. Goyal SK, *et al.* Lead thrombi associated with externalized cables on Riata ICD leads: A case series. *J Cardiovasc Electrophysiol*. 2013 Mar 11. doi: 10.1111/jce.12134.
29. Palmisano P, *et al.* Rate, causes and impact on patient outcome of implantable device complications requiring surgical revision: A retrospective, large population, bi-centre survey. *Europace*. 2013;**15**:531–40
30. Poole JE, *et al.* Complication rates associated with pacemaker or implantable cardioverter-defibrillator generator replacements and upgrade procedures: results from the replace registry. *Circulation*. 2010;**122**:1553–61
31. Baman TS, *et al.* Pacemaker reuse: an initiative to alleviate the burden of symptomatic bradyarrhythmia in impoverished nations around the world. *Circulation*. 2010;**122**:1649–56
32. Baman TS, *et al.* Safety of pacemaker reuse: a meta-analysis with implications for underserved nations. *Circ Arrhythm Electrophysiol*. 2011;**4**:318–23
33. Wazni O, *et al.* Strategic choices to reduce implantable cardioverter-defibrillator-related morbidity. *Nat Rev Cardiol*. 2010;**7**:376–83
34. Crossley GH, *et al.* The Heart Rhythm Society (HRS)/American Society of Anesthesiologists (ASA) expert consensus statement on the perioperative management of patients with implantable defibrillators, pacemakers and arrhythmia monitors: facilities and patient management this document was developed as a joint project with the American Society of Anesthesiologists (ASA), and in collaboration with the American Heart Association (AHA), and the Society of Thoracic Surgeons (STS). *Heart Rhythm*. 2011;**8**:1114–54
35. 2013 ESC Guidelines on cardiac pacing and cardiac resynchronization therapy. *Eur Heart J*. 2013. doi:10.1093/eurheartj/eht150
36. Vijgen J, *et al.* Consensus statement of the European Heart Rhythm Association: updated recommendations for driving by patients with implantable cardioverter defibrillators. *Europace*. 2009;**11**:1097–107
37. Epstein AE, *et al.* Addendum to 'personal and public safety issues related to arrhythmias that may affect consciousness: implications for regulation and physician recommendations: a medical/scientific statement from the American Heart Association and the North American Society of Pacing and Electrophysiology': public safety issues in patients with implantable defibrillators: a scientific statement from the American Heart Association and the Heart Rhythm Society. *Circulation*. 2007;**115**:1170–6
38. Thijssen J, *et al.* Driving restrictions after implantable cardioverter defibrillator implantation: an evidence-based approach. *Eur Heart J*. 2011;**32**:2678–87
39. Levine GN, *et al.* Sexual activity and cardiovascular disease: a scientific statement from the American Heart Association. *Circulation*. 2012;**125**:1058–72

Part XIV

Diseases of the aorta

Relevant guidelines

ESC 2001 Task Force report on aortic dissection

Task Force on Aortic Dissection, European Society of Cardiology. Diagnosis and management of aortic dissection. *Eur Heart J.* 2001;**22**:1642–81.

ACC/AHA 2010 guidelines on thoracic aortic disease (specific issues on pre- and post-op care have not been included. The reader should consult with the actual text for this purpose)

2010 ACCF/AHA/AATS/ACR/ASA/SCA/SCAI/SIR/STS/SVM guidelines for the diagnosis and management of patients with thoracic aortic disease. *J Am Coll Cardiol.* 2010;**55**:e27–129.

ESC 2010 guidelines on GUCH

ESC guidelines for the management of grown-up congenital heart disease (new version 2010). *Eur Heart J.* 2010;**31**:2915–57.

ESC 2012 guidelines on valve disease

Guidelines on the management of valvular heart disease (version 2012). The Joint Task Force on the Management of Valvular Heart Disease of the European Society of Cardiology (ESC) and the European Association for Cardio-Thoracic Surgery (EACTS). *Eur Heart J.* 2012;**33**:2451–96.

Chapter 70

Acute aortic syndromes

Definitions and classification

The term acute aortic syndrome includes the classic aortic dissection and conditions with a similar clinical profile, such as intramural aortic haematoma and penetrating atherosclerotic aortic ulcer. [1,2]

Aortic dissection (AoD) denotes disruption of the medial layer of the aorta, with bleeding within and along the wall, resulting in separation of the layers of the aorta (Figure 70.1). The outer part of the aortic media forms with the adventitia the false channel outside wall whereas the rest of the media and the intima constitute the inner wall, i.e. the intimomedial flap (also called intimal flap).[2] An intimal disruption is usually present (90% of cases) that results in tracking of the blood in a dissection plane within the media. This may rupture through the adventitia or back through the intima into the aortic lumen. Dissection may, and often does, occur without an aneurysm being present. The term 'dissecting aortic aneurysm' is often used incorrectly and should be reserved only for those cases where a dissection occurs in an aneurysmal aorta.[3]

Acute dissection is defined as occurring within 2 weeks of onset of pain.

Subacute dissection Between 2 and 6 weeks from onset of pain.

Chronic dissection More than 6 weeks from onset of pain.

Intramural haematoma (IMH) is characterized by the absence of an entrance tear. The false lumen is created by a haemorrhage into the aortic media, most likely after rhexis of the vasa vasorum that penetrates the outer half of the aortic media from the adventitia. An entrance tear is not visualized by the current imaging techniques but is usually found at surgery or autopsy.[3] IMH may evolve into classic dissection. Involvement of the ascending aorta and aortic diameter ≥5 cm are the most important predictors of mortality.

Penetrating atherosclerotic ulcer (PAU) is ulceration of an aortic atherosclerotic lesion that penetrates the internal elastic lamina into the media. It is usually found in the descending aorta and may precipitate IMH or classic dissection. However, the natural history of PAU is virtually unknown.[1]

Incomplete dissection refers to that situation in which there is laceration of the intima and subjacent media (dissection tear) without significant intramural (separation of the medial layers) dissection. Patients are at high risk of aortic rupture.

Classifications of aortic dissection

The **De Bakey classification** is based on the origin of the tear and the extent of the dissection:

Type I: dissection originates in the ascending aorta and propagates distally to include, at least, the aortic arch and typically the descending aorta (surgery usually recommended).

Type II: dissection originates in and is confined to the ascending aorta (surgery usually recommended).

Type III: dissection originates in the descending aorta and propagates most often distally (non-surgical treatment usually recommended). In type IIIa, the dissection is limited to the descending thoracic aorta, and, in type IIIb, it extends below the diaphragm.

The **Stanford classification** is based on the involvement of the ascending aorta vs the arch and/or descending aorta.

Type A: all dissections involving the ascending aorta, regardless of the site of origin (surgery usually recommended).

Type B: all dissections that do not involve the ascending aorta (non-surgical treatment usually recommended). Involvement of the aortic arch without involvement of the ascending aorta in the Stanford classification is labelled as type B.

Anatomy of the aorta

Aortic root includes the aortic valve annulus, the aortic valve cusps, and the sinuses of Valsalva.

Ascending aorta includes the tubular portion of the ascending aorta, beginning at the sinotubular junction and extending to the brachiocephalic artery origin.

Aortic arch from the origin of the brachiocephalic artery to the isthmus between the origin of the left subclavian artery and the ligamentum arteriosum, coursing in front of the trachea and to the left of the oesophagus and the trachea.

Descending aorta from the isthmus and through the diaphragm to the abdomen.

An acute aortic syndrome is defined as pain due to aortic pathology.[1,2] It usually occurs as an acute event in patients with hypertension and is associated with three interrelated conditions (aortic dissection, intramural haematoma, and penetrating atherosclerotic ulcer).

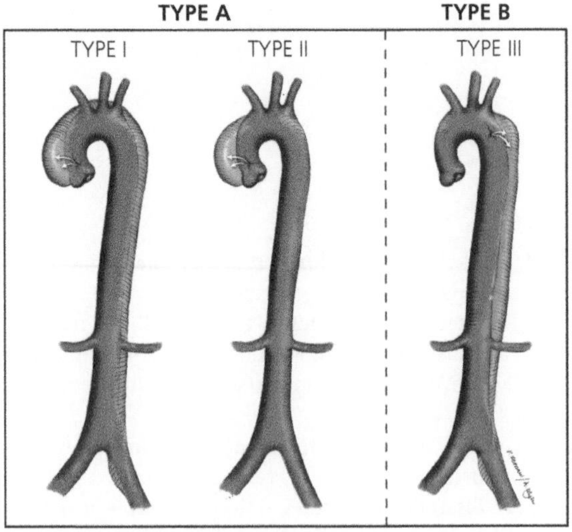

Figure 70.1 Classification schemes of acute aortic dissection.

Braverman, A. C. Acute aortic dissection: clinician update. *Circulation* 2010;**122**:184–188

Epidemiology

The true incidence of AoD is difficult to define since it leads to immediate death in 40% of patients. Estimates range from 3 to 16 cases per 100 000 persons per year, being higher in men (>40 years old) than in women.[3, 4]

Pathophysiology

Mechanisms that weaken the media layers of the aorta lead to higher wall stress, can induce aortic dilatation and aneurysm formation, eventually resulting in intramural haemorrhage, aortic dissection, or rupture. Acute aortic dissection requires a tear in the aortic intima that commonly is preceded by medial wall degeneration or cystic medial necrosis.[2] Certain genetic conditions, such as mutations in the gene **FBN1** that encodes the extracellular matrix protein fibrillin-1 and cause Marfan's syndrome, also weaken the media layers of the aorta and predispose to dissection. In addition, mutations in TGFBR1/2, ACTA2, MHY11, and S11A12 encoding transformin growth factor-beta receptors, smooth muscle a-actin, myocin heavy chain, and the proinflammatory protein S100A12, respectively, predispose humans to aortic diseases.[5]

Aetiology

Risk factors for AoD include conditions that result in aortic medial degeneration or place extreme stress on the aortic wall (Table 70.1). The main risk factor is arterial hypertension.[6] Traumatic rupture of the aorta is seen in 20% of fatal motor vehicle accidents.[3]

Table 70.1 Risk factors for development of thoracic aortic dissection

Conditions associated with increased aortic wall stress
Hypertension, particularly if uncontrolled
Phaeochromocytoma
Cocaine or other stimulant use
Weightlifting or other Valsalva manoeuvre
Trauma
Deceleration or torsional injury (e.g. motor vehicle crash, fall)
Coarctation of the aorta
Conditions associated with aortic media abnormalities
Genetic
Marfan's syndrome
Ehlers--Danlos syndrome, vascular form
Bicuspid aortic valve (including prior aortic valve replacement)
Turner syndrome
Loeys–Dietz syndrome
Familial thoracic aortic aneurysm and dissection syndrome
Inflammatory vasculitides
Takayasu arteritis
Giant cell arteritis
Behçet arteritis
Ormond's disease (retroperitoneal fibrosis)
Other
Pregnancy
Polycystic kidney disease
Chronic corticosteroid or immunosuppression agent administration
Infections involving the aortic wall, either from bacteraemia or extension of adjacent infection
Iatrogenic factors
Catheter/instrument intervention
Valvular/aortic surgery
Side or cross-clamping/aortotomy
Graft anastomosis
Patch aortoplasty

Presentation

Patients with acute aortic syndromes often present in a similar fashion, regardless of whether the underlying condition is AoD, IMH, PAU, or contained aortic rupture. **Acute chest pain** is the most common symptoms, but dissection may also occur without any symptoms or signs (6% of cases).[3] In contrast with the more gradual increasing intensity of pain due to coronary syndromes, pain from aortic dissection has a sudden onset with maximal intensity, often at the time of onset. However, coronary compression by the false lumen or extension of the dissection flap into the coronary ostium may cause **coronary ischaemia** in up 19% of cases.[3] The classic characteristics of pain are its tearing or ripping quality, and, most of the time, pain is described as sharp or stabbing, but the description can be highly variable. Chest pain irradiating to the neck, throat, or jaw indicates that the aortic segment involved is the ascending aorta whereas pain located in the back or the abdomen suggests that the diseased segment is most probably the descending aorta (Table 70.2). **Fever** may be present. **Cerebrovascular accidents** occur in up to 40% of cases and may be transient but is suggestive of arch vessel involvement. **Syncope** (13%) is an ominous sign; it may be caused by severe AR or tamponade, impaired cerebral flow, false lumen rupture into the pleural space, and vasovagal responses. Approximately 6–13% of patients present with **cardiac failure** or **shock. Death** is usually due to rupture of the false channel. Perfusion deficits and end-organ ischaemia as a result of dissection-related obstruction of aortic branch vessels are presented in Table 70.3.

Physical findings

A complete search for arterial perfusion differentials in both upper and lower extremities, evidence of visceral ischaemia, focal neurologic deficits, a murmur of aortic regurgitation, bruits, and findings compatible with possible cardiac tamponade is essential. Findings depend upon the extension of the dissection, as previously described, and the rapidity of the process.

Table 70.2 Differential diagnosis for high-risk pain or examination features

Chest pain
Acute myocardial infarction
Pulmonary embolism
Spontaneous pneumothorax
Esophageal rupture
Abdominal pain
Renal/biliary colic
Bowel obstruction/perforation
Non-dissection-related mesenteric ischaemia
Back pain
Renal colic
Musculoskeletal pain
Intervertebral disc herniation
Pulse deficit
Non-dissection-related embolic phenomena
Non-dissection-related arterial occlusion
Focal neurologic deficit
Primary ischaemic cerebrovascular accident
Cauda equina syndrome

2010 ACCF/AHA/AATS/ACR/ASA/SCA/SCAI/SIR/STS/SVM Guidelines for the diagnosis and management of patients with thoracic aortic disease *J Am Coll Cardiol*. 2010;**55**:e27–e129.

Table 70.3 End-organ complications of acute aortic dissection

Type	End-organ complication
Cardiovascular	Aortic insufficiency
	Syncope
	Pericardial tamponade
	Myocardial ischaemia or infarction
	Congestive heart failure
Neurologic	Ischaemic stroke or transient ischaemic attack
	Peripheral neuropathy
	Paraplegia/paraparesis
	Spinal ischaemia
Pulmonary	Pleural effusion
	Aortopulmonary fistula with haemorrhage
Gastrointestinal	Mesenteric ischaemia or infarction
	Aortoenteric fistula with haemorrhage
Renal	Renal failure
	Renal ischaemia or infarction
Extremities	Limb ischaemia

2010 ACCF/AHA/AATS/ACR/ASA/SCA/SCAI/SIR/STS/SVM Guidelines for the diagnosis and management of patients with thoracic aortic disease. *J Am Coll Cardiol*. 2010;**55**:e27–e129.

Aortic regurgitation (45–75% of cases) may be due to dilatation of the aortic root, disruption of the aortic valve by extension of the dissection or by the prolapsing flap. **Pulse differentials** may be present (30%). The majority of patients with acute type A aortic dissection present with **aortic diameters <5.5 cm**. Although up to 75% of patients may be hypertensive,[3] on presentation, >50% patients with type A dissection may be found **normotensive or hypotensive** (IRAD data).[7] **Ischaemic lower extremities** (30%) and **tamponade** (5–10% in proximal dissections) may also be present. Paraplegia and other neurological signs may be present in up to 40% of patients.[8]

Diagnosis

AoD should be suspected in any patient presenting with acute chest pain, especially in the context of a wide mediastinum, and usually without ECG evidence of STEMI. Recommendation for the initial evaluation of patients are presented in Figure 70.2 and Table 70.4.

Chest X-ray has low sensitivity in excluding AoD in patients with widened mediastinum or abnormal aortic contour (especially in patients with chest trauma), but a completely normal chest X-ray lowers the likelihood of AoD.

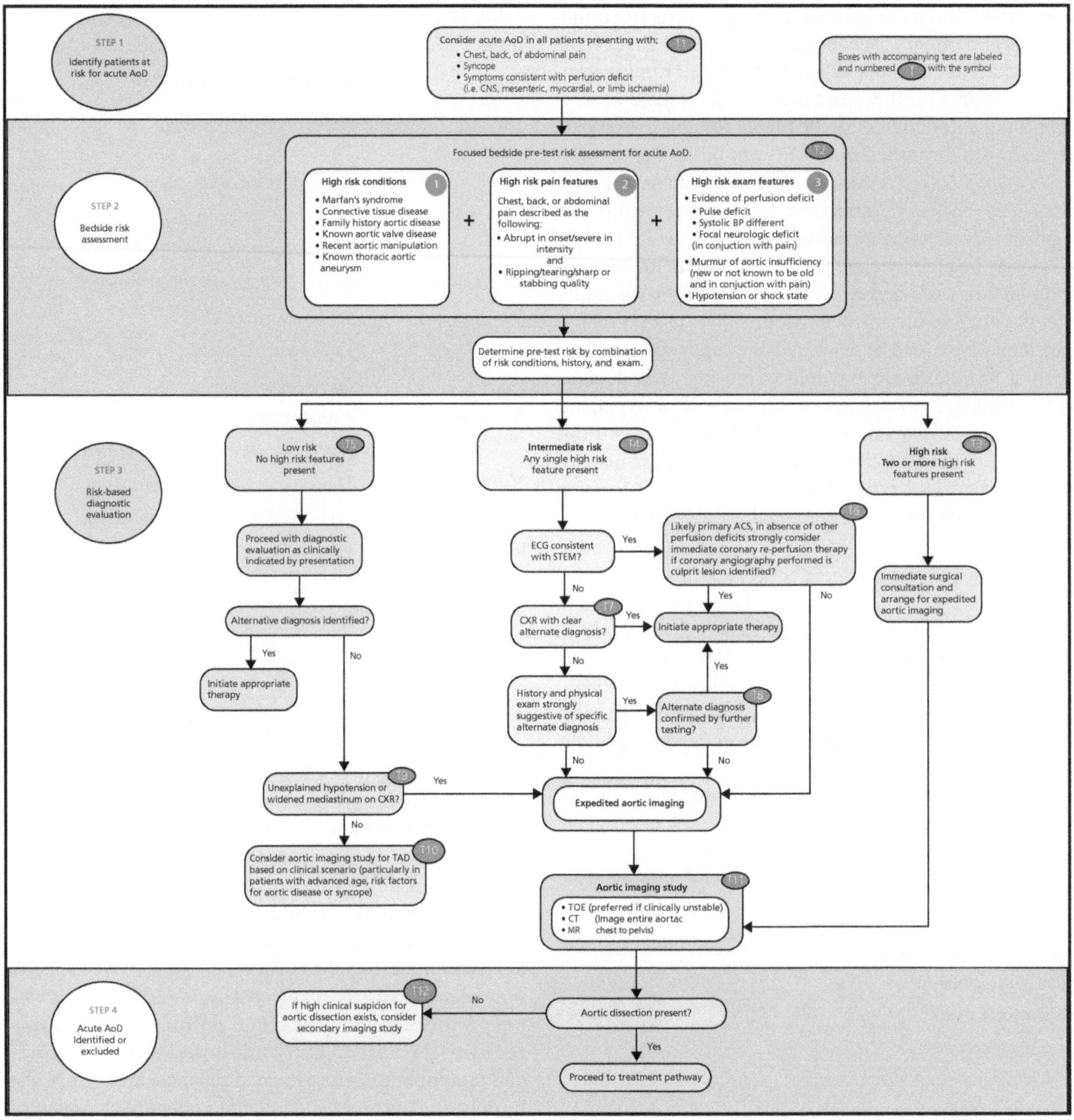

Figure 70.2 ACCF/AHA 2010 GL on thoracic aortic disease. AoD evaluation pathway.

ACS indicates acute coronary syndrome; AoD, aortic dissection; BP, blood pressure; CNS, central nervous system; CT, computed tomographic imaging; CXR, chest X-ray; EKG, electrocardiogram; MR, magnetic resonance imaging; STEMI, ST elevation myocardial infarction; TAD; thoracic aortic disease; and TOE, transoesophageal echocardiogram.

2010 ACCF/AHA/AATS/ACR/ASA/SCA/SCAI/SIR/STS/SVM Guidelines for the diagnosis and management of patients with thoracic aortic disease. *J Am Coll Cardiol*. 2010;**55**:e27–e129.

Transoesophageal echocardiography has 80% sensitivity and 95% specificity for proximal AoD. For distal AoD, sensitivity is lower, and mid-portion ascending dissections may be missed. Another disadvantage is the interference of reverberation artefacts that are produced by the echocardiography that may obscure the picture.

Multidetector helical CT with contrast (305 mL/s up to 150 mL) has excellent sensitivity and specificity (100 and 98%, respectively) in diagnosing AoD, even in trauma patients. ECG-gated tomographic images limit motion artefacts.

Magnetic resonance angiography with gadolinium is currently the imaging modality of choice. MRI or CT

Table 70.4 ACCF/AHA 2010 GL on thoracic aortic disease. Recommendations for estimation of pretest risk of thoracic aortic dissection

High-risk conditions and historical features	I-B
	• Marfan's syndrome, Loeys–Dietz syndrome, vascular Ehler–Danlos syndrome, Turner syndrome, or other connective tissue disease.
	• Patients with mutations in genes known to predispose to thoracic aortic aneurysms and dissection, such as FBN1, TGFBR1, TGFBR2, ACTA2, and MYH11.
	• Family history of aortic dissection or thoracic aortic aneurysm.
	• Known aortic valve disease.
	• Recent aortic manipulation (surgical or catheter-based).
	• Known thoracic aortic aneurysm.
High-risk chest, back, or abdominal pain features	I-B
	• Pain that is abrupt or instantaneous in onset.
	• Pain that is severe in intensity.
	• Pain that has a ripping, tearing, stabbing, or sharp quality.
High-risk examination features	I-B
	• Pulse deficit.
	• Systolic blood pressure limb differential greater than 20 mmHg.
	• Focal neurologic deficit.
	• Murmur of aortic regurgitation (new).
Recent aortic manipulation (surgical or catheter-based) or a known history of aortic valvular disease.	I-C
In patients with suspected or confirmed aortic dissection and a syncopal episode, examination to identify neurologic injury or the presence of pericardial tamponade.	I-C
Patients with acute neurologic complaints should be questioned about the presence of chest, back, and/or abdominal pain and checked for peripheral pulse deficits, as patients with dissection-related neurologic pathology are less likely to report thoracic pain than the typical aortic dissection patient.	I-C

2010 ACCF/AHA/AATS/ACR/ASA/SCA/SCAI/SIR/STS/SVM Guidelines for the diagnosis and management of patients with thoracic aortic disease. *J Am Coll Cardiol*. 2010;**55**:e27–e129.

should be combined with TOE for optimum results. Standards for measurements are presented in Table 70.5.

Angiography has lower sensitivity and specificity than the other techniques.

D-dimers elevation is very sensitive for aortic dissection but not specific since it may rise in several other conditions (see Chapter 74 on PE). A negative test (cut-off value of 500 ng/mL) performed within the first 24 hours of symptoms excludes dissection.[9] Other biomarkers are promising but have no definitive role as yet.

Therapy

Acute aortic dissection of the ascending aorta (type A) is highly lethal, with a mortality of 1–2% per hour after symptom onset. Without surgery, mortality exceeds 50% at 1 month. Uncomplicated (type B) descending dissections have a 30-day mortality of 10% and may be managed medically or by stent grafting in the future. In complicated acute type B aortic dissections, open surgery may be considered, but thoracic endovascular aortic repair (TEVAR) is the treatment of choice.[10] Intramural haematomas and penetrating ulcers are treated in the same manner as classic dissection.[2, 3] Aortic dissection with persistent patent false lumen carries a high risk of complications. Marfan's syndrome, aorta diameter, and a large entry tear located in the proximal part of the dissection indicate a high risk of complications, particularly in type B dissections.[11]

Initial management

Decreasing wall stress by lowering blood pressure and heart rate is the first step in haemodynamically stable patients (Figure 70.3 and Table 70.6). IV propranolol, metoprolol, esmolol, and especially labetalol (and alpha and beta blocker) are used.[12] If beta blockers are not tolerated or contraindicated, verapamil or diltiazem are a less well-established

Table 70.5 Imaging recommendations for aortic dissection

ACCF/AHA 2010 GL on thoracic aortic disease. Recommendations for screening tests

ECG	I-B
Given the relative infrequency of dissection-related coronary artery occlusion, the presence of ST segment elevation suggestive of myocardial infarction should be treated as a primary cardiac event without delay for definitive aortic imaging, unless the patient is at high risk for aortic dissection.	
Chest X-ray	I-C
A negative chest X-ray should not delay definitive aortic imaging in patients determined to be high-risk for aortic dissection.	III-C
Transoesophageal echocardiogram, computed tomographic imaging, or magnetic resonance imaging in patients at high risk for the disease.	I-B
Measurements of aortic diameter should be taken at reproducible anatomic landmarks, perpendicular to the axis of blood flow. For aortic root measurements, the widest diameter, typically at the mid-sinus level, should be used.	I-C
For computed tomographic imaging or magnetic resonance imaging, the external diameter should be measured perpendicular to the axis of blood flow.	I-C
For echocardiography, the internal diameter should be measured perpendicular to the axis of blood flow.	I-C

2010 ACCF/AHA/AATS/ACR/ASA/SCA/SCAI/SIR/STS/SVM Guidelines for the diagnosis and management of patients with thoracic aortic disease. *J Am Coll Cardiol*. 2010;**55**:e27–e129.

ESC 2001 on aortic dissection. Diagnostic imaging in acute aortic dissection

Transthoracic echocardiography followed by transoesophageal echocardiography	I-C
Computed tomography	I-C
• If detection of tears is crucial	IIb-C
Contrast angiography	
• To define anatomy in visceral malperfusion and to guide percutaneous interventions	I-C
• In stable patients	IIa-C
• Routine preoperative coronary angiography	III-C
• In haemodynamically unstable patients	IIb-C
Magnetic resonance imaging	IIa-C
• In haemodynamically unstable patients	III-C
Intravascular ultrasound	IIa-C
• To guide percutaneous interventions	IIb-C

ESC 2001 on aortic dissection. Imaging in chronic dissection

Magnetic resonance imaging	I-C
Transthoracic echocardiography followed by transoesophageal echocardiography	IIa-C
Computed tomography	IIa-C
Conventional angiography	
• To guide percutaneous interventions	I-C
• Preoperative diagnosis in selected patients	IIa-c
• For complete staging of the disease	IIa-C
Intravascular ultrasound	
• To guide percutaneous interventions	IIa-C

Task Force on Aortic Dissection, European Society of Cardiology. Diagnosis and management of aortic dissection. *Eur Heart J*. 2001;**22**:1642–81.

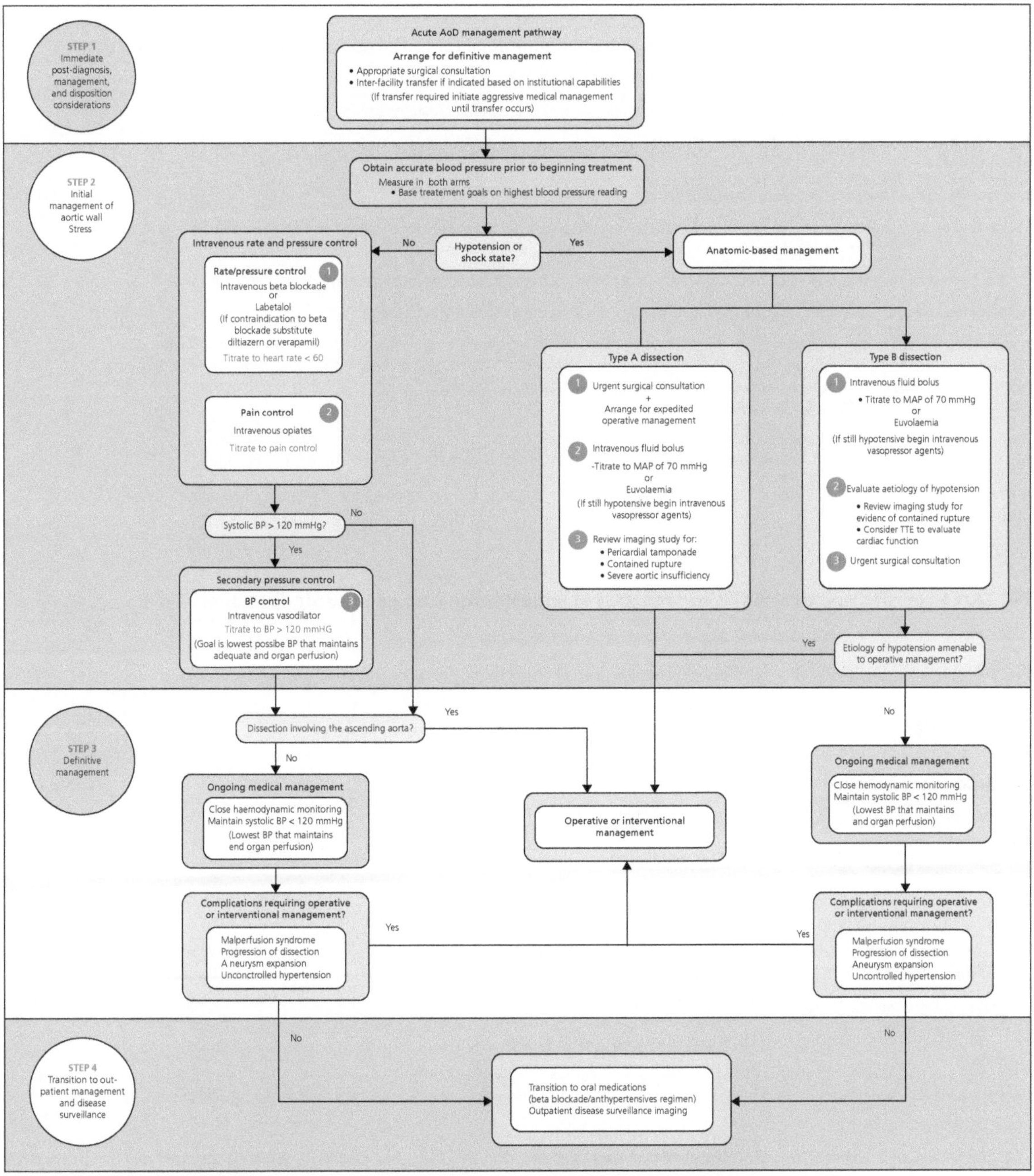

Figure 70.3 ACCF/AHA 2010 GL on thoracic aortic disease. AoD management pathway.

AoD indicates aortic dissection; BP, blood pressure; MAP, mean arterial pressure; TTE, transthoracic echocardiogram.
2010 ACCF/AHA/AATS/ACR/ASA/SCA/SCAI/SIR/STS/Sreproduced from VM Guidelines for the diagnosis and management of patients with thoracic aortic disease. *J Am Coll Cardiol*. 2010;**55**:e27–e129.

Table 70.6 Management of aortic dissection

ACCF/AHA 2010 GL on thoracic aortic disease. Recommendations for initial management of aortic dissection	
In the absence of contraindications, IV beta blockade titrated to a target heart rate ≤60 bpm.	I-C
Non-dihydropyridine calcium channel blocking agents in patients with clear contraindications to beta blockade.	I-C
If systolic blood pressures remain >120 mmHg after adequate heart rate control, ACEI and/or other vasodilators should be administered IV.	I-C
Beta blockers should be used cautiously in the setting of acute aortic regurgitation.	I-C
Vasodilator therapy should not be initiated prior to rate control so as to avoid associated reflex tachycardia that may increase aortic wall stress.	III-C
Urgent surgical consultation should be obtained, regardless of the anatomic location (ascending versus descending).	I-C
Dissection involving the ascending aorta should be urgently evaluated for emergent surgical repair.	I-B
In ascending thoracic aortic dissection, all of the aneurysmal aorta and the proximal extent of the dissection should be resected. A partially dissected aortic root may be repaired with aortic valve resuspension. Extensive dissection of the aortic root should be treated with aortic root replacement with a composite graft or with a valve sparing root replacement. If a De Bakey type II dissection is present, the entire dissected aorta should be replaced.	I-C
Dissection involving the descending aorta should be managed medically, unless life-threatening complications develop (e.g. malperfusion syndrome, progression of dissection, enlarging aneurysm, inability to control blood pressure or symptoms).	I-B

2010 ACCF/AHA/AATS/ACR/ASA/SCA/SCAI/SIR/STS/SVM Guidelines for the diagnosis and management of patients with thoracic aortic disease. *J Am Coll Cardiol*. 2010;**55**:e27–e129.

ESC 2001 on aortic dissection. Initial management of patients with suspected aortic dissection	
Detailed medical history and complete physical examination (whenever possible)	I-C
Intravenous line, blood sample (CK, TnT(I), myoglobin, WBC, D-dimer, haematocrit, LDH)	I-C
ECG: documentation of ischaemia	I-C
HR and blood pressure monitoring	I-C
Pain relief (morphine sulphate)	I-C
Reduction of systolic blood pressure using beta blockers (IV propranolol, metoprolol, esmolol, or labetalol)	I-C
Transfer to intensive care unit	I-C
In patients with severe hypertension, additional vasodilator (IV sodium nitroprusside to titrate BP to 100–120 mmHg)	I-C
In patients with obstructive pulmonary disease, blood pressure lowering with calcium channel blockers	II-C
Imaging in patients with ECG signs of ischaemia before thrombolysis if aortic pathology is suspected	II-C
Chest X-ray	III-C

Task Force on Aortic Dissection, European Society of Cardiology. Diagnosis and management of aortic dissection. *Eur Heart J*. 2001;**22**:1642–81.

ESC 2001 on aortic dissection. Management of haemodynamically unstable patients with suspected aortic dissection	
Profound haemodynamic instability: intubation and ventilation	I-C
Transoesophageal echocardiography as the sole diagnostic procedure—call surgeon	II-C
Surgery based on findings of cardiac tamponade by transthoracic echocardiography	II-C
Pericardiocentesis (lowers intrapericardial pressure (recurrent bleeding!))	III-C

Task Force on Aortic Dissection, European Society of Cardiology. Diagnosis and management of aortic dissection. *Eur Heart J*. 2001;**22**:1642–81.

Table 70.6 (Continued)

ACCF/AHA 2010 GL on thoracic aortic disease. Recommendation for surgical intervention for acute thoracic aortic dissection	
For patients with ascending thoracic aortic dissection, all of the aneurysmal aorta and the proximal extent of the dissection should be resected. A partially dissected aortic root may be repaired with aortic valve resuspension. Extensive dissection of theaortic root should be treated with aortic root replacement with a composite graft or with a valvesparing root replacement. If a DeBakey Type II dissection is present, the entire dissected aorta should be replaced.	I-C
Treat intramural hematoma similar to aortic dissection in the corresponding segment of the aorta.	IIa-C
ESC 2001 on aortic dissection. Surgical therapy of acute type A (type I and II) aortic dissection	
Emergency surgery to avoid tamponade/aortic rupture	I-C
Valve-preserving surgery—tubular graft if normal-sized aortic root and no pathological changes of valve cusps	I-C
Replacement of aorta and aortic valve (composite graft) if ectatic proximal aorta and/or pathological changes of valve/aortic wall	I-C
Valve-sparing operations with aortic root remodelling for abnormal valves	IIa-C
Valve preservation and aortic root remodelling in Marfan's patients	IIa-C

ESC 2001 on aortic dissection. Surgical therapy of acute type B (type II) aortic dissection	
Medical therapy	I-C
Surgical aortic replacement if signs of persistent or recurrent pain, early expansion, peripheral ischaemic complications, rupture	I-C
Surgical or endovascular fenestration and stenting if persisting mesenteric, renal, or limb ischaemia or neurologic deficits	IIa-C

ESC 2001 on aortic dissection. Interventional therapy in aortic dissection	
Stenting of obstructed branch origin for static obstruction of branch artery	IIa-C
Balloon fenestration of dissecting membrane plus stenting of aortic true lumen for dynamic obstruction	IIa-C
Stenting to keep fenestration open	IIa-C
Fenestration to provide reentry tear for dead-end false lumen	IIa-C
Stenting of true lumen	
• To seal entry (covered stent)	IIb-C
• Enlarge compressed true lumen	IIa-C

ESC 2001 on aortic dissection. Therapy for chronic aortic dissection	
Type A (type I, II):	
Indications for surgery as in non-dissecting aneurysm if symptoms or aortic regurgitation or aortic diameter >(5–) 6 cm	I-C
Type B (type III):	
Indications for surgery as in non-dissecting aneurysms if symptoms or progressive aortic enlargement to ≥6.0 cm	I-C
Endovascular stenting if surgical indication and suitable anatomy	IIa-C

Task Force on Aortic Dissection, European Society of Cardiology. Diagnosis and management of aortic dissection. *Eur Heart J*. 2001;**22**:1642–81.

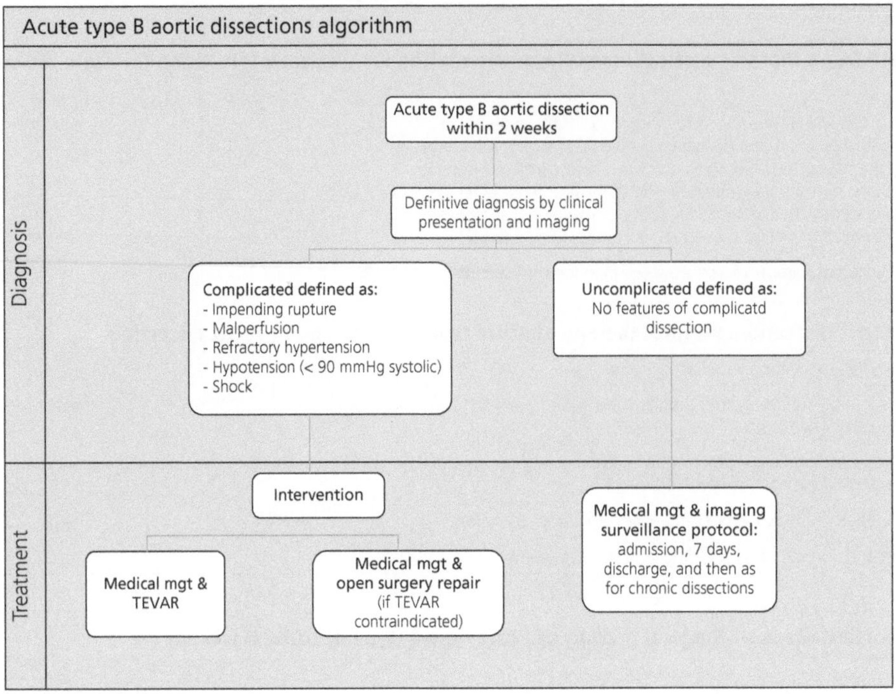

Figure 70.4 Algorithms for management of acute, subacute, and chronic type B aortic dissections. TEVAR indicates transthoracic endovascular repair.

Fattori R, *et al.* Interdisciplinary expert consensus document on management of type B aortic dissection. *J Am Coll Cardiol.* 2013;**61**:1661–78

alternative. Initial targets are a heart rate <60 bpm and a systolic blood pressure between 100 and 120 mmHg. Vasodilators, such as sodium nitroprusside, nicardipine, or nitroglycerine, may be needed after initiation of beta blockade. Pain control with opiates is essential.

Surgery

Urgent surgical consultation is vital (Table 70.6). Type A dissections are operated with implantation of a composite graft in the ascending aorta, with or without reimplantation of coronary arteries. Resecting or closing any significant communication between true and false lumina in the distal ascending aorta or aortic arch is important.[10] Patients with uncomplicated aortic dissections confined to the descending aorta are treated with medical therapy. Indications for endovascular interventions in type B dissections have been recently reviewed by an expert multidisciplinary panel (Figure 70.4).[13] For acute (first 2 weeks) type B aortic dissection, the pooled early mortality rate is approximately 6.4% with medical treatment, 10.2% with transthoracic endovascular repair (TEVAR), and 17.5% with open surgery.[13] Urgent surgical repair is recommended in traumatic aortic rupture.[3]

Follow-up

Excellent control of blood pressure and regular imaging are essential. The 10-year actuarial survival rate of patients with an aortic dissection who leave the hospital is 30% to 60%.[5]

References

1. Vilacosta I, *et al.* Acute aortic syndrome: a new look at an old conundrum. *Postgrad Med J.* 2010;**86**:52–61
2. Tsai TT, *et al.* Acute aortic syndromes. *Circulation.* 2005;**112**:3802–13
3. Hiratzka LF, *et al.* 2010 ACCF/AHA/AATS/ACR/ASA/SCA/SCAI/SIR/STS/SVM guidelines for the diagnosis and management of patients with thoracic aortic disease: a report of the American College of Cardiology Foundation/American Heart Association Task Force on practice guidelines, American Association for Thoracic Surgery, American College of Radiology, American Stroke Association, Society of Cardiovascular Anesthesiologists, Society for Cardiovascular Angiography and Interventions, Society of Interventional Radiology, Society of Thoracic Surgeons, and Society for Vascular Medicine. *Circulation.* 2010;**121**:e266–369
4. Olsson C, *et al.* Thoracic aortic aneurysm and dissection: increasing prevalence and improved outcomes reported in a nationwide population-based study of more than 14,000 cases from 1987 to 2002. *Circulation.* 2006;**114**:2611–18
5. Das D, *et al.* S100a12 expression in thoracic aortic aneurysm is associated with increased risk of dissection and perioperative complications. *J Am Coll Cardiol.* 2012;**60**:775–85
6. Howard DP, *et al.* Population-based study of incidence and outcome of acute aortic dissection and premorbid risk factor control: 10-year results from the Oxford Vascular Study. *Circulation.* 2013;**127**:2031–2037

7. Pape LA, *et al.* Aortic diameter > or = 5.5 cm is not a good predictor of type A aortic dissection: observations from the International Registry of Acute Aortic Dissection (IRAD). *Circulation.* 2007;**116**:1120–7
8. Erbel R, *et al.* Diagnosis and management of aortic dissection. *Eur Heart J.* 2001;**22**:1642–81
9. Suzuki T, *et al.* Diagnosis of acute aortic dissection by D-dimer: the International Registry of Acute Aortic Dissection Substudy on Biomarkers (IRAD-BIO) experience. *Circulation.* 2009;**119**:2702–7
10. Grabenwoger M, *et al.* Thoracic endovascular aortic repair (TEVAR) for the treatment of aortic diseases: a position statement from the European Association for Cardio-Thoracic surgery (EACTS) and the European Society of Cardiology (ESC), in collaboration with the European Association of Percutaneous Cardiovascular Interventions (EAPCI). *Eur Heart J.* 2012;**33**:1558–63
11. Evangelista A, *et al.* Long-term outcome of aortic dissection with patent false lumen: predictive role of entry tear size and location. *Circulation.* 2012;**125**:3133–41
12. Genoni M, *et al.* Chronic beta-blocker therapy improves outcome and reduces treatment costs in chronic type B aortic dissection. *Eur J Cardiothorac Surg.* 2001;**19**:606–10
13. Fattori R, *et al.* Interdisciplinary expert consensus document on management of type B aortic dissection. *J Am Coll Cardiol.* 2013;**61**:1661–78

Chapter 71

Thoracic aortic aneurysms and other conditions

Thoracic aortic aneurysms

Definitions and classification

Thoracic aortic aneurysms are classified into four general anatomical categories: ascending aortic aneurysms (60%), aortic arch aneurysms (10%), descending aortic aneurysms (40%), and thoracoabdominal aneurysms (10%).[1] The ascending aorta, and/or root, is most commonly involved while involvement of the aortic arch occurs in <10%.

Aneurysm (or true aneurysm) A permanent localized dilatation of an artery, having at least a 50% increase in diameter compared with the expected normal diameter of the artery in question. Although all three layers (intima, media, and adventitia) may be present, the intima and media in large aneurysms may be so attenuated that, in some sections of the wall, they are undetectable.[2] Normal adult thoracic aortic diameters depend on age, sex, and body surface area (BSA). Average diameters in the adult (although the aorta is not a perfect cylinder) are approximately 3.5–3.7 cm (female) and 3.6–3.9 cm (male) in the root (upper limit 2.1 cm/m^2 at the sinuses of Valsalva for both sexes) and <3 in the ascending and descending aorta.[2] MRI and CT measure the external aortic diameter which is expected to be 0.2–0.4 cm larger than the internal one as measured at echocardiography.

Annuloaortic ectasia is often used to describe root aneurysms associated with genetic conditions and usually Marfan's syndrome.

Pseudoaneurysm (or false aneurysm) Contains blood resulting from disruption of the arterial wall, with extravasation of blood contained by periarterial connective tissue and not by the arterial wall layers. Such an extravascular haematoma that freely communicates with the intravascular space is also known as a pulsating haematoma.

Ectasia Arterial dilatation less than <150% of normal arterial diameter.

Arteriomegaly Diffuse arterial dilatation involving several arterial segments with an increase in diameter greater than 50% by comparison to the expected normal arterial diameter.

Epidemiology

The incidence of thoracic aortic aneurysms is estimated to be increasing, and there are around 10.4 cases per 100 000 person-years.[3] Aneurysm disease is the 18th most common cause of death in all individuals and the 15th most common in individuals >65 years.[4]

Aetiology

Smoking, **hypertension**, and **chronic obstructive pulmonary disease** are the most important risk factors. In addition, conditions that are associated with aortic medial abnormalities (Table 70.1 of Chapter 70) may also lead to aneurysm formation. Potentially clinically significant ascending aorta (but not aortic root) dilation is present in a large proportion of paediatric patients with **isolated congenital complete heart block**, probably due to fetal exposure to maternal autoantibodies.[5] The development and expansion of an aortic aneurysm is an indolent process. The diameter of the aorta grows slowly with age at 0.12 cm/year, with the descending growing faster than the ascending aorta.[1] The average rate of expansion of thoracic aortic aneurysms is estimated to be 0.10 to 0.42 cm/y.[2]

Presentation

Many patients with a thoracic aortic aneurysm are asymptomatic and diagnosed by chest X-ray or CT scan obtained for other reasons. With large aneurysms, compressive symptoms on adjacent structures may develop: **hoarseness** from left recurrent laryngeal nerve stretching, **stridor** from tracheal or bronchial compression, **dyspnoea** from lung compression, **dysphagia**, from oesophageal compression, and **plethora and oedema** from superior vena cava compression. **AR** may develop due to aortic root or ascending aortic dilatation and result in heart failure. **Neck and jaw pain** may occur with aortic arch aneurysms whereas **back, interscapular, and/or left shoulder pain** may occur with descending thoracic aortic aneurysms. **Embolization** of atherosclerotic debris to the kidneys, mesenteric arteries, and limbs may be seen. Finally, acute syndromes, including **dissection** or **rupture without dissection**, may occur. **Chest pain and hypotension** may occur due to haemorrhage into the pleural or pericardial space. **Aorto-oesophageal fistula** and **haemoptysis** can also be seen.[1] Atherosclerotic coronary artery disease may coexist.

Diagnosis

CT or MRI is used for estimation of the external aortic diameter. All imaging modalities, including MRA, have limitations. Apart from absolute size, temporal changes and shape loss of the normal waist of the aorta at the sinotubular junction) are of importance.[4]

Therapy

Recommendations for medical management are presented in Table 71.1. Cessation of **smoking** is strongly recommended, and exertion at maximal capacity and competive, contact, and isometric sports are avoided.[6] **Beta blockers, and especially ACE/ARBs**, have been shown to inhibit aneurysm expansion.[7,8] **Statins** are also used, especially in the presence of aortic atheroma. New therapies with doxycycline or macrolide antibiotics and antioxidant agents are under study.[3]

In the ascending aorta, there is a steep increase in complication rates once the aneurysm exceeds 6 cm in diameter. Above that diameter, the rate of aortic dissection and rupture increases to >30% a year. In descending aortic aneurysms, this happens when the diameter reaches 7 cm.[1] Surgical or endovascular treatment of **ascending aortic** aneurysms is contemplated when the diameter exceeds **5.5 cm or when the growth rate exceeds 0.5 cm/year or when the diameter is >4.5 cm, but aortic valve disease or genetic syndromes associated with aneurysm are present or pregnancy** is planned (Table 71.2). Operational risk should be <5%.[2] Valve-sparing aortic root replacements are becoming more popular. Therapy of **descending aortic** aneurysms is still unsatisfactory but continues to evolve with the development of new technologies and management strategies.[9] Both surgery and endovascular stent grafts have increased mortality and morbidity, including the risk of spinal cord ischaemic injury. Open surgical repair has a surgical mortality rate of 5% to 10% for elective repair and up to twice as high for non-elective operations, with a risk of spinal cord ischaemia causing paraplegia in 5% to 10%.[1] The value of fenestrated endografts is not yet proven. Long-term treatment with beta-blockers reduces the progression of aortic dilatation.[10] In general, repair is recommended for a descending thoracic aortic at

Table 71.1 ACCF/AHA 2010 GL on thoracic aortic disease. Recommendation for medical treatment of patients with thoracic aortic diseases

Stringent control of hypertension, lipid profile optimization, smoking cessation, and other atherosclerosis risk reduction measures.	I-C
Recommendations for blood pressure control	
Antihypertensive therapy to a goal of <140/90 mmHg (patients without diabetes) or less than 130/80 mmHg (patients with diabetes or chronic renal disease).	I-B
Beta blockers to all patients with Marfan's syndrome and aortic aneurysm to reduce the rate of aortic dilatation unless contraindicated.	I-B
For patients with thoracic aortic aneurysm, reduce blood pressure with beta blockers and ACEI or ARBs to the lowest point patients can tolerate without adverse effects.	IIa-B
An angiotensin receptor blocker (losartan) is reasonable for patients with Marfan's syndrome to reduce the rate of aortic dilatation unless contraindicated.	IIa-B
Recommendation for dyslipidaemia	
Treatment with a statin to achieve a target LDL cholesterol <70 mg/dL for patients with a coronary heart disease risk equivalent, such as non-coronary atherosclerotic disease, atherosclerotic aortic aneurysm, and coexistent coronary heart disease at high risk for coronary ischaemic events.	IIa-A
Recommendation for smoking cessation	
Smoking cessation and avoidance of exposure to environmental tobacco smoke at work and home. Follow-up, referral to special programmes, and/or pharmacotherapy (including nicotine replacement, buproprion, or varenicline) are useful as is adopting a stepwise strategy aimed at smoking cessation (the 5 As are Ask, Advise, Assess, Assist, and Arrange).	I-B

2010 ACCF/AHA/AATS/ACR/ASA/SCA/SCAI/SIR/STS/SVM Guidelines for the diagnosis and management of patients with thoracic aortic disease. *J Am Coll Cardiol*. 2010;**55**:e27–e129.

Table 71.2 Surgical and endovascular treatment by location of disease

ACCF/AHA 2010 GL on thoracic aortic disease. Ascending aorta and aortic sinuses	
Surgical repair in asymptomatic patients with degenerative thoracic aneurysm, chronic aortic dissection, intramural haematoma, penetrating atherosclerotic ulcer, mycotic aneurysm, or pseudoaneurysm, with ascending aorta or aortic sinus diameter ≥5.5 cm.	I-C
In Marfan's syndrome or other genetically mediated disorders (vascular Ehlers–Danlos syndrome, Turner's syndrome, bicuspid aortic valve, or familial thoracic aortic aneurysm and dissection), operation is recommended at smaller diameters (4.0 to 5.0 cm, depending on the condition).	I-C
Patients with a growth rate of >0.5 cm/y in an aorta that is <5.5 cm in diameter should be considered for operation.	I-C
Patients undergoing aortic valve repair or replacement and who have an ascending aorta or aortic root >4.5 cm should be considered for concomitant repair of the aortic root or replacement of the ascending aorta.	I-C
Separate valve and ascending aortic replacement are recommended in patients without significant aortic root dilatation, in elderly patients, or in young patients with minimal dilatation who have aortic valve disease.	I-C
Patients with Marfan's, Loeys–Dietz, and Ehlers–Danlos syndromes and other patients with dilatation of the aortic root and sinuses of Valsalva should undergo excision of the sinuses in combination with a modified David reimplantation operation, if technically feasible, or, if not, root replacement with valved graft conduit.	I-B
Elective aortic replacement in Marfan's syndrome, other genetic diseases, or bicuspid aortic valves when the ratio of maximal ascending or aortic root area (πr^2) in cm^2 divided by the patient's height in metres exceeds 10.	IIa-C
Patients with Loeys–Dietz syndrome or a confirmed TGFBR1 or TGFBR2 mutation undergo aortic repair when the aortic diameter is ≥4.2 cm by transoesophageal echocardiogram (internal diameter) or ≥4.4–4.6 cm by computed tomographic imaging and/or magnetic resonance imaging (external diameter).	IIa-C
ACCF/AHA 2010 GL on thoracic aortic disease. Aortic arch aneurysms	
For thoracic aortic aneurysms also involving the proximal aortic arch, partial arch replacement, together with ascending aorta repair, using right subclavian/axillary artery inflow and hypothermic circulatory arrest.	IIa-B
Replacement of the entire aortic arch for acute dissection when the arch is aneurysmal or there is extensive aortic arch destruction and leakage.	IIa-B
Replacement of the entire aortic arch for aneurysms of the entire arch, for chronic dissection when the arch is enlarged, and for distal arch aneurysms that also involve the proximal descending thoracic aorta, usually with the elephant trunk procedure.	IIa-B
For patients with low operative risk in whom an isolated degenerative or atherosclerotic aneurysm of the aortic arch is present, operative treatment is reasonable for asymptomatic patients when the diameter of the arch is >5.5 cm.	IIa-B
In isolated aortic arch aneurysms <4.0 cm in diameter, reimage using computed tomographic imaging or magnetic resonance imaging at 12-month intervals.	IIa-C
In isolated aortic arch aneurysms ≥4.0 cm in diameter, reimage using computed tomographic imaging or MRI at 6-month intervals.	IIa-C
ACCF/AHA 2010 GL on thoracic aortic disease. Descending thoracic aorta and thoracoabdominal aorta	
For chronic dissection, particularly if associated with a connective tissue disorder, but without significant co-morbid disease, and a descending thoracic aortic diameter >5.5 cm, open repair is recommended.	I-B
For degenerative or traumatic aneurysms of the descending thoracic aorta exceeding 5.5 cm, saccular aneurysms, or post-operative pseudoaneurysms, endovascular stent grafting should be strongly considered when feasible.	I-B
For thoracoabdominal aneurysms, in whom endovascular stent graft options are limited and surgical morbidity is elevated, elective surgery if the aortic diameter is >6.0 cm or less if a connective tissue disorder, such as Marfan's or Loeys–Dietz syndrome, is present.	I-C
For thoracoabdominal aneurysms and with end-organ ischaemia or significant stenosis from atherosclerotic visceral artery disease, an additional revascularization procedure is recommended.	I-B

2010 ACCF/AHA/AATS/ACR/ASA/SCA/SCAI/SIR/STS/SVM Guidelines for the diagnosis and management of patients with thoracic aortic disease. *J Am Coll Cardiol*. 2010;**55**:e27–e129.

ESC 2001 on aortic dissection. Reoperation following repair of aortic dissection	
Surgical intervention for:	
• Secondary aneurysm in dissected aorta remote from initial repair	I-C
• Recurrent dissection or aneurysm formation at previous intervention site	I-C
Graft replacement for gross dehiscence or infection	I-C
Use of homografts to replace infected protheses	IIa-C
Endovascular stenting if surgical indication and suitable anatomy	IIa-C

Task Force on Aortic Dissection, European Society of Cardiology. Diagnosis and management of aortic dissection. *Eur Heart J*. 2001;**22**:1642–81.

6 cm if repaired with open surgical technique and 5.5 cm if repaired with endovascular technique (5.5 cm for Marfan's patients) or if the rate of growth is >1 cm/y.

Follow-up

Computed tomographic imaging or magnetic resonance imaging of the aorta is reasonable at 1, 3, 6, and 12 months post-dissection and, if stable, annually thereafter so that any threatening enlargement can be detected (ACC/AHA 2010 I-C). Surveillance imaging is similar in patients with intramural haematoma.

Pregnancy

Recommendations for pregnancy are presented in Tables 71.3 and 71.4.

Aortic arch and thoracic aortic atheroma and atheroembolic disease

Aortic arch atheroma and, in particular, plaques 4 mm or greater in thickness proximal to the origin of the left subclavian artery are associated with stroke and constitute one-third of patients with otherwise unexplained stroke.[11, 12] Non-calcified plaques convey a higher risk for recurrent vascular events.[13] Statins may result in regression of atheroma and are recommended (ACC/AHA 2010 IIa-C).[14, 15] They are probably more effective in combination with bisphosphonates such as etidronate.[16] Anticoagulation may also be beneficial, especially in patients with mobile lesions or aortic arch atheroma >4 cm (ACC/AHA 20101 IIb-C).[17]

Cardiovascular conditions associated with thoracic aortic disease

Bicuspid aortic valve

This is discussed in Chapter 7 on congenital conditions. Aortic aneurysms are found in 20% of patients undergoing surgery for a bicuspid valve, and 15% of patients with acute aortic dissection have bicuspid valves.[2]

Aberrant right subclavian artery

Aberrant right subclavian artery, which arises as the fourth branch from the aorta, courses behind the oesophagus in approximately 80% of patients and causes dysphagia in many patients. Dysphagia usually occurs in adults as the artery enlarges (Kommerell diverticulum).[2]

Coarctation of the aorta

This is discussed in Chapter 1 on GUCH. Approximately 25% of patients with untreated coarctation die due to aortic rupture.[2]

Right aortic arch

A right-sided aortic arch is present in approximately 0.5% of the population and rarely requires surgical repair. However, some patients present with dysphagia or asthma-like symptoms with expiratory wheezing. Diagnosis is made by CT or MR demonstrating either tracheal compression or oesophageal compression with the oesophagus enlarged and filled with gas above the level of the arch.[2]

Table 71.3 ACCF/AHA 2010 GL on thoracic aortic disease. Recommendations for counselling and management of chronic aortic diseases in pregnancy

Women with Marfan's syndrome and aortic dilatation, as well as without Marfan's syndrome but with aortic disease, should be counselled about the risk of aortic dissection, as well as the heritable nature of the disease, prior to pregnancy.	I-C
Strict blood pressure control, specifically to prevent stage II hypertension, with known thoracic aortic dilatation or a familial or genetic predisposition for aortic dissection.	I-C
Monthly or bimonthly echocardiographic measurements of the ascending aortic dimensions until birth.	I-C
MRI (without gadolinium) is recommended over computed tomographic imaging.	I-C
Transoesophageal echocardiogram is an option for imaging of the thoracic aorta.	I-C
Pregnant women with aortic aneurysms should be delivered where cardiothoracic surgery is available.	I-C
Fetal delivery via Caesarean section for patients with significant aortic enlargement, dissection, or severe aortic valve regurgitation.	IIa-C
Prophylactic surgery for progressive aortic dilatation and/or advancing aortic valve regurgitation.	IIb-C

2010 ACCF/AHA/AATS/ACR/ASA/SCA/SCAI/SIR/STS/SVM Guidelines for the diagnosis and management of patients with thoracic aortic disease. *J Am Coll Cardiol*. 2010;**55**:e27–e129.

Table 71.4 ESC 2011 GL on prenancy. Recommendations for pregnancy. Recommendations for the management of aortic disease

Women with Marfan's syndrome or other known aortic disease should be counselled about the risk of aortic dissection during pregnancy and the recurrence risk for the offspring.	I-C
Imaging of the entire aorta (CT/MRI) before pregnancy in patients with Marfan's syndrome or other known aortic disease.	I-C
Women with Marfan's syndrome and an ascending aorta >45 mm should be treated surgically pre-pregnancy.	I-C

Table 71.4 (Continued)

Strict blood pressure control in pregnant women with known aortic dilatation, (history of) type B dissection, or genetic predisposition for dissection.	I-C
Repeated echocardiographic imaging every 4 weeks during pregnancy in patients with ascending aorta dilatation.	I-C
For imaging of pregnant women with dilatation of the distal ascending aorta, aortic arch, or descending aorta, MRI (without gadolinium) is recommended.	I-C
Imaging of the ascending aorta in women with a bicuspid aortic valve.	I-C
In patients with an ascending aorta <40 mm, vaginal delivery is favoured.	I-C
Women with aortic dilatation or (history of) aortic dissection should deliver in a centre where cardiothoracic surgery is available.	I-C
In patients with an ascending aorta >45 mm, Caesarean delivery should be considered.	I-C
Surgical treatment pre-pregnancy in women with aortic disease associated with a bicuspid aortic valve when the aortic diameter is >50 mm (or >27 mm/m² BSA).	IIa-C
Prophylactic surgery during pregnancy if the aortic diameter is ≥50 mm and increasing rapidly.	IIa-C
In Marfan's and other patients with an aorta 40–45 mm, vaginal delivery with epidural anaesthesia and expedited second stage should be considered.	IIa-C
In Marfan's and other patients with an aorta 40–45 mm, Caesarean section may be considered.	IIb-C
Patients with (or history of) type B dissection should be advised against pregnancy.	III-C

ESC Guidelines on the management of cardiovascular diseases during pregnancy: the Task Force on the Management of Cardiovascular Diseases during Pregnancy of the European Society of Cardiology (ESC), *Eur Heart J*. 2011;**32**:3147–97.

References

1. Danyi P, *et al.* Medical therapy of thoracic aortic aneurysms: are we there yet? *Circulation*. 2011;**124**:1469–76
2. Hiratzka LF, *et al.* 2010 ACCF/AHA/AATS/ACR/ASA/SCA/SCAI/SIR/STS/SVM guidelines for the diagnosis and management of patients with thoracic aortic disease: a report of the American College of Cardiology Foundation/American Heart Association Task Force on practice guidelines, American Association for Thoracic Surgery, American College of Radiology, American Stroke Association, Society of Cardiovascular Anesthesiologists, Society for Cardiovascular Angiography and Interventions, Society of Interventional Radiology, Society of Thoracic Surgeons, and Society for Vascular Medicine. *Circulation*. 2010;**121**:e266–369
3. Clouse WD, *et al.* Improved prognosis of thoracic aortic aneurysms: a population-based study. *JAMA*. 1998;**280**:1926–9
4. Elefteriades JA, *et al.* Thoracic aortic aneurysm clinically pertinent controversies and uncertainties. *J Am Coll Cardiol*. 2010;**55**:841–57
5. Radbill AE, *et al.* Ascending aortic dilation in patients with congenital complete heart block. *Heart Rhythm*. 2008;**5**:1704–8
6. Cozijnsen L, *et al.* What is new in dilatation of the ascending aorta? Review of current literature and practical advice for the cardiologist. *Circulation*. 2011;**123**:924–8
7. Ahimastos AA, *et al.* Effect of perindopril on large artery stiffness and aortic root diameter in patients with Marfan syndrome: a randomized controlled trial. *JAMA*. 2007;**298**:1539–47
8. Erbel R, *et al.* Diagnosis and management of aortic dissection. *Eur Heart J*. 2001;**22**:1642–81
9. Coady MA, *et al.* Surgical management of descending thoracic aortic disease: open and endovascular approaches: a scientific statement from the American Heart Association. *Circulation*. 2010;**121**:2780–804
10. Genoni M, *et al.* Chronic beta-blocker therapy improves outcome and reduces treatment costs in chronic type B aortic dissection. *Eur J Cardiothorac Surg*. 2001;**19**:606–10
11. Amarenco P, *et al.* Atherosclerotic disease of the aortic arch and the risk of ischemic stroke. *N Engl J Med*. 1994;**331**:1474–9
12. Khatibzadeh M, *et al.* Aortic atherosclerotic plaques as a source of systemic embolism. *J Am Coll Cardiol*. 1996;**27**:664–9
13. Cohen A, *et al.* Aortic plaque morphology and vascular events: a follow-up study in patients with ischemic stroke. FAPS investigators. French Study of Aortic Plaques in Stroke. *Circulation*. 1997;**96**:3838–41
14. Corti R, *et al.* Effects of aggressive versus conventional lipid-lowering therapy by simvastatin on human atherosclerotic lesions: a prospective, randomized, double-blind trial with high-resolution magnetic resonance imaging. *J Am Coll Cardiol*. 2005;**46**:106–12
15. Yonemura A, *et al.* Effect of lipid-lowering therapy with atorvastatin on atherosclerotic aortic plaques detected by noninvasive magnetic resonance imaging. *J Am Coll Cardiol*. 2005;**45**:733–42
16. Kawahara T, *et al.* Atorvastatin, etidronate, or both in patients at high risk for atherosclerotic aortic plaques: a randomized, controlled trial. *Circulation*. 2013;**127**:2327–35
17. Ferrari E, *et al.* Atherosclerosis of the thoracic aorta and aortic debris as a marker of poor prognosis: benefit of oral anticoagulants. *J Am Coll Cardiol*. 1999;**33**:1317–22

Chapter 72

Genetic syndromes associated with thoracic aneurysm and dissection

Marfan's syndrome

Definition

Marfan's syndrome is a multisystem disease characterized by long bone overgrowth and other skeletal abnormalities, dislocation of the ocular lens, decreased skeletal muscle mass, pneumothorax, mitral valve prolapse, and dilatation of the aortic root.

Aetiology

Marfan's syndrome is an autosomal dominant condition with high penetrance, but variable expression, and represents one of the more common, potentially lethal Mendelian conditions, with an estimated prevalence of 1/3000–5000 individuals.[1] The most common mutations (>800) that cause classic Marfan's syndrome are in the gene **FBN**1 that encodes the extracellular matrix protein, fibrillin-1. Some families or sporadic patients in which some of the features of Marfan's syndrome occur, but usually without ectopia lentis and thus overlapping with the **Loyes–Dietz syndrome**, have mutations in the gene **TGFBR2** that encodes receptors for the cytokine transforming growth factor-β (TGF-β) (Table 72.1). Children of an affected parent have a 50% chance to develop the syndrome while one-third of cases represent *de novo* mutations. Approximately 25% of patients do not have a family history and represent new cases due to sporadic mutations for the condition.

Pathophysiology

Perturbation of fibrillin-1 results in degeneration of the medial layer, with disarray throughout the extracellular matrix, progressive fragmentation, and loss of elastic lamellae, and excess activation of the cytokine transforming growth factor-β (TGF-β), a potent stimulator of inflammation and fibrosis. Ongoing destruction of the elastic and collagen lamellae and medial degeneration result in progressive dilatation of proximal aortic segments, as well as a predisposition to aortic dissection from the loss of elasticity and appropriate medial layer support. Superimposed on underlying Marfan's syndrome tissue abnormalities are the normal haemodynamic stressors on the proximal aorta throughout the cardiac cycle.[1]

Presentation and physical findings

Chest pain in a person with **tall, asthenic habitus, anterior chest deformity, or a family history of aortic dissection or sudden death** should always raise the suspicion of aortic dissection. Patients with Marfan's syndrome are predisposed to thoracic aortic aneurysm or dissection, and every patient with the syndrome has evidence of aortic involvement at some point during their life. Cardiovascular, ocular, and skeletal features are presented in Table 72.1. Mitral valve prolapse, MR, and AR may also be seen. The ECG may show ST segment abnormalities, prolonged QT, and AV conduction disturbances.

Diagnosis

Major criteria for the diagnosis include aortic dilatation, family history, ectopic (dislocated) lens that differentiates Marfan's from Loeys–Dietz syndrome, identification of FBN1 mutation, and the presence of systemic features, such as wrist and thumb signs, pectus carinatum and hindfoot deformity, pneumothorax, and dural ectasia. The **revised Ghent criteria** are presented in Table 72.2.[2] They might have lower sensitivity, even in patients with aortic root >40 mmHg, due to the use of the Z-score (aortic size ratio based on gender- and body size-related norms in order to take into account that the diameter of the aorta is directly proportional to body size throughout normal growth) that seems to underestimate aortic root dilatation.[3] Disorders that are often clinically difficult to distinguish from Marfan's syndrome, such as **familial ectopia lentis, MASS phenotype** (myopia, mitral valve prolapse, aortic root dilatation, striae, skeletal findings), and **familial aortic aneurysm**, may also be associated with mutations in FBN1. Thus, for the patient being evaluated for the first time who has some, but not enough, features for a clinical diagnosis and no, or an uncertain, family history, molecular analysis is of minimal help. DNA analysis is indicated when a pathological mutation is known in a family, and relatives at risk can be screened for this mutation. Recommendations for follow-up of patients are presented in Table 72.3.

Risk stratification

Aortic size >5 cm, Z-score >3, proximal aortic ratio >1.3 (i.e. >30% enlargement of the aortic root above the mean for that patient's age and body surface area), rapid increase in aortic size (>0.5 cm/year), and family history are ominous

Table 72.1 ACCF/AHA 2010 GL on thoracic aortic disease. Genetic syndromes associated with thoracic aortic aneurysm and dissection

Genetic syndrome	Common clinical features	Genetic defect	Diagnostic test	Comments on aortic disease
Marfan's syndrome	Skeletal features (see text), Ectopia lentis, Dural ectasia,	*FBN1* mutations*	Ghent diagnostic criteria DNA for sequencing	Surgical repair when the aorta reaches 5.0 cm, unless there is a family history of AoD at <5.0 cm, a rapidly expanding aneurysm, or presence of significant aortic valve regurgitation
Loeys–Dietz syndrome	Bifid uvula or cleft palate, Arterial tortuosity, Hypertelorism, Skeletal features similar to MFS, Craniosynostosis, Aneurysms and dissections of other arteries	*TGFBR2* or *TGFBR1* mutations	DNA for sequencing	Surgical repair recommended at an aortic diameter of ≥4.2 cm by TOE (internal diameter) or 4.4 to ≥4.6 cm by CT and/or MR (external diameter)
Ehlers–Danlos syndrome, vascular form	Thin, translucent skin, Gastrointestinal rupture, Rupture of the gravid uterus Rupture of medium-sized to large arteries	*COL3A1* mutations	DNA for sequencing Dermal fibroblasts for analysis of type III collagen	Surgical repair is complicated by friable tissues Non-invasive imaging recommended
Turner's syndrome	Short stature, Primary amenorrhoea, Bicuspid aortic valve, Aortic coarctation, Webbed neck, low-set ears, low hairline, broad chest	45,X karyotype	Blood (cells) for karyotype analysis	AoD risk is increased in patients with bicuspid aortic valve, aortic coarctation, hypertension, or pregnancy

AoD indicates aortic dissection; *COL3A1*, type III collagen; CT, computed tomographic imaging; *FBN1*, fibrillin-1; MFS, Marfan's syndrome; MR, magnetic resonance imaging; TOE, transoesophageal echocardiogram; *TGFBR1*, transforming growth factor-beta receptor type I; *TGFBR2*, transforming growth factor-beta receptor type II.

* The defective gene at a second locus for MFS is *TGFBR2*, but the clinical phenotype as MFS is debated.

2010 ACCF/AHA/AATS/ACR/ASA/SCA/SCAI/SIR/STS/SVM Guidelines for the diagnosis and management of patients with thoracic aortic disease. *J Am Coll Cardiol*. 2010;**55**:e27–e129.

Table 72.2 Revised Ghent criteria

In the absence of family history
1. Ao (Z ≥2) and ectopia lentis
2. Ao (Z ≥2) and FBN1 mutation
3. Ao (Z ≥2) and systemic features (≥7 points), as presented in Table 72.1
4. Ectopia lentis and FBN1 mutation and aortic diameter at the sinuses of Valsalva above indicated Z-score or aortic root dissection
In the absence of family history
5. Ectopia lentis and family history of Marfan's
6. Systemic features (≥7 points) and family history of Marfan's
7. Ao (Z ≥2 above 20 years old, ≥3 below 20 years) and family history of Marfan's
Scoring of systemic features
Wrist AND thumb sign—3 (wrist OR thumb sign—1)
Pectus carinatum deformity—2 (pectus excavatum or chest asymmetry—1)
Hindfoot deformity—2 (plain pes planus—1)
Pneumothorax—2
Dural ectasia—2
Protrusio acetabuli—2
Reduced US/LS AND increased arm/height AND no severe scoliosis—1
Scoliosis or thoracolumbar kyphosis—1
Reduced elbow extension—1
Facial features (3/5)—1 (dolichocephaly, enophthalmos, downslanting palpebral fissures, malar hypoplasia, retrognathia)
Skin striae—1
Myopia >3 dioptres—1
Mitral valve prolapse (all types)—1

prognostic factors.[1] Identification of a FBN1 mutation, in general, denotes increased risk.[4] Apart from aortic rupture, patients with Marfan's can die from severe MR or ventricular arrhythmias that may be seen in 20% of patients, conferring a long-term risk of arrhythmic sudden death of 4%.[5]

Therapy

Beta blockers (aiming at a resting heart rate <60 bpm) should be given to all patients and may reduce mortality.[6] If contraindicated or not tolerated, **verapamil** is a second-line treatment. **ARB** may also be used in combination with beta blockers, especially for those with detected dissection. Effects of therapy should be monitored regularly (Table 72.3). Isometric static exercise, competitive contact sports, involving bodily collisions, and marked changes in ambient air pressure (as in scuba diving or sudden changes in altitude in non-pressurized aircraft that may cause pneumothorax) are avoided. Aerobic exercise allowing a heart rate <100 bpm (110 for children) is permitted under beta blockade (see also http://www.Marfan.org).

Indications for surgery Surgery with a valve conduit is recommended in patients with aortic root diameter >5 cm[7] or 4.5 cm in the presence of a family history, rapid diameter change (>0.5 cm/y), and significant AR (Table 72.3). Risk of sudden death or aortic dissection remains low in patients with Marfan's syndrome and aortic diameter between 45 and 49 mm. [8] Mortality with elective surgery is 1.5% and 11.7% with emergency root replacement. The David technique, with preservation of the native valve, is rather preferable to composite mechanical valve conduits (Bentall)

Table 72.3 Genetic syndromes

ACCF/AHA 2010 GL on thoracic aortic disease. Recommendations for genetic syndromes	
Echocardiogram at the time of diagnosis of Marfan's syndrome to determine the aortic root and ascending aortic diameters and 6 months thereafter to determine the rate of enlargement of the aorta.	I-C
Annual imaging for patients with Marfan's syndrome if stability of the aortic diameter is documented. If the maximal aortic diameter is ≥4.5 cm or if the aortic diameter shows significant growth from baseline, more frequent imaging should be considered.	I-C
Patients with Loeys–Dietz syndrome or a confirmed genetic mutation known to predispose to aortic aneurysms and aortic dissections (TGFBR1, TGFBR2, FBN1, ACTA2, or MYH11) should undergo complete aortic imaging at initial diagnosis and 6 months thereafter.	I-C
Patients with Loeys–Dietz syndrome should have yearly MRI from the cerebrovascular circulation to the pelvis.	I-B
Patients with Turner's syndrome should undergo imaging of the heart and aorta for evidence of bicuspid aortic valve, coarctation of the aorta, or dilatation of the ascending thoracic aorta. If initial imaging is normal and there are no risk factors for aortic dissection, repeat imaging should be performed every 5 to 10 years or if otherwise clinically indicated. If abnormalities exist, annual imaging or follow-up imaging should be done.	I-C
Consider surgical repair of the aorta in all adult patients with Loeys–Dietz syndrome or a confirmed TGFBR1 or TGFBR2 mutation and an aortic diameter ≥4.2 cm by transoesophageal echocardiogram (internal diameter) or ≥4.4–4.6 cm by computed tomographic imaging and/or MRI (external diameter).	IIa-C
For women with Marfan's syndrome contemplating pregnancy, prophylactically replace the aortic root and ascending aorta if the diameter is > 4.0 cm.	IIa-C
If the maximal cross-sectional area in square centimetres of the ascending aorta or root divided by the patient's height in meters exceeds a ratio of 10, surgical repair is reasonable because shorter patients have dissection at a smaller size and 15% of patients with Marfan's syndrome have dissection at a size <5.0 cm.	IIa-C
In patients with Turner's syndrome with additional risk factors, including bicuspid aortic valve, coarctation of the aorta, and/or hypertension, and in patients who attempt to become pregnant or who become pregnant, perform imaging of the heart and aorta to help determine the risk of aortic dissection.	IIb-C

2010 ACCF/AHA/AATS/ACR/ASA/SCA/SCAI/SIR/STS/SVM Guidelines for the diagnosis and management of patients with thoracic aortic disease. *J Am Coll Cardiol*. 2010;**55**:e27–e129.

ESC 2001 on aortic dissection. Prevention of aortic dissection in inherited diseases (Marfan's Syndrome, Ehlers–Danlos syndrome, annuloaortic ectasia)	
Lifelong beta adrenergic blockade	I-C
Periodic routine imaging of the aorta	I-C
Prophylactic replacement of the aortic root before diameter exceeds 5·0 cm in patients with family history of dissection	IIa-C
Prophylactic replacement of the aortic root before diameter exceeds 5·5 cm	IIa-C
Moderate restriction of physical activity	I-C

Task Force on Aortic Dissection, European Society of Cardiology. Diagnosis and management of aortic dissection. *Eur Heart J*. 2001;**22**:1642–81.

ESC 2010 GL on GUCH. Indications for surgery in Marfan's	
Aortic root maximal diameter is:	
>50 mm	I-C
46–50 mm with:	I-C
- Family history of dissection, or	
- Progressive dilation >2 mm/year as confirmed by repeated measurement, or	
- Severe AR or MR, or	
- Desire of pregnancy	
Other parts of the aorta >50 mm or dilation is progressive	IIa-C

Table 72.3 (Continued)

ESC 2012 GL on valve disease. Aortic root disease (whatever the severity of AR)	
Patients who have aortic root disease with maximal aortic diameter:	
≥50 mm for patients with Marfan's syndrome	I-C
≥45 mm for patients with Marfan's syndrome with risk factors[1]	IIa-C
≥50 mm for patients with bicuspid valves with risk factors[2]	IIa-C
≥55 mm for other patients	IIa-C

1: Family history of aortic dissection and/or aortic size increase >2 mm/year (on repeated measurements using the same imaging technique, measured at the same aorta level with side-by-side comparison and confirmed by another technique), severe AR or mitral regurgitation, desire of pregnancy.
2: Coarctation of the aorta, systemic hypertension, family history of dissection, or increase in aortic diameter >2 mm/year (on repeated measurements using the same imaging technique, measured at the same aorta level with side-by-side comparison and confirmed by another technique).

Table 72.4 Gene defects associated with familial thoracic aortic aneurysm and dissection

Defective gene leading to familial thoracic aortic aneurysms and dissection	Contribution to familial thoracic aortic aneurysms and dissection	Associated clinical features	Comments on aortic disease
TGFBR2 mutations	4%	Thin, translucent skin Arterial or aortic tortuosity Aneurysm of arteries	Multiple aortic dissections documented at aortic diameters <5.0 cm
MYH11 mutations	1%	Patent ductus arteriosus	Patient with documented dissection at 4.5 cm
ACTA2 mutations	14%	Livedo reticularis Iris flocculi Patent ductus arteriosus Bicuspid aortic valve	Two of 13 patients with documented dissections <5.0 cm

ACTA2 indicates actin, alpha 2, smooth muscle aorta; *MYH11*, smooth muscle specific beta-myosin heavy chain; and *TGFBR2*, transforming growth factor-beta receptor type II.
2010 ACCF/AHA/AATS/ACR/ASA/SCA/SCAI/SIR/STS/SVM Guidelines for the diagnosis and management of patients with thoracic aortic disease. *J Am Coll Cardiol*. 2010;**55**:e27–e129.

but requires extended experience and patients with totally normal native valves.[9] Type A dissection should be operated whereas medical therapy is preferable in type B dissection, unless the aortic diameter exceeds 5–6 cm. Stents are not recommended. Elective root replacement by a prosthesis may constitute a risk factor for downstream, type B aortic dissection (because of the loss of the elastic properties of the root or clamp injuries of the aorta) but in clinical practice this appears to be outweighed by the risk of type A dissection if timely proximal repair is not performed.[10]

Pregnancy

Pregnancy may be allowed under beta blockade, with a known small risk of small-for-dates babies, hyperbilirubinaemia, and hyperglycaemia. Pregnancy causes a slight increase in aortic root diameter and should be discouraged in women with previous aortic dissection. Dissection and rupture are more common in the third trimester, up to 2 days after uneventful delivery, and usually occurs in patients with aortic root diameters >4.5 cm. Recommendations for pregnancy are presented in Tables 71.3 and 71.4 of Chapter 71 on aortic aneurysms. AACF/AHA guidelines consider an aortic root diameter ≤40 mm to be considered safe whereas both the European and Canadian guidelines accept a limit of 45 mm, and recent evidence supports this view.[11]

Other heritable syndromes and genetic defects associated with thoracic aortic disease

Heritable disorders associated with aortic dilatation are **Loeys–Dietz syndrome**, the vascular form of **Ehlers–Danlos syndrome**, and **Turner's syndrome**. Clinical features and genetic causes are presented in Table 72.1. Genetic defects associated with **familial thoracic aortic aneurysm** and dissection that do not belong to any described syndrome are presented in Table 72.4. In addition to these, other genetic syndromes, such as **autosomal dominant polycystic kidney disease** and **Noonan's syndrome**, are also associated with aortic dissections. Recommendations for the management of these patients are presented in Table 72.5.

Table 72.5 ACCF/AHA 2010 GL on thoracic aortic disease. Recommendations for familial thoracic aortic aneurysms and dissections

Aortic imaging for first-degree relatives of patients with thoracic aortic aneurysm and/or dissection to identify those with asymptomatic disease.	I-B
If the mutant gene (FBN1, TGFBR1, TGFBR2, COL3A1, ACTA2, MYH11) associated with aortic aneurysm and/or dissection is identified in a patient, first-degree relatives should undergo counselling and testing. Then, only the relatives with the genetic mutation should undergo aortic imaging.	I-C
If one or more first-degree relatives of a patient with known thoracic aortic aneurysm and/or dissection are found to have thoracic aortic dilatation, aneurysm, or dissection, then imaging of second-degree relatives is reasonable.	IIa-B
Sequencing of the ACTA2 gene is reasonable in patients with a family history of thoracic aortic aneurysms and/or dissections to determine if ACTA2 mutations are responsible for the inherited predisposition.	IIa-B
Sequencing of other genes known to cause familial thoracic aortic aneurysms and/or dissection (TGFBR1, TGFBR2, MYH11) may be considered in patients with a family history and clinical features associated with mutations in these genes.	IIb-B
If one, or more, first-degree relatives of a patient with known thoracic aortic aneurysm and/or dissection are found to have thoracic aortic dilatation, aneurysm, or dissection, then referral to a geneticist may be considered.	IIb-C

2010 ACCF/AHA/AATS/ACR/ASA/SCA/SCAI/SIR/STS/SVM Guidelines for the diagnosis and management of patients with thoracic aortic disease. *J Am Coll Cardiol*. 2010;**55**:e27–e129.

Siblings and parents of patients should be followed with aortic imaging every 2 years.[12]

References

1. Keane MG, *et al.* Medical management of Marfan's syndrome. *Circulation*. 2008;**117**:2802–13
2. Loeys BL, *et al.* The revised Ghent nosology for the Marfan's syndrome. *J Med Genet*. 2010;**47**:476–85
3. Radonic T, *et al.* Critical appraisal of the revised Ghent criteria for diagnosis of Marfan's syndrome. *Clin Genet*. 2011;**80**:346–53
4. Detaint D, *et al.* Cardiovascular manifestations in men and women carrying a FBN1 mutation. *Eur Heart J*. 2010;**31**:2223–9
5. Yetman AT, *et al.* Long-term outcome in patients with Marfan's syndrome: is aortic dissection the only cause of sudden death? *J Am Coll Cardiol*. 2003;**41**:329–32
6. Rossi-Foulkes R, *et al.* Phenotypic features and impact of beta blocker or calcium antagonist therapy on aortic lumen size in the Marfan's syndrome. *Am J Cardiol*. 1999;**83**:1364–8
7. Genoni M, *et al.* Chronic beta-blocker therapy improves outcome and reduces treatment costs in chronic type B aortic dissection. *Eur J Cardiothorac Surg*. 2001;**19**:606–10
8. Jondeau G, *et al.* Aortic event rate in the Marfan's population: a cohort study. *Circulation*. 2012;**125**:226–32
9. Benedetto U, *et al.* Surgical management of aortic root disease in Marfan's syndrome: a systematic review and meta-analysis. *Heart*. 2011;**97**:955–8
10. Schoenhoff FS, *et al.* Acute aortic dissection determines the fate of initially untreated aortic segments in marfan syndrome. *Circulation*. 2013;**127**:1569–75
11. Donnelly RT, *et al.* The immediate and long-term impact of pregnancy on aortic growth rate and mortality in women with Marfan's syndrome. *J Am Coll Cardiol*. 2012;**60**:224–9
12. Hiratzka LF, *et al.* 2010 ACCF/AHA/AATS/ACR/ASA/SCA/SCAI/SIR/STS/SVM guidelines for the diagnosis and management of patients with thoracic aortic disease: a report of the American College of Cardiology Foundation/American Heart Association Task Force on practice guidelines, American Association for Thoracic Surgery, American College of Radiology, American Stroke Association, Society of Cardiovascular Anesthesiologists, Society for Cardiovascular Angiography and Interventions, Society of Interventional Radiology, Society of Thoracic Surgeons, and Society for Vascular Medicine. *Circulation*. 2010;**121**:e266–369

Chapter 73

Inflammatory diseases associated with thoracic aortic disease

Introduction

Inflammation of large arteries, such as the aorta and its major branches, occurs in a number of disorders, including Kawasaki syndrome, Behçet's syndrome, rheumatoid arthritis, ankylosing spondylitis, syphilis, and tuberculosis. Infected thoracic aortic aneurysms due to bacterial infections may also be seen as a complication of endocarditis or cardiac surgery or due to contiguous spread from adjacent thoracic structures. Aortitis and large-vessel arteritis are characteristics of Takayasu's arteritis and giant cell (temporal) arteritis.[1,2]

Takayasu's arteritis

Definition

Takayasu's arteritis, also known as pulseless disease, is an idiopathic arteritis involving the aorta and its branches.

Epidemiology

It mainly affects women (ten times more than men) and is usually, but not invariably, diagnosed in the third decade of life. In the USA, its prevalence is 2.6 cases/million.[3]

Pathophysiology

Takayasu's is a T cell-mediated panarteritis, the pathogenesis of which remains poorly defined. The disease proceeds from adventitial vasa vasorum involvement inward, with resultant tissue destruction that yields aneurysms and inflammatory infiltrates that cause stenosis. Coronaries are affected in <10% with the development of aneurysms. In the Japanese type, the thoracic aorta and great vessels are most commonly affected. In the Indian type, the disease most commonly affects the abdominal aorta and the renal arteries.[1]

Presentation

Fatigue, night sweats, anorexia, malaise, and weight loss characterize the acute phase of the disease. Chronic symptoms are upper extremity claudication, cerebrovascular insufficiency (vision loss, light-headedness, stroke) and carotid artery pain, and hypertension in involvement of the renal arteries.

Diagnosis

The diagnosis of Takayasu's arteritis is made by identifying, at least, three of the 1990 American College of Rheumatology criteria:[4] (1) age of onset younger than 40 years, (2) intermittent claudication, (3) diminished brachial artery pulse, (4) subclavian artery or aortic bruit, (5) systolic blood pressure variation of greater than 10 mmHg between arms, and (6) angiographic (CT, MR) evidence of aorta or aortic branch vessel stenosis. ESR and CRP are elevated in 50–70% of patients, depending on the disease phase (Table 73.1).

Therapy

Immunosuppression with steroids or agents, such as methotrexate, azathioprine, and anti-tumour necrosis factor-alpha agents, are used for 1–2 years (Table 73.2). Remissions occur in 40–60% of patients on steroids, and 40% of them respond to cytotoxic agents.[3, 5] Markers of inflammation are not indicators of disease activity under treatment. Surgical revascularization is implemented, when needed, in the non-acute phase but at an increased risk of anastomotic aneurysms. Percutaneous intraluminal angioplasty of the carotid, subclavian, and renal arteries is feasible. Surgical or percutaneous revascularization is associated with a 44% 5-year rate of complications, particularly when it is performed at time of prominent biological inflammation.[6]

Table 73.1 ACC/AHA 2010 GL on thoracic aortic disease. Inflammatory diseases associated with thoracic aortic aneurysm and dissection

Names	Criteria used in diagnosis/source	When is diagnosis established?
Takayasu's arteritis	Age of onset <40 years Intermittent claudication Diminished brachial artery pulse Subclavian artery or aortic bruit Systolic BP variation of >10 mmOHg between arms Aortographic evidence of aorta or aortic branch stenosis	≥3 criteria are present (sensitivity 90.5%; specificity 97.8%)
Giant cell arteritis	Age >50 y Recent-onset localized headache Temporary artery tenderness or pulse attenuation Elevated erythrocyte sedimentation rate >50 mm/h Arterial biopsy shows necrotizing vasculitis	≥3 criteria are present (sensitivity greater than 90%; specificity >90%)
Behçet's disease	Oral ulceration Recurrent genital ulceration Uveitis or retinal vasculits Skin lesions—erythema nodosum, pseudofolliculitis, or pathergy	Oral ulceration plus two of the other three criteria
Ankylosing spondylitis	Onset of pain <40 years Back pain for >3 mo Morning stiffness Subtle symptom onset Improvement with exercise	Four of the diagnostic criteria are present

2010 ACCF/AHA/AATS/ACR/ASA/SCA/SCAI/SIR/STS/SVM Guidelines for the diagnosis and management of patients with thoracic aortic disease. *J Am Coll Cardiol*. 2010;**55**:e27–e129.

Table 73.2 ACC/AHA 2010 GL on thoracic aortic disease. Recommendations for Takayasu's arteritis and giant cell arteritis

Corticosteroids at a high dose (prednisone 40 to 60 mg daily at initiation or its equivalent) to reduce the active inflammatory state.	I-B
The success of treatment should be periodically evaluated to determine disease activity by repeated physical examination and either an erythrocyte sedimentation rate or C-reactive protein level.	I-B
Elective revascularization should be delayed until the acute inflammatory state is treated and quiescent.	I-B
The initial evaluation should include thoracic aorta and branch vessel CT or MRI to investigate the possibility of aneurysm or occlusive disease.	I-C
Treat patients receiving corticosteroids with an additional anti-inflammatory agent if there is evidence of progression of vascular disease, recurrence of constitutional symptoms, or re-elevation of inflammatory marker.	IIa-C

Reproduced from 2010 ACCF/AHA/AATS/ACR/ASA/SCA/SCAI/SIR/STS/SVM Guidelines for the diagnosis and management of patients with thoracic aortic disease. *J Am Coll Cardiol*. 2010;**55**:e27–e129.

Giant cell (temporal) arteritis

Definition

Giant cell arteritis involves the aorta and its secondary and tertiary branches, and especially the external and internal carotids, and shares the same pathology with Takayasu's arteritis.

Epidemiology

It mainly affects patients above 50 years (with a peak at 75–85 years, women:men in a 3:2 ratio) and has a predilection for northern Europeans. Its incidence in the USA is 20/100 000.[2]

Pathophysiology

This is also a T cell-mediated arteritis that mainly involves the extracranial branches of the aorta and spares intracranial vessels. In medium-sized arteries, inflammation results in narrowing and obstruction of vessels, but, in the thoracic aorta, aneurysm formation and rupture may be caused.

Presentation

It is variable. Half of the patients report **malaise, fever, night sweats, weight loss, and depression. Headache, scalp tenderness, and abnormal temporal arteries** are present in most patients with biopsy-proven disease. Jaw claudication is common (50%), visual changes and/or neurologic symptoms and stroke develop in one-third of patients. Diplopia, amaurosis fugax, or blurriness are important to notice since, if left untreated, permanent blindness may occur. Up to 30% of patients develop large artery complications, such as aortic aneurysm/dissection and stenosis of the vertebral, subclavian, and brachial arteries.[7] Approximately 40% of patients also have polymyalgia rheumatica, which has the same genetic risk factors and acute-phase responses.[2]

Diagnosis

It is established by, at least, three of the 1990 American College of Rheumatology criteria: (1) age older than 50 years, (2) recent-onset localized headache, (3) temporal artery pulse attenuation or tenderness, (4) erythrocyte sedimentation rate greater than 50 mm/h, and (5) an arterial biopsy demonstrating necrotizing vasculitis. With intracranial disease, temporal artery biopsies (performed within 7 days of steroid initiation) are diagnostic in up to 80% of cases.[1]

Therapy

Immunosuppression with steroids and aspirin for 1 or 2 years is the treatment of choice. Steroids are essential to prevent blindness, although exacerbations of the disease may be seen in 30–59% of patients (Table 73.2).

References

1. Hiratzka LF, *et al.* 2010 ACCF/AHA/AATS/ACR/ASA/SCA/SCAI/SIR/STS/SVM guidelines for the diagnosis and management of patients with thoracic aortic disease: a report of the American College of Cardiology Foundation/American Heart Association Task Force on practice guidelines, American Association for Thoracic Surgery, American College of Radiology, American Stroke Association, Society of Cardiovascular Anesthesiologists, Society for Cardiovascular Angiography and Interventions, Society of Interventional Radiology, Society of Thoracic Surgeons, and Society for Vascular Medicine. *Circulation.* 2010;**121**:e266–369
2. Weyand CM, *et al.* Medium- and large-vessel vasculitis. *N Engl J Med.* 2003;**349**:160–9
3. Kerr GS, *et al.* Takayasu arteritis. *Ann Intern Med.* 1994;**120**:919–29
4. Arend WP, *et al.* The American College of Rheumatology 1990 criteria for the classification of Takayasu arteritis. *Arthritis Rheum.* 1990;**33**:1129–34
5. Maksimowicz-McKinnon K. New insights into the pathogenesis and treatment of Takayasu arteritis. *Expert Rev Clin Immunol.* 2009;**5**:445–9
6. Saadoun D, *et al.* Retrospective analysis of surgery versus endovascular intervention in Takayasu arteritis: a multicenter experience. *Circulation.* 2012;**125**:813–19
7. Nuenninghoff DM, *et al.* Incidence and predictors of large-artery complication (aortic aneurysm, aortic dissection, and/or large-artery stenosis) in patients with giant cell arteritis: a population-based study over 50 years. *Arthritis Rheum.* 2003;**48**:3522–31

Part XV

Venous thromboembolism

Relevant guidelines

ESC 2008 guidelines on pulmonary embolism

Guidelines on the diagnosis and management of acute pulmonary embolism: the Task Force for the Diagnosis and Management of Acute Pulmonary Embolism of the European Society of Cardiology (ESC). *Eur Heart J*. 2008;**29**:2276–315.

AHA 2011 scientific statement on pulmonary embolism, iliofemoral deep vein thrombosis, and chronic thromboembolic pulmonary hypertension

Management of massive and submassive pulmonary embolism, iliofemoral deep vein thrombosis, and chronic thromboembolic pulmonary hypertension: a scientific statement from the American Heart Association. *Circulation*. 2011;**123**:1788–830.

ACP 2011 guideline on venous thromboembolism prophylaxis in hospitalized patients

Venous thromboembolism prophylaxis in hospitalized patients: a clinical practice guideline from the American College of Physicians. *Ann Intern Med*. 2011;**155**:625–32.

ACCP 2012 guidelines on antithrombotic therapy

American College of Chest Physicians Antithrombotic Therapy and Prevention of Thrombosis Panel. Executive summary: Antithrombotic Therapy and Prevention of Thrombosis, 9th ed: American College of Chest Physicians Evidence-Based Clinical Practice Guidelines. *Chest*. 2012;**141**(2 Suppl):7S–47S. Erratum in: *Chest*. 2012;**141**:1129.

ESC 2011 guidelines on pregnancy

ESC guidelines on the management of cardiovascular diseases during pregnancy. *Eur Heart J*. 2011;**32**:3147–97.

Chapter 74

Pulmonary embolism

Definitions

Venous thromboembolism denotes pulmonary embolism and deep venous thrombosis. Pulmonary embolism (PE) refers to embolization of usually thrombotic material to pulmonary arteries, with complete or partial occlusion of one or more of their branches. Venous thromboembolism (VTE) includes PE and deep venous thrombosis (DVT).[1]

Epidemiology

Pulmonary embolism is a common, potentially life-threatening cardiopulmonary illness. The mortality rate associated with PE is 15% in the first 3 months after diagnosis and, in nearly 25% of the cases, present with sudden death.[1] The annual incidence of VTE, in general, is approximately 1.2 cases per 1000 adults.[1,2] PE usually occurs 3–7 days after the onset of DVT.[3] Blacks have a 3-fold higher incidence for PE than whites, and blacks and Hispanics suffer fatal PE at a significantly younger age than whites.[4]

Pathophysiology

Pulmonary emboli most often arise from the deep veins of the lower extremity and pelvis and, very rarely, from subclavian or arm veins. Their consequences become apparent when more than 30–50% of the pulmonary arterial bed is occluded.[3] In addition to obstruction, acute PE leads to the release of pulmonary artery vasoconstrictors and hypoxaemia, with a subsequent increase in pulmonary vascular resistance and right ventricular afterload, RV dilatation, and tricuspid regurgitation.[5] RV pressure overload can also lead to interventricular septal flattening and deviation toward the left ventricle in diastole, thereby impairing LV filling. The subsequent reduction in coronary artery perfusion pressure, in the context of the increased wall stress, leads to RV ischaemia and subsequent failure. Ventilation to perfusion mismatch, increases in total dead space, impaired transfer of carbon monoxide due to loss of gas exchange surface, and decreased pulmonary compliance caused by lung oedema result in arterial hypoxaemia and an increased alveolar-arterial oxygen gradient. Hyperventilation may contribute to hypocapnia and respiratory alkalosis. The presence of hypercapnia suggests massive PE, leading to increased anatomical and physiological dead space and impaired minute ventilation.[1,5]

Aetiology

Venous stasis, hypercoagulability, and endothelial damage predispose to VTE (Table 74.1). A **family history** of thromboembolism in ≥2 siblings is a major risk factor for venous thromboembolism.[6] **Obesity, smoking**, and **long-haul air travel** are recognized causes of PE. Thrombophilias cause impaired neutralization of thrombin or failure to control thrombin generation and thus predispose to VTE. The most common inherited thrombophilias are **factor V Leiden** (autosomal dominant single-point mutation that brings resistance to activated protein C) and a mutation in the **prothrombin gene G20210A**. Homozygous patients are at higher risk. They are difficult to identify, and the most

Table 74.1 Major risk factors for venous thromboembolism

Inherited*
Factor V Leiden mutation
Prothrombin gene (factor II) mutation (G20210A, mainly in whites and Hispanics)
Hyperhomocysteinaemia (mutation in methylene tetrahydrofolate reductase)
Deficiency of antithrombin III, protein C, or protein S
Acquired
Age
Smoking
Obesity
Malignancy
Hip frcture
Surgery (orthopedic or surgery for cancer)
Spinal cord injury
Antiphospholipid antibody syndrome
Hyperhomocysteinaemia due to folate deficiency
Hormone replacement therapy and oral contraceptive pills (including progesterone-only and, especially, third-generation pills)
Personal or family history of venous thromboembolism
Recent trauma or hospitalization
Acute infection
Long-haul air travel (flight distances >500 km)
Congestive heart failure
Pacemaker or implantable cardiac defibrillator leads and indwelling venous catheters

* A family history of VTE in siblings is a major risk factor

important action is to obtain a careful family history. Deficiencies of antithrombin 3, protein C, and protein S are very rare. The Women's Health Initiative study documented a 2-fold increase of VTE among women on combined oestrogen and progesterone preparations,[7] and a history of PE or DVT is an absolute contraindication to **oral contraceptives.** Combined oral contraceptives with levonorgestrel or norgestimate confer half the risk of venous thrombosis than oral contraceptives containing desogestrel, gestodene, or drospirenone. Progestogen-only pills do not confer an increased risk of venous thrombosis.

Women who use combined contraceptive transdermal patches containing norelgestromin (the active metabolite of norgestimate) and ethinylestradiol or vaginal rings with etonogestrel (third-generation progestogen) and ethinylestradiol are at an increased risk of venous thrombosis.[8] The risk of venous thrombosis is not significantly increased with the use of subcutaneous implants containing etonogestrel only and the levonorgestrel intrauterine system.[8] Thrombosis of the **popliteal vein or more proximally,** and especially iliofemoral deep vein thrombosis, carries a higher risk for PE than isolated calf vein thrombosis.[9] Cancer should be suspected in patients who have recurrent idiopathic VTE.[10] Female sex, lung cancer, TNM stage >1, and previous VTE indicate a higher risk of VTE in cancer patients.[11]

In 30% of cases, PE occurs in the absence of any predisposing factors.[3] Heart diseases increase the near-term risk for pulmonary embolism not associated with diagnosed peripheral vein thrombosis.[12] Acute infection that requires hospitalization, blood transfusion, and the use of erythropoiesis-stimulating agents are also possible triggers for acute VTE in non-cancer patients.[13]

Presentation

The presentation of PE ranges from mild dyspnoea to cardiogenic shock, thus making the disease difficult to diagnose. Dyspnoea is the most common symptom and tachypnoea the most common physical sign. Patients may be anxious, but otherwise completely asymptomatic, or present with hypotension and cyanosis. Pleuritic pain, cough, or haemoptysis indicate pulmonary infarction by a peripherally located PE.

Diagnosis

Pulmonary embolism should be suspected in all patients who present with new or worsening dyspnoea, chest pain, or sustained hypotension without an alternative obvious cause, but the diagnosis is confirmed by objective testing in only about 20% of patients.[14]

Chest X-ray is usually normal. Findings, such as focal oligaemia (Westermark sign), a peripheral wedge-shaped opacity, usually in the lower half of the lung field (Hampton's hump), or an enlarged right descending pulmonary artery (Pallas's sign) are rare.[1]

ECG may reveal signs of RV strain, including incomplete or complete RBBB, T wave inversion in the anterior precordium, and S wave in lead I and Q wave and T wave inversion in lead III (the $S_1Q_3T_3$ patterns), or may mimic an old inferior MI. It may be also be normal, especially in the young.

Echocardiography is insensitive for diagnosis, but the detection of RV dysfunction is an ominous prognostic factor. Regional RV dysfunction with free wall hypokinesia sparing the apex (McConnel sign) is specific for PE but seen with massive emboli.[1]

D-dimer ELISA can be used to exclude PE in patients with a low suspicion of PE. D-dimer is a degradation product of fibrin that is also produced in a wide variety of conditions, such as cancer, inflammation and dissection of the aorta, and pregnancy. The test is, therefore, of limited value in high probability of PE because co-morbid conditions may have already raised the D-dimer levels. The specificity of the test is also reduced in hospitalized or elderly patients. The usually accepted threshold level is 500 ng/mL, although a cut-off value of 750 microNewgram/L for patients aged 60 years and older has been proposed for the exclusion of deep vein thrombosis.[15]

Chest CT with a multidetector scanner (MCT) and the use of intravenous contrast are the principal diagnostic imaging modality, with a negative predictive value 95–99%.[1,14] In patients with a high clinical probability of pulmonary embolism and negative findings on MCT, the value of additional testing is controversial. Venous ultrasonography shows a deep vein thrombosis in less than 1% of such patients.[14] MCT is considered, at least, as accurate as **invasive pulmonary angiography.**[1] **Magnetic resonance** imaging is less sensitive.[5]

Ventilation perfusion (V/Q) scans are reserved for patients with renal failure, allergy to contrast dye, or when a multidetector CT scanner is not available. A normal scan rules out a PE but is diagnostic in 20–50% of patients with suspected PE.[14] MCT delivers a higher dose of radiation to the mother but a lower dose to the fetus than V/Q lung scanning. Single photo emission tomography ventilation perfusion (SPECT V/Q) is a promising new modality with better sensitivity than planar V/Q.[16]

Venous ultrasonography (compression ultrasonography), which has now replaced venography, should precede imaging tests in pregnant women and in patients with contraindication to CT scanning. Confirmed DVT in patients with suspected PE is an indication for anticoagulation therapy.[14]

A diagnostic work-up is shown in Figure 74.1. Clinical prediction scores [17,18] and diagnostic criteria are presented in Tables 74.2 and 74.3. The Revised Geneva score[17] is more comprehensive than the Wells score.[18] Detailed recommendations have also been provided by the ACCP 2012 guidelines on antithrombotic therapy.[19]

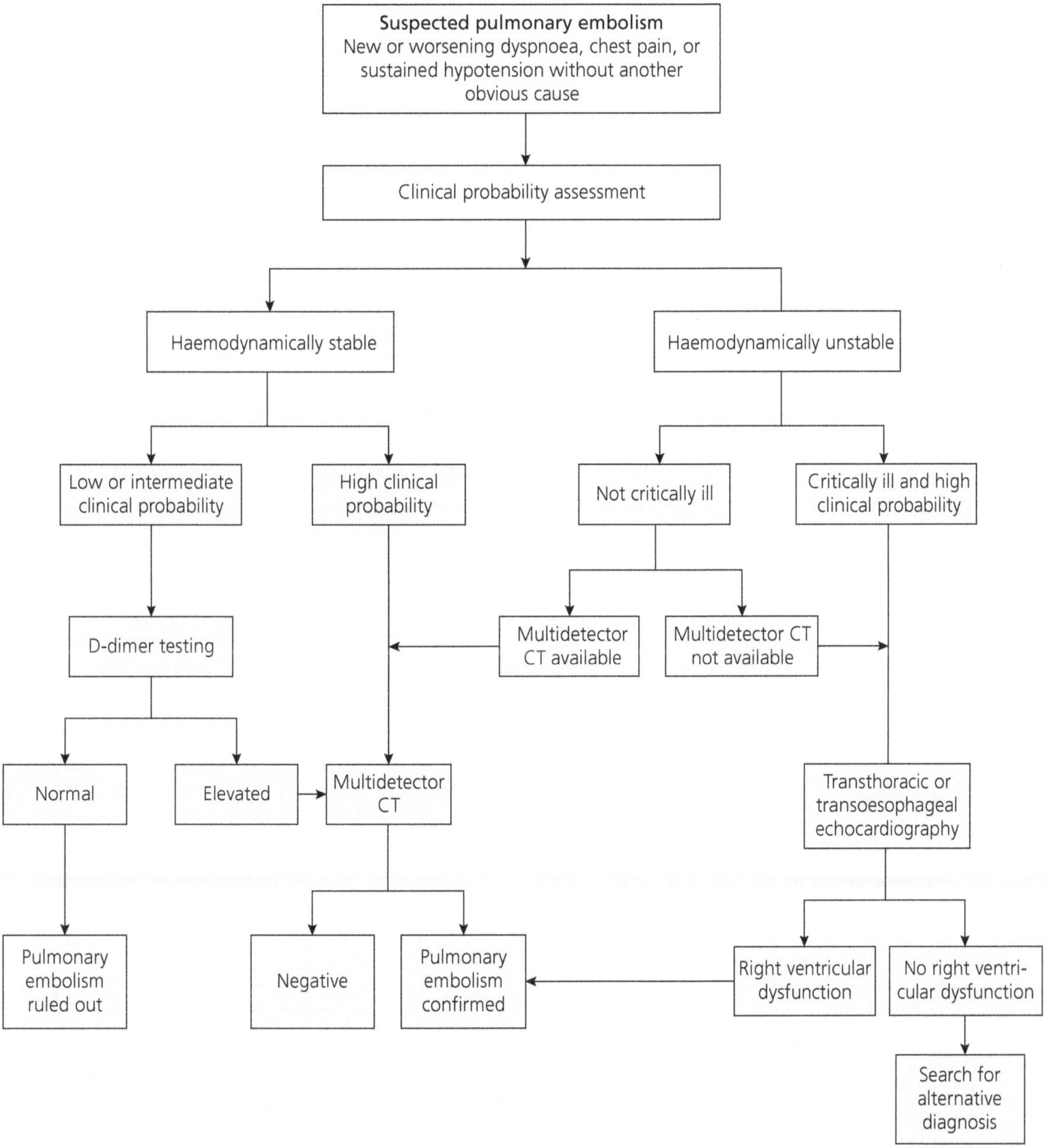

Figure 74.1 Diagnostic Workup for pulmonary embolism. The initial assessment of the clinical probability of pulmonary embolism is based on either clinical judgement or clinical decision rules (Wells and revised Geneva scores). Patients are considered to be haemodynamically unstable if they are in shock or have a systolic blood pressure of less than 90 mmHg or a drop in pressure of more than 40 mmHg for more than 15 minutes (in the absence of new-onset arrhythmia, hypovolaemia, and sepsis). In cases in which multidetector CT is not available or in patients with renal failure or allergy to contrast dye, the use of ventilation perfusion scanning is an alternative. In patients with a high clinical probability and an elevated D-dimer level, but with negative findings on multidetector CT, venous ultrasonography should be considered. Among critically ill patients with right ventricular dysfunction, thrombolysis is an option; multidetector CT should be performed when the patient's condition has been stabilized if doubts remain about clinical management. In patients who are candidates for percutaneous embolectomy, conventional pulmonary angiography can be performed to confirm the diagnosis of pulmonary embolism immediately before the procedure, after the finding of right ventricular dysfunction.
Agnelli G, Becattini C. Acute pulmonary embolism. *N Engl J Med*. 2010;**363**:266–74.

Table 74.2 Clinical prediction rules for PE

Revised Geneva score	
Variable	**Points**
Predisposing factors	
Age >65 years	+1
Previous DVT or PE	+3
Surgery or fracture within 1 month	+2
Active malignancy	+2
Symptoms	
Unilateral lower limb pain	+3
Haemoptysis	+2
Clinical signs	
Heart rate	
75–94 beats/min	+3
≥95 beats/min	+5
Pain on lower limb, deep vein at palpation, and unilateral oedema	+4
Clinical probability	**Total**
Low	0–3
Intermediate	4–10
High	≥11

Le Gal G, *et al*. Prediction of pulmonary embolism in the emergency department: the revised Geneva score. *Ann Intern Med* 2006;**144**:165–71.

Risk stratification

The simplified version of the Pulmonary Embolism Severity Index (sPESI) is a practical way for risk stratification (Table 74.4). It is based on six equally weighted variables: age >80 years; history of cancer; history of heart failure or chronic lung disease; systolic blood pressure <100 mmHg; pulse rate >110 bpm; and arterial oxyhaemoglobin saturation <90%.[20]

Shock and sustained hypotension indicate an in-hospital mortality of 58% (ICOPE Registry).[21]

RV dysfunction, detected on echocardiography or MCT (RV diameter/LV diameter >0.9), is an independent predictor of mortality.[22] RV failure with haemodynamic compromise is encountered in <5% of all patients with acute PE and is associated with an, at least, 15% risk of in-hospital death within the first hours after admission.[23]

BNP and **pro-BNP** elevated levels, as well as **troponins**, also indicate an adverse outcome, especially in the context of echocardiographic RV dysfunction.[24,25] High-sensitivity troponin (hsTnT cut-off level of 14 pg/mL) exhibits a high prognostic sensitivity for excluding early PE-related death, and combination of hsTnT with sPESI (Table 74.2) improves the prediction of both acute and long-term outcome.[26]

Classification of PE

The recent AHA classification[9] is:

Massive PE

Acute PE with sustained hypotension (systolic blood pressure <90 mmHg for, at least, 15 minutes or requiring inotropic support, not due to a cause other than PE, such as arrhythmia, hypovolaemia, sepsis, or left ventricular dysfunction), pulselessness, or persistent profound bradycardia (heart rate <40 bpm with signs or symptoms of shock).

Submassive PE

Acute PE without systemic hypotension (systolic blood pressure <90 mmHg) but with either RV dysfunction or myocardial necrosis.

RV dysfunction is defined by the presence of, at least, one of the following:

- RV dilation (apical 4-chamber RV diameter divided by LV diameter >0.9) or RV systolic dysfunction on echocardiography
- RV dilation (4-chamber RV diameter divided by LV diameter >0.9) on CT
- Elevation of BNP (>90 pg/mL) or of N-terminal pro-BNP (>500 pg/mL)
- Electrocardiographic changes (new complete or incomplete RBBB, anteroseptal ST elevation or depression, or anteroseptal T wave inversion)

Myocardial necrosis is defined as elevation of troponin I (>0.4 ng/mL) or of troponin T (>0.1 ng/mL)

Low-risk PE

Acute PE and the absence of the clinical markers of adverse prognosis that define massive or submassive PE.

Acute therapy

Haemodynamically stable patients

Acute pulmonary embolism requires initial short-term therapy with **heparin (UFH or LMWH) or fondaparinux** for, at least, 5 days, followed by therapy with a vitamin K antagonist for, at least, 3 months, depending on the risk of recurrence (Tables 74.4 and 74.5). In patients with a high clinical probability of pulmonary embolism, anticoagulant treatment should be initiated while diagnostic confirmation is awaited. LMWH are, at least, as efficacious and safe as UFH.[27] Dose adjustment is needed in renal failure (see Chapter 27 on UA/NSTEMI). Fondaparinux is also efficacious and safe, compared to UFH,[28] and may be used in heparin-induced thrombocytopenia (although not approved for this purpose) but is contraindicated in creatinine clearance <20 mL/min.

Table 74.3 ESC 2008 guidelines on PE. Diagnosis of PE

Suspected high-risk PE	
Emergency CT or bedside echocardiography, as indicated by the presence of shock or hypotension.	I-C
Suspected non-high-risk PE	
Diagnostic strategy is based on clinical probability, assessed either implicitly or using a validated prediction rule.	I-A
Plasma D-dimer measurement in emergency department patients to reduce the need for unnecessary imaging and irradiation, preferably using a highly sensitive assay.	I-A
Lower limb compression venous ultrasonography (CUS) in search of DVT in selected patients with suspected PE to obviate the need for further imaging tests if the result is positive.	IIb-B
Systematic use of echocardiography for diagnosis in haemodynamically stable, normotensive patients is not recommended.	III-C
Pulmonary angiography when there is discrepancy between clinical evaluation and results of non-invasive imaging tests.	IIa-C
The use of validated criteria for diagnosing PE is recommended. Validated criteria, according to clinical probability of PE (low, intermediate, or high), are detailed below.	I-B
Suspected non-high-risk PE	
Low clinical probability	
Normal D-dimer level using either a highly or moderately sensitive assay excludes PE	I-A
Normal perfusion lung scintigraphy excludes PE	I-A
Non-diagnostic (low or intermediate probability) V/Q scan may exclude PE:	IIa-B
Particularly when combined with negative proximal CUS	I-A
Negative MDCT safely excludes PE	I-A
Negative SDCT only excludes PE when combined with negative proximal CUS	I-A
High-probability V/Q scan may confirm PE but:	IIa-B
Further testing may be considered in selected patients to confirm PE	IIb-B
Compression venous ultrasonograph showing a proximal DVT confirms PE	I-B
If compression venous ultrasonograph shows only a distal DVT, further testing to confirm PE	IIa-B
SDCT or MDCT showing a segmental or more proximal thrombus confirms PE	I-A
Further testing to confirm PE if SDCT or MDCT shows only subsegmental clots	IIa-B
Suspected non-high-risk PE	
Intermediate clinical probability	
Normal D-dimer level using a highly sensitive assay excludes PE	I-A
Further testing if D-dimer level is normal when using a less sensitive assay	IIa-B
Normal perfusion lung scintigraphy excludes PE	I-A
In non-diagnostic V/Q scan, further testing to exclude or confirm PE	I-B
Negative MDCT excludes PE	I-A
Negative SDCT only excludes PE when combined with negative proximal CUS	I-A
High-probability ventilation perfusion lung scintigraphy confirms PE	I-A
CUS showing a proximal DVT confirms PE	I-B
If CUS shows only a distal DVT, further testing should be considered	IIa-B
SDCT or MDCT showing a segmental or more proximal thrombus confirms PE	I-A
Further testing may be considered in case of subsegmental clots to confirm PE	IIb-B
Suspected non-high-risk PE	
High clinical probability	
D-dimer measurement is not recommended in high clinical probability patients, as a normal result does not safely exclude PE, even when using a highly sensitive assay	III-C
In patients with a negative CT, further tests should be considered in selected patients to exclude PE	IIa-B
High-probability ventilation perfusion lung scintigraphy confirms PE	I-A

(Continued)

Table 74.3 (Continued)

CUS showing a proximal DVT confirms PE	I-B
If CUS shows only a distal DVT, further testing should be considered	IIb-B
SDCT or MDCT showing a segmental or more proximal thrombus confirms PE	I-A
Further testing where there are subsegmental clots to confirm PE	IIb-B

CUS, Newcompression venous ultrasonography.

Guidelines on the diagnosis and management of acute pulmonary embolism: the Task Force for the Diagnosis and Management of Acute Pulmonary Embolism of the European Society of Cardiology (ESC). *Eur Heart J*. 2008;**29**:2276–315.

The risk of major bleeding with these agents is 3–6%. For heparin-induced thrombocytopenia, see also Chapter 27 on UA/NSTEMI.

- UFH: IV bolus 80 IU/kg (or 5000 IU), followed by continuous infusion 18 IU/kg/h (or 1000 IU/h), aiming at aPTT 1.5–2.5 control (measured 4–6 h after bolus and 3 h after each dose adjustment.
- Enoxaparin: 1 mg/kg/12 h SC (or 1.5 mg/kg/24 h in the USA)
- Fondaparinux: 5g SC (body weight <50 mg)
  - 7.5 mg SC (body weight 50–100 kg)
  - 10 mg SC (body weight >100 kg).

Stable, low-risk patients might be managed on an outpatient basis after discharge < or 24 h after diagnosis, with instructions on self-performed SC injections,[29] but more data are certainly needed.

Fibrinolysis confers no benefit over conventional anticoagulation in stable, low-risk patients with PE (Tables 74.4, 74.6).[30,31] In patients with submassive PE and pulmonary hypertension or RV dysfunction, fibrinolysis with alteplase and heparin thrombolysis reduces the rate of clinical deterioration albeit without reducing mortality,[32] and may also decrease the incidence of subsequeny chronic thromboembolic pulmonary hypertension. In intermediate-risk, normotensive patients, fibrinolysis with tenecteplace and heparin has conferred a reduction in death or hemodynamic collapse at 7 days, but at a significant excess in hemorrhagic stroke, especially in those >=75 years old (PEITHO trial).[33] Fibrinolysis is recommended in hypotensive patients (SBP<90 mm Hg) by the ACCP 2012 GL (2C). **Streptokinase** (250 000 IU over 30 min, followed by 100 000 IU/h over 12–24 h, or preferably 1.5 million IU over 2h), **urokinase** (4400 IU/kg over 10 min, then 4400 IU/kg/h over 12–24 h, or 3 million IU over 2 h), and **alteplase** (tPA, 100 mg over 2 h or 0.6 mg/kg over 15 min up to 50 mg) are the approved agents. UFH heparin is discontinued before thrombolysis and restarted when the aPTT is <80 s, but it can be continued with alteplase or tenecteplace.[3,32] Tenecteplase and rateplase have also been tried successfully. All thrombolytics should be given intravenously since direct administration into the pulmonary artery has not been found superior. The greatest benefit is observed when treatment is initiated within 48 h of symptom onset, but thrombolysis can still be useful in patients who have symptoms for 6–14 days.[3] A rate of 9% major bleeding and <0.5% intracranial haemorrhage has been reported in recent trials.[32] Contraindications to thrombolysis, such as intracranial disease, uncontrolled hypertension, ischaemic stroke in previous 6 months, major surgery or trauma within the last 3 weeks, and gastrointestinal bleeding within the last month, are discussed in Chapter 26 on MI.

Table 74.4 Risk stratification in PE. **Simplified pulmonary embolism severity index (sPESI)**

Variable	Score
Age >80 y	1
History of cancer	1
History of heart failure or chronic lung disease	1
Pulse ≥110 bpm	1
Systolic BP <100 mmHg	1
SaO_2 <90%	1

Total score 0, low risk; ≥1, high risk.

Jimenez D, *et al*. Simplification of the pulmonary embolism severity index for prognostication in patients with acute symptomatic pulmonary embolism. *Arch Intern Med*. 2010;**170**:1383–9.

The short-acting oral Xa inhibitor **rivaroxaban** (15 mg twice daily for 3 weeks, followed by 20 mg once daily without initial heparin) was recently found to treat equally well PE compared to enoxaparin followed by a vitamin K antagonist, albeit with less bleeding risk.[34] Apixaban (10 mg bd for 7 days, followed by 5 mg bd for 6 months) was also equally effective to conventional therapy but with significantly less bleeding in patients with PE or DVT.[35]

Haemodynamically unstable patients

They should be treated with pharmacological or mechanical thrombolysis.

Modest fluid challenge (500 mL dextran) may increase cardiac index. Aggressive volume expansion may worsen RV function. Nasal oxygen should be given for hypoxia.

Table 74.5 ESC 2008. Therapy of PE

ESC 2008 guidelines on PE. Acute therapy of PE	
High-risk pulmonary embolism	
Anticoagulation with unfractionated heparin initiated without delay	I-A
Systemic hypotension is corrected to prevent progression of RV failure and death	I-C
Vasopressive drugs for hypotensive patients	I-C
Dobutamine and dopamine in low cardiac output and normal blood pressure	IIa-B
Aggressive fluid challenge is not recommended	III-B
Oxygen in patients with hypoxaemia	I-C
Thrombolytic therapy in cardiogenic shock and/or persistent arterial hypotension	I-A
Surgical pulmonary embolectomy if thrombolysis is absolutely contraindicated or has failed	I-C
Catheter embolectomy or fragmentation of proximal pulmonary arterial clots as an alternative to surgical treatment when thrombolysis is absolutely contraindicated or has failed	IIb-C
Non-high-risk pulmonary embolism	
Anticoagulation initiated without delay while diagnostic work-up is still ongoing	I-C
LMWH or fondaparinux as initial treatment	I-A
In patients at high risk of bleeding and in those with severe renal dysfunction, unfractionated heparin (UFH) with an aPTT 1.5–2.5 times normal as initial treatment	I-C
Initial treatment with UFH, LMWH or fondaparinux for, at least, 5 days and replaced by vitamin K antagonists only after achieving target INR levels,	I-A
For, at least, 2 consecutive days	I-C
Routine use of thrombolysis in non-high-risk PE patients is not recommended, but it may be considered in selected patients with intermediate-risk PE	IIb-B
Thrombolytic therapy should be not used in patients with low-risk PE	III-B
ESC 2008 guidelines on PE. Acute and long-term therapy of PE	
For PE secondary to a transient (reversible) risk factor, treatment with a VKA for 3 months	I-A
For unprovoked PE, treatment with a VKA for, at least, 3 months	I-A
Long-term oral anticoagulation after a first episode of unprovoked PE and low risk of bleeding and when stable anticoagulation can be achieved	IIb-B
Long-term treatment for patients with a second episode of unprovoked PE recommended	I-A
In patients on long-term anticoagulants, the risk/benefit ratio of continuing such treatment should be reassessed at regular intervals	I-C
For patients with PE and cancer, LMWH should be considered for the first 3–6 months,	IIa-B
After this period, VKA or LMWH should be continued indefinitely or until the cancer is considered cured	I-C
VKA to maintain INR of 2.5 (range 2.0–3.0), regardless of treatment duration	I-A

Guidelines on the diagnosis and management of acute pulmonary embolism: the Task Force for the Diagnosis and Management of Acute Pulmonary Embolism of the European Society of Cardiology (ESC). *Eur Heart J*. 2008;**29**:2276–315.

Table 74.6 AHA 2011 scientific statement

Recommendations for initial anticoagulation for acute PE	
Subcutaneous LMWH, intravenous or subcutaneous UFH with monitoring, unmonitored weight-based subcutaneous UFH, or subcutaneous fondaparinux in patients with objectively confirmed PE.	I-A
Therapeutic anticoagulation during the diagnostic work-up to patients with intermediate or high clinical probability of PE and no contraindications to anticoagulation.	I-C

SC LMWH (one daily double dose) or fondaparinux are preferred to UFH by the ACCP 2012 GL (2C).

AHA 2011 scientific statement on pulmonary embolism, iliofemoral deep vein thrombosis, and chronic thromboembolic pulmonary hypertension. *Circulation*. 2011;**123**:1788–830.

Table 74.7 AHA 2011 scientific statement

Recommendations for fibrinolysis for acute PE	
Patients with massive acute PE and acceptable risk of bleeding complications.	IIa-B
Patients with submassive acute PE and adverse prognosis (new haemodynamic instability, worsening respiratory insufficiency, severe RV dysfunction, or major myocardial necrosis) and low risk of bleeding complications.	IIb-C
Patients with low-risk PE, submassive acute PE with minor RV dysfunction, minor myocardial necrosis, and no clinical worsening.	III-B
Undifferentiated cardiac arrest.	III-B

AHA 2011 scientific statement on pulmonary embolism, iliofemoral deep vein thrombosis, and chronic thromboembolic pulmonary hypertension. *Circulation*. 2011;**123**:1788–830.

If mechanical ventilation is necessary, positive end-expiratory pressure should be applied with caution since it may worsen RV failure.

Dobutamine and **epinephrine** in case of hypotension are the agents of choice if inotropic support is needed.[3] Cardiac index should not be raised above physiological values without proper reperfusion therapy since this may aggravate the ventilation perfusion mismatch.

Fibrinolysis offers a 50% reduction in mortality and is clearly indicated in patients with haemodynamic instability.[31] Percutaneous mechanical thrombectomy (thrombus fragmentation and aspiration) and surgical embolectomy are offered to high-risk patients with contraindication to thrombolytic treatment and those in whom thrombolytic treatment has not improved haemodynamic status.

Percutaneous mechanical thrombectomy confers a clinical success in 86.5% of cases at a rate of major procedural complications of 2.4% (Table 74.7).[36] Three main categories exist:

1. Aspiration thrombectomy through a dedicated sunction catheter.
2. Thrombus fragmentation through a balloon, manually rotating pigtail, or a dedicated device.
3. Rheolytic thrombectomy through high-velocity jet sunction catheters.

Practical aspects have been recently reviewed.[37,38]

Pharmacomechanical therapy, i.e. low-dose, local fibrinolysis, combined with thrombus fragmentation or aspiration, may also be used in massive, centrally located thrombi.[30] Ultrasound accelerated thrombolysis via a dedicated catheter is a new option for life-threatening conditions.[39]

Surgical embolectomy may be now performed off bypass and without aortic cross-clamping, with a <10% intraoperative mortality in experienced centres.

Table 74.8 AHA 2011 scientific statement

Recommendations for catheter embolectomy and fragmentation	
Depending on local expertise, either catheter embolectomy and fragmentation or surgical embolectomy is reasonable for patients with massive PE and contraindications to fibrinolysis.	IIa-C
Catheter embolectomy and fragmentation or surgical embolectomy for patients with massive PE who remain unstable after receiving fibrinolysis.	IIa-C
Transfer patients with massive PE who cannot receive fibrinolysis or who remain unstable after fibrinolysis to an institution experienced in either catheter embolectomy or surgical embolectomy if these procedures are not available locally and safe transfer can be achieved.	IIa-C
Catheter embolectomy or surgical embolectomy for patients with submassive acute PE judged to have clinical evidence of adverse prognosis (new haemodynamic instability, worsening respiratory failure, severe RV dysfunction, or major myocardial necrosis).	IIb-C
Catheter embolectomy or surgical thrombectomy for patients with low-risk PE or submassive acute PE with minor RV dysfunction, minor myocardial necrosis, and no clinical worsening.	III-C

AHA 2011 scientific statement on pulmonary embolism, iliofemoral deep vein thrombosis, and chronic thromboembolic pulmonary hypertension. *Circulation*. 2011;**123**:1788–830.

Long-term therapy

Vitamin K antagonists are started at the first day of IV/SC anticoagulation, with a target of INR 2–3. In patients with pulmonary embolism secondary to a temporary (reversible) risk factor, therapy with vitamin K antagonists should be given for 3 months (ACCP 2012 1B). The risk of recurrent pulmonary embolism is less than 1% per year on anticoagulation and 2 to 10% per year after the discontinuation of such therapy.[14] Thus, the duration of long-term anticoagulation should be based on the risk of recurrence after cessation of treatment with vitamin K antagonists and the risk of bleeding during treatment.[40] Male sex, proximal DVT, elevated D-dimer levels after discontinuing anticoagulation[41] as well as cancer, inherited thrombophilia (factors V and II—Table 74.1, obesity, and unprovoked pulmonary embolism indicate candidates for indefinite anticoagulation with periodic reassessment of the risk-benefit ratio. An INR of

2–3 is recommended during the first 3 to 6 months after the acute event. After an initial course, low-intensity therapy (INR 1.5–1.9) may be an option.[42] **Rivaroxaban** (15 mg twice daily for 3 weeks, followed by 20 mg once daily) has also been tried for acute and long-term therapy.[34] In acutely ill medical patients, rivaroxaban (10 mg daily for 35 days) reduced the risk of venous thromboembolism but with an increased risk of bleeding.[43] The oral antithrombin **dabigatran** (see Chapter 52 on AF) has also been shown not inferior to warfarin in patients with PE or deep vein thrombosis, without increasing the risk of bleeding.[44] In patients who had already completed a 3-month course of anticoagulation with either warfarin or dabigatran, continuation of dabigatran 150 mg bd was as effective and carried a lower risk of bleeding than warfarin, although there was increased incidence of acute coronary syndromes.[45] In the recent ACCP 2012 guidelines, a weak recommendation is given in favour of VKA and LMWH therapy over dabigatran and rivaroxaban due to lack of post-marketing safety data at the time of manuscript preparation, but it is mentioned that these agents are more convenient for the patients and may be associated with improved clinical outcomes.[19] The FDA has approved rivaroxaban for treatment and prophylaxis of both DVT and PE. Extended anticoagulation with **apixaban** for 12 months at 5 or 2.5 mg bd in patients who had already completed a 6–12 months course of anticoagulation with warfarin or apixaban, has also reduced the risk of recurrent venous thromboembolism without increasing the rate of major bleeding.[46] Following anticoagulation therapy for 3–6 months, aspirin administration reduces the rate of venous thromboembolism and major vascular events.[47,48] **Statin** therapy decreases the risk of recurrent PE, irrespective of VKA.[49]

Retrievable vena cava filters should be reserved for patients with contraindications to anticoagulation (Tables 74.8 and 74.9). Permanent vena cava filters increase the risk of DVT.[50]

Special conditions

PE in heart failure

The relative risk of PE doubles in patients with heart failure.[51] Diagnosis may be difficult and is based on the presence of dyspnoea and hypoxaemia out of proportion to findings of vascular congestion, new or worsened right greater than left heart failure (especially high JVP in the absence of pulmonary rales), and demonstration of new or worsened RV dilatation and dysfunction on echocardi-

Table 74.9 ESC 2008 guidelines on PE

Recommendations for venous filters	
IVC filters when there are absolute contraindications to anticoagulation and a high risk of venous thromboembolism recurrence.	IIb-B
The routine use of IVC filters is not recommended.	III-B

Guidelines on the diagnosis and management of acute pulmonary embolism: the Task Force for the Diagnosis and Management of Acute Pulmonary Embolism of the European Society of Cardiology (ESC). *Eur Heart J.* 2008;**29**:2276–315.

Table 74.10 AHA 2011 scientific statement . Recommendations on IVC filters in the setting of acute PE

IVC filter to patients with any confirmed acute PE (or proximal DVT) and contraindications to anticoagulation or with active bleeding complication.	I-C
Resume anticoagulation in patients with an IVC filter once contraindications to anticoagulation or active bleeding complications have been resolved.	I-C
Patients with retrievable IVC filters should be evaluated periodically for filter retrieval within the specific filter's retrieval window.	I-C
IVC filter to patients with recurrent acute PE despite therapeutic anticoagulation.	IIa-C
Permanent IVC filter device for DVT or PE patients who will require permanent IVC filtration (e.g. those with a long-term contraindication to anticoagulation).	IIa-C
Retrievable IVC filter device or DVT or PE patients with a time-limited indication for an IVC filter (e.g. those with a short-term contraindication to anticoagulation therapy).	IIa-C
IVC filter for patients with acute PE and very poor cardiopulmonary reserve, including those with massive PE.	IIb-C
Routine use of IVC filter as an adjuvant to anticoagulation.	III-C

AHA 2011 scientific statement on pulmonary embolism, iliofemoral deep vein thrombosis, and chronic thromboembolic pulmonary hypertension. *Circulation*. 2011;**123**:1788–830.

Table 74.11 AHA 2011 scientific statement. Recommendations on PFO in the face of a PE

Screening for PFO with an echocardiogram with agitated saline bubble study or transcranial Doppler study in patients with massive or submassive PE.	IIb-C
Surgical embolectomy for patients with any type of PE found to have impending paradoxical embolism (thrombus entrapped within a PFO).	IIb-C

AHA 2011 scientific statement on pulmonary embolism, iliofemoral deep vein thrombosis, and chronic thromboembolic pulmonary hypertension. *Circulation*. 2011;**123**:1788–830.

ography or chest CT. Elevated biomarkers and D-dimers are of no help. Oral anticoagulation is more difficult to manage due to stasis and concomitant medications (amiodarone and clopidogrel potentiate the effect of warfarin whereas spironolactone accelerates its metabolism). VTE prophylaxis with stockings, pneumatic compression devices, or LMWH or warfarin are indicated in all hospitalized patients with heart failure.[51]

Right heart thrombi

Thrombolysis is also indicated in the presence of right heart thrombi (in <4% of patients with PE), although surgical embolectomy may be required in the presence of massive thrombi, especially those straddling the interatrial septum through the foramen ovale. Conventional anticoagulation is not effective.[3]

Non-thrombotic PE

Air embolism may occur during catheterization procedures. Haemodynamic consequences depend on the amount injected. Nasal oxygen is the treatment of choice. **Fat** embolism occurs after fracture of long bones and, rarely, with liposuction, lipid and propofol infusions, and hepatic necrosis. **Septic, tumour, and talk** (drug abusers) emboli may also occur. Amniotic fluid embolism is rare but potentially catastrophic (1/8000–1/80 000 pregnancies). Treatment is supportive.[3]

PFO in the presence of PE

This is discussed in the Chapter on cardiomyopathies. Recommendations of AHA are presented in Table 74.10.

References

1. Piazza G, *et al.* Acute pulmonary embolism: part I: epidemiology and diagnosis. *Circulation*. 2006;**114**:e28–32
2. Heit JA. The epidemiology of venous thromboembolism in the community. *Arterioscler Thromb Vasc Biol.* 2008;**28**:370–2
3. Torbicki A, *et al.* Guidelines on the diagnosis and management of acute pulmonary embolism: the Task Force for the diagnosis and management of acute pulmonary embolism of the European Society of Cardiology (ESC). *Eur Heart J.* 2008;**29**:2276–315
4. Tang Y, *et al.* Ethnic differences in out-of-hospital fatal pulmonary embolism. *Circulation*. 2011;**123**:2219–25
5. Goldhaber SZ. Pulmonary embolism. *Lancet.* 2004;**363**:1295–305
6. Zoller B, *et al.* Age- and gender-specific familial risks for venous thromboembolism: a nationwide epidemiological study based on hospitalizations in Sweden. *Circulation.* 2011;**124**:1012–20
7. Rossouw JE, *et al.* Risks and benefits of estrogen plus progestin in healthy postmenopausal women: principal results from the Women's Health Initiative randomized controlled trial. *JAMA*. 2002;**288**:321–33
8. Lidegaard O, *et al.* Venous thrombosis in users of non-oral hormonal contraception: follow-up study, Denmark 2001–10. *BMJ*. 2012;**344**:e2990
9. Jaff MR, *et al.* Management of massive and submassive pulmonary embolism, iliofemoral deep vein thrombosis, and chronic thromboembolic pulmonary hypertension: a scientific statement from the American Heart Association. *Circulation*. 2011;**123**:1788–830
10. Prandoni P, *et al.* Deep-vein thrombosis and the incidence of subsequent symptomatic cancer. *N Engl J Med.* 1992;**327**:1128–33
11. Louzada ML, *et al.* Development of a clinical prediction rule for risk stratification of recurrent venous thromboembolism in patients with cancer-associated venous thromboembolism. *Circulation*. 2012;**126**:448–54
12. Sorensen HT, *et al.* Heart disease may be a risk factor for pulmonary embolism without peripheral deep venous thrombosis. *Circulation*. 2011;**124**:1435–41
13. Rogers MA, *et al.* Triggers of hospitalization for venous thromboembolism. *Circulation*. 2012;**125**:2092–9
14. Agnelli G, *et al.* Acute pulmonary embolism. *N Engl J Med.* 2010;**363**:266–74
15. Schouten HJ, *et al.* Validation of two age dependent D-dimer cut-off values for exclusion of deep vein thrombosis in suspected elderly patients in primary care: retrospective, cross sectional, diagnostic analysis. *BMJ.* 2012;**344**:e2985
16. Le Duc-Pennec A, *et al.* Diagnostic accuracy of single-photon emission tomography ventilation/perfusion lung scan in the diagnosis of pulmonary embolism. *Chest.* 2012;**141**:381–7
17. Le Gal G, *et al.* Prediction of pulmonary embolism in the emergency department: the revised Geneva score. *Ann Intern Med.* 2006;**144**:165–71
18. Wells PS, *et al.* Use of a clinical model for safe management of patients with suspected pulmonary embolism. *Ann Intern Med.* 1998;**129**:997–1005
19. Guyatt GH, *et al.* Introduction to the ninth edition: Antithrombotic therapy and prevention of thrombosis, 9th ed: American College of Chest Physicians evidence-based clinical practice guidelines. *Chest.* 2012;**141**:48S–52S
20. Lankeit M, *et al.* A strategy combining imaging and laboratory biomarkers in comparison with a simplified clinical score for risk stratification of patients with acute pulmonary embolism. *Chest.* 2012;**141**:916–22

21. Goldhaber SZ, *et al.* Acute pulmonary embolism: Clinical outcomes in the International COoperative Pulmonary Embolism Registry (ICOPER). *Lancet.* 1999;**353**:1386–9
22. Becattini C, *et al.* Multidetector computed tomography for acute pulmonary embolism: diagnosis and risk stratification in a single test. *Eur Heart J.* 2011;**32**:1657–63
23. Konstantinides S, *et al.* Pulmonary embolism: risk assessment and management. *Eur Heart J.* 2012;**33**:3014–22
24. Becattini C, *et al.* Prognostic value of troponins in acute pulmonary embolism: a meta-analysis. *Circulation.* 2007;**116**:427–33
25. Klok FA, *et al.* Brain-type natriuretic peptide levels in the prediction of adverse outcome in patients with pulmonary embolism: a systematic review and meta-analysis. *Am J Respir Crit Care Med.* 2008;**178**:425–30
26. Lankeit M, *et al.* Predictive value of the high-sensitivity troponin T assay and the simplified pulmonary embolism severity index in haemodynamically stable patients with acute pulmonary embolism: a prospective validation study. *Circulation.* 2011;**124**:2716–24
27. Quinlan DJ, *et al.* Low-molecular-weight heparin compared with intravenous unfractionated heparin for treatment of pulmonary embolism: a meta-analysis of randomized, controlled trials. *Ann Intern Med.* 2004;**140**:175–83
28. Buller HR, *et al.* Subcutaneous fondaparinux versus intravenous unfractionated heparin in the initial treatment of pulmonary embolism. *N Engl J Med.* 2003;**349**:1695–702
29. Aujesky D, *et al.* Outpatient versus inpatient treatment for patients with acute pulmonary embolism: an international, open-label, randomised, non-inferiority trial. *Lancet.* 2011;**378**:41–8
30. Piazza G, *et al.* Management of submassive pulmonary embolism. *Circulation.* 2010;**122**:1124–9
31. Wan S, *et al.* Thrombolysis compared with heparin for the initial treatment of pulmonary embolism: A meta-analysis of the randomized controlled trials. *Circulation.* 2004;**110**:744–9
32. Konstantinides S, *et al.* Heparin plus alteplase compared with heparin alone in patients with submassive pulmonary embolism. *N Engl J Med.* 2002;**347**:1143–50
33. Pulmonary Embolism Thrombolysis (PEITHO) trial. Abstract. *ACC.* 2013
34. Buller HR, *et al.* Oral rivaroxaban for the treatment of symptomatic pulmonary embolism. *N Engl J Med.* 2012;**366**:1287–97
35. Agnelli G, *et al.*, for the AMPLIFY Investigators. Oral apixaban for the treatment of acute venous thromboembolism. *NEJM.* 2013:July 1, 2013. doi: 2010.1056/NEJMoa1302507
36. Kuo WT, *et al.* Catheter-directed therapy for the treatment of massive pulmonary embolism: systematic review and meta-analysis of modern techniques. *J Vasc Interv Radiol.* 2009;**20**:1431–40
37. Engelberger RP, *et al.* Catheter-based reperfusion treatment of pulmonary embolism. *Circulation.* 2011;**124**:2139–44
38. Sobieszczyk P. Catheter-assisted pulmonary embolectomy. *Circulation.* 2012;**126**:1917–22
39. Uktima trial. *ACC.* 2013
40. Goldhaber SZ, *et al.* Optimal duration of anticoagulation after venous thromboembolism. *Circulation.* 2011;**123**:664–7
41. Eichinger S, *et al.* Risk assessment of recurrence in patients with unprovoked deep vein thrombosis or pulmonary embolism: the Vienna prediction model. *Circulation.* 2010;**121**:1630–6
42. Ridker PM, *et al.* Long-term, low-intensity warfarin therapy for the prevention of recurrent venous thromboembolism. *N Engl J Med.* 2003;**348**:1425–34
43. Cohen AT, *et al.* Rivaroxaban for thromboprophylaxis in acutely ill medical patients. *N Engl J Med.* 2013;**386**:513–23
44. Schulman S, *et al.* Dabigatran versus warfarin in the treatment of acute venous thromboembolism. *N Engl J Med.* 2009;**361**:2342–52
45. Schulman S, *et al.* Extended use of dabigatran, warfarin, or placebo in venous thromboembolism. *N Engl J Med.* 2013;**368**:709–18
46. Agnelli G, *et al.* Apixaban for extended treatment of venous thromboembolism. *N Engl J Med.* 2013;**368**:699–708
47. Becattini C, *et al.* Aspirin for preventing the recurrence of venous thromboembolism. *N Engl J Med.* 2012;**366**:1959–67
48. Brighton TA, *et al.* Low-dose aspirin for preventing recurrent venous thromboembolism. *N Engl J Med.* 2012;**367**:1979–87
49. Biere-Rafi S, *et al.* Statin treatment and the risk of recurrent pulmonary embolism. *Eur Heart J.* 2013;**34**:1800–6
50. Qaseem A, *et al.* Venous thromboembolism prophylaxis in hospitalized patients: a clinical practice guideline from the American College of Physicians. *Ann Intern Med.* 2011;**155**:625–32
51. Piazza G, *et al.* Pulmonary embolism in heart failure. *Circulation.* 2008;**118**:1598–601

Chapter 75

Deep vein thrombosis

Overview

Diagnosis is made by D-dimer test (moderately or highly sensitive) and compression ultrasound of proximal veins. The AHA 2011 recommendations for management are presented in Table 75.1.[1] The American College of Physicians (ACP) has also released recommendations.[2] ACP recommends pharmacological prophylaxis with LMW or UF heparin or a related drug in medical (including stroke) patients and against the use of mechanical prophylaxis with graduated compression stockings for prevention of venous thromboembolism. The most detailed guidelines on prevention of thrombosis in both medical and surgical patients and various clinical settings have been published by the American College of Chest Physicians (ACCP).[3] ACCP recommends graduated compression stockings only in medical patients who are bleeding or are at high risk for major bleeding. Recommendations on the management of patients with established DVT are provided in Chapter 74.

Thromboembolism in pregnancy

Pregnant women have a 4- to 5-fold increased risk of thromboembolism compared with non-pregnant women. Approximately 80% of thromboembolic events in pregnancy are venous, with a prevalence of 0.5–3/1000 pregnant women. Specific guidelines have been published by the American College of Obstetrics And Gynecology and Royal College of Obstetricians and Gynaecologists in the UK.[4] Compression ultrasonography of the proximal veins should be considered when new-onset deep venous thrombosis is suspected. When using anticoagulants, heparin compounds are preferred. Recommendations by the ESC are provided in Tables 75.2 to 75.4.[5]

Table 75.1 AHA 2011 scientific statement. Iliofemoral deep vein thrombosis

Recommendations for initial anticoagulation for patients with iliofemoral deep vein thrombosis (IFDVT)	
In the absence of suspected or proven heparin-induced thrombocytopenia, patients with IFDVT should receive therapeutic anticoagulation with either:	
IV UFH, or	I-A
UFH by subcutaneous injection, or	I-B
LMWH, or	I-A
Fondaparinux	I-A
Patients with suspected or proven heparin-induced thrombocytopenia should receive a direct thrombin inhibitor	I-B
Recommendations for long-term anticoagulation therapy for patients with IFDVT	
Warfarin overlap with initial anticoagulation therapy for a minimum of 5 days and until the INR is >2.0 for, at least, 24 hours, and then targeted to an INR of 2.0 –3.0.	I-A
Patients with first-episode IFDVT related to a major reversible risk factor should have anticoagulation stopped after 3 months.	I-A
Patients with recurrent or unprovoked IFDVT should have, at least, 6 months of anticoagulation and be considered for indefinite anticoagulation, with periodic reassessment of the risks and benefits of continued anticoagulation.	I-A
Cancer patients with IFDVT should receive LMWH monotherapy for, at least, 3 to 6 months or as long as the cancer or its treatment (e.g. chemotherapy) is ongoing.	I-A
LMWH monotherapy in children with DVT.	IIb-C
Recommendations for use of compression therapy for patients with IFDVT	
30 to 40 mmHg knee-high graduated elastic compression stockings (ECS) on a daily basis for, at least, 2 years.	I-B
Daily use of 30 to 40 mmHg knee-high graduated ECS in patients with prior IFDVT and symptomatic post-thrombotic syndrome (PTS).	IIa-C
Intermittent sequential pneumatic compression, followed by daily use of 30 to 40 mmHg knee-high graduated ECS in patients with prior IFDVT and severe oedema.	IIb-B

(Continued)

Table 75.1 (Continued)

Recommendations for filters for patients with IFDVT (as described in Chapter 74 on PE)	
Recommendations for endovascular thrombolysis and surgical venous thrombectomy for patients with IFDVT	
Catheter-directed thrombolysis (CDT) or pharmacomechanical CDT (PCDT) to patients with IFDVT associated with limb-threatening circulatory compromise (i.e. phlegmasia cerulea dolens).	I-C
Transfer to a centre with expertise in endovascular thrombolysis if indications for endovascular thrombolysis are present.	I-C
CDT or PCDT for patients with IFDVT associated with rapid thrombus extension despite anticoagulation, and/or	IIa-C
Symptomatic deterioration from the IFDVT despite anticoagulation	IIa-B
CDT or PCDT as first-line treatment of patients with acute IFDVT to prevent PTS in selected patients at low risk of bleeding complications.	IIa-B
Surgical venous thrombectomy by experienced surgeons in patients with IFDVT.	IIb-B
Systemic fibrinolysis routinely to patients with IFDVT.	III-A
CDT or PCDT to most patients with chronic DVT symptoms (>21 days) or patients who are at high risk for bleeding complications.	III-B
Recommendations for percutaneous transluminal venous angioplasty and stenting for patients with IFDVT	
Stent placement in the iliac vein to treat obstructive lesions after CDT, PCDT, or surgical venous thrombectomy.	IIa-C
Percutaneous transluminal angioplasty without stenting for isolated obstructive lesions in the common femoral vein.	IIa-C
Iliac vein stents to reduce PTS symptoms and heal venous ulcers in patients with advanced PTS and iliac vein obstruction.	IIa-C
After venous stent placement, the use of therapeutic anticoagulation after venous stent placement; similar dosing, monitoring, and duration as without stents.	IIa-C
Use of antiplatelet therapy with concomitant anticoagulation in patients perceived to be at high risk of rethrombosis.	IIb-C

AHA 2011 scientific statement on pulmonary embolism, iliofemoral deep vein thrombosis, and chronic thromboembolic pulmonary hypertension. *Circulation*. 2011;**123**:1788–830.

Table 75.2 ESC 2011 on pregnancy. Checklist for risk factors for venous thromboembolism, modified according to Royal College of Obstetricians and Gynaecologists

Pre-existing risk factors
Previous recurrent VTE[a]
Previous VTE unprovoked or oestrogen-related[2]
Previous VTE provoked
Family history of VTE
Known thrombophilia
Medical co-morbidities, e.g. heart or lung diseases, SLE, cancer, inflNewammatory conditions, nephritic syndrome, sickle cell disease, IV drug use
Age >35 years
Obesity, BMI >30 kg/m[b]
Parity ≥3
Smoker
Gross varicose veins
Obstetric risk factors
Pre-eclampsia
Dehydration/hyperemesis/ovarian hyperstimulation syndrome
Multiple pregnancy or assisted reproductive therapy
Emergency Caesarean section
Elective Caesarean section
Mid-cavity or rotational forceps
Prolonged labour (>24 hours)
Peripartum haemorrhage (>1 L or transfusion)

(Continued)

Table 75.2 (Continued)

Transient risk factors
Current systemic infection
Immobility
Surgical procedure in pregnancy or <6 weeks post-partum
Patients with previous recurrent VTEs (1) or those with (2) a previous unprovoked or oestrogen-related VTE belong to the high risk group.

a: Patients with previous recurrent VTEs (>1), or those with a previous unprovoked or oestrogen-related VTE belong to the high risk group
b: Obesity based on booking weight
Example: in a pregnant woman with a family history of VTE, age >35 years, and obesity (BMI >30 kg/m^2), the total number of risk factors is 3. This patient belongs to the intermediate-risk group and requires VTE prophylaxis accordingly.
ESC guidelines on the management of cardiovascular diseases during pregnancy. *Eur Heart J.* 2011;**32**:3147–97.

Table 75.3 ESC 2011 on pregnancy Risk groups according to risk factors, definition, and preventive measures, modified according to Royal College of Obstetricians and Gynaecologists

Risk groups	Definition according to risk factors	Preventive measures according to risk group
High risk	Patients with:	
	(i) Previous recurrent VTE (>1), or	High-risk patients should receive antenatal prophylaxis with
	(ii) VTE unprovoked/oestrogen-related, or	LMWH as well as post-partum for the duration of 6 weeks
	(iii) Single previous VTE + thrombophilia or family history	Graduated compression stockings are also recommended during pregnancy and post-partum
Intermediate risk	Patients with:	In intermediate-risk patients, antenatal prophylaxis with LMWH should be considered
	(i) 3 or more risk factors other than those listed above as high risk	Prophylaxis is recommended post-partum for, at least, 7 days or longer, if >3 risk factors persist
	(ii) 2 or more risk factors other than those listed as high risk if patient is admitted to hospital	Graduated compression stockings should be considered during pregnancy and post-partum.
Low risk	Patients with: <3 risk factors	In low-risk patients, early mobilization and avoidance of dehydration is recommended

Several risk scores for the identification of patients at different risk levels have been developed, yet all risk scores, including the above, still need validation in prospective studies.
ESC guidelines on the management of cardiovascular diseases during pregnancy. *Eur Heart J.* 2011;**32**:3147–97.

Table 75.4 ESC 2011 on pregnancy. Recommendations for the prevention and management of venous thromboembolism in pregnancy and puerperium

Assessment of risk factors for VTE in all women who are pregnant or consider pregnancy	I-C
Mothers should be informed about the signs and symptoms of VTE in pregnancy and the necessity to contact the physicians if they occur	I-C
Antenatal prophylaxis with LMWH as well as post-partum for 6 weeks in high-risk patients	I-C
Post-partum prophylaxis with LMWH for, at least, 7 days or longer if >3 risk factors persist in intermediate-risk patients	I-C
Early mobilization and avoidance of dehydration in low-risk patients	I-C
Graduated compression stockings antepartum and post-partum in all women at high risk	I-C
D-dimer measurement and compression ultrasonography in patients with suspected VTE during pregnancy	I-C
For acute VTE during pregnancy, UFH in high-risk and LMWH in non-high-risk patients	I-C
Graduated compression stockings in women with intermediate risk during pregnancy and post-partum	IIa-C
Antenatal prophylaxis with LMWH in intermediate-risk patients	IIa-C
Routine screening for thrombophilia should not be performed	III-C

ESC guidelines on the management of cardiovascular diseases during pregnancy. *Eur Heart J.* 2011;**32**:3147–97.

References

1. Jaff MR, *et al.* Management of massive and submassive pulmonary embolism, iliofemoral deep vein thrombosis, and chronic thromboembolic pulmonary hypertension: a scientific statement from the American Heart Association. *Circulation.* 2011;**123**:1788–830
2. Qaseem A, *et al.* Venous thromboembolism prophylaxis in hospitalized patients: a clinical practice guideline from the American College of Physicians. *Ann Intern Med.* 2011;**155**:625–32
3. Guyatt GH, *et al.* Introduction to the ninth edition: Antithrombotic therapy and prevention of thrombosis, 9th ed: American College of Chest Physicians evidence-based clinical practice guidelines. *Chest.* 2012;**141**:48S–52S
4. Chauhan SP HN, Berghella V, Siddiqui D. Comparison of two national guidelines in obstetrics: American versus Royal College of Obstetricians and Gynaecologists. *Am J Perinatol.* 2010;**27**:763–70.
5. Regitz-Zagrosek V, *et al.* ESC guidelines on the management of cardiovascular diseases during pregnancy: the Task Force on the management of cardiovascular diseases during pregnancy of the European Society of Cardiology (ESC). *Eur Heart J.* 2011;**32**:3147–97

Part XVI

Pulmonary hypertension

Relevant guidelines

ACCF/AHA 2009 guidelines on pulmonary hypertension

ACCF/AHA 2009 expert consensus document on pulmonary hypertension. *Circulation*. 2009;**119**:2250–94.

ESC 2009 guidelines on pulmonary hypertension

ESC guidelines for the diagnosis and treatment of pulmonary hypertension. *Eur Heart J*. 2009;**30**:2493–537.

AHA 2011 scientific statement on management of submassive pulmonary embolism, iliofemoral deep vein thrombosis, and chronic thromboembolic pulmonary hypertension

Management of massive and submassive pulmonary embolism, iliofemoral deep vein thrombosis, and chronic thromboembolic pulmonary hypertension: a scientific statement from the American Heart Association. *Circulation*. 2011;**123**:1788–830.

Chapter 76

Definitions and classification of pulmonary hypertension

Definition and classification

Pulmonary hypertension (PH) is defined as a mean PA pressure ≥25 mmHg at rest, as assessed by right heart catheterization.[1,2] The recent clinical classification of pulmonary hypertension is presented in Table 76.1.[3] Pulmonary veno-occlusive disease and/or pulmonary capillary haemangiomatosis represent a distinct category, but not completely separated, from pulmonary arterial hypertension and have been designated as clinical group 1. The key haemodynamic feature that differentiates group 2 PH is wedge pressure elevation >15 mmHg (post-capillary pulmonary hypertension).

Table 76.1 Updated classification of PH (Dana Point 2008)[3]

1 Pulmonary arterial hypertension (PAH)
1.1 Idiopathic
1.2 Heritable:
1.2.1 BMPR2
1.2.2 ALK1, endoglin (with or without hereditary haemorrhagic telangiectasia)
1.2.3 Unknown
1.3 Drugs and toxins induced
1.4 Associated with (APAH):
1.4.1 Connective tissue diseases
1.4.2 HIV infection
1.4.3 Portal hypertension
1.4.4 Congenital heart disease
1.4.5 Schistosomiasis
1.4.6 Chronic haemolytic anaemia
1.5 Persistent pulmonary hypertension of the newborn
1′ Pulmonary veno-occlusive disease and/or pulmonary capillary haemangiomatosis
2 Pulmonary hypertension due to left heart disease
2.1 Systolic dysfunction
2.2 Diastolic dysfunction
2.3 Valvular disease
3 Pulmonary hypertension due to lung diseases and/or hypoxia
3.1 Chronic obstructive pulmonary disease
3.2 Interstitial lung disease
3.3 Other pulmonary diseases with mixed restrictive and obstructive pattern
3.4 Sleep-disordered breathing
3.5 Alveolar hypoventilation disorders
3.6 Chronic exposure to high altitude
3.7 Developmental abnormalities
4 Chronic thromboembolic pulmonary hypertension
5 PH with unclear and/or multifactiorial mechanisms
5.1 Haematological disorders: myeloproliferative disorders, splenectomy.
5.2 Systemic disorders: sarcoidosis, pulmonary Langerhans cell histiocytosis, lymphangioleiomyomatosis, neurofibromatosis, vasculitis
5.3 Metabolic disorders: glycogen storage disease, Gaucher's disease, thyroid disorders
5.4 Others: tumoural obstruction, fibrosing mediastinitis, chronic renal failure on dialysis

(Continued)

ALK1, activin receptor-like kinase type 1; BMPR2, bone morphogenetic protein receptor type 2; HIV, human immunodeficiency virus; APAH, associated pulmonary arterial hypertension.
Simonneau G, *et al*. Updated clinical classification of pulmonary hypertension. *J Am Coll Cardiol*. 2009;**54**(1 Suppl):S43–54.

References

1. Galie N, *et al.* Guidelines for the diagnosis and treatment of pulmonary hypertension: the Task Force for the diagnosis and treatment of pulmonary hypertension of the European Society of Cardiology (ESC) and the European Respiratory Society (ERS), endorsed by the International Society of Heart and Lung Transplantation (ISHLT). *Eur Heart J.* 2009;**30**:2493–537
2. McLaughlin VV, *et al.* ACCF/AHA 2009 expert consensus document on pulmonary hypertension: a report of the American College of Cardiology Foundation Task Force on expert consensus documents and the American Heart Association: developed in collaboration with the American College of Chest Physicians, American Thoracic Society, Inc., and the Pulmonary Hypertension Association. *Circulation.* 2009;**119**:2250–94
3. Simonneau G, *et al.* Updated clinical classification of pulmonary hypertension. *J Am Coll Cardiol.* 2009;**54**:S43–54

Chapter 77

Pulmonary arterial hypertension and hypertension associated with pulmonary venous abnormalities

Pulmonary arterial hypertension

Definition

Pulmonary arterial hypertension (PAH) is a syndrome due to restricted flow through the pulmonary arterial circulation, resulting in increased pulmonary vascular resistance and ultimately in right heart failure.

Epidemiology

The prevalence of PAH is estimated to 15 per million.[1]

Aetiology

Causes are presented in Table 76.1 of Chapter 76 on the classification of pulmonary hypertension. **Idiopathic pulmonary arterial hypertension**, the most common type of PAH (6 per million), is more prevalent in women. **Heritable forms** of PAH (<10%) include clinically sporadic idiopathic PAH, with germline mutations mainly of bone morphogenetic protein receptor 2 (BMPR2) gene, as well as the activin receptor-like kinase type 1 gene (ALK1) or the endoglin gene, and clinical familial cases with or without identified mutations.[2,3] PAH due to BMPR2 mutations is inherited as an autosomal dominant disease with incomplete penetrance and genetic anticipation. **Drugs** that may cause PAH are presented in Table 77.1. Several conditions are also associated with PAH as shown in Table 77.1. Pulmonary hypertension, in the context of **congenital heart disorders**, may lead to Eisenmenger's syndrome, as discussed in Chapter 1 on GUCH (Table 77.2). The mechanism of PAH in patients with **schistosomiasis** is probably multifactorial and includes portal hypertension and local vascular inflammation. **Chronic haemolytic anaemia**, such as sickle cell disease, thalassaemia, hereditary spherocytosis, stomatocytosis, and microangiopathic haemolytic anaemia, may result in PAH. The mechanism of PAH in chronic haemolysis is related to a high rate of nitric oxide (NO) consumption, leading to a state of resistance to NO bioactivity.[4]

Pathophysiology

PAH is a panvasculopathy, predominantly affecting small pulmonary arteries (<500 μm) that regulate regional blood flow in the lung (resistance arteries) whereas pulmonary veins are unaffected. Intimal hyperplasia, medial hypertrophy, adventitial proliferation, thrombosis *in situ*, varying degrees of inflammation, and plexiform arteriopathy are histological characteristics.[4,5] Multiple pathogenic pathways have been implicated in the development of PAH, including those at the molecular and genetic levels and in the smooth muscle and endothelial cells and adventitia. Excessive cell proliferation and reduced rates of apoptosis, as well as excessive vasoconstriction in 20% of patients, induce vascular remodelling with loss of vascular luminal cross section.[5] Excessive vasoconstriction has been related to abnormal function or expression of potassium channels in the smooth muscle cells and to endothelial dysfunction that leads to chronically impaired production of vasodilator and antiproliferative agents, such as NO and prostacyclin, along with overexpression of vasoconstrictor and

Table 77.1 ESC 2009 guidelines on pulmonary hypertension. Drugs associated with PAH

Definite
Aminorex
Fenfluramine
Dexfenfluramine
Toxic rapeseed oil
Benfluorex
Likely
Amphetamines
L-tryptophan
Meta-amphetamines
Possible
Cocaine
Phenylpropanolamine
St John's Wort
Chemotherapeutic agents
Selective serotonin reuptake inhibitors
Pergolide

Recent evidence also indicates that 3-kinase inhibitors, such as dasatinib, used for chronic myeloid leukaemia, may also cause precapillary pulmonary hypertension (Montani D, *et al.* Pulmonary arterial hypertension in patients treated by dasatinib. *Circulation*. 2012;**125**:2128–37).
ESC Guidelines for the diagnosis and treatment of pulmonary hypertension. *Eur Heart J*. 2009;**30**:2493–537

Table 77.2 ESC 2009 guidelines on pulmonary hypertension

Clinical classification of congenital, systemic-to-pulmonary shunts associated with pulmonary arterial hypertension.
A. Eisenmenger's syndrome
Eisenmenger's syndrome includes all systemic-to-pulmonary shunts due to large defects, leading to a severe increase in PVR and resulting in a reversed (pulmonary-to-systemic) or bidirectional shunt. Cyanosis, erythrocytosis, and multiple organ involvement are present.
B. Pulmonary arterial hypertension associated with systemic-to-pulmonary shunts
In these patients with moderate to large defects, the increase in PVR is mild to moderate; systemic-to-pulmonary shunt is still largely present, and no cyanosis is present at rest.
C. Pulmonary arterial hypertension with small[a] defects
In cases with small defects (usually ventricular septal defects <1 cm and atrial septal defects <2 cm of effective diameter assessed by echocardiography), the clinical picture is very similar to idiopathic PAH.
D. Pulmonary arterial hypertension after corrective cardiac surgery
In these cases, congenital heart disease has been corrected, but PAH is either still present immediately after surgery or has recurred several months or years after surgery in the absence of significant post-operative residual congenital lesions or defects that originate as a sequela to previous surgery.

[a] The size applies to adult patients.
PAH, pulmonary arterial hypertension; PVR, pulmonary vascular resistance.
ESC Guidelines for the diagnosis and treatment of pulmonary hypertension. *Eur Heart J*. 2009;**30**:2493–537.

proliferative substances, such as thromboxane A2 and endothelin-1.[4] Eventually, pathological increases in PVR cause right heart failure.

Presentation

Patients initially present with dyspnoea and fatigue. Peripheral oedema and other signs of RV failure follow. Syncope in PAH is associated with worsening right heart function and is an independent predictor of a poor prognosis.[6]

Physical examination

Initial findings are **S_3** (right ventricular), accentuated **P_2**, **early systolic click** from PV, pansystolic murmur of **TR**, diastolic murmur of **PR**, and **left parasternal lift**.

Jugular vein distension, hepatomegaly, peripheral oedema, ascites, and cool extremities characterize patients in a more advanced state (Table 77.3).[4]

Lung sounds are usually normal. Signs of associated disorders may be also seen.

Investigations

Chest X-ray is abnormal in 90% of patients and typically displays decreased peripheral lung vascular markings (pruning) and hilar pulmonary artery prominence due to central pulmonary arterial dilatation (Figure 77.1). Right atrium and RV enlargement may be seen in more advanced cases.

ECG may reveal right atrial enlargement, right ventricular hypertrophy and strain, and right axis deviation of the QRS complex. A normal ECG does not exclude PAH.

Echocardiography shows right atrial and right ventricular enlargement, abnormal contour, flattening, or reverse curvature of the interventricular septum, TR, and underfilled left heart chambers (Table 77.4). The Doppler echocardiographic index (Tei index or myocardial performance index), an index of combined RV systolic and diastolic function obtained by dividing the sum of both isovolumetric contraction and relaxation intervals by the ejection time, appears to be predictive of an adverse outcome.[1] Doppler measurements of the PA pressure, however, may be significantly inaccurate (by as much as 38 mmHg).[7]

Cardiac catheterization It is necessary to establish the diagnosis and allow vasodilator testing (Table 77.5). Typically, there is a mean pulmonary artery pressure (mPAP) >25 mmHg (and usually >42 mmHg); a pulmonary capillary wedge pressure (PCWP), left atrial pressure, or left ventricular end-diastolic pressure (LVEDP) ≤15 mmHg; and a pulmonary vascular resistance (PVR) greater than 3 Wood units. Associated mortality of the procedure is 0.05%.

Lung function tests There is decreased lung diffusion capacity for carbon monoxide (typically in the range of 40–80% predicted) and mild to moderate reduction of lung volumes. Mild peripheral airway obstruction can also be detected. PO_2 is usually normal and PCO_2 low due to hyperventilation.

High-resolution CT is important to exclude interstitial lung disease and emphysema. The presence of interstitial markings similar to those seen with advanced left ventricular failure, such as diffuse central (as opposed to panlobular that is seen with PAH) ground glass opacification and thickening of interlobular septa, suggest ***pulmonary veno-occlusive disease***. Diffuse bilateral thickening of the interlobular septae and the presence of small, centrilobular, poorly circumscribed nodular opacities suggest ***pulmonary capillary haemangiomatosis***.

MRI is the image modality of choice for assessment of RV function. Poor RV function, including stroke volume ≥25 mL/m², RV end-diastolic volume ≥84 mL/m², and LV end-diastolic volume ≤40 mL/m², are independent predictors of mortality and treatment failure.[8]

Specific blood tests may be needed for diagnosis (Figures 77.2 and 77.3).

Lung biopsy is not generally indicated.

Table 77.3 ACCF/AHA 2009 consensus document on pulmonary hypertension. Physical examination in pulmonary hypertension

Sign	Implication
Physical signs that reflect severity of PH	
Accentuated pulmonary component of S_2 (audible at apex in over 90%)	High pulmonary pressure increases force of pulmonic valve closure
Early systolic click	Sudden interruption of opening of pulmonary valve into high-pressure artery
Mid-systolic ejection murmur	Turbulent transvalvular pulmonary outflow
Left parasternal lift	High right ventricular pressure and hypertrophy present
Right ventricular S_4 (in 38%)	High right ventricular pressure and hypertrophy present
Increased jugular a wave	Poor right ventricular compliance
Physical signs that suggest moderate to severe PH	
Moderate to severe PH	
Holosystolic murmur that increases with inspiration	Tricuspid regurgitation
Increased jugular v waves	
Pulsatile liver	
Diastolic murmur	Pulmonary regurgitation
Hepatojugular reflux	High central venous pressure
Advanced PH with right ventricular failure	
Right ventricular S_3 (in 23%)	Right ventricular dysfunction
Distension of jugular veins	Right ventricular dysfunction or tricuspid regurgitation or both
Hepatomegaly	Right ventricular dysfunction or tricuspid regurgitation or both
Peripheral oedema (in 32%)	
Ascites	
Low blood pressure, diminished pulse pressure, cool extremities	Reduced cardiac output, peripheral vasoconstriction
Physical signs that suggest possible underlying cause or associations of PH	
Central cyanosis	Abnormal V/Q, intra-pulmonary shunt, hypoxaemia, pulmonary-to-systemic shunt
Clubbing	Congenital heart disease, pulmonary venopathy
Cardiac auscultatory findings, including systolic murmurs, diastolic murmurs, opening snap, and gallop	Congenital or acquired heart or valvular disease
Rales, dullness, or decreased breath sounds	Pulmonary congestion or effusion or both
Fine rales, accessory muscle use, wheezing, protracted expiration, productive cough	Pulmonary parenchymal disease
Obesity, kyphoscoliosis, enlarged tonsils	Possible substrate for disordered ventilation
Sclerodactyly, arthritis, telangiectasia, Raynaud phenomenon, rash	Connective tissue disorder
Peripheral venous insufficiency or obstruction	Possible venous thrombosis
Venous stasis ulcers	Possible sickle cell disease
Pulmonary vascular bruits	Chronic thromboembolic PH
Splenomegaly, spider angiomata, palmar erythema, icterus, caput medusa, ascites	Portal hypertension

ACCF/AHA 2009 expert consensus document on pulmonary hypertension. *Circulation*. 2009; **119**:2250–94.

Genetic counselling and recommendation for BMPR2 genotyping might be indicated in first-degree relatives of patients with this mutation or within pedigree of two or more patients with a diagnosis of PAH.[4]

Diagnosis strategies are presented in Figures 77.2 and 77.3.

Risk stratification

The prognosis of PAH is poor, with an approximately 15% mortality within 1 year on modern therapy. Predictors of a poor prognosis include: advanced functional class (Table 77.6), poor exercise capacity as measured by 6-minute

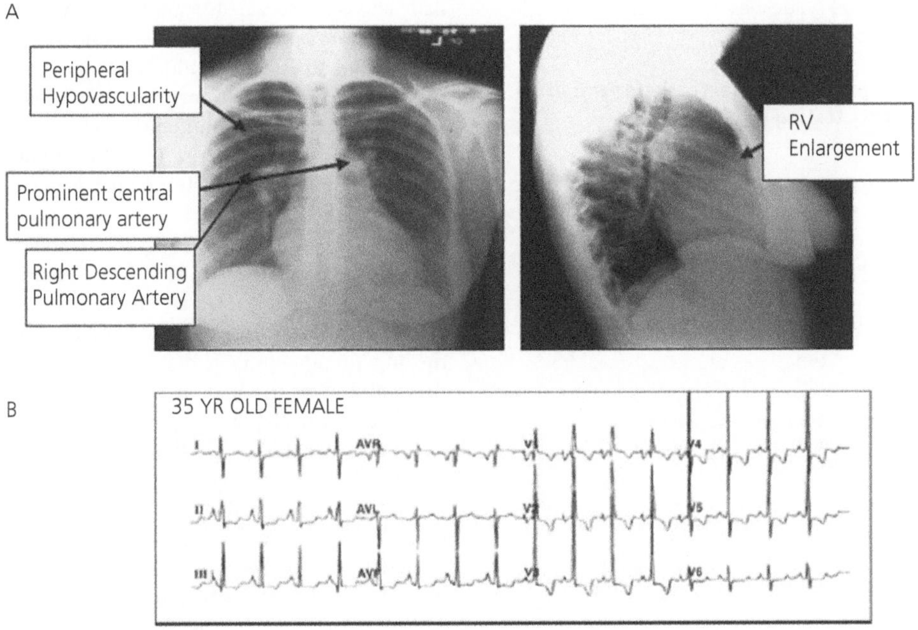

Figure 77.1 Chest X-ray (A) and ECG (B) from a patient with PAH.

ACCF/AHA 2009 expert consensus document on pulmonary hypertension. *Circulation*. 2009;**119**:2250–94.

Table 77.4 ESC 2009 guidelines on pulmonary hypertension

Arbitrary criteria for estimating the presence of PH based on tricuspid regurgitation peak velocity and Doppler-calculated PA systolic pressure at rest (assuming a normal right atrial pressure of 5 mmHg) and on additional echocardiographic variables suggestive of PH	
Echocardiographic diagnosis: PH unlikely	
Tricuspid regurgitation velocity ≤2.8 m/s, PA systolic pressure ≤36 mmHg, and no additional echocardiographic variables suggestive of PH	I-B
Echocardiographic diagnosis: PH possible	
Tricuspid regurgitation velocity ≤2.8 m/s, PA systolic pressure ≤36 mmHg, but presence of additional echocardiographic variables suggestive of PH	IIa-C
Tricuspid regurgitation velocity 2.9–3.4 m/s, PA systolic pressure 37–50 mmHg, with/without additional echocardiographic variables suggestive of PH	IIa-C
Echocardiographic diagnosis: PH likely	
Tricuspid regurgitation velocity >3.4 m/s, PA systolic pressure >50 mmHg, with/without additional echocardiographic variables suggestive of PH	I-B
Exercise Doppler echocardiography is not recommended for screening of PH	III-C

ESC Guidelines for the diagnosis and treatment of pulmonary hypertension. *Eur Heart J*. 2009;**30**:2493–537.

walk test or cardiopulmonary exercise test, high right atrial pressure, tricuspid annular displacement (TAPSE), significant RV dysfunction or failure, low cardiac index, elevated BNP, and underlying diagnosis of scleroderma spectrum of diseases (Table 77.7).[9,10]

Therapy

Treatment (as well as diagnosis) of PAH is not easy.[7] Acute vasodilator testing to test the presence of pulmonary vasoreactivity has prognositic value and should be performed in all patients with idiopathic PAH who might be considered potential candidates for long-term calcium channel blocker therapy (Table 77.8). Those with overt right heart failure or haemodynamic instability should not undergo acute vasodilator testing. The definition of an acute responder is a reduction in mPAP of at least 10 mmHg to an absolute mPAP of less than 40 mmHg without a decrease in cardiac output.[4]

General measures that should be addressed include diet, exercise, appropriate vaccinations, and avoidance of pregnancy. In-flight O_2 administration (2 L/min) should be considered for patients in WHO-FC III and IV and those with arterial blood O_2 pressure consistently <8 kPa (60 mmHg). Patients should avoid going to altitudes above 1500–2000 m without supplemental O_2. If AF intervenes, rhythm control is recommended.[4]

Table 77.5 ESC 2009 guidelines on pulmonary hypertension

Recommendations for right heart catheterization (A) and vasoreactivity testing (B)	
A	
In all patients with PAH to confirm the diagnosis, to evaluate the severity, and when PAH-specific drug therapy is considered	I-C
For confirmation of efficacy of PAH-specific drug therapy	IIa-C
For confirmation of clinical deterioration and as baseline for the evaluation of the effect of treatment escalation and/or combination therapy	IIa-C
B	
Vasoreactivity testing in patients with IPAH, heritable PAH, and PAH associated with anorexigen use to detect patients who can be treated with high doses of a CCB	I-C
A positive response to vasoreactivity testing is defined as a reduction of mean PAP ≥10 mmHg to reach an absolute value of mean PAP ≤40 mmHg with an increased or unchanged cardiac output	I-C
Vasoreactivity testing should be performed only in referral centres	IIa-C
Vasoreactivity testing should be performed using nitric oxide as vasodilator	IIa-C
Vasoreactivity testing in other types of PAH	IIb-C
Vasoreactivity testing using IV epoprostenol or IV adenosine	IIb-C
The use of an oral or IV CCB in acute vasoreactivity testing is not recommended	III-C
Vasoreactivity testing to detect patients who can be safely treated with high doses of a CCB is not recommended in patients	III-C

ESC Guidelines for the diagnosis and treatment of pulmonary hypertension. *Eur Heart J*. 2009;**30**:2493–537.

Oxygen is recommended to maintain oxygen saturation greater than 90%.

Warfarin anticoagulation is recommended in all patients with idiopathic PAH, heritable PAH, PAH due to anorexigens, and those receiving therapy with long-term IV prostaglandins (Figures 77.4 and 77.5).

Diuretics are used for symptomatic management of RV volume overload.

Calcium channel blockers (diltiazem up to 720 mg daily, long-acting nifedipine up to 240 mg daily, and amlodipine up to 20 mg daily, in all starting with low doses, but not the more potent negative inotropic verapamil) are indicated only for patients who have a positive acute vasodilator response (Tables 77.9 and 77.10). Patients treated with calcium channel blockers, as with other vasodilators, should be followed closely for both the safety and efficacy of this therapy.

Endothelin receptor antagonists are oral therapies that improve exercise capacity in PAH. **Bosentan** (62.5 mg twice daily and uptitrated to 125 mg twice daily after 4 weeks)[11] and the more selective antagonists **ambrisentan** (5–10 mg daily)[12] and **sitaxsentan** (100 mg daily) [13] have been successfully tried in various forms of PAH (Table 77.9). Liver function tests must be monitored indefinitely on a monthly basis. Aminotransferase rise (3–10%) might be less with ambrisentan. Drug interactions have been summarized in the ESC guidelines.[5]

Prostanoids Continuous intravenous **epoprostenol** improves exercise capacity and haemodynamics (and survival in idiopathic PAH)[14] and is the preferred treatment option for the most critically ill patients. Epoprostenol is the only therapy for PAH that has been shown to prolong survival, but its use may be prohibited by its high cost. Treatment is initiated at a dose of 2–4 ng/kg/min, with doses increasing at a rate limited by side effects (flushing, headache, diarrhoea, leg pain). The optimal dose varies between individual patients, ranging in the majority between 20 and 40 ng/kg/min. Serious adverse events related to the delivery system include pump malfunction, local site infection, catheter obstruction, and sepsis. Abrupt interruption of the epoprostenol infusion should be avoided as, in some patients, this may lead to death.[4,5]

Treprostinil, a prostanoid, may be delivered via either continuous intravenous or subcutaneous infusion.[15] Initial dose is 1–2 ng/kg/min, with doses increasing at a rate limited by side effects (local site pain, flushing, headache), up to 20 and 80 ng/kg/min. Oral and inhaled formulations that avoid Gram-negative infections induced by IV administration are promising. Recently, oral treprostinil diolamine was shown to improve exercise capacity in PAH patients not receiving other treatment. Therapy was generally well tolerated; the most common adverse events were headache (69%), nausea (39%), diarrhea (37%), and pain in jaw (25%).[16]

Iloprost is a prostanoid delivered by an adaptive aerosolized device six times daily (2.5–5 mg/inhalation). Inhaled iloprost is well tolerated, with flushing and jaw pain being the most frequent side effects.[17]

Phosphodiesterase (PDE)-5 inhibitors (sildenafil and tadalafil) also improve exercise capacity and haemodynamics in PAH.[18,19] Side effects are mild to moderate and mainly related to vasodilation (headache, flushing, epistaxis). Recently, a possible association of sildenafil with deafness has been reported.[20]

Atrial septostomy and **lung transplantation** are options for selected patients who progress despite optimal medical management.

Treatment response is assessed by improvement in exercise capacity (6-minute walk test, cardiopulmonary exercise test, treadmill test) and haemodynamics. Treatment of specific groups is presented in Tables 77.11, 77.12, and 77.13.

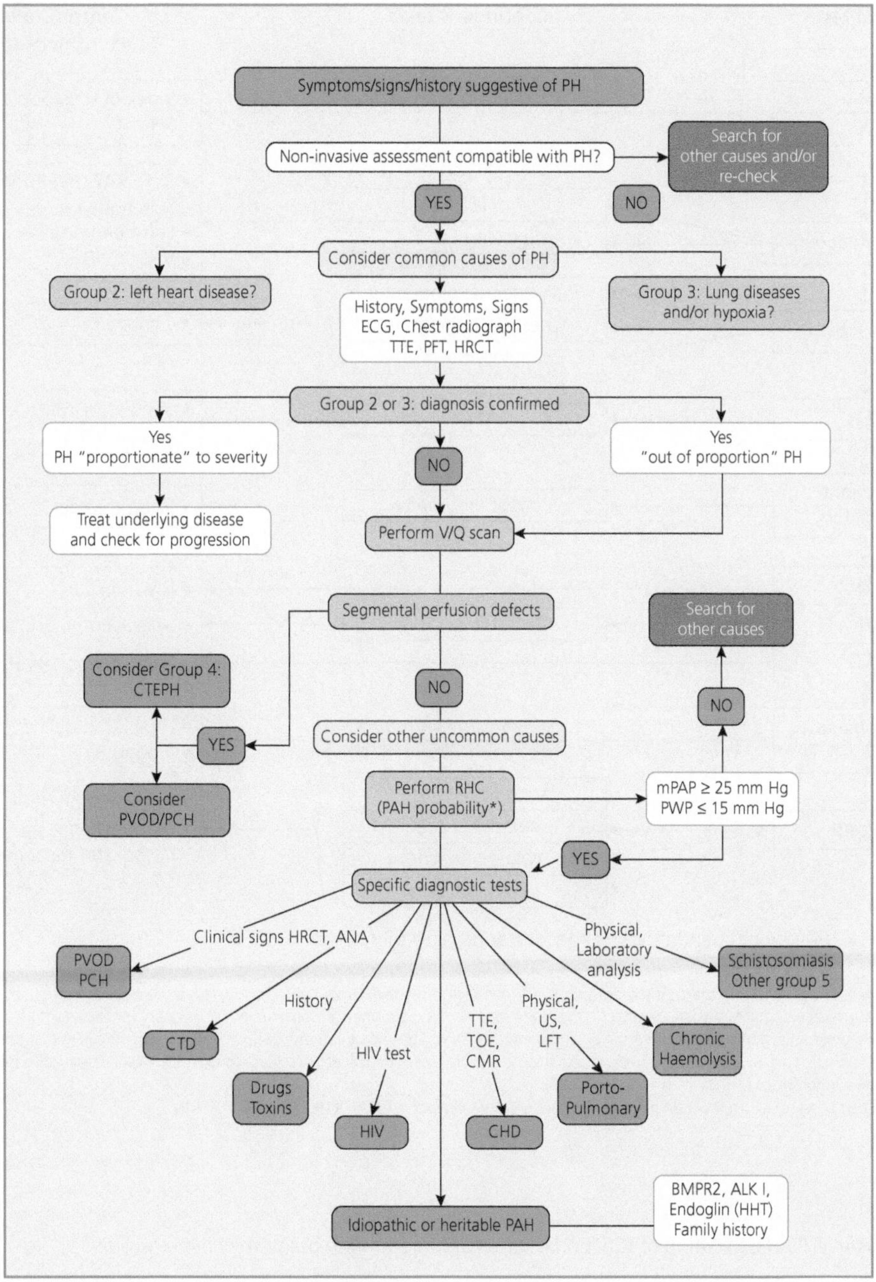

Figure 77.2 ESC 2009 guidelines: diagnostic algorithm.

ALK-1, activin receptor-like kinase; ANA, antinuclear antibodies; BMPR2, bone morphogenetic protein receptor 2; CHD, congenital heart disease; CMR, cardiac magnetic resonance; CTD, connective tissue disease; HHT, hereditary haemorrhagic telangiectasia; HIV, human immunodeficiency virus; HRCT, high-resolution computed tomography; LFT, liver function tests; mPAP, mean pulmonary arterial pressure; PAH, pulmonary arterial hypertension; PCH, pulmonary capillary haemangiomatosis; PFT, pulmonary function test; PH, pulmonary hypertension; PVOD, pulmonary veno-occlusive disease; PWP, pulmonary wedge pressure; RHC, right heart catheterization; TOE, transoesophageal echocardiography; TTE, transthoracic echocardiography; US, ultrasonography; V/Q scan, ventilation/perfusion lung scan.

ESC Guidelines for the diagnosis and treatment of pulmonary hypertension. *Eur Heart J*. 2009;**30**:2493–537

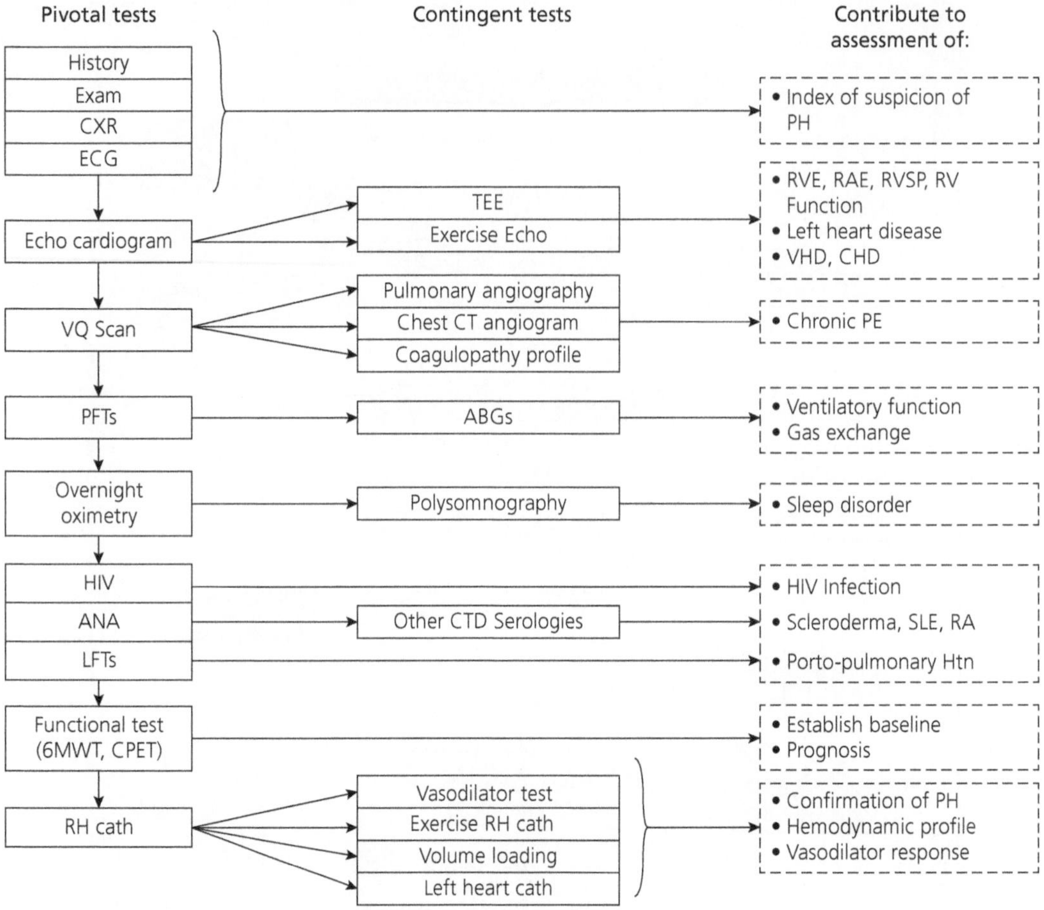

Figure 77.3 AHA 2009 recommendations: diagnostic approach to PAH.

6MWT indicates 6-minute walk test; ABGs, arterial blood gases; ANA, antinuclear antibody serology; CHD, congenital heart disease; CPET, cardiopulmonary exercise test; CT, computerized tomography; CTD, connective tissue disease; CXR, chest X-ray; ECG, electrocardiogram; HIV, human immunodeficiency virus screening; Htn, hypertension; LFT, liver function test; PE, pulmonary embolism; PFT, pulmonary function test; PH, pulmonary hypertension; RA, rheumatoid arthritis; RAE, right atrial enlargement; RH Cath, right heart catheterization; RVE, right ventricular enlargement; RVSP, right ventricular systolic pressure; SLE, systemic lupus erythematosus; TEE, transesophageal echocardiography; VHD, valvular heart disease; and VQ Scan, ventilation-perfusion scintigram.
ACCF/AHA 2009 expert consensus document on pulmonary hypertension. *Circulation*. 2009; **119**:2250–94.

Table 77.6 NYHA/WHO classification of functional status of patients with pulmonary hypertension

I	Patients with pulmonary hypertension in whom there is no limitation of usual physical activity; ordinary physical activity does not cause increased dyspnoea, fatigue, chest pain, or presyncope.
II	Patients with pulmonary hypertension who have mild limitation of physical activity. There is no discomfort at rest, but normal physical activity causes increased dyspnoea, fatigue, chest pain, or presyncope.
III	Patients with pulmonary hypertension who have a marked limitation of physical activity. There is no discomfort at rest, but less-than-ordinary activity causes increased dyspnoea, fatigue, chest pain, or presyncope.
IV	Patients with pulmonary hypertension who are unable to perform any physical activity and who may have signs of right ventricular failure at rest. Dyspnoea and/or fatigue may be present at rest, and symptoms are increased by almost any physical activity (ESC).

Table 77.7 ESC 2009 guidelines on pulmonary hypertension. Parameters with established importance for assessing disease severity, stability, and prognosis in PAH

Better prognosis	Determinants of prognosis	Worse prognosis
No	Clinical evidence of RV failure	Yes
Slow	Rate of progression of symptoms	Rapid
No	Syncope	Yes
I, II	WHO-FC	IV
Longer (>500 m)[a]	6MWT	Shorter (<300 m)
Peak O_2 consumption >15 mL/min/kg	Cardiopulmonary exercise testing	Peak O_2 consumption <12 mL/min/kg
Normal or near-normal	BNP/NT-pro-BNP plasma levels	Very elevated and rising
No pericardial effusion TAPSE[b] >2.0 cm	Echocardiographic findings[b]	Pericardial effusion TAPSE[b] <1.5 cm
RAP <8 mmHg and CI ≥2.5 L/min/m²	Haemodynamics	RAP >15 mmHg or CI ≤2.0 L/min/m²

* Depending on age.
[b] tricuspid annular displacement (TAPSE) and pericardial effusion have been selected because they can be measured in the majority of the patients.
BNP, brain natriuretic peptide; CI, cardiac index; 6MWT, 6-minute walking test; RAP, right atrial pressure; TAPSE, tricuspid annular plane systolic excursion; WHO-FC, WHO functional class.
ESC Guidelines for the diagnosis and treatment of pulmonary hypertension. *Eur Heart J*. 2009;**30**:2493–537.

Table 77.8 Vasodilator therapy. ACCF/AHA 2009 consensus document on pulmonary hypertension. Agents for acute vasodilator testing

	Epoprostenol	Adenosine	Nitric oxide
Route of administration	Intravenous infusion	Intravenous infusion	Inhaled
Dose titration	2 ng/kg/min every 10 to 15 min	50 micrograms/kg/min every 2 min	None
Dose range	2 to 10 ng/kg/min	50 to 250 micrograms/kg/min	10 to 80 ppm
Side effects	Headache, nausea, light-headedness	Dyspnoea, chest pain, AV block	Increased left heart filling pressure in susceptible patients

ACCF/AHA 2009 expert consensus document on pulmonary hypertension. *Circulation*. 2009; **119**:2250–94.

ESC 2009 guidelines: route of administration, half-life, dose ranges, increments, and duration of administration of the most commonly used agents for pulmonary vasoreactivity tests

Drug	Route	Half-life	Dose range[a]	Increments[b]	Duration[c]
Epoprostenol	Intravenous	3 min	2–12 ng/kg/min	2 ng/kg/min	10 min
Adenosine	Intravenous	5–10 s	50–350 micrograns/kg/min	50 micrograms/kg/min	2 min
Nitric oxide	Inhaled	15–30 s	10–20 ppm	–	5 min[d]

* Initial dose and maximal tolerated dose suggested (maximal dose limited by side effects, such as hypotension, headache, flushing, etc.).
[b] Increments of dose by each step.
[c] Duration of administration on each step.
[d] For NO, a single step within the dose range is suggested.
ESC Guidelines for the diagnosis and treatment of pulmonary hypertension. *Eur Heart J*. 2009;**30**:2493–537.

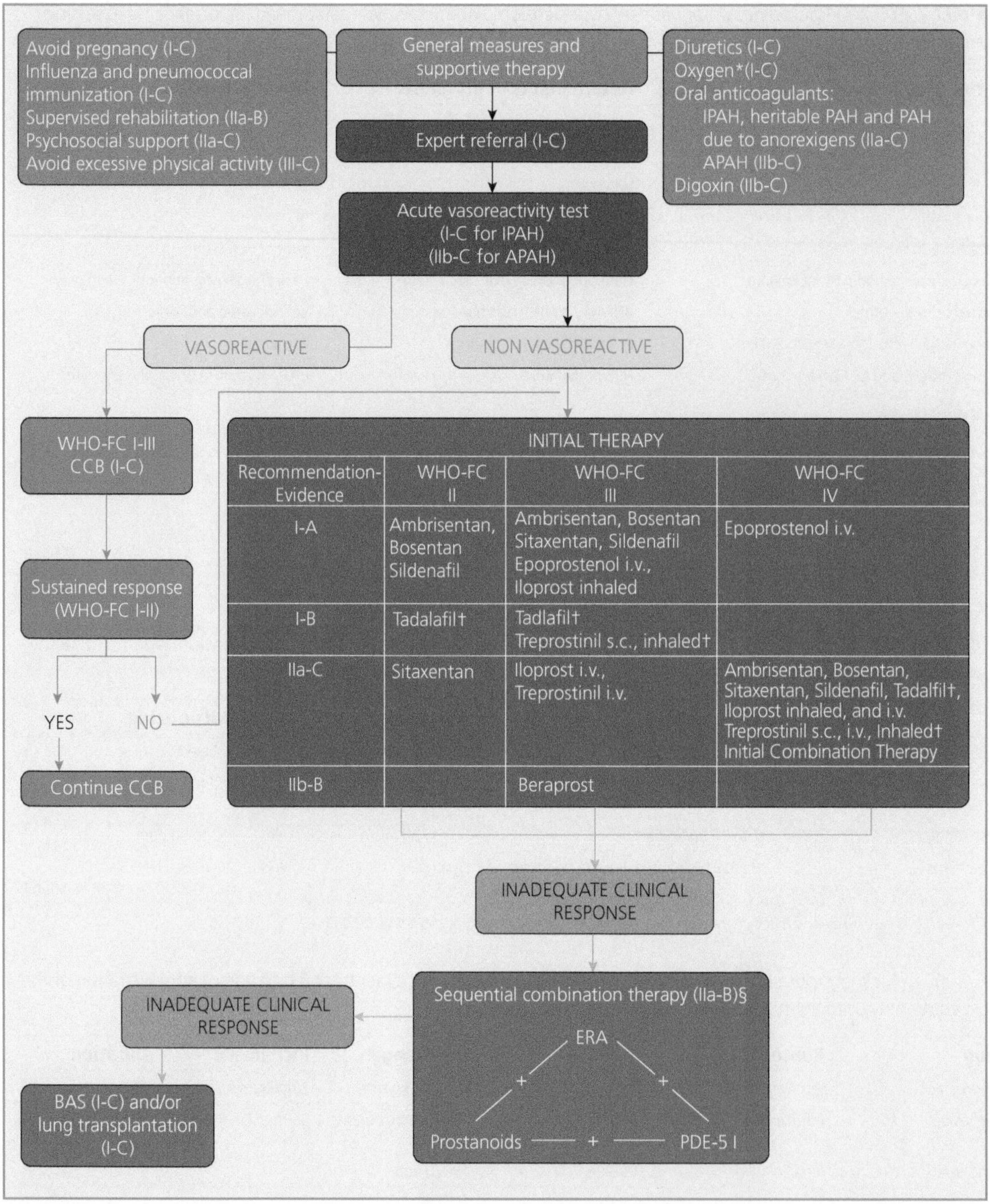

Recommendation-Evidence	WHO-FC II	WHO-FC III	WHO-FC IV
I-A	Ambrisentan, Bosentan Sildenafil	Ambrisentan, Bosentan Sitaxentan, Sildenafil Epoprostenol i.v., Iloprost inhaled	Epoprostenol i.v.
I-B	Tadalafil†	Tadlafil† Treprostinil s.c., inhaled†	
IIa-C	Sitaxentan	Iloprost i.v., Treprostinil i.v.	Ambrisentan, Bosentan, Sitaxentan, Sildenafil, Tadalfil†, Iloprost inhaled, and i.v. Treprostinil s.c., i.v., Inhaled† Initial Combination Therapy
IIb-B		Beraprost	

Figure 77.4 ESC 2009 guidelines: evidence-based treatment algorithm for pulmonary arterial hypertension patients (for group 1 patients only).

* To maintain arterial blood O_2 pressure ≥8 kPa (60 mmHg). † Under regulatory review in the European Union. § IIa-C for WHO-FC II. APAH, associated pulmonary arterial hypertension; BAS, balloon atrial septostomy; CCB, calcium channel blocker; ERA, endothelin receptor antagonist; IPAH, idiopathic pulmonary arterial hypertension; PDE5 I, phosphodiesterase type-5 inhibitor; WHO-FC, World Health Organization functional class.

ESC Guidelines for the diagnosis and treatment of pulmonary hypertension. *Eur Heart J.* 2009;**30**:2493–537

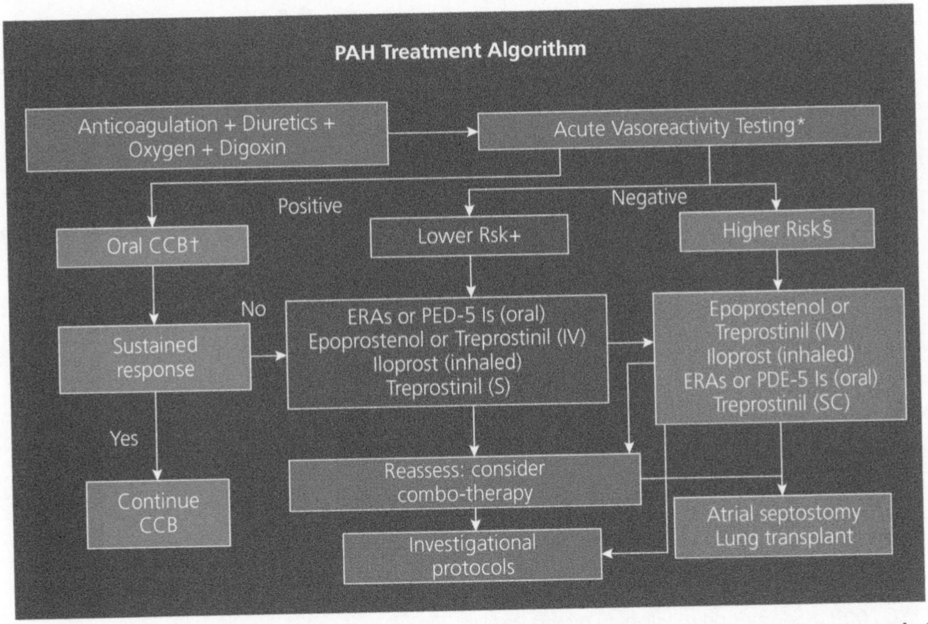

Figure 77.5 AHA 2009 recommendations: treatment algorithm for PAH. Background therapies include warfarin anticoagulation, which is recommended in all patients with IPAH without contraindication. Diuretics are used for management of right heart failure. Oxygen is recommended to maintain oxygen saturation greater than 90%.

* Acute vasodilator testing should be performed in all IPAH patients who may be potential candidates for long-term therapy with calcium channel blockers (CCBs). Patients with PAH due to conditions other than IPAH have a very low rate of long-term responsiveness to oral CCBs, and the value of acute vasodilator testing in such patients needs to be individualized. IPAH patients in whom CCB therapy would not be considered, such as those with right heart failure or haemodynamic instability, should not undergo acute vasodilator testing. † CCBs are indicated only for patients who have a positive acute vasodilator response, and such patients need to be followed closely both for safety and efficacy. ‡ For patients who did not have a positive acute vasodilator testing and are considered lower risk based on clinical assessment, oral therapy with ERA or PDE-5I would be the first line of therapy recommended. If an oral regimen is not appropriate, the other treatments would need to be considered, based on the patient's profile and side effects and risk of each therapy. § For patients who are considered high risk based on clinical assessment, continuous treatment with intravenous (IV) prostacyclin (epoprostenol or treprostinil) would be the first line of therapy recommended. If a patient is not a candidate for continuous IV treatment, the other therapies would have to be considered, based on the patient's profile and side effects and risk of each treatment. Combination therapy should be considered when patients are not responding adequately to initial monotherapy. Timing for lung transplantation and/or atrial septostomy is challenging and is reserved for patients who progress despite optimal medical treatment.

ACCF/AHA 2009 expert consensus document on pulmonary hypertension. *Circulation*. 2009; **119**:2250–94.

Table 77.9 ESC 2009 guidelines on pulmonary hypertension. Recommendations for efficacy of specific drug therapy, balloon atrial septostomy, and lung transplantation for pulmonary arterial hypertension (group 1) according to WHO functional class (WHO-FC)

		WHO-FC II	WHO-FC III	WHO-FC IV
Calcium channel blockers		I-C[a]	I-C[a]	–
Endothelin receptor antagonists	Ambrisentan	I-A	I-A	IIa-C
	Bosentan	I-A	I-A	IIa-C
	Sitaxentan	IIa-C	I-A	IIa-C
Phosphodiesterase type-5 inhibitors	Sildenafil	I-A	I-A	IIa-C
	Tadalafil[b]	I-B	I-B	IIa-C

(Continued)

Table 77.9 (Continued)

		WHO-FC II	WHO-FC III	WHO-FC IV
Prostanoids	Beraprost	–	IIb-B	–
	Epoprostenol (intravenous)	–	I-A	I-A
	Iloprost (inhaled)	–	I-A	I-A
	Iloprost (intravenous)	–	IIa-C	IIa-C
	Treprostinil (subcutaneous)	–	I-B	IIa-C
	Treprostinil (intravenous)	–	IIa-C	IIa-C
	Treprostinil (inhaled)[b]	–	I-B	IIa-C
Initial drugs combination therapy		–	–	IIa-C
Sequential drugs combination therapy		IIa-C	IIa-B	IIa-B
Balloon atrial septostomy		–	I-C	I-C
Lung transplantation		–	I-C	I-C

[a] Only in responders to acute vasoreactivity tests. I for idiopathic PAH heritable PAH, and PAH due to anorexigens: IIa for APAH conditions.
[b] Under regulatory review in the European Union.
ESC Guidelines for the diagnosis and treatment of pulmonary hypertension. *Eur Heart J*. 2009;**30**:2493–537.

Table 77.10 ESC 2009 guidelines on pulmonary hypertension

Recommendations for PAH associated with congenital cardiac shunts	
Bosentan in WHO-FC III patients with Eisenmenger's syndrome	I-B
Other endothelin receptor antagonists, phosphodiesterase type-5 inhibitors, and prostanoids in patients with Eisenmenger's syndrome	IIa-C
In the absence of significant haemoptysis, oral anticoagulant treatment in patients with PA thrombosis or signs of heart failure	IIa-C
Supplemental O_2 therapy when it produces a consistent increase in arterial oxygen saturation and reduces symptoms	IIa-C
If symptoms of hyperviscosity are present, phlebotomy with isovolumic replacement usually when the haematocrit is >65%	IIa-C
Combination therapy in patients with Eisenmenger's syndrome	IIb-C
CCBs are not recommended in Eisenmenger's syndrome	III-C

ESC Guidelines for the diagnosis and treatment of pulmonary hypertension. *Eur Heart J*. 2009;**30**:2493–537.

Table 77.11 ESC 2009 guidelines on pulmonary hypertension

Recommendations for PAH associated with connective tissue disease (CTD)	
The same treatment algorithm as in patients with idiopathic PAH is recommended	I-A
Echocardiographic screening for the detection of PH in symptomatic patients with scleroderma spectrum of diseases	I-B
Echocardiographic screening for the detection of PH in symptomatic patients with all other CTDs	I-C
Right heart catheterization in all cases of suspected PAH associated with CTD, in particular if specific drug therapy is considered	I-C
Oral anticoagulation should be considered on an individual basis	IIa-C
Echocardiographic screening for the detection of PH in asymptomatic patients with the scleroderma spectrum of disease	IIb-C

ESC Guidelines for the diagnosis and treatment of pulmonary hypertension. *Eur Heart J*. 2009;**30**:2493–537.

Table 77.12 ESC 2009 guidelines on pulmonary hypertension

Recommendations for PAH associated with portal hypertension	
Echocardiographic screening for the detection of PH in symptomatic patients with liver diseases and/or in candidates for liver transplantation	I-B
The same treatment algorithm as in patients with idiopathic PAH is recommended, taking into consideration co-morbidities	IIa-C
Anticoagulation in patients with increased risk of bleeding	III-C
Significant PAH is a contraindication to liver transplantation if mean PAP is ≥35 mmHg and/or PVR is ≥250 dynes.s.cm^{-5}	III-C

ESC Guidelines for the diagnosis and treatment of pulmonary hypertension. *Eur Heart J*. 2009;**30**:2493–537.

Table 77.13 ESC 2009 guidelines on pulmonary hypertension

Recommendations for PAH associated with HIV infection	
Echocardiography in patients with unexplained dyspnoea to detect HIV-related cardiovascular complications	I-C
The same treatment algorithm as in patients with idiopathic PAH is recommended, taking into consideration co-morbidities and drug-drug interactions	IIa-C
Anticoagulation in patients with increased risk of bleeding	III-C

ESC Guidelines for the diagnosis and treatment of pulmonary hypertension. *Eur Heart J*. 2009;**30**:2493–537.

Table 77.14 ESC 2009 guidelines on pulmonary hypertension

Recommendations for pulmonary veno-occlusive disease	
Referral of patients with PVOD to a transplant centre for evaluation as soon as the diagnosis is established	I-C
Patients with PVOD should be managed only in centres with extensive experience in PAH due to the risk of lung oedema after the initiation of PAH-specific drug therapy	IIa-C

ESC Guidelines for the diagnosis and treatment of pulmonary hypertension. *Eur Heart J*. 2009;**30**:2493–537.

Pulmonary hypertension associated with pulmonary venous capillary abnormalities

In rare instances, the typical histological findings of PAH are associated with an occlusive venopathy (**pulmonary veno-occlusive disease**, PVOD) or a microvasculopathy (**pulmonary capillary haemangiomatosis**). In addition to the histology of PAH, these entities also exhibit the findings of pulmonary venous hypertension, including pulmonary haemosiderosis, interstitial oedema, and lymphatic dilation. Although the clinical presentation is usually indistinguishable from PAH, rapid development of pulmonary oedema after administration of vasodilators, such as epoprostenol, has been reported in both entities and is often a clue to the appropriate diagnosis.[5]

In pulmonary veno-occlusive disease, intimal fibrosis and thrombosis originate in the small pulmonary veins and venules.[21] The pathogenesis is unknown, but mutations in the bone morphogenetic protein receptor II (BMPR2) gene have been identified as also happens with idiopathic pulmonary hypertension.[22] Patients with PVOD are more severely hypoxaemic and have a much lower diffusion capacity of carbon monoxide than in other forms of PAH. High-resolution CT scanning is the investigation of choice. Typical findings suggestive of PVOD are the presence of **subpleural thickened septal lines**, **centrilobular ground glass opacities** (contrasting with a panlobular distribution found in idiopathic PAH), and **mediastinal lymphadenopathy**. Changes consistent with pulmonary oedema may also be seen on CT imaging in patients with PVOD. **Wedge pressure** is normal in veno-occlusive disease. Pulmonary capillary haemangiomatosis is difficult to differentiate from PVOD, and the diagnostic and therapeutic aspects are very similar. Medical therapy is unsatisfactory, and lung transplantation is the only curative option. Therapy is undertaken in specializing centres (Table 77.14).

References

1. Humbert M, *et al.* Pulmonary arterial hypertension in France: results from a national registry. *Am J Respir Crit Care Med*. 2006;**173**:1023–30
2. Lane KB, *et al.* Heterozygous germline mutations in BMPR2, encoding a TGF-beta receptor, cause familial primary pulmonary hypertension. *Nat Genet*. 2000;**26**:81–4
3. Trembath RC, *et al.* Clinical and molecular genetic features of pulmonary hypertension in patients with hereditary haemorrhagic telangiectasia. *N Engl J Med*. 2001;**345**:325–34
4. McLaughlin VV, *et al.* ACCF/AHA 2009 expert consensus document on pulmonary hypertension: a report of the American College of Cardiology Foundation Task Force on expert consensus documents and the American Heart Association: developed in collaboration with the American College of Chest Physicians, American Thoracic Society, Inc., and the Pulmonary Hypertension Association. *Circulation*. 2009;**119**:2250–94
5. Galie N, *et al.* Guidelines for the diagnosis and treatment of pulmonary hypertension: the Task Force for the diagnosis and treatment of pulmonary hypertension of the European Society of Cardiology (ESC) and the European Respiratory Society (ERS), endorsed by the International Society of Heart and Lung Transplantation (ISHLT). *Eur Heart J*. 2009;**30**:2493–537
6. Le RJ, *et al.* Syncope in adults with pulmonary arterial hypertension. *J Am Coll Cardiol*. 2011;**58**:863–7
7. Ghofrani HA, *et al.* Uncertainties in the diagnosis and treatment of pulmonary arterial hypertension. *Circulation*. 2008;**118**:1195–201
8. van Wolferen SA, *et al.* Prognostic value of right ventricular mass, volume, and function in idiopathic pulmonary arterial hypertension. *Eur Heart J*. 2007;**28**:1250–7

9. Forfia PR, *et al.* Tricuspid annular displacement predicts survival in pulmonary hypertension. *Am J Respir Crit Care Med.* 2006;**174**:1034–41
10. McLaughlin VV, *et al.* Pulmonary arterial hypertension. *Circulation.* 2006;**114**:1417–31
11. Provencher S, *et al.* Long-term outcome with first-line bosentan therapy in idiopathic pulmonary arterial hypertension. *Eur Heart J.* 2006;**27**:589–95
12. Galie N, *et al.* Ambrisentan for the treatment of pulmonary arterial hypertension: results of the ambrisentan in pulmonary arterial hypertension, randomized, double-blind, placebo-controlled, multicenter, efficacy (ARIES) study 1 and 2. *Circulation.* 2008;**117**:3010–19
13. Barst RJ, *et al.* Treatment of pulmonary arterial hypertension with the selective endothelin-a receptor antagonist sitaxsentan. *J Am Coll Cardiol.* 2006;**47**:2049–56
14. McLaughlin VV, *et al.* Survival in primary pulmonary hypertension: the impact of epoprostenol therapy. *Circulation.* 2002;**106**:1477–82
15. Simonneau G, *et al.* Continuous subcutaneous infusion of treprostinil, a prostacyclin analogue, in patients with pulmonary arterial hypertension: a double-blind, randomized, placebo-controlled trial. *Am J Respir Crit Care Med.* 2002;**165**:800–4
16. Jing Z-C, *et al.* Efficacy and safety of oral treprostinil monotherapy for the treatment of pulmonary arterial hypertension: A randomized, controlled trial. *Circulation.* 2013;**127**:624–33
17. Opitz CF, *et al.* Clinical efficacy and survival with first-line inhaled iloprost therapy in patients with idiopathic pulmonary arterial hypertension. *Eur Heart J.* 2005;**26**:1895–902
18. Galie N, *et al.* Tadalafil therapy for pulmonary arterial hypertension. *Circulation.* 2009;**119**:2894–903
19. Hoeper MM, *et al.* Sildenafil citrate therapy for pulmonary arterial hypertension. *N Engl J Med.* 2006;**354**:1091–3; author reply 1091–3
20. Khan AS, *et al.* Viagra deafness—sensorineural hearing loss and phosphodiesterase-5 inhibitors. *Laryngoscope.* 2011;**121**:1049–54
21. Detsky ME, *et al.* Clinical problem-solving. Under pressure. *N Engl J Med.* 2010;**362**:449–54
22. Rich S, *et al.* Diagnosis and treatment of secondary (non-category 1) pulmonary hypertension. *Circulation.* 2008;**118**:2190–9

Chapter 78

Pulmonary hypertension associated with left heart disease and lung disease, and chronic thromboembolic pulmonary hypertension

Pulmonary hypertension associated with left heart disease

Definition

Patients have elevated pulmonary venous pressure (as reflected by a pulmonary capillary wedge pressure ≥15 mmHg), usually as a consequence of either mitral valve disease or LV diastolic dysfunction.[1] It is, therefore, a **post-capillary pulmonary hypertension**, as opposed to the other pre-capillary forms.

Pathophysiology

Chronic elevation of the LA or diastolic LV filling pressure causes a backward transmission of the pressure to the pulmonary venous system that triggers vasoconstriction in the arterial pulmonary bed. For reasons that remain unclear, some patients do not progress to reactive pulmonary vasoconstriction despite the presence of chronic advanced heart failure.[1]

Diagnosis

Exertional dyspnoea is the most common symptom. Diagnostic tests may reveal the causative condition and differentiate pulmonary venous hypertension from pulmonary arterial hypertension (PAH).

ECG LV, rather than RV, hypertrophy may be present.

Chest X-ray Pulmonary vascular congestion, pleural effusions, and, on occasion, pulmonary oedema.

Echocardiography Valve disease and reduced LV function can be detected. Left atrial enlargement, concentric remodelling of the LV (relative wall thickness >0.45), LV hypertrophy, and the presence of echocardiographic indicators of elevated LV filling pressure suggest PH due to left heart disease rather than PAH. However, in the absence of detectable significant valve disease, Doppler echocardiography alone may not exclude PAH since pulmonary hypertension itself produces diastolic filling abnormalities in the LV.[2]

Chest CT Ground glass opacities and a mosaic perfusion pattern, consistent with chronic pulmonary oedema, that are not seen in PAH.

Cardiac catheterization An elevated wedge pressure at end-expiration establishes the diagnosis but may not always be accurately measured and may be normal due to the use of diuretics. Exercise or inotropic challenges may increase cardiac output and expose increased wedge pressure. Short-acting pulmonary vasodilators may also be used in cases with low wedge pressure and normal cardiac output.

Prognosis

Prognosis of these patients is poor, with >50% mortality in 2 years.[3] An elevated transpulmonary gradient (mean PAP minus mean PWP) >12 mmHg is suggestive of progressive intrinsic changes in the pulmonary circulation overriding the passive increase in PWP.[1] This progressed form is also called **reactive PH** and resembles pre-capillary forms.

Therapy

It is targeting the underlying condition (Tables 78.1 and 78.2). No heart failure drugs are contraindicated because of PH. Although preliminary results with phosphodiesterase type-5 inhibitors have been promising,[4,5] pulmonary vasodilators may be harmful. The potential role of vasodilators, in cases where the pulmonary hypertension is clearly disproportionate to the extent of underlying left heart disease, is also under investigation.[6]

Pulmonary hypertension associated with lung disease

Chronic obstructive pulmonary disease and interstitial lung disease are the most common causes.

Pathophysiology

Hypoxia induces muscularization of distal vessels and medial hypertrophy of more proximal arteries as well as a loss of vessels, which is compounded by a loss of lung parenchyma in the setting of lung disease.[2] In patients with mild pulmonary hypertension in association with smoking, severe fibroproliferative neointimal formation can also be seen but not the development of plexiform lesions. A marked reduction in diffusing capacity for carbon monoxide is a consistent feature of the patients with connective tissue diseases who have pulmonary hypertension.

Table 78.1 ESC 2009 guidelines on pulmonary hypertension

Recommendations for PH due to left heart disease	
Optimal treatment of the underlying left heart disease	I-C
Patients with 'out of proportion' PH should be enrolled in RCTs targeting PH-specific drugs	IIa-C
Increased left-sided filling pressures may be estimated by Doppler echocardiography	IIb-C
Invasive measurements of PWP or LV end-diastolic pressure to confirm the diagnosis of PH due to left heart disease	IIb-C
Right heart catheterization in patients with echocardiographic signs suggesting severe PH	IIb-C
The use of PAH-specific drug therapy is not recommended	III-C

ESC Guidelines for the diagnosis and treatment of pulmonary hypertension. *Eur Heart J*. 2009;**30**:2493–537.

Clinical forms

Chronic obstructive pulmonary disease

Patients present with **dyspnoea and RV failure** in the setting of marked **hypoxaemia**. The typical ECG pattern of **cor pulmonale** is tall, pointed P waves in leads II, III, and aVF, and right axis deviation with RV hypertrophy pattern or simply rS complexes across the precordium. Pulmonary hypertension is usually mild but still predictive of the prognosis. Severe pulmonary hypertension may be seen in genetically predisposed patients (<5%). COPD, as a cause of hypoxic PH, is diagnosed on the evidence of irreversible airflow obstruction, together with increased residual volumes and reduced diffusion capacity for carbon monoxide and normal or increased carbon dioxide tension. The only effective treatment is supplemental oxygen. Pulmonary vasodilators may worsen the ventilation perfusion mismatch (Tables 78.2 and 78.3).

Interstitial lung disease

This can be due to either a connective tissue disorder or to idiopathic pulmonary fibrosis. Pulmonary hypertension is relatively mild (**mean <40 mmHg**). Results with pulmonary vasodilators have not been consistent, and the only treatment of severely symptomatic patients is lung transplantation.[7] A decrease in **lung volume**, together with a decrease in **diffusion capacity for carbon monoxide**, may indicate a diagnosis of interstitial lung disease.

Chronic thromboembolic pulmonary hypertension

Definition

Chronic thromboembolic pulmonary hypertension is defined as mean PA pressure >25 mmHg that persists 6 months after PE is diagnosed.[8] It is differentiated by recurrent pulmonary embolism by a gradual progression of symptoms and signs of pulmonary hypertension, as opposed to profound episodic exacerbations, and a lack of response to fibrinolytic therapy or at least 6 months of antithrombotic therapy.[8]

Table 78.2 ACCF/AHA consensus document 2009 on PH

Summary of recommendations in PH
1. Patients with PH require a thorough diagnostic evaluation to elucidate the roles of pulmonary venous hypertension, chronic lung disease with hypoxaemia, and/or pulmonary thromboembolism to the pathogenesis of their disease. Accordingly, right heart catheterization, lung function and imaging studies, determination of arterial oxygen saturation (at rest, with activity, and overnight), and ventilation perfusion scanning are all mandatory elements of the assessment of these patients.
2. Patients with PH related to pulmonary venous hypertension may be considered for PAH-specific therapy provided:
a. The cause of the pulmonary venous hypertension is first optimally treated; and
b.The PCWP is normal or only minimally elevated; and
c. The transpulmonary gradient (TPG) and PVR are significantly elevated; and
d. The patient's symptoms suggest that PAH-specific therapy may yield clinical benefit.
3. Patients with PH related to chronic lung disease and hypoxAemia may be considered for PAH-specific therapy provided:
a. The chronic lung disease and hypoxaemia are first optimally treated; and
b. The TPG and PVR are significantly elevated; and
c. The patient's symptoms suggest that PAH-specific therapy may yield clinical benefit.
4. Patients with chronic thromboembolic PH may be considered for PAH-specific therapy provided:
a. Appropriate secondary preventative measures, including anticoagulation, have been instituted; and
b. PTE has been performed or is not indicated; and
c. The TPG and PVR are significantly elevated; and
d. The patient's symptoms suggest that PAH-specific therapy may yield clinical benefit.
5. Patients with PH following cardiac surgery may be considered for PAH-specific therapy provided:
a. The surgery and concomitant medical therapy provide optimal treatment of the underlying cardiac disease; and
b. The surgery and concomitant medical therapy result in a normal or only minimally elevated PCWP; and
c. The TPG and PVR remain significantly elevated; and
d. The patient's clinical condition suggests that PAH-specific therapy may yield clinical benefit.

Treatment of such patients with PAH-specific therapy should be undertaken with great care, as these treatments may result in an increase in fluid retention, left-sided cardiac filling pressures, and pulmonary oedema and result in clinical deterioration. Decisions about whether and how to treat such patients should be made on a case-by-case basis by experienced PH caregivers.

ACCF/AHA 2009 expert consensus document on pulmonary hypertension. *Circulation*. 2009; **119**:2250–94

Table 78.3 ESC 2009 guidelines on pulmonary hypertension

Recommendations for PH due to lung diseases	
Echocardiography as a screening tool for the assessment of PH	I-C
Right heart catheterization for a definite diagnosis of PH	I-C
Optimal treatment of the underlying lung disease including long-term O_2 therapy in patients with chronic hypoxaemia	I-C
Patients with 'out of proportion' PH should be enrolled in RCTs targeting PAH-specific drugs	IIa-C
PAH-specific drug therapy is not recommended	III-C

ESC Guidelines for the diagnosis and treatment of pulmonary hypertension. *Eur Heart J*. 2009;**30**:2493–537

Epidemiology

Its occurs in 1–3% of acute pulmonary embolism cases,[9,10] but its true incidence is unknown.

Aetiology

Predisposing factors are presented in Table 78.4.[11,12] Patients usually, but not invariably, present in their 40s, and the disease is twice as common in women. Microemboli of tumour cells may also cause pulmonary hypertension and right heart failure in patients with breast cancer or other types of carcinoma (pulmonary tumour thrombotic microangiopathy). Mediastinal fibrosis secondary to tuberculosis, sarcoidosis, histoplasmosis, and radiation therapy may resemble chronic thromboembolic disease, although the typical thromboembolic lesions on high-resolution CT are missing.

Pathophysiology

Within months or years after PE, the original embolic material is replaced by fibrous tissue that is incorporated in the intima and media of the PAs. Abnormal degradation of fibrinogen, autoimmunity, and chronic staphylococcal infections are proposed mechanisms of ineffective fibrinolysis. Neurohumoral factors, such as endothelin-1, induce additional vasoconstriction, with resultant small-vessel arteriopathy, intimal proliferation, microvascular thrombosis, and plexiform lesion formation.

At least 60–70% of pulmonary vasculature must be occluded before pulmonary hypertension develops. Four types of disease have been described.[12]

Presentation and physical findings

Exercise intolerance and dyspnoea are the most common presenting symptoms. Peripheral oedema, syncope, and haemoptysis may be late findings. Careful history reveals previous PE in up to 75% of the cases (Table 78.5).[13]

Table 78.4 Risk factors of CTPE

Unprovoked and recurrent venous thromboembolism
PA pressure >50 mmHg at PE or 6 months after therapy
Ventriculo-atrial shunts and infected pacemakers
Splenectomy
Sickle cell disease
Blood groups other than O
Lupus anticoagulant/antiphospholipid antibodies
Thyroid disease and thyroid replacement therapy
History of malignancy
Dysfibrinogenaemia
Chronic inflammatory disorders (osteomyelitis, inflammatory bowel disease)

Table 78.5 AHA 2011 scientific statement on PE, IDVT, and CTEPH

Recommendations for diagnostic evaluation of CTEPH	
Patients presenting with unexplained dyspnoea, exercise intolerance, or clinical evidence of right-sided heart failure, with or without prior history of symptomatic VTE, should be evaluated for CTEPH.	I-C
It is reasonable to evaluate patients with an echocardiogram 6 weeks after an acute PE to screen for persistent pulmonary hypertension that may predict the development of CTEPH.	IIa-C

Management of massive and submassive pulmonary embolism, iliofemoral deep vein thrombosis, and chronic thromboembolic pulmonary hypertension: a scientific statement from the American Heart Association. *Circulation*. 2011;**123**:1788–830.

A loud **P_2**, with reduction of the respiratory variation of the **S_2 splitting**, and **palpable RV** are the initial findings, followed by typical RV failure signs (right S_3, TR, hepatomegaly and ascites, and peripheral oedema) and bruits over the peripheral lungs due to turbulent pulmonary flow.

A thrombophilic disorder can be found in 30% of patients and splenectomy in 3% of them.[11]

Diagnosis

Chest X-ray is usually unremarkable. Hilar fullness due to enlarged PAs is a late finding, and peripheral lung opacities due to scarring from previous PE are rare.

Echocardiography reveals pulmonary hypertension and RV dysfunction.

Arterial blood oxygen levels may show hypoxaemia or be normal.

Lung function tests are necessary to exclude obstructive or fibrotic lung disease.

V/Q scanning typically shows multiple bilateral perfusion defects. A normal scan rules out the disease. It has a higher sensitivity that CT for diagnosis of CTEPH.[14]

Contrast-enhanced CT may show central pulmonary artery dilatation, abrupt narrowing or tapering of peripheral pulmonary vessels, right ventricular hypertrophy, right ventricular and atrial enlargement, dilated bronchial arteries, and a ground glass or mosaic pattern of attenuation due to variable lung perfusion. Microemboli of tumour cells are beyond the resolution of the CT pulmonary angiogram.

MRI may also be used but has less sensitivity in diagnosing PE.

Right heart catheterization with pulmonary angiography still remains the standard for establishing the diagnosis and assessing operability. Systolic and mean PA pressures are >40 mmHg and 25 mmHg, respectively, and PVR >3 Wood units. Capillary wedge pressure is <15 mmHg (excluding left-sided heart disease). In some patients, the wedge pressure may be higher because of severe RV dilation, interventricular dependence, and resultant LV diastolic dysfunction; in these cases, the PVR is usually high (>600 dyn.s.cm–^{5}).[13] Specific angiographic patterns include pulmonary artery webs or bands, intimal irregularities, abrupt stenoses of major pulmonary arteries, and obstruction of lobar or segmental arteries at their origins. Pulmonary angioscopy may also be performed.[13]

Therapy

Chronic anticoagulation is recommended in all patients (Tables 78.6 and 78.7). The value of specific medical therapy is limited, and the most effective therapy is

Table 78.6 ESC 2009 guidelines on pulmonary hypertension

Recommendations for chronic thromboembolic pulmonary hypertension (CTEPH)	
The diagnosis is based on the presence of pre-capillary PH (mean PAP ≥25 mmHg, PVR >2 Wood units) in patients with multiple chronic/organized occlusive thrombi/emboli in the elastic pulmonary arteries (main, lobar, segmental, subsegmental)	I-C
Lifelong anticoagulation is indicated	I-C
Surgical pulmonary endarterectomy is the recommended treatment	I-C
Once perfusion scanning and/or CT angiography show signs compatible with CTEPH, the patient should be referred to a centre with expertise in surgical pulmonary endarterectomy	IIa-C
The selection of patients for surgery should be based on the extent and location of the organized thrombi, on the degree of PH, and on co-morbidities	IIa-C
PAH-specific drug therapy in selected CTEPH patients, such as patients not candidates for surgery or patients with residual PH after pulmonary endarterectomy	IIb-C

ESC Guidelines for the diagnosis and treatment of pulmonary hypertension. *Eur Heart J*. 2009;**30**:2493–537.

Table 78.7 AHA 2011 scientific statement on PE, IDVT, and CTEPH

Recommendations for medical therapy and pulmonary endarterectomy in patients with CTEPH	
Patients with objectively proven CTEPH should be promptly evaluated for pulmonary endarterectomy, even if symptoms are mild.	I-B
Patients with objectively proven CTEPH should receive indefinite therapeutic anticoagulation in the absence of contraindications.	I-C
PAH (WHO group I)-specific medical therapy for patients with CTEPH who are not surgical candidates (because of co-morbidities or patient choice) or who have residual pulmonary hypertension after operation not amenable to repeat pulmonary endarterectomy at an experienced centre	IIb-B
PAH (WHO group I)-specific medical therapy should not be used in lieu of pulmonary endarterectomy or delay evaluation for pulmonary endarterectomy for patients with objectively proven CTEPH who are or may be surgical candidates at an experienced centre.	III-B

Management of massive and submassive pulmonary embolism, iliofemoral deep vein thrombosis, and chronic thromboembolic pulmonary hypertension: a scientific statement from the American Heart Association. *Circulation*. 2011;**123**:1788–830.

pulmonary thromboendarterectomy.[15] Preoperative predictors of a favourable outcome are PVR <1200 dyn.s.cm^{-5} and the absence of co-morbid conditions. A reduction in PA pressure after administration of inhaled nitric oxide is also indicative of a response to pulmonary thromboendarterectomy. In experienced centres, the intraoperative mortality is 5–10%.

In inoperable patients, the endothelin receptor antagonist bosentan, the phosphodiesterase inhibitor sildenafil, and prostacyclin analogues, such as treprostinil, have been used with clinical improvement.[16–18] New agents are also under investigation. The role of balloon angioplasty is not established. There is no specific treatment for (the usually fatal) pulmonary tumour thrombotic microangiopathy, apart from that directed at the underlying cancer.[19]

References

1. Guazzi M, *et al.* Pulmonary hypertension due to left heart disease. *Circulation*. 2012;**126**:975–90
2. Rich S, *et al.* Diagnosis and treatment of secondary (non-category 1) pulmonary hypertension. *Circulation*. 2008;**118**:2190–9
3. Grigioni F, *et al.* Prognostic implications of serial assessments of pulmonary hypertension in severe chronic heart failure. *J Heart Lung Transplant*. 2006;**25**:1241–6
4. Guazzi M, *et al.* Pulmonary hypertension in heart failure with preserved ejection fraction: a target of phosphodiesterase-5 inhibition in a 1-year study. *Circulation*. 2011;**124**:164–74
5. Lewis GD, *et al.* Sildenafil improves exercise capacity and quality of life in patients with systolic heart failure and secondary pulmonary hypertension. *Circulation*. 2007;**116**:1555–62
6. McLaughlin VV, *et al.* ACCF/AHA 2009 expert consensus document on pulmonary hypertension: a report of the American College of Cardiology Foundation Task Force on expert consensus documents and the American Heart Association: developed in collaboration with the American College of Chest Physicians, American Thoracic Society, Inc., and the Pulmonary Hypertension Association. *Circulation*. 2009;**119**:2250–94
7. King TE, Jr., *et al.* BUILD-1: A randomized placebo-controlled trial of bosentan in idiopathic pulmonary fibrosis. *Am J Respir Crit Care Med*. 2008;**177**:75–81
8. Piazza G, *et al.* Chronic thromboembolic pulmonary hypertension. *N Engl J Med*. 2011;**364**:351–60
9. Becattini C, *et al.* Incidence of chronic thromboembolic pulmonary hypertension after a first episode of pulmonary embolism. *Chest*. 2006;**130**:172–5
10. Pengo V, *et al.* Incidence of chronic thromboembolic pulmonary hypertension after pulmonary embolism. *N Engl J Med*. 2004;**350**:2257–64
11. Bonderman D, *et al.* Risk factors for chronic thromboembolic pulmonary hypertension. *Eur Respir J*. 2009;**33**:325–31
12. Jaff MR, *et al.* Management of massive and submassive pulmonary embolism, iliofemoral deep vein thrombosis, and chronic thromboembolic pulmonary hypertension: a scientific statement from the American Heart Association. *Circulation*. 2011;**123**:1788–830
13. Pepke-Zaba J, *et al.* Chronic thromboembolic pulmonary hypertension (CTEPH): results from an international prospective registry. *Circulation*. 2011;**124**:1973–81
14. Tunariu N, *et al.* Ventilation-perfusion scintigraphy is more sensitive than multidetector CTPA in detecting chronic thromboembolic pulmonary disease as a treatable cause of pulmonary hypertension. *J Nucl Med*. 2007;**48**:680–4
15. Jensen KW, *et al.* Pulmonary hypertensive medical therapy in chronic thromboembolic pulmonary hypertension before pulmonary thromboendarterectomy. *Circulation*. 2009;**120**:1248–54
16. Jais X, *et al.* Bosentan for treatment of inoperable chronic thromboembolic pulmonary hypertension: BENEFIT (bosentan effects in inoperable forms of chronic thromboembolic pulmonary hypertension), a randomized, placebo-controlled trial. *J Am Coll Cardiol*. 2008;**52**:2127–34
17. Toshner MR, *et al.* Pulmonary arterial size and response to sildenafil in chronic thromboembolic pulmonary hypertension. *J Heart Lung Transplant*. 2010;**29**:610–15
18. Voswinckel R, *et al.* Favorable effects of inhaled treprostinil in severe pulmonary hypertension: results from randomized controlled pilot studies. *J Am Coll Cardiol*. 2006;**48**:1672–81
19. Ross JJ, *et al.* Interactive medical case. Breathless. *N Engl J Med*. 2011;**365**:e47

Part XVII

Infective endocarditis

Relevant guidelines

AHA 2005 statement on endocarditis

Infective endocarditis: diagnosis, antimicrobial therapy, and management of complications: a statement for healthcare professionals from the Committee on Rheumatic Fever, Endocarditis, and Kawasaki Disease, Council on Cardiovascular Disease in the Young, and the Councils on Clinical Cardiology, Stroke, and Cardiovascular Surgery and Anesthesia, American Heart Association: endorsed by the Infectious Diseases Society of America. *Circulation.* 2005;**111**:e394–434.

ESC 2009 guidelines on infective endocarditis

Guidelines on the prevention, diagnosis, and treatment of infective endocarditis (new version 2009): the Task Force on the Prevention, Diagnosis, and Treatment of Infective Endocarditis of the European Society of Cardiology (ESC). Endorsed by the European Society of Clinical Microbiology and Infectious Diseases (ESCMID) and the International Society of Chaemotherapy (ISC) for Infection and Cancer. *Eur Heart J.* 2009;**30**:2369–413.

ACC/AHA 2008 guidelines of valve disease

2008 focused update incorporated into the ACC/AHA 2006 guidelines for the management of patients with valvular heart disease. *J Am Coll Cardiol.* 2008;**52**:e1–142.

Chapter 79

Infective endocarditis

Definition

Infective endocarditis (IE) denotes infection of the endocardial surface of the heart. It most commonly involves heart valves (especially mitral and aortic) but may also occur at the site of a septal defect, on the chordae tendineae, or on the mural endocardium.[1–3] The characteristic lesion, a vegetation, is composed of a collection of platelets, fibrin, microorganisms, and inflammatory cells.[2] IE is either acute or subacute-chronic, and is usually classified in four categories: native valve endocarditis, prosthetic valve endocarditis, infective endocarditis in intravenous drug users, and nosocomial infective endocarditis (Table 79.1).

Epidemiology

The incidence of IE ranges within 3–10 episodes/100 000 person-years[4] and has not changed over the past two decades.[1,2] In the western world, there is an increasing incidence of IE associated with a prosthetic valve and a possible decrease in patients with underlying rheumatic heart disease,[5] which is more frequent in underdeveloped countries.[4] New at-risk groups in developed countries include injection drug addicts, elderly with valvular sclerosis, people with prosthetic valves, patients on haemodialysis, and those with nosocomial exposure. IE is now more often an acute disease; most cases occur in patients over 60 years old, and men are more likely to be affected than women.[4,5] Although endocarditis is an uncommon coexisting condition in bacterial meningitis (in 2% of patients and usually due to *Streptococcus pneumoniae* and *Staphylococcus aureus*), it is associated with a high rate of unfavorable outcome.[6]

Aetiology

According to the International Collaboration on Endocarditis Prospective Cohort Study, a multinational and multicentre study of 2781 adults with IE conducted at 58 sites in 25 countries, *Staphylococcus aureus* is now the most common cause of IE in much of the world, followed by *viridans streptococci*, enterococci, and coagulase-negative staphylococcus.[5] This finding was confirmed by the recent French AEPEI report.[7] Gram-positive organisms account for >80% of all cases (Figure 79.1). Candida is the most frequent cause of fungal endocarditis, and culture-negative IE comprise 5–12% of all cases.

Cardiac abnormalities that are associated with high risk of IE are prosthetic cardiac valves or prosthetic material used for cardiac valve repair, previous infective endocarditis, congenital conditions unrepaired or repaired with prosthetic material, and cardiac transplant recipients with valve regurgitation due to a structurally abnormal valve (see Prophylaxis). However, 50% of cases of infective endocarditis develop in patients with no known history of valve disease.[1]

Pathophysiology

The primary event is bacterial adherence to damaged endocardium. Excoriation of the endothelium triggers coagulation, and is colonized by bacteria that attract monocytes to produce tissue factor and cytokines. Cytokines and procoagulant factors contribute to continuing enlargement of the infected coagulum that eventually creates the vegetation. Organisms, such as *Staphylococcus (S.) aureus*, streptococci, and enterococci, have surface adhesins that mediate attachment to the vegetation. *S. aureus* also carries fibronectin-binding proteins on its surface that are adhered to the endothelium through the affinity of integrins, proteins that are produced as a response of endothelial cells to local inflammation.[2] Microorganisms become enveloped within the vegetation and trigger further tissue factor production and platelet activation that both kill bacteria through microbicidal proteins and have procoagulant effects. Tissue invasion and abscess formation then follows. Infective endocarditis is more often due to Gram-positive than Gram-negative bacteria possibly because of differences in adherence to damaged valves or because of differences in their susceptibility to serum-induced killing.[2] Bacterial adherence is completed within minutes during transient bacteraemia that can be caused by various activities. There is now evidence that most cases of infective endocarditis are not attributable to an invasive procedure, and bacteraemia resulting from daily activities is much more likely to cause infective endocarditis than bacteraemia associated with a dental, or other, procedure. Thus, antibiotic prophylaxis in this setting is no longer mandatory.

Presentation

More than 90% of patients present with **fever**, often associated with systemic symptoms of malaise, anorexia,

Table 79.1 ESC 2009 GL on endocarditis. Classification and definitions of IE

IE according to localization of infection and presence or absence of intracardiac material	
• Left-sided native valve IE	
• Left-sided prosthetic valve IE (PVE)	
- Early PVE: <1 year after valve surgery	
- Late PVE: >1 year after valve surgery	
• Right-sided IE	
• Device-related IE (permanent pacemaker or cardioverter-defibrillator)	
IE according to the mode of acquisition	
• Healthcare-associated IE	
- Nosocomial	IE developing in a patient hospitalized >48 hours prior to the onset of signs/symptoms consistent with IE
- Non-nosocomial	Signs and/or symptoms of IE starting <48 hours after admission in a patient with healthcare contact defined as: 1) Home-based nursing or intravenous therapy, haemodialysis, or intravenous chemotherapy <30 days before the onset of IE; or 2) Hospitalized in an acute care facility <90 days before the onset of IE; or 3) Resident in a nursing home or long-term care facility
• Community-acquired IE	Signs and/or symptoms of IE starting <48 hours after admission in a patient not fulfilling the criteria for healthcare-associated infection
• Intravenous drug abuse-associated IE	IE in an active injection drug user without alternative source of infection
Active IE	
• IE with persistent fever and positive blood cultures, *or*	
• Active inflammatory morphology found at surgery, *or*	
• Patient still under antibiotic therapy, *or*	
• Histopathological evidence of active IE	
Recurrence	
• Relapse	Repeat episodes of IE caused by the same microorganism <6 months after the initial episode
• Reinfection	Infection with a different microorganism Repeat episode of IE caused by the same microorganism >6 months after the initial episode

Guidelines on the prevention, diagnosis, and treatment of infective endocarditis (new version 2009). *Eur Heart J*. 2009;**30**:2369–413.

myalgias, and weight loss. Fever may be absent or minimal in patients with congestive heart failure, chronic renal or liver failure, previous use of antimicrobial drugs, or infective endocarditis caused by less virulent organisms, in the elderly, and in immunocompromised patients. **Embolic events** to the brain (>50% of emboli), spleen, or lung occur in 15–30% of patients with IE and may be the presenting feature.[4]

Native valve endocarditis Degenerative lesions, such as mitral regurgitation and senile aortic stenosis, are present in up to 50% of patients with IE older than 60 years.[2] Mitral valve prolapse predisposes patients to IE, with an estimated incidence of 0.01% per patient-year of follow-up. The risk is significantly higher in the presence of flail leaflets and MR (1.5% per year).[8]

Prosthetic valve endocarditis is found in 5–25% of patients with IE.[3,5] It is **early** (within 2 months post-operatively, usually due to *S. aureus*) or **late** (typically >12 months post-operatively), often due to streptococci and Gram-negative bacteria of the **HACEK** group. Although mechanical valves probably have a higher rate of infection during the first 3 months after surgery, similar rates with bioprostheses are seen later.[3] Prosthetic valve endocarditis may be manifested as an indolent illness with low-grade fever or it can be acute with new or changing murmurs and congestive heart failure. Unexplained fever in a patient with a prosthetic valve should prompt careful evaluation for prosthetic valve endocarditis.

In patients with **implanted devices**, clinical manifestations of pocket infection are present in the majority of patients with early lead-associated endocarditis (<6 months after device implantation). However, late lead-associated endocarditis should be considered in any patient who presents with fever, bloodstream infection, or signs of sepsis, even if the device pocket appears uninfected. Prompt recognition and management may improve outcomes.[9]

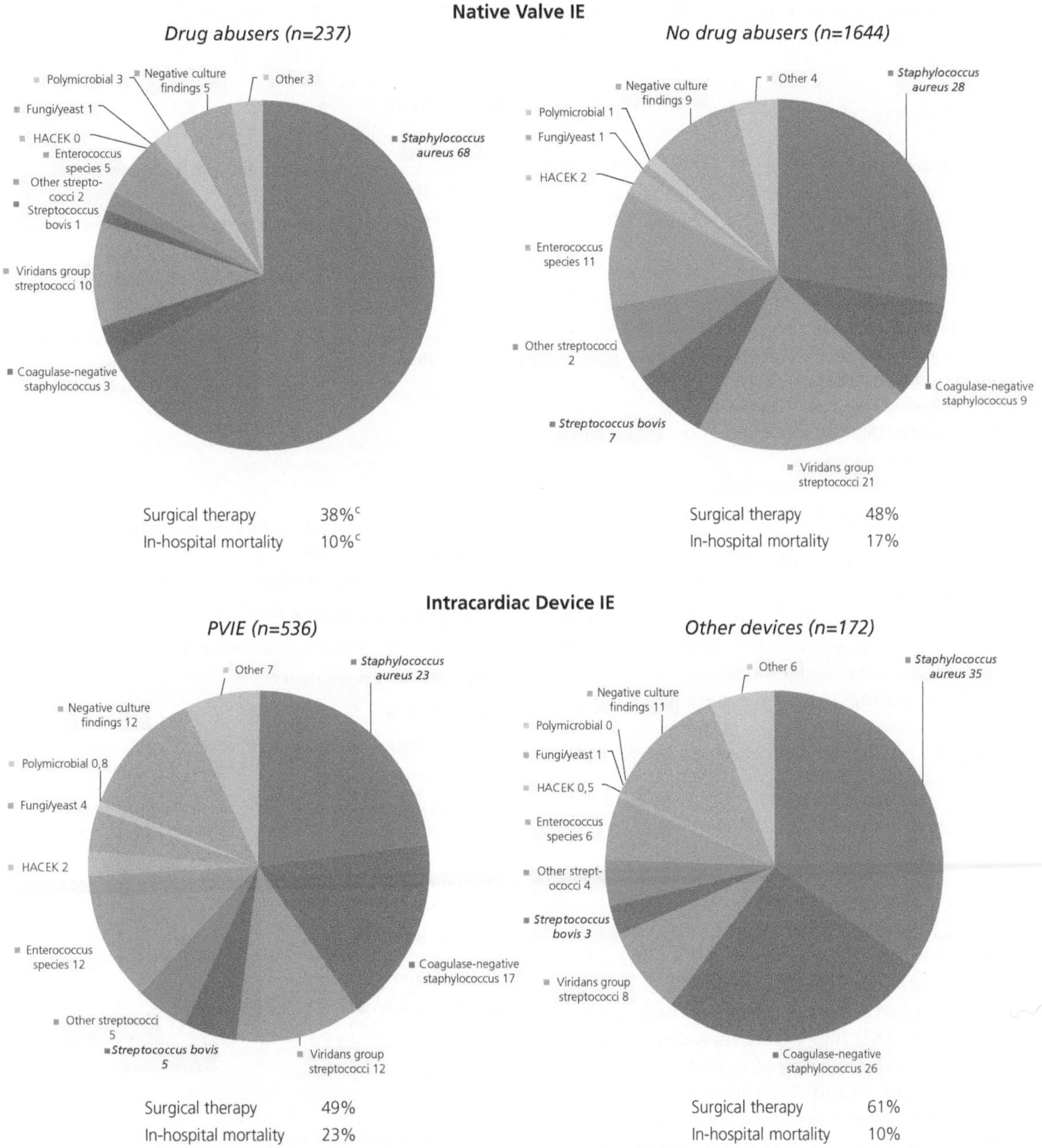

Figure 79.1 Microbiology of IE.

Numbers indicate percentages of patients. HACEK, bacteria consisting of *Haemophilus* species, *Aggregatibacter* (formerly *Actinobacillus*) *actinomycetemcomitans, Cardiobacterium hominis, Eikenella corrodens,* and *Kingella* species; IE, infective endocarditis; PVIE, prosthetic valve IE.
Data from Murdoch DR, *et al*. Clinical presentation, etiology, and outcome of infective endocarditis in the 21st century: the International Collaboration on Endocarditis-Prospective Cohort Study. *Arch Intern Med* 2009;**169**:463–732

In **IV drug addicts**, IE usually occurs in the absence of pre-existing valve lesions. The tricuspid valve is affected in >50% of cases, but only one-third of patients have a murmur on admission.[10] *S. aureus* is the most common pathogen (up to 70%), followed by streptococci, *Pseudomonas aeruginosa*, and **polymicrobial** causes (including **anaerobes**). In HIV-positive IV drug abusers, the risk is inversely related to the CD4 count (4-fold higher if CD4 <200 cells/μL).[11]

Nosocomial endocarditis is defined as IE developing in patients hospitalized >48 h prior to the onset of symptoms or signs of IE.

Clinical features

Heart murmurs are found in up to 50% of patients while worsening of **old murmurs** is found in 20% of patients.[5]

Myoskeletal symptoms (arthralgia, myalgia, back pain) may appear early with the disease.

Peripheral stigmata of IE are increasingly uncommon (2–8%), as patients generally present at an early stage of the disease, are not pathognomonic, and are virtually absent in tricuspid valve endocarditis.

- **Splinter haemorrhages** (linear petechiae in the mid-nailbed).
- **Osler's nodes** (tender, raised nodules on the pads of fingers or toes).
- **Janeway's lesions** (non-tender, slightly raised haemorrhages on palms and soles).
- **Conjunctival haemorrhage.**
- **Roth's spots** (haemorrhagic spots with a central white area in the retina).

Systemic embolism usually occurs to the **brain, spleen,** and **kidneys** or other organs in left-sided IE, and to **lungs** in right-sided IE (see Complications).

Neurological findings may be due to embolism or intracranial haemorrhage.

Heart failure may be seen with ensuing valve destruction or chordal rupture.

Diagnosis

The currently used **modified Duke criteria** are presented in Table 79.2. The usefulness of Duke criteria has been validated in many studies worldwide.[12]

Transthoracic echocardiography has a sensitivity of 60–70% for detecting vegetations (Table 79.3).

Transoesophageal echocardiography is the first-line imaging modality (ESC 2009 I-B). It increases sensitivity to 75–95% while maintaining specificity of 85–98%.[3] It is also more sensitive for detecting perivalvular extension of the infection, valve perforations, and myocardial abscess.

Cerebral angiography or **magnetic resonance angiography** is used for detection of intracranial mycotic aneurysms.

CT or **MRI** are also used for detection of cerebral bleeding or splenic emboli and abscess.

ESR and **CRP** (elevated in >60% of patients), as well as **leukocytosis, anaemia,** and **microscopic haematuria,** may be present but are not specific.

Blood cultures In patients with possible infective endocarditis, three, or at least two, sets of cultures of blood (one aerobic and one anaerobic), collected by separate venepunctures, should be obtained within the first 1 to 2 hours of presentation. Patients with cardiovascular collapse should have three cultures of blood obtained at 5-to-10-minute intervals and thereafter receive empirical antibiotic therapy. For the main causative agents, the first

Table 79.2 ESC 2009 GL on endocarditis. Definition of infective endocarditis according to the proposed modified Duke criteria

Major criteria
Blood cultures positive for IE
• **Typical microorganisms consistent with IE from two separate blood cultures:**
Viridans streptococci, *Streptococcus bovis,* HACEK group, *Staphylococcus aureus*; or
Community-acquired enterococci, in the absence of a primary focus;
or
• **Microorganisms consistent with IE from persistently positive blood cultures:**
At least two positive blood cultures of blood samples drawn >12 h apart; or
All of three or a majority of ≥4 separate cultures of blood (with first and last sample drawn at least 1h apart)
or
• **Single positive blood culture for *Coxiella burnetii* or phase I IgG antibody titre >1:800**
Evidence of endocardial involvement
• **Echocardiography positive for IE**
Vegetation; abscess; new partial dehiscence of prosthetic valve
• **New valvular regurgitation**
Minor criteria
• **Predisposition:** predisposing heart condition, injection drug use
• **Fever:** temperature >38°C
• **Vascular phenomena:** major arterial emboli, septic pulmonary infarcts, mycotic aneurysm, intracranial haemorrhages, conjunctival haemorrhages, Janeway lesions
• **Immunological phenomena:** glomerulonephritis, Osler's nodes, Roth's spots, rheumatoid factor
• **Microbiological evidence:** positive blood culture but does not meet a major criterion or serological evidence of active infection with organism consistent with IE
Diagnosis of IE is definite in the presence of:
2 major criteria, or
1 major and 3 minor criteria, or
5 minor criteria
Diagnosis of IE is possible in the presence of:
1 major and 1 minor criteria, or
3 minor criteria

Guidelines on the prevention, diagnosis, and treatment of infective endocarditis (new version 2009). *Eur Heart J.* 2009;**30**:2369–413.

Table 79.3 Use of echocardiography during diagnosis and treatment of endocarditis

Echocardiography as soon as possible (<12 h after initial evaluation)
TOE recommended in patients with clinical suspicion of IE and normal TTE
TOE after positive TTE as soon as possible in patients at high risk for complications
TOE 7–10 d after initial TOE if suspicion exists without diagnosis of IE or with worrisome clinical course during early treatment of IE
Intraoperative TOE is recommended in all patients requiring surgery for:
Identification of vegetations, mechanism of regurgitation, abscesses, fistulas, and pseudoaneurysms
Confirmation of successful repair of abnormal findings
Assessment of residual valve dysfunction
Elevated afterload, if necessary, to avoid underestimating valve insufficiency or presence of residual abnormal flow
TTE after completion of therapy to assess valve function and morphology and ventricular size and function (TTE usually adequate; TOE or review of intraoperative TOE may be needed for complex anatomy to establish new baseline)

TOE: transoesophageal echocardiography, TTE: transthoracic echocardiography. Modified from ACC/AHA 2005 statement, and ESC 2009 GL.

two blood cultures may be positive in more than 90% of cases. Sampling from central venous catheters carries a high risk of contaminants (mainly staphylococci).

Culture-negative endocarditis occurs in 10–20% of IE patients. It is often associated with antibiotic use within the previous 2 weeks and fastidious (Bartonella, *Coxiella burnetii*, *HACEK* group, fungi) or intracellular pathogens (*Brucella, Rickettsiae, Chlamydia, Tropheryma whipplei*) that are not easily detected by standard culture conditions. Subacute right-sided IE, mural IE, and uraemia are other causes. Serologic testing, **polymerase-chain-reaction (PCR)** assay on valve samples or blood, and highly specialized microbio- logic techniques lead to the identification of the pathogen in up to 60% of cases.[1]

HACEK group are fastidious, Gram-negative bacilli that grow slowly in standard blood culture media, and recovery may require prolonged incubation. Thus, the microbiology laboratory should be asked to retain blood cultures for ≥2 weeks in all patients suspected of having IE but whose blood cultures are initially negative. Bacteraemia caused by HACEK microorganisms in the absence of an obvious focus of infection is highly suggestive of endocarditis, even in the absence of typical physical findings. HACEK IE is very uncommon in North America.[2]

Q fever IE *(Coxiella burnetii)* and **Bartonella IE** are also more common in Europe than in North America.[4] Q fever IE (a zoonosis) is one of the most common causes of culture-negative IE. Serology (IgG phase 2 >1:800), tissue culture and immunohistology, and PCR of surgical material are needed for diagnosis of Q fever IE.

Bartonella species *(B. quintana* and *B. henselae)* IE is a subacute form that may present with heart failure due to AR. Predisposing factors are alcoholism, homelessness, and exposure to body lice. Blood cultures, serology, culture and immunohistology, and PCR of surgical material are needed for identification of Brucella or Bartonella or Legionella species.

Serology, culture and immunohistology, and PCR of surgical material are needed for Mycoplasma species and histology and PCR of surgical material for identification of *Tropheryma whippelii.* PCR amplification of the 16S ribosomal RNA gene that is specific for bacteria in tissue samples,[13] including valves and peripheral emboli, but it can remain positive, even after long-term treatment with antibiotics.

Therapy

Detailed antibiotic schemes have been published by the ACC/AHA and ESC (see Appendix 2). Therapy of IE is mostly based on expert opinion since no large randomized studies exist. Bactericidal antibiotics are indicated, and the choice of an optimum regimen is based on antibiotic susceptibility testing and minimum inhibitory concentrations (MIC) of the principal drugs for the infecting pathogens. Prolonged therapy (4–6 weeks) is usually necessary for the avoidance of relapses. Therapy can be switched to oral route once fever has subsided and blood cultures are negative.[4]

Streptococci are becoming increasingly resistant to penicillin and other beta lactams (intermediate resistance MIC: 0.1–1 mg/L; high resistance MIC: >1 mg/L). Combination with an aminoglycoside increases their activity. Groups B, C, and G Streptococci are generally more resistant than viridans group streptococci (a-haemolytic) and *S. bovis* (a non-enterococcal group D Streptococcus). **Pneumococcal** endocarditis is often seen in patients with HIV and as a complication of alcoholism. It can follow a fulminant course with concurrent meningitis, and early surgery may be required to prevent complications.[14]

Traditionally, coagulase-positive **staphylococci** (*S. aureus*) cause primarily native valve endocarditis whereas coagulase-negative staphylococci (*S. epidermidis* and various other species) cause primarily prosthetic valve endocarditis, but considerable overlap exists. *S. aureus* is now the most common cause of IE in the developed world.[5] **Methicillin-resistant staphylococci** (MRSA) are also resistant to most other antibiotics (including quinolones), and vancomycin resistance is also beginning to develop[15] Therapy of IE due to vancomycin-resistant MRSA is not established. Daptomycin is an effective alternative to vancomycin/gentamicin for MRSA endocarditis.[15] Linezolid, and quinupristin-dalfopristin may be effective.[4,10]

Enterococcal IE typically occurs in older male patients with urinary tract infection or instrumentation. The morbidity and mortality of enterrococcal endocarditis are high with increasing resistance to aminoglycosides. Recent evidence indicates that with strains highly resistant to both streptomycin and gentamicin, ampicillin plus ceftriaxone for 6 weeks should be the regimen of choice. In patients with non-highly resistant enterococci there are 2 options: If treatment with ampicillin plus gentamicin is chosen, gentamicin can be shortened to 2 weeks and simplified to once-daily dosing to avoid nephrotoxicity; conversely, ampicillin plus ceftriaxone are also safe and effective.[16] Multidrug-resistant enterococci are also resistant to vancomycin and cause infections of increased morbidity and mortality. Specialist infectious diseases advice is needed in these cases.

HACEK group become increasingly resistant to beta lactam antibiotics but are susceptible to fluoroquinolones, trimethoprim-sulfamethoxazole, and azthreonam.[4]

Candida IE is treated with amphotericin B (3–5 mg/kg), with or without fluctytosine (5-FC) (25 mg/kg/6 h).[17] Alternative regimens include amphotericin B deoxycholate (0.6–1 mg/kg daily), with or without 5-FC, or an echinocandin, such as caspofungin (50–150 mg), micafungin (100–150 mg), or anidulafungin (100–200 mg), each given as a single daily dose. Step-down therapy to fluconazole 400–800 mg (6–12 mg/kg) daily is advised only for a susceptible organism in a stable patient whose blood cultures have become negative. Valve replacement is usually needed. In treated cases, chronic lifelong suppression with fluconazole 400–800 mg (6–12 mg/kg) daily is recommended, especially in patients who were not suitable for valve replacement.[17]

The management of **culture-negative IE** is presented in Table 79.4.

The management of **IE related to cardiac devices** is discussed in Chapter 68 on cardiac devices.

Criteria for outpatient therapy are presented in Table 79.5.

Complications

Heart failure due to valve destruction, **uncontrolled infection**, and **embolic phenomena** are the most common complications of IE, and constitute indications for valve replacement. Indications for surgery are presented in Tables 79.6 and 79.7. Other indications for surgery are IE due to organisms that are difficult to eradicate, such as *Pseudomonas aeruginosa*, Brucella, *Coxiella burnetii*, and fungi, and IE on prosthetic valves. Surgical mortality in active IE is 6–25%. Improved outcomes with surgery have been unequivocally proved only with hemodynamic deterioration due to valvular regurgitation.[18] When surgery is performed within the first week of antibiotic treatment, there may be increased risks of relapse and prosthetic-valve dysfunction.[19] However, in the recent randomized EASE trial, early surgery was beneficial in patients with left-sided infective endocarditis, severe valve disease, and large vegetations.[20] Valvular surgery should be deferred when hemorrhage is present.[21] In mitral valve IE, repair is feasible, but in the aortic position valve replacement is usually needed. Mechanical and biological prostheses have similar outcome.[4] If blood cultures are still negative at the time of surgery, a sample of valve tissue should be obtained for culture, and a broad-range PCR assay should be performed to help identify the causative microorganism.

Heart failure may be seen in up to 40% of IE cases and is most commonly associated with aortic than mitral regurgitation. Urgent surgery is indicated in unstable patients; otherwise, stable AR or MR are dealt with after eradication of the infection.

Uncontrolled infection Fever associated with infective endocarditis often resolves within 2 to 3 days after the start of appropriate antimicrobial treatment in patients with less virulent pathogens, and defervescence occurs in the majority of patients by the end of the second week of treatment. The most common causes of persistent fever (>14 days) are infection due to resistant organisms, extension of infection beyond the valve (often with myocardial abscess, pseudoaneurysm, or fistula), other nosocomial infection, pulmonary embolism, and drug hypersensitivity (particularly if the fever resolves and then recurs). Perivalvular extension is suspected in cases of persistent fever or new AV block. Perivalvular abscess is more common in aortic IE, and especially in prosthetic valve IE (50–100%).[4] The presence of persistent positive blood cultures is an independent risk factor for in-hospital mortality which doubles the risk of death of patients with left-sided endocarditis.[22]

Embolic events are related to migration of vegetations. They are more often seen with large vegetations (>10 mm) and *S. aureus* or Candida IE. Reported incidence is 20–40% but much lower after initiation of suitable antibiotic therapy (6–12%). Aspirin does not reduce the risk of embolization.[17] The risk is higher during the first 2 weeks of treatment and with large (>10 mm and especially >15 mm) and mobile vegetations. The role of anticoagulants in IE is controversial. Temporary discontinuation of anticoagulation until the septic phase of the disease is overcome may be useful in cases of *S. aureus* endocarditis.[21] Recommendations are provided in Table 79.8.

Neurological complications may be due to emboli (usually middle cerebral artery), intracranial haemorrhage due to mycotic aneurysms that result from septic embolization of vegetations to the arterial vasa vasorum, or due to rupture of an artery related to septic arteritis at the site of embolism. Vegetation size ≥3 cm, *Staphylococcus aureus* as the causative microorganism, and involvement of the mitral valve are risk factors related to the development of neurological complications, whereas early and appropriate antimicrobial treatment reduced their incidence.[21] Unruptured aneurysms may resolve with antibiotic therapy alone, and patients should be followed with serial angiography performed to document the resolution of the aneurysm. Endovascular treatment should be pursued only if the aneurysm is very large (e.g., >10 mm) or if it is not resolving or is enlarging despite treatment with antibiotics.[1] The management of neurological complications is presented in Table 79.9.

Table 79.4 ESC 2009 GL on endocarditis. Empirical antibiotic treatment of IE before or without pathogen identification

Antibiotic	Dosage and route	Duration (weeks)	Level of evidence	Comments
Native valves				
Ampicillin-sulbactam	12 g/day IV in 4 doses	4–6	IIb-C	Patients with blood culture-negative IE should be treated in consultation with an infectious disease specialist
or				
Amoxicillin-clavulanate	12 g/day IV in 4 doses	4–6	IIb-C	
with				
Gentamicin[a]	3 mg/kg/day IV or IM in 2 or 3 doses.	4–6		
Vancomycin[b]	30 mg/kg/day IV in 2 doses	4–6	IIb-C	For patients unable to tolerate beta lactams
with				
Gentamicin[a]	3 mg/kg/day IV or IM in 2 or 3 doses	4–6		
with				
Ciprofloxacin	1000 mg/day orally in 2 doses or 800 mg/day IV in 2 doses	4–6		Ciprofloxacin is not uniformly active on Bartonella spp. Addition of doxycycline (see Appendix 2) is an option if Bartonella spp. is likely
Prosthetic valves (early, <12 months post-surgery)				
Vancomycin[b]	30 mg/kg/day IV in 2 doses	6	IIb-C	If no clinical response, surgery and maybe extension of the antibiotic spectrum to Gram-negative pathogens must be considered
with				
Gentamicin[a]	3 mg/kg/day IV or IM in 2 or 3 doses	2		
with				
Rifampin	1200 mg/day orally in 2 doses			
Prosthetic valves (late, ≥12 months post-surgery)				
Same as for native valves				

ESC 2009 GL on endocarditis. Antibiotic treatment of blood culture-negative IE according to suspected cause

Pathogens	Proposed therapy[a]	Treatment outcome
Brucella spp.	Doxycycline (200 mg/24h), plus co-trimoxazole (960 mg/12h), plus rifampin (300–600 mg/24h) for ≥3 months[b] orally	Treatment success defined as an antibody titre <1:60
***Coxiella burnetii* (agent of Q fever)**	Doxycycline (200 mg/24h), plus hydroxychloroquine (200–600 mg/24h)[c] orally *or* Doxycycline (200 mg/24h), plus quinolone (ofloxacin 400 mg/24h) orally (>18 months treatment)	Treatment success defined as anti-phase I IgG titre <1:200 and IgA and IgM titres <1:50
Bartonella spp.	Ceftriaxone (2 g/24h) or ampicillin (or amoxicillin) (12 g/24h) IV *or* Doxycycline (200 mg/24h) orally for 6 weeks *plus* Gentamicin (3 mg/24h), or netilmicin IV (for 3 weeks)[d]	Treatment success expected in ≥90%
***Legionella* spp.**	Erythromycin (3 g/24h) IV for 2 weeks, then orally for 4 weeks, *plus* Rifampin (300–1200 mg/24h) *or* Ciprofloxacin (1.5 g/24h) orally for 6 weeks	Optimal treatment unknown. Because of high susceptibility, quinolones should probably be included.

(*Continued*)

Table 79.4 (Continued)

Pathogens	Proposed therapy[a]	Treatment outcome
Mycoplasma spp.	Newer fluoroquinolones[e] (>6 months treatment)	Optimal treatment unknown
***Tropheryma whippelii*[f] (agent of Whipple's disease)**	Co-trimoxazole, penicillin G (1.2 MU/24h), and streptomycin (1 g/24h) IV for 2 weeks, then co-trimoxazole orally for 1 year *or* Doxycycline (200 mg/24h) plus hydroxychloroquine (200–600 mg/24h)[c] orally for ≥18 months	Long-term treatment, optimal duration unknown

[a] Due to the lack of large series, optimal duration of treatment of IE due to these pathogens is unknown. The presented durations are based on selected case reports.
[b] Addition of streptomycin (15 mg/kg/24 h in two doses) for the first few weeks is optional in Brucella IE.
[c] Doxycycline plus hydroxychloroquine (with monitoring of serum hydroxychloroquine levels) is superior to doxycycline alone and to doxycycline + fluoroquinolone for Q fever IE.
[d] Several therapeutic regimens were reported for Bartonella IE, including aminopenicillins and cephalosporins combined with aminoglycosides, doxycycline, vancomycin, and quinolones.
[e] Newer fluoroquinolones are more potent than ciprofloxacin against intracellular pathogens, such as Mycoplasma spp., Legionella spp., and Chlamydia spp.
[f] Treatment of Whipple IE remains highly empirical. Successes have been reported with long-term (>1 year) co-trimoxazole therapy.γ-interferon plays a protective role in intracellular infections and has been proposed as adjuvant therapy in Whipple's disease.

Table 79.5 ESC 2009 GL on endocarditis. Criteria which determine suitability of outpatient parenteral antibiotic therapy (OPAT) for infective endocarditis

Phase of treatment	Guidelines for use
Critical phase (weeks 0–2)	Complications occur during this phase. Preferred inpatient treatment during this phase. **Consider OPAT**: if oral streptococci, patient stable, no complications.
Continuation phase (beyond week 2)	**Consider OPAT:** if medically stable. **Do not consider OPAT:** if heart failure, concerning echocardiographic features, neurological signs, or renal impairment
Essential for OPAT	Educate patient and staff. Regular post-discharge evaluation (nurses 1/day, physician in charge 1–2/week). Prefer physician-directed programme, not home infusion model.

Guidelines on the prevention, diagnosis, and treatment of infective endocarditis (new version 2009): *Eur Heart J*. 2009;**30**:2369–413.

Table 79.6 AHA 2008 GL on VD. Surgery for endocarditis

Native valve	
Patients with valve stenosis or regurgitation resulting in heart failure.	I-B
Patients with AR or MR with haemodynamic evidence of elevated LV end-diastolic or left atrial pressures (e.g. premature closure of MV with AR, rapid decelerating MR signal by continuous wave Doppler (v wave cut-off sign), or moderate or severe pulmonary hypertension).	I-B
Endocarditis caused by fungal or other highly resistant organisms.	I-B
Endocarditis complicated by heart block, annular or aortic abscess, or destructive penetrating lesions (e.g. sinus of Valsalva to right atrium, right ventricle, or left atrium fistula; mitral leaflet perforation with aortic valve endocarditis; or infection in annulus fibrosa).	I-B
Patients with recurrent emboli and persistent vegetations despite appropriate antibiotic therapy.	IIa-C
Patients with mobile vegetations >10 mm with or without emboli.	IIb-C
Prosthetic valve	
Consultation with a cardiac surgeon is indicated for infective endocarditis of a prosthetic valve.	I-C
Patients who present with heart failure.	I-B
Surgery is indicated for patients with infective endocarditis of a prosthetic valve who present with dehiscence of a prosthetic valve evidenced by cine fluoroscopy or echocardiography.	I-B
Evidence of increasing obstruction or worsening regurgitation.	I-C
Complications (e.g. abscess formation).	I-C
Evidence of persistent bacteraemia or recurrent emboli despite appropriate antibiotic treatment.	IIa-C
Relapsing infection.	IIa-C
Uncomplicated infective endocarditis of a prosthetic valve caused by first infection with a sensitive organism.	III

ACC/AHA 2008 focused update incorporated into the ACC/AHA 2006 guidelines for the management of patients with valvular heart disease. *J Am Coll Cardiol*. 2008;**52**:e1–142.

Table 79.7 ESC 2009 GL on endocarditis. Surgery for endocarditis

Indications and timing of surgery in left-sided native valve infective endocarditis	
Heart failure	
Emergency:[1] Aortic or mitral IE with severe regurgitation or valve obstruction causing refractory pulmonary oedema or cardiogenic shock	I-B
Emergency: Aortic or mitral IE with fistula into a cardiac chamber or pericardium causing refractory pulmonary oedema or shock	I-B
Urgent: Aortic or mitral IE with severe regurgitation or valve obstruction and persisting heart failure or echo signs of poor haemodynamic tolerance (early mitral closure or pulmonary hypertension)	I-B
Elective: Aortic or mitral IE with severe regurgitation and no heart failure	IIa-B
Uncontrolled infection	
Urgent: Locally uncontrolled infection (abscess, false aneurysm, fistula enlarging vegetation)	I-B
Urgent: Persisting fever and positive blood cultures >7–10 days	I-B
Urgent/elective: Infection caused by fungi or multiresistant organisms	I-B
Prevention of embolism	
Urgent: Aortic or mitral IE with large vegetations (>10 mm) following one or more embolic episodes despite appropriate antibiotic therapy	I-B
Urgent: Aortic or mitral IE with large vegetations (>10 mm) and other predictors of complicated course (heart failure, persistent infection, abscess)	I-C
Urgent: Isolated very large vegetations (>15 mm)[2]	IIb-C

[1] Emergency surgery: surgery performed within 24 h; urgent surgery: within a few days; elective surgery: after at least 1 or 2 weeks of antibiotic therapy.
[2] Surgery may be preferred if procedure preserving the native valve is feasible.

Indications and timing of surgery in prosthetic valve IE	
Heart failure	
Emergency:[1] Severe prosthetic dysfunction (dehiscence or obstruction) causing refractory pulmonary oedema or cardiogenic shock	I-B
Emergency: Fistula into a cardiac chamber or pericardium causing refractory pulmonary oedema or shock	I-B
Urgent: Severe prosthetic dysfunction and persisting heart failure	I-B
Elective: Severe prosthetic dehiscence without heart failure	I-B
Uncontrolled infection	
Urgent: Locally uncontrolled infection (abscess, false aneurysm, fistula enlarging vegetation)	I-B
Urgent/elective: Infection caused by fungi or multiresistant organisms	I-B
Urgent: Persisting fever and positive blood cultures >7–10 days	I-B
Urgent/elective: Infection caused by staphylococci or Gram-negative Bacteria (most cases of early prosthetic valve IE)	IIa-C
Prevention of embolism	
Urgent: Recurrent emboli despite appropriate antiobiotic therapy	I-B
Urgent: Large vegetations (>10 mm) and other predictors of complicated course (heart failure, persistent infection, abscess)	I-C
Urgent: Very large vegetations (>15 mm)	IIb-C

[1] Emergency surgery: surgery performed within 24 h; urgent surgery: within a few days; elective surgery: after at least 1 or 2 weeks of antibiotic therapy.

Indications and timing of surgery for right-sided IE	
Microorganisms difficult to eradicate (e.g. persistent fungi) or bacteraemia for >7 days (e.g. *S. aureus*, *P. aeruginosa*) despite appropriate antimicrobial therapy, or persistent tricuspid vegetations >20 mm after recurrent pulmonary emboli, with or without concomitant right heart failure, or right heart failure secondary to severe TR with poor response to diuretics.	IIa-C

Guidelines on the prevention, diagnosis, and treatment of infective endocarditis (new version 2009): *Eur Heart J*. 2009;**30**:2369–413.

Table 79.8 ESC 2009 GL on endocarditis. **Management of antithrombotic therapy in IE**

Interruption of antiplatelet therapy only with major bleeding	I-B
In ischaemic stroke without cerebral haemorrhage, replacement of oral anticoagulation with UFH, with close monitoring of aPTT or ACT	I-C
In intracranial haemorrhage, interruption of all anticoagulation	I-C
In intracranial haemorrhage and a mechanical valve, UFH (with close monitoring of aPTT or ACT) reinitiated as soon as possible following multidisciplinary discussion	IIa-C
In the absence of stroke, replacement of oral anticoagulation with UFH during 2 weeks in case of *S. aureus* IE, with close monitoring of aPTT or ACT	IIb-C

Guidelines on the prevention, diagnosis, and treatment of infective endocarditis (new version 2009): the Task Force on the Prevention, Diagnosis, and Treatment of Infective Endocarditis of the European Society of Cardiology (ESC). *Eur Heart J*. 2009;**30**:2369–413.

Table 79.9 ESC 2009 GL on endocarditis. **Management of neurological complications**

After a silent cerebral embolism or transient ischaemic attack, surgery without delay if an indication remains.	I-B
Following intracranial haemorrhage, surgery must be postponed for at least 1 month.	I-C
Neurosurgery or endovascular therapy for very large, enlarging, or ruptured intracranial aneurysm.	I-C
After stroke, surgery indicated for heart failure, uncontrolled infection, abscess, or persistent high embolic risk should not be delayed. Surgery should be considered as long as coma is absent and cerebral haemorrhage has been excluded by cranial CT.	IIa-B
Look for intracranial aneurysm in any patient with IE and neurological symptoms (CT or MR angiography).	IIa-B
Conventional angiography when non-invasive techniques are negative and the suspicion of intracranial aneurysm remains.	IIa-B

Guidelines on the prevention, diagnosis, and treatment of infective endocarditis (new version 2009): *Eur Heart J*. 2009;**30**:2369–413.

Glomerulonephritis is immune complex-mediated (15% of patients with IE). Renal embolism may cause haematuria (25% of patients) but rarely azotaemia. Antibiotic-induced interstitial nephritis (mainly with aminoglycosides and vancomycin), or severe haemodynamic impairement may also contribute.

Pyogenic spondylodiscitis, peripheral arthritis, and **myopericarditis** may also be seen. Splenic emboli are common, but **splenic abscess** is rare.

Prognosis

Increased age, pulmonary oedema, paravalvular complications, prosthetic valve IE, and staphylococcal IE are prognostic factors for in-hospital mortality.[2] Mortality rates vary according to the offending organism and range from approximately 10% with viridans streptococci, 25–45% with *S. aureus*, to >50% with fungi (mainly Candida and Aspergillus) and *P. aeruginosa*. Q fever IE also carries a high mortality. Overall mortality is 17–23% for left-sided IE and 10% for right-sided IE.[5] Operative mortality is 5–15%.[3] Relapses usually occur within 2 months of discontinuation of therapy in 2–20% of patients.[4] Risk factors are inadequate duration of antibiotic therapy or the presence of resistant organisms, persistent focus of infection (i.e. abscess), and prosthetic valve endocarditis.

Pregnancy

The incidence of IE during pregnancy has been reported to be 0.006%[3] and is either a complication of a pre-existing cardiac lesion or the result of intravenous drug abuse. Maternal mortality approaches 33%, most deaths relating to heart failure or an embolic event, while fetal mortality is 29%.[3] Close attention should be paid to any pregnant woman with unexplained fever and a cardiac murmur since rapid detection and appropriate treatment are important in reducing the risk of both maternal and fetal mortality.

Prophylaxis

Turbulent blood flow produced by congenital or valve disease may traumatize the endocardium and endothelial surfaces. Invasion of the bloodstream by microbes that can colonize this damaged site may result in clinical infection. Transient bacteraemia may occur after invasive procedures, such as gastrointestinal and genitourinary, particularly at a site of pre-existing infection. It is also very common during dental procedures and during daily activities, such as toothbrushing or defecation. Oral mucosal surfaces, and particularly the gingival crevice around teeth, are populated by a dense endogenous microflora, including species, such as streptococci, and at least 126 individual bacteria have been isolated in blood cultures after extractions or toothbrushing.[24,25] The rationale for endocarditis prophylaxis, therefore, was that antibiotics by limiting bacteraemia should be effective in preventing infective endocarditis following invasive procedures.

However, up to now, there has been no consistent association between interventional procedures, dental or non-dental, and the development of IE, and no controlled, randomized study has proven the efficacy of prophylaxis. Recent studies have shown that most cases of infective endocarditis are not attributable to an invasive procedure and that the protective efficacy of antibiotic prophylaxis was not significant.[26,27] Bacteraemia resulting from daily activities, such as chewing food, brushing teeth, flossing, use of water irrigation devices and other activities, is much more likely to cause infective endocarditis than bacteraemia associated with a dental procedure.[19] The presence of dental disease may increase the risk of bacteraemia associated with these routine activities. Maintenance of optimal oral health and hygiene may reduce the incidence of bacteraemia from daily activities and is more important than prophylactic antibiotics for a dental procedure in reducing the risk of infective endocarditis.[28] Finally, the risk of a serious allergic reaction to amoxicillin may be greater than the risk of contracting infective endocarditis. For these reasons, both the ACC/AHA[29] and the ESC [4] recommend that prophylaxis is no longer mandatory in any patient. It is still recommended as a Class IIa in high-risk patients only, as indicated in Table 79.10. Recommended antibiotics are presented in Table 79.11.

Thus, antibiotic infective endocarditis prophylaxis should be given only to high-risk patients prior to dental procedures that involve manipulation in gingival tissue or periapical region of the teeth or perforation of the

Table 79.10 IE prophylaxis

ACC/AHA 2008 GL on valve disease. Recommendations for IE prophylaxis		
Prophylaxis against infective endocarditis is reasonable for the following patients at highest risk for adverse outcomes from infective endocarditis who undergo dental procedures that involve manipulation of either gingival tissue or the periapical region of teeth or perforation of the oral mucosa:		
Patients with prosthetic cardiac valves or prosthetic material used for cardiac valve repair	IIa-B	
Patients with previous infective endocarditis	IIa-B	
Patients with CHD	IIa-B	
	Unrepaired cyanotic CHD, including palliative shunts and conduits	
	Completely repaired congenital heart defect with prosthetic material or device, whether placed by surgery or by catheter intervention, during the first 6 months after the procedure Repaired CHD with residual defects at the site or adjacent to the site of a prosthetic patch or prosthetic device (both of which inhibit endothelialization)	
Cardiac transplant recipients with valve regurgitation due to a structurally abnormal valve	IIa-C	
Prophylaxis against infective endocarditis is not recommended for non-dental procedures (such as transoesophageal echocardiogram, oesophagogastroduodenoscopy, or colonoscopy) in the absence of active infection	III-B	
ESC 2009 GL on endocarditis. Cardiac conditions at highest risk of infective endocarditis for which prophylaxis is recommended when a high risk procedure is performed		
Antibiotic prophylaxis should only be considered for patients at highest risk of IE	IIa-C	
	1. Patients with a prosthetic valve or a prosthetic material used for cardiac valve repair	
	2. Patients with previous IE	
	3.Patients with congenital heart disease	
	a. Cyanotic congenital heart disease, without surgical repair or with residual defects, palliative shunts, or conduits	
	b. Congenital heart disease with complete repair with prosthetic material, whether placed by surgery or by percutaneous technique, up to 6 months after the procedure	
	c. When a residual defect persists at the site of implantation of a prosthetic material or device by cardiac surgery or percutaneous technique	
Antibiotic prophylaxis is no longer recommended in other forms of valvular or congenital heart disease	III-C	

(Continued)

Table 79.10 (Continued)

ESC 2009 GL on endocarditis. Recommendations for prophylaxis of infective endocarditis in highest risk patients according to the type of procedure at risk	
Dental procedures	
Antibiotic prophylaxis should only be considered for dental procedures requiring manipulation of the gingival or periapical region of the teeth or perforation of the oral mucosa	IIa-C
Antibiotic prophylaxis is not recommended for local anaesthetic injections in non-infected tissue, removal of sutures, dental X-rays, placement or adjustment of removable prosthodontics or orthodontic appliances or braces. Prophylaxis is also not recommended following the shedding of deciduous teeth or trauma to the lips and oral mucosa	III-C
Respiratory tract procedures	
Antibiotic prophylaxis is not recommended for respiratory tract procedures, including bronchoscopy or laryngoscopy, transnasal or endotracheal intubation	III-C
Gastrointestinal or urogenital procedures	
Antibiotic prophylaxis is not recommended for gastroscopy, colonoscopy, cystoscopy, or transoesophageal echocardiography	III-C
Skin and soft tissue	
Antibiotic prophylaxis is not recommended for any procedure	III-C

2008 focused update incorporated into the ACC/AHA 2006 guidelines for the management of patients with valvular heart disease. *J Am Coll Cardiol.* 2008;**52**:e1–142.
Guidelines on the prevention, diagnosis, and treatment of infective endocarditis (new version 2009). *Eur Heart J.* 2009;**30**:2369–413.

Table 79.11 Regimens for endocarditis prophylaxis before dental procedure

ACC/AHA 2008 GL on valve disease
Amoxicillin 2 g po (50 mg/kg po) or ampicillin 2 g IM or IV (50 mg/kg IM or IV)
or
Cefazolin or ceftriaxone 1 g IM or IV (50 mg/kg IM or IV)
Allergy to penicillins
Cephalexin 2 g po (50 mg/kg po)*
or
Clindamycin 600 mg po (20 mg/kg po) or clindamycin 600 mg IM or IV (20 mg/kg IM or IV)
or
Azithromycin or clarithromycin 500 mg po (15 mg/kg po)
or
Cefazolin or ceftriaxone 1 g IM or IV 50 mg/kg IM or IV
Antibiotic regimens administered 30–60 min before dental procedures that involve manipulation in gingival tissue or periapical region of the teeth or perforation of the oral mucosa.
In brackets are paediatric doses.
IM or IV should be given only if the patient is unable to take oral medication.
* Or other first- or second-generation cephalosporins
Cephalosporins should not be used in patients with a history of anaphylaxis, angioedema, or urticaria with penicillins or ampicillin.
ESC 2009 GL on endocarditis
Amoxicillin or ampicillin 2 g po or IV (50 mg/kg po or IV)
Or
Cephalexin 2 g po (50 mg/kg IV) or cefazolin or ceftriaxone 1 g IV (50 mg/kg IV)

(*Continued*)

Table 79.11 (Continued)

Allergy to penicillins
Clindamycin 600 mg po or IV (20 mg/kg po or IV)
Antibiotic regimens administered 30–60 min before dental procedures that involve manipulation in gingival tissue or periapical region of the teeth or perforation of the oral mucosa.

In brackets are paediatric doses.
IM or IV should be given only if the patient is unable to take oral medication.
Cephalosporins should not be used in patients with a history of anaphylaxis, angioedema, or urticaria with penicillins or ampicillin.

ACC/AHA guidelines of valve disease of 2008. 2008 focused update incorporated into the ACC/AHA 2006 guidelines for the management of patients with valvular heart disease. *J Am Coll Cardiol*. 2008;**52**:e1–142.

ESC guidelines on endocarditis 2009. Guidelines on the prevention, diagnosis, and treatment of infective endocarditis (new version 2009). *Eur Heart J*. 2009;**30**:2369–413.

oral mucosa. Prophylaxis is no longer needed for routine anaesthetic injections through non-infected tissue, dental radiographs, placement of removable prosthodontic or orthodontic appliances, adjustment of orthodontic appliances, placement of orthodontic brackets, shedding of deciduous teeth, or bleeding from trauma to the lips or oral mucosa.

Antibiotic infective endocarditis prophylaxis is also no longer indicated in patients with native valve disease, such as aortic stenosis, mitral stenosis, or mitral valve prolapse. However, for patients with cardiac conditions about which data are virtually lacking, such as bicuspid aortic valves, coarctation of the aorta, significant native valve disease, or severe hypertrophic obstructive cardiomyopathy, and who are subjected to dental procedures as indicated, or to other procedures in the presence of active infection, or before vaginal delivery, the situation should be discussed and patient preferences should be assessed. If doctors and patients feel more comfortable, they can continue using prophylaxis with the antibiotic schemes proposed by ACC/AHA and ESC. These new recommendations have not resulted in a higher incidence of streptococcal endocarditis.[7]

References

1. Hoen B, Duval X. Infective endocarditis. *N Engl J Med*. 2013;**368**:1425–33
2. Moreillon P, *et al*. Infective endocarditis. *Lancet*. 2004;**363**:139–49
3. Mylonakis E, *et al*. Infective endocarditis in adults. *N Engl J Med*. 2001;**345**:1318–30
4. Habib G, *et al*. Guidelines on the prevention, diagnosis, and treatment of infective endocarditis (new version 2009): the Task Force on the prevention, diagnosis, and treatment of infective endocarditis of the European Society of Cardiology (ESC). Endorsed by the European Society of Clinical Microbiology and Infectious Diseases (ESCMID) and the International Society of Chemotherapy (ISC) for infection and cancer. *Eur Heart J*. 2009;**30**:2369–413
5. Murdoch DR, *et al*. Clinical presentation, etiology, and outcome of infective endocarditis in the 21st century: the International Collaboration on Endocarditis-Prospective Cohort Study. *Arch Intern Med*. 2009;**169**:463–73
6. Lucas MJ, *et al*. Endocarditis in adults with bacterial meningitis. *Circulation* 2013;**127**:2056–2062
7. Duval X, *et al*. Temporal trends in infective endocarditis in the context of prophylaxis guideline modifications: three successive population-based surveys. *J Am Coll Cardiol*. 2012;**59**:1968–76
8. Foster E. Clinical practice. Mitral regurgitation due to degenerative mitral-valve disease. *N Engl J Med*. 2010;**363**:156–65
9. Greenspon AJ, *et al*. Timing of the most recent device procedure influences the clinical outcome of lead-associated endocarditis results of the MEDIC (Multicentre Electrophysiologic Device Infection Cohort). *J Am Coll Cardiol*. 2012;**59**:681–7
10. Baddour LM, *et al*. Infective endocarditis: diagnosis, antimicrobial therapy, and management of complications: a statement for healthcare professionals from the Committee on Rheumatic Fever, Endocarditis, and Kawasaki Disease, Council on Cardiovascular Disease in the Young, and the Councils on Clinical Cardiology, Stroke, and Cardiovascular Surgery and Anesthesia, American Heart Association: Endorsed by the Infectious Diseases Society of America. *Circulation*. 2005;**111**:e394–434
11. Wilson LE, *et al*. Prospective study of infective endocarditis among injection drug users. *J Infect Dis*. 2002;**185**:1761–6
12. Li JS, *et al*. Proposed modifications to the Duke criteria for the diagnosis of infective endocarditis. *Clin Infect Dis*. 2000;**30**:633–8
13. Houpikian P, *et al*. Diagnostic methods current best practices and guidelines for identification of difficult-to-culture pathogens in infective endocarditis. *Infect Dis Clin North Am*. 2002;**16**:377–92, x
14. Lefort A, *et al*. Comparison between adult endocarditis due to beta-haemolytic streptococci (serogroups A, B, C, and G) and *Streptococcus milleri*: a multicentre study in France. *Arch Intern Med*. 2002;**162**:2450–6
15. Rehm SJ, *et al*. Daptomycin versus vancomycin plus gentamicin for treatment of bacteraemia and endocarditis due to *Staphylococcus aureus*: subset analysis of patients infected with methicillin-resistant isolates. *J Antimicrob Chemother*. 2008;**62**:1413–21
16. Hospital Clinic Endocarditis Study Group. A new era for treating enterococcus faecalis endocarditis: Ampicillin plus short-course gentamicin or ampicillin plus ceftriaxone: That is the question! *Circulation*. 2013;**127**:1763–66

17. Pappas PG, *et al.* Clinical practice guidelines for the management of candidiasis: 2009 update by the Infectious Diseases Society of America. *Clin Infect Dis.* 2009;**48**:503–35
18. Prendergast BD, *et al.* Surgery for infective endocarditis: who and when? *Circulation.* 2010;**121**:1141–52
19. Thuny F, *et al.* The timing of surgery influences mortality and morbidity in adults with severe complicated infective endocarditis: A propensity analysis. *Eur Heart J.* 2011;**32**:2027–33
20. Kang DH, *et al.* Early surgery versus conventional treatment for infective endocarditis. *N Engl J Med.* 2012;**366**:2466–73
21. García-Cabrera E, *et al.* on behalf of the Group for the Study of Cardiovascular Infections of the Andalusian Society of Infectious Diseases (SAEI) and the Spanish Network for Research in Infectious Diseases (REIPI). Neurological complications of infective endocarditis: Risk factors, outcome, and impact of cardiac surgery: A multicenter observational study. *Circulation.* 2013;**127**:2272–84
22. López J, *et al.* Prognostic role of persistent positive blood cultures after initiation of antibiotic therapy in left-sided infective endocarditis. *Eur Heart J.* 2012 Nov 9. [Epub ahead of print] PubMed PMID: 23144047.
23. Chan KL, *et al.* A randomized trial of aspirin on the risk of embolic events in patients with infective endocarditis. *J Am Coll Cardiol.* 2003;**42**:775–80
24. Hill EE, *et al.* Infective endocarditis: changing epidemiology and predictors of 6-month mortality: a prospective cohort study. *Eur Heart J.* 2007;**28**:196–203
25. Lockhart PB, *et al.* Bacteremia associated with toothbrushing and dental extraction. *Circulation.* 2008;**117**:3118–25
26. Lacassin F, *et al.* Procedures associated with infective endocarditis in adults. A case control study. *Eur Heart J.* 1995;**16**:1968–74
27. Van der Meer JT, *et al.* Efficacy of antibiotic prophylaxis for prevention of native-valve endocarditis. *Lancet.* 1992;**339**:135–9
28. Tsolka P, *et al.* Infective endocarditis prophylaxis for dental procedures in 2009: what has changed? *Hellenic J Cardiol.* 2009;**50**:493–7
29. Bonow RO, *et al.* 2008 focused update incorporated into the ACC/AHA 2006 guidelines for the management of patients with valvular heart disease: a report of the American College of Cardiology/American Heart Association Task Force on practice guidelines (Writing Committee to revise the 1998 guidelines for the management of patients with valvular heart disease). Endorsed by the Society of Cardiovascular Anesthesiologists, Society for Cardiovascular Angiography and Interventions, and Society of Thoracic Surgeons. *J Am Coll Cardiol.* 2008;**52**:e1–142

Part XVIII

Rheumatic fever

Relevant guidelines

AHA 1992 guidelines for diagnosis of rheumatic fever

Guidelines for the diagnosis of rheumatic fever. Jones Criteria, 1992 update. Special Writing Group of the Committee on Rheumatic Fever, Endocarditis, and Kawasaki Disease of the Council on Cardiovascular Disease in the Young of the American Heart Association. *JAMA*. 1992;**268**:2069–73.

ACC/AHA 2009 statement on prevention of rheumatic fever

AHA scientific statement: prevention of rheumatic fever and diagnosis and treatment of acute streptococcal pharyngitis. *Circulation*. 2009;**119**:1541–51.

Chapter 80

Rheumatic fever

Definition

Acute rheumatic fever (ARF) results from an autoimmune response to infection with group A streptococcus. Although the acute illness causes considerable morbidity and even mortality, the major clinical and public health effects derive from the long-term damage to heart valves, i.e. rheumatic heart disease.[1]

Epidemiology

In developing areas of the world, acute rheumatic fever and rheumatic heart disease are estimated to affect nearly 20 million people, with an incidence exceeding 50 per 100 000 children, and are the leading causes of cardiovascular death during the first five decades of life. In contrast, the incidence of acute rheumatic fever has decreased dramatically in most developed countries.[2] The prevalence of rheumatic heart disease increases with age, peaking in adults aged 25–34 years and being higher in women.

Aetiology

Infections of the pharynx with group A *beta-haemolytic streptococci* (GAS) are the precipitating cause of rheumatic fever. Streptococcal skin infections (impetigo or pyoderma) have not been proven to lead to acute rheumatic fever, at least in non-tropical countries. Some strains of group A streptococci belonging to certain M serotypes are more likely to cause rheumatic fever, and HLA types and B cell alloantigens have been associated with increased susceptibility to rheumatic fever and rheumatic carditis.[1] In the past, approximately 3% of untreated streptococcal pharyngitis were followed by rheumatic fever. Appropriate therapy prevents rheumatic fever, but at least one-third of episodes of ARF result from inapparent streptococcal infections.[2]

Pathophysiology

The autoimmune response that causes ARF is supposed to be triggered by molecular mimicry between epitopes on the pathogen (group A streptococcus) and specific human tissues. The structural and immunological similarities between streptococcal M protein and myosin are essential to the development of rheumatic carditis. The initial damage to the valve might be due to laminin that is present in the valvular basement membrane and around endothelium, and which is recognized by T cells against myosin and M protein.[3]

In young patients, mitral valve regurgitation is the predominant cardiac lesion, but mitral stenosis becomes progressively more common with increasing age.[1]

Presentation

Group A streptococcal pharyngitis is primarily a disease of children 5–15 years of age, usually occuring in winter and early spring. Acute pharyngitis is caused considerably more often by viruses than by bacteria. Viruses that commonly cause pharyngitis include influenza virus, parainfluenza virus, rhinovirus, coronavirus, adenovirus, respiratory syncytial virus, Epstein–Barr virus, enteroviruses, and herpesviruses. Other causes of acute pharyngitis include *groups C and G streptococci, Neisseria gonorrhoeae, Mycoplasma pneumoniae, Chlamydia pneumoniae, Arcanobacterium haemolyticum*, and human immunodeficiency virus (HIV).[2]

There is typically sudden-onset sore throat, pain on swallowing, fever, headache, and possibly nausea or vomiting. Polyarthralgia and carditis follow afterwards.

Clinical forms

The main features of ARF are described in the modified Jones criteria,[4] as presented, together with the WHO criteria,[5] in Table 80.1.

Carditis, associated with a murmur of valvulitis, occurs in 50–70% of patients and is the most specific manifestation of ARF.

Polyarthritis is the most common, but least specific, major manifestation. The classic migratory polyarthritis of the major joints of rheumatic fever should be distinguished from the post-streptococcal reactive arthritis of the small joints of the hand that does not carry a risk of carditis.

Chorea (Sydenham's chorea, St. Vitus dance, or chorea minor) occurs in about 20% of cases. It is a delayed manifestation of ARF, usually appearing ≥3 months after the onset of the precipitating streptococcal infection.

Erythema marginatum and **subcutaneous nodules** in the elbows, knees, and the occipital portion of the scalp are rare (<5%).

Table 80.1 Diagnosis of ARF

Jones criteria (1992)
Two major or one major and two minor manifestations must be present, plus evidence of antecedent group A Streptococcus infection
Chorea and indolent carditis do not require evidence of antecedent group A Streptococcus infection
Recurrent episode requires only one major or several minor manifestations, plus evidence of antecedent group A Streptococcus infection
Major manifestations
Carditis
Polyarthritis
Chorea
Erythema marginatum
Subcutaneous nodules
Minor manifestations
Arthralgia
Fever
Raised erythrocyte sedimentation rate or C-reactive protein concentrations
Prolonged PR interval on electrocardiogram
Evidence of antecedent group A Streptococcus infection
Positive throat culture or rapid antigen test for group A Streptococcus
Raised or rising streptococcal antibody titre
WHO criteria (2001)
Chorea and indolent carditis do not require evidence of antecedent group A Streptococcus infection
First episode
As per Jones criteria
Recurrent episode
In a patient without established RHD: as per first episode
In a patient with established RHD: requires two minor manifestations, plus evidence of antecedent group A Streptococcus infection. Evidence of antecedent group A Streptococcus infection as per Jones criteria, but with addition of recent scarlet fever

Table 80.2 AHA 2009 statement on rheumatic fever prevention

Clinical and epidemiological findings and diagnosis of GAS pharyngitis
Features suggestive of GAS as causative agent
Sudden-onset sore throat
Pain on swallowing
Fever
Scarlet fever rash
Headache
Nausea, vomiting, and abdominal pain
Tonsillopharyngeal erythema
Tonsillopharyngeal exudates
Soft palate petechiae ('doughnut' lesions)
Beefy, red, swollen uvula
Tender, enlarged anterior cervical nodes
Patient 5–15 years of age
Presentation in winter or early spring (in temperate climates)
History of exposure
Features suggestive of viral origin
Conjunctivitis
Coryza
Hoarseness
Cough
Diarrhoea
Characteristic exanthems
Characteristic enanthems

AHA scientific statement: Prevention of rheumatic fever and diagnosis and treatment of acute Streptococcal pharyngitis. *Circulation*. 2009;**119**:1541–51.

Diagnosis

Differentiation of group A streptococcal pharyngitis from pharyngitis caused by other pathogens is impossible on clinical grounds. However, several clues may be helpful (Table 80.2).

Throat culture

Microbiological confirmation, with either a throat culture or a rapid antigen detection test (RADT), is required for the diagnosis (Class I-B, AHA 2009).[2] In untreated patients with GAS pharyngitis, a properly obtained throat culture (by vigorous swabbing of both tonsils and posterior pharynx) is almost always positive. A positive throat culture may reflect chronic colonization by GAS and cannot be used to differentiate carriage from infection. A negative throat culture permits the physician to withhold antibiotic therapy from the large majority of patients with sore throats.

When deciding whether to perform a microbiological test for a patient with acute pharyngitis, the clinical and epidemiological findings in Table 80.2 need to be considered (Class I-B, AHA 2009).

For patients with acute pharyngitis and clinical and epidemiological findings suggestive of a viral origin, the pretest probability of GAS is low, and testing usually does not need to be performed (Class IIb-B, AHA 2009).

The use of a clinical algorithm without microbiological confirmation has been recently recommended as an acceptable strategy for diagnosing GAS pharyngitis in adults. This approach could result in the receipt of inappropriate antimicrobial therapy by an unacceptably large number of adults with non-streptococcal pharyngitis and is not recommended (Class III-B, AHA 2009).

Antigen detection tests

Most of these tests have a high degree of specificity, but their sensitivity in clinical practice can be unacceptably low. Treatment is indicated for the patient with acute pharyngitis who has a positive RADT (Class I-B, AHA 2009). However, as with the throat culture, a positive test may reflect chronic colonization instead of active infection. A negative test does not exclude the presence of GAS, and a throat culture should be performed (Class I-B, AHA 2009).

Newer tests with improved sensitivity are developed. Physicians who use newer tests without culture backup in children and adolescents should compare the results of that specific RADT with those of blood agar plate cultures to confirm adequate sensitivity in their practice (Class IIa-C, AHA 2009). However, because of the low incidence of GAS infections and extremely low risk of acute rheumatic fever in adults, diagnosis of GAS pharyngitis on the basis of an antigen detection test alone, without confirmation of negative RADT results by a negative throat culture, is reasonable and an acceptable alternative to diagnosis on the basis of throat culture results (Class IIa-C, AHA 2009).

Streptococcal antibody tests

Anti-streptococcal antibody titres reflect past, and not present, immunological events and, therefore, cannot be used to determine whether an individual with pharyngitis and GAS in the pharynx is truly infected or merely a streptococcal carrier.

Therapy

The 2009 AHA recommendations are presented in Table 80.3.[2] Streptococcal infections that occur in family members of patients with current or previous rheumatic fever should also be treated promptly (Class I-B, AHA 2009).

Prophylaxis

An individual with a previous attack of rheumatic fever in whom GAS pharyngitis develops is at high risk for a recurrent attack of rheumatic fever. A recurrent attack can be associated with worsening of the severity of rheumatic heart disease that developed after a first attack or, less frequently, with the new onset of rheumatic heart disease in individuals who did not develop cardiac manifestations during the first attack.[2,6]

Continuous prophylaxis is recommended for patients with well-documented histories of rheumatic fever (including cases manifested solely by Sydenham chorea) and those with definite evidence of rheumatic heart disease (Class I-A, AHA 2009). Antibiotics and duration of prophylaxis recommendations are presented in Tables 80.4 and 80.5. Such prophylaxis should be initiated as soon as acute rheumatic fever or rheumatic heart disease is diagnosed. A full therapeutic course of penicillin first should be given to patients with acute rheumatic fever to eradicate residual GAS, even if a throat culture is negative at that time.

Table 80.3 AHA 2009 statement on rheumatic fever prevention.* Primary prevention of rheumatic fever (treatment of streptococcal tonsillopharyngitis)

Agent	Dose	Mode	Duration	Rating
Penicillins				
Penicillin V (phenoxymethyl penicillin)	Children: 250 mg 2–3 times daily for ≤27 kg (60 lb); children >27 kg (60 lb), adolescents, and adults: 500 mg 2–3 times daily	Oral	10 days	I-B
	Or			
Amoxicillin	50 mg/kg once daily (maximum 1 g)	Oral	10 days	I-B
	Or			
Benzathine penicillin G	600 000 U for patients ≤27 kg (60 lb); 200 000 U for patients >27 kg (60 lb)	Intramuscular	Once	I-B
For individuals allergic to penicillin				
Narrow-spectrum cephalosporin† (cephalexin, cefadroxil)	Variable	Oral	10 days	I-B
	Or			
Clindamycin	20 mg/kg per day divided in three doses (maximum 1.8 g/d)	Oral	10 days	IIa-B
	Or			

(Continued)

Table 80.3 (Continued)

Agent	Dose	Mode	Duration	Rating
Azithromycin	12 mg/kg once daily (maximum 500 mg)	Oral	5 days	IIa-B
	Or			
Clarithromycin	15 mg/kg per day divided bd (maximum 250 mg bd)	Oral	10 days	IIa-B

† To be avoided in those with immediate (type I) hypersensitivity to a penicillin.
Sulfonamides, trimethoprim, tetracyclines, and fluoroquinolones are not acceptable alternatives.
* Similar recommendations have been provided by ACC/AHA GL on valve disease.
AHA scientific statement: Prevention of rheumatic fever and diagnosis and treatment of acute Streptococcal pharyngitis. *Circulation*. 2009;**119**:1541–51.

Table 80.4 AHA 2009 statement on rheumatic fever prevention. Secondary prevention of rheumatic fever (prevention of recurrent attacks)

Agent	Dose	Mode	Rating
Benzathine penicillin G	600 000 U for children ≤27 kg (60 lb), 1 200 000 U for those >27 kg (60 lb) every 4 wk* 250 mg twice daily	Intramuscular	I-A
Penicillin V		Oral	I-B
Sulfadiazine	0.5 g once daily for patients ≤27 kg (60 lb), 1.0 g once daily for patients >27 kg (60 lb)	Oral	I-B
For individuals allergic to penicillin and sulfadiazine			
Macrolide or azalide	Variable	Oral	I-C

* In high-risk situations, administration every 3 weeks is justified and recommended.
AHA scientific statement: Prevention of rheumatic fever and diagnosis and treatment of acute Streptococcal pharyngitis. *Circulation*. 2009;**119**:1541–51.

Table 80.5 AHA 2009 statement on rheumatic fever prevention** Duration of secondary rheumatic fever prophylaxis

Category	Duration after last attack	Rating
Rheumatic fever with carditis and residual heart disease (persistent valvular disease*)	10 years or until 40 years of age (whichever is longer), sometimes lifelong prophylaxis (see text)	I-C
Rheumatic fever with carditis but no residual heart disease (no valvular disease*)	10 years or until 21 years of age (whichever is longer)	I-C
Rheumatic fever without carditis	5 years or until 21 years of age (whichever is longer)	I-C

* Clinical or echocardiographic evidence.
** Similar recommendations have been provided by ACC/AHA GL on valve disease.
AHA scientific statement: Prevention of rheumatic fever and diagnosis and treatment of acute Streptococcal pharyngitis. *Circulation*. 2009;**119**:1541–51.

References

1. Carapetis JR, *et al.* Acute rheumatic fever. *Lancet*. 2005;**366**:155–68
2. Gerber MA, *et al.* Prevention of rheumatic fever and diagnosis and treatment of acute streptococcal pharyngitis: a scientific statement from the American Heart Association Rheumatic Fever, Endocarditis, and Kawasaki Disease Committee of the Council on Cardiovascular Disease in the Young, the Interdisciplinary Council on Functional Genomics and Translational Biology, and the Interdisciplinary Council on Quality of Care and Outcomes Research: endorsed by the American Academy of Pediatrics. *Circulation*. 2009;**119**:1541–51
3. Galvin JE, *et al.* Cytotoxic mAb from rheumatic carditis recognizes heart valves and laminin. *J Clin Invest*. 2000;**106**:217–24
4. Guidelines for the diagnosis of rheumatic fever. Jones criteria, 1992 update. Special Writing Group of the Committee on Rheumatic Fever, Endocarditis, and Kawasaki Disease of the Council on Cardiovascular Disease in the Young of the American Heart Association. *JAMA*. 1992;**268**:2069–73
5. WHO. Rheumatic fever and rheumatic heart disease: report of a WHO Expert Consultation, Geneva, 29 October–1 November 2001. Geneva: World health Organization, 2004.
6. Bonow RO, *et al.* 2008 focused update incorporated into the ACC/AHA 2006 guidelines for the management of patients with valvular heart disease: a report of the American College of Cardiology/American Heart Association Task Force on practice guidelines (Writing Committee to revise the 1998 guidelines for the management of patients with valvular heart disease). Endorsed by the Society of Cardiovascular Anesthesiologists, Society for Cardiovascular Angiography and Interventions, and Society of Thoracic Surgeons. *J Am Coll Cardiol*. 2008;**52**:e1–142

Part IXX

Athlete's heart

Chapter 81

Athlete's heart

Exercise-induced cardiac remodelling

Isotonic exercise, i.e. endurance exercise with activities, such as long-distance running, cycling, and swimming, results in sustained elevations in cardiac output, with normal or reduced peripheral vascular resistance. It represents primarily a volume challenge for the heart that affects all four chambers.[1]

Isometric exercise, i.e. strength training, results in increased peripheral vascular resistance and normal, or only slightly elevated, cardiac output. This increase in peripheral vascular resistance causes transient, but potentially marked, systolic hypertension and LV afterload.[1]

LV hypertrophy and dilatation in isotonic and hypertrophy in isometric exercise. Mild reductions of LVEF might be seen, although there is evidence that both systolic and diastolic LV function may improve with exercise.

RV dilatation and increased free wall thickness have been seen in athletes with isotonic or isometric exercise. Recently, intensive endurance exercise of increased duration (i.e. marathon runners) was reported to result in transient RV dysfunction that is usually reversible, although septal fibrosis was seen in athletes with intensive training for prolonged periods.[2] The clinical significance of this observation is uncertain. In black athletes without concomitant symptoms or family history, T-wave inversion and RV enlargement may be a bening finding.[3]

Aortic root may be slightly dilated (up to 1.6 mm compared to controls), but marked aortic root dilatation represents a pathological process and not a physiological adaptation to exercise.[4] Slightly larger **left atrium** has also been detected in in trained athletes.

Common cardiovascular conditions associated with sudden death in athletes are presented in Table 81.1.

Table 81.1 Common cardiovascular conditions associated with sudden death in athletes

HCM
Congenital coronary anomalies
Genetic channelopathies (Brugada, early repolarization syndrome, LQTS, SQTS, CPVT)
Blunt trauma
Commotio cordis
Coronary artery disease
ARVC
Myocarditis
Bicuspid aortic valve with stenosis or dilated aortic root
WPW

Interpretation of the ECG in athletes

Differentiation between adaptive and pathological ECG changes in athletes is not always easy. Recommendations have been published by the ESC5 and a group of US experts.[6]

ECG patterns seen in athletes are presented in Table 81.2. Points for differentiating between adaptive changes and truly pathological findings are:[5,6]

Table 81.2 Classification of abnormalities of the athlete's electrocardiogram

Group 1: common and training-related ECG changes	Group 2: uncommon and training-unrelated ECG changes
Sinus bradycardia	T wave inversion
First-degree AV block	ST segment depression
Incomplete RBBB	Pathological Q waves
Early repolarization	Left atrial enlargement
Isolated QRS voltage criteria for left ventricular hypertrophy	Left axis deviation/left anterior hemiblock
	Right axis deviation/left posterior hemiblock
	Right ventricular hypertrophy
	Ventricular pre-excitation
	Complete LBBB or RBBB
	Long or short QT interval
	Brugada-like early repolarization

European Association of Cardiovascular Prevention and Rehabilitation. Recommendations for interpretation of 12-lead electrocardiogram in the athlete. *Eur Heart J*. 2010;**31**:243–59

1. Sinus bradycardia is normal. Only heart rates <30 bpm and pauses ≥3 s during wake suggest sick sinus syndrome.
2. First- and second-degree type 1 (Wenckebach) blocks are benign and usually resolve with hyperventilation or exercise.

3. Axis between −30 and +115 degrees is normal.
4. LV hypertrophy needs further evaluation only in the presence of family history of sudden cardiac death or non-voltage ECG criteria suggesting pathological ECG hypertrophy.
5. Q waves >3 mm in depth and/or >40 ms duration in any lead, except aVR, III, and V_1, suggest hypertrophic cardiomyopathy (HCM) (Figure 81.1). Standard criteria for MI in athletes should also be considered in those >40 years of age.
6. Inferolateral early repolarization patterns may be seen in young athletes and is a dynamic phenomenon caused by exercise.[7] Two types predominate (Figure 81.2). An elevated ST segment with upward concavity and positive T wave is seen in Caucasians, and an elevated ST segment with upward convexity and negative T wave in African-Caribbean athletes (Figure 81.3). It should be noted that African athletes display large proportion of ECG abnormalities, including an increase in R/S wave voltage, ST segment elevation, and inverted or diffusely flat T waves.[8] Pathological early repolarization patterns are discussed in Chapter 56 on inherited channelopathies.
7. Incomplete RBBB (QRS <120 ms) is common. However, it should be differentiated from ARVC and Brugada syndrome (Figure 81.4). Complete LBBB or RBBB with hemiblock necessitates cardiological work-up, including myocardial imaging. ECG of siblings should also be obtained to exclude genetically determined AV conduction disease.

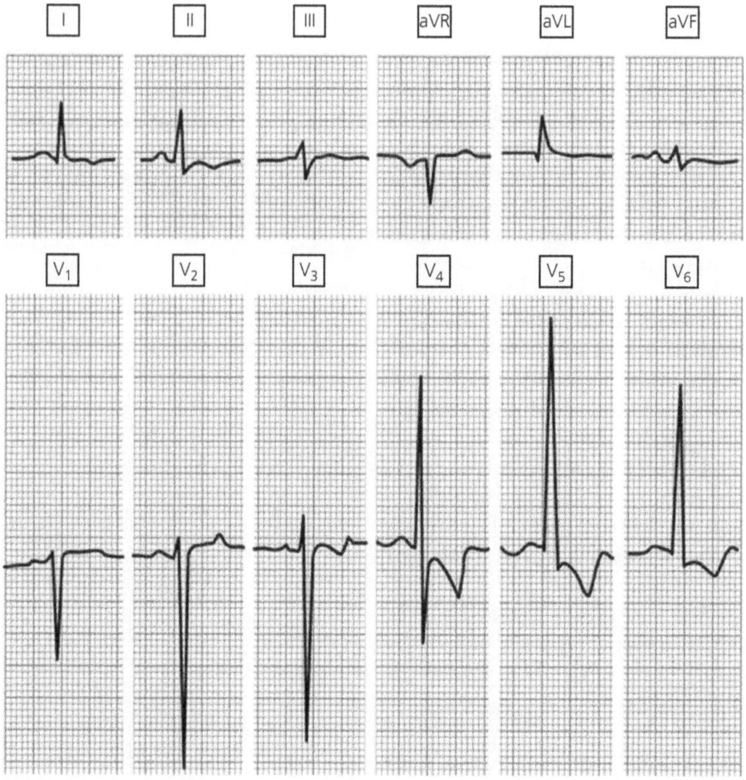

Figure 81.1 Twelve-lead ECG of an asymptomatic athlete with HCM. The disease was suspected at pre-participation evaluation from ECG abnormalities consisting of increased QRS voltages and inverted T waves in lateral leads. HCM was diagnosed by echocardiography afterwards.

European Association of Cardiovascular Prevention and Rehabilitation. Recommendations for interpretation of 12-lead electrocardiogram in the athlete. *Eur Heart J*. 2010;**31**:243–59.

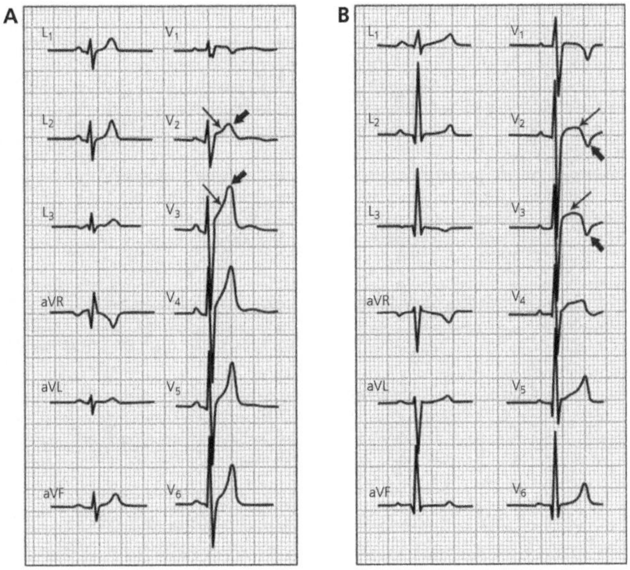

Figure 81.2 Different patterns of precordial early repolarization in two healthy athletes. (A) ST segment elevation with upward concavity (arrows), followed by a positive T wave (arrowheads). (B) ST segment elevation with upward convexity (arrows), followed by a negative T wave (arrowheads). European Association of Cardiovascular Prevention and Rehabilitation. Recommendations for interpretation of 12-lead electrocardiogram in the athlete. *Eur Heart J*. 2010;**31**:243–59.

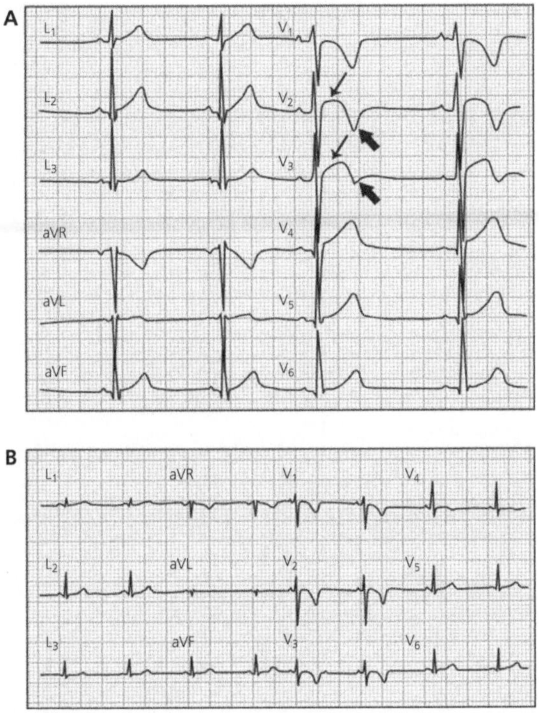

Figure 81.3 (A) Early repolarization pattern in a healthy black athlete characterized by right precordial T wave inversion (arrowhead), preceded by ST segment elevation (arrow). (B) Right precordial T wave inversion in a patient with ARVC. Note that, unlike early repolarization, in ARVC, the right precordial leads do not demonstrate any elevation of the ST segment. European Association of Cardiovascular Prevention and Rehabilitation. Recommendations for interpretation of 12-lead electrocardiogram in the athlete. *Eur Heart J*. 2010;**31**:243–59.

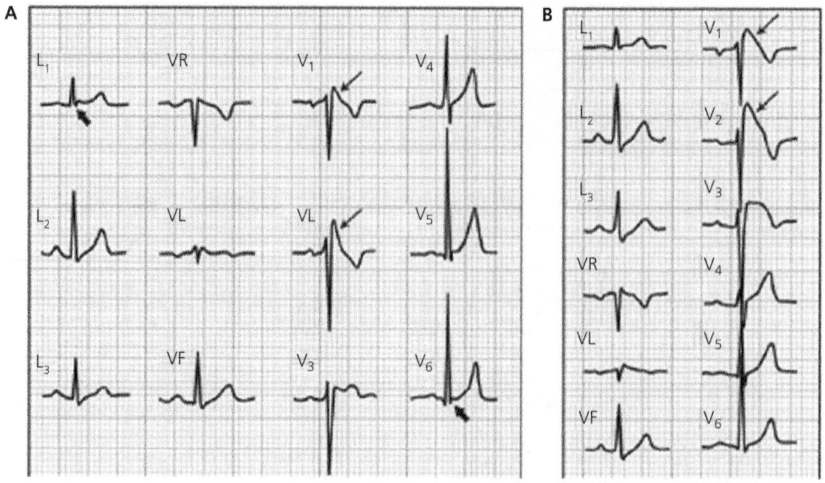

Figure 81.4 (A) Borderline Brugada ECG pattern mimicking incomplete RBBB. Unlike the 'R wave' of RBBB, the 'J wave' (arrows) of Brugada ECG is confined to right precordial leads (V_1 and V_2) without reciprocal 'S wave' (of comparable voltage and duration) in leads V_1 and V_6 (arrowhead). (B) In this case, definitive diagnosis of Brugada ECG was achieved by a drug challenge with sodium channel blockers which unmasked diagnostic 'coved-type' (arrows) pattern (V_1 and V_2). European Association of Cardiovascular Prevention and Rehabilitation.

Recommendations for interpretation of 12-lead electrocardiogram in the athlete. *Eur Heart J*. 2010;**31**:243–59.

ECG abnormality	Criteria for further evaluation	Example
Q waves	>3 mm in depth or >40 ms duration in any lead except III, aVR, aVL and V_1	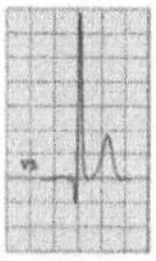
ST depression	>0.5 mm below PR isoelectric line between J-junction and beginning of T waves in V_4, V_5, V_6, I, aVL >1 mm in any lead	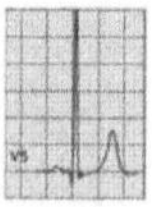
T wave inversion	>1 mm in leads other than III, aVR and V_1 (except V_2 and V_3 in women <25 years)	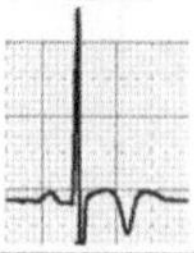
Atrial abnormalities	Right: P wave amplitude >2.5 mm Left: i) Negative portion of P wave in V_1, V_2 of >40 ms duration and 1 mm in depth; or ii) total P wave duration >120 ms	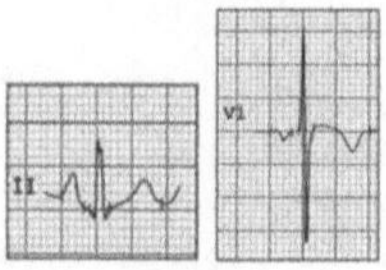
Right ventricular hypertrophy	>30 years: i) R wave >7 mm in V_1; or ii) R/S ration >1 in V_1; or iii) sum of R wave in V_1 and S wave in V_5 or V_6 >10.5 mm <30 years: above plus right atrial enlargement, T wave inversion in V_2, V_3, or right axis deviation >115°	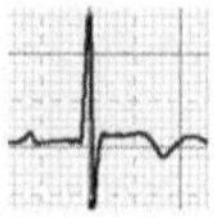

Figure 81.5 Summary of recommendations for pre-participation examination in ECG screening. RAA, right atrial abnormality; LAA, left atrial abnormality; RVH, right ventricular hypertrophy; RAD, right axis deviation; RBBB, right bundle branch block; TWI, T wave inversion; and QTc, heart rate correction of the QT interval.

Uberoi A, *et al*. Interpretation of the electrocardiogram of young athletes. *Circulation*. 2011;**124**:746–57.

8. Suspicion of long QT (>470 ms in men and >480 ms in women) or short QT (<340 ms) should lead to evaluation by a specialist. A QTC ≤380 ms may also be a marker of abuse of anabolic androgenic steroids.
9. WPW needs ablation for the elimination of the very low risk of sudden death, particularly since athletes may develop AF. Exclusion of conditions, such as Ebstein disease, HCM, and glycogen storage cardiomyopathy, should be undertaken.

A summary of recommendations for pre-participation examination in ECG screening are presented in Figure 81.5.

Arrhythmias in athletes

Sudden cardiac death and arrhythmias in athletes (SVT, AF, VT) are discussed in the relevant chapters.

Classification of sports

Classification of sports from the 36th Bethesda Conference and by the ESC are presented in Figures 81.6 and 81.7.[9–11]

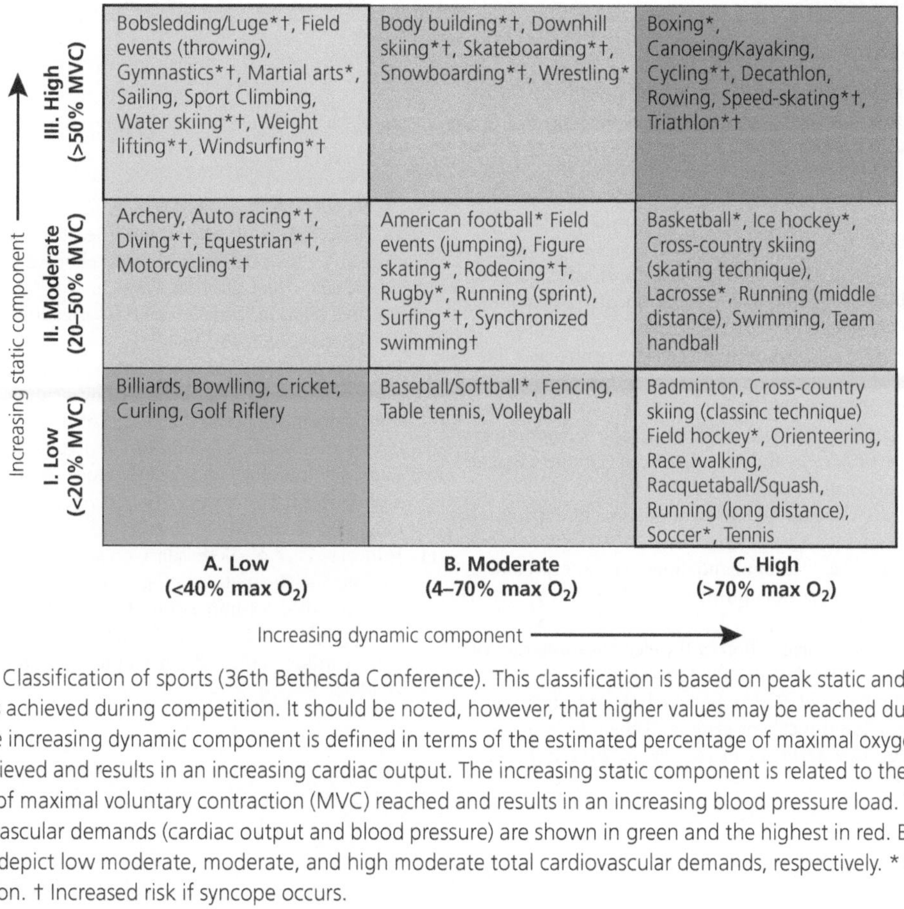

Figure 81.6 Classification of sports (36th Bethesda Conference). This classification is based on peak static and dynamic components achieved during competition. It should be noted, however, that higher values may be reached during training. The increasing dynamic component is defined in terms of the estimated percentage of maximal oxygen uptake ($MaxO_2$) achieved and results in an increasing cardiac output. The increasing static component is related to the estimated percentage of maximal voluntary contraction (MVC) reached and results in an increasing blood pressure load. The lowest total cardiovascular demands (cardiac output and blood pressure) are shown in green and the highest in red. Blue, yellow, and orange depict low moderate, moderate, and high moderate total cardiovascular demands, respectively. * Danger of bodily collision. † Increased risk if syncope occurs.

Mitchell JH, *et al*. Task Force 8: classification of sports. *J Am Coll Cardiol*. 2005;**45**:1364–7.

	A. Low dynamic	B. Moderate dynamic	C. High dynamic
I. Low static	Bowling Cricket Golf Riflery	Fencing Table tennis Tennis (doubles) Volleyball	Badminton Race walking Running (marathon) Cross-country skiing (classic)
II. Moderater static	Auto racing[a,b] Diving[b] Equestrian[a,b] Motorcycling[a,b] Gymnastics[a] Karate/Judo[a] Sailing Archering	Baseball[a]/softball[a] Field events (jumping) Figure skating[a] Lacrosse[a] Running (sprint)	Squash[a] Basketball[a] Biathlon Ice hockey[a] Field hockey[a] Rugby[a] Soccer[a] Cross-country skiing (skating) Running (mid/long) Swimming Tennis (single) Team handball[a]
III. High static	Bobsledding[a,b] Field events (throwing) Luge[a,b] Rock Climbing[a,b] Waterskiing[a,b] Weight lifting[a] Windsurfing[a]	Body building[a] Downhill skiing[a,b] Wrestling[a] Snow boarding[a,b]	Boxing[a] Canoeing, Kayaking Cycling[a,b] Decathlon Rowing Speed skating Triathlon[a,b]

Figure 81.7 Classification of sports (ESC).

[a] Danger of bodily collision. [b] Increased risk if syncope occurs.

Pelliccia A, *et al*; Study Group of Sports Cardiology of the Working Group of Cardiac Rehabilitation and Exercise Physiology; Working Group of Myocardial and Pericardial Diseases of the European Society of Cardiology. *Eur Heart J*. 2005;**26**:1422–45.

References

1. Baggish AL, *et al.* Athlete's heart and cardiovascular care of the athlete: scientific and clinical update. *Circulation*. 2011;**123**:2723–35
2. La Gerche A, *et al.* Exercise-induced right ventricular dysfunction and structural remodelling in endurance athletes. *Eur Heart J*. 2012;**33**:998–1006
3. Zaidi A, *et al.* Physiological right ventricular adaptation in elite athletes of African and Afro-Caribbean origin / clinical perspective. *Circulation*. 2013;**127**:1783–92
4. Iskandar A, Thompson PD. A meta-analysis of aortic root size in elite athletes. *Circulation*. 2013;**127**:791–8
5. Corrado D, *et al.* Recommendations for interpretation of 12-lead electrocardiogram in the athlete. *Eur Heart J*. 2010;**31**:243–59
6. Uberoi A, *et al.* Interpretation of the electrocardiogram of young athletes. *Circulation*. 2011;**124**:746–57
7. Noseworthy PA, *et al.* Early repolarization pattern in competitive athletes: clinical correlates and the effects of exercise training. *Circ Arrhythm Electrophysiol*. 2011;**4**:432–40
8. Di Paolo FM, *et al.* The athlete's heart in adolescent Africans: an electrocardiographic and echocardiographic study. *J Am Coll Cardiol*. 2012;**59**:1029–36
9. Mitchell JH, *et al.* Task Force 8: classification of sports. *J Am Coll Cardiol*. 2005;**45**:1364–7
10. Pelliccia A, *et al.* Recommendations for competitive sports participation in athletes with cardiovascular disease: a consensus document from the Study Group of Sports Cardiology of the Working Group of Cardiac Rehabilitation and Exercise Physiology and the Working Group of Myocardial and Pericardial Diseases of the European Society of Cardiology. *Eur Heart J*. 2005;**26**:1422–45
11. Pelliccia A, *et al.* Bethesda Conference #36 and the European Society of Cardiology Consensus Recommendations revisited a comparison of U.S. and European criteria for eligibility and disqualification of competitive athletes with cardiovascular abnormalities. *J Am Coll Cardiol*. 2008;**52**:1990–6

Part XX

Cardiac tumours and pseudoaneurysms

Chapter 82

Cardiac tumours

Primary cardiac tumours

Primary cardiac tumours are a rare entity across all age groups, with a reported prevalence of 0.001–0.03% in autopsy series.[1] Primary tumours consist 0.3% to 0.7% of all cardiac tumours, whereas metastasis to the heart from other primary cancers is 30 times more common.[2] Approximately 75% of primary cardiac tumours are benign, and, of those, the majority are myxomas.[3,4] Cardiac lipomas and papillary fibroelastomas occur in adults and are usually asymptomatic. Of the malignant tumours which often occur in the young, 75% are sarcomas.[2] Malignant primary cardiac sarcomas are usually located in the right atrium and are most commonly angiosarcomas. In the left atrium, the most common malignant tumours are pleomorphic sarcoma (also known as malignant fibrous histiocytoma) and leiomyosarcoma.[2] Rhabdomyomas and fibromas are seen in infants.

Aetiology

The genetics of primary cardiac tumours is poorly understood, especially for those that occur sporadically. Myxomas are familial in 10% of cases. Carney's syndrome (or complex) is an autosomal dominant syndrome characterized by familial recurrent cardiac and mucocutaneous myxomas arising from mesenchymal cells, pigmented lesions over the lips, conjunctiva, and genitalia, adenomas of the breast and thyroid, and endocrine abnormalities, including Cushing's syndrome and acromegaly. Genetic studies have identified mutations in the gene encoding protein kinase A, regulatory subunit 1-α (PRKAR1α).[5] There are no demonstrable associations with malignant sarcomas.

Presentation

Systemic or pulmonary embolization, congestive heart failure from intracardiac obstruction, and arrhythmias may occur. Cardiac myxoma is the most common primary cardiac tumour to produce emboli to virtually any organ or tissue. Cerebral aneurysm, secondary to embolic tumour fragments, is a life-threatening complication. Left atrial sarcomas tend to be more solid and less infiltrative than right-sided sarcomas, and they tend to metastasize later. They usually present with symptoms of blood flow obstruction and severe congestive heart failure. Right-sided cardiac tumours are usually malignant and appear as bulky, infiltrative masses that grow in an outward pattern. These are usually fast-growing tumours that metastasize early and do not present with congestive heart failure until late in the disease.[2]

Investigations

Cardiac MRI and 3D echocardiography are the investigations of choice for intracardiac tumours.[4] A CT of the chest with contrast agent is needed to exclude lung metastasis of malignant tumours. Two-dimensional transthoracic and transoesophageal echocardiography underestimate tumour mass by as much as 24%.[2]

Therapy

Myxomas are completely excised under cardiopulmonary bypass; this may not always be feasible.[3] Recurrence occurs in 3% of the cases and may be local or in extracardiac locations, such as the brain, lung, and other tissues. Thus, follow-up for more than 10 years is advisable.[1] Malignant primary cardiac tumours have a dismal prognosis, and, without surgical resection, the survival rate at 9 to 12 months is only 10%.[2]

Cardiac metastases

Cardiac metastases are much more common than primary tumours. In a recent post-mortem survey of 7289 malignant neoplasms, an incidence of 9.1% of heart metastases was found. The highest rate was reported in pleural mesothelioma (48.4%), melanoma (27.8%), lung adenocarcinoma (21%), undifferentiated carcinoma (19.5%), lung squamous cell carcinoma (18.2%), and breast carcinoma (15.5%).[6]

References

1. McManus B, *et al.* Primary tumours of the heart. In: Libby P, Bonow RO, Mann DL, Zipes DP (Eds). Heart disease. pp. 1815–28, Saunders, Phliadelphia, 2008
2. Leja MJ, *et al.* Primary cardiac tumours. *Tex Heart Inst J.* 2011;**38**:261–2
3. Pacini D, *et al.* Primary benign cardiac tumours: long-term results. *Eur J Cardiothorac Surg.* 2012;**41**:812–19
4. Hoey ET, *et al.* MRI and CT appearances of cardiac tumours in adults. *Clin Radiol.* 2009;**64**:1214–30
5. Shetty Roy AN, *et al.* Familial recurrent atrial myxoma: Carney's complex. *Clin Cardiol.* 2011;**34**:83–6
6. Bussani R, *et al.* Cardiac metastases. *J Clin Pathol.* 2007;**60**:27–34

Chapter 83

Pseudoaneurysms of the heart

Introduction

A pseudoaneurysm is a rupture of a blood vessel or of the myocardial wall that is contained by pericardium, thrombus, or adhesions and has typically a narrow neck.[1] A true aneurysm is contained by all layers of the myocardium or vessel and displays a paradoxical movement, bulging outward during systole. Although their natural history is not well defined, pseudoaneurysms usually have a greater risk of rupture (30–45%) and should thus be considered for immediate repair.[2]

Aetiology

Myocardial infarction is the most common cause of LV pseudoaneurysms. Aortic valvular surgery and endocarditis (pseudoaneurysms at the mitral-aortic intervalvular fibrosa), blunt or penetrating trauma, and radiofrequency ablation are less common causes.[1, 2] Pseudoaneurysms of the native coronary arteries may occur after stenting or after spontaneous coronary arterial dissection whereas pseudoaneurysms of bypass grafts tend to occur at suture line sites or after stenting.[1, 2]

Diagnosis

Patients may be asymptomatic or present with a murmur and/or heart failure. Systemic embolism may also occur. Rupture results in tamponade, shock, or sudden death. Transthoracic echocardiography has low sensitivity to detect pseudoaneurysms; transoesophageal echocardiography, cardiac CT, and MRI offer a higher diagnostic yield.[3]

Treatment

Ventricular pseudoaneurysms are more likely to rupture when they are relatively acute (<3 months), large, or located within the anterior or lateral ventricular wall.[4] Saphenous vein graft pseudoaneurysm should be considered for repair if large (>1 cm) or if associated with symptoms.[5] Surgical repair or percutaneous closure may be used.[6] Conservative management may be considered in high-risk patients with chronic pseudoaneurysms. The use of anticoagulation is controversial since it may increase the risk of rupture.

References

1. Hulten EA, *et al.* Pseudoaneurysms of the heart. *Circulation.* 2012;**125**:1920–5
2. Frances C, *et al.* Left ventricular pseudoaneurysm. *J Am Coll Cardiol.* 1998;**32**:557–61
3. Brown SL, *et al.* Distinguishing left ventricular aneurysm from pseudoaneurysm: a review of the literature. *Chest.* 1997;**111**:1403–9
4. Yeo TC, *et al.* Clinical profile and outcome in 52 patients with cardiac pseudoaneurysm. *Ann Intern Med.* 1998;**128**: 299–305
5. Sareyyupoglu B, *et al.* Surgical treatment of saphenous vein graft aneurysms after coronary artery revascularization. *Ann Thorac Surg.* 2009;**88**:1801–5
6. Dudiy Y, *et al.* Percutaneous closure of left ventricular pseudoaneurysm. *Circ Cardiovasc Interv.* 2011;**4**:322–6.

Part XXI

Cardiovascular disease in pregnancy

Chapter 84

Cardiovascular disease in pregnancy

Overview

General issues on cardiovascular disease in pregnancy are discussed. The implications of pregnancy for individual disease entities are also discussed in relevant chapters.

Pregnancy is associated by an increase in blood volume (50%), cardiac output, and heart rate, combined with a decrease in systemic vascular resistance.[1] Risk factors (before pregnancy) have been estimated by the CARPEG score (heart disease in general) and the ZAHARA and Khairy *et al.* studies (Table 84.1).[2–4]

In general they are:

- LVEF <40%
- NYHA >II or cyanosis
- Left heart obstruction (mitral valve area <2 cm^2, aortic valve area <1.5cm^2 with gradient >30 mmHg)
- Prior cardiac event or arrhythmia and use of cardiac medication
- Mechanical valve replacement
- Systemic or pulmonary AV valve regurgitation.

The most prevalent cardiac complications during pregnancy are arrhythmias and heart failure and hypertensive complications. Neonatal complications increase with:

- Poor functional class or cyanosis
- Left heart obstruction
- Anticoagulation
- Smoking
- Mechanical valve replacement
- Multiple gestations.

Women experiencing common pregnancy complications, such as gestational diabetes mellitus, preeclampsia and other hypetensive disorders, intrauterine growth restriction, and preterm delivery, are at increased risk of cardiovascular disease.[5] These complications are prevalent (36%), and provide an opportunity for early identification of women at increased risk of cardiovascular disease later in life.

Tables 84.2 and 84.3 present the WHO classification of associated risks.[1,6]

Table 84.1 Predictors of maternal cardiovascular events

CARPREG study. Predictors of maternal cardiovascular events and risk score in patients with cardiovascular disease
Prior cardiac event (heart failure, transient ischaemic attack, stroke before pregnancy or arrhythmia).
Baseline NYHA functional class >II or cyanosis.
Left heart obstruction (mitral valve area <2 cm^2, aortic valve area <1.5 cm^2, peak LV outflow tract gradient >30 mmHg by echocardiography).
Reduced systemic ventricular systolic function (ejection fraction <40%).
CARPREG risk score: for each CARPREG predictor that is present, a point is assigned. Risk estimation of cardiovascular maternal complications
0 point 5%
1 point 27%
>1 point 75%
Predictors of maternal cardiovascular events identified in congential heart diseases
ZAHARA study predictors
History of arrhythmia event.
Baseline NYHA functional class >II.
Left heart obstruction (aortic valve peak gradient >50 mm Hg).
Mechanical valve prosthesis.
Moderate/severe systemic atrioventricular valve regurgitation (possibly related to ventricular dysfunction).
Moderate/severe subpulmonary atrioventricular valve regurgitation (possibly related to ventricular dysfunction).
Use of cardiac medication pre-pregnancy.
Repaired or unrepaired cyanotic heart disease.
Khairy study predictors
Smoking history.
Reduced subpulmonary ventricular function and/or severe pulmonary regurgitation.

Table 84.2 ESC 2011 GL on pregnancy. Modified World Health Organization (WHO) classification of maternal cardiovascular risk: principles

Risk class	Risk of pregnancy by medical condition
I	No detectable increased risk of maternal mortality and no/mild increase in morbidity.
II	Small increased risk of maternal mortality or moderate increase in morbidity.
III	Significantly increased risk of maternal mortality or severe morbidity. Expert counselling required. If pregnancy is decided upon, intensive specialist cardiac and obstetric monitoring needed throughout pregnancy, childbirth, and the puerperium.
IV	Extremely high risk of maternal mortality or severe morbidity; pregnancy contraindicated. If pregnancy occurs, termination should be discussed. If pregnancy continues, care as for class III.

ESC Guidelines on the management of cardiovascular diseases during pregnancy. *Eur Heart J*. 2011;**32**:3147–97.

Table 84.3 ESC 2011 GL on pregnancy. Modified World Health Organization (WHO) classification of maternal cardiovascular risk: application

Conditions in which pregnancy risk is WHO I
Uncomplicated, small, or mild
Pulmonary stenosis
Patent ductus arteriosus
Mitral valve prolapse
Successfully repaired simple lesions (atrial or ventricular septal defect, patent ductus arteriosus, anomalous pulmonary venous drainage)
Atrial or ventricular ectopic beats, isolated
Conditions in which pregnancy risk is WHO II or III
WHO II (if otherwise well and uncomplicated)
Unoperated atrial or ventricular septal defect
Repaired tetralogy of Fallot
Most arrhythmias
WHO II–III (depending on individual)
Mild left ventricular impairment
Hypertrophic cardiomyopathy
Native or tissue valvular heart disease not considered WHO I or IV
Marfan's syndrome without aortic dilatation
Aorta <45 mm in aortic disease associated with bicuspid aortic valve
Repaired coarctation
WHO III
Mechanical valve
Systemic right ventricle
Fontan circulation
Cyanotic heart disease (unrepaired)
Other complex congenital heart disease
Aortic dilatation 40–45 mm in Marfan's syndrome
Aortic dilatation 45–50 mm in aortic disease associated with bicuspid aortic valve
Conditions in which pregnancy risk is WHO IV (pregnancy contraindicated)
Pulmonary arterial hypertension of any cause
Severe systemic ventricular dysfunction (LVEF <30%, NYHA III/IV)
Previous peripartum cardiomyopathy with any residual impairment of left ventricular function
Severe mitral stenosis, severe symptomatic aortic stenosis
Marfan's syndrome with aorta dilated >45 mm
Aortic dilatation >50 mm in aortic disease associated with bicuspid aortic valve
Native severe coarctation

ESC Guidelines on the management of cardiovascular diseases during pregnancy. *Eur Heart J*. 2011;**32**:3147–97.

Table 84.4 ESC 2011 on pregnancy. General recommendations

Pre-pregnancy risk assessment and counselling in all women with known or suspected congenital or acquired cardiovascular and aortic disease.	I-C
Risk assessment in all women with cardiac diseases of childbearing age and after conception.	I-C
High-risk patients should be treated in specialized centres by a multidisciplinary team.	I-C
Genetic counselling to women with congenital heart disease or congenital arrhythmia, cardiomyopathies, aortic disease or genetic malformations associated with CVD.	I-C
Echocardiography should be performed in any pregnant patient with unexplained or new cardiovascular signs or symptoms.	I-C
Before cardiac surgery, a full course of corticosteroids should be administered to the mother, whenever possible.	I-C
For the prevention of infective endocarditis in pregnancy, the same measures as in non-pregnant patients should be used.	I-C
Vaginal delivery is recommended as first choice in most patients.	I-C
MRI (without gadolinium) should be considered if echocardiography is insufficient.	IIa-C
In patients with severe hypertension, vaginal delivery with epidural analgesia and elective instrumental delivery should be considered.	IIa-C
When gestational age is at least 28 weeks, delivery before necessary surgery should be considered.	IIa-C
Caesarean delivery for obstetric indications or for patients with dilatation of the ascending aorta >45 mm, severe aortic stenosis, preterm labour while on oral anticoagulants, Eisenmenger's syndrome, or severe heart failure.	IIa-C
Caesarean delivery in Marfan's patients with an aortic diameter 40–45 mm.	IIb-C
A chest radiograph, with shielding of the fetus, may be considered if other methods are not successful in clarifying the cause of dyspnoea.	IIb-C
Cardiac catheterization may be considered with very strict indications, timing, and shielding of the fetus.	IIb-C
CT and electrophysiological studies, with shielding of the fetus, may be considered in selected patients for vital indications.	IIb-C
CABG or valvular surgery may be considered when conservative and medical therapy has failed, in situations that threaten the mother's life and that are not amenable to percutaneous treatment.	IIb-C
Prophylactic antibiotic therapy during delivery is not recommended.	III-C

CT, computed tomography; CVD, cardiovascular disease; MRI, magnetic resonance imaging.

ESC Guidelines on the management of cardiovascular diseases during pregnancy. *Eur Heart J*. 2011;**32**:3147–97

Table 84.5 ESC 2011 on pregnancy. Estimated fetal and maternal effective doses for various diagnostic and interventional radiology procedures

Procedure	**Fetal exposure**		**Maternal exposure**	
Chest radiograph (PA and lateral)	<0.01 mGy	<0.01 mSv	0.1 mGy	0.1 mSv
CT chest	0.3 mGy	0.3 mSv	7 mGy	7 mSv
Coronary angiography[a]	1.5 mGy	1.5 mSv	7 mGy	7 mSv
PCI or radiofrequency catheter ablation[a]	3 mGy	3 mSv	15 mGy	15 mSv

[a] Exposure depends on the number of projections or views.

CT, computed tomography; PA, posteroanterior; PCI, percutaneous coronary intervention.

ESC Guidelines on the management of cardiovascular diseases during pregnancy. *Eur Heart J*. 2011;**32**:3147–97.

The ESC general recommendations are presented in Table 84.4. Recommendations for specific disorders are presented in the relevant chapters. Table 84.5 presents estimated fetal and maternal effective doses for various diagnostic and interventional radiology procedures, and Appendix 3 the ESC 2011 recommendations on drug use in pregnancy and breastfeeding.

References

1. Regitz-Zagrosek V, *et al.* ESC guidelines on the management of cardiovascular diseases during pregnancy: the Task Force on the management of cardiovascular diseases during pregnancy of the European Society of Cardiology (ESC). *Eur Heart J*. 2011;**32**:3147–97
2. Drenthen W, *et al.* Predictors of pregnancy complications in women with congenital heart disease. *Eur Heart J*. 2010;**31**:2124–32
3. Khairy P, *et al.* Pregnancy outcomes in women with congenital heart disease. *Circulation*. 2006;**113**:517–24
4. Siu SC, *et al.* Prospective multicenter study of pregnancy outcomes in women with heart disease. *Circulation*. 2001;**104**:515–21
5. Fraser A, *et al.* Associations of pregnancy complications with calculated cardiovascular disease risk and cardiovascular risk factors in middle age: the AVON longitudinal study of parents and children. *Circulation*. 2012;**125**:1367–80
6. Thorne S, *et al.* Risks of contraception and pregnancy in heart disease. *Heart*. 2006;**92**:1520–5

Part XXII

Cardiovascular drugs

Chapter 85

Cardiovascular drugs

Antiarrhythmic drugs

Beta blockers are discussed in Chapter 24 on hypertension and Chapter 31 on heart failure. Other antiarrhythmic agents are discussed in Chapter 49 on tachycarrhythmias.

Antiplatelet agents

Aspirin and $P2Y_{12}$ receptor blockers are discussed mainly in Chapter 27 on UA/NSTEMI.

Anticoagulants

Heparins, warfarin, and new anticoagulants, such as thrombin and Xa inhibitors, are mainly discussed in Chapter 27 on UA/NSTEMI, Chapter 22 on valve disease, and Chapter 52 on AF.

Beta blockers, diuretics, ACEIs, ARBs, CCBs

They are discussed in the Chapter 24 on hypertension and Chapter 31 on heart failure.

Statins, fibrates

They are mainly discussed in Chapter 29 on stable CAD.

Drugs for erectile dysfunction

Erectile dysfunction is a predictor of coronary artery disease, especially in men >60 years of age.[1] Phosphodiesterase-5 inhibitors (PDE5Is) (sildenafil [Viagra], vardenafil [Levitra], and tadalafil [Cialis]) are used for erectile dysfunction. Sildenafil (Revatio) and tadalafil (Adcirca) are also prescribed for pulmonary hypertension (see Chapter 77). There is now evidence that PDE5Is do not significantly affect the incidence of adverse cardiovascular events.[2] Tadalafil, in particular, has fewer effects on the cardiovascular system than the other PDE5Is, as exemplified by its minimal effects on BP in healthy control subjects.

Sildenafil (50–100 mg) and vardenafil (10–20 mg) lead to peak plasma levels in 60 min and have a half-life of 3–5 hours. Tadalafil (10–20 mg) peaks at 2 hours and has a half-life of 17.5 h, and its absorption is not influenced by food. Reduced initial doses are required for patients with hepatic impairment, creatinine clearance <30 mL/min, and age >65 years.

PDE5Is improve erectile function by enhancing nitric oxide availability in the penis and its supplying vasculature, resulting in vasodilation and increased blood flow. Since phosphodiesterase-5 is also located elsewhere in the body, including the pulmonary and systemic vasculature, and in hypertrophied myocardium, PDE5Is are also used for pulmonary arterial hypertension. Initial evidence also suggests beneficial effects in congestive heart failure, secondary pulmonary hypertension, high-altitude pulmonary oedema, high-altitude pulmonary hypertension, and Raynaud's phenomenon.[3]

Side effects and precautions

Most common side effects are mild headache and flushing. A direct link between PDE5Is and optic neuropathy could not be established, but a possible link between these drugs, especially sildenafil, and hearing impairment has been reported.[4] Priapism is rare.

PDE5I can be safely given with antihypertensive medications.

Care is needed with nitrates and alpha blockers (Table 85.1).[5]

Nitrates

Penile erections and endothelium-mediated vasodilation are mediated through cGMP, which promotes trabecular and vascular smooth muscle relaxation. PDE5Is prevent the breakdown of cGMP. Nitric oxide donors (i.e. nitrates) increase the production of cGMP. Because both PDE5Is and nitrates increase cGMP, co-administration can generate excess accumulation of cGMP and can trigger marked vasodilation and severe hypotension. Thus, all nitrates are contraindicated for at least 24 h after sildenafil/vardenafil and 48 h after tadalafil.

In case of hypotension due to concomitant administration of nitrates, placing the patient in the Trendelenburg position, aggressive fluid resuscitation, and, if necessary, an α-agonist (phenylephrine) or a β-agonist (norepinephrine) are recommended.[3] There is no antidote to PDE5Is.

α-blockers

'Uroselective' α-blockers (tamsulosin, alfuzosin) preferentially inhibit $\alpha 1_A$ and $\alpha 1_D$ receptors, found primarily in the prostate, and benefit patients with benign prostatic hypertrophy. Other α-blockers (terazosin) are less selective, and

Table 85.1 AHA statement on sexual activity and cardiovascular disease 2012. Use of PDE5 inhibitors

PDE5 inhibitors are useful for the treatment of erectile dysfunction in patients with stable CVD.	I-A
The safety of PDE5 inhibitors is unknown in patients with severe aortic stenosis or HCM.	IIb-C
PDE5 inhibitors should not be used in patients receiving nitrate therapy.	III-B
Nitrates should not be administered to patients within 24 hours of sildenafil or vardenafil administration or within 48 hours of tadalafil administration.	III-B

Sexual Activity and Cardiovascular Disease: A Scientific Statement From the American Heart Association. *Circulation*. 2012;**125**:1058–1072

some (doxazosin) are used as third-line agents for hypertension because of their higher affinity for $\alpha 1_B$ receptors, which are abundant in the peripheral vasculature. All α-blockers can cause vasodilation and orthostatic hypotension, and co-administration with PDE5Is increases the risk of a clinically significant decrease in BP. This risk is reduced with tadalafil, with uroselective α-blockers, when low doses of α-blockers are used, when dosing is separated by several hours (instead of simultaneously), and when patients are on stable therapy with one agent before the other drug class is administered.[1]

Other drug interactions

PDE5I are metabolized mainly by the cytochrome P450 (mainly 3A4 cytochrome) pathway, and their concentrations may be increased by drugs, such as cimetidine, erythromycin, clarithromycin, and ciprofloxacin (mainly sildenafil), ketoconazole (mainly vardenafil and tadalafil), and ritonavir (all of them). Rifampin and bosentan may reduce their levels. QT prolongation is minimal with PDE5Is. Vardenafil and sildenafil have been studied and produced no increase of absolute QT and only similar, small increases of the QTc interval, with a shallow dose-response curve.[6]

References

1. Schwartz BG, *et al.* Clinical cardiology: physician update: erectile dysfunction and cardiovascular disease. *Circulation*. 2011;**123**:98–101
2. Schwartz BG KR. Drug interactions with phosphodiesterase-5 inhibitors used for the treatment of erectile dysfunction or pulmonary hypertension. *Circulation*. 2010;**122**:88–95
3. Schwartz BG, *et al.* Cardiac uses of phosphodiesterase-5 inhibitors. *J Am Coll Cardiol*. 2012;**59**:9–15
4. Shamloul R, *et al.* Erectile dysfunction. *Lancet*. 2013;**381**:153–65.
5. Levine GN, *et al.* Sexual activity and cardiovascular disease: a scientific statement from the American Heart Association. *Circulation*. 2012;**125**:1058–72
6. Morganroth J, *et al.* Evaluation of vardenafil and sildenafil on cardiac repolarization. *Am J Cardiol*. 2004;**93**:1378–83

Appendix 1

Recommendation classes and levels of evidence used in guidelines

Class I Evidence and/or general agreement that a given treatment or procedure is beneficial, useful, and effective (**recommended/indicated**).
Class II Conflicting evidence and/or a divergence of opinion about the usefulness/efficacy of a given treatment or procedure.
Class IIa Weight of evidence/opinion is in favour of usefulness/efficacy (**should be considered**).
Class IIb Usefulness/efficacy is less well established by evidence/opinion (**may be considered**).
Class III Evidence or general agreement that the given treatment or procedure is not useful/effective, and in some cases may be harmful (**is not recommended**).

Level of evidence A Data derived from multiple randomized clinical trials or meta-analyses.
Level of evidence B Data derived from a single randomized clinical trial or large non-randomized studies.
Level of evidence C Consensus of opinion of the experts and/or small studies, retrospective studies, registries.

Conversion of units

Cholesterol	mg/dL	x 0.026	to	mmol/L
Creatinine	mg/dL	x 88.4	to	µmol/L
Digoxin	ng/mL	x 1.28	to	nmol/L
Glucose	mg/dL	x 0.055	to	mmol/L

Appendix 2

Therapy of endocarditis

ACC/AHA GL 2008 on valve disease. Therapy of native valve endocarditis caused by viridans group streptococci and *Streptococcus bovis*

Regimen	Dosage and route	Duration (week)	Comments
Aqueous crystalline penicillin G sodium	12–18 million U per 24 h IV, either continuously or in 4 or 6 equally divided doses	4	Preferred in most patients greater than 65 years of age or patients with impairment of 8th cranial nerve function or renal function
or			
Ceftriaxone sodium	2 g per 24 h IV/IM in 1 dose	4	
	Paediatric dose: penicillin 200 000 U per kg per 24 h IV in 4–6 equally divided doses; ceftriaxone 100 mg per kg per 24 h IV/IM in 1 dose (not to exceed adult dose)		
Aqueous crystalline penicillin G sodium	12–18 million U per 24 h IV, either continuously or in 6 equally divided doses	2	Two-week regimen not intended for patients with known cardiac or extracardiac abscess or for those with creatinine clearance of less than 20 mL per min, impaired 8th cranial nerve function, or Abiotrophia, Granulicatella, or Gemella spp. infection. Gentamicin dosage should be adjusted to achieve peak serum concentration of 3–4 microgram per mL and trough serum concentration of less than 1 microgram per mL when 3 divided doses are used; nomogram used for single daily dosing
or			
Ceftriaxone sodium	2 g per 24 h IV/IM in 1 dose	2	4 weeks for strains resistant to penicillin
plus			
Gentamicin sulfate	3 mg per kg per 24 h IV/IM in 1 dose	2	Other potentially nephrotoxic drugs (e.g. non-steroidal anti-inflammatory drugs) should be used with caution in patients receiving gentamicin therapy
	Paediatric dose: penicillin 200 000 U per kg per 24 h IV in 4–6 equally divided doses; ceftriaxone 100 mg per kg per 24 h IV/IM in 1 dose; gentamicin 3 mg per kg per 24 h	2	
	IV/IM in 1 dose or 3 equally divided doses		
Vancomycin hydrochloride	30 mg per kg per 24 h IV in 2 equally divided doses not to exceed 2 g per 24 h, unless concentrations in serum are inappropriately low PAediatric dose: 40 mg per kg per 24 h IV in 2–3 equally divided doses	4	Vancomycin therapy recommended only for patients unable to tolerate penicillin or ceftriaxone; vancomycin dosage should be adjusted to obtain peak (1 h after infusion completed) serum concentration of 30–45 microgram per mL and a trough concentration range of 10–15 microgram per mL. Vancomycin dosages should be infused during course of at least 1 h to reduce risk of histamine release 'red man' syndrome

ACC/AHA 2008 focused update incorporated into the ACC/AHA 2006 guidelines for the management of patients with valvular heart disease. *J Am Coll Cardiol*. 2008;**52**:e1–142.

ESC 2009 GL on endocarditis. Antibiotic treatment of IE due to oral streptococci and group D streptococci

Antibiotic	Dosage and route	Duration (weeks)	Level of evidence
Strains fully susceptible to penicillin (MIC <0.125 mg/L)			
Standard treatment			
Penicillin G[b]	12–18 million U/day IV in 6 doses	4[c]	I-B
or			
Amoxicillin[d]	100–200 mg/kg/day IV in 4–6 doses	4[c]	I-B
or			
Ceftriaxone[e]	2 g/day IV or IM in 1 dose	4[c]	I-B
	Paediatric doses:[f] Penicillin G 200 000 U/kg/day IV in 4–6 divided doses Amoxicillin 300 mg/kg/day IV in 4–6 equally divided doses Ceftriaxone 100 mg/kg/day IV or IM in 1 dose		
Two-week treatment[g]			
Penicillin G	12–18 million U/day IV in 6 doses	2	I-B
or			
Amoxicillin[d]	100–200 mg/kg/day IV in 4–6 doses	2	I-B
or			
Ceftriaxone[e]	2 g/day IV or IM in 1 dose	2	I-B
with			
Gentamicin[h]	3 mg/kg/day IV or IM in 1 dose	2	I-B
or			
Netilmicin	4–5 mg/kg/day IV in 1 dose	2	I-B
	Paediatric doses:[f] Penicillin, amoxicillin, and ceftriaxone as above Gentamicin 3 mg/kg/day IV or IM in 1 dose or in 3 equally divided doses		
In beta lactam-allergic patients			
Vancomycin[i]	30 mg/kg/day IV in 2 doses ***Paediatric doses:***[f] Vancomycin 40 mg/kg/day IV in 2–3 equally divided doses	4[c]	I-C
Strains relatively resistant to penicillin (MIC 0.125–2 mg/L)			
Standard treatment			
Penicillin G	24 million U/day IV in 6 doses	4[c]	I-B
or			
Amoxicillin[d]	200 mg/kg/day IV in 4–6 doses	4[c]	I-B
with			
Gentamicin[h]	3 mg/kg/day IV or IM in 1 dose	2	
In beta lactam-allergic patients			
Vancomycin[i]	30 mg/kg/day IV in 2 doses ***Paediatric doses:***[f] As above	4[c]	I-C
with			
Gentamicin[h]	3 mg/kg/day IV or IM in 1 dose	2	

[a] See text for other streptococcal species.
[b] Preferred in patients 65 years or with impaired renal function.
[c] 6-week therapy in PVE.
[d] Or ampicillin, same dosages as amoxicillin.
[e] Preferred for outpatient therapy.
[f] Paediatric doses should not exceed adult doses.
[g] Only if non-complicated native valve IE.
[h] Renal function and serum gentamicin concentrations should be monitored once a week. When given in a single daily dose, pre-dose (trough) concentrations should be <1 mg/L and post-dose (peak; 1 h after injection) serum concentrations should be approximately 10–12 mg/L.
[i] Serum vancomycin concentrations should achieve 10–15 mg/L at pre-dose (trough) level and 30–45 mg/L at post-dose level (peak; 1 h after infusion is completed).

2009 ESC guidelines on endocarditis 2009. Guidelines on the prevention, diagnosis, and treatment of infective endocarditis (new version 2009).

ACC/AHA 2008 on valve disease. Therapy for endocarditis caused by staphylococci in the absence of prosthetic materials

Regimen	Dosage and route	Duration	Comments
Oxacillin-susceptible strains			
Nafcillin or oxacillin	12 g per 24 h IV in 4–6 equally divided doses	6 wk	For complicated right-sided IE and for left-sided IE; for uncomplicated right-sided IE, 2 wk (see full text) Penicillin G 24 million U per 24 h IV in 4 to 6 equally divided doses may be used in place of nafcillin or oxacillin if strain is penicillin susceptible (minimum inhibitory concentration less than or equal to 0.1 μg per ml) and dose does not produce beta lactamase.
with			
Optional addition of gentamicin sulfate	3 mg per kg per 24 h IV/IM in 2 or 3 equally divided doses	3–5 d	Clinical benefit of aminoglycosides has not been established Gentamicin should be administered in close temporal proximity to vancomycin, nafcillin, or oxacillin dosing
	Pediatric dose: Nafcillin or oxacillin 200 mg per kg per 24 h IV in 4–6 equally divided doses; gentamicin 3 mg per kg per 24 h IV/IM in 3 equally divided doses		
Penicillin-allergic (nonanaphylactoid type) patients			Consider skin testing for oxacillin-susceptible staphylococci and questionable history of immediate-type hypersensitivity to penicillin
Cefazolin	6 g per 24 h IV in 3 equally divided doses	6 wk	Cephalosporins should be avoided in patients with anaphylactoid-type hypersensitivity to beta lactams; vancomycin should be used in these cases
with			
Optional addition of gentamicin sulfate	3 mg per kg per 24 h IV/IM in 2 or 3 equally divided doses	3–5 d	Clinical benefit of aminoglycosides has not been established
	Pediatric dose: cefazolin 100 mg per kg per 24 h IV in 3 equally divided doses; gentamicin 3 mg per kg per 24 h IV/IM in 3 equally divided doses		
Oxacillin-resilient strains			
Vancomycin	30 mg per kg per 24 h IV in 2 equally divided doses	6 wk	Adjust vancomycin dosage to achieve 1-h serum concentration of 30–45 μg per ml and trough concentration of 10–15 μg per ml Vancomycin dosages should be infused during course of at least 1 h to reduce risk of histamine-release "red man" syndrome

ACC/AHA 2008 focused update incorporated into the ACC/AHA 2006 guidelines for the management of patients with valvular heart disease. *J Am Coll Cardiol*. 2008;**52**:e1–142.

ACC/AHA GL 2008 on Valve Disease: Therapy of Native Valve Endocarditis Caused by Viridans Group Streptococci and *Streptococcus bovis*

Regimen	Dosage and Route	Duration, wk	Comments
Aqueous crystalline penicillin G sodium	12–18 million U per 24 h IV either continuously or in 4 or 6 equally divided doses	4	Preferred in most patients greater than 65 y of age or patients with impairment of 8th cranial nerve function or renal function
or			
Ceftriaxone sodium	2 g per 24 h IV/IM in 1 dose	4	
	Pediatric dose: penicillin 200 000 U per kg per 24 h IV in 4–6 equally divided doses; ceftriaxone 100 mg per kg per 24 h IV/IM in 1 dose (not to exceed adult dose)		
Aqueous crystalline penicillin G sodium	12–18 million U per 24 h IV either continuously or in 6 equally divided doses	2	Two-week regimen not intended for patients with known cardiac or extracardiac abscess or for those with creatinine clearance of less than 20 ml per min, impaired 8th cranial nerve function, or *Abiotrophia*, *Granulicatella*, or *Gemella* spp infection.

(Continued)

Regimen	Dosage and Route	Duration, wk	Comments
			Gentamicin dosage should be adjusted to achieve peak serum concentration of 3–4 micrograms per ml and trough serum concentration of less than 1 microgram per ml when 3 divided doses are used; nomogram used for single daily dosing.
or			
Ceftriaxone sodium	2 g per 24 h IV/IM in 1 dose	2	4 weeks for strains resistant to penicillin
plus			
Gentamicin sulfate	3 mg per kg per 24 h IV/IM in 1 dose	2	Other potentially nephrotoxic drugs (e.g., nonsteroidal anti-inflammatory drugs) should be used with caution in patients receiving gentamicin therapy.
	Pediatric dose: penicillin 200 000 U per kg per 24 h IV in 4–6 equally divided doses; ceftriaxone 100 mg per kg per 24 h IV/IM in 1 dose; gentamicin 3 mg per kg per 24 h	2	
Vancomycin hydrochloride	IV/IM in 1 dose or 3 equally divided doses 30 mg per kg per 24 h IV in 2 equally divided doses not to exceed 2 g per 24 h unless concentrations in serum are inappropriately low	4	Vancomycin therapy recommended only for patients unable to tolerate penicillin or ceftriaxone; vancomycin dosage should be adjusted to obtain peak (1 h after infusion completed) serum concentration of 30–45 micrograms per ml and a trough concentration range of 10–15 micrograms per ml
	Pediatric dose: 40 mg per kg per 24 h IV in 2–3 equally divided doses		Vancomycin dosages should be infused during course of at least 1 h to reduce risk of histamine-release "red man" syndrome.

ACC/AHA 2008 focused update incorporated into the ACC/AHA 2006 guidelines for the management of patients with valvular heart disease. *J Am Coll Cardiol.* 2008;**52**:e1–142.

ESC 2009 GL on endocarditis. Antibiotic treatment of IE due to *Staphylococcus* spp.

Antibiotic	Dosage and route	Duration (weeks)	Level of evidence
Native valves			
Methicillin-susceptible staphylococci			
(Flu)cloxacillin	12 g/day IV in 4–6 doses	4–6	I-B
or			
Oxacillin			
with			
Gentamicin[a]	3 mg/kg/day IV or IM in 2 or 3 doses	3–5 days	
	Paediatric doses:[b]		
	Oxacillin or (flu)cloxacillin 200 mg/kg/day IV in 4–6 equally divided doses		
	Gentamicin 3 mg/kg/day IV or IM in 3 equally divided doses		
Penicillin-allergic patients or methicillin-resistant staphylococci			
Vancomycin[c]	30 mg/kg/day IV in 2 doses	4–6	I-B
with			
Gentamicin[a]	3 mg/kg/day IV or IM in 2 or 3 doses	3–5 days	
	Paediatric doses:[b]		
	Vancomycin 40 mg/kg/day IV in 2–3 equally divided doses		
Prosthetic values			
Methicillin-susceptible staphylococci:			
(Flu)cloxacillin	12 g/day IV in 4–6 doses	≥ 6	I-B

(Continued)

Antibiotic	Dosage and route	Duration (weeks)	Level of evidence
or			
Oxacillin			
with			
Rifampin[d]	1200 mg/day IV or orally in 2 doses	≥ 6	
and			
Gentamicin[a]	3 mg/kg/day IV or IM in 2 or 3 doses	2	
	Paediatric doses:[b]		
	Oxacillin and (flu)cloxacillin as above		
	Rifampin 20 mg/kg/day IV or orally in 3 equally divided doses		
Penicillin-allergic patients and methicillin-resistant staphylococci			
Vancomycin[c]	30 mg/kg/day IV in 2 doses	≥6	I-B
with			
Rifampin[d]	1200 mg/day IV or orally in 2 doses	≥6	
and			
Gentamicin[a]	3 mg/kg/day IV or IM in 2 or 3 doses	2	
	Paediatric doses:[b]		
	As above		

[a] The clinical benefit of gentamicin addition has not been formally demonstrated. Its use is associated with increased toxicity and is, therefore, optional.
[b] Paediatric doses should not exceed adult doses.
[c] Serum vancomycin concentrations should achieve 25–30 mg/L at pre-dose (trough) levels.
[d] Rifampin increases the hepatic metabolism of warfarin and other drugs. Rifampin is believed to play a special role in prosthetic device infection because it helps eradicate bacteria attached to foreign material. Rifampin should always be used in combination with another effective anti-staphylococcal drug to minimize the risk of resistant mutant selection.
[e] Although the clinical benefit of gentamicin has not been demonstrated, it remains recommended for PVE. Renal function and serum gentamicin concentrations should be monitored once/week (twice/week in patients with renal failure). When given in three divided doses, pre-dose (trough) concentrations should be <1 mg/L and post-dose (peak; 1 h after injection) concentrations should be between 3–4 mg/L.
2009 ESC guidelines on endocarditis 2009. Guidelines on the prevention, diagnosis, and treatment of infective endocarditis (new version 2009).

ACC/AHA 2008 GL on valve disease. Therapy for native valve or prosthetic valve enterococcal endocarditis

Regimen	Dosage and Route	Duration, wk	Comments
Ampicillin sodium	12 g per 24 h IV in 6 equally divided doses	4 to 6	Native valve: 4-wk therapy recommended for patients with symptoms of illness less than or equal to 3 mo; 6-wk therapy recommended for patients with symptoms greater than 3 mo
or			
Aqueous crystalline penicillin G sodium	18–30 million U per 24 h IV either continuously or in 6 equally divided doses	4 to 6	Prosthetic valve or other prosthetic cardiac material: minimum of 6-wk therapy recommended
or Ampicillin-sulbactam *if the strain produces beta-lactamase* *plus*	12 g/24 h IV in 4 equally divided doses	6	Unlikely that the strain will be susceptible to gentamicin; if strain is gentamicin resistant, then >6 wk of ampicillin-sulbactam therapy will be needed
Gentamicin sulfate	3 mg per kg per 24 h IV/IM in 3 equally divided doses	4 to 6	Dosage of gentamicin should be adjusted to achieve peak serum concentration of 3 to 4 μg per ml and a trough concentration of less than 1 μg per ml. Patients with a creatinine clearance < 50 ml/min should be treated in consultation with an infectious diseases specialist Streptomycin sulfate 15 mg/kg/24h IV or IM in 2 doses if strain resistant to gentamicin Minimum 6 weeks for prosthetic valve IE

(*Continued*)

Regimen	Dosage and Route	Duration, wk	Comments
Vancomycin hydrochloride	30 mg per kg per 24 IV in 2 equally divided doses	6	Vancomycin therapy is recommended only for patients unable to tolerate penicillin or ampicillin
plus			
Gentamicin sulfate	3 mg per kg per 24 h IV/IM in 3 equally divided doses Pediatric dose: vancomycin 40 mg per kg per 24 h IV in 2 or 3 equally divided doses; gentamicin 3 mg per kg per 24 h IV/IM in 3 equally divided doses	6	6 wk of vancomycin therapy recommended because of decreased activity against enterococci

ACC/AHA 2008 focused update incorporated into the ACC/AHA 2006 guidelines for the management of patients with valvular heart disease. *J Am Coll Cardiol.* 2008;**52**:e1–142.

AHA 2005 statement on endocarditis. Therapy for native valve or prosthetic valve enterococcal endocarditis with strains resistant to penicillin, aminoglycoside, and vancomycin

Patients with endocarditis caused by these strains should be treated in consultation with an infectious diseases specialist; cardiac valve replacement may be necessary for bacteriologic cure; cure with antimicrobial therapy alone may be <50%; severe, usually reversible thrombocytopenia may occur with use of linezolid, especially after 2 wk of therapy; quinupristin-dalfopristin only effective against *E faecium* and can cause severe myalgias, which may require discontinuation of therapy; only small no. of patients have reportedly been treated with imipenem/cilastatin-ampicillin or ceftriaxone + ampicillin.

E faecium	Linezolid 600 mg/14 h IV/PO or quinupristin-dalfopristin 7.5 mg/kg /8 h IV for 8 weeks.
E faecalis	Imipenem/cilastatin 500 mg/6 h IV plus ampicillin 2 g/4h IV, or ceftriaxone 2 g IV/IM plus ampicillin 2 g/4h IV for 8 weeks.

ESC 2009 GL on Endocarditis. Antibiotic treatment of IE due to Enterococcus spp.

Antibiotic	Dosage and route	Duration (weeks)	Level of evidence
Beta lactam and gentamicin susceptible strain (for resistant isolates, see a, b, c)			
Amoxicillin	200 mg/kg/day IV in 4–6 doses	4–6[d]	I-B
with			
Gentamicin[e]	3 mg/kg/day IV or IM in 2 or 3 doses	4–6	
	Paediatric doses:[f]		
	Amoxicillin 300 mg/kg/day IV in 4–6 equally divided doses		
	Gentamicin 3 mg/kg/day IV or IM in 3 equally divided doses		
or			
Ampicillin	200 mg/kg/day IV in 4–6 doses	4–6[d]	I-B
with			
Gentamicin[e]	3 mg/kg/day IV or IM in 2 or 3 doses	4–6	
	Paediatric doses:[f]		
	Ampicillin 300 mg/kg/day IV in 4–6 equally divided doses		
	Gentamicin as above		
or			
Vancomycin[g]	30 mg/kg/day IV in 2 doses	6	I-C
with			
Gentamicin[e]	3 mg/kg/day IV or IM in 2 or 3 doses	6	
	Paediatric doses:[f]		
	Vancomycin 40 mg/kg/day IV in 2–3 equally divided doses		
	Gentamicin as above		

[a] High-level resistance to gentamicin (MIC 500 mg/L): if susceptible to streptomycin, replace gentamicin with streptomycin 15 mg/kg/day in two equally

(Continued)

divided doses (I, A). Otherwise, use more prolonged course of beta lactam therapy. The combination of ampicillin with ceftriaxone was recently suggested for gentamicin-resistant *E. faecalis* (IIa, B).

[b] Beta lactam resistance: (i) if due to beta lactamase production, replace ampicillin with ampicillin-sulbactam or amoxicillin with amoxicillin-clavulanate (I, C); (ii) if due to PBP5 alteration, use vancomycin-based regimens.

[c] Multiresistance to aminoglycosides, beta lactams, and vancomycin: suggested alternatives are (i) linezolid 2 × 600 mg/day IV or orally for ≥8 weeks (IIa, C) (monitor haematological toxicity); (ii) quinupristin-dafopristin 3 × 7.5 mg/kg/day for ≥8 weeks (IIa, C); (iii) Beta lactam combinations, including imipenem plus ampicillin or ceftriaxone plus ampicillin for ≥8 weeks (IIb, C).

[d] 6-week therapy recommended for patients with >3 months of symptoms and in PVE.

[e] Monitor serum levels of aminoglycosides and renal function as indicated in previous tables of this appendix.

[f] Paediatric doses should not exceed adult doses.

[g] In beta lactam-allergic patients. Monitor serum vancomycin concentrations as indicated in previous tables of this appendix.

2009 ESC guidelines on endocarditis 2009. Guidelines on the prevention, diagnosis, and treatment of infective endocarditis (new version 2009).

ACC/AHA 2008 GL on valve disease. Therapy for both native and prosthetic valve endocarditis caused by HACEK

Regimen	Dosage and route	Duration, wk	Comments
Ceftriaxone sodium	2 g per 24 h IV/IM in 1 dose	4	Cefotaxime or another third- or fourth-generation cephalosporin may be substituted
or			
Ampicillin-sulbactam	12 g per 24 IV in 4 equally divided doses	4	
or			
Ciprofloxacin	1000 mg per 24 h PO or 800 mg per 24 h IV in 2 equally divided doses	4	Fluoroquinolone therapy recommended only for patients unable to tolerate cephalosporin and ampicillin therapy; levofloxacin, gatifloxacin, or moxifloxacin may be substituted; fluoroquinolones generally not recommended for patients less than 18 y old
	Pediatric dose: Ceftriaxone 100 mg per kg per 24 h IV/IM once daily; ampicillin-sulbactam 300 mg per kg per 24 h IV divided into 4 or 6 equally divided doses; ciprofloxacin 20 to 30 mg per kg per 24 h IV/PO in 2 equally divided doses		Prosthetic valve: patients with endocarditis involving prosthetic cardiac valve or other prosthetic cardiac material should be treated for 6 wk

HACEK group: Haemophilus parainfluenzae, Haphrophilus, Actinobacillus actinomycetemcomitans, Cardiobacterium hominis, Eikenella corrodens, and *Kingella kingae.*

Patients should be informed that intramuscular injection of ceftriaxone is painful.

Fluoroquinolones are highly active in vitro against HACEK microorganisms.
Published data on use of fluoroquinolone therapy for endocarditis caused by HACEK are minimal.

ACC/AHA 2008 focused update incorporated into the ACC/AHA 2006 guidelines for the management of patients with valvular heart disease. *J Am Coll Cardiol.* 2008;**52**:e1–142.

ACC/AHA 2008 GL on valve disease. therapy for culture-negative endocarditis including *Bartonella* endocarditis

Regimen	Dosage* and Route	Duration, wk	Comments
Native valve			
Ampicillin-sulbactam	12 g per 24 h IV in 4 equally divided doses	4–6	Patients with culture-negative endocarditis should be treated with consultation with an infectious diseases specialist
plus			
Gentamicin sulfate	3 mg per kg per 24 h IV/IM in 3 equally divided doses	4–6	
Vancomycin	30 mg per kg per 24 h IV in 2 equally divided doses	4–6	Vancomycin recommended only for patients unable to tolerate penicillins
plus			
Gentamicin sulfate	3 mg per kg per 24 h IV/IM in 3 equally divided doses	4–6	
plus			
Ciprofloxacin	1000 mg per 24 h PO or 800 mg per 24 h IV in 2 equally divided doses	4–6	

(*Continued*)

Regimen	Dosage* and Route	Duration, wk	Comments
	Pediatric dose: ampicillin-sulbactam 300 mg per kg per 24 h IV in 4–6 equally divided doses; gentamicin 3 mg per kg per 24 h IV/IM in 3 equally divided doses; vancomycin 40 mg per kg per 24 h in 2 or 3 equally divided doses; ciprofloxacin 20–30 mg per kg per 24 h IV/PO in 2 equally divided doses		
Prosthetic valve (early-less than or equal to 1 y)			
Vancomycin	30 mg per kg per 24 h IV in 2 equally divided doses	6	
plus			
Gentamicin sulfate	3 mg per kg per 24 h IV/IM in 3 equally divided doses	2	
plus			
Cefepime	6 g per 24 h IV in 3 equally divided doses	6	
plus			
Rifampin	900 mg per 24 h PO/IV in 3 equally divided doses	6	
	Pediatric dose: vancomycin 40 mg per kg per 24 h IV in 2 or 3 equally divided doses; gentamicin 3 mg per kg per 24 h IV/IM in 3 equally divided doses; cefepime 150 mg per kg per 24 h IV in 3 equally divided doses; rifampin 20 mg per kg per 24 h PO/IV in 3 equally divided doses		
Prosthetic valve (late-greater than 1 y)		6	Same regimens as listed above for native valve endocarditis
Suspected Bartonella, culture negative			
Ceftriaxone sodium	2 g per 24 h IV/IM in 1 dose	6	Patients with *Bartonella* endocarditis should be treated in consultation with an infectious diseases specialist
plus			
Gentamicin sulfate	3 mg per kg per 24 h IV/IM in 3 equally divided doses	2	
with/without			
Doxycycline	200 mg per kg per 24 h IV/PO in 2 equally divided doses	6	
Documented Bartonella, culture positive			
Doxycycline	200 mg per 24 h IV or PO in 2 equally divided doses	6	If gentamicin cannot be given, then replace with rifampin, 600 mg per 24 h PO/IV in 2 equally divided doses
plus			
Gentamicin sulfate	3 mg per kg per 24 h IV/IM in 3 equally divided doses	2	
	Pediatric dose: ceftriaxone 100 mg per kg per 24 h IV/IM once daily; gentamicin 3 mg per kg per 24 h IV/IM in 3 equally divided doses; doxycycline 2–4 mg per kg per 24 h IV/PO in 2 equally divided doses; rifampin 20 mg per kg per 24 h PO/IV in 2 equally divided doses		

*: dosages recommended for patients with normal renal function.

ACC/AHA 2008 focused update incorporated into the ACC/AHA 2006 guidelines for the management of patients with valvular heart disease. *J Am Coll Cardiol*. 2008;**52**:e1–142.

ESC 2011 on pregnancy

Recommendations on drug use in pregnancy and breastfeeding

A The Guideline Committee added acenocoumarol and phenprocoumon in analogy to warfarin to this list. The necessity for risk assessment also applies to these two OAC. Previously, the risk category X was attributed to warfarin. In the opinion of the Task Force, available evidence suggests that risk category D is more appropriate for warfarin and other vitamin K antagonists.
B Adenosine: most of the experiences with this drug are in the second and third trimesters. Its short half-life may prevent it from reaching the fetus.
C Atenolol is classified D by FDA; nevertheless, some authors classify it as C.
D The available data on first-trimester use do not strongly support teratogenic potential.

Because ACE inhibitors, angiotensin II receptor blockers, aldosterone antagonists, and renin inhibitors should be avoided during pregnancy and breastfeeding, the risk category is D. Positive outcomes with ACE inhibitors have been described, and pregnancy does not have to be terminated if the patient was exposed to these medications but should be followed up closely.
E Breastfeeding is possible if the mother is treated with the drug.
F Digoxin: the experience with digoxin is extensive, and it is considered to be the safest antiarrhythmic drug during pregnancy. A prophylactic antiarrhythmic efficacy has never been demonstrated.
G Statins: should not be prescribed in pregnancy and during breastfeeding since their harmlessness is not proven, and disadvantages to the mother are not to be expected by a temporary interruption of the therapy for the time period of pregnancy.

Drugs	Classfication (Vaughan Williams for AA drugs)	FDA category	Placenta permeable	Transfer to breast milk (fetal dose)	Adverse effects
Abciximab	Monoclonal antibody with antithrombotic effects	C	Unknown	Unknown	Inadequate human studies; should be given only if the potential benefit outweighs the potential risk to the fetus
Acenocoumarol[a]	Vitamin K antagonist	D	Yes	Yes (no adverse effects reported)	Embryopathy (mainly first trimester), bleeding
Acetylsalicylic acid (low dose)	Antiplatelet drug	B	Yes	Well-tolerated	No teratogenic effects known (large datasets)
Adenosine[b]	Antiarrhythmic	C	No	No	No fetal adverse effects reported (limited human data)
Aliskiren	Renin inhibitor	D	Unknown	Unknown	Unknown (limited experience)
Amiodarone	Antiarrhythmic (class III)	D	Yes	Yes	Thyroid insufficiency (9%), hyperthyroidism, goitre, bradycardia, growth retardation, premature birth
Ampicillin, amoxicillin, cephalosporins, erythromycin, mezlocillin, penicillin	Antibiotics	B	Yes	Yes	No fetal adverse effects reported
Imipenem, rifampicin, telcoplanin, vancomycin	Antibiotics	C	Unknown	Unknown	Risk cannot be excluded (limited human data)
Aminoglycosides, quinolones, tetracyclines	Antibiotics	D	Unknown	Unknown	Risk to the fetus exists (reserved for vital indications)
Atenolol[c]	β-blocker (class II)	D	Yes	Yes	Hypospadias (first trimester); birth defects, low birthweight, bradycardia, and hypoglycaemia in fetus (second and third trimester)

Drugs	Classfication (Vaughan Williams for AA drugs)	FDA category	Placenta permeable	Transfer to breast milk (fetal dose)	Adverse effects
Benazepril[d]	ACE inhibitor	D	Yes	Yes[e] (maximum 1.6%)	Renal or tubular dysplasia, oligohydramnios, growth retardation, ossification disorders of skull, lung hypoplasia, contractures, large joints, anaemia, intrauterine fetal death
Bisoprolol	β-blocker (class II)	C	Yes	Yes	Bradycardia and hypoglycaemia in fetus
Candesartan	Angiotensin II receptor blocker	D	Unknown	Unknown; not recommended	Renal or tubular dysplasia, oligohydramnios, growth retardation, ossification disorders of skull, lung hypoplasia, contractures, large joints, anaemia, intrauterine fetal death
Captopril[d]	ACE inhibitor	D	Yes	Yes[e] (maximum 1.6%)	Renal or tubular dysplasia, oligohydramnios, growth retardation, ossification disorders of skull, lung hypoplasia, contractures, large joints, anaemia, intrauterine fetal death
Clopidogrel	Antiplatelet drug	C	Unknown	Unknown	No information during pregnancy available
Colestipol, cholestyramine	Lipid-lowering drugs	C	Unknown	Yes, lowering fat-soluble vitamins	May impair absorption of fat-soluble vitamins, e.g. vitamin K > cerebral bleeding (neonatal)
Danaparoid	Anticoagulant	B	No	No	No side effects (limited human data)
Digoxin[f]	Cardiac glycoside	C	Yes	Yes[e]	Serum levels unreliable, safe
Diltiazem	Calcium channel blocker (class IV)	C	No	Yes[e]	Possible teratogenic effects
Disopyramide	Antiarrhythmic (class IA)	C	Yes	Yes[e]	Uterus contraction
Enalapril[d]	ACE inhibitor	D	Yes	Yes[e] (maximum 1.6%)	Renal or tubular dysplasia, oligohydramnios, growth retardation, ossification disorders of skull, lung hypoplasia, contractures, large joints, anaemia, intrauterine fetal death
Eplerenone	Aldosterone antagonist	–	Unknown	Unknown	Unknown (limited experience)
Fenofibrate	Lipid-lowering drug	C	Yes	Yes	No adequate human data
Flecainide	Antiarrhythmic (class IC)	C	Yes	Yes[e]	Unknown (limited experience)
Fondaparinux	Anticoagulant	–	Yes (maximum 10%)	No	New drug, (limited experience)
Furosemide	Diuretic	C	Yes	Well-tolerated; milk production can be reduced	Oligohydramnios
Gemfibrozil	Lipid-lowering drug	C	Yes	Unknown	No adequate human data
Glyceryl trinitrate	Nitrate	B	Unknown	Unknown	Bradycardia, tocolytic
Heparin (low molecular weight)	Anticoagulant	B	No	No	Long-term application: seldom osteoporosis and markedly less thrombocytopenia than UF heparin
Heparin (unfractionated)	Anticoagulant	B	No	No	Long-term application: osteoporosis and thrombocytopenia
Hydralazine	Vasodilator	C	Yes	Yes[e] (maximum 1%)	Maternal side effect: lupus-like symptoms; fetal tachyarrhythmias (maternal use)
Hydrochlorothiazide	Diuretic	B	Yes	Yes, milk production can be reduced	Oligohydramnios

Drugs	Classfication (Vaughan Williams for AA drugs)	FDA category	Placenta permeable	Transfer to breast milk (fetal dose)	Adverse effects
Irbesartan[d]	Angiotensin II receptor blocker	D	Unknown	Unknown	Renal or tubular dysplasia, oligohydramnios, growth retardation, ossification disorders of skull, lung hypoplasia, contractures, large joints, anaemia, intrauterine fetal death
Isosorbide dinitrate	Nitrate	B	Unknown	Unknown	Bradycardia
Isradipine	Calcium channel blocker	C	Yes	Unknown	Potential synergism with magnesium sulfate may induce hypotension
Labetalol	-/-blocker	C	Yes	Yes[e]	Intrauterine growth retardation (second and third trimester), neonatal bradycardia and hypotension (used near term)
Lidocaine	Antiarrhythmic (class IB)	C	Yes	Yes[e]	Fetal bradycardia, acidosis, central nervous system toxicity
Methyldopa	Central -agonist	B	Yes	Yes[e]	Mild neonatal hypotension
Metoprolol	-blocker (class II)	C	Yes	Yes[e]	Bradycardia and hypoglycaemia in fetus
Mexiletine	Antiarrhythmic (class IB)	C	Yes	Yes[e]	Fetal bradycardia
Nifedipine	Calcium channel blocker	C	Yes	Yes[e] (maximum 1.8%)	Tocolytic; sublingual application and potential synergism with magnesium sulfate may induce hypotension (mother) and fetal hypoxia
Phenprocoumon[a]	Vitamin K antagonist	D	Yes	Yes (maximum 10%), well tolerated as inactive metabolite	Coumarin embryopathy, bleeding
Procainamide	Antiarrhythmic (class IA)	C	Yes	Yes	Unknown (limited experience)
Propafenone	Antiarrhythmic (class IC)	C	Yes	Unknown	Unknown (limited experience)
Propranolol	-blocker (class II)	C	Yes	Yes[e]	Bradycardia and hypoglycaemia in fetus
Quinidine	Antiarrhythmic (class IA)	C	Yes	Yes[e]	Thrombopenia, premature birth, 8th cranial nerve toxicity.
Ramipril[d]	ACE inhibitor	D	Yes	Yes (maximum 1.6%)	Renal or tubular dysplasia, oligohydramnios, growth retardation, ossification disorders of skull, lung hypoplasia, contractures, large joints, anaemia, intrauterine fetal death
Sotalol	Antiarrhythmic (class III)	B	Yes	Yes[e]	Bradycardia and hypoglycaemia in fetus (limited experience)
Spironolactone	Aldosterone antagonist	D	Yes	Yes[e] (maximum 1.2%); milk production can be reduced	Antiandrogenic effects, oral clefts (first trimester)
Statins	Lipid-lowering drugs	X	Yes	Unknown	Congenital anomalies
Ticlopidine	Antiplatelet	C	Unknown	Unknown	Unknown (limited experience)
Valsartan[d]	Angiotensin II receptor blocker	D	Unknown	Unknown	Renal or tubular dysplasia, oligohydramnios, growth retardation, ossification disorders of skull, lung hypoplasia, contractures, large joints, anaemia, intrauterine fetal death
Verapamil oral	Calcium channel blocker (class IV)	C	Yes	Yes[e]	Well tolerated (limited experience during pregnancy)

Drugs	Classfication (Vaughan Williams for AA drugs)	FDA category	Placenta permeable	Transfer to breast milk (fetal dose)	Adverse effects
Verapamil IV	Calcium channel blocker (class IV)	C	Yes	Yes[e]	Intravenous use may be associated with a greater risk of hypotension and subsequent fetal hypoperfusion
Vernakalant	Antiarrhythmic (class III)	–	Unknown	Unknown	No experience of use in pregnancy
Warfarin[a]	Vitamin K antagonist	D	Yes	Yes (maximum 10%), well tolerated as inactive metabolite	Coumarin embryopathy, bleeding

ACE, angiotensin-converting enzyme; UF, unfractionated.

ESC Guidelines on the management of cardiovascular diseases during pregnancy. *Eur Heart J*. 2011;**32**:3147–97.

[a]The Guideline Committee added acenocoumarol and phenprocoumon in analogy to warfarin to this list. The necessity for risk assessment also applies to these two OAC. Previously the risk category X was attributed to warfarin. In the opinion of the Task Force available evidence suggests that risk category D is more appropriate for warfarin and other vitamin K antagonists (see references and discussion in Section 5.5).

[b]Adenosine: most of the experiences with this drug are in the second and third trimesters. Its short half-life may prevent it from reaching the fetus

[c]Atenolol is classified D by FDA, nevertheless some authors classify as C.

[d]The available data on first-trimester use do not strongly support teratogenic potential. Because ACE inhibitors, angiotensin II receptor blockers, aldosterone antagonists, and renin inhibitors should be avoided during pregnancy and breastfeeding the risk category is D. Positive outcomes with ACE inhibitors have been described and pregnancy does not have to be terminated if the patient was exposed to these medications, but should be followed-up closely.

[e]Breastfeeding is possible if the mother is treated with the drug.

[f]Digoxin: the experience with digoxin is extensive, and it is considered to be the safest antiarrhythmic drug during pregnancy. A prophylactic antiarrhythmic efficacy has never been demonstrated.

[g]Statins: should not be prescribed in pregnancy and during breastfeeding since their harmlessness is not proven and disadvantages to the mother are not to be expected by a temporary interruption of the therapy for the time period of pregnancy.

Index

A

B

D

E

F

I

S

U

V

W